F

RODALE'S BASIC
Natural Foods Cookbook

Editor: Charles Gerras

**Collaborating Editors and Text Authors:
Camille Cusumano and Carol Munson**

Editorial Assistant: Camille Bucci

A Fireside Book
Published by Simon & Schuster Inc.
New York London Toronto Sydney Tokyo

A Fireside Book
Simon & Schuster Building
Rockefeller Center
1230 Avenue of the Americas
New York, New York 10020

Copyright © 1984 by Rodale Press, Inc.
All rights reserved
including the right of reproduction
in whole or in part in any form
First Fireside Edition, 1989
Published by arrangement with Rodale Press, Inc.
FIRESIDE and colophon are registered trademarks
of Simon & Schuster Inc.
Manufactured in the United States of America
10 9 8 7 6 5 4 3 2   Pbk.
Library of Congress Cataloging in Publication Data
Rodale's basic natural foods cookbook / editor, Charles Gerras ;
    collaborating editors and text authors, Camille Cusumano and Carol
    Munson; editorial assistant, Camille Bucci.
        p.   cm.
    1. Cookery (Natural foods)   I. Gerras, Charles.   II. Cusumano,
Camille.   III. Munson, Carol.
TX741.R625 1989
641.5′637—dc19   88-21256
                                                            CIP

ISBN 0-671-67338-6 Pbk.

Recipe Development

Faye Martin	Dolores Riccio	Sheryl London	Anita Hirsch
Joan Bingham	Dora Jonassen	Annemarie Colbin	Camille Cusumano
Gretel Ruppert	Jeanne Cimino	Marion Gorman	Debra Deis
Maggie Oster	Diana Resek	Margaret Linder	Susan Hercek

and Linda Gilbert, Rhonda Diehl, JoAnn Coponi, Carol Munson, Camille Bucci, Louise Gainfort, Phoebe Brooks, Marie Harrington, and Brenda Gracely

Recipe Testing in the Rodale Test Kitchen

Supervisor of Publication Testing: Anita Hirsch
Testers: Karen Haas, JoAnn Coponi, Rhonda Diehl, and Pat Singley

Copy Coordinators: Dolores Plikaitis with Barbara Nykoruk

Copy Editors: Jan Barckley, Judy Camarda, and Louise Doucette

Book Designers: Jerry O'Brien and Anita Groller

Illustrator: Janet Bohn

Project Assistant: Gregory Paulnack

Contents

Acknowledgments

This book was completed only through the hard work and dedication of many people. Now that the job is done, I welcome the opportunity to credit those who made it possible.

Camille Cusumano and Carol Munson concentrated their considerable culinary skills and nutritional backgrounds on meeting the monumental mandate to create the text for "the most complete all-purpose cookbook available." They accomplished the task with an enthusiasm and energy that never flagged. The extras they provided would warm any editor's heart—food discussions more thorough than the other books of this kind, unique checklists and tables, and careful coverage of numerous uncommon foodstuffs omitted from other publications. No one could have worked harder or to better effect.

Camille Bucci was a part of this project from its initial planning stages to its conclusion. Her primary responsibility was to deal with the vast number of recipes—researching the basic dishes, checking with the testers about the quality of submitted recipes, going over all 1,500 recipes for sense and basic style. In the course of developing the book, she unhesitatingly absorbed an ever-ballooning variety of other duties and served as a most valued member of the core group.

Faye Martin is an inventive food expert to whom we turned early on for ideas on what unique values we could bring to our book. Her wise observations helped us in forming the basic plan and attitude we used throughout.

Dorothy Smickley and Bobbie Hartranft are two experts at divining what editors really intend when they cross out words or pencil in sentences that run around the page. They deciphered and typed numerous complicated tables, dozens of chapters in rough draft, and scores of recipes precisely, speedily, and willingly.

We were fortunate, indeed, in acquiring the services of some very imaginative cooks to contribute the hundreds of appetizing recipes in the book. These clever women provided just the kind of exciting new ideas we wanted, using natural foods in new and irresistible combinations. They met every Rodale request with grace and with dispatch. They establish, once and for all, the fact that healthful dishes and exciting dining can be one.

The staff of Rodale's test kitchen is never less than wonderful, no matter what we ask of them. They do not panic and they do not complain, but they do deliver. Admirably. Anita Hirsch, who supervised this project, is knowledgeable about every aspect of food and food preparation. Her comments and those of the other testers concerning recipes and the text were especially helpful.

We also turned to Linda Gilbert for help in developing some new ideas in such areas as food preservation and using certain grains. She always provided a thorough and professional answer to every request.

X

Paul Rubinstein generously shared his impressive expertise as a chef and food writer by means of an in-depth commentary on every chapter of the original manuscript. His suggestions aided us in making some critical decisions about the tone and content of the book. Lorraine Mairiello, a home economist, also checked the manuscript for culinary accuracy.

Joan Bingham and Jane Kinderlehrer generously evaluated the manuscript as a personal favor. As cookbook authors in their own right, the objective comments they offered gave us some valuable insights concerning the best way to present certain points of information.

Until Dolores Plikaitis came on the scene, our book seemed doomed to sink in a mire of stylistic problems. She took on the job of sorting out the inconsistencies and making every recipe presentation, every usage, every cross-reference as one throughout. As copy coordinators, she and Barbara Nykoruk led three copy editors in deciding whether a recipe would call for "chick-peas" or "garbanzos"; "oil," "vegetable oil," or "salad oil"; and exactly how recipe directions would be worded. Dolores and Barbara set rules for hyphenations, use of italics, and literally hundreds of similar fine points that can surface in a large reference work. Aside from that, good copy editors (and these are the best) helpfully suggest more felicitous wording, point out redundancies, ask editors for clarifications, and make inquiries to ensure accuracy. Although the deadline was tight, nothing was left to chance, no point was passed over, all in pursuit of the perfect result. Throughout the intense effort, courtesy and patience never faltered. The contribution this group made to the quality of this book was a major one.

Jerry O'Brien started us off with a charming and distinctive jacket design that won everyone from the start. Jerry also set the preliminary design for the book's interior before other duties pulled him away from the project. Fortunately for us, Anita Groller was able to take over. She fleshed out the basic design and followed through brilliantly. She found us an ideal illustrator in Janet Bohn, and they worked beautifully together to produce the fine artwork you see throughout the book. Anita quietly performed miracles every day.

In the end, most books are chasing the calendar. If manuscript is late, if art is lost or must be redone, if the editor calls for last-minute changes, the production coordinator has to figure out how to make everything come out on time just the same. Barbara Herman is a master of this sleight of hand, and she used all of her powers to pull this one off. Our deep gratitude to Barbara, who never settles for "it can't be done."

These are but a few of the people who gave of themselves in bringing this book to completion. To one degree or another, it has involved all department heads and staff in Rodale's Book Division, everybody in the test kitchen, and artists and copy writers in the company's promotion department and marketing area.

As you can see, we required—and received—plenty of help in putting this book between covers. My warm thanks to each person for his or her contribution to the work. May it fulfill our fondest hopes.

C. G.

Introduction

This is a book designed to make you comfortable with natural foods. It is a cooking encyclopedia created especially for people who want to prepare dishes that are not only delicious but also free from both artificial ingredients and products that have been more than minimally processed.

Our interest in natural foods comes out of a basic Rodale tradition: Natural Is Better. There is no mystery in that. It is an incontrovertible truth that Nature knows more about the best composition of food and how it should taste than any manufacturer does.

A good cook chooses food in its freshest, least-tampered-with state—fresh fruits simply cut and served, not sweetened, colored, or canned; a freshly caught fish, herbed and broiled, not one ground up and pressed into flavorless, breaded squares; a home-baked, whole grain, firm-textured bread, not a bleached white, cotton experience. Of course, the natural product is miles ahead nutritionally, but even if it were not, think of its marvelous flavor compared with the processed version!

Natural foods cooks are determined to have both good taste and nutritional riches, so they insist on full control over what they serve. Each dish will be as fresh as the season and the circumstances permit, and the ingredients in it will be real, not man-made approximations. If a food is to have any flavorings, the cook will decide which and how much; no more of the surprise sugar or salt in processed products for them.

Until now many of these cooks found it necessary to keep two cookbooks handy—one to use as a basic cooking reference and a second for cooking with natural foods. They learned through experience that a cookbook featuring cakes and pies sweetened with honey, instead of sugar, was an unlikely source for information on the classic sauces. Conversely, cooks who treasured a cookbook for its quick-reference list of equivalents and substitutions or its foolproof guide to broiling meats soon discovered that they must look elsewhere for soyfoods recipes or tips on whole grain piecrusts. *Rodale's Basic Natural Foods Cookbook* brings these two types of cooking information together.

From the beginning our efforts to produce this book were sparked by a fantasy we pursued: Mother is handing *our* book to a young home-maker. "You will need an all-purpose cookbook," she says. "I chose this one because it has all the basic information the classics have, *and* it provides valuable guidance for cooking with natural foods as well." The fantasy has materialized. This is that book.

Fitness House, the company dining room that opened at Rodale in 1970, laid the foundation for this project through the practical experience gained there. Its original mandate was to provide a wholesome, full course midday meal for Rodale employees, but that role expanded quickly. Within weeks of its opening, the Fitness House kitchen also became an experimental laboratory and clearinghouse for natural foods cooking techniques and information.

The regular diners instigated the unplanned transformation. They had questions about how to use honey to the best advantage as a sweetener and how to add more nutrition to basic recipes. They also wanted the original Fitness House recipes for such favorites as Cold Melon Soup (a sure sellout on hot summer days), Fitness House Sautéed Liver (people who bragged they "*never eat liver!*" were the first to sign up for that specialty), Whole Wheat Crescent Rolls, and Carob Brownies so they could make these treats at home.

Early on, Fitness House cooks acceded to requests for a nonmeat menu once a week (a custom that then provided many fine recipe ideas, and still does). They instituted salad days in summer—with sometimes a dozen salads to choose from! A series of low-cost menus presented loads of ideas for employees anxious to cut family grocery expenses.

Before long the editors of the Rodale magazines were tapping Fitness House for a new kind of service: "We need recipe ideas for an article on soy flour." "Can you provide material for a piece on baking various whole grain breads?" "Will you test these four varieties of green beans for texture and flavor and choose the best for a gardening report we're doing—and we could use a couple of recipes featuring the winner."

When local home economists visited Fitness House, they stayed long after lunch, pumping the staff with technical questions and gathering recipes. Writers from national publications came to do stories about the Rodale approach to foods and food preparation. Internationally known gourmets came to Emmaus, Pennsylvania, especially to dine at Fitness House. Food manufacturers began to see Rodale recipes as potential commercial products, and they began to call.

Lessons, hints, tips, and techniques for cooking with natural foods were coming out of Fitness House in a steady stream. It was time to pull the information together for the general public. The result, *The Rodale Cookbook,* was published in 1972. It has sold over 500,000 copies.

New responsibilities came with the enviable reputation Fitness House built. Resources were strained by the ever-increasing requests for original recipes to illustrate the popular food articles in the magazines; the Rodale experimental farms wanted ideas for dishes using new crops such as amaranth; *Prevention* magazine wanted an herbal granular substitute for salt. Some of the recipes in cookbook manuscripts submitted by free-lance authors required conversion to all-natural ingredients. Of course, everybody turned to the Fitness House cooks.

It became obvious that a formal, separate test kitchen would have to be created so Fitness House could resume its original role as a dining room. Special units were set up in the test kitchen for experiments—recipes for new condiments to be made at home; special soy product development; healthful candies in bar form, using only nutritious ingredients; and a syrup to use instead of chocolate syrup.

A distinct group (with its own staff) was installed to implement the company policy that calls for testing every recipe slated to appear in any Rodale book or magazine. We want to be sure each one can be followed as written and will result in a quality product.

This is the kind of background and experience that lies at the core of this book. It is the key to our confidence in presenting the definitive natural foods cookbook.

Open this book to any section and you will also find the kind of extensive general reference material and instruction you require from any of the best all-purpose cookbooks. It tells you everything from how to carve a turkey and how big a roast it takes to serve eight, to how to rescue a curdled hollandaise sauce or turn out a crystal-clear consommé. Dozens of tables provide quick access to food basics, and step-by-step illustrations and directions help you to master the more complicated cooking skills. Cooks stumped for new ideas will delight in page after page of marvelous menus for quick-to-make family meals, dinner parties, no-meat meals, brunches, and low-cost meals.

However, we believe the special value of this book is in the extraordinary information and cooking ideas it contains. For example, a complete chapter on legumes covers virtually every kind of bean and features an extensive overview of various soybean products, including tofu. Readers can choose from dozens of recipes that feature soy-foods, a new taste experience for many families.

The Breads chapter is much concerned with the baking properties and nutritional values of whole grains. It includes a list of suggested whole grain combinations intended to increase the vitamin value of your loaves and to introduce your family to new flavors and textures in all sorts of breads.

Nuts and seeds contain superior food value, but more than that, they offer a largely unexplored versatility. Aside from the usual, our book shows cooks how to use nuts and seeds in interesting new ways as butters, meals, and milks.

Sprouts, whose value is universally recognized by knowledgeable cooks and nutritionists, rarely get serious attention in any but oriental cookbooks. We believe they merit every cook's careful consideration so we devote a full chapter to sprouts and sprouting and recipes that feature sprouts.

Sea vegetables, basic to the diets of many sophisticated cultures throughout the world, are a mystery to most Americans. However, the variety and taste appeal of these low-cost, mineral-rich foods are so impressive that we have set aside a chapter to introduce them. Readers learn the characteristics of various types, how to shop for them, and how to use them in cooking.

Desserts are the biggest challenge for the health-conscious cook. We present practical alternatives to such items as sugar, chocolate, and white flour, and we offer recipes that use nutritious whole grain flours, wheat germ, nuts, yogurt, and fruits as ingredients in irresistible sweets.

Our Beverages chapter stresses wholesome fruit and vegetable juices as bases for delicious and refreshing drinks. It also presents the opportunity to turn from the ever-present coffee and tea to a wide selection of herb drinks that can soothe you or energize you, depending on your mood.

The more than 1,500 recipes in this book prove that natural ingredients can be used to create every kind of dish from a homey Fresh Tomato Soup to a glamorous Orange-Almond Bavarian Cream. With this book you can please plain eaters with simple Corn Muffins or Apple Pie, or you can impress sophisticated diners with Miso-Egg Drop Soup or Apricot Soufflé.

These few examples can only hint at the fresh attitudes toward food and food preparation that have inspired this book. The resources of the Rodale Test Kitchen are devoted to the proposition that the purest, most nutritious food is also the best tasting. We believe that the information and the recipes in this book will convince any cook that this is true.

Rodale's Basic Natural Foods Cookbook is a totally new concept in cookbooks. Its range is unprecedented. With pride and confidence we invite you to use and enjoy it.

Before You Start to Cook

To be a good cook and to use any cookbook with confidence, you must understand the basics of food preparation. It is important to feel comfortable about meal planning and knowledgeable when selecting equipment for a specific kitchen task. It is essential to be aware of correct measuring techniques and cooking terms and to be familiar with equivalent measures and ingredients. This chapter provides that kind of general information. It is an excellent reference for all your cooking questions. (Refer to specific chapters for cooking instructions and information regarding particular food groups, such as meats, fruits, vegetables, or grains.)

Meal Planning

Whether cooking just for yourself, your family, or for company, plan meals in advance to make the most of the time, energy, and resources available to you. This will also help your food shopping excursions become more efficient.

Of course, your primary concern is to provide nutritionally balanced meals that the entire household will enjoy. In general, choosing foods for variety—foods with contrasting colors and textures and complementary flavors—usually ensures a good nutritional mix (see Appendix 1).

For household members with allergies, special health needs, or other dietary restrictions, however, meal planning may also involve omitting certain foods or whole food groups. Take these needs into account when shopping and cooking in order to make necessary substitutions.

Budget limitations and the seasonal availability of foods will affect your meal planning as well. If money is a problem, plan dishes that do not require exotic ingredients or others that are expensive. Follow tips on making meat go further and using less expensive cuts of meat, especially if your household consumes a great deal of it. For a cheaper (and often more healthful) alternative protein source, incorporate vegetarian meals into your diet and build them around fruits and vegetables most plentiful at that time of year (see Meatless Cooking, page 10).

Food Shopping

Like most activities food shopping is a skill that can be perfected with experience and the use of a few basic considerations. Here is some information that will give you a head start.

Some foods deteriorate quickly so they must be purchased in amounts that will be used up fast. Fish, meats, eggs, dairy foods, and fresh produce, for example, lose quality within a few days of purchase. What is not used by then is wasted. Other foods have a long storage life and may be bought in bulk for savings and convenience. Dried foods such as grains, beans, and flours can be kept for months if stored properly.

Of course, the quantity of any foods you buy also depends on the number of people in the household.

Here are several hints to help you plan your food shopping trips most efficiently:

• To help in making the list of items to buy, decide which recipes you want to make in the coming week. Try to plan on recipes that will use up the foods you already have on hand and that feature foods that are currently in abundance. Emphasize dishes that are favorites at your house.

• Now estimate how much of each ingredient you must buy. Be sure to consult the yield or number of servings of the recipes you intend to make, so you can plan on using leftovers. Consider whether the leftovers can be stored or if they must be used up the next day.

• Know the storing properties of all ingredients in a recipe before you decide how much to buy or make. Sometimes it is better to cut a recipe and store the remaining uncooked ingredients for another time. In other cases it is more efficient to cook a full recipe and store the excess for a future meal.

Coordinating the Parts of a Meal

To have the various elements of a meal ready at the proper time, yet done to perfection, is a challenge for every cook. A plan, however simple, is the only way to ensure success. Though experienced cooks may have invisible, seemingly effortless plans, new cooks and those having invited guests for a meal will probably find that written plans work best.

Start by setting up a table similar to the one below. Then fill in the columns (your own work pace determines much of this). After deciding how much time is needed for each task, relist the items, starting with those that require the most time to complete. Figure on at least 15 minutes extra for interruptions, then figure backward from the time you wish to serve the meal and insert the approximate starting times next to each item.

Menu Item	Preparation Time (min)	Cooking Time (min)	Preparation for Serving (min)	Total (min)
Macaroni and cheese	15	20	1	36
Green peas	15	6	1	22
Tossed garden salad	10	. . .	5	15
Fresh fruit cup (dessert)	10	50 (chilling)	3	63

Then relist items in the order of preparation and include times.

4:55 P.M.: Prepare fruit cup and refrigerate.
5:05 P.M.: Prepare macaroni and cheese and set aside.
5:20 P.M.: Shell peas and set aside.
5:35 P.M.: Put macaroni and cheese in oven; prepare salad.
5:45 P.M.: Toss salad.
5:50 P.M.: Put peas on to cook.
5:55 P.M.: Macaroni and cheese done.
5:56 P.M.: Peas done.
6:00 P.M.: Serve dinner.

With the scheduling done thoughtfully, meal preparation can proceed with ease, and the cook can announce confidently when dinner will be served.

Label Reading

Although the recipes in this book aim to avoid canned, processed, or premixed foods, there may be times when it is necessary to buy such foods. It is wise to develop the habit of reading labels before you purchase. They provide much important information for consumers—some of which is required by the federal Food and Drug Administration—concerning quality and hidden ingredients in the packaged product. Although many commercial products have words like "natural" or "organic" on their labels, such foods are still not federally or legally defined in terms of standards for quality. "Natural" might mean simply that all the ingredients in the product were derived from nature, including chemicals in the additives. Reading the ingredients list is really the only way to know what you are buying.

Most packaged food products must have an ingredients list on the label. (Exceptions include those with standards of identity, such as mayonnaise, jellies, chocolate products, macaroni, noodles, cheese and cheese products, milk, cream, ice cream, frozen desserts, margarine, canned tomatoes, nut products, and fish). The ingredients are listed in descending order of weight. Additives must be listed. If flavors or colors are artificial, this must be stated.

Foods that have added nutrients or whose manufacturers make nutritional claims (such as "low cholesterol" or "low fat") must bear the nutritional contents on their labels. The nutritional information provided includes the number of calories and the amount of grams of protein, carbohydrate, and fat contained in each serving of the product. It also includes the percentage of U.S. Recommended Daily Allowances of protein and several important vitamins and minerals in each serving. The label should also give the serving size and state how many servings there are per container.

The following information must also be on all food labels: the name of the product, the net contents or net weight—including liquid and dry weight; and the name and place of business of the manufacturer.

Choosing and Using Vegetable Oils

The popularity of vegetable oils as a replacement for butter, lard, and other similar shortenings in cooking has increased steadily in recent years. Not only are fats from nonanimal sources more healthful due to their lower cholesterol content, but oils are easier to manage when measuring exact amounts. They also offer a wide choice of flavorings, ranging from the rich and assertive quality olive oil lends to hearty Mediterranean favorites to the virtually imperceptible essence of safflower oil or corn oil in baked goods and sautéed dishes. *In this book "vegetable oil" given as a recipe ingredient refers to safflower or corn oil; any other oil needed will be specified by name.*

Those new to buying and using vegetable oils for cooking might be puzzled by the many types of these oils offered for sale at the market. Here is an overview of the designations and hints on which type of oil is best suited to the purpose at hand.

Oils are refined by means of chemicals and high heat to remove solids, color, flavor, and aroma and to prolong shelf life. Cooks use refined oils for preparing dishes in which a strong flavor from the oil is undesirable—eggs, seafood, and cakes, for example.

Few vegetable oils are sold in unrefined form; that is, extracted by cold pressing. (It does not follow that all cold-pressed oils are unrefined.) Despite the name, the cold-pressing process calls for heating oils to 150 to 240°F. Still, these unrefined, cold-pressed oils retain most of their natural flavor and aroma. They also keep more of their vitamin E, which is heat sensitive, although refined oils do retain a significant amount of vitamin E as well.

Unrefined oils have a deeper color and may darken even more at high cooking temperatures. Cold-pressed, unrefined oils tend to become rancid quickly, so store them in the refrigerator. Some clouding under refrigeration is normal. As a rule, it is better not to use the rich-colored, strong-flavored oils for deep frying, for sautéing, in baked goods, or for greasing pans. They are more suitable for marinades or salad dressings and sauces in which you wish to accent the taste of a particular oil.

Healthful Replacements for Commonly Used Foods

It is often as easy to use healthful ingredients in a dish as it is to use the less desirable processed, fatty, or salty items. Consult the list below when assembling recipe ingredients, and consider using yogurt in place of sour cream, vegetable oil in place of lard, for example. It is simple and wise.

Commonly Used Food	Replacement	Commonly Used Food	Replacement
Bread crumbs, white	wheat germ whole grain bread crumbs	Gelatin, artificially flavored and sweetened	agar unflavored, unsweetened gelatin
Chocolate	carob	Graham crackers, crushed	wheat germ whole grain bread crumbs
Corn flakes, crushed	wheat germ whole grain bread crumbs	Lard	butter chicken fat vegetable oil
Cream		Milk, whole	low-fat yogurt low-fat or skim milk
Sour	yogurt	Pancake syrup, commercial	honey molasses pure maple syrup
Whipped	yogurt		
Flour		Pasta, white	whole wheat pasta
White, as a thickener	barley, oat, rye, or whole wheat pastry flour brown rice flour cornstarch	Rice, white	brown rice buckwheat groats bulgur
White, in making breads	barley, brown rice, buckwheat, millet, oat, rye, soy (in combination with another whole grain flour), or whole wheat flour finely ground cornmeal ground nuts	Salt	herbs spices
		Shortening, hydrogenated	butter chicken fat vegetable oil
White, in making cookies and cakes	barley, brown rice, buckwheat, millet, oat, rye, soy (in combination with another whole grain flour), or whole wheat pastry flour finely ground cornmeal ground nuts	Sugar, brown or white	diastatic malt fruit juice honey maple syrup molasses

Cooking for a Few

The meal planning and shopping guidelines given earlier apply to any size household. However, you must be particularly careful not to overbuy for small households. When cooking for a few:

• Consider the storage space and keeping facilities you have before you buy large quantities of any item.

• When possible, avoid shopping in supermarkets that specialize in large economy packages of many foods. Instead, buy from shops such as natural foods stores, small groceries, or farmers' markets where foods are sold loose and you can buy in quantities that suit your needs.

• Check the dating code on perishable goods to be sure they can be stored in your refrigerator for several days after purchase.

• When buying chicken, it is cheaper to buy a whole chicken and then cut it into parts for freezing. (Be sure to label the parts with a name and date.) If you use only white meat, buy chicken breasts—one breast will usually serve two persons. Cooked chicken can be stored for several days in the refrigerator to be used in recipes such as chicken salad or casseroles.

• If you buy your meat in a supermarket, ask the meat counter personnel to break up the large packages of meats such as steaks and chops. Ground beef can be stored safely in the refrigerator for several days to be used in a few different recipes.

• Buy only enough fresh fruits and vegetables for about three days at a time.

• Whenever possible, cook foods in bulk (it can save you time) and freeze them in serving-size portions. For example, dried beans, most stocks, and some soups take a long time to cook. Therefore, it is wise to make large amounts of these, then break them down to smaller portions for freezing. Most grains and fresh vegetables cook quickly but also can be cooked ahead of time and frozen.

• If it is not possible to cut a recipe or to freeze the leftover portion, consider ways to serve what remains in other forms throughout the week. Leftover meat can be made into sandwiches, hot or cold—or mixed with vegetables, beans, or grains for casseroles. Leftover vegetables, grains, pasta, and beans can be mixed with savory dressings for cold salads. They also can be made into quick-cooking casseroles or added to soups or stews just before serving. Reheating foods will cause some nutrient loss so heat cooked foods as little as possible. A wok is a good utensil for reheating cooked meats, grains, and vegetables because it does the job so quickly. A steamer also may be used.

• Make easy, uncomplicated dishes. Use as many fresh ingredients as possible. For a quick, nutritious dessert or snack, simply serve fresh fruits and cheeses or dried fruit and nut mixes.

• When making a salad dressing, prepare enough dressing for several uses throughout the rest of the week. Bake full recipes of muffins and other quick breads; what is not needed immediately can be frozen, then oven-heated in about 20 minutes right out of the freezer.

For menu suggestions using recipes from this book, see page 12.

Fixing Foods Children Like

The fact that children—even very young ones—often have definite preferences concerning food can complicate family meal planning. In the search for dishes that might please your children, consider that most youngsters like:

• the mild, delicate flavors found in young carrots, new potatoes, custards, and bananas;

• foods that are easily chewed, such as tuna and meat patties;

• warm foods but not hot or cold ones (ice cream is an obvious exception) and bland foods, not spicy ones;

• simple dishes and not complex casseroles and sophisticated sauces;

• the bright colors of carrots, oranges, peas, and tomatoes;

• textures that are easy to deal with—such as the smoothness of puddings and the consistent texture of scrambled eggs—not foods they consider dry, rough, or stringy.

A list of the recipes that will especially appeal to children is given on page 16. Recipes are grouped by course so that you can select one recipe or plan entire meals that will be a hit with your youngsters.

Preparing Quick Meals

Preparing meals that not only feature nutrient-packed whole foods but also are ready in just minutes need not be difficult nor worrisome. The key lies in planning sensible menus. Here are some helpful suggestions:

• Save both time and energy by planning an entire meal that can be baked in the oven.

• Choose substantial casseroles made with whole grains or legumes.

• Consolidate each menu into two courses: a hearty main course and a refreshing dessert of fresh fruits.

• Work up a repertoire of recipes that can be cooked rapidly in a pressure cooker or that will cook untended in a slow cooker. Stews and other dishes that call for braised meats or poultry are good choices.

• Be on the lookout for recipes that use uncooked fruits or vegetables.

• Keep your favorite quick-to-prepare selections in a handy card file. Limit these to recipes that take no longer than 20 minutes to prepare and can be cooked in less than an hour.

• During the actual preparation of a quick meal, efficiency is a plus. When possible, mix and bake foods in dishes that can double as serving dishes. Organize ingredients so that you can do all the measuring and chopping at once. If you use garlic frequently, invest in a good garlic press.

• Whenever feasible, cook, grate, or chop more food than is needed for the current meal, and freeze the extras for use in other dishes. Foods such as cooked legumes, cooked barley, cooked rice, grated cheese, diced onions, chopped green peppers, and sautéed mushrooms are ideal for doing this since they freeze very nicely and thaw quickly.

• Cooking sauces, soups, and casseroles in quantity and then freezing them is another time-saver. Reheat these at the same temperatures called for in the original recipes. If you have leftover meat, vegetables, and rolls, freeze them on a small tray or plate as a complete meal and reheat in the oven as a convenience dinner.

For menus that feature dishes from this book and illustrate the variety of fare and taste combinations that can be prepared even when you are in a hurry, see page 13. They can be used as a start for your collection of ideas for fast meals.

Planning Meals for Guests

Happily, it is possible to entertain, have time to visit with the guests, and still serve an impressive meal. The price for the freedom to enjoy your own parties is careful planning. That means considering everything from the season of the year to your guests' food preferences—or, in some cases, requirements. If the weather is wintery, you will want to match their expectation for hearty, hot dishes such as roasts, stews, and casseroles. When it is warm outside, light, simple dishes, refreshing salads, and cold soups are often most appropriate. Maybe a guest simply has a distaste for fish or red meat; another might be bound by special food restrictions—dietary or religious. You should take these factors into account if the group is small.

When you are actually ready to decide on the menu, choose simple but varied dishes that you know will work. It is dangerous to experiment with dishes that are new to you when guests are coming. (Save your recipe tests for family meals, when a ruined dish will not mean a ruined party.) Most of all, be on the lookout for recipes that can wait without a loss of quality or ones that reheat readily at the last minute. A meal built around such dishes gives you the opportunity to enjoy your guests instead of being tied up in the kitchen until it is time to serve the food.

If you are having a crowd for dinner, the best course is to use recipes designed to serve large numbers. If such recipes are not available to you, the volume of other recipes can be increased, though it is generally better to cook several batches of the recipe as given. Few recipes can be multiplied without limit and still turn out well.

When you do increase a recipe, remember to adjust the seasonings for the added volume and to compensate for the increased preparation time. You must also remember to compensate for longer heating and chilling times. From the standpoints of flavor and safety, the quicker cooking and cooling characteristics of small batches are preferable since bacteria breed rapidly in food that is just lukewarm.

The number of courses you choose to serve depends on your preferences and the formality of the meal. Three courses—appetizer, entrée, and dessert—are the usual choice, but for a very formal occasion the number might be six. The early course (or courses) should be light, to whet appetites for the main course. Fresh fruits, a juice, or a consommé are good starters for the meal. Then serve a substantial main course that does not repeat the flavor or texture of the first. The final course is usually something sweet and can range from an elaborate carob mousse or cherry custard pie to the fresh sweetness of sliced fruit, perhaps heightened by the sharp bite of a cheese.

For menu suggestions when entertaining, see page 14. The recipes noted there offer a touch of elegance combined with simplicity, the type of meal that is welcomed by guests at any luncheon or dinner.

Meatless Cooking

Planning some of your meals without meat not only will introduce family and guests to refreshing dining experiences but also will offer them many potential health benefits. The wide variety of vegetables, fruits, whole grains, dried beans, and various dairy foods finds limitless interpretations in meatless dishes for any course. The range of textures and flavors among these foods, accented by vibrant colors and attractive shapes, ensures sustained interest throughout the meal.

Merely substituting plant and vegetable protein for some of the meat in your diet immediately translates into reduced consumption of saturated fat and a higher intake of valuable dietary fiber. Those who eat well-planned meatless meals also tend to consume fewer calories, yet they feel satisfied.

The major protein sources for meatless meals are grains, legumes (dried beans, peas, and lentils), nuts and seeds, and dairy products. However, dairy products also contain some of the saturated fat of meat products, so many people choose to limit their consumption of these. Many fresh vegetables contain some quality protein, but the amounts are minimal so it is best to come to vegetables primarily for their rich vitamin and mineral content and the necessary roughage they contribute to our diets.

Preparation Time for Meatless Meals

Most grains and many legumes cook in less than an hour. Some may take longer, but these can be cooked in large quantities, frozen in serving portions, and used as needed. Most fresh vegetables take no longer than 30 minutes to cook, and many less than half that time. Raw vegetable salads require only some peeling, cutting, and chopping. Fruits, nuts, and seeds are staples of meatless diets that require no cooking at all and can serve as substantial and healthy snack foods. They are also welcome additions to soups and casseroles for added nutrition.

A cook in a hurry has a wide choice among meatless soups, salads, and casseroles that are quick and easy. Vegetable stocks cook up in 30 to 60 minutes and are a good staple that can be stored in abundance for use in many types of dishes.

Flavoring Meatless Dishes

Those new to meatless cooking are sure to notice that flavors are a departure from the very pronounced tastes of meat dishes. Each type of grain has its own subtle flavor—nutty and sweet, creamy, earthy, tangy, or any combination of these. Various legumes also have mild but distinct flavors and aromas when cooked. Fresh fruits and vegetables are often used to complement dishes featuring beans or grains. Legumes and grains also lend themselves to just about any kind of seasoning, including sauces and fresh or dried herbs and spices.

If you do a lot of meatless cooking, it is a good idea to keep plenty of homemade condiments on hand. Homemade catsup, tomato sauce, mayonnaise, mustard, chutney, and relish are sources of highly concentrated flavor that can liven up grain or bean dishes as well as steamed vegetables and hot or cold salads.

Experienced cooks know that there are several foods besides fresh herbs and spices that are considered indispensable aromatics. They have very concentrated flavors and often are used to season mild foods such as grains, legumes, or even fish, fowl, or meats. Some of the most commonly used aromatics include garlic, the onion family, mushrooms, celery, carrots, hot and sweet peppers, tomatoes, and eggplant. These ingredients can add zest to meatless dishes and may be used in combination or separately.

The Concept of Complementary Protein

Grains and legumes are the major plant sources of protein, but the protein they contain (like some animal protein sources) is deficient in certain of the "essential" amino acids that make up the protein capable of sustaining human life. However, if these foods are combined with each other at the same meal, each supplements the limiting amino acids of the other, thus improving the quality of protein consumed at the meal. This complementary relationship also exists between grains and milk products, legumes and seeds, and for some of the food combinations between grains and seeds, milk products and legumes, and milk products and seeds. This concept seems to have been instinctive to many cultures where meat has been a small part of the diet or totally absent from it. Consider the traditional black beans and rice of South America, corn tortillas and pinto beans of Mexico, polenta (cornmeal and cheese) of Italy, as well as pasta (wheat) dishes that include beans or cheese. In the Middle East this complementarity is represented by *dal* (lentils or dried peas) with rice and by hummus (sesame seeds and chick-peas).

Soyfoods

Soyfoods have assumed an especially important role in meatless diets because they are just about the best concentrated nonmeat protein sources. Like other legumes, soybeans should be eaten with a grain or dairy food at the same meal, to enhance protein value. Certain soyfoods have served as the "meat" of Eastern diets for centuries. Easy preparation and limitless culinary possibilities have increased the popularity of tofu among Western cooks in recent years. Tempeh (fermented soybeans) has a taste and texture akin to meat and it is even richer in protein than tofu or soybeans. It also has a good fiber content. Other important soyfoods include soymilk, soy flour, and soy grits and flakes. (See Legumes chapter for a complete discussion of soy products.)

To help plan your vegetarian meals, see page 16 for a listing of menu suggestions based on recipes in this book.

Menu Suggestions

It is an awesome challenge to come up with an appealing meal plan three times a day, seven days a week. Every cook has days when inspiration is elusive. Here is some help for getting over those times.

Family Menus

Beef and Barley Bake, page 488
Polynesian Vegetable Medley, page 214
Tossed Green Salad, page 166
Whole Wheat Popovers, page 390
Peach-Almond Frozen Yogurt, page 645

Stuffed Peppers, page 494
Mellow Wax Beans and Mushrooms, page 216
Sautéed Corn with Sour Cream, page 226
Fresh Fruit Ambrosia, page 641

Lamb Curry with Condiments, page 498,
with cooked bulgur
Braised Peas and Lettuce, French Style, page 234
Orange Custard, page 642

Southern-Style Pork Chop Casserole, page 505
Zucchini Italiano, page 240
Fresh Mushroom Salad, page 168
Apple Pie, page 719

Walnut and Herb-Stuffed Meat Loaf, page 494
Ratatouille, page 227
Spinach Salad, page 167, with Sour Cream and
Vinegar Dressing, page 184
Herb-Roasted Potatoes and Onions, page 237,
or baked potatoes
Angel Food Cake, page 674

Veal and Chicken Paprikash, page 510
Parslied Carrots and Zucchini Julienne, page 223
Chick-pea and Savoy Cabbage Salad, page 173
Buttermilk Biscuits, page 390
Blueberry Buckle, page 640

Baked Chicken Cacciatore, page 530,
with whole wheat pasta or
Polenta Cheese Squares, page 302
Eggplant Salad, page 168
Fennel Cookies, page 702, or Lemon Cookies,
page 704

Chicken with Vegetables and Tofu, page 538
Brown Rice Salad with Radishes and
Snow Pea Pods, page 308
Carob Bread Pudding, page 652

Turkey Tetrazzini, page 546
Brussels Sprouts in Walnut-Brown Butter Sauce,
page 219
Mexican Tomatoes, page 243
Golden Almond Shortcake, page 678

Broiled Codfish, page 578
Broccoli, Mushroom, and Pasta Salad, page 173
Lemon Chiffon Pie, page 726

Tuna Frittata, page 590
Stuffed Vegetables, page 210
Red Lentils and Red Onion Salad
with Tangy Mustard Dressing, page 177
Rice Custard, page 651, or Carrot Cake, page 677

Crab Cakes, Southern Style, page 592
Steamed Peas Piquant, page 234
Twice-Baked Potatoes, page 236,
or cooked brown rice
Butterscotch Brownies, page 709

Low-Cost and Low-Meat Menus

Chilled Mint-Pea Soup, page 128
Baked Zucchini Boats Stuffed with Bulgur and
Ground Lamb, page 314
Pita Butter Crisps, page 91
Poached Pears, page 628

linguine with Fish Sauce with Lemon, Parsley, and Tomato, page 327
steamed asparagus with Basil Butter, page 148
Three-Bean Salad, page 169
Honey-Baked Apples, page 620

Lasagna, page 331
Fresh Raw Vegetables with Vinaigrette Sauce, page 168
Baked Pears with Almonds and Yogurt, page 628

South of the Border Casserole, page 340
Tossed Green Salad, page 166
Crème Caramel, page 661

Black Bean Soup, page 116
Sea Shells with Avocado or Chili Sauce, page 334
Trout Salad with Mediterranean Dressing, page 178
Pumpkin Pie, page 729

Cheese and Pasta Casserole with Tuna Cakes, page 335
Zucchini Pancakes, page 241
Caesar Salad, page 165
Basic Vanilla Ice Milk, page 644

Cashew-Rice Casserole, page 308
Brussels Sprouts Kabobs, page 219
Norwegian Fish Salad, page 176
Yogurt Coffee Cake, page 684

Menus for Quick Meals

Beef Liver, Italian Style, page 510, with whole wheat noodles
Roasted Eggplant, page 227
Cucumber Salad, page 167
fresh fruit

Oven-Baked Beef-Mushroom Frittata, page 436
Waldorf Salad, page 171
Hash-Brown Potatoes, page 235
fresh pineapple with unsweetened shredded coconut

Ratatouille, page 227, with cooked brown rice or other whole grain
Spinach Salad, page 167
fresh fruit and cheese

Fillets of the Sea with Cream, page 571, on whole wheat toast points
steamed asparagus
fruit-flavored yogurt

Pork Chops with Pineapple, page 504
Turnips with Apples en Casserole, page 244
Summer Rice Salad, page 175
yogurt flavored with maple syrup and cinnamon

Codfish with Cheese Sauce, page 578, with cooked whole grains
steamed string beans
Sautéed Radishes and Cucumbers, page 237
apple slices dusted with cinnamon

Macaroni and Cheese, page 338
Sweet and Sour Red Cabbage, page 221
sliced kiwi fruit and orange segments with sour cream

Burritos, page 278, with cooked brown rice
Tossed Green Salad, page 166
Basic Vanilla Ice Cream, page 643

Tofu Stroganoff, page 286
Curried Eggs and Avocados, page 428
Peanut Butter-Stuffed Prunes, page 713

Menus for Entertaining

Baba Ghannouj, page 78, with raw
vegetable dippers
Lamb Stew with Artichoke Hearts, page 499
Bulgur, Fresh Beans, and Chick-peas
in Basil-Tomato Puree, page 315
Peachy Parfaits, page 642

Nachos, page 90, or Pizzaritas, page 91
Chili con Carne, page 490
Chili-Cheese Skillet Corn Bread, page 386
Raw Vegetable Salad, page 169
Melon Melba, page 647

Greek Lemon Soup, page 116
Leg of Lamb with Nut-Herb Stuffing, page 494
Spanakopeta, page 228
sliced fresh tomatoes and feta cheese
with Vinaigrette, page 184
Greek Walnut Cake, page 661

Supplì al Telefono, page 91
Spinach Lasagna, page 332
Celery Parmesan and Fennel, page 227
Stuffed Artichokes, page 212,
or Skewered Vegetable Antipasto, page 232
Biscotti, page 700, with French Carob Ice Cream,
page 644

Oriental Shrimp Nuggets with Hot Mustard,
page 95, or Shrimp Egg Rolls, page 97
Sukiyaki, page 487, with cooked brown rice
Lalap, page 169
Chinese Almond Cookies, page 702

Savory Broccoli Cocktail Cubes, page 88
Cheese and Cornmeal Gems, page 84
Red Snapper with Black Butter, page 579
Saffron Rice, page 312
Jerusalem Artichokes with Stir-Fry Vegetables,
page 212
Tossed Green Salad, page 166,
with Horseradish-Yogurt Dressing, page 182
Trifle, page 662

Cucumber Canapés, page 77
Veal Roast Stuffed with Sweetbreads, page 514
Basil Asparagus with Pasta, page 213
Orange, Fennel, and Watercress Salad, page 170
Pecan Pie, page 728, with Crème Chantilly,
page 695

Bite-Size Quiches, page 89
Elegant Poached Fillet of Sole, page 571
Marinated Millet Salad
with Layered Vegetables and Bean Sprouts,
page 303
Herb Casserole Bread, page 367
Orange-Almond Bavarian Cream, page 625

Artichoke Heart Soufflettes, page 86
Paella, page 604
Saffron Rice, page 312
Peas and Cheese Salad, page 176
Spanish Cream, page 648

Brunch Menus

Cheese-Mushroom Quiche, page 442
Apple-Honey-Oatmeal Muffins, page 388
sliced fresh honeydew melon
Carob Demitasse, page 748

Creamy Scrambled Eggs with Sweet Pepper,
page 432
Crusty Brown Bread, page 385, with honey or jam
Baked Pears with Almonds and Yogurt, page 628
Camomile-Peppermint Tea, page 750

Fruited French Toast, page 434, with butter
and jam or maple syrup
White Grape–Mint Mold, page 181
Honey Eggnog, page 749

Cheese-Mustard Soufflé, page 438
Pineapple and Curried Seafood Salad
in Pineapple Shells, page 630
Bagels, page 362, with cream cheese
Raspberry Shrub, page 743

Eggs and Broccoli Scramble, page 433
Sticky Cinnamon Buns, page 376
Spicy Peaches with Strawberry Hearts,
page 627
Hot Carob-Granola Drink, page 749

Liver, Buckwheat, and Onions in Potato Nests,
page 300
Whole Wheat Crescent Rolls, page 378
sliced fresh fruit with Cardamom-Yogurt Sauce,
page 149
Emerald Isle, page 746

Eggs, Chantilly Style, page 430
Blueberry Muffins, page 387
Hungarian Cold Sour Cherry Soup, page 623
herb tea

Eggs Chanticleer, page 430
Cheese-Herb Twist, page 363
sliced fresh tomatoes
Carob Demitasse, page 748

Blini with Raspberries, page 620
Three-Fruit Fish Salad with Ginger Sauce,
page 176
Applesauce-Raisin Muffins, page 387
Spiced Mint Tea, page 751

All-Corn Waffles, page 395, with fresh strawberries
or peaches and whipped cream or yogurt
Tropical Beet and Tuna Salad, page 177
Orange-Cashew Cooler, page 743

Fluffy Cottage Cheese Pancakes, page 394,
with raspberry jam
Cauliflower Omelet Mornay, page 435
Hot Carob-Granola Drink, page 749

Spinach Frittata, page 437
Hash-Brown Potatoes, page 235
Steamed Brown Bread, page 385
orange juice

Picnic Menus

Tofu Meat Loaf, page 287,
on Pumpernickel Bread, page 372
Curried Melon Salad, page 170
Cool Coleslaw, page 165
Peanut Butter Cookies, page 706

Sorrel-Stuffed Eggs, page 230
Ratatouille, page 227
Peas and Cheese Salad, page 176
Angel Food Cake, page 674

Wheat Berry, Spiced Cauliflower, and
Onion Salad, page 317
Tofu-Tuna Bake, page 286
Sweet and Sour Beans, page 280
Fresh Fruit Ambrosia, page 641

South Seas Chicken Salad, page 176
Peas and Shrimp Salad, page 234
Tofu-Guacamole Deviled Eggs, page 286
Pound Cake, page 682, and fresh fruit

Chili con Carne Salad, page 174
Kefir Potato Salad, page 168
Gazpacho, page 128
Banana Drops, page 700

Tortellini, Pimiento, and Sausage Salad, page 340
Raw Vegetable Salad, page 169
Pickled Green Peppers, page 235
Old-fashioned Rice Pudding, page 311

Curried Chicken and Corn Salad, page 174
Tabbouleh Salad, page 317
Pignoli Dip, page 82,
with Bran-Sesame Crackers, page 391
Carob Brownies, page 709

Deviled Eggs, page 428
Hummus, page 81, with raw carrot and
celery dippers
Mexi-Bean Salad, page 272
Zucchini-Raisin Quick Bread, page 387

Vegetarian Menus

Dutch Sour Cream-Bean Soup, page 116
Millet-Stuffed Peppers, page 303
Vegetables with Oriental Sauce, page 229
Tofu Cheese Pie, page 731

Chilled Broccoli Soup, page 127
Brown Rice and Eggplant with Cheese Custard,
page 308
Fresh Fruit Ambrosia, page 641

Bulgur Confetti Salad
with Sesame Seed Dressing, page 314
Jamaican Sweet Potatoes, page 242
Maple Mousse, page 648

Whole Garden Soup with Rice and Pesto,
page 122
Vegetable-Bean Patties, page 279
Carob Mousse, page 648

Tofu Lasagna, page 286
Spinach Salad, page 167
Apricot Upside-Down Skillet Cake, page 675

Creole Frittata, page 436, with cooked brown rice
Mexi-Bean Salad, page 272
Pecan Cookies, page 706

Corn Chowder, page 118
Chinese Stir-Fried Vegetables
with Tofu and Millet, page 302
Carrot Cookies with Orange Frosting, page 701

Soupe au Pistou, page 121
Vegetable Soufflé, page 440
Oatmeal-Honey Wafers, page 705

Summer Rice Salad, page 175
Tempeh Burgers, page 284
Summer Dessert Omelet, page 643

Menus for Children

To create menus that will please your children,
select recipes from several of the following
groupings.

Appetizers

Bite-Size Quiches, page 89
Caribbean Chicken, page 93
Fruited Cheese Log, page 84
Miniature Pizzas, page 90
Parmesan Pita Puffs, page 90

Soups

Cream of Chicken Soup, page 123
Fresh Tomato Soup, page 119
Old-fashioned Chicken-Rice Soup, page 115

About Kitchen Equipment

The tools you need for cooking and baking in your kitchen need not be elaborate. Relatively few of the many items available are actually necessary. Choose kitchen tools that have multiple uses and obviate the need for a larger repertoire of equipment, thus saving on space, clean-up work, and money. This applies to electric appliances as well, which often represent a considerable investment.

Evaluate how often you really will need the tool or utensil you are considering. Can a tool you already own do the same job? Specialized equipment is nice to own once you have the basics, but remember that each new item will require storage space and, often, extra care.

Selecting Cookware and Bakeware

Cookware and bakeware may be made of ceramic, glass, or one or several of various metals. Each material has its own characteristics and particular responses to different kinds of heat used in the kitchen. When selecting cooking and baking vessels, you should know the qualities of the various materials used and understand what to look for in good construction—and always keep in mind the particular role the vessel will have in your kitchen.

Here are some basic pointers to help you in shopping for cookware and bakeware:

• Inspect the construction. Covers should fit snugly; look for covers with skirts (rims that fit inside the vessels).

• Look for crevices at joints and seams where food might lodge, and check for imperfections in the surface.

• Flat bottoms or concave bottoms designed to flatten on heating are best in cookware.

• Utensils should be good conductors of heat (see Guide to Materials table, page 19).

• The heavier the pot, the better it is for cooking. A thick iron pot retains heat better and diffuses it more economically than a lightweight one. Cheap, thin, enameled pots heat up more rapidly and unevenly, so food is more likely to burn and stick.

• Choose materials that will not affect color, flavor, or nutritive values of food (see Guide to Materials table, below).

• No part of a pot or pan should be inaccessible to a mixing spoon.

• Handles and knobs (preferably heat resistant) should be sturdy with a comfortable grip that will keep your hand a safe distance from hot metal. Rivets are good fasteners for handles to pots; they should be flush to the surface. Screws are less secure. Spot welding, often used for spouts, is a good fastening method, as is brazing (the handle is bonded to the pot with copper or brass).

• Cooking and baking utensils should be easy to clean, with no interior seams, crevices, or rough edges.

• For pots and skillets choose versatile sizes to accommodate several cooking tasks (see Basic Cookware, page 22).

Energy-Saving Tips

The scarcity of fuel, and its consequent high cost, has made all of us conscious of the value of conserving energy whenever possible. Here are some easy ways to do so:

• Cover metal utensils when possible during cooking. Turn the heat off a few minutes before the food is done. Retained heat, especially in the heating elements of electric ranges, will finish the cooking. Low heat and snugly fitting covers save on energy.

• Pots and pans should fit the surface heating unit. Flames or the heating element should not extend beyond the bottom of the pot.

• Select the right size pot for the amount of food you are cooking.

• Pressure cookers cook faster and save energy.

• Portable electric appliances—skillets, slow cookers, and toaster-ovens—may use less energy than an electric range unit.

Guide to Materials for Cookware and Bakeware

Material	Heating Properties	Response to Foods	Use and Care	Type of Equipment Suitable For
Aluminum	Good, even heat conduction; cools quickly.	Will discolor foods and affect taste of foods left in pan for more than 15 minutes. Acid foods will also discolor pan's surface.	Cool before washing in warm, soapy water—dry immediately. Undissolved salt may cause pitting—add salt to hot liquid and stir in before adding liquid to pot.	soup pots, frying pans, bakeware, measuring utensils, cooking utensils
Cast-iron	Good conductor of heat, but is slow and may be uneven causing "hot spots." Good conductor of radiant (oven) heat.	May transfer some residual flavors and odors to, and cause discoloration of, foods, especially acid foods.	Must be seasoned according to manufacturer's instructions to prevent rusting. Wash with water or in a light, soapy solution; scrub with a brush only if necessary. Never soak; always dry immediately.	skillets, muffin tins, roasting pans, Dutch ovens, griddles

[continued]

Guide to Materials for Cookware and Bakeware—*Continued*

Material	Heating Properties	Response to Foods	Use and Care	Type of Equipment Suitable For
Copper	Excellent, uniform heat conduction; cools quickly.	Reacts with all foods, creating a potentially poisonous substance, thus copper utensils must be lined with another metal, often tin. Exception: copper bowls used for beating egg whites.	Wash lining with soapy water; polish copper with commercial copper cleaner or with mixture of flour, salt, lemon juice, and ammonia.	pots, saucepans, casseroles, teapots, molds, mixing bowls
Earthenware	Absorbs heat slowly, but well; retains heat for a long time.	May retain tastes and odors and transfer them to foods unless utensil is glazed.	Cool before washing with warm water and abrasive scrubber. Soap alone may be used to clean glazed surfaces.	casseroles, slow cookers
Glass	Absorbs heat very slowly, but retains for a long time.	May cook or bake foods faster on the outside unless temperature is adjusted.	Cool before washing in warm, soapy water with abrasive scrubber.	baking dishes, casseroles, pie plates
Nonstick finish	Depends on metal of vessel or utensil.	None, unless it chips or peels.	Season if manufacturer's instructions say to do so. Wash in hot, soapy water using soft sponge or dishcloth. Do not use sharp or rough-edged utensils on nonstick surfaces. Avoid high heat.	most cookware, bakeware, and cooking utensils
Porcelain enamel	Absorbs heat very slowly, but retains for a long time. Absorbs radiant (oven) heat particularly well.	None.	Cool before washing with warm, soapy water. Avoid use of harsh abrasives. Soak to loosen cooked-on food. Clean stained surface with baking soda.	baking pans, casseroles, bakeware
Stainless steel	Good heat conduction if combined with aluminum or copper.	May cause slight discoloring of highly acid foods.	Wash with warm, soapy water. Avoid use of harsh, abrasive cleaners. Soak briefly to remove burned-on food. Dry immediately after cleaning.	frying pans, bakeware

Types of Kitchen Equipment

Like any other job, cooking is easiest and most efficient when the proper tools are used. Choose each kind of knife, pan, or electrical appliance for optimal usefulness. The information below will help you in your selection.

Knives

Experienced cooks believe a set of good, sharp knives is the cook's most indispensable tool. Good knives are expensive but well worth it, for they perform many vital functions. With proper care knives will serve you well and last a long time.

Shopping for Knives

When shopping for a set of knives, look for the best quality possible. Check to see if the manufacturer's name is engraved on the blade; this is usually a sign of good workmanship. Hold the knife in your hand. It should feel comfortable to you, and the blade should seem well anchored in the handle. Depending on what you will use the knife for, you should also note the weight, balance, flexibility, and sharpness of each knife in a set. Some of the things to observe or inquire about upon closer inspection are:

The type of material(s) used: Forged carbon steel knives, among the most expensive, are the choice of most professional chefs. High-carbon steel is generally regarded as the most satisfactory material for knives because it takes a good, sharp edge most efficiently and keeps it for a long time. The knife requires more care, however, than other materials, and acid foods will discolor it.

Stainless steel knives may be cheaper than carbon steel knives. They are harder than carbon steel and keep their sharpness even longer, but they are more difficult to sharpen when they do dull. However, stainless steel has the advantage of being rustproof, and it will not affect the flavor and color of food as carbon steel will if not properly cared for.

An intermediate choice for quality and budget purposes is stainless steel with a high percentage of carbon. This alloy combines some of the best qualities of both carbon and steel. Knives of tempered stainless steel with a high carbon content are considered among the best.

The grind of the blade: Most professional knives are taper ground, or forged in one piece from bar steel with all parts of the knife shaped in a series of processes. The handle is added before the edge is ground. The blade is machine ground with a taper from back to edge and from handle to blade tip. Carbon and stainless steel knives may both be taper ground.

Hollow ground knives have broad, concave cutting surfaces. They are very good for slicing but are easily damaged. Most of the cheaper knives cut from thin strips of stainless steel are hollow ground.

The handle material: The handle should be made from a material that does not absorb moisture and that resists shrinking and warping. The best handles are made from close-grained hardwood or plastic-wood laminates. High-quality plastic is good but may be slippery when wet. Maple and walnut, rosewood, bone ivory, hard rubber, steel, and aluminum may also be used for knife handles.

The way the knife is put together: Examine the way the handle is secured to the knife. The tang, or the part of the blade that extends into the handle, may run the full length or part of the length of the handle, depending on the type of knife. The tang on good knives is forged from the same piece of metal as the blade, which lends strength to the knife. It should be securely fastened inside the handle, ideally with two or three good-size rivets. Small nails, brads, or a metal collar are not sturdy enough and will not hold a knife together for very long.

The type of cutting edge: The cutting edges of knives vary in shape and thickness, depending on the blade's intended use. When choosing knives for the various cutting jobs in food preparation, consider the length, shape, and degree of flexibility of the entire blade as well as the type of cutting edge.

The following are the most commonly needed knives:

paring knife—a small, usually 2½- to 3-inch blade; gives leverage without unnecessary strain on the fingers; used for turning, paring, and trimming small and light vegetables

utility knife (sometimes called a French knife or a chef's knife)—a larger blade, 6 to 8 inches; similar to a paring knife but used to cut large vegetables and to slice, cube, and mince vegetables, nuts, and herbs; may also be used to trim meat, slice cold poultry, clean fish, or do anything for which a paring knife is too short

serrated knife—a fine-toothed knife with sawlike points cut into the blade edge; used to cut smooth, soft foods such as bread, tomatoes, grapefruits, and cucumbers. A serrated bread knife, which is most useful, should be fairly rigid and long, to slice across large loaves. A grapefruit knife is small, with a curved, double-edged serrated blade, to cut away sections of grapefruit halves

carving knife—should be very sharp, slightly flexible, and long, to cut hot, yielding meats; should have a long, thin point that curves in order to cut around bones

boning knife—used for removing bones from raw meat and poultry; should have a rigid, narrow, broad-backed blade with a sharp point

filleting knife—should be strong, thin-backed, and have a pointed, sharp, and flexible blade

butcher knife—a thick and heavy knife with a long, about 5¼- to 10-inch, firm blade for cutting, trimming, and finishing cuts of meat

cleaver—a strong and heavy knife used to cut through bone and to tenderize meat; also good for light chopping, mincing, dicing, scraping, and shredding of meats, fish, and vegetables

Caring for Knives

The life of a knife can be extended impressively through good care. Follow the tips below to maintain the like-new quality of a fine knife.

• Always chop on a wooden or polypropylene surface to preserve the knife's edge. Hard surfaces dull the edge.

• Do not place knives in a dishwasher. Wash them by hand in hot, soapy water and dry immediately. All knives should be cleaned and wiped dry right after being used. High-carbon steel knives especially demand immediate care, as they discolor and stain quickly. Clean stained blades with a cork sprinkled with an abrasive cleaning powder.

• Do not store kitchen knives in drawers or jars where the blades will hit against other utensils. The best way to store them is to slot them in a knife box or in a wall-fixed rack within easy reach of the work surface.

Sharpening Knives

Sharpen knives with a hand-held steel or a sharpening stone. To use a sharpening steel: Draw the knife blade lightly down the steel at a shallow (20-degree) angle. Repeat, putting the knife first to the front of the steel, then to the back.

To use a sharpening stone: Place the stone on a flat surface, with a damp cloth underneath to keep it secure. Support the stone with one hand and gently draw the knife blade across its length at a shallow angle. Do this several times. Then turn the blade over and repeat in the opposite direction. If the stone has both a coarse and a fine surface, run each side of the blade over the coarse surface first.

Basic Cookware

crepe/omelet pan—a shallow pan with sloping sides (an omelet pan may be slightly deeper than a crepe pan)

pots—having several sizes useful, preferably two-quart, four-quart, and eight-quart pots with covers (see Guide to Materials table, page 19) pressure cooker—an airtight pot that cuts cooking time by about 50 to 70 percent; suitable for cooking stocks, soups, dried beans, grains, and for blanching vegetables; also useful for canning and preserving

saucepan or double boiler—a two- to four-cup capacity best

skillets—a 7-inch, 10-inch, and a 12-inch skillet useful

steamer—an expanding metal basket that fits inside different-shaped pots; used to cook fresh vegetables or to reheat foods

wok—a bowl-shaped pan of light metal used in Chinese cooking for rapid stir-frying of vegetables and other foods

Electrical Appliances

blender—good for blending liquids, grinding, pureeing foods finely, and for making sauces

food processor—takes the tedium out of chopping, mincing, slicing, and shredding normally done by hand with a sharp knife; with the proper attachments can also knead dough, puree, and beat batters, thus replacing the need for a blender or electric mixer. (Many cooks feel it is an adequate replacement for these and similar appliances; others feel the original appliances meet their needs more efficiently.)

griddle—good for cooking pancakes evenly and in quantity

hand-held mixer—useful for blending sauces and other foods, especially as they cook on the stove

slow cooker—an electric pot that cooks soups, stews, and similar dishes very slowly; especially helpful to working cooks who wish to leave meals to cook slowly throughout the day

table mixer—valuable to those who bake often; frees the cook to do other jobs as the batter is blending

toaster-oven—more useful than a regular toaster; especially good for grilling sandwiches; toasting thicker, more fragile, home-baked goods; reheating foods; and for cooking small casseroles

Crushing and Grinding Utensils

food mill—a mechanical-type sieve with three different cutting disks to puree food from fine to coarse (often replaced today by an electric food processor)

garlic press—a utensil held like a pair of scissors and squeezed to release the crushed garlic clove or its juice through tiny holes in the utensil's head

juice extracter—many designs available—manual or electric—but should release juice from citrus fruits without the pulp and seeds

masher—a hand-held utensil with either a coiled metal base or a flat, slotted one for mashing and pureeing cooked potatoes and other root vegetables right in the pan in which they are cooked

meat grinder—a hand-operated machine, usually of cast-iron framework and attached to a table by clamps, into which meat is dropped and then hand-cranked through a disk for the desired coarseness

meat tenderizer—a hand-held utensil of various designs—usually a fluted, steel face on a hammerhead, or a pyramid-shaped, spiky-headed wood, plastic, or metal hammer—with which meat is pounded until tender

mortar and pestle—a primitive but efficient instrument consisting of a smooth, regularly curved bowl (mortar), usually of marble or wood, and a compatibly shaped grinder (pestle) of the same material; very useful for pulverizing nuts and seeds, garlic, herbs, and whole spices

nut and shellfish cracker—a sturdy, steel utensil that should permit some control over pressure to crack nuts and shellfish shells without crushing their contents

pepper mill—a hand-held wooden or plastic container with a grinding mechanism in its base for grinding whole peppercorns when freshly ground pepper is called for in a recipe

ricer—a cone-shaped metal container with a compatibly shaped wooden pestle that forces cooked foods such as chestnuts, potatoes, apples, or other fruit or root vegetables through the container's tiny perforations to obtain dry, ricelike grains of these foods

spice grinder—an instrument similar to a pepper mill for grinding up whole spices and, in some cases, whole dried herbs

Cutting Utensils Other Than Knives

apple corer—a circular, stainless steel blade surrounded by blades set like wheel spokes that, when pressed down on an apple, divide it into neatly cored sections

cheese wire—a stainless steel wire and roller with a plastic handle, used to slice hard and semihard cheeses as thin or thick as needed

cutting board—a block of wood or polyethylene plastic used to protect counters and tabletops as well as knife blades when chopping meats and vegetables or slicing bread and other foods

egg slicer—a slicer, consisting of fine wires stretched across a slotted base, that can slice peeled, hard-cooked eggs into neat, uniform slices for garnishes or other purposes

grater—a box with four variously perforated sides used to grate foods from fine to coarse, or a flat sheet with two types of surfaces and a slicing blade

peeler/parer—used to thinly peel or shave the skins of fresh vegetables to minimize nutrient loss; can be of various designs, but the most popular one has a fluted blade that can be used to core or to scoop out blemishes from vegetables

scissors—a good, sharp pair useful for cutting paper and for jobs for which shears may be too awkward

shears—used to cut through tough materials such as small bones, poultry joints, shellfish, and raw meat; the cutting edges need not be as sharp as those of scissors

zester—an instrument with a curved blade containing five little holes that, when drawn firmly across the skin of a citrus fruit, pares the skin but not the pith

Draining Utensils

colander—a bowl-shaped container with many small holes for draining pasta and vegetables

salad spinner—a more efficient version of a salad shaker, consisting of a plastic container with an inner, rotating plastic basket that, when spun quickly, forces excess water from lettuce and other leafy vegetables into the outer container

Skimming, Lifting, and Turning Utensils

fork—a long-handled metal utensil useful for lifting and turning meat or fowl, to steady a roast being carved, or to lift large vegetables from water or from a steamer

skimmer or slotted spoon—a large, metal, flat spoon with holes, used to lift food from boiling water or to skim grease or scum from soups and stocks

spatula—a flat wooden, metal, or plastic utensil for lifting and turning omelets and other frying foods

tongs—a flexible, metal grabber for turning frying foods, serving spaghetti, and lifting vegetables and other foods out of hot water

Thermometers

candy thermometer—made of glass and stainless steel with a clip for attaching it to the side of a pan; gradations up to 350°F; increases accuracy in determining the stages of sugar in candy making

dairy thermometer—a glass alcohol thermometer in a plastic case; used for checking the temperature of yogurt or cheese

deep frying thermometer—made of glass and stainless steel with a clip for attaching it to the side of a pan; gradations from 100 to 500°F; aids in determining the oil temperature for frying foods

freezer thermometer—made of glass and plastic; used to measure the coldness of a freezer

meat thermometer—made of stainless steel; used to check the internal temperatures of meats

multipurpose thermometer—measures from 40 to 220°F; good for checking room temperatures when making yogurt or bread

oven thermometer—a glass mercury tube set in stainless steel; used to determine the accuracy of any oven's thermostat

Measuring Utensils

measuring cups—liquid and dry measuring cups available in metal, plastic, or glass; liquid measuring cups have graduated markings and a pouring spout; dry measuring ones come in a nestled set of four that each measure flush to the rim

measuring spoons—a set of spoons made of plastic or metal that come in four sizes—one-quarter teaspoon, one-half teaspoon, one teaspoon, and one tablespoon—for accurately measuring wet and dry ingredients

scale—used to measure by weight instead of volume; available in either balance or spring models

Mixing Utensils

bowls—various sizes for mixing; preferably made of glass or stainless steel

rotary beater—a hand-held utensil with two four-bladed beaters operated by a small hand-turned crank; useful for mixtures that may be too heavy for a wire whisk

rubber spatula—a flexible piece of rubber (preferably heatproof) attached to a wooden or plastic handle for scraping batter and dough mixtures from mixing bowls and remaining condiments from jars

wire whisk—a hand-held, metal utensil with looped, springy wires ideal for stirring sauces and beating egg whites

wooden spoon—useful for mixing, stirring where a large metal spoon is undesirable

Basic Bakeware

Baking pan sizes may vary; standard sizes are listed below.

angel food (tube)—10 × 4-inch

baking sheet—14 × 10-inch with or without rim

jelly-roll pan—15½ × 10½ × 1-inch

loaf pans—8½ × 4½-inch and 9 × 5-inch

muffin/cupcake tins—2½ × 1¼-inch

ovenproof casseroles—2-quart and 10-inch-square

pie plates—9 × 1¼-inch; also 8-inch and 10-inch

rectangular cake pans—10 × 6 × 1½-inch and 13 × 9½ × 2-inch

round cake pans—9 × 1½-inch

springform pan—8-inch or 10-inch

square cake pans—9 × 9 × 1¾-inch

Special Bakeware

mold for cakes or gelatins—a pan decoratively shaped for special cakes, gelatins, and aspics

quiche dish—a porcelain pie plate with straight sides and fluted edges ramekin—a small, often round or oval, ovenproof dish that is made of earthenware or porcelain and used as a mold or individual serving dish

soufflé dish—a round, deep, straight-sided, ovenproof dish

terrine—a straight-sided clay, porcelain, or cast-iron pot with a lid, for making pâtés or terrines

Baking and Oven Utensils

baster—a syringelike plastic tube with a rubber bulbous end, for drawing up the juices of a cooking meat or fowl for basting

cake rack—a metal grate used to allow air to circulate freely around cooling cakes, breads, and other baked goods

cookie cutters—variously shaped metal cutters for shaping rolled cookie dough quickly

insulated gloves or pot holders—useful to protect hands when they are in contact with hot objects

metal skewers—long, needlelike, steel pins used to hold meat and poultry firmly in shape during cooking

pastry bag—a canvas or nylon bag that is cone shaped with a plain tip or decorative pastry tips for piping whipped cream, icing, and various fillings

pastry blender—a utensil consisting of five or six steel-wire cutters fastened in arclike fashion to both ends of a wooden handle; used for quickly cutting fat into flour in pastry making

pastry brush—a brush resembling a small house-painting brush; used to apply washes of beaten egg, milk, or syrup to dough or pastries before or after baking

roasting rack—a metal, gratelike stand used to keep roasting meat or poultry raised above the fat or juices dripping from it

rolling pin—a wooden or plastic cylinder with handles, for rolling out dough

sieve—a bowl or drum-shaped utensil with a metal mesh bottom used for separating fine particles from coarse ones or straining solids from liquids or as a flour sifter

sifter—a utensil similar to a sieve but deeper and with an oscillating mechanism for sifting flour for cakes and other baked goods or for dredging

trivet—a metal or ceramic stand for use under hot dishes and baking utensils to protect counters and table surfaces

trussing needle—a large sewing needle for sewing up poultry or stuffed meats; comes in various lengths

Measuring Accurately

In the preparation of recipes, accurate measuring of ingredients often makes the difference between success and failure. Use these basic tools to simplify measuring: a liquid measuring cup, a set of dry measuring cups, and a set of measuring spoons.

Liquid measuring cups are generally made of clear glass or plastic and have visible markings for every one-quarter and one-third cup. Select a cup that has the last marking far enough below the rim so that when it contains a full cup of liquid you can still pick it up without spilling it. The cup should have a handle and a pouring spout.

Dry measuring cups, which come as a set of four cups that nestle one inside the other, are made of metal or plastic. The cups range in size from one-quarter cup to one cup, and each measures flush to the rim. This feature enables you to level the ingredients with the flat edge of a knife or spatula.

Both dry and liquid ingredients are measured with the same type of measuring spoon. The spoons come in sizes from one-quarter teaspoon to one tablespoon. Like dry measuring cups, they are flush so that you can level off dry ingredients with a knife or spatula.

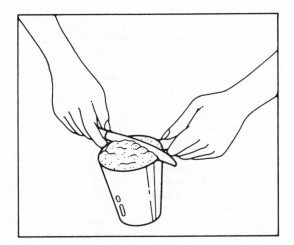

Measurements for recipes in this book and others are, as a rule, level unless a recipe states differently. When a measure is not level, directions will state, for example, a scant one-half cup or a heaping teaspoon.

To measure dry ingredients such as flour, bread crumbs, or minced or grated foods: Either stir the ingredient lightly with a fork, to break up

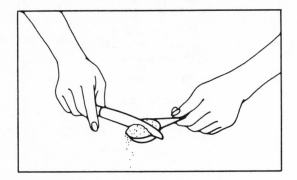

lumps and introduce air, or, if flour, sift before measuring. Spoon the ingredient lightly into the measuring cup or measuring spoon until it is overflowing; then level off (scrape off) the excess with the flat edge of a knife or spatula. Do not tap the cup, shake down the contents, or pack the ingredients, unless the recipe instructs otherwise.

To measure liquid ingredients: Place the cup on a level surface; do not hold it over the mixture to which you are adding the liquid (you may spill some). Fill the cup slowly to the desired level; then, without lifting the cup, check the amount at eye level. When measuring sticky ingredients such as syrup, honey, or molasses, oil the cup lightly before adding the ingredient, and scrape out the measure well with a spatula. Use spoons to measure less than one-quarter cup, and fill them to the brim without spilling the liquid over.

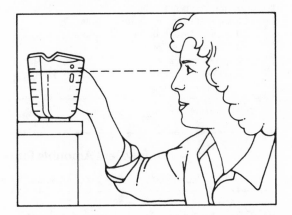

To measure shortening: Measure oil and melted butter (melt an approximate amount before measuring) by the same method as for other liquids. But pack softened (room temperature) butter firmly into a dry measuring cup, pressing out the pockets of air. Level off the butter with a knife or spatula to remove the excess, then scrape out the cup well with a spatula. If the butter is packaged in sticks with marked amounts, use a sharp knife to cut chilled, firm butter at the appropriate marking.

Equivalent Measures

Cooks are constantly being called upon to make decisions and to improvise. If a recipe calls for two cups of honey, the cook must decide if a jar marked "eight fluid ounces" will fill the requirement. If a recipe calls for one-quarter liter of oil, does that translate to one cup of oil? Will a one-pound head of cabbage yield three cups of shredded cabbage for a coleslaw recipe? Some of these answers come with experience, but the handy tables below will resolve many doubts quickly.

Equivalent Weights and Measures

Pinch or dash = less than ⅛ teaspoon
3 teaspoons = 1 tablespoon
2 tablespoons = 1 fluid ounce
1 jigger = 1½ fluid ounces
4 tablespoons = ¼ cup or 2 fluid ounces
5 tablespoons + 1 teaspoon = ⅓ cup
8 tablespoons = ½ cup or 4 fluid ounces
10 tablespoons + 2 teaspoons = ⅔ cup
12 tablespoons = ¾ cup
16 tablespoons = 1 cup or 8 fluid ounces
1 cup = ½ pint
2 cups = 1 pint or 16 fluid ounces
4 cups = 1 quart or 32 fluid ounces
4 quarts = 1 gallon
8 quarts = 1 peck
4 pecks = 1 bushel
1 pound = 16 ounces

NOTE: All measures are level.

Metric Equivalents for Dry and Liquid Measures

Dry Ingredients	Liquid Ingredients
1 gram = 0.035 ounce	1 deciliter = 6 tablespoons + 2 teaspoons
5 grams = approximately 1 teaspoon	¼ liter = 1 cup + 2¼ teaspoons
28.35 grams = 1 ounce	
50 grams = 1¾ ounces	½ liter = 1 pint + 4½ teaspoons
100 grams = 3½ ounces	
227 grams = 8 ounces	1 liter = 1 quart + scant ¼ cup
1,000 grams (1 kilogram) = 2 pounds, 3¼ ounces	4 liters = 1 gallon + 1 scant cup
	10 liters = approximately 2½ gallons + 2½ cups

Equivalent Amounts for Common Recipe Ingredients

Ingredient	Amount	Equals	Equivalent Amount
Almonds			
Unshelled	1 pound	=	1¼ cups nutmeats
Shelled	1 pound	=	4-4½ cups nutmeats
Apples	1 pound	=	3 cups raw, sliced
	1 pound	=	1 ⅔ cups cooked, chopped
	1 pound	=	1¼ cups pureed
Apricots, dried	1 pound	=	3¼ cups dried
Bananas	1 pound (3-4 medium)	=	1¾ cups mashed

Equivalent Amounts for Common Recipe Ingredients—*Continued*

Ingredient	Amount	Equals	Equivalent Amount
Beef	1 pound	=	3 cups minced
	1 pound	=	2 cups ground
Blue cheese	4 ounces	=	1 cup crumbled
Brazil nuts			
Unshelled	1 pound	=	1½ cups nutmeats
Shelled	1 pound	=	3 cups nutmeats
Bread			
Dry	1 slice	=	1/3 cup fine crumbs
Fresh	1 slice	=	½ cup soft crumbs
Brown rice, raw	1 cup	=	4 cups cooked
Buckwheat groats, raw	1 cup	=	4 cups cooked
Bulgur, raw	1 cup	=	4 cups cooked
Butter	1 stick	=	8 tablespoons
	1 stick	=	½ cup
	1 stick	=	4 ounces
Whipped	1 pound	=	3 cups
Cabbage	1 pound	=	4½ cups shredded
Carrots	1 pound	=	3 cups shredded
Cheddar cheese	½ pound	=	2 cups grated
Coconut	3½ ounces	=	1 1/3 cups flaked
	3½ ounces	=	1 cup grated
Cornmeal	1 pound	=	3 cups
Cottage cheese	½ pound	=	1 cup
Cream cheese	3 ounces	=	6 tablespoons
Cream, heavy	1 cup	=	2 cups whipped
Garlic	1 small clove	=	⅛ teaspoon powder
Gelatin	¼-ounce envelope	=	1 tablespoon
Kidney beans, dry	1 pound	=	2½ cups dry
	1 pound	=	6 cups cooked
Lemon	1 medium	=	1 teaspoon grated rind
	1 medium	=	3 tablespoons juice

[*continued*]

Equivalent Amounts for Common Recipe Ingredients—*Continued*

Ingredient	Amount	Equals	Equivalent Amount
Lentils, dry	1 pound	=	2¼ cups dry
	1 pound	=	5 cups cooked
Lima beans, dry	1 pound	=	2½ cups dry
	1 pound	=	6 cups cooked
Navy beans, dry	1 pound	=	2 cups dry
	1 pound	=	5 cups cooked
Macaroni, raw	1 pound	=	4 cups raw
	1 pound	=	8 cups cooked
Mushrooms	½ pound	=	3 cups sliced
Noodles	1 pound	=	6 cups raw
	1 pound	=	7 cups cooked
Oats, rolled	1 pound	=	6¼ cups raw
	1 pound	=	8 cups cooked
Onion	1 medium	=	½ cup minced
Orange	1 medium	=	2½ tablespoons grated rind
	1 medium	=	⅓ cup juice
Peanuts			
Unshelled	1 pound	=	2 cups nutmeats
Shelled	1 pound	=	4-4½ cups nutmeats
Pecans			
Unshelled	1 pound	=	2¼ cups nutmeats
Shelled	1 pound	=	4-4½ cups nutmeats
Pepper, sweet	1 large	=	1 cup minced
Potatoes	3 medium	=	1¾ cups mashed
Raisins, seedless	1 pound	=	2¾ cups
Spaghetti, raw	1 pound	=	4 cups raw
	1 pound	=	7-8 cups cooked
Spinach	1 pound	=	1½ cups cooked, chopped
Strawberries	1 pint	=	1½ cups sliced
Walnuts			
Unshelled	1 pound	=	1¾ cups nutmeats
Shelled	1 pound	=	4-4½ cups nutmeats
Wheat germ	12 ounces	=	3 cups
Whole wheat flour	1 pound	=	3¾ cups
Yeast	1 package	=	1 tablespoon dry
	1 package	=	1 cake compressed

Substitute Ingredients

Of course, a wise cook plans ahead before starting to prepare a dish, but even the best sometimes turns to the cupboard for a vital ingredient and finds it bare. If there is no time to run to the store, substitutions are often possible. Oil can replace butter in many recipes; raisins may be used in place of prunes, and so forth. Here are some simple substitutes that might save you in a pinch.

Recipe Ingredient Substitutes

Ingredient	Amount	Equals	Equivalent Amount	Substitute Ingredient
Arrowroot	1½ teaspoons	=	1 tablespoon	flour
	2 teaspoons	=	1 tablespoon	cornstarch
Baking powder	1 teaspoon	=	¼ teaspoon	baking soda plus ⅝ teaspoon cream of tartar
	1 teaspoon	=	¼ teaspoon	baking soda plus ½ cup buttermilk or yogurt
	1 teaspoon	=	¼ teaspoon	baking soda plus ¼ cup molasses
Butter	1 cup	=	⅞ cup	vegetable oil
Buttermilk	1 cup	=	1 cup	plain yogurt
	1 cup	=	1 cup	skim milk plus 1 tablespoon lemon juice or vinegar
Cayenne pepper	⅛ teaspoon	=	3-4 drops	liquid hot pepper
Chocolate	1 ounce	=	3 tablespoons	carob plus 2 tablespoons water
Cracker crumbs	¾ cup	=	1 cup	whole grain bread crumbs
Cream				
Heavy	1 cup	=	⅓ cup	butter plus ¾ cup milk
Sour	1 cup	=	1 cup	yogurt
Flour	1 tablespoon	=	1½ teaspoons	cornstarch
	1 tablespoon	=	1 tablespoon	quick-cooking tapioca
	1 tablespoon	=	1 tablespoon	corn flour
	1 tablespoon	=	1 tablespoon	potato flour
Lemon juice	1 teaspoon	=	½ teaspoon	vinegar
Milk, whole	1 cup	=	1 cup	reconstituted nonfat dry milk plus 2½ teaspoons butter
Mustard, prepared	1 tablespoon	=	1 teaspoon	dry mustard
Prunes, pitted and minced	½ cup	=	½ cup	raisins
Tomatoes, chopped	1 cup	=	½ cup	tomato sauce plus ½ cup water

Food and Cooking Terms

New cooks, as well as experienced ones, are frequently confronted in recipes with terms they have never seen before—terms that are critical to the success of the dish. How does one cook in a *bain-marie,* temper eggs, butterfly a fish fillet? What is bolted grain, a galantine, a jellmeter? This listing explains these and hundreds of other words and phrases that pertain to food and cooking.

acid food: a food with a high acid content, such as all fruits, tomatoes, and pickled foods

acidophilus milk: a cultured milk with a sharp, acid taste often taken for its easy digestibility and its live culture, which helps promote a healthy intestinal tract

acidulate: to make water acidic by adding lemon juice or vinegar

-ade: a sweetened drink made from water and fruit juice that may contain high percentages of water and sweetener when made commercially

agar: a gelatinous extract of red algae used as a jelling or stabilizing agent in foods such as molded salads

aïoli: a garlic-mayonnaise dressing

à la nappe **(coat a spoon):** just thick enough to coat a spoon; refers to the consistency of a sauce

al dente: literally "to the teeth," or cooked just firm to the bite; refers to pasta and sometimes vegetables

amaranth: a food plant grown for its spinachlike leaves and for its seeds, which can be ground into flour

amorphous candy: see **noncrystalline candy**

antipasto: an appetizer salad, of Italian character, consisting of tidbits of various hot or cold foods such as sardines, olives, cheeses, marinated salads, meats, eggs, and fresh vegetables arranged on a platter

arrowroot: a starch from the root of a tropical plant used to thicken sauces and soups; virtually interchangeable with cornstarch

aspic: a savory molded salad made with stock from meat, fish, poultry, or vegetables; also, the savory jelly used to garnish meat or fish

au gratin: covered with bread crumbs, butter, or cheese, then baked or broiled until a golden, crisp crust results

backfin: the crab meat, usually in small chunks, from various parts of the crab's body

bain-marie: a water bath in which containers of custard may be placed to help prevent curdling during cooking

bake: to cook by dry heat in an oven in containers that may or may not be covered; generally called roasting when referring to meats; the pan is never covered during roasting

baking powder: a powder used as a leavening agent in making baked goods (usually quick breads) that consists of a carbonate, an acid substance, and a starch or flour

baking soda: a white, crystalline, alkaline substance used as a leavening in quick breads with a high content of acid ingredients

ballotine: a bird that has been fully or partially boned, stuffed, reshaped, and then roasted or steamed; usually served hot

bar cookie (sheet cookie): a cookie similar to a drop cookie in consistency, made by spreading the batter in a shallow pan, baking it, and then cutting it into individual bars

bard: to tie sheets or strips of fat around lean cuts of meat so that the meat stays moist during cooking

barley sugar: granulated sugar that has been heated to form a mass without any crystals, then cooled into a hard cake; in candy making, barley sugar occurs just before caramelization

baste: to spoon melted fat, meat drippings, fruit juice, sauce, or water over meat or another food so that the food retains moisture during cooking; basting also adds flavor

batter: an uncooked mixture of egg, flour, leavening, and liquid that is thin enough to be poured or dropped from a spoon

bean curd: see **tofu**

bean flour: a meal or powder produced by grinding uncooked, dried legumes

bean puree: a paste or thick pulp produced by grinding cooked legumes, usually with small amounts of liquid

beat: to smooth a mixture or to introduce air into it

using a brisk, circular motion that lifts the mixture over and over

béchamel: a basic white sauce made from a white roux and milk or cream

berry: a fruit in which numerous tiny seeds are scattered throughout the edible flesh

beurre composé: see **compounded butter**

beurre manié: see **kneaded butter**

bind: to use egg, sauce, moistened bread crumbs, or other ingredients to hold a mixture together

biscuit: a small quick bread made from dough that has been rolled and cut or dropped from a spoon

bisque: a slightly thick, creamy soup made from shell-fish or poultry

bivalve: a shellfish with a two-valved shell, such as a mussel, clam, or scallop

black butter: clarified butter cooked slowly until a very dark, almost black color results

blackstrap molasses: a product that remains after commercial extraction of sugar from the sugar-cane plant

blanc, blond, and *brun:* the colors of the various roux — white, golden, and brown — used to make a sauce

blanch: to steam or boil food very briefly, then cool it rapidly in cold water; used mainly for preparing vegetables for freezing or drying; also used to remove the skins from nut kernels

bleached flour: a freshly milled flour that has been treated with oxidizing agents to remove its yellow pigment and make it considered more suitable for bread making

blend: to combine two or more ingredients thoroughly

blossom end: the slightly round end opposite the stem on fruits and vegetables

boil: to heat water or another liquid until bubbles rise continually and break on the surface; also, to cook food in water or another liquid

bolted: processed by mechanical sifting applied to whole grains to remove the bran and germ, hence some of the original food value

bone: to remove the major bones from poultry parts or whole poultry or meats

bouillon (broth or stock): a liquid obtained by cooking meat or poultry, bones, and vegetables together

bouquet garni: a combination of fresh or dried herbs, usually parsley, thyme, and bay leaf, used to flavor soups and stewed meats; for easy retrieval from the pot, fresh herbs are tied together with string, dried herbs are wrapped in cheesecloth

braise: to cook meat slowly in a covered saucepan with a small amount of liquid; the meat is often browned first in a small amount of fat

bran: the coat of the seed of cereal grain that is separated from flour or meal by sifting or bolting

bread: to coat with bread crumbs or other similar ingredients; the food is often dipped in milk or beaten egg before being breaded

brewer's yeast: a nonactive yeast, high in protein and B vitamins, which can be used as a nutritional supplement in baking and cooking

broil: to cook over or under direct heat

broth: see **bouillon**

brown: to darken the surface of a food (usually meat) by cooking — baking, roasting, frying — with moderate to high heat

brown butter: clarified butter cooked until a rich, brown color results

brown sauce: a basic sauce made from a brown roux and usually a brown stock

bulb vegetable: an edible, fleshy vegetable with overlapping leaves, such as garlic, leek, and onion plants, found underground

bulgur: wheat that has been cracked by parboiling, then dried

butter: cream that is skimmed from the top of whole milk, then churned or agitated until it forms a solid mass that can be spread; called sweet butter when unsalted

butter, fruit: a very thick, smooth spread made from fruit pulp and a sweetener; the ingredients are cooked together, sometimes with spices, and usually strained

butter cake (creamed cake): a cake that is raised by the addition of a chemical leavener such as baking powder or soda

butterfly: to slice boneless meat, such as a chop or leg roast, horizontally through the center but not quite to the edge, so that the cut of meat can be opened flat like a book

butterfly fillets: two fish fillets that are connected by the fish's belly skin, forming the shape of a butterfly

butterfly shrimp: a shrimp that is sliced in half vertically so that it lies open for broiling, baking, or stuffing

buttermilk: originally the liquid left from butter making; today it is generally a cultured milk

butter swirl: a piece of butter melted in a spiral in a sauce to finish the sauce just before serving it

canapé: an appetizer of bread, toast, or crackers topped with a savory spread

caramel: a firm, chewy candy of the noncrystalline type

carob (Saint John's bread): a naturally sweet powder or chip resembling chocolate in appearance and taste; used in baked goods and beverages

carrageenan: an extract of Irish moss seaweed used as a suspending agent

caviar: the processed, salted roe of certain large fish, such as sturgeon; usually used as an appetizer

cereal: a plant that produces grain for food, or its grain; also, a prepared foodstuff of grain

cereal cream: see **light cream**

certified milk: raw milk handled and bottled under strict sanitary conditions

chapon: a piece of bread rubbed with garlic and placed in a salad for flavor

chiffonade: shredded or finely cut vegetables or herbs used to garnish soups and salads

chiffon cake: a foam cake similar to sponge cake except that the fluid batter includes shortening as well as egg yolk

chop: to cut into pieces with a sharp knife or in a blender or food processor

chou pastry: a very light but rich pastry made from a soft, batterlike dough that may be shaped with spoons or a pastry bag and is fried or baked

chunk fish: a common market form of fish appearing as a cross section of a fish after it has been dressed, usually with some backbone remaining

churned ice cream: ice cream made in a hand-crank or an electric-crank freezer

chutney: a sweet and sour relish of fruits, herbs, spices, and other seasonings

citrus fruit: a fruit with a tough peel and with flesh that can be divided into segments; usually contains a large amount of vitamin C

clarified butter (drawn butter or ghee): butter that has been melted and strained to separate the milk solids from the butterfat

clarify: to remove all impurities and specks of grease from a strained stock by meticulously mixing egg white and crushed eggshell with the stock

coagulate: to clot or congeal into a thickened mass

coat a spoon: see *à la nappe*

coddled egg: an unshelled egg lowered into boiling water, with the pan then covered, removed from the heat, and allowed to stand until the egg is set

coffee cream: see **light cream**

cold pack (raw pack): to pack vegetables, uncooked, in canning jars for processing in a pressure canner

combine: to stir two or more ingredients until mixed

compounded butter *(beurre composé)*: butter that is creamed with herbs, seasonings, or other flavorings and used to dress fish, meat, or hors d'oeuvres

concentrate: a thick juice that has had a large portion of its water removed

conserve: a jamlike mixture of two or more fruits to which nuts or raisins are usually added

consommé: a clear soup made from clarified stock

coral: the bright, reddish, edible roe of the lobster, crab, or scallop

core: to remove the core from a fruit; also, the inedible central part of an apple, pear, pineapple, or grapefruit

court bouillon: a liquid for poaching fish, obtained by simmering vegetables and seasonings in water to which wine or vinegar has been added

cream: to blend one or more foods, usually butter and honey or sugar, until soft and creamy

creamed cake: see **butter cake**

cream of tartar: an acidic chemical, acid potassium tartrate, added to beaten egg whites to stabilize them and added to fondant-type candies to prevent the growth of crystals during storage (fondant made with cream of tartar is usually pure white)

cream sauce: see **white sauce**

crème fraîche: a cultured dairy product made from heavy cream and buttermilk

crisp-tender: tender but still retaining some crispness; refers to cooked vegetables

croquette: minced poultry, meat, fish, or vegetables blended with seasonings, a small amount of liquid, and often bread crumbs, then pressed into a small cone or round shape, usually coated with egg and bread crumbs, and fried or, occasionally, baked

crudité: the French word for raw vegetable, usually referring to an array of sliced, cut, or chopped vegetables served as an appetizer, often with a dip

crumb: to coat a food with crumbs; also, to break crackers or cookies into small particles

crustacean: a member of a large class of mostly aquatic arthropods such as lobster, shrimp, or crab

crystalline candy: a type of candy, including fondant, fudge, and penuche, made by carefully heating sugar to a syrup consistency that must be closely monitored for proper crystal growth

cube: to cut food into cubes or chunks usually one inch on a side

curd: the soft mass of lumps resulting from the coagulation of milk, containing most of the protein, butterfat, and other nutrients of milk; also, the thick, protein-rich part of coagulated soymilk from which tofu is made

curdle: to separate into liquids and solids; egg and milk dishes tend to curdle during excess heating or when an acid is added

cure: to preserve beef, fish, or pork by salting, drying, pickling, and sometimes smoking; cured meats have a reddish pink color from the addition of sodium nitrate

custard: a pudding made with eggs, milk, and often a sweetener

cut in: to distribute butter or other solid fat in dry ingredients by chopping the fat into small pieces with two knives, a fork, or a pastry blender until the pieces are evenly divided and very small

dash: a small, quick shake of (usually) dried spices or herbs

date sugar: a sugar made from ground dried dates

debone: to remove meat from bones

decoction: the process of making a concentrated herb tea by steeping roots, seeds, or stems in hot, freshly boiled water

degerm: to remove the germ portion of grains in the milling process

deglaze: to add a small amount of liquid (usually water) to a pan in which some food has been sautéed or browned, then to scrape loose the particles from the pan's bottom and stir them into the liquid in order to extract all residual flavors from the pan; liquid and particles are then added to the sauce, stock, or dish being prepared

degrease: to remove the fat that collects on the surface of stock or sauce by various skimming methods such as blotting, spooning off, or chilling until the grease floats to the top and can be lifted off

devein: to remove the intestine that runs along the back or outer section of shrimp

devil: to season highly; usually applies to foods such as eggs or crab meat; mustard is a popular seasoning in deviled foods

diastatic: with its starch converted into sugar (for example, diastatic malt)

dice: to cut food into small cubes usually one-half inch on a side or less

dilute: to weaken the flavor or strength of a mixture, usually by adding water

dip: to immerse briefly to moisten, cool, or coat; also, a creamy mixture based on cheese, other dairy products, or pureed beans and used as a dipping sauce for crackers, bread, or vegetables

disjoint: to cut up poultry by severing it at the joints

dough: a mixture of flour and other ingredients stiff enough to be kneaded, rolled, or shaped by hand

draw: to remove the organs from the body cavity of meat or poultry

drawn butter: see **clarified butter**

dredge: to coat a food with flour or other dry ingredients such as cornmeal or fine, toasted bread crumbs

dressed fish (pan-dressed fish): a common market form of fish that has been gutted and has had its head, tail, and fins removed

dressing: a seasoned sauce generally based on oil and vinegar and used to add flavor to salads; also a stuffing for poultry

dried milk: either whole or nonfat milk with 95 percent of its moisture removed

drink: a commercially prepared beverage of juice, water, and sweetener, such as orange drink, which may have as little as 10 to 35 percent juice; an orange-*flavored* drink may have anywhere from no juice to 10 percent juice

drippings: the juices that are released from meat during cooking

drop cookie: a cookie made from a soft dough that is dropped from a spoon

drupe: a fruit with a single seed surrounded by edible flesh, such as a peach, plum, or cherry

du corps: of the proper thickness or consistency; refers to sauces

dumpling: a small piece of dough or batter leavened by steam in simmering liquid

durum wheat: a hard wheat that yields a glutenous flour used especially in pasta and bread making

dust: to coat a food lightly with dry ingredients

duxelle: a garnish or sauce whose principal ingredient is minced mushrooms

emulsion sauce: a sauce such as mayonnaise, béarnaise, or hollandaise, whose thickening depends on the emulsifying quality of egg yolk mixed with oil

en brochette: on a skewer

endosperm: the heart or nutritive tissue of the grain, formed within the embryo (germ) sack

enrich: to improve the nutritive value of food by artificially adding nutrients to bring them to levels established by enrichment standards

espagnole: a brown sauce variation

evaporated milk: canned milk with 40 to 50 percent of its water removed; reconstituted by adding one-half cup of water to the milk from one small (5⅓ ounces) can

exhaust: to let steam and air escape from the petcock (steam valve) of a pressure canner; exhausting permits the temperature to rise from 212 to 240°F

—a very important step that can result in seal failures or later spoilage if not carried out

extract: an essence in concentrated form used for flavoring foods

fell: a thin, papery covering on the outer layer of fat on lamb

fiber: the indigestible part of food that aids the body's intestinal tract

fillet: to remove bones from small pieces of meat such as steaks and chops; also, a piece or slice of boneless fish or meat

fin: that part of the fish's body used for propelling it through water

fines herbes: a finely chopped mixture of herbs, usually fresh but sometimes dried

fin fish: a name applied to true fish, which have fins, to distinguish them from shellfish

finie au beurre: see **finish a sauce**

finish a sauce *(finie au beurre):* to enrich a sauce, usually with butter swirls or kneaded butter

flake: to break pieces of fish or other appropriate food into small pieces with a fork

flaked meat: the crab meat, from various parts of the crab's body, that does not include lump meat

flour: to coat with flour; also, the finely ground meal of a grain, dried fruit, or dried vegetable

flower vegetable: an edible blossom such as cauliflower, broccoli, or artichoke

flute: to make a decorative crimp on the edge of pastry; also, to cut small vegetables such as mushrooms into scalloped shapes

foam cake: a cake such as angel food, sponge, or chiffon that derives a large portion of its leavening and light, airy structure from the incorporation of beaten egg white into the batter

fold: to blend together a light, airy mixture with a heavier one by a gentle lifting and turning-over motion, done carefully so that a minimum of air is lost from the light mixture

fondant: a soft, creamy preparation of sugar, water, and flavorings that is used as a basis for candies or icings

fonds de cuisine: a basic stock made from meat or fish, bones, skins of fish, and vegetables and used as a base for soups and sauces

fondue: a hot, thick dipping sauce, often cheese-based, served with chunks of bread, meat, or fruit to be dipped

fortified: enriched by the addition of certain nutrients that may or may not have been present in the original food; refers to cereals and other foods

fortified milk: whole or skim milk enriched with vitamins A and D and sometimes with minerals and protein

frappé: a flavored liquid served over or blended with cracked ice, or partially frozen

freezer burn: the dry, unpalatable spots on food caused by improper wrapping of food put in the freezer

French: to remove meat from the rib ends of lamb, pork, or veal chops, or crown roasts, and garnish the bone tips with small fruits or paper frills

freshwater fish: a fish that thrives in a lake, river, stream, or any body of water other than the ocean

fricassee: to cook by braising fowl, rabbit, or veal that has been cut into pieces

frittata: an omeletlike dish in which diced vegetables, meat, poultry, or fish are mixed with the egg before it is placed in the pan, browned on both sides, and served without being folded

fritter: a vegetable, fruit, or meat dipped in batter and fried in deep, hot oil

fruit vegetable: a heavy, succulent fruit, such as a tomato, eggplant, green pepper, cucumber, okra, or squash, that is commonly eaten as a vegetable

fry: to cook in fat; also referred to as sautéing or pan-frying when a small amount of fat is used or as deep frying when a large quantity of fat is used (in deep frying, the food is actually submerged in hot fat)

fudge: a soft, creamy candy of the crystalline type, made from sugar, milk, butter, and flavoring

fumet: a liquid obtained by simmering the heads, bones, and skins of fish with vegetables

galantine: a bird that has been completely boned, stuffed, and shaped into a roll like a plump sausage and usually poached, chilled, glazed with aspic, decorated, and served cold

garnish: to decorate food to increase its visual appeal; parsley, watercress, and chopped nuts are common garnishes

gelatin: a clear, tasteless protein obtained by boiling meat and bones; when chilled it becomes jelled and gives form to aspics and other molded salads

germ: the embryo portion of cereal grains that is often separated from the starchy endosperm during milling; wheat germ, which is sold as a cereal, is high in vitamin E and the B vitamins and is a popular and tasty addition to many foods

ghee: see **clarified butter**

giblets: the gizzard, heart, and liver of poultry

gill: that part of the fish used for obtaining oxygen from water

glace de viande: see **glaze**

glaze *(glace de viande):* a stock, bouillon, or broth that has been reduced to a very thick, syrupy liquid

gluten: a tenacious, elastic protein substance, especially of wheat flour, that gives cohesiveness to dough and allows dough to rise

grain: the seeds or fruits of one of various food plants, including the cereal grasses

granola: a mixture of grains, dried fruits, nuts, and/or seeds, toasted and eaten as a cereal or snack

grate: to pulverize a food by scraping it over a grater

gravy: a brown sauce whose flavor is usually derived from the meat, game, or poultry that it will season

greens: the green leaves of lettuce, spinach, kale, turnips, and other leafy vegetables, used in making salads

grind: to crush or cut food until it is in very fine particles

grits: coarsely ground hulled grain (hominy grits are the most common)

groats: a coarser grind of hulled grain than grits

gut: to remove the bowels and entrails of fish

half-and-half: a mixture of half milk and half cream that contains approximately 12 percent butterfat

hand-crank freezer: an ice cream maker that is operated by a handle that must be turned manually to churn the cream mixture

hard-cooked egg: an unshelled egg cooked in gently simmering water until the yolk is set

hard wheat flour: a flour milled from spring wheat, containing a high quantity of protein (gluten) that gives bread good volume, texture, and grain

headspace: the amount of space left in the top of a canning or freezing jar after the jar has been packed with food and liquid

heavy cream (whipping cream): cream that contains 36 to 40 percent butterfat, which makes it possible to whip it to twice its volume

hominy: hulled corn

homogenized milk: fresh fluid whole milk that has been processed to break up the particles of butterfat so that the fat remains evenly distributed throughout the milk and no longer rises to the top to form a cream line

hors d'oeuvre: any savory food served as a snack with drinks, usually when a larger meal is not planned to follow

hot pack: to precook food and pack it hot into canning jars

hull: the outer seed coat of any nut, grain, or legume

hulled bean: a bean that has had its seed coat or outer covering removed, usually by some form of light cooking

ice glazing: a process of coating fish in successive layers of ice in order to preserve it longer

infusion: the process of making herb tea by steeping leaves or flowers in hot, freshly boiled water

Irish moss: a sea vegetable used most often as an agent for thickening or emulsifying

jam: a condiment made from crushed or chopped fruit preserved in a sweetener; jam has a softer consistency than jelly

jellmeter: a glass tube through which extracted juice is passed in order to measure pectin levels

jelly: a condiment made from fruit juice preserved in a sweetener; it is clear and firm enough to hold its shape

juice: the extractable liquid in fruits and vegetables; a commercially prepared orange juice *blend* has 70 to 95 percent orange juice

juice drink: a juice with water and sweetener added that may contain only 35 to 70 percent juice when commercially prepared

julienne: cut into match-size pieces

kasha: a Russian dish of cooked buckwheat; also, whole, husked buckwheat grains before cooking

keel: the sharp, ridged center breastbone in poultry

kefir: a cultured milk with a somewhat tart taste

kernel: a nutmeat or the inner, softer part of a seed or nut

knead: to make dough smooth and elastic by pressing, folding, and stretching either by hand or with an electric mixer

kneaded butter *(beurre manié):* unmelted butter that has been mixed in pastry fashion with an equal part of flour and is used to thicken and enrich a sauce

koji: an inoculated grain used in the fermentation process for tamari

kudzu: a high-quality imported cooking starch, used to thicken sauces and soups

lard: a soft, white fat rendered from the fatty tissues of the hog

lattice-top pie: a pie with a fancy top made by crisscrossing strips of piecrust dough across the pie's filling

leaf vegetable: a thick foliage plant whose leaves are commonly eaten as a vegetable, such as lettuce, spinach, kale, kohlrabi, cabbage, collard greens, beet greens, and turnip greens

leaven, leavening: a substance or process—yeast, bicarbonate of soda, beaten egg white, or steam— used to raise breads or cakes

lecithin: a substance that is composed of two B vitamins and oil and that occurs naturally in soybeans; available in natural foods stores in both oil and granular form; lecithin oil may be used lightly to coat baking pans to prevent sticking

legume: a family of food plants, including beans, peas, and peanuts, which provide high-quality protein

liaison: a mixture of heavy cream, milk, or crème fraîche and egg or egg yolks, used as a thickener for sauces and soups

light cream (table cream or **coffee cream):** cream that contains 18 to 30 percent butterfat

light whipping cream: cream that contains 30 to 36 percent butterfat

low-acid food: any vegetable (except tomato), any meat, fish, or poultry

low-fat milk: milk skimmed of all but 1 to 2 percent of the butterfat; the small percentage retained works to imitate the flavor and texture of whole milk

low-methoxyl pectin: a type of pectin that sets up with calcium salts instead of sugar

low-sodium milk: whole or skim milk in which 90 percent of the sodium has been replaced by potassium

lump meat: the large, white chunks of crab meat considered to be the choicest selection

macédoine: a mixture of raw or cooked fruits or vegetables

malt: a grain softened by being steeped in water and allowed to germinate

marbling: the small streaks and flecks of fat found in the lean of meat

margarine: a butterlike spread made from churned vegetable oils and skim milk; much lower in saturated fats than butter, much higher in polyunsaturated ones

marinade: a seasoned, often spicy liquid in which meats, poultry, fish, or vegetables are soaked in order to tenderize or to enrich flavor (or both)

marmalade: a tender jelly containing pieces of fruit or fruit peel, commonly citrus

masa harina: finely ground flour made from hominy; used in making tortillas

mash: to reduce to a pulp

mayonnaise: a salad dressing made with beaten egg, oil, and vinegar or lemon juice

melon: a family of fruits that is divided into two groups: muskmelons and watermelons; the rinds of both groups are inedible; in muskmelons the numerous seeds are clustered in the center of the edible flesh; in watermelons the seeds are scattered throughout the edible flesh

melt: to heat a food until it liquefies

meringue: a dessert topping, or a shell, made from stiffly beaten egg white and a sweetener

mill: to grind a grain into a flour

mince: to chop food into very small pieces

mirepoix: a mixture of finely diced carrot, onion, and celery, cooked in butter and used as a foundation for seasoning sauces for meat and fish

miso: a fermented seasoning made from soybeans, having the consistency of peanut butter and used as a condiment

mix: to stir ingredients until all pieces are evenly distributed or mixture is thoroughly blended

mold: to put into a specified shape; also, a gelatin containing meats, fish, vegetables, fruits, or other savory or sweet ingredients; see **aspic**

molded dessert: a dessert such as a bombe, cold soufflé, or gelatin that is made by chilling a mixture until firm in a decorative mold from which the dessert is usually removed before serving

mollusk: a shellfish with a soft, unsegmented body enclosed in a calcareous shell

mortar and pestle: a thick, heavy bowl and the pounding instrument used for crushing herbs, spices, and other condiments

mousse: a light, spongy mold that contains gelatin or egg white to suspend its savory or sweet ingredients

muffin: a quick bread made from a batter containing egg and baked in a muffin tin

nectar: a beverage of fruit juice and pulp that may also contain water and sweeteners when commercially made

netting: the lines running across the rind of some cantaloupes

noncrystalline candy (amorphous candy): a type of candy, which includes caramels, taffies, and toffees, that is made from a syrup and requires careful heating and some stirring to ensure even heat distribution until the process of caramelization occurs

nonfat milk: fluid milk or dry milk solids that contain less than 0.5 percent butterfat

nut flour: see **nut meal**

nut meal (nut flour): coarsely or finely ground nuts with a dry, fluffy texture, most often used in recipes in a mixture with regular flour

nut milk: ground nuts or nut butter blended with water, milk, or cream

okara: literally "honorable hull"; the fibrous, insoluble by-product of soymilk and tofu, left behind after the soymilk has been extracted from the ground soybean puree

omelet: a dish made from beaten egg that is fried without being stirred, then folded in half; it may or may not have a filling placed on top of the egg as it begins to set in the pan

open-faced sandwich: a canapélike appetizer consisting of a single cracker, slice of bread, or toast topped with a savory spread

pan: see **stir-fry**

panade: a soup made with a bread base, such as onion soup

panbroil: to cook meat uncovered in a hot skillet, pouring off fat as it accumulates

pan-dressed fish: see **dressed fish**

panfry: to cook a meat or vegetable in a small amount of fat

papain: an enzyme extracted from papaya and used to tenderize meats

parboil: to boil or simmer food until partially cooked

parboiled or **parcooked grain:** grain that can be bought already partially cooked by boiling or steaming, requiring less cooking time at home

pare: to cut off the outermost covering of a fruit or vegetable with a knife

paste: a blend of flour (or other starch) and fat used as a thickener for sauces

pasteurize: to heat milk for a period of time at a temperature that destroys harmful bacteria without drastically changing the taste or texture of the milk

pastry blender: a utensil, usually having a wooden handle and three or four arched metal prongs, used for blending fat into flour in pastry making

pastry cloth: a large cloth, usually made of heavy linen with a coarse weave, on which pastry is rolled; the cloth holds flour and keeps pastry from sticking

pâté: a rich spread of finely mashed or pureed meat (usually) that is highly seasoned and spiced

pectin: a fiber that occurs naturally in the cell walls of fruits and that forms a gel when mixed with acids and sweeteners; used to thicken cooked fruits and fruit juices to make jams and jellies

peel: to remove the outer covering of a fruit or vegetable

penuche: a fudge candy of the crystalline type, made from brown sugar, butter, cream or milk, and nuts

petcock: a valve on a pressure canner that allows air and steam to escape when opened and pressure to build up when closed

petite marmite: a consommé made of a combination of beef and chicken broth and finely cut vegetables; *petite* suggests that the vegetables are cut very small; *marmite* is the earthenware container

phyllo: a paper-thin pastry dough used frequently in Middle Eastern cooking for dessert and main course dishes

pickle: a fruit or vegetable preserved in a strong vinegar solution or in a brine

pignoli: pine nuts

piima: a cultured milk that ferments at room temperature and has a mildly tart taste

pinch: the small amount of spice or herb that can be squeezed between the index finger and thumb

pinfeathers: the coarse feathers on an unplucked bird

pistou: a sauce made from basil, garlic, tomato, olive oil, and Parmesan cheese and used to garnish soups

pit: to remove the pit from fruit

pluck: to pull pinfeathers from poultry

plump: to soak raisins or other dried fruits in liquid until they are soft and puffy

poach: to cook food in a hot liquid, taking care to retain the shape of the food

poached egg: a shelled whole egg cooked in a hot liquid

polish: the inner layer of bran, left over in the refining process, that gives brown rice its characteristic color

pome: a fruit such as an apple or pear with a core and several small seeds surrounded by edible flesh

potage: a thick soup made from pureed vegetables

potato water: water in which potatoes have been boiled; often used as a liquid for activating yeast because of its starch content

pot-au-feu: a soup, based on beef stock, that can be served thick (with vegetables) or thin (as a consommé)

poultry: all domesticated birds used as food

prawn: a large shrimp

precook: to boil, steam, bake, or fry food for a few minutes before final cooking

preserve: a condiment made from whole or large pieces of fruits preserved in a thick, jellylike syrup

pressure gauge: a dial that indicates the steam pressure inside a pressure canner

process: to combine or blend foods in a food processor or a blender

proofing: the process of allowing yeast to activate in a warm, moist environment in order to produce a risen dough for bread making

puff pastry: a very delicate dough made from a high-gluten flour to give it its characteristic elasticity; puff pastry is often filled or layered with different sweet fillings

punch: a blend of several fruit juices that may contain a high percentage of water and sweeteners when commercially prepared

puree: to grind food to a pulp or paste in a food processor, a blender, a sieve, or a food mill; also, a smooth, thick or thin soup made from vegetables, legumes, poultry, or fish

quenelle: a dumpling made with finely chopped, highly seasoned fish or meat bound with egg and cooked in boiling water or stock

quick bread: a bread such as a muffin, biscuit, pancake, or scone that is leavened quickly by bicarbonate of soda, steam, or beaten egg white instead of yeast

ragout: a French vegetable and meat stew

rancid: having an unpleasant, strong smell or taste due to the decomposition of oils or fats in nuts, seeds, meats, or other fatty foods from prolonged exposure to the air

rapid boil: a full, rolling boil that covers the entire surface and cannot be stirred down

raw pack: see **cold pack**

reconstitute: to restore a concentrated food such as dry milk, juice, or soup to its original state by adding liquid (usually water)

reduce: to boil a liquid rapidly until much of its water evaporates and its flavor becomes concentrated

refine: to remove varying amounts of the original structure (hull, bran, or germ) from a grain or grain flour in the milling process

refrigerator cookie (rolled cookie): a cookie made from a dough that is refrigerated until stiff, then rolled and cut into desired shapes

refrigerator-tray ice cream: see **still-freeze ice cream**

rehydrate: to soak or cook dried food to replace the water lost during drying

relish: a savory blend of pickled vegetables with other condiments; also, a sweet blend of several chopped fruits

restore: to return selected nutrients to cereals to approximate the original nutrient levels of the whole grain

rind: the tough outer skin of a lemon, lime, orange, grapefruit, tangelo, tangerine, or melon

rise: to increase in volume because of the action of fermenting yeast, steam, or the chemical reaction between a liquid and baking powder

roast: to cook meat or poultry uncovered in hot, dry air

roe: the eggs of fish, usually still enclosed in the ovarian membrane

rolled cookie: see **refrigerator cookie**

rolled oats: oats that have been mechanically rolled in order to expand their surface and shorten their cooking time

roller stocking: a cloth stocking that fits over a rolling pin and is used to roll sticky pastry dough to keep it from needing additional flour

roll out: to use a rolling pin to roll a dough into a thin sheet

root vegetable: an underground, fleshy enlargement of a plant, such as a beet, carrot, parsnip, turnip, or rutabaga, that is eaten as a vegetable

round fish: see **whole fish**

roux: a cooked mixture of flour and butter or oil that serves as a base for thickened brown and white sauces

russeting: a lacelike, brownish patch on the skin of a fruit

safety valve: an emergency steam release that "blows" when pressure overbuilds in a pressure canner

Saint John's bread: see **carob**

salad: a dish made with one or more foods (meats, fruits, vegetables, grains, fish, nuts, cheeses, eggs) coated with a dressing

saltwater fish: a fish that thrives in the ocean's salty water

sashimi: a Japanese dish made with raw fish fillets

sauce: a fluid topping or dressing that adds flavor to a dish

sauté: to brown or cook food lightly in a small amount of fat

savarin: a cake made with a yeast mixture, baked in a ring mold, and usually soaked in flavored syrup

savory: a nonsweet sauce or dish

scald: to heat milk until tiny bubbles form around the edges of the pan in order to kill any bacteria that may inhibit the action of yeast in bread making or of a culture in making a fermented milk; also, a brownish discoloration that develops on the skins of apples and other fruits in cold storage

scale: a small, flattened, rigid plate forming part of the external body of a fish

scallop: to bake a food in a sauce, often with the ingredients layered and the top covered with bread crumbs; also, one of a family of bivalves

score: to make shallow cuts in a crisscross pattern across the surface of a food

scrambled egg: a beaten egg stirred occasionally while it is cooking

seal: to make a canning jar airtight

sear: to brown the outside of meat quickly with intense heat

seasoned flour: a flour mixed with dried herbs and spices; usually used to coat a meat, fish, fowl, or vegetable before baking or frying

seasoned lard: see *sofrito*

seed: a grain or ripened ovule of a plant capable of germinating to produce a new plant; nuts, grains, and legumes are all seeds

seed vegetable: an edible pod and its seeds from a bean or pea plant

semolina: a high-gluten flour milled from the heart or endosperm of hard durum wheat from which the bran and germ have been removed completely

sheet cookie: see **bar cookie**

shellfish: an aquatic invertebrate animal with a shell covering its body

shirred egg: a shelled, baked egg, often cooked with cream and bread crumbs

short crust: a pastry dough crust that is tender and flaky due to the high proportion of fat to flour in it

shoyu: a naturally fermented soy sauce made over a period of a year from soybeans, cracked and roasted wheat, and a mold starter; commonly misnamed tamari

shred: to cut into thin strips, usually with a grater

shrub: a concentrated fruit mixture made from berries, honey, and often vinegar, diluted with cold water, then served over ice

sieve: to strain food through a strainer

sift: to introduce air into flour; to separate fine particles from coarse ones

simmer: to cook in a liquid that is heated to just below the boiling point; bubbles form slowly and break below the surface

singe: to burn off the fine hairs that remain on a bird after it has been plucked

skim: to spoon fat from the surface of a soup or sauce

skim milk: liquid nonfat milk; vitamins A and D are often added to skim milk

slash: to cut the outer fat on a steak or chop at regular intervals so that the meat will not curl during cooking

sliver: to cut into long, thin pieces

snip: to cut into very small pieces using scissors

soba: thin buckwheat noodles (Japanese)

sofrito **(seasoned lard):** a highly spiced sauce made from a large proportion of pork fat, plus garlic, hot peppers, and various herbs and spices

soft-cooked egg: an unshelled egg cooked in gently simmering water for a brief time

soft wheat flour: a flour milled from winter wheat, containing a low quantity of protein (gluten) and used for cakes, cookies, biscuits, and pastry

solidifier: an agent, usually a mineral-rich salt of seaweed origin, used in tofu making to draw out the soymilk protein and to gather it into curds separate from the whey liquid

soufflé: either an entrée or a dessert made with a sauce, egg yolk, stiffly beaten egg white, seasonings, and an optional filling

sour cream: cream soured by culturing

sour milk: raw whole or skim milk that soured from fermentation

sponge cake: a cake based on a very thick egg yolk foam and leavened with beaten egg white

spread: a savory mixture based on cheese, hard-cooked egg, bean puree, meat, poultry, or fish, usually served with crackers or bread

springform pan: a round pan with sides that detach from the bottom when a metal clasp is loosened

sprouted wheat: whole grains of wheat that have been allowed to germinate fully or partially

sprouting: the process of allowing seeds to germinate and grow into edible shoots

steak: a common market form of fish appearing as a crosscut section of a large, firm-fleshed fish; also, a slice of meat cut from a fleshy part of a beef carcass or pork ham

steam: to cook in steam, with or without pressure

steam-leaven: to raise or lighten by the action of steam any product such as a popover, cream puff, or dumpling

steel-cut oats: oats that have been cut by a mechanical process with steel rollers

steep: to soak tea leaves, herbs, or coffee grounds in hot water to extract flavor and color

stem end: the spot where the fruit was attached to the stem, usually identified by a scar or the remains of the stem

stem vegetable: a thick, succulent stem of a plant, such as celery or asparagus, that is eaten as a vegetable

still-freeze ice cream (refrigerator-tray ice cream): ice cream made by a method using a refrigerator tray or other uncovered vessel; the freezing mixture is stirred periodically with a rotary beater to keep large ice crystals from forming

stir: to mix foods using a circular motion

stir-fry (pan): to toss and cook rapidly in hot oil small pieces of vegetable, meat, fish, or poultry

stock: see bouillon

stone-ground grain, flour: a grain or its flour ground in a mill using special stone rollers called buhrstones instead of using modern steel rollers and methods that usually remove too much of the nutritious part of the grain

strain: to pass food or liquid through a filtering surface, such as a sieve or cheesecloth, in order to make it finer in consistency or to remove undesired elements

strudel pastry: a very pliable dough similar to phyllo but made from melted fat added to flour along with some egg and milk

stuff: to fill a meat, fish, large vegetable, or the body and neck cavities of a bird with a savory dressing

sulfured molasses: a by-product of sugar refining that is available after the sugar has been crystallized; lighter in color than unsulfured and blackstrap molasses, it also contains fewer nutrients

sushi: a popular Japanese dish consisting of vinegar-rice or chopped vegetables wrapped in the sea vegetable nori

sweet acidophilus milk: a cultured milk with a taste similar to whole milk; it has the same benefits as acidophilus milk

sweetened condensed milk: canned milk that has had 50 percent of its water removed and cane sugar or corn syrup added

table cream: see light cream

taffy: a boiled, noncrystalline candy, usually made with molasses or brown sugar, that is pulled until porous and light in color

tahini: a butter made from either toasted or raw sesame seeds and used as a condiment or spread

tamari: a fermented condiment made from soybeans and inoculated grain (koji); contains no wheat

tart: a small pastry made from the same dough and in the same shape as a pie; usually filled with fresh or cooked fruit

tempeh: a traditional, fermented food of Indonesia made from cooked soybeans inoculated with a mold starter

temper: to warm beaten eggs slightly by adding a small amount of hot liquid to them in order to prevent them from curdling when combined with all of the hot liquid

tempura: a Japanese dish consisting of vegetables or seafood dipped in batter and fried

terrine: a peasant-style pâté usually made in an earthenware crock (terrine originally referred to the crock in which the pâté was made)

timbale: a creamy custard entrée baked in a mold; also, a small pastry shell filled with a custard mixture

toast: to brown in an oven or toaster in dry heat

toffee: a noncrystalline candy with a brittle but tender texture made from a boiled sugar-and-butter mixture

tofu (bean curd): a firm, custardlike cheese made from soybeans, water, and a solidifier

tomalley: the liver of the lobster

torte: a very light cake raised by egg white and made with ground nuts, cake crumbs, or bread crumbs in place of flour

toss: to mix by turning food gently over and over

trichina: a microscopic parasite, found in pork, that can be transmitted to humans and result in the disease trichinosis

trim: to cut excess fat from the outer side of a steak or chop, usually to a thickness of one-quarter inch

triticale: a high-yield, high-protein hybrid of wheat and rye

truss: to tie the legs and wings of poultry close to the body for oven roasting

tuber vegetable: a large, underground, edible portion of a plant, such as a potato or Jerusalem artichoke, that is eaten as a vegetable

tucked bird: a bird made compact by tucking the legs under a flap of skin

turkey ham: thigh meat of turkey that is processed commercially and flavored to simulate ham

ultra high temperature milk: whole milk that has been processed at 280 to 300°F (instead of the usual 160°F), then sealed in a sterilized container; unopened, UHT milk will keep up to four months without refrigeration

unbleached flour: a white flour that has been allowed to mature naturally over a period of about 30 days for better handling

velouté: a basic white sauce made from a white roux and poultry, veal, or fish stock

vinaigrette: a salad dressing made with oil, vinegar, and seasonings

vinegar: a sour liquid that results from the fermentation of wine, cider, beer, fruit, or grain by acetic acid bacteria

wax: a coating usually made from a combination of carnauba wax, beeswax, or paraffin and emulsifiers that is added to some vegetables and fruits to keep them bright and plump

wheat germ: see **germ**

whey: the liquid residue resulting from the coagulation of milk; contains mostly water and some milk sugar, minerals, protein, and butterfat; also, the watery residue that is left behind in tofu making when the soymilk coagulates into curds

whip: to beat egg white, heavy cream, or another food rapidly to introduce air into it

whipping cream: see **heavy cream**

whisk: to beat egg, cream, or egg white with a wire whisk (a utensil made of looped wires held together by a handle) until well mixed

white cake: a butter or creamed cake that does not use the egg yolk but only the egg white beaten and folded into the batter before it is baked; its white color can be achieved only with white flour

white sauce (cream sauce): a basic sauce made from a white roux and a poultry or veal stock, milk, or cream

whole dressed fish: a common market form of fish that is whole but has been scaled and gutted and has had its fins removed

whole fish (round fish): a common market form of fish that is sold as it was when taken from the water

whole milk: pasteurized milk with its full complement of butterfat; when unhomogenized whole milk is left undisturbed, the fat rises to the top and forms a cream line

whole wheat pastry flour: a whole wheat flour milled from soft wheat, containing little gluten; good for use in cookies, cakes, pastries, and quick breads

wishbone: a thin, V-shaped breastbone that is attached to the neck end of the keel in poultry

wok: a broad, round-bottom Chinese cooking utensil, used especially for stir-frying

Worcestershire sauce: a highly spiced sauce originally manufactured in Worcester, England

yeast: the living, single-celled fungus whose fermenting property is used to leaven bread dough

yellow cake: a butter or creamed cake that is yellow in color due to the incorporation of whole egg into the batter; its yellow color can be achieved only with white flour

yogurt: a custardlike, tangy, cultured dairy product; it makes an excellent substitute for sour cream

zest: the grated outer peel (rind) of a citrus fruit, usually an orange or lemon, used to flavor foods; care is taken not to include any of the bitter white membrane that lies directly below the rind

Herbs, Spices, and Condiments

Many ethnic cuisines are defined by the frequent use of a particular herb or spice. Indian cooking is known for its cardamom and its ginger; Spanish cooking was among the first to exploit the flavoring and tinting properties of golden saffron; chilies are a familiar component of many Latin American dishes; and basil and oregano are practically synonymous with Mediterranean cookery. For centuries, clever cooks have used small amounts of fresh herbs and fragrant spices to add new tastes to familiar dishes or to heighten the good flavors already present in foods. For this reason herbs and spices are especially valuable allies to the cook who doesn't use salt.

Herbs and spices can have a happy influence on the character of all foods. The same type of meat, fish, or vegetable may be prepared and presented in a variety of ways when you learn to use these seasonings. Although a few herbs and spices are rather costly, the contribution they make to a dish is always worth the price, and they are usually needed only in small amounts.

Seasoning Food with Herbs and Spices

Using herbs and spices is neither tricky nor mysterious, but a cook's effective use of them does involve a certain amount of experience and discretion. Because individual tastes differ so much, it is difficult to give precise directions for seasoning with herbs and spices. Enhancement to one person may be ruination to another. However, there are standard combinations that seem to please most people, such as tomatoes and basil, chicken and rosemary, cucumbers and dill. If you are unsure about how to use herbs and spices, start with such surefire classics and experiment with new ideas when you feel more confident.

The flavor in herbs and spices is concentrated, so it is best to find your way to the ideal measurement by starting with small amounts to avoid overseasoning food. It is especially important to use some restraint when combining herbs and spices. Many work well together and some can even be substituted for each other, but some herbs and spices present contradictory flavors and are never paired in the same dish. The table on page 54 will give you some ideas for the most effective use of herbs and spices to season foods.

To sample an herb before you season an entire dish with it, remove a small amount of the dish you are preparing and season it proportionately. If this is not possible, mix a little bit of the herb or spice with some cottage or cream cheese, or some melted butter. Let it stand at room temperature several minutes before tasting.

Developing the Most Flavor from Herbs and Spices

• To develop the flavor of dried herbs, soak them for several minutes in a liquid that can be used in the recipe—stock, oil, lemon juice, or vinegar.
• When using herbs and spices in salad dressings, allow the flavor of the combination to develop by soaking for 15 minutes to an hour.
• Work the flavors of herbs and spices into meat, poultry, and fish by rubbing them in with your hands before cooking.
• For steamed or boiled vegetables, add the herbs or spices to melted butter and allow to stand for ten minutes before seasoning the vegetables.
• To intensify the flavors of whole spices, toast them briefly in a dry, heavy skillet.
• Dried and fresh herbs may be used interchangeably in most recipes. Use three to five times more fresh herbs than dried, depending on the strength of the herb.

The flavoring power of herbs and spices may vary slightly with each batch you buy. Like any other plant or vegetable, the quality of herbs and spices depends on growing, harvesting, and storage conditions. Unless you grow your own, you cannot be really sure about these factors nor of the freshness of dried herbs and spices. A good clue to whether an herb or spice is fresh: You can smell its aroma as soon as the container is opened. If you have to sniff, it is probably stale or too old.

When to Add Herbs and Spices

Most meats may be seasoned before, during, or after their cooking period. Steaks and chops may be marinated and seasoned before cooking or marinated before and seasoned after cooking. To get the most flavor from roasted meat or poultry, rub its surface well with seasoning before cooking. Poultry absorbs flavors better if the seasoning is rubbed directly into the flesh, rather than the skin. However, soups and stews develop their best flavors when herbs and spices are added during cooking. If they are long-cooking soups or stews, wait until the last 30 minutes to add the seasonings because prolonged cooking in liquid can dissipate the pungency. The same is true for savory sauces.

What to Do When You Have Overseasoned

Because many herbs and spices are quite powerful, it is wise to add them with some restraint. If, however, you do find you have underestimated the power of a seasoning, this may be remedied in a number of ways.

• Strain as much of the herbs and spices as possible out of the dish.
• Add a peeled, whole, raw potato to the dish to absorb some of the flavor. Remove the potato just before serving.
• If possible, add more of the blander ingredients, or make a second unseasoned batch of the recipe and combine with the overseasoned one.
• Serve the dish chilled to blunt the taste of overseasoning.

Storing Herbs and Spices

Fresh herbs are more flavorful than dried herbs. Unless you grow your own, you will be lucky to find a variety of fresh ones throughout the year. Parsley is one of the few herbs that can usually be bought fresh in most places in every season. Others, such as fresh basil, have a short season and only appear briefly in supermarkets.

Fresh herbs should be stored in the refrigerator with the same care you would give other leafy green vegetables. Wash fresh herbs gently and pat them dry with paper towels or twirl them dry in a salad spinner. Be sure they are as dry as possible before refrigerating them since moisture invites mold growth. Then wrap herbs in paper toweling to absorb excess moisture and place them loosely in a plastic bag. They will keep this way for three to four days.

If you find you have an overabundance of fresh herbs and want to store them for longer than a few days, snip the leaves from their stem with scissors (after you have rinsed and drained them). Place the leaves—chopped or whole—in plastic sandwich bags and store them in the freezer. They will retain most of their fresh flavor this way and can be used directly from the freezer for cooking. For additional information see Freezing Herbs, page 755.

Drying Fresh Herbs

To dry fresh herbs, either hang them in a dry, airy room for several days until they are crumbly, or heat them in a shallow baking pan in a low oven (200°F) until completely dried (about 15 minutes to an hour, depending on the herb). Test the leaves often for crispness.

Although they do not possess the same rich quality as fresh herbs, dried herbs may be stored considerably longer. When dried, herbs retain the oils that convey their characteristic aromas and flavors, so they still have a good deal of seasoning power. These values diminish with time, so try to purchase dried herbs in small amounts as needed. If you buy them loose, store them immediately in small jars or bottles with tight-fitting caps. Label and date the bottles and store them in a cool dry place away from direct sunlight and moisture. If you use a spice rack, hang the rack away from the stove and the kitchen sink. Do not keep dried herbs for more than a year since their seasoning power will be greatly diminished after that.

Whole or Ground Herbs and Spices

Is it better to use whole or ground herbs and spices? Usually one may be substituted for the other freely, allowing 1½ times more whole spice and herbs for the ground. You may want to make a bouquet garni by wrapping the ground spices in cheesecloth for easy retrieval when substituting them for whole ones in sauces, soups, or stews. Of course, freshly grated or ground spices will be more aromatic, so do stock them whole whenever possible.

Tools for Crushing Herbs and Spices

An electric spice grinder is very handy for grinding whole spices. Small spice graters for whole nutmeg or allspice are also useful, and come in handy for grating lemon and orange peel also. For crushing herbs and spices and blending them into other ingredients, a mortar and pestle are very efficient.

If you use a blender to grind spices and herbs try this method: A pint canning jar with a standard-size mouth will fit perfectly into many blender bases. Just put the spices in the jar, place the blade, rubber, and screw bottom of the blender container onto the jar as you would a lid. Turn the jar upside down, place in the blender base, and proceed with grinding.

Herb and Spice Blends

A number of herb and spice blends are classic and nice to have around premixed for convenience. Traditional mixtures such as curry or chili powder might have 6 to 20 different ingredients. Versions of these blends are commonly available commercially, but these may not offer the exact balance of flavors you desire. It might be more satisfying to make your own at home where you can control the degree of fire. The table on page 51 lists some commonly used herb and spice blends. Specific recipes for these and other herb and spice blends begin on page 62. As with any seasoning, you should freely vary the amounts of each herb or spice to suit your own taste. Use the same precautions to store these blends as you would all herbs and spices.

Growing Herbs at Home

Starting an herb garden indoors is very easy. Any window that gets bright sun for at least six hours of the day will serve well as a growing area. Here are just a few rules.

• Herbs started indoors for later transplanting out in the garden are best started from seed no earlier than March; otherwise they will not grow into strong, healthy plants.

• Seed each variety in a separate container to allow for the varying length of time each needs to germinate. Some herbs, for example, germinate within 48 hours, while others might take three weeks or longer.

• Choose a container that will make it possible to plant the seeds in rows rather than having to scatter them over the whole surface area. The rows should be at least one inch apart and about one-quarter inch deep, the growing medium itself one inch below the rim of the container.

• After the seeds have been thinly sown in the row or rows, water them with a fine mist of water and cover the container with two sheets of newspaper. Place the container in a warm area—preferably 70°F or a little warmer—just until the seeds germinate. Then keep the growing seedlings at 60 to 65°F to keep them from shooting up too rapidly. From then on the seeds need misting with water only enough to keep the soil constantly moist but not soggy.

• Once the seedlings develop their first seed leaves, usually in seven to ten days, transplant into 2¼-inch pots, one to a pot, or into flats with a minimum spacing of 1¼ inches. The seedlings should have a single root. Set the plant itself into the soil deeper than it grew in the seed flat. The soil into which these little plants are set may be regular potting soil or at least a richer medium than that of the seed flat.

• After four weeks the plants will be ready for transplanting into three-inch pots and from there, after another three to four weeks, the plants may be planted outside any time depending on variety and weather.

• Clip the sprigs or leaves as you need them. The plants will grow more if they are trimmed often, so use herbs whenever possible. Cut them fresh with scissors, always snipping from the top of the plant.

In the fall, repot the herbs, then bring them indoors to extend the growing season. These general rules will help ensure success with an indoor windowsill herb garden:

• Use a potting mix of equal parts of peat moss, perlite, and good potting soil.

• Keep the herbs in a sunny window where they will get at least six hours of sun a day. And, protect them from drafts in extremely cold weather.

• Arrange the pots on a tray containing pebbles and a small amount of water to keep the humidity level constant around the plants, and water the plants often enough to keep the soil moist but not soggy.

• Fertilize about every two weeks with deodorized fish emulsion.

• Clip sprigs and leaves from tops regularly to encourage new growth and use them to enhance your favorite recipes.

Some of the Less Common Herbs

Here is a brief introduction to some of the more unusual herbs and suggestions for their use.

Borage: This plant produces beautiful blue flowers. It must be used fresh or washed and frozen in plastic bags since its flavor diminishes quickly. Its light, refreshing flavor (reminiscent of cucumber) is most welcome in fish dishes, soups, and salad dressings. You may also cook it as you would other greens.

Burnet: A perennial herb, burnet contributes a hint of cucumber to fresh salads; its leaves may also be floated in iced beverages.

Camomile: This fragrant herb is most often imbibed as a tisane; a small amount may also be added to meat stocks for a light, lemony flavor.

Costmary: Its leaves may be steeped to make a tea with a light mint flavor. Costmary is also good in soups, sauces, green salads, chicken, and fish dishes.

Filé powder: Derived from crushing the leaves of the sassafras tree, this licorice-tasting herb is most often used to thicken and flavor Creole dishes such as gumbo.

Horehound: This plant's curly leaves are most often made into an extract used to flavor candy.

Horseradish: This flavoring should be used sparingly because it is bitter. Horseradish sauce is made from the ground root and white vinegar. Fresh, peeled horseradish may also be ground with lemon juice as well as white vinegar. Use immediately after preparing or its flavor will diminish. Horseradish's peppery flavor may also be mixed with mayonnaise. It is most often used with cold meats, fish, and shellfish.

Hyssop: The minty leaves of hyssop may be used in vegetable or fruit salads. Its flowers are also used for a tisane.

Lemon balm: This herb has fragrant leaves and is most often used in tisanes. The leaves may also be used to garnish fruit punches.

Lemon verbena: This sweet, lemon-flavored herb is best used in teas, but may also be used to garnish fruit salads and desserts.

Lovage: The flavor of lovage is so close to that of celery that its leaves and stalks are often substituted for it. A tea may be made from lovage leaves. The seeds of this plant may be used in cakes and cookies, or pickled like capers.

Sorrel: It has a tart flavor that is often used in soups and salads, or to counterbalance sweetness. Sorrel soup is a gourmet specialty in France.

Sweet cicely: Its sweet-smelling leaves and green seeds may be added to salads or vegetables.

The dried seeds may be used to flavor cakes and confections.

Woodruff: The Germans celebrate the advent of spring with *Maibowle,* a wine punch flavored with this sweet woodland herb. Fresh woodruff leaves may also be floated in other cold punches.

Herb Vinegars

Fresh herbs soaked in vinegar result in sweet, aromatic infusions. You may use a sprig of any fresh herb—or combine several with wine vinegar and allow the herbs to exude their delicate tastes. Herb vinegars may be used in salad dressings, or to marinate meat, fish, or cooked vegetables.

Store herb vinegars at room temperature. If a vinegar becomes too strong after standing, dilute with the same type of vinegar from which it was made.

Herb Vinegar

2 cups white wine vinegar
   sprig of any fresh herb or herbs
      (tarragon, basil, dill, chervil,
      or thyme)
1 clove garlic, halved (optional)

Place ingredients in a small saucepan and heat, but do not boil. Remove garlic clove. Place fresh herb sprig and vinegar in a sterile jar or the bottle in which vinegar was purchased. Allow vinegar to cool before capping container.

Yields 2 cups

NOTE: For a heartier blend use red wine vinegar; for a tart-sweet one use cider vinegar.

Variation:
   Add any of the following combinations to vinegar in place of fresh herb and garlic:

   peppercorns, basil, parsley, and chervil
   tarragon, thyme, mint, and oregano
   lemon peel, garlic, and mint
   rosemary, garlic, and thyme

Popular Herb and Spice Blends

Blend	Usual Ingredients	Popular Uses
Apple pie spice	allspice, cinnamon, nutmeg	apple pies, applesauce, baked apples, dumplings, strudels
Barbecue spice	cayenne pepper, cloves, cumin, garlic, paprika	broiled steaks, cheese, chickens, chops, eggs, hamburgers, meat loaves, potatoes, salad dressings
Bouquet garni	bay leaf, parsley, thyme	sauces, soups, stews, stocks
Chiffonade of fresh herbs	blend of fresh herbs: basil, chervil, chives, parsley	salad dressings, soups, stews, stocks
Chili powder	allspice, chili peppers, cloves, cumin, garlic, onion, oregano	cheese and egg dishes, salads, savory sauces, soups
Chinese five-spice powder	cinnamon, cloves, fennel, pepper, star anise	meat stews, poultry, roasted meats
Crab boil	bay leaf, ginger, mustard seeds, pepper	beans, fish, poultry, rice, vegetable dishes; coating or marinating meats
Curry powder	combination of some or all of the following: allspice, cardamom, cayenne pepper, cinnamon, coriander, cumin, fennel seeds, fenugreek, ginger, mace, turmeric	bean or vegetable dishes, fish, poultry, rice; coating or marinating meats
Fines herbes	chervil, chives, parsley, tarragon, (sometimes basil, marjoram, sage, thyme)	cheese and egg dishes, salads, savory sauces, soups
Pickling spice	allspice, bay leaves, cinnamon, cloves, coriander, ginger root, mustard, pepper (sometimes anise, dill)	condiments, pickling vegetables, preserves
Pizza seasoning (Italian seasoning)	basil, chili peppers, garlic, onion, oregano, pepper, thyme	chicken cacciatore, gravies, lasagna, meat loaves, pizza, pot roasts, ravioli, sauces, spaghetti, stews
Poultry seasoning	marjoram, pepper, sage, savory, thyme, (sometimes rosemary)	dumplings, fish, ground meats, poultry
Pumpkin pie spice	cinnamon, ginger, mace, nutmeg	breads, cookies, pies, pumpkin cakes, spice cakes
Quatre epices (spice parisienne)	cinnamon, clove, ginger, nutmeg (sometimes pepper)	carrots, meats, parsnips, sauces, soups, turnips

Flowers

Usually flowers are considered strictly ornamental, but many are edible and may be used in cooking to add exotic flavors and color. The petals are the most flavorful part of the flower. Rinse the flowers before eating them. (Of course, flowers that have been chemically sprayed should not be consumed at all.) The more fragrant a flower, the more flavor it will impart to a dish.

Not all flowers may be eaten; some are unpalatable and others are poisonous. The wisest course is to eat only those you are familiar with or those approved by a recognized authority. Wild plants such as clover, dandelion, daisy, and yarrow all have edible parts. Chrysanthemums, marigolds, lilies, nasturtiums, carnations, violets, roses, gardenias, gladiolus, pansies, peonies, and tulips also have edible flowers.

Use the flowers as fresh as possible. Store fresh-cut flowers in covered containers in the refrigerator. Do not store them longer than one day, because they will acquire an unpleasant taste after that.

Some flowers, such as honeysuckle and carnations, are sweet; while others, such as nasturtiums and marigolds, have pungent and peppery flavors. Use nasturtium leaves to add a peppery taste to soups and salads. To acquaint yourself with the specific flavor a flower will impart to other foods, mix the petals with cream cheese or cottage cheese; let sit at room temperature for 15 minutes and taste.

To dry flowers for winter use, the same method applies as for drying herbs (see page 48). The young seed pods may also be pickled like capers, and the flowers themselves are tasty when added as a garnish to salads.

Try some of these easy uses for flowers:

• Float whole blossoms on cold soups or punches.

• Toss with salads, or sprinkle the chopped petals over entrées just before serving.

• Add the flavors you like to egg dishes, and to pancake and cake batters.

• Add sweet-scented flowers to pound cakes, jellies, compotes, custards, and other baked goods.

Other Natural Flavorings

The juices of citrus fruits provide a convenient source of flavoring for all types of foods. Lemon and lime juice are particularly welcome for their zesty character. Before cutting and squeezing a citrus fruit, roll it back and forth on a hard surface several times, pushing down with the palms of your hands. This makes for easier juicing.

The rinds of lemons, limes, oranges, and tangerines, called zests, are also used to add flavoring to many foods, particularly baked goods. The oils contained in the skins of these citrus fruits are potent, concentrated flavoring. Usually only a small amount of the zest is necessary in a recipe. Be sure to use unsprayed fruits, and before grating them, make sure the rind has been cleaned well. Grate only the colored portion of the fruit, avoiding the bitter white skin underneath.

Some stores carry natural flavorings in the form of extracts that do not contain alcohol, unlike most commercial brands. Almond, coconut, and vanilla are usually included in this selection.

If you bake often, you may want to make your own vanilla extract from the vanilla bean. The following recipe yields a vanilla extract strong enough to replace the commercial brand on a one-to-one ratio. Vanilla beans are available at some supermarkets, at natural foods stores, and at coffee, tea, and spice shops. Store vanilla beans in a cool dark place.

Natural Vanilla Extract

1 vanilla bean
¼ cup boiling water
1 tablespoon honey
1 tablespoon sunflower or soy oil
1 tablespoon liquid lecithin

Cut the vanilla bean into small pieces and place in a small bowl. Pour boiling water over bean pieces, cover, and allow mixture to steep overnight.

Place mixture in a blender and process at medium speed until bean pieces are pulverized. Strain mixture through cheesecloth and then return liquid to the blender.

Add honey, oil, and lecithin and blend at medium speed until thoroughly combined. Pour extract into a small bottle, cap tightly, and store in the refrigerator. Shake well before using.

Yields about 1/3 cup

Condiments

Any spice, herb, or aromatic seed is by definition a condiment. But more commonly a condiment refers to any pungent, prepared mixture used in small amounts. A condiment may be anything from simple soy sauce to fancy relishes and pickles. The idea of serving condiments as an accompaniment to foods is usually to accent the taste of the food it dresses—lamb and mint jelly, turkey and cranberry relish, boiled beef and horseradish, for example. Mustard, catsup, and mayonnaise are among the most commonly used condiments in American cuisine. These may all be made at home, as can other more exotic blends, without the extra salt and preservatives characteristic of commercial brands.

Fresh and dried fruits, honey, molasses, vinegar, and different flavored oils mixed with herbs and spices are the basis for very sharp condiments such as chutney, a popular Indian relish. This blend is a traditional accompaniment for meat and vegetable meals in India. Other parts of the world have also contributed distinctive delicacies that provide refreshing alternatives to the standard American condiments. Try a savory Latin-American chili sauce in place of commercial catsup or steak sauce, or Corn Relish (page 65) in place of hot dog relish.

Storing Condiments

Most condiments keep well if stored in the refrigerator in tightly sealed jars. Vinegar as an ingredient helps to preserve some condiments, but others are highly perishable, so be sure to refrigerate these and use them quickly. Some condiments do not spoil easily but their flavor may change or deteriorate with time. For example, horseradish turns brown and loses its zip if kept for a long period. It is best to use unpreserved condiments within a month of making them.

Chilies

The classification of the chili as a fruit belies its truly volatile nature. Fresh and dried chilies are a favorite ingredient in Mexican dishes and the so-called "Tex-Mex" cooking of the West and Southwest. Their red-hot presence is also an integral part of many authentic Mexican bean and meat dishes, sauces, and condiments. Chilies appear in spicy dishes of India, and they are used in some types of Chinese cooking. It is the characteristic bite and zing of chilies (due to a chemical called capsaicin) that people either relish or avoid with equal passion.

The interest in foods common to the Latin culture is growing steadily in this country, and the increased use of chilies is just one manifestation of this newfound enthusiasm. As cooks experience the new taste values chilies can impart to an ordinary dish, they are frequently inspired to try other foods that spring from the exciting cuisine of Spanish-speaking nations.

Chilies have varying degrees of heat, so people who would otherwise abstain can savor some chili dishes without the risk of a fire-eating experience. Although climate, soil, and similar variables dictate the pungency of all types of chilies, you can look to appearance as a clue to the degree of heat. Contrary to what one might expect, size and shape, not color, are most telling. In general, the smaller the chili is, the hotter it is. Chilies with narrow tops and pointed tips are the most pungent; the broad-topped, rounded-end ones are milder.

Color does indicate ripeness and, to some extent, spiciness. Red chilies, despite their flamboyant color, may be milder than green chilies. That is because red chilies are riper and their sweetness masks some of the heat. The pale green chilies are the most immature and they are milder than the riper dark green ones. Dark green chilies that are just streaked with light red are generally seething with spiciness and fire.

Buying Chilies

The fresh (as opposed to dried) chilies most commonly known and used are *jalapeños* and *serranos;* they are interchangeable in recipes. You can usually also find chilies frozen or canned in most Mexican and oriental markets. Fresh chilies are available from midsummer through fall. Dried chilies available in cellophane packages may be found year-round (though they may be less prevalent in the eastern part of the country).

When buying fresh chilies, look for firm, smooth, blemish-free chilies. Avoid any that look mushy, have blackened skins or stems, or have begun to shrivel. Dried chilies should be dark red (almost maroon) and have long uniform pods. Avoid any gnarled or withered ones that display signs of mold or decay from improper drying.

Storing Chilies

Store fresh chilies in the refrigerator wrapped in absorbent paper for up to four days. Dried cellophane-packed chilies may be stored in your kitchen cabinet for up to six months.

Preparing Fresh Chilies

When handling fresh (or dried hot) chilies, it is a good idea to protect your hands from the

Herb and Spice Reference Table

Herbs are the aromatic leaves of seed-producing annuals, biennials, or perennials that grow in temperate climates. Spices are generally the more pungent substance from the bark, root, fruit, bud, berry, or leaf of perennial plants that are usually tropical. Aromatic seeds, the seeds or fruits of annual plants, are of temperate origin, but may also come from warmer climates. Both herbs and spices may produce aromatic seeds.

Herb or Spice	Sources	Appearance and Flavor
Allspice	West Indies, Central America	spice reddish brown berry; pungent blend of cinnamon, nutmeg, cloves
Anise*	Spain, Mexico	aromatic seed small, grayish brown, oval-shaped seed
Basil (sweet)	India, North Mediterranean shore	herb bright, green leaves when fresh; brownish olive when dried; sweetly pungent
Bay leaf (laurel)	Mediterranean region	herb long, green leaves; woody, menthol flavor (bitter if used too freely)

NOTE: When substituting one herb or spice for another, keep in mind that the flavor will be slightly altered and also that the herb or spice substituted may be milder or stronger than the one it is replacing. Thus, you may have to adjust the amount of seasoning called for. Unless you are absolutely certain of the potency of an herb or spice, taste a little first. When substituting cayenne pepper for any spice, use only about one-quarter to one-third the amount called for in the recipe since this is a powerful and piquant spice.

*Star anise, a star-shaped seed, formerly imported from China, has a similar flavor and use. It is currently available in limited quantities.

potentially irritating effects of capsaicin by wearing gloves.

Rinse the chilies under cold water and slit them at the stem with a knife tip. Spread them on a baking sheet. Place under the broiler as close to the heat source as possible until the skin parches and blisters, about ten minutes. Remove the chilies from the baking sheet, place them in a bowl, and cover with a cool, damp towel. Allow to stand for about ten minutes.

To peel the chili's outer skin, begin at the stem end pulling it downward. You may then chop the whole peeled chili for use in a recipe or, to lessen the piquancy, remove the veins and seeds first.

Preparing Dried Chilies

When using dried chilies, rinse them first to remove any dust that may have accumulated in storage. You may add chopped dried chilies directly to soups, stews, or moist meat mixtures or casseroles that will cook for at least 30 minutes —long enough for the chilies to rehydrate. You may also rehydrate dried chilies before adding them to a dish by chopping them and placing them in a bowl with enough water to cover. Drain and use after one hour.

A potent chili sauce for tacos and other Mexican favorites may be made simply by pureeing the rehydrated chilies with the soak water and a garlic clove in a blender until smooth.

Available Forms	Popular Uses	Readily Grown at Home	Substitute With
whole seeds; ground	apple dishes, applesauce, chutneys, cookies, fish, fruits, pickling spice, pot roasts, pumpkins, shellfish, spice cakes, squash, Swedish meatballs, sweet potatoes	no	cinnamon, cloves, nutmeg
whole seeds; ground	beef stews, cakes, fish, fruit pies, fruit salads, Italian coffee, liqueurs, pickles, sausage, shellfish, sweet rolls	no	fennel
fresh; dried, crushed leaves	egg dishes, fish, fowl, French dressing, green salads, herb breads, meats, tomatoes, vegetables	yes	marjoram, oregano, thyme
dried whole leaves; ground	fish, meats (particularly lamb), pickling spices, sauces, soups, stews	yes	mint

[continued]

Herb and Spice Reference Table—*Continued*

Herb or Spice	Sources	Appearance and Flavor	
Capers	mountainous parts of Africa, Italy, France, Spain	spice small, olive greenish pods; sharp, pungent, briny flavor	
Caraway	central Europe	aromatic seed small, brown, crescent-shaped seed, slight licorice taste	
Cardamom	India, Guatemala, Sri Lanka	spice small, dark-colored pods; gingery-lemon, aromatic flavor	
Cayenne (*Capsicum*)	Latin American countries	spice plump, sweet, scarlet fruit of tropical capsicum plant; very piquant	
Celery seed†	southern France, India	aromatic seed small, light brown seeds; celery taste	
Chervil	North America	herb delicate, feathery leaves; light licorice, parsley taste	
Chive	United States	herb long, green, tubular leaves; delicate onion flavor	
Cilantro	Spain, Mexico, China, Italy	herb short stemmed with thin, round, slightly fringed leaves; pungent and peppery smell and taste	
Cinnamon‡ (bark of *Cinnamomum zeylanicum*)	southern China, Indochina, Java, Sumatra, Sri Lanka	spice reddish brown, rolled-up quill-like sticks; sweet, mildly hot	
Clove	Moluccas Islands (Indonesia)	spice dried, unopened buds of a tropical evergreen; strong, sweet, and pungent	
Coriander	Yugoslavia, French Morocco	aromatic seed dried, ripe berries of cilantro plant; almost round with straight and wavy ridges; flavor of lemon peel and sage	

†Celery seed is a member of the parsley family—not identical to the plant which is used for the vegetable celery.
‡True cinnamon is light brown and has a subtle flavor. Most of the cinnamon used in the United States is *Cassia* which has a strong flavor.

Available Forms	Popular Uses	Readily Grown at Home	Substitute With
packed in salt or vinegar	beef gravies, canapés, fish, salads, sauces, tomato and eggplant dishes	no	pickled green peppers
whole, dried seed	cabbage, cheeses, meats, onions, pickling spices, rye breads, soups, stews, turnips	yes	anise
whole seeds; ground	curry powders, fruit punches, pickling spices, puddings, Scandinavian breads and baked goods, sweet potatoes	no	coriander, ginger
ground	curries, Mexican and Indian dishes, omelets, sauces, stews	no	ground dried chili pepper, paprika
whole seeds; ground	cabbage, coleslaw, pickles, potatoes, poultry stuffings, salad dressings, soups, steak sauces	no	finely chopped celery leaves
dried whole or ground leaves	component of cream sauces, fines herbes, green salads, seafoods	yes	tarragon
fresh; minced, dried, or frozen	baked potatoes, cheeses, cottage cheese, fish, omelets, salads, soups, sour cream dips and dressings	yes	scallions
fresh	Chinese dishes, Italian salads and casseroles, Spanish and Latin American ground meat and bean dishes	no	Italian parsley
sticks; ground	breads, cakes, cookies, custards, hot apple ciders, hot carob drinks, meatballs, pies, pork roasts	no	allspice, nutmeg
whole dry buds; ground	cakes, hot spice beverages, meat gravies, pickled fruits, pies, pork dishes, puddings, stews, sweet sauces	no	cinnamon, ginger
whole seeds; ground	buns, cakes, cookies, curry powder, pastries, pickling spice blends	yes	cardamom, ginger

[continued]

Herb and Spice Reference Table—*Continued*

Herb or Spice	*Sources*	*Appearance and Flavor*
Cumin	Iran, French Morocco	aromatic seed long thin seed, yellow brown in color, dry earthy taste
Dill	California	herb small tan seeds or feathery light leaves (weed), tangy taste resembling caraway
Fennel	India, Rumania	herb watermelon-shaped, chartreuse seeds or fresh, short, celerylike bulbs; licorice flavor
Fenugreek	Asia	aromatic seed smooth, red brown, unevenly shaped seeds
Ginger	southern Asia, West Indies, Africa	spice gnarl-shaped, light brown root; sweet, piquant, peppery
Mace	Moluccas Islands (Indonesia)	spice lacy, fibrous covering around the nutmeg shell; flavor of nutmeg but milder
Marjoram	France, Portugal	herb gray green leaves; musky, slight oregano bouquet
Mint	Belgium, France, Germany	herb dark emerald leaves, warm menthol flavor
Mustard	Asia	spice tiny, white, yellow, or brown seeds; sharp, tangy, biting
Nutmeg	Java, Malaya, Granada	spice very hard, brown, ovular seed pods; spicy, mellow, nutty
Oregano	Sicily, Greece, Morocco	herb grayish green leaves; strong, aromatic, slightly menthol
Paprika (mild *Capsicum*)	Central America, southern Europe, California	spice scarlet pods (only sold ground in this country); mild, slightly piquant

Available Forms	Popular Uses	Readily Grown at Home	Substitute With
whole seeds; ground	cabbage, chili powders, cream and vegetable soups, curry powders, meat loaves, spicy sauces	no	turmeric
whole seeds; ground; weed (dried leaves)	breads, cucumbers, egg and cheese dishes, fish and shellfish, meats, pickling spices, salads, sauces, sour cream	yes	caraway
whole seeds; ground fresh stalks	chicken, fish, Italian breads and rolls, Italian sausage, roast duck, other sausage, seafood casseroles, sweet pickles	yes	anise
whole seeds; ground	artificial maple flavoring, chutneys, curry powders	no	anise, caraway, fennel
whole and cracked roots; ground; crystallized	cakes, cookies, custards, fish, meats, oriental stir-fry dishes, pastries, pickling spices, pies, poultry	no	cardamom, coriander
dried blades; ground	cherry pies, fish sauces, pound cakes, puddings, pumpkin breads, and other baked goods	no	nutmeg
dried whole leaves; ground	green vegetables such as lima beans, peas, string beans; lamb; poultry; salads; stuffings	yes	basil, oregano, thyme
whole; crushed and ground leaves; fresh; oil; extract	bean and fish soups, candies, chilled fruits, cold beverages, desserts, hot teas, jellies, lamb, peas	yes	bay leaf
whole seeds; ground; prepared	beets, Chinese egg rolls, deviled eggs, gingerbread, pickling spice, salad dressings, zesty sauces	yes	prepared mustard
whole seeds; ground	cream sauces, eggnogs, puddings, quiches, soufflés, spice cakes, steamed vegetables	no	cinnamon, mace
dried whole leaves; ground	cheese fillings, fish sauces, meatballs, meat loaves, minestrone soups, omelets, pasta sauces, stuffings, tomato-based dishes	yes	basil, marjoram, thyme
ground	cream sauces, eggs, fish, flavoring for potatoes, garnishes, salads, soups	no	cayenne pepper

[continued]

Herb and Spice Reference Table—*Continued*

Herb or Spice	Sources	Appearance and Flavor	
Parsley	California, Texas, Arizona	herb curly small or flat green leaves; herbal, sweet flavor	
Pepper§	India, Indonesia	spice round, black, shriveled berries; hot, biting, pungent taste	
Rosemary	Yugoslavia, France, Spain, Portugal	herb gray green, curved, pine needle leaves; sweet, minty taste (perfumy if overused)	
Saffron	Spain	spice delicate, orange yellow filaments; pleasantly bitter	
Sage	Albania, Yugoslavia	herb silver-tipped, gray green leaves; strong, astringent, slightly bitter flavor	
Savory	Mediterranean countries	herb dried, brownish green leaves; aromatic, piquant	
Tarragon	Europe, California	herb long, thin, green leaves; sweet, slight licorice taste	
Thyme	France, United States	herb gray green, curly leaves; warm, slightly lemony	
Turmeric	Malabar, India	spice yellow orange root; similar to ginger root in shape; musky, slightly bitter	
Vanilla bean	Malagasy Republic, Réunion, Comoro	aromatic seed capsule very dark, long, slender seed pods; sweet, pleasantly perfumy flavor	

§Ground black pepper composed of both dark and light particles is made by grinding the entire pepper berry or corn. White pepper, obtained from the same vine is processed differently so that the black hull is removed before grinding. White pepper is milder than black and somewhat musty. White pepper is preferred for light soups and sauces. Green peppercorns, simply the unripe berry, is also from the same vine and is available water packed. Crushed red pepper, not as hot as cayenne pepper, is ground from dried red chili peppers (see Chilies, page 53).

Available Forms	Popular Uses	Readily Grown at Home	Substitute With
flakes; dried leaves; fresh	fish, meats, meat and cheese fillings, purees, salads, sauces, soups, vegetables	yes	basil
whole, dried peppercorns; ground	eggs, fish, meats, meat sauces, salads, soups, vegetable soups	no	cayenne pepper or red pepper
whole, dried leaves; ground	beef, boiled vegetables, chicken, lamb, pork, poultry stuffings, soup, stews	yes	mint, sage
whole stigmata; ground	*arroz con pollo,* bouillabaisse and other French dishes, curried dishes, fish sauces, paella, Spanish cakes and breads	no	turmeric
whole leaves; ground	baked fish, cheeses, chowders, pork, poultry, salad dressings, stuffings, veal	yes	rosemary, savory
whole leaves; ground	beans, cabbage, eggs, fish, hamburgers, lentils, meat loaves, meat stuffings, peas, poultry, sauces, stews, tomatoes	yes	sage
whole dried leaves; ground	egg and tomato dishes, mayonnaise dressings, meats, pickles, poultry, prepared mustards, salads, sauces	yes	chervil
whole dried leaves; ground	bouquet garni, clam chowder, clam juice, croquettes, fish, meats, poultry, stewed and fresh tomatoes	yes	basil, marjoram, oregano
ground	chicken and fish dishes, cream sauces, curries, egg dishes, noodles, pickles, relish, rice dishes, soups	no	cumin
whole beans; pure extract	sweet foods such as cakes, cookies, custards, eggnog, frostings, ice cream, milk, pastries, puddings, rice, shakes, soufflés, sweet sauces, whipped cream	no	. . .

Herb and Spice Blends

Barbecue Spice

2 tablespoons chili powder
2 tablespoons dry mustard
1 tablespoon paprika
1 tablespoon garlic powder
1 tablespoon ground cumin
½ teaspoon cayenne pepper
½ teaspoon ground cloves (optional)

Combine all ingredients, blend, and store in an airtight container. To use, sprinkle on meats before baking or broiling, or add to flour or breading mixtures for chicken or fish.

Yields ⅓ cup

Bouquet Garni

The bouquet garni is a traditional combination of herbs that is added to soups, stews, or sauces to enhance their flavor.

1 bay leaf
2 sprigs parsley or 1½ teaspoons dried parsley
1 sprig thyme or 1 teaspoon dried thyme

Gather herbs together, tie with string, or place them in a piece of cheesecloth, tied closed, or place the herbs in a metal tea ball. For even more flavor tie herbs between 2 stalks of celery. When desired flavor has been obtained, remove and discard bouquet garni.

Chiffonade of Fresh Herbs

3 tablespoons chopped fresh parsley
1 teaspoon chopped fresh thyme
1 teaspoon chopped fresh basil
1 teaspoon chopped fresh chervil
2 teaspoons chopped fresh chives

Mix fresh herbs together until well blended. This amount flavors a stew, a soup, or a fresh green salad made to serve 4.

Yields ⅓ cup

Chinese Five-Spice Powder

2 teaspoons star anise*
2 teaspoons fennel seeds
2 teaspoons peppercorns
2 teaspoons whole cloves
1 stick of cinnamon, 2 inches long

Grind all ingredients in a blender or electric grinder until mixture is a powder. Store in an airtight container. Add 1 tablespoon or to taste, to meat dishes made to serve 6.

Yields ¼ cup

*Star anise is available in coffee, tea, and spice shops or in oriental grocery stores.

Classic Fines Herbes

1 tablespoon chopped fresh chervil
1 tablespoon chopped fresh chives
1 tablespoon chopped fresh basil, marjoram, rosemary, tarragon, or thyme (or combination of two or more)

Mix herbs together. Add mixture to appropriate sauces, soups, and egg dishes made to serve 6.

Yields 3 tablespoons

Crab Boil

8 bay leaves, crumbled
2 teaspoons peppercorns
2 teaspoons mustard seeds
2 teaspoons ground ginger
2 teaspoons dill seeds
2 teaspoons whole allspice
1 teaspoon crushed red pepper
1 teaspoon whole cloves
1 teaspoon Hungarian paprika (optional)

Mix all ingredients together until well blended.

For every 6 cups of water needed, add 1 tablespoon crab boil and simmer for 15 minutes before cooking crab or shrimp according to recipe directions.

Yields ¼ cup

Garam Masala
(Indian Spice Mixture)

4 sticks of cinnamon, 3 inches long
¾ cup cardamom pods
3 tablespoons whole cloves
6 tablespoons cumin seeds
3 tablespoons coriander seeds
3 tablespoons peppercorns

Preheat oven to 200°F.

Spread out spices in one layer on a baking sheet and roast for 20 minutes in oven. Shake pan every 5 minutes to keep spices from browning. Cool.

Break open cardamom pods, remove seeds, and discard pods. Place all spices in a blender or electric grinder, and grind until spices are a powder. Stop blender every 30 seconds or so to stir spice mixture, then grind again until mixture is uniformly ground. Store in an airtight jar. Use in recipes as directed.

Yields about 1 cup

Curry Powder

1 stick of cinnamon, 3 inches long, or 2
    teaspoons ground cinnamon
10 cardamom pods or ½ teaspoon ground
    cardamom
8 whole cloves or ½ teaspoon ground cloves
3 teaspoons cumin seeds or ground cumin
2 teaspoons peppercorns or 1 teaspoon pepper
2 teaspoons coriander seeds or ½ teaspoon
    ground coriander
1 teaspoon turmeric
3 teaspoons fenugreek seeds or 2 teaspoons
    ground fenugreek

If using whole spices, combine all ingredients, except cardamom pods and coriander seeds. Grind and sift cardamom pods and coriander seeds separately; then add to other spices and grind in a blender or electric grinder. If using ground spices, mix all together. Store in an airtight jar.

Yields ¼ cup

Variation:

Hot Curry Powder: Add 1 teaspoon cayenne pepper to mixture.

Chili Powder

2 tablespoons cumin seeds or 2 tablespoons
    ground cumin
4 dried hot chili peppers, ground,* or 2
    teaspoons crushed red pepper
2 teaspoons dried oregano
2 teaspoons garlic powder
2 teaspoons onion powder
1 teaspoon ground allspice
⅛ teaspoon ground cloves

Combine all ingredients in a blender or electric grinder and grind until mixture is a coarse powder. Use in recipes as directed.

Yields ¼ cup

*If using dried hot chili peppers, remove the seeds before grinding or the mixture will be too hot.

Herbal Seasoning

¼ teaspoon garlic powder
½ teaspoon onion powder
1 tablespoon dried parsley
½ teaspoon paprika
⅛ teaspoon cayenne pepper
½ teaspoon dried thyme
½ teaspoon dried marjoram
1 teaspoon ground toasted sesame seeds

Blend all ingredients in a blender for a few minutes. Use in a shaker as a seasoning in place of salt.

Yields about ⅓ cup

Pumpkin Pie Spice

2 teaspoons ground nutmeg
2 teaspoons ground cinnamon
1 teaspoon ground ginger
½ teaspoon ground mace
½ teaspoon ground cloves

Combine all ingredients and blend. Store in a tightly covered jar until needed.

Yields 2 tablespoons

Pickling Spice

    3 bay leaves, crumbled
    1 tablespoon mustard seeds
    1 tablespoon whole allspice
    1 tablespoon dill seeds (optional)
    1 teaspoon fenugreek seeds
    1 teaspoon coriander seeds
    1 teaspoon peppercorns
    1 teaspoon whole cloves
    1 teaspoon ground ginger
    ½ teaspoon crushed red pepper

Combine ingredients, blend, and store in an air-tight container. To use for pickling, add 2 tablespoons to every quart of pickling liquid.

    Yields ⅓ cup

Pizza Seasoning

    ¼ cup dried oregano
    2 tablespoons dried basil
    2 teaspoons onion powder
    1½ teaspoons garlic powder
    ¼ teaspoon crushed red pepper

Combine all ingredients in a jar and shake until well blended. Sprinkle on top of pizza before baking or add 1 tablespoon to every quart of tomato sauce as a seasoning.

    Yields ⅓ cup

Poultry Seasoning

    4 teaspoons dried marjoram
    4 teaspoons onion powder
    2 teaspoons dried thyme
    2 teaspoons dried sage
    2 teaspoons dried savory
    1 teaspoon celery seeds
    1 teaspoon white pepper

Combine all ingredients in a blender or electric grinder, and grind until mixture is a powder. Store in an airtight container. Sprinkle on poultry before cooking, or add 2 teaspoons to poultry, soups, stews, or casseroles made to serve 4 to 6.

    Yields ¼ cup

Quatre Epices (Spice Parisienne)

    ¼ teaspoon ground cloves
    ½ teaspoon ground ginger
    ½ teaspoon ground nutmeg
    1 teaspoon ground cinnamon
        dash of pepper

Combine all ingredients and blend. Store in a tightly covered jar. Use pinches to season meats, vegetables, soups, and sauces to taste while cooking.

    Yields 1 tablespoon

Fresh Chutneys and Relishes

Apricot Chutney

        2 cups dried apricots
    2 to 2½ cups boiling water
        3 tablespoons honey
        1½ tablespoons vinegar
        1 teaspoon minced peeled ginger root or ½
            teaspoon ground ginger
        ½ teaspoon ground coriander
            cayenne pepper, to taste
        ½ cup raw cashews
        ½ cup raisins

Place apricots in a small bowl and add enough boiling water to cover. Allow to sit until soft, about 30 minutes. Drain and chop apricots.

Combine apricots with all but the cashews and raisins. Mix well. Add cashews and raisins and mix well again.

Serve with chicken, curry dishes, or any cold meats.

    Yields about 3 cups

Date Chutney

    1½ cups sliced dates
    1 cup water
    3 tablespoons lemon juice
    ½ cup sliced fresh coconut or ¼ cup
        unsweetened shredded coconut

2 tablespoons chopped peeled ginger root or
   2 teaspoons ground ginger
   freshly ground black pepper, to taste

Combine all ingredients, except pepper, in a blender and process to a puree. Add a bit more water if necessary. Season with pepper. Store in refrigerator. Serve with curry dishes or other spicy Indian dishes.

Yields about 2 cups

Cantaloupe Relish

2 medium-size onions, sliced
¼ cup vegetable oil
1 teaspoon ground coriander
½ teaspoon ground mace
½ teaspoon ground cumin
½ teaspoon ground ginger
   pepper, to taste
4 cups cubed cantaloupe

In a large skillet sauté onions in oil for about 1 minute. Add spices and cook another minute, stirring frequently. Add cantaloupe and sauté, covered, over low heat for 20 minutes, or until cantaloupe is tender. Serve warm or cold as a relish with meat dishes. Store in refrigerator.

Yields about 2 cups

Corn Relish

6 ears of corn
1 green pepper, diced
1 sweet red pepper, diced
2 medium-size onions, minced
1⅓ tablespoons dry mustard
⅓ teaspoon turmeric
⅓ cup honey
½ cup vinegar

Remove corn from cobs and combine with diced green and red peppers and onions.

Combine remaining ingredients in medium-size saucepan. Add corn mixture and simmer slowly for 6 to 8 minutes.

Chill and serve with poultry or meat dishes.

6 servings

Fresh Cranberry Relish

4 cups fresh cranberries (about 1 pound)
2 medium-size unpeeled red apples, cored
1 large or 2 medium-size unpeeled navel
   oranges, quartered
⅔ cup honey

Alternately put cranberries, apples, and orange quarters through coarse blade of food mill. Blend in honey and combine thoroughly.

Refrigerate, covered, several hours or overnight before serving as accompaniment to poultry.

Yields 1 quart

Condiments

Sweet Catsup

2 cups tomato puree
2 cups tomato juice
1 cup cider vinegar
½ cup honey
1 teaspoon dry mustard
1 stick of cinnamon, 2 inches long
½ teaspoon whole allspice or ½ teaspoon
   ground allspice
2 stalks celery with leaves
2 medium-size onions

In a heavy saucepan, combine tomato puree, tomato juice, vinegar, honey, and mustard. Place over medium heat and bring to a boil.

Place cinnamon and allspice in a clean, thin, white cloth. Tie top tightly. Add to catsup mixture. Then add celery and onions. Bring to a boil, reduce heat, and cook, uncovered, until catsup is thick, about 3 hours. Stir occasionally during cooking.

Remove spices with a slotted spoon, remove celery and onions. Pour catsup into a heated glass container with tight-fitting lid, cool at room temperature, and then store in refrigerator.

Yields about 1 pint

Spicy Catsup

5 to 6 pounds tomatoes (15 to 17
      medium-size), peeled and sliced
¾ cup chopped onions
1 stick of cinnamon, about 3 inches long
1 large clove garlic, chopped
1 teaspoon whole cloves
1 cup vinegar
1 teaspoon paprika
dash of cayenne pepper

Simmer tomatoes and onions together for 20 to
30 minutes. Press through a sieve.

Place cinnamon, garlic, and cloves loosely in a
clean, thin, white cloth. Tie top tightly. Combine with
vinegar and simmer for 30 minutes. Remove spices.

Boil sieved tomatoes rapidly until reduced to one-
half original volume. Stir frequently to prevent sticking. Add spiced vinegar, paprika, and cayenne to
tomato mixture. Boil rapidly, stirring constantly, about
10 minutes, or until slightly thickened.

Pour into clean, hot, sterilized pint jars, leaving
a ¼-inch headspace. Adjust seals and process for 5
minutes in a boiling water bath (see Using a Water
Bath Canner, page 768).

Yields about 2 pints

Cranberry Catsup

1 pound fresh cranberries
½ cup cider vinegar
½ cup water
¾ cup honey
2 tablespoons molasses
½ teaspoon ground cinnamon
½ teaspoon ground cloves
½ teaspoon ground ginger
dash of pepper

Place cranberries in a medium-size pot with
vinegar and water, bring to a boil, and cook over
medium heat for a few minutes. Allow to cool slightly.
Then pour into blender and process until smooth.

Add remaining ingredients, one at a time, processing at the lowest speed, until mixture is very
smooth.

Pour mixture back into pot and simmer gently
for 5 minutes, stirring once or twice. Pour into glass
jars and store in refrigerator.

Serve as condiment for hot or cold poultry.

Yields about 1 quart

Chili Sauce

8 pounds tomatoes (about 25 medium-size),
      peeled and sliced
2 cups chopped sweet red peppers
2 cups chopped onions
2 cloves garlic, minced
1 hot chili pepper, chopped
2 tablespoons celery seeds
1 tablespoon mustard seeds
1 bay leaf
1 teaspoon whole cloves
1 teaspoon ground ginger
1 teaspoon ground nutmeg
2 sticks of cinnamon, 3 inches long
½ cup honey
3 cups vinegar

Combine tomatoes, sweet red peppers, onions,
garlic, and hot pepper in a large stainless steel or
enameled pot.

Place celery and mustard seeds, bay leaf, cloves,
ginger, nutmeg, and cinnamon in a cloth bag and tie
shut. Add to tomato mixture and boil until volume is
reduced to one-half, 2 to 3 hours. Stir frequently
to prevent sticking. Remove spice bag.

Add honey and vinegar. Bring to a rapid boil,
stirring constantly. Allow to simmer about 5 minutes.

Pour into clean, hot, sterilized pint jars, leaving
¼-inch headspace. Adjust seals and process for 10
minutes in a boiling water bath (see Using a Water
Bath Canner, page 768).

Yields 8 or 9 pints

Creamed Horseradish

2/3 cup freshly grated horseradish
1/3 cup white vinegar
1/3 cup mayonnaise
1 tablespoon vegetable oil

Combine horseradish and vinegar together in a blender and process at high speed. Add mayonnaise and blend well. Add oil and continue blending at high speed until fairly smooth. Cover and refrigerate.

Yields 1 cup

Extra-Rich Creamed Horseradish

3 tablespoons freshly grated horseradish
1 teaspoon lemon juice
1/4 cup sour cream
3 tablespoons light cream

Mix all ingredients well. Cover and refrigerate.

Yields 1/2 cup

Prepared Horseradish

1 cup freshly grated horseradish
1/2 cup white wine vinegar

Combine ingredients. Pack into clean jars. Seal tightly and store in refrigerator.

Yields about 1 1/4 cups

French-Style Mustard

1/4 cup ground brown mustard seeds
5 tablespoons dry mustard
1/2 cup hot water
3/4 cup champagne vinegar
2 tablespoons cold water
2 large slices onion
2 teaspoons honey
1 teaspoon molasses
2 cloves garlic, halved
1/4 teaspoon dill seeds
1/4 teaspoon ground cinnamon
1/4 teaspoon ground allspice

1/4 teaspoon dried tarragon
1/8 teaspoon ground cloves

Soak ground mustard seeds and dry mustard in water and 1/4 cup of the vinegar at room temperature at least 3 hours.

Combine remaining vinegar and ingredients in a small saucepan. Bring to a boil, boil 1 minute, remove from heat, cover, and let stand for 1 hour.

Transfer soaked mustard mixture to a blender. Strain spice mixture into mustard mixture. Press spices against the sides of the strainer to extract all the flavor. Process until mixture is the consistency of a coarse puree.

Pour mixture into the top of a double boiler, set pan over simmering water, and cook until thickened, about 20 to 25 minutes. (Mustard will thicken a bit more when chilled.)

Remove mustard from heat and pour into a jar. Let cool, uncovered. Then replace lid and store in refrigerator.

Yields 1 cup

Prepared Mustard

1/4 cup dry mustard
1/4 cup hot water
3 tablespoons white wine vinegar
1/8 teaspoon garlic powder
pinch of dried tarragon
1/4 teaspoon molasses

Soak mustard in water and 1 tablespoon of vinegar at least 2 hours.

Combine remaining vinegar, garlic, and tarragon in a separate bowl and let stand for 30 minutes. Strain tarragon from mixture and add liquid to mustard mixture. Stir in molasses.

Pour mustard into the top of a double boiler and set pan over simmering water. Cook until thickened, about 15 minutes. (Mustard will thicken a bit more when chilled.)

Remove mustard from heat and pour into a jar. Let cool, uncovered. Then replace lid and store in refrigerator.

Yields 1/2 cup

Steak Sauce

1 cup water
3 tablespoons tomato paste
2 tablespoons cider vinegar
1 tablespoon molasses
1 tablespoon soy sauce
1 teaspoon orange juice
  grated rind of 1 lemon
⅛ teaspoon cayenne pepper
1 teaspoon cornstarch
1 small onion, quartered
1 small clove garlic, minced

Combine all ingredients in a blender and blend until smooth. Transfer to a small saucepan, cover, and simmer for 20 minutes. Pour into a bottle or jar, cover, and store in refrigerator.

Yields 1½ cups

Tomato Paste

24 pounds very ripe tomatoes (about 48 large)
3 sweet red peppers, chopped
2 bay leaves, crumbled
1 clove garlic, finely minced

Combine tomatoes, peppers, and bay leaves in a large, heavy pot and cook, uncovered, over low heat for 1 hour.

Puree mixture in a food mill and then through a fine sieve. Add garlic. Return to pot and continue to cook slowly until thick enough to be mounded on a spoon. Stir often while cooking to prevent tomatoes from sticking to bottom of pan.

Spoon into ½-pint containers and freeze (or freeze in ice cube trays for small amounts).

Yields about eighteen ½ pints

Tartar Sauce

½ cup finely chopped cucumbers
¼ cup finely minced onions
2 tablespoons finely minced green peppers
3 tablespoons vinegar
2 tablespoons honey
  dash of ground allspice
  dash of turmeric
  dash of ground cloves
⅛ teaspoon celery seeds
¾ cup mayonnaise

In a small saucepan, combine cucumbers, onions, green peppers, vinegar, honey, spices, and celery seeds. Cook for 10 minutes or until vegetables are soft and dark yellow from the turmeric, and most of the liquid has evaporated. Cool.

Combine with mayonnaise, blend, and refrigerate for at least 1 hour to meld flavors. Keeps for about 1 week.

Yields 1 cup

Flowers

Lemon Nasturtium Salad

2 tablespoons minced red onions
½ teaspoon celery seeds
1¼ cups water
1 envelope unflavored gelatin
¼ cup lemon juice
¼ cup orange juice
2 tablespoons honey
½ teaspoon grated lemon rind
12 whole small nasturtium flowers
½ cup nasturtium petals
1 small cucumber, thinly sliced

In a small saucepan, simmer onions and celery seeds in 1 cup of the water, covered, for 5 minutes.

Soften gelatin in remaining water. Strain hot water into gelatin. Add lemon and orange juices, honey, and lemon rind.

Use a chilled, clear, 1-quart glass bowl as a mold. Ladle ½ cup of gelatin mixture into the mold. Swirl it around to coat inside of mold. Place whole nasturtium flowers, facing down, in a single layer over bottom of mold. Refrigerate, uncovered, until almost set. Refrigerate remaining gelatin, but don't let it become solid.

Ladle in another ½ cup of gelatin. Lay some of the cucumber slices in a single layer. Press nasturtium petals onto side of mold. Refrigerate until almost set.

Sprinkle petals over last layer and add more gelatin, topping this layer with cucumber slices. Mix any remaining cucumber and nasturtium petals into unused gelatin, and fill mold. Chill thoroughly before unmolding onto a serving plate.

6 servings

Pickled Nasturtium Buds

Pickled nasturtium buds have a peppery taste, and the liquid becomes a velvety red. Use the pickled buds in recipes requiring capers, such as sauces for fish, and in cheese spreads.

  1 cup unopened nasturtium buds
  ¼ teaspoon cumin seeds
  ¼ teaspoon fennel seeds
  3 tablespoons white vinegar
  3 tablespoons lemon juice
  ¼ cup water
  1 teaspoon honey

Scald a 1-cup jelly jar and a canning lid band. Pack buds, cumin and fennel seeds in the jar.

Bring vinegar, lemon juice, water, and honey to a boil. Stand the jar in hot water. Pour the boiling liquid over buds leaving ½-inch headspace at top of jar. Screw on canning lid, cool jar on a wire rack, and store in refrigerator for at least 1 week before using to allow flavors to blend. Use within 2 months.

  Yields 1 cup

Sweet Pansy Paperweights

Pansies have a delicate taste and texture. This dessert, which is made in individual molds (glass custard cups), looks like Victorian glass paperweights. If the pansy harvest is ample, consider doubling the recipe.

  1¼ cups water
  1 envelope unflavored gelatin
  ¼ cup lemon juice
  ¼ cup plus 2 tablespoons honey
  4 ounces cream cheese, softened
  1 tablespoon yogurt or light cream
  8 whole, small, perfect pansies
  ½ cup pansy petals

Pour ½ cup cold water over gelatin to soften it. Bring remaining water to a boil and pour over softened gelatin. Stir in lemon juice and ¼ cup of honey. Refrigerate until syrupy.

Meanwhile, beat remaining honey into cream cheese. Thin with yogurt or cream until cream cheese mixture is still thick, but will pour.

Rinse 4 glass custard cups with very cold water and spoon 1 tablespoon of syrupy gelatin in each cup. Float 2 pansies, face down, in each. Keep flowers away from sides of cup. Place cups on a small tray and refrigerate, uncovered, until firm.

Add 2 more tablespoons of gelatin to each cup. Refrigerate. When firm, place a few petals, face down, on last layer. Add cream cheese, taking care not to let cheese mixture touch sides of cups. Stir remaining petals into remaining gelatin and then fill cups with this mixture. Chill completely before unmolding each custard cup onto a serving plate.

  4 servings

Nasturtium Plum Soup

When lightly sweetened, this thick soup makes a good summertime appetizer or snack. With a little more honey, it becomes an elegant dessert.

  1 pound ripe purple or red plums, quartered
  ½ teaspoon fennel seeds
  ½ teaspoon coriander seeds
  4 whole cloves
  ¼ teaspoon whole allspice
  1 teaspoon grated orange rind
  3 cups water
  2 tablespoons cornstarch
2 to 4 tablespoons honey
  ½ cup nasturtium petals
  ¼ cup sour cream
  ¼ cup yogurt
  8 whole small nasturtium flowers

Simmer plums, fennel seeds, coriander seeds, cloves, allspice, and orange rind in 2¾ cups of the water, covered, for about 1 hour, or until plums are completely soft.

Dissolve cornstarch in remaining ¼ cup of water in a 2-quart pot. Pour in plum mixture through a large wire strainer. Press plums gently to force out juice but not pulp. Simmer, stirring, for another 5 minutes. Add 2 tablespoons of the honey. Taste soup and add more, if desired. Chill soup.

When cold, stir in nasturtium petals. Ladle soup into individual bowls.

Mix sour cream and yogurt together well, then swirl 2 tablespoons through each bowl of soup without mixing thoroughly. Top each serving with 2 whole flowers.

  4 servings

Appetizers

Just about any savory dish that can be eaten as "finger food" or in small quantities can be served as an appetizer. The light dish—a soup, salad, or pâté, for instance—served as a first course at sit-down meals is also considered an appetizer. In this section we are primarily concerned with finger foods. However they are served, appetizers are among the most seductive mediums creative cooks can use to stimulate appetites.

The range is up to you, but the occasion often dictates what should be served, from simple nibblers such as mixed nuts and raw vegetables (called "crudités") to elaborate preparations such as fancy aspics and miniature pastries. Fondues, pastries, and certain meat morsels are served piping hot, while others—aspics, pâtés, and crudités—must be well chilled. The flavors of some dips and spreads, especially those based on pungent cheeses, develop best at room temperature. It is wise to keep these temperature requirements in mind when planning the types of appetizers to serve. A good general rule is to offer just one or two types of hot appetizers and the rest cold, thus avoiding extra kitchen work after the guests have arrived. You can remove the steaming hot appetizers from the oven at the last minute. Serve them in a chafing dish or in a casserole that holds heat. When the hot items are gone, the guests can continue to help themselves to an array of cold ones.

Though appetizers are not intended as the nutritional foundation of a meal, they offer plenty of opportunity for incorporating good-tasting, nutritious ingredients, including nuts, cheeses, fresh fruits and vegetables, meats, fish, and poultry. For those who want to reduce the fat and calorie content of appetizer recipes that call for butter, mayonnaise, or cream cheese, it is a simple thing to use less butter and lighter ingredients—yogurt, sour cream, and cottage

Tips and Suggestions for Appetizers

• Fruit makes a refreshing light appetizer and can be an attractive part of the table setting. It requires little work, just some chopping or slicing. For ideas on serving fruit, see Fruits chapter.

• For some especially healthful hors d'oeuvres, serve baked or sautéed cubes of tempeh and tofu with a dipping sauce of your choice.

• Make miniature bean patties for appetizers (see Legumes chapter for recipes); serve them with creamy dips.

• See Breads chapter for different types of crackers and biscuits to serve with dips or spreads or as canapés.

• Allow for a variance in guests' tastes; along with the very spicy appetizers serve some mild-flavored ones.

• Freshen hot appetizers quickly by heating them in a toaster-oven.

• For less fat in dips and spreads, replace some or all of the cheese or dairy ingredients with crumbled, firm tofu.

• Cut garnishes at the last minute so they remain fresh-looking.

• Allow watery ingredients such as tomatoes and cucumbers to drain well before adding them to canapés or little sandwiches.

cheese or ricotta cheese. For flavor, aromatic seasonings and spices can often replace fat-rich ingredients.

When deciding which appetizers to serve, consider the content of the meal that will follow. Avoid any flavors or ingredients planned for the main course. If fondue or cheese and egg pastries are included among the appetizers, for example, these dairy products should not reappear in the entrée. How rich are the appetizers in relation to the dinner? Serve light appetizers before heavy meals and richer ones before light meals. It is a mistake to be too generous with appetizers. Although there is usually some time for socializing between serving the appetizers and the main course, a lavish array of appetizers will dull, not enhance, your guests' enjoyment of the meal to follow. Figure about four to five small pieces per person.

Preparing Ahead and Storing Appetizers

With a kitchen blender it is easy to puree the ingredients used in preparing dips and spreads. Most foods of this type may be prepared ahead and refrigerated for two or three days. Store them and all other appetizers in tightly covered containers. Trays of canapés or open-faced sandwiches may be stored for several hours in the refrigerator if wrapped carefully in moisture-proof plastic wrap. If kept much longer than that, they may become soggy and unappetizing. Allow canapés, dips, and spreads to reach room temperature before serving.

For appetizers that include pastry, the dough may be made, rolled, and shaped (and baked if necessary) in advance, and refrigerated or frozen. The filling, if made in advance, should be stored separately and added just before the pastries are baked. Before freezing any appetizers, check into the freezing qualities of their ingredients (see Freezing, page 752).

Presenting Appetizers

Of course, all food should be served invitingly, but artful presentation of appetizers is especially important. Be creative in arranging them on trays or in bowls. Consider textures, colors, and shapes—bright orange carrot curls, rosy radish petals, and crimson bell pepper rings are all alluring—and edible—garnishes.

When appropriate, use fresh, fragrant herbs to decorate appetizers. Put sprigs of fresh basil, parsley, chervil, or thyme on individual canapés. For deviled eggs, pipe the filling through a pastry bag with a decorative tip, then sprinkle the eggs

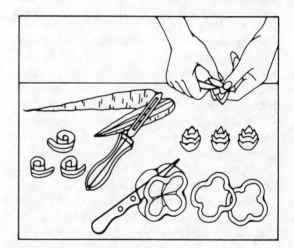

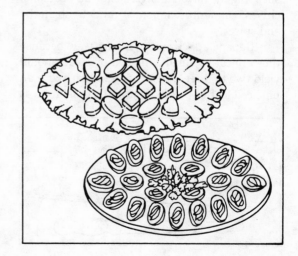

lightly with paprika and/or chopped parsley. Use the various tips of a pastry bag to spread the filling on open-faced sandwiches. Sliced hard-cooked eggs are an attractive and versatile garnish. Arrange them on trays with a sprig of fresh herb, or a dab of savory dip or spread. Spread them on top of molds and aspics for color contrasts.

Serve spreads and dips in several small bowls of varying shapes, colors, and materials, instead of one large one.

Canapés and Open-faced Appetizers

Canapés are small hot or cold bite-size appetizers consisting of bread, toast, or crackers topped with a savory spread. They may also be filled miniature sandwiches of several tiers, spreads rolled in thin bread, or filled two-toned triangles. Canapés lend themselves to numerous geometric shapes that invite a variety of attractive garnishings.

Among the scores of fillings and spreads appropriate for canapés, cheese is particularly popular as a base, but mashed eggs and ground or pureed meat, fish, and chicken are also used in this way. The fillings should be tangy, featuring such highly flavored ingredients as scallions, chives, pimientos, mustard, and fresh herbs and spices.

Canapé appetizers go a long way, because they are cut so small. One loaf of bread should yield two to three dozen canapés. Start with an unsliced loaf of bread; remove the crust (unless

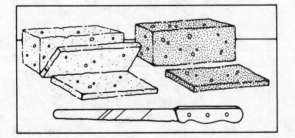

working with long round loaves) and use it later in stuffings or breadings. Cut even slices and spread them with filling; then cut, roll, or slice these. For different-shaped canapés, slice the loaf horizontally and apply the spread to the entire slice, then cut to desired shapes.

Fine-grained bread works best for rolled canapés and day-old bread holds its shape better than fresh. Chill or freeze the bread for about a half hour before spreading fillings; the firmed bread resists tearing. Use a sharp, hot knife to cut bread as cleanly as possible. Spreads are easiest to work with at room temperature. When making canapés several hours before serving, spread a thin layer of butter on the bread. The butter will keep the bread from absorbing the filling's moisture.

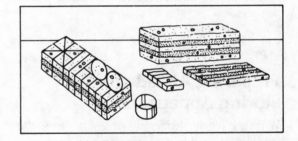

For open-faced or several-tiered sandwiches, use an assembly line procedure. Line up the bread, toast, or crackers. Apply the spread to all slices, then cut to desired shapes and sizes and garnish.

For added flavor use different whole grain breads, crackers, and flatbreads. For a two-toned effect in tiered sandwiches, use light and dark wheat and rye breads. Experiment with different shapes—square, oblong, round, triangular, diamond.

Crepes and tortillas of corn or whole wheat are perfect wraps for canapé fillings. After spreading them with filling, roll and cut them into smaller bite-size morsels that can be pierced with a wooden pick for serving. Or stack them up, layered with various fillings, then cut into wedges.

Dips and Spreads

Dips and spreads for crackers, bread, or raw vegetables are easy-to-do party appetizers. Blends with sour cream, yogurt, and cottage, ricotta, or cream cheese may be seasoned with scores of tangy flavors, then chilled. A delicious alternative to these dairy-based dips are bean dips. Just about any dried bean can be cooked, pureed (for pureeing directions, see page 262), and then seasoned to make a zesty vegetable pâté or dip. Chick-peas, soybeans, lima beans, and pinto beans are especially good choices for bean dips. Guacamole—seasoned, mashed avocado—is a good accompaniment with pinto bean dip. Both are favorites of Mexican cuisine.

Cheese and Egg Appetizers

Cheese and crackers, like deviled eggs prepared with a varying degree of spiciness, are perennial favorites. Quiche, cheese balls, and fondues are elegant preparations with a universal appeal. Quiche may be prepared in an 8- or 9-inch piecrust, then cut into uniform, bite-size pieces. For an added festive touch, prepare miniature quiches in 2-inch fluted tart shells.

Hard-cooked eggs may be sliced or halved, then garnished, or they may be diced or crumbled and used as a garnish for bigger appetizers. Omelets and frittatas filled with spinach, broccoli, cauliflower, or other tasty vegetables can be cooked, then cut into morsels and served with wooden picks.

Vegetable Appetizers

Vegetable appetizers are effective appetite enhancers. They are tasty yet light. Besides their popular role as dippers or crudités, they can be prepared numerous ways to serve as appetizers. Serve steamed whole artichokes with melted butter as a dip or with garlic mayonnaise for a different attraction. Large vegetables such as eggplant, squash, or bell pepper may be hollowed

out and used as containers for dips and spreads. Stuff celery stalks and mushroom caps with cheese spreads and chill well.

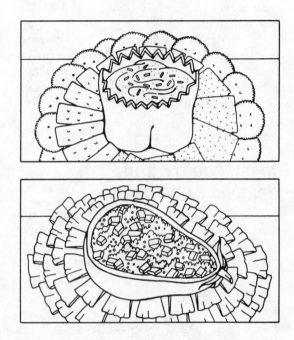

Marinated vegetables are nice predinner nibbles. Steep carrots, cauliflower and broccoli florets, and other crisp vegetables in your favorite marinade for a few hours, and serve in a wide, shallow casserole dish. Supply guests with small plates and forks so they can serve themselves.

For more formal meals, you might prepare a vegetable stew such as ratatouille. It may be served very hot in a hollowed-out eggplant half or in a large chafing dish.

Pastry Appetizers

The same pastry doughs used to make pies, tarts, cream puffs, turnovers, and strudels can be used to make elegant miniature appetizers. Prepare the usual recipes for these doughs, then cut into small triangles, crescent shapes, spirals, or any other desired shapes. Use pastry doughs to encase fillings as basic as cheese or as exotic as curried shrimp or chicken croquette mixture. In most cases, the filling is baked with the pastry. Cream puffs are an exception; the filling is piped into the baked pastry.

The dough required for a single 9-inch piecrust will yield 15 to 20 2-inch tart shells that can be used for small hand-held quiches or for holding other mixtures. (For guidelines about working with pastry doughs, see Pies and Pastries chapter.)

Meat, Poultry, and Seafood Appetizers

Mouth-watering tidbits of meat, poultry, and seafood are always welcome. Just a tray or bowl of them alongside the canapés or cheese and crackers is plenty and adds sufficient variety.

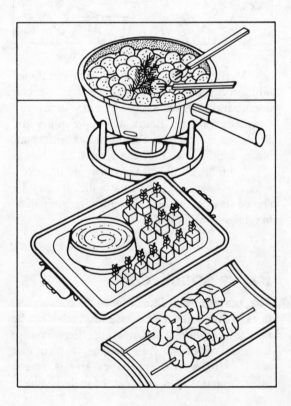

Serve these cooked morsels skewered with other edible extras such as fruits or vegetables, steeped in piquant sauces or glazes, or offered with dipping sauces such as soy sauce or a zesty mustard sauce.

Small meatballs can be made ahead of time, then reheated with a sauce just before serving. Some exotic appetizers consist of chicken or beef cubes marinated and then broiled.

The tender white meat of broiler-fryers or roasters is ideal for chicken appetizers. If time permits, buy whole chicken breasts and debone them yourself (for deboning directions, see page 524). Leftover poultry can be used to make salads and fillings for appetizers.

Fresh seafood is always a treat as an appetizer and need not be expensive. Shrimp, crab meat, and lobster can be chopped and stretched with mayonnaise, yogurt, or cottage cheese to serve as spreads on canapé rounds of bread, crackers, or toast. Large shrimp may be served as finger food with a dipping sauce.

Fresh fish is equally tantalizing. Build an appetizer buffet spread around a salmon or tuna mousse. Any filleted fish may also be used in canapé spreads.

Pâtés and Molds

Pâtés and molds are often the eye-catching centerpiece of the buffet table. At formal or informal affairs surround these fancy preparations with trays or bowls of the smaller appetizers.

Pâté, very similar to meat loaf in preparation, is made from a smooth mixture with highly seasoned ingredients. Chicken liver is probably the most common type of pâté, but a number of other meats can be used as well. Veal and pistachio nuts are the basis for a delicious rich gourmet pâté (see Pistachio and Veal Country Pâté recipe, page 99). All-vegetable pâtés can be served to guests who prefer to avoid meat (see Vegetable Terrine recipe, page 99).

Pâtés may be made in crocks or bowls that lend their attractive shapes. Terrine, a peasant-style pâté, is usually baked in an earthenware dish, traditionally lined with bacon and compacted with a heavy object on top of the meat to make it easier to slice.

Although molds require time for the gelatin to set, they are ideal because they can be made two or three days in advance and chilled until needed (see Molded Salads, page 160). Jellied

meat or fish stocks are a flavorful basis for salad aspics. Vegetable stock mixed with gelatin or agar may also be used.

Choose interesting mold shapes to complement your arrangement, such as a fish mold for seafood. A ring mold can be made very attractive with a creative garnish and salad-filled center. In clear molds, the many ingredients suspended in gelatin—diced meat, fresh vegetable or fruit salads, eggs, or nutmeats—lend an intriguing aspect.

Appetizers for Ethnic Cuisine

When serving ethnic meals, serve appetizers that coordinate with the theme.

Some suggestions:

Mexican
Mexican-Style Baked Fondue, page 84
Pizzaritas, page 91
Guacamole, page 80, with corn chips
Chili-Cheese Fritters, page 83
Nachos, page 90
Chili con Carne, page 490

French
Bite-Size Quiches, page 89
Brie or Camembert cheese with warmed
    French bread rounds
Cut-up raw vegetables (crudités) with
    Crunchy Toasty Onion Dip, page 79, or
    Aïoli Sauce, page 144
Gruyère Canapés, page 77
Ratatouille, page 227
Vegetable Terrine, page 99

Italian
Antipasto of any combination of the following:

Tomato slices
Roasted Eggplant, page 227
Mellow Wax Beans and Mushrooms, page
    216, chilled

Celery and fennel stuffed with ricotta cheese
Celery Parmesan and Fennel, page 227
Roasted and Marinated Peppers, page 88
Cubes of provolone or mozzarella cheese
    with small slices of Italian bread
Skewered Vegetable Antipasto, page 232

Suppli al Telefono, page 91
Miniature Pizzas, page 90

Middle Eastern
Baba Ghannouj, page 78
Hummus, page 81
Falafel with Tahini Sauce, page 271
Spanakopeta, page 228
Pita bread, warmed and cut into triangles
Feta cheese with tomato and cucumber slices

Oriental
Kakiage (Tempura Vegetables) with Oriental
    Dipping Sauce, page 252
Bean and Rice Balls, page 272
Fresh tofu cubes with soy sauce for dipping
Shrimp Egg Rolls, page 97
Vegetables with Oriental Sauce, page 229

Antipasto

Antipasto, which literally means "before the meal," is an Italian tradition that refers to appetizers served before the main course. The various

components of an antipasto are attractively served, often in separate little bowls, or they may be compartmentalized on a large tray. The original Italian version includes some extremely spicy condiments—anchovies, sardines, capers with eggplant salad, marinated mushrooms, artichoke hearts, carrots and cauliflower in brine, hot and sweet peppers, cured black and green olives, provolone cheese, and Genoa or Sicilian salami. Fresh celery, fennel, and tomato slices are also part of this potpourri. The high salt and/or oil content of some of these foods limits their inclusion in the antipasto recipes of health-conscious cooks, but many tasty variations are possible.

Appetizers in Other Chapters

Canapés

Crespelle Wedges

Crespelle
½ cup cold water
¾ cup nonfat dry milk
1 tablespoon grated Parmesan cheese
3 eggs
2 teaspoons cornstarch

Filling
2 tablespoons butter
1 clove garlic, crushed

1 cup finely chopped mushrooms
2 hard-cooked eggs, finely chopped
1 can (6 to 7 ounces) water-packed tuna
1 tablespoon grated onions
¼ to ½ cup mayonnaise
½ cup shredded cooked chicken breast
1 large green pepper
1 large sweet red pepper
3 slices provolone cheese

Dressing
¼ cup mayonnaise
¼ cup sour cream

Garnish
chopped fresh parsley
chopped sweet red and green peppers
chopped carrots

To make the crespelle: Combine water, dry milk, Parmesan, eggs, and cornstarch in a small bowl. Beat until perfectly smooth. Allow to stand at room temperature for about ½ hour. Brush a 7-inch crepe pan lightly with oil and heat over moderately high heat. Pour about 3 tablespoons batter into pan. Brown well on one side, carefully peel from crepe pan, turn over, and brown lightly on other side. Remove crepe and stack between sheets of wax paper. Repeat process, being certain to brush pan lightly with additional oil before each crepe is made, to prevent sticking. You should have about 8 crepes.

To make the filling and assemble: In a small skillet melt butter and add garlic and mushrooms. Sauté over moderate heat until mushrooms are soft, about 5 minutes. Drain and place in a small bowl to cool.

Combine eggs with 2 teaspoons mayonnaise. Set aside. Combine tuna with onions and 2 teaspoons mayonnaise. Set aside. Combine chicken with 1 tablespoon mayonnaise. Set aside.

Roast red and green peppers (see Using Vegetables table, page 204), then mince them separately.

Place 1 crepe on a serving plate. Spread with thin layer of mayonnaise. Cover with cheese slices. Place second crepe on cheese. Spread with thin layer of mayonnaise, then green peppers. Continue to stack alternate layers of crepes and remaining fillings in this order: chicken, red peppers, tuna, egg mixture, mushroom mixture.

Be careful that layers are kept even, with no hump in the center. When final crepe has been added, cover with square of wax paper and weight down with another plate. Cover the whole assembly with plastic wrap to seal and refrigerate several hours or overnight.

To make the dressing: Just before serving, combine mayonnaise and sour cream and frost the stacked crepes with mixture. Garnish with chopped parsley, peppers, and carrots, if desired. To serve, slice with a sharp knife into about 20 wedges and spear each with a wooden pick.

Makes about 20

Cucumber Canapés

¼ cup plus 2 tablespoons butter, softened
1 tablespoon minced fresh parsley
1 tablespoon minced watercress
6 slices whole grain bread, with crusts removed
1 large unpeeled cucumber, thinly sliced
    freshly ground pepper, to taste

Combine butter with parsley and watercress and spread mixture on bread.

Arrange cucumber slices on buttered bread in overlapping pattern and sprinkle with pepper. Cut bread into triangles or rectangles and serve.

Makes about 2 dozen

Egg Canapés Parmesan

2 tablespoons butter
4 eggs
4 slices whole wheat toast
¼ cup Parmesan cheese

Preheat oven to 375°F.

In a small skillet, melt butter and scramble eggs. Divide scrambled eggs between slices of toast and spread evenly. Sprinkle each piece of toast with 1 tablespoon cheese. Place canapés on an ungreased baking sheet and bake for 10 minutes. Remove from oven, cut into triangles, and serve immediately.

Makes 16

Gruyère Canapés

6 slices whole grain toast
¾ cup thick Béchamel Sauce (page 141)
½ cup grated Gruyère cheese
¼ cup grated Parmesan cheese
    cayenne pepper

Preheat oven to 375°F.

Quarter toast into desired shapes. Combine sauce and Gruyère and spread thickly on toast pieces. Sprinkle Parmesan and dash of cayenne over each canapé. Place canapés on an ungreased baking sheet and bake for 10 minutes, or until tops are golden brown.

Makes 2 dozen

Hard-Cooked Egg Canapés

8 hard-cooked eggs
1 cup thick Béchamel Sauce (page 141)
6 slices whole grain toast
½ cup whole grain bread crumbs
2 tablespoons butter

Preheat oven to 375°F.

Finely chop 2 eggs and blend with sauce. Slice remaining eggs into 4 slices each and set aside.

Quarter toast into triangles. Spread each triangle with sauce-egg mixture, then top each with 2 slices of egg.

In a small skillet sauté bread crumbs in butter for 3 minutes, then sprinkle over canapés. Place canapés on an ungreased baking sheet and bake for 10 to 15 minutes, or until lightly browned.

Makes 2 dozen

Lobster Canapés

1 cup diced lobster meat
½ cup sliced mushrooms
¾ cup thick Béchamel Sauce (page 141)
¼ cup shredded cheddar cheese
16 whole grain toast rounds
½ cup whole grain bread crumbs
2 tablespoons butter

Preheat oven to 375°F.

Combine lobster, mushrooms, sauce, and cheese. Spread mixture evenly over toast rounds.

In a small skillet sauté bread crumbs in butter for 3 minutes, then sprinkle over canapés. Place canapés on an ungreased baking sheet and bake for 5 minutes, or just until hot.

Makes 16

Sardine Canapés

2 cans (3¾ ounces) sardines, drained
2 tablespoons olive oil
2 hard-cooked eggs, chopped
4 slices whole wheat bread
¼ cup whole grain bread crumbs
2 tablespoons butter
cayenne pepper

Preheat oven to 350°F.

Using a blender or sieve, puree 1 can sardines together with olive oil. Mix with eggs, then rub mixture through a sieve. Spread evenly over bread slices and top with whole sardines.

In a small skillet sauté bread crumbs in butter for 3 minutes. Sprinkle 1 tablespoon crumbs over each sardine-topped slice. Bake for 7 to 10 minutes, or until heated through. Sprinkle each slice with a pinch of cayenne, then cut into triangles and serve warm.

Makes 16

Spinach Canapés

1 pound spinach
¾ cup thick Béchamel Sauce (page 141)
6 slices whole grain toast
¼ cup grated Parmesan cheese

Preheat oven to 375°F.

Steam spinach for 3 minutes. Drain well, squeezing out all excess moisture.

Using a blender or sieve, puree spinach together with sauce.

Quarter each slice of toast into squares or rectangles. Spread each piece with spinach mixture, then sprinkle with cheese. Place canapés on an ungreased baking sheet and bake for 10 minutes, or until lightly browned.

Makes about 2 dozen

Watercress and Mushroom Canapés

1 loaf whole wheat bread, sliced
½ cup butter, softened
1 small bunch watercress
¼ pound mushrooms, sliced
1 tablespoon lemon juice
1 small jar (4 ounces) pimientos

Cut bread slices into rounds with a cookie cutter. Butter each round. Place sprig of watercress, slice of mushroom dipped in lemon juice, and piece of pimiento on top of each round of bread.

10 servings

Dips and Spreads

Baba Ghannouj
(Eggplant Appetizer)

1 large eggplant
¼ cup sesame oil
juice of 1 lemon, or to taste
1 clove garlic, minced
¼ teaspoon cayenne pepper
¼ cup chopped fresh parsley

Preheat oven to 350°F.

Broil or bake eggplant for about 45 minutes, or until tender, turning occasionally. Allow it to cool, then peel and discard skin and cut pulp into chunks.

In a blender or food processor, puree eggplant and then combine with oil, lemon juice, garlic, and cayenne. Add more lemon juice, if desired. Garnish with parsley. Serve with whole wheat pita bread, cut into wedges, and thin slices of Bermuda onion.

Yields about 2¼ cups

Blue Cheese Dip

4 ounces blue cheese (about 1 cup crumbled)
½ cup sour cream
1 small onion, grated
1 teaspoon pepper
chopped fresh chives

In a small bowl mix together cheese, sour cream, onions, and pepper. Sprinkle with chives. Serve with crackers or raw vegetable dippers.

Yields about 1½ cups

Cheddar Cheese Dip or Spread

1 pound sharp cheddar cheese, finely grated
1½ cups yogurt
½ cup finely chopped walnuts
2 teaspoons dry mustard
walnut pieces

Combine cheese, yogurt, finely chopped walnuts, and mustard in a small bowl. Mix well, then place in a serving bowl and garnish with walnut pieces. Chill thoroughly before serving. Serve with crackers or raw vegetable dippers.

Yields about 3 cups

Creamy Cheese-Mint Dip

    8 ounces cream cheese
    1 cup apple-mint jelly
    3 tablespoons yogurt
    ½ cup heavy cream, whipped
       mint sprigs

In a small bowl beat together cream cheese, ¾ cup jelly, and yogurt until smooth and creamy. Coarsely break up remaining jelly and carefully fold into cream cheese mixture. Fold in whipped cream, then place in a serving bowl and garnish with mint. Refrigerate several hours. Serve well chilled with assorted pieces of fresh fruit, such as strawberries, melon, plums, apricots, peaches, and pears.

Yields about 2 cups

Creamy Liptauer Spread with Accompaniments

    Spread
    1 pound cream cheese
    2 tablespoons yogurt
    ¼ cup butter, softened
    2 tablespoons paprika

    Accompaniments
    ½ cup sliced scallions
    ½ cup chopped radishes
    ½ cup finely chopped green peppers
    ½ cup chopped cucumbers
       thin slices of dark whole grain bread

To make the spread: Combine cheese, yogurt, butter, and paprika in a small bowl and blend until creamy and light.

Arrange spread in mound in center of a serving platter. Arrange chopped vegetables in mounds around cheese. Accompany with bread slices. Each person spreads a bit of cheese on a small slice of bread and piles on the vegetables to taste.

Yields about 2½ cups

Crunchy Toasty Onion Dip

    1 medium-size Bermuda onion
    8 ounces cream cheese or low-fat cottage cheese
    1½ teaspoons soy sauce
    3 tablespoons yogurt, or more if needed
    2 teaspoons onion powder
    ¼ teaspoon ground thyme

Preheat oven to 250°F.

Peel onion and slice from top to bottom into fine slivers. Spread onion slivers on a large ungreased baking sheet in one layer. Place in oven for about 1 hour, stirring at frequent intervals to ensure even toasting. Allow onion slivers to remain in oven until lightly browned and crisped. The length of time for this will vary, so watch carefully to prevent overbrowning. Remove toasted onion slivers from baking sheet and set aside.

Process cream cheese or cottage cheese in an electric mixer until smooth. Add remaining ingredients and beat until light, creamy, and of dipping consistency. (Add additional yogurt if necessary.) Stir in toasted onions. Refrigerate in a tightly covered container for several hours or overnight. Serve with raw vegetables or crackers.

Yields 1 cup

Curry Dip

    ½ cup mayonnaise
    ½ cup yogurt
    1 teaspoon tarragon vinegar
    ½ teaspoon grated horseradish
       (optional)
    1 teaspoon grated onions
    ½ teaspoon soy sauce
    ¼ teaspoon garlic powder
    1 tablespoon curry powder

Combine all ingredients in a small bowl and mix well. Chill. Serve with raw vegetables, such as broccoli and cauliflower florets, celery sticks, and carrot sticks.

Yields 1 cup

Florentine Dip for Fresh Vegetables

1 pound spinach, steamed, chopped, and
squeezed dry
1 cup mayonnaise
½ cup finely chopped scallions
2 tablespoons grated Parmesan or
Romano cheese
½ teaspoon grated nutmeg
1 to 2 tablespoons minced fresh herbs (optional)
milk or heavy cream, for thinning

Combine spinach, mayonnaise, scallions, cheese, nutmeg, and herbs (if used) in a small bowl. Add just enough milk or cream to create a thick dipping consistency. Chill at least 1 hour to mellow flavors. Serve with cucumber or zucchini spears or other raw vegetable dippers.

Yields about 2 cups

Guacamole

1 medium-size avocado, chopped
1 medium-size tomato, chopped
½ small onion, chopped
2 tablespoons lemon juice
dash of crushed red pepper

In a blender, process all ingredients at low speed. Serve with Tortilla Chips (page 80) or crackers.

Yields 1¾ cups

Hearty and Hot Stroganoff Dip

1 pound lean ground beef
1 cup coarsely chopped mushrooms
½ cup chopped onions
1 large clove garlic, minced
1 teaspoon paprika
½ teaspoon pepper
1 tablespoon whole wheat flour
¾ cup rich Beef Stock (page 110)
¾ cup sour cream

Place beef in a deep saucepan. Top with mushrooms, then onions and garlic. Cover tightly and cook over moderate heat, allowing ingredients to steam in rendered juices until beef is thoroughly cooked, but not browned, and vegetables are tender. Remove lid. Add paprika and pepper and stir, breaking meat into small bits. Drain excess fat. Sprinkle flour over ingredients in saucepan and gradually stir in stock. Bring to a hard simmer and cook until thickened. Remove from heat.

Just before serving, bring ingredients to a hard simmer again, remove from heat, and add sour cream. Serve in a warming dish along with a utensil to spoon dollops onto toast or bread triangles.

Yields about 3 cups

Hot Cheese and Avocado Dip with Tortilla Chips

1 hot green chili pepper
2 avocados, mashed
3 tablespoons lemon juice
½ cup chopped canned tomatoes, mashed
1 teaspoon vinegar
1 tablespoon minced onions
1 large clove garlic, crushed
dash of cayenne pepper
1½ cups grated Havarti cheese
Tortilla Chips (see below)

Roast, peel, and seed chili (see page 54), then mince and combine with avocados, lemon juice, tomatoes, vinegar, onions, garlic, and cayenne. Blend well (mixture will not be perfectly smooth), then fold in 1 cup cheese. Place mixture in a well-greased 7 × 11-inch baking dish. Decoratively place several tortilla chips around edge of mixture, sticking them in partway. Sprinkle mixture with remaining ½ cup cheese. Bake at 375°F for about 30 minutes, or until bubbly and hot. Serve immediately with remaining crisp tortilla chips to be used for dipping.

Yields about 3½ cups

Tortilla Chips

vegetable oil, for frying
12 Corn Tortillas (page 392)

Pour ½ inch oil into a skillet just larger than diameter of tortilla. Heat oil to 375°F. Cut almost to center of each tortilla, forming 6 wedges with sections still connected at center. Drop into hot oil, one at a time, and crisp quickly on each side. Remove from oil and drain well on paper towels. Repeat until all tortillas are crisped. When cool, break apart into wedges.

Makes 6 dozen

Hummus

½ cup dried chick-peas
½ cup tahini (sesame butter)
1 clove garlic
3 tablespoons lemon juice
dash of cayenne pepper
chopped fresh parsley

Soak chick-peas (see page 261 for soaking directions). Drain. Add fresh water to cover and cook until tender, about 2 hours. Drain, reserving cooking water.

Puree chick-peas (save a few for garnish) in a blender, adding a little reserved cooking water, or mash them with a fork. Add tahini, garlic, and lemon juice. Process until smooth.

Spread on a flat platter and garnish with cayenne, parsley, and a few cooked chick-peas. Serve with Indian puri or chapati.

Yields 2 cups

Lima Bean and Sesame Dip

½ cup sesame seeds, toasted
1½ cups cooked lima beans, drained
½ small onion, quartered
1 tablespoon vegetable oil
¼ cup mayonnaise
¼ cup yogurt
2 teaspoons lemon juice

Grind toasted sesame seeds to a meal in blender. Remove from blender and set aside.

Combine lima beans and onion pieces and puree in blender, adding a little water if necessary to blend evenly. Transfer to a small bowl. Add ground sesame seeds and remaining ingredients to lima bean puree. Stir until well combined. Serve as a dip for crackers or cut-up raw vegetables.

Yields about 2½ cups

Low-Cal Dunk for Veggies

2 cups low-fat cottage cheese
2 cloves garlic, crushed
2 tablespoons minced scallions
1 tablespoon minced fresh chives
2 tablespoons minced fresh parsley
1 tablespoon minced fresh oregano or 1 teaspoon dried oregano
½ teaspoon minced fresh thyme or ¼ teaspoon dried thyme
2 tablespoons lemon juice

Finely sieve cottage cheese until smooth and creamy. Fold in garlic, scallions, herbs, and lemon juice. Cover and refrigerate several hours to allow flavors to blend. Serve well chilled surrounded with assorted fresh vegetables cut into strips or slices (such as celery, carrots, radishes, scallions, green peppers, zucchini, and cucumbers).

Yields about 2 cups

Pinto Bean Dip

1 large tomato, coarsely chopped
1 medium-size onion, coarsely chopped
1 hot chili pepper, halved
2 cloves garlic
2 tablespoons soy sauce
4 teaspoons chili powder
2 teaspoons ground cumin
2 cups cooked pinto beans, drained (kidney beans or soybeans may be substituted)

Place tomato, onions, pepper, garlic, soy sauce, chili powder, and cumin in a blender. Process on medium speed until smooth. Add 1 cup beans and process on medium speed until blended. Add remaining beans and blend again until smooth. Serve with Tortilla Chips (page 80) or crackers.

Yields 2 cups

Sardine Dip

1 can undrained sardines
2 hard-cooked eggs
1 teaspoon lemon juice
1 teaspoon dry mustard
several sprigs fresh parsley or 1 teaspoon dried parsley
½ teaspoon dried tarragon or oregano
2 scallions, halved, or ½ small onion

Combine all ingredients in a blender and process until smooth. Serve with crackers or strips of whole grain bread.

Yields about 1½ cups

Pignoli Dip

1 cup slivered almonds, roasted
½ cup pine nuts, roasted
½ cup olive or vegetable oil
1 clove garlic
¾ teaspoon dried basil
⅓ cup coarsely chopped fresh parsley
½ cup farmer cheese or cottage cheese
3 to 4 tablespoons yogurt
    roasted sesame seeds (optional)

Place almonds and pine nuts in a blender with 1 tablespoon oil, garlic, and basil. Process on high speed until smooth, scraping down sides of container occasionally. Gradually add remaining oil and blend until mixture is creamy. Add parsley. Blend in cheese and yogurt on medium speed.

Scrape into bowl and chill. Sprinkle sesame seeds (if used) over top before serving. Use as a dip for raw vegetables.

Yields 2 cups

Svengali Spread

2 tablespoons vegetable oil
1 cup chopped mushrooms
¼ cup chopped scallions
¼ cup chopped fresh parsley
    pinch each of ground coriander, cumin,
        turmeric, cloves, and cinnamon
2 tablespoons lemon juice
¼ cup mayonnaise
⅓ cup peanut butter
1 teaspoon soy sauce
    dash of crushed red pepper, or to taste
½ cup chopped roasted peanuts

Heat oil in a medium-size skillet. Add mushrooms, scallions, parsley, and spices. Cook over moderately high heat until mushrooms cook quite dry and excess liquid evaporates. Remove from heat and allow to cool to room temperature.

In a small bowl blend together lemon juice, mayonnaise, peanut butter, soy sauce, and crushed red pepper until well mixed. Add cooled mushroom mixture. Pack into a crock, top with peanuts, and chill. Serve with crackers or toast points.

Yields about 1½ cups

Swiss-Almond Cheese Spread

3 ounces cream cheese, softened
4 to 6 tablespoons buttermilk, at room
        temperature
4 ounces Swiss cheese, finely grated
4 ounces Muenster cheese, finely grated
¾ cup sliced almonds, toasted

Using an electric mixer, blend cream cheese with 4 tablespoons buttermilk. Beat in grated cheeses. Add more buttermilk as necessary until mixture is of spreading consistency. Stir in toasted almonds. Pack into crock and refrigerate at least overnight. Return to room temperature before serving with toast points or crackers.

Yields 1½ cups

Tuna-Yogurt Dip

1 cup yogurt
1 can (6 to 7 ounces) water-packed tuna
2 scallions, halved
1 ripe avocado, peeled and cut into chunks
2 teaspoons honey
2 teaspoons vinegar
    juice of 1 lime
1 cup chopped fresh parsley
    avocado slices or green grapes

Place all ingredients in a blender and process until almost smooth. Serve as a dip for raw vegetables or as a dressing for tossed salads. Garnish with avocado slices or green grapes. (Use within 1 day.)

Yields 2 cups

Walnut-Cheese Spread

7 ounces Gouda cheese, finely grated
1 cup finely chopped walnuts
1 tablespoon butter
1 teaspoon minced garlic
1 tablespoon chopped fresh coriander or parsley

Combine cheese, nuts, butter, garlic, and coriander or parsley in a small bowl and beat until smooth. (This spread can be refrigerated until needed.) Serve at room temperature, with crackers or bread rounds.

Yields about 2 cups

Cheese and Egg Appetizers

Blue Cheese Flan

 ¾ cup fine whole grain cracker crumbs
 ¼ cup butter, melted
 2 tablespoons water
 1 envelope unflavored gelatin
 2 tablespoons lemon juice
 8 ounces blue cheese
 3 ounces cream cheese
   dash of cayenne pepper
 ½ cup heavy cream, whipped
 2 pears, cut into wedges
 2 apples, cut into wedges

Combine cracker crumbs and butter and pat on bottom and partway up sides of a 9-inch springform pan. Place water in a small saucepan, sprinkle gelatin over water, and allow to stand 3 minutes to soften gelatin. Add lemon juice and heat gently until gelatin has dissolved.

Place blue cheese and cream cheese in a medium-size bowl. Beat gelatin mixture into cheeses until very smooth. Season with cayenne. Carefully fold in whipped cream, then pour into prepared pan and refrigerate several hours, or overnight, until firm. When ready to serve, run a knife around edge of pan to loosen sides, and unmold onto serving plate. Garnish with wedges of apples and pears.

10 servings

Cheese Ball

 ½ cup crumbled blue cheese or Roquefort cheese
 ½ cup cream cheese, softened
 2 tablespoons butter, softened
 1 teaspoon Hungarian paprika
 ½ cup finely ground walnuts

Combine blue cheese or Roquefort, cream cheese, butter, and paprika. Mix together very well. On a piece of wax paper, form cheese mixture into a ball. On another piece of wax paper, sprinkle walnuts. Roll ball in nuts, coating all surfaces.

Wrap ball first in wax paper and then in plastic wrap. Refrigerate overnight or up to 2 days, to allow flavors to blend. Serve with crackers.

Makes one 4-inch-diameter, 12-ounce ball

Cheese Fondue

 2 cups shredded Gruyère cheese
   (about 8 ounces)*
 2 cups shredded Swiss cheese (about 8 ounces)*
 1 tablespoon cornstarch
 1 clove garlic
 1 cup apple juice
 1 tablespoon lemon juice
 3 ounces cream cheese, cut into chunks
   apple and pear wedges
   whole grain bread, cut into large cubes

Toss Gruyère and Swiss cheeses with cornstarch until coated.

Slice garlic in half and rub all around inside of top of double boiler, then discard.

Pour apple juice and lemon juice into double boiler top and place over simmering water. Gradually add cheese and cornstarch mixture, stirring until cheeses are melted. Swirl cream cheese into mixture. Remove from heat. Serve warm with apple and pear wedges and bread cubes for dipping.

4 to 6 servings

*Be certain that cheeses contain at least 45 percent butterfat to ensure they will melt well.

Chili-Cheese Fritters

 2 eggs, separated
 1 cup diced zucchini
 1 small onion, finely chopped
 2 teaspoons chili powder
 ⅔ cup shredded Monterey Jack cheese or
   medium-sharp cheddar cheese
 ¼ cup whole grain bread crumbs
   corn oil, for frying

In a medium-size bowl, beat egg yolks with a wire whisk or electric mixer until thick and lemon colored. Stir in zucchini, onions, chili powder, cheese, and bread crumbs, one item at a time in that order.

Beat egg whites until stiff but not dry, then gradually fold them into zucchini mixture. Do not overstir.

Heat ¼ inch oil in a small skillet. Pour ¼ cup batter into skillet for each fritter and brown fritters on both sides. Drain well on paper towels and serve warm.

Makes 8

Cheese and Cornmeal Gems

½ cup cornmeal
½ cup triticale flour
2 teaspoons baking powder
3 tablespoons butter
½ cup diced mild cheddar cheese
¼ cup corn
1 tablespoon chopped red sweet peppers
1 tablespoon chopped scallions
¼ cup plus 2 tablespoons milk
   dash of cayenne pepper
1 egg

Preheat oven to 400°F.

In a small bowl combine cornmeal, flour, and baking powder and blend well. Cut in butter. Toss cheese, corn, chopped peppers and scallions in flour mixture until coated and well distributed.

In a separate bowl mix together milk, cayenne, and egg until blended, then quickly stir into dry ingredients. Drop by rounded tablespoons onto a well-greased baking sheet, placing gems several inches apart. Bake for 15 to 20 minutes, or until browned.

4 servings

Cheesy Toast Treats

2 tablespoons butter
2 tablespoons whole wheat flour
½ teaspoon dry mustard
1½ teaspoons onion powder
1⅔ cups milk
1½ cups grated English cheddar cheese
   (about 1 pound)
5 tablespoons tomato paste
8 slices whole wheat toast
   small tomato slices
½ cup Date Chutney (page 64)

Melt butter in a 2-quart saucepan. Add flour and cook until foamy. Add dry mustard and onion powder, then whisk in milk. Cook over medium heat, stirring constantly, until thickened. Remove from heat and stir in cheese and tomato paste. Blend well until cheese is melted. (Heat slowly, if necessary; be careful not to overheat or mixture will curdle.)

Slice toast into triangles and arrange on a platter. Spoon warm cheese mixture over toast and garnish with tomato slices. Serve chutney separately as a condiment to add to each bite.

4 to 6 servings

Fruited Cheese Log

⅓ cup unsweetened crushed pineapple, well drained
⅓ cup pineapple juice
½ cup finely chopped dried apricots
⅓ cup chopped dates
8 ounces cream cheese, softened
1 pound Monterey Jack cheese or cheddar cheese, grated
⅔ cup chopped walnuts

Combine pineapple, pineapple juice, apricots, and dates in a small bowl. Set aside until juice has been absorbed by fruits.

In a larger bowl blend together cream cheese and Monterey Jack or cheddar cheese, then blend in fruits mixture. Chill in refrigerator for several hours or overnight.

When thoroughly chilled, form into a log. Sprinkle walnuts on a sheet of wax paper and carefully roll log in walnuts until all surfaces are coated. Serve as a spread with crackers.

Makes one 2-pound log

Mexican-Style Baked Fondue

12 slices whole grain bread
2 tablespoons butter, softened
1 package (10 ounces) frozen corn, thawed
1 can (7 ounces) green chili peppers, seeded and cut into strips
2 cups grated Monterey Jack cheese
4 eggs, beaten
4 cups milk

Grease a 9 × 13-inch baking dish.

Butter one side of each slice of bread and cut slices in half. Arrange ½ of the slices, butter-side up, on bottom of baking dish. Cover with ½ of the corn and ½ of the chili strips. Sprinkle with ½ of the cheese. Repeat layer, using remaining bread, corn, chili strips, and cheese.

Combine eggs and milk and pour over casserole. Allow to stand for 30 minutes.

Preheat oven to 350°F.

Place casserole in oven and bake for 40 minutes. Cut into small squares and serve piping hot on small warm plates.

10 to 12 servings

Oven-Browned Cheese

6 pounds ricotta cheese, well drained
3 tablespoons coarsely ground pepper

Preheat oven to 400°F.

Butter a 9-inch stoneware pie plate.

Mound ricotta cheese into pie plate. With fingers, force black pepper randomly into sides and top of ricotta cheese about 1 inch deep. Sprinkle top and sides with additional pepper.

Bake for 2 to 3 hours, or until cheese is dark brown. (Darkness enhances flavor.) Store in a cool place. To serve, slice into thin wedges and accompany with unpeeled apple slices.

30 servings

Stuffed Gouda

7 ounces Gouda cheese (in red paraffin)
2 tablespoons chopped green peppers
2 tablespoons chopped tart crisp red apple
1 teaspoon caraway seeds
3 tablespoons mayonnaise

Carefully cut star shape into top of paraffin. Remove star and set aside. Use serrated grapefruit knife to carefully remove cheese, leaving wax bowl intact. Set bowl aside.

Finely grind or grate cheese, then mix with remaining ingredients. Pile cheese mixture back into reserved wax bowl and top with cut-out star. Serve with crisp apple or pear wedges.

Yields about 1½ cups

Swiss-Stuffed Eggs

6 small hard-cooked eggs
2 tablespoons butter
⅔ cup minced mushrooms
2 shallots, minced
    dash of cayenne pepper

⅔ cup finely grated Swiss cheese
    mayonnaise
12 mushroom caps, lightly sautéed (optional)

Split eggs in half horizontally. Pass yolks through a sieve into a small bowl. Reserve whites.

Melt butter in a small skillet and sauté mushrooms and shallots until tender. Cool slightly, then add to sieved egg yolks. Season with cayenne and blend in cheese.

Remove small slice from bottom of reserved egg white "cups" so that they stand upright. Fill with egg yolk mixture. Garnish each with dab of mayonnaise. (If used, set mushroom caps upside down and place an egg half into each cap.) Serve eggs cold or place under a broiler using moderate heat until just heated and mayonnaise is puffy.

Makes 1 dozen

Triple-Tier Cheese

8 ounces cream cheese, softened
¼ cup cottage cheese, blended or sieved until
    smooth
¼ cup grated Romano cheese
1 teaspoon minced fresh sage or ½ teaspoon
    ground sage
2 tablespoons minced fresh parsley
¼ cup crumbled blue cheese
1 teaspoon tomato paste
1 clove garlic, crushed and minced to a pulp

Line a 1½-cup rectangular or round mold with plastic wrap.

Cream together cream cheese and cottage cheese until light and fluffy. Blend in Romano, then divide mixture into thirds. Pack first third into prepared mold. To next third, add sage, parsley, and blue cheese. Beat vigorously until mixture becomes tinted with green. Pack on top of first layer in mold. To last third, add tomato paste and garlic. Pack on top of second layer. Chill mold several hours or overnight in refrigerator. Unmold onto serving plate and serve with crackers or toast points.

4 servings

NOTE: When fresh herbs are in season, prepare a minced mixture of 1 tablespoon each parsley, basil, and sage, and sprinkle a layer between each flavor of cheese.

Vegetable Appetizers

Artichoke Heart Soufflettes

   1 jar (9 ounces) artichoke hearts (6 to 8),
       quartered
   Mustard Vinaigrette (page 185)
   8 slices whole wheat bread
   2 eggs, separated
   2 tablespoons mayonnaise
   ¼ cup finely grated cheddar cheese
   ½ teaspoon dry mustard
       dash of cayenne pepper

Place artichoke hearts in a shallow bowl. Cover with vinaigrette and toss. Allow to marinate for at least 1 hour, tossing occasionally, or overnight, refrigerated. Drain, quarter each heart, and set aside.

Preheat oven to 300°F.

Butter both sides of bread slices, remove crusts, and cut bread into 24 to 30 circles or squares. Place on a baking sheet and bake for about 15 minutes, or until crisp. Leave on baking sheet and place 1 marinated artichoke heart quarter on each.

Beat egg yolks with a wire whisk or electric mixer until thick. Fold mayonnaise, cheese, mustard, and cayenne into yolks. Beat egg whites until stiff but not dry. Carefully fold egg yolk mixture into beaten egg whites. Top each artichoke heart portion with a spoonful of soufflé mixture. Bake at 400°F for about 15 minutes, or until puffed and golden. Serve immediately.

Makes 2 to 2½ dozen

Avocado and Mushroom Hors d'Oeuvres

   1 pound medium-size mushrooms
   ⅔ cup olive oil
   ¼ cup white wine vinegar
10 to 12 sprigs parsley, minced
   1 clove garlic, minced
       pepper, to taste
   2 ripe avocados
       juice of 1 lemon
   ½ teaspoon soy sauce
   1 small bunch watercress
       lemon wedges

Break stems off mushrooms and reserve for other use. Set caps aside.

Combine olive oil, vinegar, parsley, garlic, and pepper and mix well. Add mushroom caps and turn to coat each cap with marinade. Cover and refrigerate overnight.

Just before serving, cut avocados into halves, remove seeds, and scoop out flesh. Using a fork, mash flesh together with lemon juice and soy sauce until smooth, or puree in a blender. Remove mushroom caps from marinade. (Reserve marinade for other vegetables or use as a salad dressing.) Fill each cap with puree. Arrange on a serving platter lined with a bed of watercress and garnish with lemon wedges. Serve with homemade toasted bread.

   6 to 8 servings

Fried Zucchini Flowers

   1¾ cups whole wheat flour
   ¼ cup olive oil
   1 egg
       pinch of freshly grated nutmeg
   2 tablespoons champagne vinegar
   1½ cups cold water
   16 zucchini flowers
   ½ cup combination peanut oil and olive oil

Sift flour into a small bowl. Add olive oil, egg, nutmeg, vinegar, and water, mixing thoroughly after each addition. Stir until batter is smooth.

Remove stems and pistils from flowers, then wash flowers gently in cold water. Dry on paper towels.

Heat peanut and olive oil in a small skillet. Prepare a serving dish lined with paper towels.

Dip each flower into batter and then place in hot oil. Cook for 1 minute on each side, or until golden brown. Remove from skillet and place on prepared serving dish. Discard paper towels and serve flowers immediately.

   Makes 16

Lima Bean Hors d'Oeuvres

   1 tablespoon butter
   1 cup chopped onions
   2 cloves garlic, minced
   2 cups cooked lima beans, drained
   3 tablespoons chopped fresh parsley
   1 tablespoon dried thyme
   1 tablespoon dried oregano

1 teaspoon grated lemon rind
3 tablespoons lemon juice

Heat butter in a large skillet over medium heat. Add onions and garlic and sauté lightly until onions are translucent.

In a large bowl, combine beans, 2 tablespoons parsley, thyme, oregano, lemon rind, and juice. Add sautéed onions and garlic and toss gently until ingredients are well combined. Chill.

Transfer to a serving dish, garnish with remaining parsley, and serve accompanied with small plates and cocktail forks.

4 servings

Nut-Stuffed Mushrooms

16 to 20 medium-size mushrooms
    2 cloves garlic, minced
    3 tablespoons chopped shallots or scallions
    3 tablespoons chopped fresh parsley
    ¼ cup walnuts, ground
    4 tablespoons butter

Carefully remove stems from mushrooms. Set caps aside. Chop stems and mix with garlic, shallots or scallions, parsley, and nuts.

Melt 1 to 2 tablespoons butter in a small skillet. Add nut mixture and sauté for 3 to 4 minutes. Cool slightly.

Cream remaining butter in a small bowl, then stir in nut mixture. Place mushroom caps in a baking dish and fill each with a spoonful of mixture. Place under broiler for about 5 minutes, or until very hot and bubbly.

Makes 16 to 20

Pickled Pickup Stix

These marinated carrot sticks make a colorful addition to an hors d'oeuvre tray or relish dish. The turmeric brings an exotic note to the blend.

2 to 3 carrots
    ½ cup white or cider vinegar
    ½ cup water
    5 tablespoons honey

    1 clove garlic
    ½ teaspoon turmeric
    1 piece dried hot chili pepper, 1 to 2 inches long

Cut carrots into ½-inch strips about 5 inches long. Cook or steam for 3 to 4 minutes, or until just slightly tender. Remove from heat and plunge into cold water. Drain.

In a small saucepan boil remaining ingredients together for 5 minutes.

Place crisp-tender carrot sticks in a glass or earthenware container. Pour hot mixture through a sieve over carrots, to cover them completely. Cover container and refrigerate several hours or overnight.

Makes 8 to 12

Red Pepper Rosebuds

    2 large sweet red peppers
    ¼ cup water
    2 tablespoons vinegar
    2 tablespoons butter
    2 tablespoons vegetable oil
    ½ pound finely chopped mushrooms
    1 large clove garlic
    1 tablespoon Worcestershire sauce
    2 tablespoons cream cheese or butter, softened
      watercress leaves

Cut tops from peppers and slice peppers into halves from stem end to blossom end. Place water and vinegar in a large skillet, add pepper halves, cover, and cook for 15 to 20 minutes, or until very tender. Allow to cool in liquid, then drain and carefully peel off tough outer skin. Cut each peeled pepper half into 4 to 6 wedges.

Heat 2 tablespoons butter and oil in skillet. Add mushrooms, garlic, and Worcestershire sauce and cook over moderately high heat until mixture is very dry, stirring continuously with a wooden spoon. Remove from heat and allow to cool. When cool, mix with cream cheese or butter.

Spread each peeled pepper slice with a thin layer of mushroom paste and roll, jelly-roll fashion, beginning at wide end. Secure each with a wooden pick. Set upright on an hors d'oeuvre tray and apply small bits of watercress leaves so that they resemble rosebuds.

Makes 16 to 24

Plantain Snacks

2 firm plantains*
¼ cup cornstarch
2 teaspoons ground cinnamon
2 tablespoons vegetable oil
¼ cup butter
  lime wedges

Peel outside skin off plantains. Thinly slice fruit on the diagonal.

Combine cornstarch and cinnamon and then dust plantain slices with this mixture.

Heat oil and butter in a large skillet to 350°F (moderate heat). Sauté plantains until crispy and golden. Serve warm or cool in a napkin-lined basket, accompanied with wedges of lime to squeeze on as desired.

4 servings

*Plantains, related to bananas, are a popular fruit in tropical countries. They are available in this country in Spanish grocery stores and in supermarkets near Spanish-speaking communities.

Roasted and Marinated Peppers

1 large green pepper
1 large sweet red pepper
1 clove garlic, minced
  olive oil
  chopped fresh basil, to taste
  wine vinegar (optional)
  whole wheat toast

Place whole peppers under preheated broiler until skins are black. Remove from oven and cover with a linen towel, or place in an airtight plastic bag. Allow to cool.

When peppers are cool, carefully remove skins and tops, along with seeds. Rinse with cold water. Slice into strips and place in a flat dish. Sprinkle generously with garlic, olive oil, basil (reserving a little basil for garnish), and vinegar (if used). Let marinate a few hours, or overnight.

Arrange on a platter and garnish with reserved basil. Serve with whole wheat toast.

4 servings

Savory Broccoli Cocktail Cubes

2 tablespoons vegetable oil
1 small head broccoli, finely chopped; or
  ½ small head broccoli, finely chopped,
  and 2 small zucchini, shredded
½ cup minced onions
¼ cup minced green peppers
2 tablespoons chopped fresh parsley
1½ teaspoons minced fresh savory
1 teaspoon minced fresh thyme
2 teaspoons Worcestershire sauce
4 eggs, beaten
⅔ cup milk
  dash of ground nutmeg
2 cups cooked brown rice
6 ounces cheddar cheese, shredded
¼ cup grated Parmesan cheese

Heat oil in a large saucepan. Add broccoli (and zucchini, if used), onions, peppers, and parsley and sauté lightly, tightly covered, until vegetables are tender, 7 to 10 minutes. Add savory, thyme, and Worcestershire sauce to vegetables and stir to blend.

Preheat oven to 350°F.

Beat eggs and milk together. Add to vegetable mixture along with nutmeg, rice, and cheddar cheese. Stir to blend well. Pour into well-buttered or oiled 7 × 11-inch baking dish. Sprinkle top with Parmesan. Bake for 40 to 50 minutes, or until well set and very brown. Allow to cool at least 30 minutes before cutting into 24 2-inch squares. Serve warm in small petit four cups.

Makes 2 dozen

Snappy Snap-Peas

18 fresh sugar pea pods
3 ounces cream cheese
3 tablespoons butter
1 teaspoon tomato paste
1 dried hot chili pepper, ground (1½ to 2½
  teaspoons)

Split pea pods along one side. Beat together cream cheese, butter, and tomato paste until fluffy.

Add ground chili to taste. (The flavor and hotness will intensify upon standing.)

Spoon or pipe a heaping teaspoon of cheese filling into each pea pod. Chill before serving.

Makes 1½ dozen

Variation:

Snappy Cucumber Rounds: Instead of using sugar pea pods, sandwich ½ teaspoon filling between unpeeled cucumber slices.

Spicy Sesame-Eggplant Bits

2 teaspoons sesame seeds
½ cup cornmeal
½ teaspoon curry powder
2 egg whites
¼ cup vegetable oil
1 medium-size eggplant, cut into 1½-inch cubes (about 2 cups)
yogurt (optional)

Preheat oven to 400°F.

In a small bowl stir together sesame seeds, cornmeal, and curry powder until well blended.

Place egg whites in another small bowl and whisk in vegetable oil until foamy and slightly thickened.

Dip each eggplant cube into egg white mixture, then coat with cornmeal mixture. Place coated cubes on well-greased baking sheet and bake for 15 minutes. Serve as is or accompanied with a small bowl of yogurt.

4 servings

Pastry Appetizers

Bite-Size Quiches

1 cup whole wheat pastry flour
3 tablespoons vegetable oil
2 tablespoons cold water
¼ cup shredded Swiss cheese
1 egg
¼ cup light cream
1 teaspoon chopped fresh chives

dash of white pepper
½ teaspoon ground nutmeg

Preheat oven to 400°F.

Place flour in a medium-size bowl. Add oil and toss lightly with a fork. Sprinkle flour with cold water, a tablespoon at a time, and toss with a fork. Dough particles should stick together when pressed between your fingers. Divide into 12 uniform pieces and press each piece into one cup of a lightly oiled miniature muffin tin, forming a little pastry shell. Build up edge.

Divide cheese evenly among miniature quiche shells.

Lightly beat together egg, cream, chives, and pepper. Carefully spoon about 1 tablespoon of mixture into each shell. Sprinkle with nutmeg. Bake for 15 minutes, or until set.

Makes 1 dozen

Malfatti Dumplings

3 cups cooked spinach, well drained
3 cups ricotta cheese
3 eggs, beaten
2¾ cups grated Parmesan cheese
½ teaspoon ground cinnamon
¼ cup whole wheat flour
⅓ cup whole grain bread crumbs
pepper, to taste
butter

Mince drained spinach finely and combine with ricotta, eggs, 2¼ cups Parmesan, cinnamon, flour, bread crumbs, and pepper. Mix thoroughly. With floured hands, use 1 tablespoon of mixture to form a little oval about 1½ inches long and ½ inch wide. Repeat until all dumplings are formed.

Bring 4 quarts of water to a rapid boil, reduce heat, and add dumplings one at a time. When they rise to the surface, they are cooked. Remove with a slotted spoon and place on a warm serving platter.

When layer of dumplings covers bottom of platter, dot with butter and some of remaining Parmesan cheese. Keep warm in oven. Repeat layers. Serve immediately on warm plates.

8 servings

Miniature Pizzas

Crust
1½ teaspoons dry yeast
½ cup warm water
1 teaspoon honey
1 tablespoon olive oil
2 cups whole wheat pastry flour

Filling
2 tablespoons olive oil
1 medium-size onion, minced
1 green pepper, minced
1 clove garlic, minced
½ pound lean ground beef
⅔ cup tomato paste
½ cup water
½ teaspoon ground sage
½ teaspoon dried basil
¼ teaspoon dried oregano
⅛ teaspoon anise seeds
⅛ teaspoon crushed red pepper (optional)
1 cup grated mozzarella cheese

To make the crust: In a mixing bowl, dissolve yeast in warm water and honey. Set aside for 5 minutes to proof. Then add olive oil and 1¼ cups flour. Mix thoroughly. Add enough remaining flour to form a soft dough. Knead on floured surface for 5 minutes. Cover and let rise in a warm place for 45 minutes.

Preheat oven to 375°F and prepare filling while dough rises.

To make the filling: Heat 1 tablespoon olive oil in a heavy skillet. Sauté onions, green peppers, and garlic until tender but not brown. Add beef and sauté until cooked. Drain excess fat and set beef aside.

In a small saucepan, stir together tomato paste, water, remaining oil, sage, basil, oregano, anise seeds, and crushed red pepper (if used). Add cooked beef and vegetables and simmer gently for 5 to 10 minutes, stirring occasionally. Mixture will be quite thick. Allow to cool to lukewarm.

To assemble: Punch down dough and roll out to a thickness of ³⁄₁₆ inch on a floured surface. Cut into 18 circles about 2¾ inches in diameter. Turn up tiny edge of dough around perimeter of each circle. Place on lightly oiled baking sheet.

Spoon filling onto dough circles, dividing evenly. Top with mozzarella. Bake for 15 minutes, or until cheese is bubbly and slightly browned. Serve hot or cold. Store in refrigerator if not served immediately.

Makes 1½ dozen

Nachos

Salsa
¾ cup finely chopped green tomatoes or green peppers
½ cup finely chopped scallions
1 hot green chili pepper, seeded and finely chopped
1 tablespoon vinegar

24 to 36 Tortilla Chips (page 80)
1½ cups shredded colby cheese

To make the *salsa:* In a small glass bowl combine tomatoes or green peppers, scallions, chili, and vinegar. Blend well and set aside at room temperature for 1 hour.

When *salsa* is ready, spread tortilla chips on a heatproof serving platter in a single layer, overlapping slightly and at random. Distribute cheese over top. Place in a 350°F oven for several minutes, or until cheese has melted. Remove from oven and sprinkle small amount of *salsa* over nachos. Serve extra *salsa* in a little bowl with a small spoon to add additional bite to nachos.

6 to 8 servings

Parmesan Pita Puffs

2 tablespoons butter, softened
2 pita bread pockets, split into single rounds
1 cup mayonnaise
½ cup grated Parmesan cheese
1 tablespoon minced onions
1 tablespoon minced green or sweet red peppers

Preheat oven to 400°F.

Lightly butter cut sides of pita bread rounds and place on a baking sheet cut-side up. Combine mayonnaise, Parmesan, onions, and peppers. Divide mixture among buttered pita rounds. Bake about 10 minutes, or until puffy. To serve, divide each pita round into 6 wedges.

Makes 2 dozen

Pita Butter Crisps

These garlicky crisps are a delicious alternative to crackers, for use with dips and spreads or to enjoy on their own.

⅓ cup butter
1 clove garlic, crushed to a pulp
½ teaspoon dried oregano
    pinch of crushed red pepper
2 pita bread pockets, split into single rounds

Preheat oven to 300°F.

In a small saucepan, melt together butter, garlic, oregano, and red pepper. Simmer slowly for several minutes to blend flavors.

Brush mixture generously on both sides of pita rounds. Place on a baking sheet and bake for 30 to 45 minutes, or until completely dry and crisp. Cool.

Break each round into 6 to 8 irregularly shaped pieces. Store in a tightly covered container.

Makes 24 to 32

Pizzaritas

1 cup peeled, seeded, and chopped Italian-style tomatoes
1 clove garlic, crushed
¼ teaspoon dried oregano
⅛ teaspoon ground cumin
½ teaspoon chopped fresh coriander or ⅛ teaspoon dried coriander
    dash of ground cloves
    dash of ground cinnamon
    pinch of crushed red pepper, or to taste
1½ cups cooked kidney beans, drained and coarsely chopped
1 mild green chili pepper
1 tablespoon soy sauce
1 tablespoon vegetable oil
4 Corn Tortillas (page 392)
1 cup shredded Monterey Jack cheese

Combine tomatoes, garlic, oregano, cumin, coriander, cloves, cinnamon, and red pepper in a small saucepan. Simmer over moderate heat until quite thick, about 10 minutes. Remove from heat and add beans. Set aside.

Roast, peel, and seed chili (see page 54), then cut into slivers and place in a small shallow container.

Combine soy sauce and oil. Pour mixture over chili slivers and marinate for 15 to 20 minutes at room temperature.

Heat a large griddle to about 375°F. Oil griddle lightly and place tortillas on it. Toast one side of tortillas until lightly flecked with brown. Turn over. Place ¼ of the tomato mixture on toasted side of each tortilla. Top each with ¼ of the cheese. Arrange marinated chili slivers decoratively on each. Cover griddle with a large lid until tortillas are heated through and cheese is melted. Cut each tortilla into 4 wedges and serve warm.

Makes 16

Supplì al Telefono

These Italian-style cheese and rice bits may also be served as a first course with a tablespoon of tomato sauce over each appetizer.

2 cups hot cooked brown rice
2 eggs, beaten
¼ cup grated Romano cheese
4 ounces mozzarella cheese, cut into ½-inch cubes
1 cup fine whole grain bread crumbs
½ teaspoon dried oregano
½ teaspoon dried basil
¼ teaspoon dried thyme
¼ teaspoon onion powder
2 tablespoons vegetable oil

Combine rice, eggs, and Romano. Set aside to cool to room temperature. When rice mixture has cooled, use about 1½ tablespoons to form a ball around a cube of mozzarella, completely covering the cheese. (Moistened hands will be helpful.) Pack rice against cheese as if making a snowball. (There will be about 12, the size of golf balls.) Allow balls to chill on wax paper in refrigerator about 1 hour.

Preheat oven to 400°F.

Combine remaining ingredients in a shallow bowl. Carefully roll balls in bread crumb mixture until completely coated. Place on a greased baking sheet and bake for about 20 minutes. (Do not overbake or cheese will bubble out, breaking the rice balls.) Serve warm.

4 servings

Shrimp Custard Squares

Crust
1 cup fine whole grain bread crumbs or
   cracker crumbs
2 tablespoons grated Parmesan cheese
¼ cup butter, melted

Filling
1 cup shredded Swiss cheese or Gruyère cheese
1 cup thinly sliced scallions
1½ cups small cooked shrimp
1½ cups milk
6 eggs, beaten
1 teaspoon cornstarch
   dash of grated nutmeg
   dash of cayenne pepper
1 tablespoon grated Parmesan cheese

Garnish
cherry tomato slices
parsley sprigs
small cooked shrimp

To make the crust: Blend all ingredients well and pat firmly into bottom of well-buttered 7 × 11-inch baking pan.

To make the filling: Pat Swiss cheese or Gruyère cheese over prepared crust. Steam scallions until tender. Spread cooked scallions over cheese. Distribute shrimp over scallions.

Preheat oven to 400°F.

Beat together milk, eggs, cornstarch, nutmeg, and cayenne. Pour over shrimp. Sprinkle top with Parmesan. Bake for 15 minutes, then reduce oven temperature to 350°F and continue to bake for about 15 minutes longer, or until custard is set, golden brown, and puffy. Remove from oven and set aside for 15 to 20 minutes to cool. When cool, cut into 24 squares. Serve warm in flattened fluted paper baking cups. If desired, decorate top of each square with slice of cherry tomato, sprig of parsley, and/or small whole shrimp.

Makes 2 dozen

Spinach and Chicken-Filled Party Pie

Crust
½ loaf dry whole grain bread, crumbled
¼ to ½ cup warm water
½ cup minced onions
1 clove garlic, crushed to a pulp
1 egg, beaten
¼ cup chopped fresh parsley
¼ cup grated Romano cheese

Filling
1 pound fresh spinach, cooked, or 1 package
   (10 ounces) frozen spinach, thawed
1 tablespoon plus 2 teaspoons vegetable oil
1 cup coarsely chopped mushrooms
1 cup chopped cooked chicken
½ teaspoon dried thyme
¼ teaspoon grated nutmeg
1 teaspoon soy sauce
3 ounces cream cheese, softened
2 teaspoons grated Parmesan cheese or Romano
   cheese

To make the crust: Generously butter or oil a 9-inch glass pie plate. Place crumbled bread in a mixing bowl and pour enough warm water over bread to moisten all. Squeeze out excess moisture with hands, and crumble into bowl again. Add onions, garlic, egg, parsley, and Romano cheese. Pat ½ of the mixture into bottom and up sides of pie plate.

To make the filling: Drain spinach well, then squeeze out all excess moisture. Distribute spinach evenly over bottom layer of crust.

Preheat oven to 425°F.

In a small skillet heat 1 tablespoon oil and sauté mushrooms until tender. Add chicken, thyme, and nutmeg. Cool slightly. Blend in soy sauce and cream cheese. Pour chicken mixture on top of spinach layer.

With moist hands, pat remaining bread mixture over top to cover chicken layer completely. Brush with remaining 2 teaspoons oil and sprinkle Parmesan or Romano over the top. Bake for 15 minutes. Reduce oven temperature to 350°F and bake about 20 minutes longer, or until top is firm and lightly browned. Cool almost to room temperature before cutting into 20 small wedges.

Makes 20

Meat, Poultry, and Seafood Appetizers

Mex-Tex Meatballs

Meatballs
¼ cup hot rich Beef Stock (page 110)
½ cup cornmeal
¼ cup grated Monterey Jack cheese
¼ cup minced onions
1 pound lean ground beef
1 egg, beaten

Sauce
1 tablespoon vegetable oil
¼ cup chopped onions
1 clove garlic, minced
2 tablespoons finely chopped green peppers
1 teaspoon dried oregano
½ teaspoon ground cumin
1 teaspoon chopped fresh coriander or ¼ teaspoon dried coriander
2 cups tomato puree
2 teaspoons soy sauce
½ teaspoon crushed red pepper, or to taste

To make the meatballs: In a small bowl pour hot stock over cornmeal and let sit for 15 minutes. Place mixture in a small saucepan over moderate heat and cook, stirring constantly, until mixture is as thick as mashed potatoes. Cool slightly. Mix in cheese, onions, beef, and egg and blend well. Form into 24 walnut-size meatballs. Set aside.

To make the sauce: Heat oil in a deep saucepan. Add onions, garlic, chopped peppers, oregano, cumin, and coriander and cook until vegetables are tender but not browned. Add remaining ingredients and simmer for 10 minutes. Drop in prepared meatballs. Cover and continue to simmer for 30 minutes. Serve hot on wooden picks.

Makes 2 dozen

Caribbean Chicken

4 whole chicken breasts, boned and skinned (about 2 pounds boneless)
1 teaspoon ground ginger
2 teaspoons paprika
⅓ cup lemon juice
½ cup vegetable oil
½ cup Poultry Stock (page 110)
4 medium-size onions, thinly sliced
½ cup finely chopped sweet red peppers
⅓ cup dried currants
2 cups grated unsweetened coconut
⅓ cup chopped fresh parsley

Cut chicken breasts in half, place between sheets of wax paper, and pound to ½-inch thickness. Sprinkle both sides with ginger, paprika, and 3 tablespoons lemon juice. Let stand for 20 minutes.

In a large skillet place ¼ cup oil and ¼ cup stock. Add chicken and cook over medium heat for about 7 minutes, or until cooked through. Remove chicken from pan, and cut into bite-size pieces. Arrange pieces in a single layer in a shallow 9 × 13-inch baking dish.

Preheat oven to 375°F.

Sauté onions in remaining ¼ cup oil until tender but not browned. Stir in peppers, currants, remaining lemon juice, and remaining stock. Blend well, then spoon over chicken.

Combine coconut and parsley and sprinkle over chicken. Bake for 10 to 15 minutes, or until coconut is lightly toasted. Serve hot with wooden picks.

10 servings

Olde Dutch *Bitter-Ballen* with Horseradish-Dill Dip

1 pound lean ground beef
2 medium-size potatoes, thinly sliced
½ cup minced onions
¼ cup minced celery
2 tablespoons grated carrots
2 tablespoons minced fresh parsley
1 teaspoon ground sage
½ teaspoon dried thyme
1 teaspoon Worcestershire sauce
1 egg, beaten
½ cup milk
1½ to 2 cups well-seasoned whole grain bread
　　　crumbs
　　vegetable oil, for frying (optional)
　　Horseradish-Dill Dip (see below)

Crumble ground beef in bottom of a deep sauce-pan. Layer potatoes, onions, celery, carrots, and parsley on top of meat. Cover tightly and cook over moderate heat until beef is cooked and vegetables are very tender. Spoon off any excess fat that has accumulated. Add sage, thyme, and Worcestershire sauce, and mash ingredients with a slotted spoon until well blended but not perfectly smooth. Allow to cool to room temperature and then form into 36 walnut-size balls. Chill thoroughly in refrigerator.

In a small bowl, beat together egg and milk. Place bread crumbs in another bowl. Dip balls in egg mixture and then roll in bread crumbs until well coated. Allow to chill for 1 hour.

In a large skillet heat ½ inch oil to 375°F. Fry balls on all sides, then drain on paper towels. Or, place balls on a baking sheet and brown in 400°F oven for 15 to 20 minutes. Serve warm on wooden picks accompanied by a bowl of dip.

Makes 3 dozen

Horseradish-Dill Dip

1 cup sour cream
1½ teaspoons chopped fresh dill
2 tablespoons grated horseradish

Combine all ingredients in a small bowl and blend well.

Yields 1 cup

Chicken-Eggplant Sate

⅓ cup plus 2 tablespoons vegetable oil
½ cup minced onions
1 hot chili pepper, seeded and minced
1 clove garlic, minced
½ cup tomato paste
½ cup peanut butter
½ cup water, Poultry Stock (page 110), or
　　Vegetable Stock (page 111)
1 small eggplant
1 teaspoon soy sauce
　juice of ½ lemon
1 whole chicken breast, boned and skinned

Heat 2 tablespoons oil in a small saucepan. Add onions, chili pepper, and garlic and slowly sauté until vegetables are tender but not browned. Stir in tomato paste, peanut butter, and water or stock. (Sauce will be rather thick.) Heat slightly. (Overheating will cause sauce to separate.)

Peel eggplant and cut into about 24 cubes. Combine remaining ⅓ cup oil, soy sauce, and lemon juice in a small bowl. Toss eggplant cubes in oil mixture until most of the oil has been absorbed.

Cut chicken into about 24 cubes and place in another bowl. Add ½ cup peanut butter sauce to chicken and toss cubes until well coated. Allow to stand 30 minutes.

Spear 1 cube of eggplant and 1 cube of chicken on a wooden pick. Repeat until all cubes are used. Place on a broiler pan and broil rather slowly, about 8 to 10 inches from heat, for about 20 minutes, turning often to brown evenly. Serve hot with a bowl of remaining warm sauce for dipping.

Makes about 2 dozen

Infernal Wings

½ cup tomato sauce
¼ cup vinegar
¼ cup maple syrup
¼ teaspoon ground cloves
1 teaspoon onion powder
　dash of cayenne pepper, or to taste
1 pound chicken wings (8 to 10)

Combine all ingredients except wings in a small saucepan. Stir to blend and bring to a boil. Remove from heat to cool slightly.

Prepare wings by first removing "finger" (or largest bone) of each. Then separate each wing at "elbow." The small portion will have 2 small bones. Remove the smaller of these. Using a sharp paring knife, scrape meat back from end of each portion, turning it inside out, to form miniature drumstick. Place chicken in shallow glass baking pan and pour sauce over. Allow to marinate several hours or overnight in refrigerator.

Preheat oven to 400°F.

Spread wings in single layer in a greased 9 × 13-inch baking pan. Bake for 30 to 40 minutes. Just before serving, brown quickly under broiler.

Makes 16 to 20

Madras Chicken Balls

    2 teaspoons vegetable oil
    ¼ cup minced onions
    ¼ cup minced green peppers
    ½ cup finely chopped peeled tart apples
    1 clove garlic, minced
    ¼ teaspoon turmeric
    ⅛ teaspoon ground allspice
      pinch of ground cloves
    1 lime
    1 tablespoon honey
    1 tablespoon butter
    ½ cup coarsely chopped almonds
    ½ teaspoon curry powder
      dash of cayenne pepper
    1 cup ground or minced cooked chicken
    3 ounces cream cheese, softened
  2 to 3 teaspoons vinegar
    1⅓ cups unsweetened flaked coconut
    36 small melon balls or fresh pineapple chunks

Heat oil in a small saucepan and gently sauté onions, green peppers, apples, and garlic. Cover tightly and cook over low heat until very tender. Uncover and season with turmeric, allspice, and cloves and stir over heat until well blended.

Grate rind of lime, then add to sautéed vegetables along with lime's juice and honey. Stir well and cook a few minutes longer, if necessary, until mixture is quite dry and excess moisture has evaporated. Set aside to cool to room temperature.

Melt butter in a small skillet. Gently sauté almonds, curry powder, and cayenne until almonds are toasted. Set aside to cool to room temperature.

Combine cooled vegetable mixture, cooled almonds, chicken, cream cheese, and vinegar. Form mixture into 36 small balls (about 1 scant tablespoon per ball). Roll balls in coconut until well coated. Place in single layer on a flat dish, cover, and chill well. Spear each ball on a wooden pick along with melon ball or pineapple chunk.

Makes 3 dozen

Oriental Shrimp Nuggets with Hot Mustard

    2 cups chopped cooked shrimp
    ½ cup chopped Jerusalem artichokes
    ¼ cup minced scallions
  1½ tablespoons cornstarch
    2 teaspoons lemon juice
    1 teaspoon soy sauce
    ½ teaspoon grated peeled ginger root
    1 egg, beaten
      cornstarch, for dusting
      vegetable oil, for frying
      Hot Mustard (see below)

Mix together shrimp, artichokes, scallions, cornstarch, lemon juice, soy sauce, ginger root, and egg until mixture will squeeze into balls. Use heaping teaspoon of mixture to form 36 to 40 balls and dust lightly with additional cornstarch. Place nuggets on wax paper and refrigerate for at least 1 hour.

Heat ½ inch oil in a small skillet to 375°F. Drop shrimp nuggets one by one into hot oil and brown lightly. Drain excess oil by rolling lightly on paper towels. Serve immediately with a bowl of Hot Mustard for dipping.

Makes 36 to 40

NOTE: Shrimp nuggets may be refrigerated or frozen and then reheated in a 400°F oven for several minutes just before serving.

Hot Mustard

    ¼ cup dry mustard
    2 teaspoons vinegar
    ¼ cup boiling water

Combine mustard and vinegar. Gradually stir in water. Allow to stand at room temperature for at least 15 minutes before using.

Yields about ⅓ cup

Sausage-Stuffed Prunes

½ pound lean ground beef
½ pound lean ground pork
1 clove garlic, crushed to a pulp
1 tablespoon orange juice, or more if needed
¼ teaspoon dried thyme
¼ teaspoon ground sage
   pinch each of ground nutmeg, allspice,
     and cloves
½ teaspoon pepper
½ cup whole grain bread crumbs
12 ounces pitted dried prunes (about 42)

Preheat oven to 400°F.

Combine all ingredients except prunes in a medium-size bowl and mix until well blended. Use fingers to form a pocket in each prune. (If prunes are too dry, soak a short while in extra orange juice.) Use about 1½ tablespoons meat mixture to overstuff each prune. Round tops nicely.

Stand stuffed prunes upright in a greased 9 × 13-inch baking pan and bake for about 20 minutes. Serve hot on wooden picks.

Makes about 42

Monkfish Cocktail Picks
with Seafood Cocktail Sauce

½ cup water
1 bay leaf
   dash of crushed red pepper
   juice of ½ lemon, with squeezed rind reserved
   pinch of dried tarragon
3 or 4 celery leaves
1 small slice onion
1½ pounds monkfish fillet
18 to 20 cherry tomatoes
   salad greens
   lemon wedges
   Seafood Cocktail Sauce (see opposite)

Combine water, bay leaf, red pepper, lemon juice and rind, tarragon, celery leaves, and onion slice in a large saucepan or fish poacher. Bring mixture to a boil, reduce heat, cover, and simmer for 5 minutes.

Peel off tough outer membrane of monkfish if necessary. Place fish in 1 whole piece in simmering liquid. Cover tightly and poach for 15 to 20 minutes,

or until cooked through. Cool fish in poaching liquid. Then remove from liquid and discard any bits of seasoning clinging to it. Cut the fish into 18 to 20 cubes, as evenly shaped as possible. Arrange a fish cube and a cherry tomato on individual wooden picks and serve on a bed of fresh greens garnished with lemon wedges. Serve cocktail sauce in a separate bowl for dipping.

Makes 18 to 20

Seafood Cocktail Sauce

½ cup mayonnaise
2 teaspoons tomato paste
2 tablespoons tarragon vinegar
1 tablespoon horseradish, drained
1 teaspoon Worcestershire sauce
   dash of ground cloves
   dash of cayenne pepper
   dash of ground allspice
½ cup heavy cream, whipped

Combine mayonnaise, tomato paste, vinegar, horseradish, Worcestershire sauce, and spices. Blend well, then fold in whipped cream. Chill.

Yields about 1¾ cups

Salmon Croquettes

1 medium-size onion, chopped
4 scallions, chopped
1 tablespoon butter
1 pound salmon fillets, cooked, then flaked
1 cup cottage cheese
3 eggs
2 egg yolks
2 cups whole grain bread crumbs
1 tablespoon minced fresh chives or 1½
   teaspoons dried chives
1 tablespoon minced fresh dill or 1½ teaspoons
   dillweed
1 tablespoon minced fresh parsley or 1½
   teaspoons dried parsley
¼ teaspoon paprika

Preheat oven to 350°F.

Sauté onions and scallions in butter until onions are translucent. Transfer to a large bowl. Add salmon, cottage cheese, eggs, egg yolks, bread crumbs, chives, dill, parsley, and paprika and mix well. With lightly oiled hands, press 1 tablespoon of mixture into a croquette (cone shape). Place croquettes with point up (you will have about 38 in all) on greased baking sheet and bake for 15 minutes if croquettes are to be reheated, or 20 minutes if they are to be served immediately. (Croquettes are done when firm to the touch.) Or, if you prefer, sauté in butter on both sides until browned.

Makes about 38

Sautéed Bay Scallops

1½ pounds small bay scallops
½ cup whole wheat pastry flour
¼ cup plus 2 tablespoons butter
    freshly ground pepper, to taste
¼ cup chopped fresh parsley
    juice of ½ lemon

Dry scallops well and dust lightly with flour.

Melt butter in a large skillet, add scallops, and brown lightly. Add pepper and sprinkle with parsley and lemon juice. Place on a heated platter. Serve at once with wooden picks or provide small plates and forks.

6 servings

Shrimp Egg Rolls

3 dried shiitake mushrooms*
½ cup lukewarm water
1 pound Chinese cabbage
2 tablespoons vegetable oil
½ pound uncooked medium-size shrimp, peeled and deveined
8 fresh mushrooms, thinly sliced
1 cup mung bean sprouts or soy sprouts
½ cup chopped scallions
2 cloves garlic, minced
1 teaspoon minced peeled ginger root
2 teaspoons soy sauce
1 tablespoon whole wheat flour
2 tablespoons water
12 large egg roll skins
    vegetable oil, for frying
    Sesame Ginger Sauce (page 151)
    Hot Mustard (page 95)

Soak shiitake mushrooms in lukewarm water for 30 minutes. Remove mushrooms, discard hard stems, and cut mushrooms into ½-inch pieces.

Remove tough stalk portions from cabbage leaves. Cut stalks across fiber, at a slight angle, into thin slices and set aside. Chop leaves into ½-inch squares and set aside separately.

Place a wok over high heat and add 1 tablespoon oil. When hot, add shrimp and stir-fry for about 2 minutes, or until shrimp is opaque. Remove shrimp from wok, cool slightly, and chop into small pieces. Set aside.

Add remaining 1 tablespoon oil to wok and heat again over high heat. Add cabbage stalks and sliced fresh mushrooms. Stir-fry for 1 minute. Then, stirring after each addition, add sprouts, shiitake mushrooms, scallions, garlic, and ginger root. Add cabbage leaves and stir until completely wilted. It is important that the filling be dry. If a bit more cooking will evaporate accumulated liquid, cook further. If not, drain everything in a colander to remove excess liquid. Add shrimp and soy sauce. Cool.

Make a paste to seal the loose ends of the egg rolls by mixing flour with water. Spread 6 egg roll skins on a flat surface. Place ¼ cup filling on each skin. Roll, tucking in ends and sealing edge with flour paste. Repeat with remaining skins.

Preheat oven to 300°F. Place a 9 × 13-inch baking pan in oven while heating.

Put enough oil in a clean wok so that 2 egg rolls can be shallow-fried at one time. Heat oil until scallion ring dropped in it dances in circles. Fry egg rolls, two at a time, turning with tongs to brown both sides. Drain on paper towels and then transfer to pan in oven. Bake each egg roll at least 10 minutes before serving. Serve hot with Sesame Ginger Sauce and Hot Mustard for dipping.

Makes 1 dozen

NOTE: Varying the fillings for egg rolls is easy. The only rule is that the filling must be very dry and cooled to room temperature. Have 3 cups of filling for 12 fat egg rolls.

*Shiitake mushrooms are commonly available in oriental grocery stores.

Variation:

Carrot-Tofu Egg Roll: Replace shrimp with 4 ounces crumbled firm tofu and ½ cup diced lightly cooked carrots.

Tuna-Pecan Ovenhot

If you prefer to serve this dish as a first course, simply bake it in four small ramekins.

1 tablespoon finely chopped pecans
2 tablespoons whole grain bread crumbs
1 tablespoon grated Parmesan cheese
¼ teaspoon dried oregano
8 ounces cream cheese, softened
2 tablespoons yogurt
2 tablespoons minced onions
1 tablespoon minced green or sweet red peppers
¼ cup coarsely chopped pecans
   dash of cayenne pepper
1 can (6 to 7 ounces) water-packed tuna, flaked
   pecan halves

Preheat oven to 350°F.
Generously butter a 2-cup baking dish.
Combine 1 tablespoon finely chopped pecans with bread crumbs, Parmesan, and oregano. Reserve about 1 tablespoon of mixture to be used for topping. Use remainder to coat buttered baking dish.

In a small bowl beat cream cheese and yogurt until light and fluffy. Blend in onions, peppers, chopped pecans, and cayenne. Lightly stir in tuna. Pile mixture into prepared baking dish and sprinkle with reserved topping. Bake about 20 minutes, or until bubbly. Serve with whole wheat crackers or toast points. Garnish with several pecan halves just before serving.

4 servings

Young *Calamari* Salad

This high-protein, low-calorie salad is a delicious way to introduce squid, or calamari as the Italians call it, to those who have never tried it.

4 pounds baby squid
½ cup olive oil
   juice of 3 lemons
10 slivers pimiento
2 tablespoons minced green peppers
1 cup croutons
2 teaspoons chopped fresh parsley
1 teaspoon finely chopped garlic
   pepper, to taste

Wash squid, then cut main body into ¼-inch rings. Cut tentacles and legs into small pieces. Place squid in a large pot, cover with water, add 1 table-

spoon olive oil, and cook for 10 minutes. When done, drain; then mix together with remaining olive oil and other ingredients.

Arrange squid on a serving dish and let cool for at least 1 hour. Refrigerate and serve chilled.

12 servings

Pâtés

Chicken Pâté

¼ cup almonds
2 tablespoons vegetable oil
1 chicken (roaster, about 3 pounds), boned and skinned
2 tablespoons soy sauce
2 tablespoons wine vinegar
½ teaspoon garlic powder

Grind the almonds coarsely in a blender at high speed. Set aside.

Place oil in a large skillet. Cut chicken into 1-inch pieces and place in skillet. Add soy sauce and vinegar and sprinkle garlic powder over all. Sauté for a few minutes, uncovered, over high heat, stirring and turning until the chicken is just done. (Do not over-cook or it will get dry.)

Remove from heat and allow to cool for a few minutes. With a fork, pick out pieces of chicken and drop into blender through opening in blender top, with machine going at highest speed, until all is ground. Add 3 tablespoons of cooking liquid and reserved nuts and blend until well distributed. Serve with crackers and celery and carrot sticks.

Yields about 3 cups

Herb-Liver Pâté

1 tablespoon vegetable oil
1 small onion, coarsely chopped
1 clove garlic, chopped
¼ teaspoon dried savory
¼ teaspoon dried thyme
½ pound chicken livers
1 hard-cooked egg
   pepper, to taste

Heat oil in a small skillet. Add onions, garlic, savory, and thyme and sauté until onions are translucent.

Add chicken livers and cook over medium heat until just done. Remove skillet from heat and allow livers to cool for a few minutes. Blend by dropping into a blender through opening in blender top, one liver at a time, with motor going at high speed. Blend in egg and pepper. Serve with crackers and cucumber and tomato slices.

Yields 1 cup

Vegetable Terrine

Serve this terrine cold with crackers and French bread as a first course or at a buffet table. Although it takes a little extra time to make, the terrine looks and tastes impressive.

2 cups cooked brown rice, at room temperature
1 cup shredded Jarlsberg cheese
6 tablespoons grated Parmesan cheese
¼ teaspoon pepper
2 eggs, beaten
2 scallions, finely chopped
1 pound Chinese cabbage (about 1½ large heads)
¼ cup butter
1 large onion, finely chopped
2 cloves garlic, minced
1 teaspoon chopped fresh thyme or ½ teaspoon dried thyme
¼ cup fine whole grain bread crumbs
3 carrots, cooked until tender
Yogurt-Tahini Dressing (page 185)

Mix rice with ½ cup Jarlsberg, 3 tablespoons Parmesan, ⅛ teaspoon pepper, 2 tablespoons beaten egg, and scallions. Press ½ of the rice mixture into bottom of a generously buttered hinged pâté mold (10 × 3-inch) or an 8½ × 4½-inch loaf pan. Reserve remaining rice mixture.

Remove heavy ribs from cabbage and chop into ½-inch squares. (This will yield about 4 quarts, chopped.) In a large pot melt 2 tablespoons butter and sauté cabbage with onions, garlic, and thyme until quite dry. Transfer to a bowl and set bowl in cold water. Stir occasionally to cool quickly. When cool, stir in 2 tablespoons beaten egg, 2 tablespoons bread crumbs, ¼ cup Jarlsberg, and 3 tablespoons Parmesan. Press evenly over rice layer in pâté mold or loaf pan.

Mash carrots together with 2 tablespoons beaten egg, 2 tablespoons bread crumbs, remaining pepper, and ¼ cup of Jarlsberg. Spread over cabbage layer. Preheat oven to 350°F.

Press remaining rice mixture firmly over carrot layer. Dot with remaining butter. Cover pan loosely with foil and bake for 1 to 1¼ hours, or until terrine is firm and begins to brown at edges. If in doubt, insert a small thin knife into center of terrine for 20 seconds. When terrine is done, the knife will come out very hot to the touch. Chill completely.

To serve unmold terrine onto a cutting board. Cut into ¾-inch-thick slices. Serve slices on their sides with dressing.

8 to 16 servings

Pistachio and Veal Country Pâté

1 cup finely chopped mushrooms
2 tablespoons butter
1 pound lean ground veal
1 pound ground pork shoulder, with some fat
2 eggs
¼ cup plus 1 tablespoon heavy cream or milk
½ cup chopped fresh parsley
¼ cup plus 1 tablespoon finely chopped shallots
1 teaspoon grated lemon rind
1 teaspoon dried basil
¼ teaspoon dried thyme
¾ teaspoon pepper
½ teaspoon ground allspice
¾ to 1 cup pistachios
2 bay leaves
lemon wedges

In a small skillet sauté mushrooms in hot butter for 5 minutes. Remove from heat and let cool. Combine remaining ingredients, except bay leaves and lemon wedges, in a mixing bowl. Add cooled mushrooms. Mix well with wooden spoon or by hand.

Line a 9 × 5-inch loaf pan or straight-sided baking dish with foil. Fill with pâté mixture, packing down firmly. Place bay leaves on top and cover with foil. Preheat oven to 325°F.

Bake pâté for 1 hour. Uncover and bake 1 hour longer, or until juices run clear. Remove from oven and let cool. After 30 minutes, weight down top of pâté. Let cool completely at room temperature and then chill for 24 hours.

Serve directly from pan or dish, or unmold onto a serving plate or board. Garnish with lemon wedges. Serve thinly sliced with toasted bread and lettuce leaves.

10 servings

Soups

Almost everyone seems to find comfort in a steaming bowl of soup. Perhaps this stems from its association with olden days and a slow-simmering kettle of soup over the hearth—it meant daily sustenance in lean times. Today, many of us associate soup with grandmother's constant nurturing. She always had a delicious soup handy to cure our colds and fevers. It is no wonder soup has the power to make people feel good. It has a homey, comforting aura about it that restores the spirit as well as the body. Soups are the most fundamental kind of nourishment.

Just about every culture affirms the restorative quality of soup. Italian minestrone, made with kidney or navy beans, pasta, and as many as eight or nine different vegetables, is a savory, tomato-rich soup, as delicious and health-giving as it sounds. *Soupe au pistou, potage,* and *pot-au-feu* are all French variations on this same theme. The ingredients for these hearty soups might be leftover vegetables, pureed and filled out with a rich stock, or they may be peasant-style soups with chunky vegetables in a thin, flavorful broth. The Spanish version of these soups is even heartier; a blend of cabbage, haricot beans, fresh peas, and seasonal vegetables is enriched with the flavors of pork, garlic, and thyme. This type of soup, cooked in an earthenware casserole, is so rich in good taste that it is often savored over several days as the flavors mingle and intensify.

It is no wonder that soup is so prevalent in every type of cuisine—the principle for making it is so simple. Any well-chosen combination of nutritious ingredients, simmered in a liquid until the good flavors and nutrients are absorbed into it, becomes a good-tasting soup. Most soups are made this way.

This procedure is very similar to that used to make stocks. The simmering time for stocks is longer and the solid ingredients are eventually strained from the liquid and discarded. Stocks represent the flavor and goodness from which many tasty soups originate.

Stocks

Stocks are called *fonds de cuisine*—foundations of cooking. They are the very basis of a good soup and they do require some time, but little work, as a rule. Stocks, delicious by themselves, also serve as a base for other dishes. Many soups, sauces, casseroles, and stews take their theme from an amplified stock.

A meat-based broth may be made a day ahead and refrigerated overnight. In the morning, all the fat will have collected on the surface and solidified so that it can be lifted off easily, a process called "degreasing." If you intend to keep the stock refrigerated several days, the fat on top will help to preserve it, so do not remove the fat until the day the stock is to be used.

Long, slow cooking is a cardinal requirement for meat stocks. Whereas fish and vegetable stocks may require as little as 30 to 60 minutes of cooking, warm-blooded meat must be cooked

Equipment for Making Soups and Stocks

The equipment needed for making stocks and soups is so basic to all types of cooking that you probably have it in your kitchen already. Check this list if you want to be sure you have everything necessary for the various steps involved in making soups and stocks:

Large heavy pot (four- to six-quart capacity, preferably stainless steel or enameled)
Slotted spoon, large spatula, or stock skimmer
Large strainer
Cheesecloth or loosely woven dish towel (for straining)
Ladle
Storage containers with tightly fitting lids
Wire whisk (to clarify)
Asbestos burner pad (to diffuse heat evenly under the stockpot)

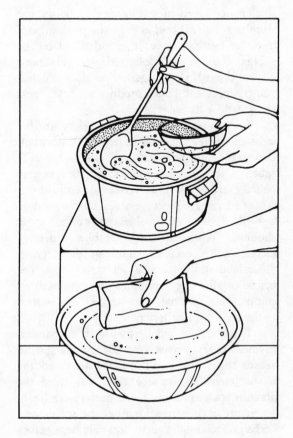

slowly. An asbestos heating pad over your stove's burner helps to control the temperature and prevent burning. Placing the meat bones on a wire rack in the pot can also prevent the pot's contents from sticking.

A stock is made by gently simmering nutrient- and flavor-rich ingredients such as bones, meat, vegetables, poultry, or fish. (Broth and bouillon are also terms for this same preparation.) For meat, poultry, and fish stocks, the pot should never be completely covered during this process.

The gentle simmer cannot be overemphasized — small bubbles should barely ripple on the surface of the liquid. A rolling boil will encourage an overabundance of scum to collect on the surface of the stock. This occurrence is due to albumin, a protein secretion from the meat bones. Nutritionists point out that the unattractive scum is rich in protein, and worth retaining with the stock. However, skimming with a slotted spoon or large spatula is a traditional procedure during the first half hour of simmering, when the scum appears. You may also wrap a piece of cheesecloth around the utensil to facilitate skimming.

Any tiny beads of grease that remain may be skimmed from the surface with a paper towel. A clear and appetizing broth will result from this careful procedure.

Stockpot Ingredients

Bones provide the natural gelatinous quality for stock. Any cooked or uncooked bones with some meat remaining make good soup bones, but you can get equally good results from bare bones coupled with an inexpensive piece of stew meat. When possible, have your butcher chop large bones into smaller pieces — about two inches long — to expose the interior goodness and to fit into the pot more easily.

Pork, lamb, and ham bones in the stockpot produce a dominating flavor, so unless a meat stock recipe specifically calls for such bones, use them sparingly. If beef is to be the predominant flavor of broth, it may be rounded out by the subtlety of chicken and bolstered by the gelatinous texture of veal. Used together or alone, veal or poultry meat and bones produce a white stock, so named for its pale color.

Carrots, onions, leeks, and celery are the most common aromatics added to the stockpot. Beware of vegetables such as asparagus, broccoli, cabbage, and turnips, whose strong flavors may be too overbearing if used in large quantities. It is not necessary to peel vegetables, but they should be well scrubbed and any blemishes or bad spots should be removed. Cut vegetables into large pieces; small pieces tend to mush and disintegrate, thus clouding the stock. Adding the vegetables before or after the skimming process has been completed is optional. Experienced cooks attest to the success of either choice.

Fresh spices and herbs—such as parsley, thyme, and bay leaves—may be used to further season the stockpot. When herbs are dried, the flavor intensifies, so use about one-third the amount you would use if the herbs were fresh. To ensure easy retrieval, gather the spices and herbs into a bouquet garni. If whole large leaves or fresh sprigs are used to make the bouquet, fasten them all together with a string tied to a stalk of celery or a leek leaf. Smaller fragments, such as seeds, crumbled herbs, and ground spices, may be tied into a piece of cheesecloth and anchored down beneath a soup bone.

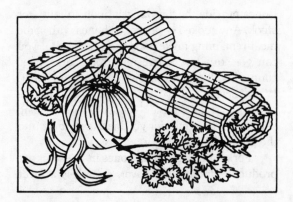

When you have placed the necessary ingredients in the stockpot, add cold water (never hot) until it covers everything by about 1½ inches. Hot water tends to sear the ingredients, sealing in flavorful juices; cold water drains the juices from the ingredients soaking in it. Hot water may be added during cooking if the liquid in the stockpot gets too low. The amount of liquid suggested in a recipe is only an approximation; if you find that too much water has been used, it can always be reduced through longer cooking. It is essential to keep the ingredients in the pot covered by water at all times.

Brown Stock

Browning stock elements before adding them to the water caramelizes the vegetables and meat juices. A brown stock, or *fond brun,* is made by browning the meat, bones, and vegetables in the oven before adding them to the water to simmer. The appetizing hue and rich flavor that result are a generous bonus for this simple extra step.

Use beef or veal bones, or knuckles sawed into three- or four-inch pieces. Chicken wings or backs may be used to enhance the flavor. Roast the bones and meat in a hot oven (425°F) for one hour, or until nicely colored. Turn the bones occasionally to promote even cooking. During the final half hour of roasting, add carrots cut into large pieces and unpeeled onions. Leaving skins on the onions adds sweetness and color to the broth. Transfer the roasted bones, meat, and vegetables to the stockpot.

The next step is to degrease and deglaze the pan. To do this, spoon any fat out of the roasting pan (use a syringe if necessary), leaving behind any juices. Add a little cold water and scrape the brown caramelized particles from the pan's bottom with a wooden spoon. Pour all this into the stockpot.

Add water and seasonings to the pot and leave it to simmer gently for five to six hours or longer, skimming as necessary.

Browned Poultry Stock

A browned poultry stock is made almost the same way as a basic brown stock, but only requires three to four hours of simmering. The poultry bones, which tend to burn easily, are browned in a skillet on top of the stove. Generous amounts of oil should coat the skillet in which the three- to four-inch pieces are sautéed until browned.

Place the browned parts in the stockpot. Sauté the vegetables — large pieces of unpeeled onions and carrots — in the pan drippings. When they are sufficiently browned, transfer them to the stockpot. Degrease the drippings, then deglaze the skillet with a little cold water and add the particles to the pot. Skim the simmering stock as necessary.

White Stock

A white stock, or *fond blanc,* is made from veal or poultry meat and bones that have not been browned. It may be the base for a cream or velouté soup or sauce, as its paleness works well with the pure white of dairy products. Onion skins, often added to brown stocks, are not used with a white stock. Vegetables are added to the broth only after the bones and water have come to a boil and the broth has been skimmed.

A white stock requires about 3½ hours of slow simmering. Once the veal knuckles and bones are in place, a few chicken parts may be added for additional flavor. Veal bones exude a lot of albuminous scum, so frequent skimming may be necessary.

Poultry Stock

Poultry stock is economical and easy to make. Collect leftover poultry bones and carcasses (raw or cooked), hack them into small pieces, and freeze them until you are ready to make the stock. Place the frozen bones in the pot; they will defrost as you bring the water to a rolling boil. Drain and rinse the bones and the pot, getting rid of surface scum. Then cover bones, vegetables, and seasonings with fresh cold water and simmer for three to four hours.

Chicken stock may be made from virtually all parts of the chicken — wing tips, carcasses, gizzards, hearts, backs, and necks — except the liver. Never use liver for chicken stock; it gives off an unpleasant flavor and darkens the liquid. Chicken feet are rich in the natural gelatin that gives body to the broth. (If your butcher doesn't stock them, poultry farms and Jewish neighborhood shops are good sources for chicken feet.) Blanch them in boiling water for five minutes and peel or rub off the yellow skin before adding them to the stockpot.

Vegetable Stock

A vegetable broth may be made with any combination of fresh vegetables or leftover vegetable trimmings. Unlike meat and poultry stocks, vegetable stocks seldom require skimming, and the cooking time is much shorter — 30 to 60 minutes of simmering. You need only remember a few basic precepts. Strong vegetables yield strong stock, so use only a touch of them to strengthen the broth. Starchy vegetables such as corn, peas, and potatoes tend to cloud the stock, so it is best to use them in small quantities. Parsnips and carrots sweeten the liquid. If you want to intensify the broth's flavor, sauté vegetables lightly in a little butter before adding them.

Vegetable stock lacks the gelatinous quality of meat stock and has less body. You can give the broth more substance by adding a tablespoon of agar flakes, a sea vegetable with natural gelatinous quality (see How to Firm Up Limp Stock, page 106).

Fish Stock

Fish stock is easy and quick to make. Everything may be put into the pot and simmered for one hour, then strained and reduced. Longer cooking would yield a bitter, disagreeable taste. A good fish stock, also called *fumet,* can be made from parts of the fish that are usually discarded. Fish heads, carcasses, trimmings of lean white fish — all can be used. Do not use fatty or oily fish such as salmon, mackerel, or herring, for they flavor the broth too strongly. A fish stock will not be as clear as one made from meat or vegetables, and will be much less gelatinous than meat stock.

Fresh fish is essential in making fish stock. When buying fish in the market, look for clear, unglazed, bulging eyes and bright red or pinkish gills. If a fresh fish is not to be used at once, remove the gills at the earliest opportunity, as this is the first part of the fish to become strong tasting.

Straining and Reducing

When all the ingredients in the stockpot have yielded their goodness and flavors to the cooking liquid, it is time to strain it to separate liquid from solids. In some cases, that of consommé, for example, this straining must be quite meticulous.

To strain stock, line a large sieve or colander with a damp, loosely woven cloth, and place it over a clean bowl or pan. Ladle the broth into the strainer, then wash out the pot used to cook the stock. The strained stock may be returned to the pot for further reducing, if desired. The solid ingredients may be discarded.

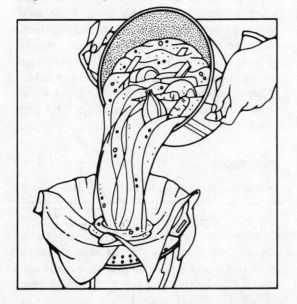

Reducing the stock concentrates its body and flavor into a smaller volume, as with a *glace de viande,* or meat glaze. To reduce stock, boil it vigorously, uncovered, until the volume is decreased by one-third to one-half. Skim, if necessary.

To discourage unwelcome bacteria from growing in the warm liquid, the strained and reduced stock should be cooled, uncovered, as quickly as possible. This is done before refrigerating the stock. To cool quickly, place the pot in a larger basin or bowl, surround it with ice, and stir the broth until it is completely cool, or set the pot on blocks in a sink filled with cold water.

Storage

The cooled stock, stored in covered containers, should be refrigerated at once. It will keep under refrigeration for about a week. If you wish to keep stock on hand longer, freeze it in small covered containers or in ice cube trays. The frozen cubes can be unmolded and stored in sealed plastic bags, then used as needed, without having to thaw a large quantity of stock. Label and date the stock you freeze. It will keep for up to a year. Before using any stock that has been frozen, bring it to a full rolling boil to kill any harmful bacteria.

Soups should be stored with the same precautions used for stocks. Soups made with cream, milk, or eggs should not be kept refrigerated for longer than two days. All soups may be frozen, but those made with cream, milk, or eggs tend to separate when thawed. As with stock, reheat to the boiling point before serving.

Jellied Stock

Jellied stock may be served hot or cold, plain or embellished with garnishes such as chopped chives or a dollop of yogurt.

The way cold jellied stocks are to be used determines how firm they should be. To be eaten as an appetizer, jellied stock should be firm enough to break into soft lumps. If it is to be used as an aspic set in a decorative mold, it must be somewhat firmer in order to retain its shape when unmolded; too much rigidity, however, is undesirable. Aspics used for coating or decorating must be gelatinous enough to hold foods in place (see Molded Salads, page 160).

The classic jellied soup is based on a homemade stock made with bones, which give off natural gelatin. Veal knuckles, calf's feet, and chicken feet are well suited for this, but do not use too much gelatinous food or the stock will be too viscous. Long, slow simmering (at least six hours) is essential for drawing out the gelatin from the bones. Fast boiling will cause albumin and fat to incorporate themselves into the liquid, giving thickness and pastiness instead of richness and clarity.

A brilliant sparkle marks the perfect gelatin. Meticulously skimming and straining the stock will promote this essential translucent quality. Clarifying (see Consommé, below) is usually done, unless opaque ingredients such as yogurt, cream, or mayonnaise are to be mixed in.

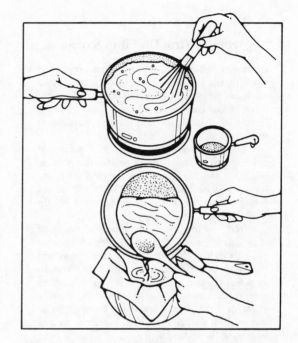

Consommé

A consommé is made by carefully clarifying a jellied stock. The stock is clarified with egg whites and crushed egg shells which attract and trap food particles that are too fine to be strained out.

To clarify: Place well-degreased stock in a large (four-quart capacity), clean enameled or stainless steel saucepan, and slowly heat until melted (if it has jelled) and warm.

At this point, fold or whisk egg whites and crushed shells into the stock so that they come in contact with all the liquid in the pan. (Use one egg white and shell per quart of stock.) The egg matter will form a crust like a dome. Reduce the heat and allow the stock to barely simmer, undisturbed, until clear (five to ten minutes). To check clarity and to ensure that the stock never goes beyond a gentle simmer, gently push the

coagulated egg whites aside several times during clarifying process.

When the stock looks clear, turn off the heat and let stand for at least ten minutes. Wring out a clean dish towel in cold water and arrange it in a large strainer placed over a deep bowl. Holding the egg white crust back with a spoon, carefully strain the clarified stock into the bowl. Do not wring out the cloth into the stock.

A delicious, healthful, low-calorie consommé may be served hot, garnished with scallions or chives. Yogurt and/or any chopped vegetable make a nutritious garnish when the consommé is chilled.

Meat Glaze *(Glace de Viande)*

When meat stock is strained and reduced until very thick and syrupy, it becomes a highly concentrated essence that may be used in small quantities to flavor soups, sauces, or casseroles. This concentration of meat flavor is called a meat glaze, or *glace de viande*. When cool, the firm gelatinous texture of the glaze permits conve-

How to Firm Up Limp Stock

Unflavored gelatin may be used to firm up a jellied stock that is too limp. To set a very thin liquid stock, use about two tablespoons of gelatin for every three to four cups of liquid. To set or firm up a loosely jelled stock, use half these proportions of unflavored gelatin.

Measure out one-quarter to one-half cup of cold stock for each tablespoon of gelatin that will be used. Sprinkle the gelatin over the cold stock and let it stand for five minutes to soften. Heat the remaining stock and stir in the softened gelatin until dissolved.

You may test the setting power of the stock after gelatin powder has been added by pouring one-half inch of the stock into a small bowl and placing it in the refrigerator until set (about 15 minutes). If the jelled stock is too soft, more gelatin powder should be added and the mixture retested. If the jelled stock is too firm, it can be diluted with a small amount of unjellied stock or water and then retested.

Vegetable stock may also be set to any desired consistency with agar. Measure agar in the same amount specified for gelatin powder, and test its setting power as described.

nient handling and storage. Two quarts of stock will condense into approximately one cup of glaze. This rendering may seem meager considering the time and effort involved, but it is used in very small amounts. Half a teaspoon can enrich a sauce or a soup, a stew or a casserole. It may be reconstituted in hot water and used in place of stock.

To make a glaze: Place two quarts of any meat stock in a medium-size saucepan. Bring the stock to a boil and cook it, uncovered, over medium heat for about one hour, or until it is reduced by half. Strain this through a fine sieve into a smaller pan and continue to cook until this is reduced by half, about 30 minutes or longer. Strain once more into an even smaller pan, and turn the heat down to very low. Continue to cook about 20 minutes longer.

At this point it is absolutely essential to maintain the stock at a low temperature and to keep a close watch on the pan so that the reduced stock does not stick to the bottom or burn. It will become thick and syrupy with bubbles on the surface. When the stock will lightly coat a metal spoon, transfer it to a heatproof bowl and let it stand until cool.

Cover the cooled glaze and store it in the refrigerator; it will keep there for weeks. The glaze can also be frozen; it will keep that way for about a year.

If you decide to freeze it, the best way is to turn out the cooled glaze when it has hardened into a firm jelly, and cut it into small pieces. Arrange the pieces on a baking sheet and place in the freezer until frozen. Then transfer the cubes to a covered container or a plastic bag for freezer storage.

Purees

Gourmet cooks adore the simplicity of a puree. Legumes, vegetables, poultry, or fish all provide a delectable base for a smooth, appetizing puree. A basic puree is simple to make. The ingredients are first cooked, then processed in a food processor or blender. Sometimes a sieve is also used after pureeing, to ensure the proper uniform texture. A puree may be enriched with cream, milk, or eggs for a more-filling soup.

The texture and consistency of a puree may vary—starchy vegetables such as peas, potatoes, and beans possess a grainy thickness that needs no further enrichment. Thinner-bodied purees may be thickened with cream, flour, or both. A puree is usually limited to the flavor of one ingredient, sometimes two. A muddied or unwelcome taste may result from too many different ingredients. Stringy vegetables such as celery, or those with skin such as peas, may be blanched before being pureed, and then sieved or put through a food mill to ensure smoothness.

When pureeing in a blender, moisten the contents with some of the cooking liquid and scrape down the sides of the blender each time you blend. Blend small quantities at a time for best results. If using a food processor, strain off the liquid first, then recombine after pureeing. Never boil a puree soup after cream, butter, or eggs have been added, or it may curdle.

Velouté-Thickened Soups

Velouté-thickened soups are prepared from a white roux (see White and Brown Sauces, page 135). Broth or stock is added to the flour-butter combination. This method is used to make cream soups. Or, it may be used to thicken purees made with vegetables that lack the ability to thicken on their own, such as mushrooms, spinach, tomatoes, and onions.

The same methods used to thicken sauces may be used to thicken and enrich soups. The addition of barley, oatmeal, and other grains will also add body to a soup. Nut flours and cooked beans provide another nutritious means of thickening soups.

Panades

Bread, often the mere rudiment of a meal, may form the body of some soups. Old or stale bread may be used. A delicious Provençale panade consists of bread steeped in boiling water or broth, mashed to a puree, then enriched with butter and eggs. A crusty onion soup is probably the most renowned of panades. Thick rounds of coarse bread are drenched in broth that has been flavored with the sweetness of onions sautéed in butter. The garnish, grated Swiss and Parmesan gratiné, is an integral part of this dish.

Panades are quite variable, and provide a creative, tasty receptacle for leftover breads. Coarse-textured peasant-type bread is the best; finer-grained breads cannot stand up to the liquid used.

Chilled Soups

A chilled soup can be just as appealing as a hot one. It satisfies on a hot summer day the way a steaming bowl of soup does in winter. The preparation is just as easy, with some slight differences—less fat (if any) is used and, of course, less cooking may be involved.

The roster of famous chilled soups includes vichyssoise, the classic chilled puree of leek and potato, and gazpacho, a raw vegetable soup favored in the torrid sections of Spain and Latin America. When heavier foods are undesirable, such savory soups are excellent substitutes.

Many cold vegetable purees may become re-vivifying cocktails. Sour cream, yogurt, or cream is the best means of enriching these healthful chilled soups.

Sweet and tart are the characteristic flavors of fruit soups. Many types of fruits may serve as the basis of tangy, delicious cold soups, their sweetness heightened or rounded off with contrasting ingredients. For example, lemon or lime juice can enliven many fruit-based soups. In making fruit soups, the fruit may be left raw or it may be lightly cooked. The liquid used can also add some flavor to the soup. Many broths and stocks are quite suitable for fruit soups.

Fish Soups

Soups made with fish as the main ingredient are often full meals that provide good-tasting nutrition. Fish is high in protein, and the many vegetables and herbs with which it may be cooked result in endless versions of fish soups, stews, bisques, and chowders. It is best to make fish soups with whatever is regional and seasonal. The freshest fish naturally offers the most delicate taste.

A New England or Manhattan chowder can be made with almost any fish. Whether it is creamy or tomato-based, the fish stock used will provide robustness. Different in texture and appearance from a chunky chowder, but equally alluring, is a bisque. A bisque is a creamed soup that often has shellfish as the main ingredient.

The fishermen of Marseilles are perhaps most responsible for bouillabaisse, the renowned Provençale fish stew. Traditionally made from whatever fish or shellfish the fishermen brought in each day, the recipe may vary accordingly. Vegetables and a tomato-seasoned broth add up to a harmonious blend of zesty flavors. Large crusts of bread to sop up the broth that remains are a gastronomic mandate.

Soup Enhancers

In addition to the traditional stocks and meat glaze used to give soups flavor, there are several useful condiments and sauces that you can make in your kitchen. You can keep these on hand and use them to season many different soups.

Garlic Stock

Garlic stock is a savory liquid that may be used as a base for tomato or vegetable soups. Lengthy cooking subdues the garlic's pungency without diminishing its distinct flavor. A large head of garlic will subtly season two to three quarts of stock.

Soy Seasonings

Soy sauce (or tamari) and miso (see Soy Products, page 263) provide a rich flavor for nonmeat soups. Soy sauce may be mixed with vegetable stock in a ratio of one to eight (more or less according to taste). Quick-cooking vegetables may then be added for a satisfying soup.

Miso broth is a mineral supplement containing calcium, copper, iron, magnesium, phosphorus, and potassium. It also contains some protein. Never boil a liquid to which miso has been added; the heat will destroy its "friendly" bacteria.

To make miso broth: Mix about one teaspoon of miso with approximately one-quarter cup of hot water until the paste is dissolved. Then add three-quarter cup more hot water and stir well. Drink while hot.

As a soup enhancer, dilute several tablespoons of miso in enough water to form a thin paste, then add it to a simple vegetable soup after you have removed the pot from the heat.

Sea vegetable soups are particularly good with miso.

Sauce Seasonings

Among the more unusual additions to soup are several sauces which are familiar in European kitchens. Made with strong and aromatic ingredients, these should be spooned gingerly over each individual serving of soup.

A mortar and pestle blend of hot chilies, basil, and garlic transforms into a fiery Mediterranean sauce called *rouille* that may be used to enhance fish soups. Another rich sauce pounded from similar ingredients is *pistou*. *Pistou* is a classic sauce spooned over rustic-style vegetable soups. *Aïoli* sauce, a garlic mayonnaise, is used as the base and final touch for a fish soup called *bourride*.

Garnishes

Although the primary consideration is always taste, garnishes that add both texture and color are welcome enhancements for soups. Herbs and vegetables, chopped, sliced, or grated, are the usual choices for garnishing soups. But sometimes a garnish may also add body or depth to a soup. Clear broths or consommés may host a variety of pasta shapes, dumplings, or quenelles. Cheese-, spinach-, or meat-filled pasta served in *brodo,* or in broth, complement the broth's lightness.

A garnish can be simply an edible extra added to improve appearance, though not all soups require this. Sprigs of basil, chopped chives, chervil, watercress leaves, and strips of celery stimulate the appetite and set off a soup's fixed appearance. Julienne vegetables or meat can also enliven a delicate, clear broth. Crisp croutons provide a contrasting texture and flavor for creamy smooth purees.

Some cooks prefer to allow each guest to garnish his or her own soup. In this case, trim and slice vegetables—pepper, carrot, tomato, onion—into small, even pieces and place them in separate bowls on the table.

The world of herbs is almost boundless, but several seem to be particularly popular for garnishing soups. A few peppery leaves of watercress can point up the fine flavor and color of a white cream soup. A sprig of mint may enliven bean or fish soups. And, while the anise flavor of fennel is also used quite often with fish soups, a few basil or parsley leaves can enhance most vegetable soups or purees. Simple soups accept more complex garnishes, but there is no special secret to garnishing properly. Often the cook may decide what flavors to match up based on personal preference.

"Egg rain" adds substance and richer taste to a clear broth. To make egg rain: Mix every two eggs with one tablespoon of whole wheat flour. Beat the batter until very smooth, then drizzle the mixture through a wide, perforated

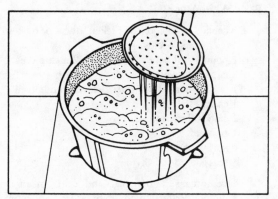

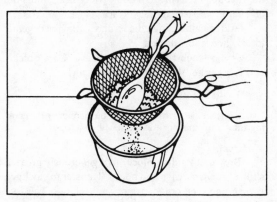

spoon into one quart of simmering broth. Continue to cook for four to five minutes.

Egg garnishings, such as a poached egg floating in a clear broth, sometimes serve as enrichment. Color contrast should be kept in mind, however. Hard-cooked yolk, finely sieved, may be used as a garnish for a simple lentil soup, but it would be lost on a rich cream soup.

Serving Soup

The way a soup is presented often establishes the mood of the meal. In America, deep round soup bowls are most often used. A hearty peasant soup may be ladled directly from the pot into these heavy bowls. A hot luncheon soup may be appropriately served in hand-warming mugs.

In Europe, where soup more often forms part of the supper meal, wide flat soup plates are more prevalent. Soup cools faster in these and they are better suited to the very wide flat soupspoons used there. This European usage also encourages the slurping of soup, a custom not fully embraced by American etiquette.

In most Italian and French homes, a soup tureen is an indispensable piece of kitchenware. This may be of heavy painted pottery or a delicate porcelain such as the legendary *capodimonte* from Naples. These vessels usually hold soups that form the body of a meal—a vegetable puree, fish stew, or potage. They may be placed in the center of the table and each guest served with a wide porcelain ladle.

Soup intended as an appetizer for a meal of several courses would naturally be served in a smaller quantity and in smaller bowls. A rust-colored consommé or stock may be served hot or cold in small crystal or glass bowls to elucidate the theme of an elegant dinner. In Japanese restaurants, garnished clear broths are often served in bright-colored lacquered bowls from which one sips directly.

Chilled soups, such as fruit soups and cold consommés, may be served in small crystalware also, but are equally appealing in double-handled china cups. Serve these soups from a large crystal or glass punch bowl set in a bed of ice to keep them chilled. A bright-hued gazpacho may also be served this way. As a brunch appetizer or summer evening refreshment, this cold vegetable puree should be served in a tall, chilled cocktail glass and garnished with a stalk of celery.

Stocks

Beef Stock

> 3 pounds shin beef, trimmed of fat and cut into chunks
> 5 large onions, halved
> 10 medium-size carrots, halved
> 8 medium-size tomatoes, quartered
> 16 cups cold water
> ½ pound mushrooms
> pepper, to taste

Combine all ingredients in a 6- to 8-quart soup pot. Bring to a boil, reduce heat to low, and simmer for 2 hours, uncovered.

Let sit for 30 minutes, then strain stock through a fine sieve. Cool quickly and refrigerate. When cold, remove fat from top of liquid.

> Yields 4 quarts

NOTE: A richer stock may be made by increasing the cooking time until the stock is reduced by ⅓ to ½.

Basic Brown Stock

> 2 pounds meaty beef bones, sawed into small pieces
> 2 pounds veal shanks, sawed into small pieces
> 1 pound chicken wings
> 3 unpeeled medium-size onions, quartered
> 2 carrots, cut into large pieces
> 20 cups cold water
> 5 sprigs parsley
> 2 sprigs thyme
> 1 leek, cut into large pieces
> 1 stalk celery, cut into large pieces

Preheat oven to 425°F.

Spread bones, shanks, and wings in a shallow 18 × 12-inch roasting pan. Roast until brown, about

1 hour. Turn occasionally to promote even browning. During last 30 minutes of roasting, add onions and carrots.

Transfer bones and vegetables to an 8-quart soup pot. Degrease roasting pan drippings, then add 2 cups water to pan and deglaze it over high heat, scraping up brown bits. Add this liquid to stockpot along with parsley, thyme, leek, celery, and remaining water. Bring to a boil, reduce heat, and simmer very gently, uncovered or partially covered, for 6 hours. Skim off any surface froth that accumulates during first 30 minutes of simmering.

Strain stock through a fine sieve. Cool quickly, then chill in refrigerator. Remove fat that forms on surface of cold stock.

> Yields about 2 quarts

NOTE: A richer stock may be made by increasing the cooking time until the stock is reduced by ⅓ to ½.

Poultry Stock
(Basic White Stock)

> 1 cooked or uncooked chicken, duck, or turkey carcass, broken apart
> 1 pound veal bones, sawed into 2-inch pieces
> 12 cups cold water
> 1 large onion, stuck with 2 cloves and halved
> 1 carrot, halved
> 1 stalk celery, halved
> 1 bay leaf
> 6 sprigs parsley
> ½ teaspoon dried thyme

Place carcass, veal bones, and water in an 8-quart soup pot. Bring to a boil, reduce heat, and skim off scum that rises to the surface.

Add remaining ingredients and simmer very gently for 3½ hours, uncovered.

Strain stock through a fine sieve. Cool quickly and refrigerate. When cold, remove surface fat.

> Yields 5½ to 6 cups

NOTE: A richer stock may be made by increasing the cooking time until the stock is reduced by ⅓ to ½.

Variation:

Browned Poultry Stock: In a generously greased skillet brown carcass and bones. Transfer to stockpot. Brown unpeeled onion, carrot, and celery halves in pan drippings, then transfer these to stockpot. Degrease drippings. Add 1 cup water to skillet and deglaze. Pour brown particles and liquid into stockpot, along with remaining water. Then proceed as above.

Vegetable Stock

    5 large onions, halved
    10 medium-size carrots, halved
    8 medium-size tomatoes, quartered
    1 clove garlic, minced
    5 stalks celery, halved
    1 bunch parsley
    16 cups cold water

Combine all ingredients in a 6- to 8-quart soup pot. Bring to a boil, reduce heat to low, cover, and simmer for 1 hour.

Let sit for 30 minutes and then strain broth through a large sieve. Cool stock, then refrigerate or freeze it.

   Yields 4 quarts

NOTE: A richer stock may be made by continuing to simmer the stock (uncovered), after straining, until it is reduced by $1/3$ to $1/2$.

Court Bouillon

    8 cups cold water
    2 carrots, quartered
    1 large onion or 4 shallots, chopped
    4 scallions or 2 small leeks, chopped
    2 sprigs tarragon or ½ teaspoon dried tarragon
    2 sprigs thyme or ¼ teaspoon dried thyme
    2 bay leaves
    4 sprigs parsley
    10 peppercorns
       juice of 2 lemons

Combine all ingredients except lemon juice. Bring to a boil, then reduce heat and cover pot. Simmer for 30 minutes. Strain broth through a large sieve and add lemon juice. Chill, then refrigerate or freeze.

   Yields about 2 quarts

NOTE: Traditionally, the French replace 1½ cups water with dry white wine in this recipe.

Fish Stock

    2 pounds fish heads, backs, and bones*
    6 cups cold water
       juice of 1 large lemon
    2 large onions, quartered
    3 stalks celery, quartered
    3 carrots, quartered
    1 bay leaf
    10 peppercorns
    3 sprigs parsley
    1 sprig thyme

Place all ingredients in a 5-quart soup pot. Bring to a boil, reduce heat, and simmer, uncovered, for 1 hour. Skim scum off surface if necessary.

Soak a 3-layer piece of cheesecloth in cold water, wring out, and line a large sieve with it. Strain broth through cheesecloth into another large clean pot.

Cool stock and refrigerate or freeze until needed. If large fish heads are used, remove the meat to use in fish soup or salad.

   Yields about 1½ quarts

NOTE: A richer stock may be made by continuing to simmer the stock (uncovered), after straining, until it is reduced by $1/3$ to $1/2$.

*Do not use fatty or oily fish such as salmon, mackerel, or herring.

Garlic Stock

    16 cups cold water
    24 unpeeled cloves garlic, crushed
    4 medium-size carrots, halved
    4 stalks celery, halved
    2 large onions, quartered
    2 turnips, peeled and quartered
    2 sprigs parsley

Combine all ingredients in a 6- to 8-quart soup pot. Bring to a boil, then reduce heat, cover, and simmer for 1 hour. Strain stock through a large sieve. Cool, then refrigerate or freeze it.

   Yields 3 quarts

NOTE: A richer stock may be made by continuing to simmer the stock (uncovered), after straining, until it is reduced by $1/3$ to $1/2$.

Meat and Poultry Soups

Chicken Gumbo

         1 small stewing hen
         8 cups cold water
         1 medium-size onion, chopped
    4 or 5 green shallots
         2 cloves garlic, minced
         1 cup chopped okra
         ½ cup chopped celery leaves
         4 bay leaves
         1 sprig thyme
         2 cups chopped peeled tomatoes
         2 tablespoons chopped fresh parsley

Place chicken and water in a large soup pot. Bring to a boil, then reduce heat, cover, and simmer for 1 to 2 hours, skimming off foam as necessary. Strain stock into a large bowl and skim off all surface fat.

Remove meat from cooked chicken, chop it, and return to pot, along with stock. Add onions, shallots, garlic, okra, celery leaves, bay leaves, and thyme and simmer for 45 minutes. Then add tomatoes and parsley and simmer a few minutes more. Remove bay leaves and serve.

    8 servings

Chicken Soup Julienne

         1 chicken (broiler-fryer), cut into pieces
     6½ cups cold water
         1 large onion, quartered
         2 large carrots
         1 leek
         1 large stalk celery
         1 small zucchini
           pepper, to taste
         ¼ cup chopped fresh parsley

Place chicken in a 4-quart soup pot with water and quartered onion. Slice 1 carrot and add to pot. Bring to a boil, then reduce heat, cover, and simmer for about 3 hours, skimming off foam as necessary.

Remove chicken from pot and reserve. Skim fat from surface of stock. Or, place stock in refrigerator overnight and remove hardened fat from surface the next day. Pour stock (about 5½ cups) into a large clean pot.

Cut leek, celery, and carrot into thin julienne strips about 2 inches long. Do same with zucchini, using only outside part with green skin (discard inner seed section). Add to stock along with pepper. Bring to a boil and simmer, covered, about 10 minutes, or until carrot is almost soft.

Remove meat from ½ of the reserved chicken and chop it into small pieces. Add to stock and heat until hot. Stir in parsley and serve.

    4 to 6 servings

Chunky Beef Soup

         4 cups Beef Stock (page 110)
         ½ cup diced onions
         ½ cup diced celery
         ½ cup diced carrots
         1 cup chopped peeled tomatoes
         1 clove garlic, minced
         1 teaspoon minced fresh oregano
         1 teaspoon minced fresh thyme
         1 tablespoon minced fresh parsley
         1 bay leaf
         ½ cup sliced fresh green beans (1-inch lengths)
         ½ cup fresh corn, cut from the cob
         1 cup diced cooked beef
           minced fresh parsley
           grated cheddar cheese

Combine stock, onions, celery, carrots, tomatoes, garlic, oregano, thyme, parsley, and bay leaf in a large saucepan and place over medium heat. Cover pot and bring to a boil. Reduce heat and simmer for 30 minutes.

Add green beans, corn, and beef. Cover and continue to simmer for 20 minutes longer, or until all vegetables are tender. Remove bay leaf. Serve garnished with parsley and cheese.

    4 servings

Chunky Chicken Soup with Summer Vegetables

         4 cups Poultry Stock (page 110) or Vegetable
           Stock (page 111)
         ½ cup diced onions
         ½ cup diced celery
         ¼ cup diced green peppers
         1 cup chopped peeled tomatoes
         1 tablespoon minced fresh parsley

1 teaspoon minced fresh dill
½ cup fresh corn, cut from the cob
½ cup fresh green peas
2 cups diced green and yellow summer squash
1 cup diced cooked chicken
grated Parmesan cheese
minced fresh dill

Combine stock, onions, celery, green peppers, tomatoes, parsley, and dill in a large saucepan and place over medium heat. Cover pot and bring to a boil. Reduce heat and simmer for 30 minutes.

Add corn. Cover and continue simmering for another 20 minutes. Stir in peas, squash, and chicken. Cover and continue to simmer 10 minutes longer, or until all vegetables are tender. Serve garnished with cheese and dill.

4 to 6 servings

Chunky Turkey Soup with Winter Vegetables

4 cups Poultry Stock (page 110) or Vegetable
Stock (page 111)
1 cup apple juice
½ cup diced peeled sweet potatoes
½ cup diced winter squash
½ cup diced peeled turnip
½ cup diced celery
½ cup diced onions
1 clove garlic, minced
1 tablespoon minced fresh parsley
2 teaspoons minced fresh thyme
1 teaspoon minced fresh rosemary
1 cup broccoli florets
½ cup cooked baby lima beans, drained
1 cup diced cooked turkey
grated Gruyère or Swiss cheese

Combine stock and apple juice in a large saucepan and place over medium heat. Add sweet potatoes, winter squash, turnip, celery, onions, garlic, parsley, thyme, and rosemary. Cover pot and bring to a boil. Reduce heat and simmer for 30 minutes.

Add broccoli, lima beans, and turkey. Cover again and continue simmering for another 20 minutes, or until all vegetables are tender. Serve garnished with cheese.

4 servings

Consommé Madrilene

8 cups rich Beef Stock (page 110) or Poultry
Stock (page 110), or a combination of these
2 egg whites, slightly beaten
2 egg shells, crumbled
3 to 4 medium-size tomatoes (about 1 pound),
diced
¼ teaspoon cayenne pepper (optional)
minced fresh herbs (parsley, tarragon,
and thyme)
peeled, seeded, and finely chopped tomatoes

Using stock, egg whites, and egg shells, prepare a consommé (for directions, see page 105). Add the diced tomatoes and cayenne (if used) to the stock after the egg matter has formed the crustlike dome. Simmer and strain consommé as instructed in consommé directions, then cover and chill. Serve garnished with fresh herbs and chopped tomatoes.

6 to 8 servings

Variation:

Consommé Espagnole: Add ¼ cup minced sweet red or pimiento peppers to the stock, along with the tomatoes. Add minced red or pimiento peppers to the garnish as well.

Egg Drop Soup

2 cups Poultry Stock (page 110) or Vegetable
Stock (page 111)
2 teaspoons soy sauce
1 egg, beaten
½ teaspoon sesame oil
1 tablespoon rice vinegar
2 teaspoons finely sliced scallions

Combine stock and soy sauce in a small saucepan and bring to a boil. Remove from heat. Pour egg very slowly in a thin stream into hot soup. When egg has coagulated, stir slowly. Add oil and vinegar. Serve garnished with scallions.

2 servings

Variation:

Miso-Egg Drop Soup: Blend 1 tablespoon miso in 1 teaspoon water and stir into stock before adding egg.

Mulligatawny Soup

This soup of India came to Western menus by way of the English who once ruled there. The name means "pepper water," a description that can be validated by the intensity and the amount of curry added.

      1 chicken (broiler-fryer)
      ¼ cup plus 2 tablespoons butter
      1 medium-size onion, finely chopped
      1 large carrot, finely chopped
      4 large stalks celery, finely chopped
      1 green pepper, finely chopped
      ½ clove garlic, minced
      ½ cup whole wheat pastry flour
      1 teaspoon curry powder
      4 medium-size tomatoes, chopped
      7 cups Poultry Stock (page 110)
      ¾ cup uncooked brown rice

Debone chicken and cut meat into small pieces. Discard bones and skin.

In a 4-quart heavy-bottom soup pot melt ¼ cup butter. Add chicken meat and brown quickly over high heat. Remove chicken and set aside.

Add remaining butter to pot and sauté onions, carrots, celery, green peppers, and garlic until slightly brown and soft. Remove from heat and add flour, curry powder, tomatoes, and stock. Return to heat and bring to a boil, stirring constantly. Reduce heat, cover, and simmer for 1 hour.

Add rice and bring to a boil, stirring occasionally. Stir in chicken, cover tightly, and simmer for 45 minutes without removing the cover.

      4 to 6 servings

Peanut Butter Soup

      2 tablespoons vegetable oil
      1 medium-size onion, chopped
      1 cup chopped celery
      ¼ cup peanut butter
      2½ cups Poultry Stock (page 110)
      1 cup tomato juice
      ⅛ teaspoon white pepper
      ½ teaspoon ground coriander
      1 cup yogurt

In a medium-size saucepan heat oil and sauté onions and celery until tender. Stir peanut butter into

sautéed mixture. Add stock, tomato juice, pepper, and coriander. Bring to a boil, then reduce heat, cover, and simmer for 10 minutes. Just before serving, stir in yogurt and heat through, but do not boil. Serve hot.

      4 to 6 servings

Garbure
(Bean Soup with Vegetables)

The French word for "bunch" suggested the apt name for this traditional thick soup of southwestern France. It contains cabbage and a bunch of whatever vegetables are at hand, plus almost any kind of available meat for added flavor.

      1 cup dried navy or pea beans
      8 cups water
      2 medium-size potatoes, sliced
      2 medium-size onions, sliced
   1 or 2 leeks, sliced
      2 medium-size turnips, peeled and sliced
      2 medium-size carrots, sliced
      ½ cup dried split peas
      1 bay leaf
      1 teaspoon dried thyme
      1 teaspoon dried marjoram
      ¼ cup minced fresh parsley or 2 tablespoons
         dried parsley
      3 cloves garlic, minced
      1 hot chili pepper
      ½ small head cabbage (about ½ pound),
         shredded
   ½ to 1 pound roasted pork, chicken, goose,
         duck, beef, or other meat (optional)
   8 to 12 cooked pork sausage links, drained
         (optional)
   ⅔ to ¾ cup coarsely chopped roasted chestnuts
         (page 402)
         grated Gruyère or Swiss cheese

Soak navy or pea beans (see page 261 for soaking directions). Drain and set aside.

Bring water to a boil in a large heavy-bottom soup pot. Add potatoes, onions, leeks, turnips, carrots, split peas, bay leaf, thyme, marjoram, parsley, garlic, chili, and soaked beans. Cover and bring quickly to a boil again. Reduce heat and simmer for 1 hour.

Add cabbage and (if used) roasted meat and sausages. Cover and bring quickly to a boil once more, then reduce heat and simmer for 30 minutes.

Discard bay leaf and pepper. Remove meat and sausage (if used), slice it, and put a serving in each bowl. Add soup. Garnish with chestnuts and cheese. Serve with whole wheat or rye bread.

4 to 6 servings

Variation:

Garbure Gratiné: Omit dried beans, split peas, and chestnuts. At the same time cabbage is added to soup, add 1½ cups each fresh fava or lima beans, fresh peas, and sliced fresh green beans (1-inch lengths) as well as ¾ cup diced green peppers. Before serving, pour soup into a large ovenproof casserole or individual ovenproof soup crocks. Place slices of whole grain bread on top of soup and sprinkle with cheese. Set under broiler until cheese is melted and golden.

Turkey and Bean Soup

This soup is a tasty way to use the leftover meat, carcass, and pan drippings from a roasted turkey.

1 cup dried navy beans
½ cup dried black beans
1 roasted turkey carcass
　leftover pan drippings, degreased
2 medium-size onions, quartered
3 stalks celery, with leaves, sliced
3 carrots, sliced
16 cups cold water
¼ cup tomato paste
4 cups chopped cooked turkey
¼ cup plus 1 tablespoon chopped fresh parsley
　pepper, to taste
3 large carrots, diced

In separate bowls, soak navy and black beans (see page 261 for soaking directions). Drain.

In a large heavy-bottom soup pot, place turkey carcass, leftover drippings, onions, celery, and carrots. Add water, and more if necessary, to cover. Bring to a boil, reduce heat, and simmer for 3 hours.

Remove bones and strain stock. Pour stock back into pot and add tomato paste, chopped turkey, parsley, pepper, carrots, and soaked beans. Cook over low heat for at least 3 hours, or until beans are soft.

8 servings

Old-fashioned Chicken-Rice Soup

1 chicken (roaster, 3½ pounds)
12 cups cold water
3 peppercorns
¼ bay leaf
2 sprigs parsley
4 medium-size carrots, cubed
1 stalk celery, with leaves, halved
1 medium-size onion, stuck with 2 cloves
½ cup uncooked brown rice
　chopped fresh parsley

In a large heavy-bottom soup pot, place chicken, water, peppercorns, bay leaf, and parsley sprigs. Bring to a boil and skim foam from surface.

Reduce heat and add carrots, celery, and onion. Cover and simmer for 1 hour, or until chicken is tender.

Lift out chicken and set aside. Remove celery, onion with cloves, and bay leaf and discard. Skim fat from surface of stock, then add rice, cover, and simmer slowly until tender, 30 to 35 minutes.

Meanwhile, remove chicken from bones and cut meat into bite-size pieces. Return chicken to stock and heat thoroughly, about 20 minutes. Garnish with chopped parsley before serving.

6 to 8 servings

Turkey and Zucchini Soup

1 medium-size baking potato, diced
1 large onion, chopped
3 medium-size zucchini, cut into chunks
4 cups Poultry Stock (page 110)
　pepper, to taste
½ teaspoon ground ginger
1¼ cups minced cooked turkey
¼ cup milk

Place potatoes, onions, zucchini, and stock in a large soup pot. Stir in pepper and ginger and bring to a boil. Cover pot and cook over low heat for about 15 minutes, or until potatoes are soft.

Puree soup in a food processor or blender, then return to pot. Add turkey and milk and heat slowly until hot. (Do not allow to boil.)

4 to 6 servings

Legume and Grain Soups

Black Bean Soup

1 cup dried black beans
3 tablespoons vegetable oil
1 medium-size onion, chopped
1 green pepper, chopped
1 stalk celery, chopped
1 carrot, chopped
2 cloves garlic, chopped
2 cups Poultry Stock (page 110)
lemon juice, to taste
chopped fresh chives

Soak beans (see page 261 for soaking directions). Drain, then place in a 4-quart heavy-bottom saucepan and add fresh water to cover. Cover pan and simmer until beans are almost tender, about 2 hours. Drain.

In a large skillet heat oil and add onions, green peppers, celery, carrots, and garlic. Sauté until vegetables are almost tender, then add to beans in pan. Add stock, cover, and simmer until beans are tender, 45 to 60 minutes. Remove from heat and cool slightly.

Puree soup using sieve or food mill, then return to pan. Add lemon juice and heat slowly until hot. Garnish with chives before serving.

6 to 8 servings

German Lentil Soup

3 cups dried lentils
8 cups cold water
1 meaty beef bone
2 medium-size onions, diced
2 medium-size carrots, diced
½ cup diced celery
1 medium-size potato, grated
2 bay leaves
¼ teaspoon dried thyme
½ teaspoon pepper (optional)
2 teaspoons lemon juice

Place lentils in a large heavy-bottom soup pot. Add water, beef bone, vegetables, bay leaves, thyme, and pepper (if used). Bring to a boil over medium heat, then reduce heat, cover, and simmer until lentils and vegetables are tender, about 45 minutes.

Remove bone (do not discard) and bay leaves and skim excess fat from soup.

Remove meat from bone, dice it, and return beef to pot. Slowly stir in lemon juice, then serve immediately.

6 to 8 servings

Greek Lemon Soup
(Avgolemono)

6 cups rich Poultry Stock (page 110)
½ cup uncooked brown rice
1 egg
2 egg yolks
¼ cup lemon juice
2 tablespoons chopped fresh parsley
⅛ teaspoon cayenne pepper
chopped fresh dill

Place stock in a medium-size heavy-bottom saucepan and bring to a boil. Add rice, reduce heat to low, cover, and cook until tender, 30 to 35 minutes.

Place egg and egg yolks in a medium-size bowl and beat with a rotary beater or wire whisk until light and frothy. Slowly add lemon juice, beating thoroughly.

Just before serving, dilute egg-lemon mixture with 1 cup hot stock, beating constantly with a wire whisk until well blended. Then gradually add mixture to remaining hot soup, stirring constantly. Bring almost to the boiling point, but do not boil or the soup will curdle. Stir in parsley and cayenne. Remove from heat and serve immediately, garnished with dill.

4 to 6 servings

Dutch Sour Cream-Bean Soup

4 cups cooked white beans, drained with liquid reserved
1 large onion, grated
⅛ teaspoon pepper
1 tablespoon soy sauce
¾ cup sour cream, at room temperature
¼ cup chopped fresh parsley

Place beans in a large heavy-bottom saucepan and mash lightly. Add 2 cups reserved bean liquid (adding water if necessary to make the full amount). Stir in onions, pepper, and soy sauce and bring to a boil. Remove from heat and fold in sour cream. Garnish with parsley and serve in well-heated soup bowls.

4 servings

Lentil-Sausage Soup

12 ounces fresh pork sausage, cut into bite-size chunks
1 cup chopped leeks
2 cups cooked lentils, drained with liquid reserved
1 teaspoon dried basil
1 cup reserved lentil liquid and/or Vegetable Stock (page 111)
2 cups chopped escarole
1 tablespoon lemon juice

Brown sausage in a large heavy-bottom soup pot. Add leeks and sauté for about 7 minutes. Add lentils, basil, and 1 cup reserved lentil liquid, adding stock if necessary to make the full amount. Cover and simmer for 30 minutes.

Add escarole and cook 10 minutes longer. Just before serving, add lemon juice.

4 to 6 servings

Provençale Bean Stew

2 tablespoons vegetable oil
1 cup chopped onions
2 cups sliced carrots
3 leeks, sliced
1 teaspoon minced garlic
4 cups cooked white beans, drained with liquid reserved
4 cups reserved bean liquid and/or Vegetable Stock (page 111), Poultry Stock (page 110), or water
½ cup chopped fresh parsley
2 bay leaves
1 teaspoon dried thyme
3 whole cloves
2 cups cubed peeled sweet potatoes
2 cups cubed peeled turnips
1 cup cubed peeled kohlrabi
2 cups shredded cabbage, Swiss chard, or spinach
1 teaspoon soy sauce

In a large heavy-bottom soup pot, heat oil. Add onions, carrots, leeks, and garlic and sauté for about 7 minutes. Add beans and reserved liquid, stock, or water, parsley, bay leaves, thyme, cloves, sweet potatoes, turnips, and kohlrabi. Cover and cook slowly for 1 hour, or until vegetables are tender. During cooking, add more liquid if needed to thin stew.

Add cabbage, chard, or spinach, and then soy sauce. Simmer for another 20 minutes. Remove bay leaves and serve.

6 servings

Scotch Broth

4 cups Beef Stock (page 110) or Poultry Stock (page 110)
¾ cup barley
½ cup fresh or frozen peas
2 large carrots
1 small turnip, peeled and diced
1 leek or medium-size onion, chopped
2 cups chopped kale
3 sprigs parsley
pepper, to taste

Place stock in a 4-quart heavy-bottom soup pot and bring to a boil. Add barley and peas, then reduce heat to a simmer.

Coarsely slice 1 carrot and grate the other. Add carrots and remaining ingredients to stock, cover, and simmer for 45 to 60 minutes.

8 servings

Split Pea Soup

2 cups dried split peas
1 meaty beef bone
10 cups cold water
½ cup chopped onions
1 cup diced celery
2 cups finely diced carrots
2 tablespoons vegetable oil
pepper, to taste
1 tablespoon chopped fresh parsley

Place split peas, beef bone, and water in a 4-quart heavy-bottom soup pot. Bring to a boil over medium heat. Reduce heat to low, cover, and simmer.

Meanwhile, sauté onions, celery, and carrots in oil and then stir into soup. Simmer, covered, for 1½ hours, or until split peas are very tender. Season with pepper during last hour of cooking.

Remove beef bone and cut meat from it. Return beef to soup. Garnish with parsley before serving.

6 to 8 servings

Russian Barley Soup

1 small onion, minced
1 tablespoon butter
2 cups Poultry Stock (page 110)
½ cup barley, cooked
¼ teaspoon dillweed
¼ teaspoon ground coriander
½ teaspoon dried mint
1 tablespoon rye or whole wheat flour
2 eggs, beaten
1 cup yogurt
2 tablespoons lemon juice
 chopped fresh parsley
 chopped fresh mint

Sauté onions in butter.

In a large heavy-bottom saucepan bring stock to a boil and stir in onions, cooked barley, and dried herbs. Reduce heat.

In a small bowl, blend flour into eggs, then carefully stir in yogurt. Add a little hot soup to egg and yogurt mixture, gradually stirring it in to avoid "scrambling" the eggs. Pour mixture into pan of hot soup, then stir in lemon juice. Keep hot but do not permit to boil. Add fresh parsley and mint just before serving.

6 servings

Lima Bean Chowder

5 cups cooked lima beans, drained
3 tablespoons butter
1 cup chopped onions
1 cup chopped celery
⅛ to ¼ teaspoon cayenne pepper
2 cups coarsely chopped peeled tomatoes
2 cups fresh or frozen corn
1 tablespoon soy sauce
3 cups milk
3 ounces Monterey Jack cheese, grated

Puree 1 cup of the lima beans in a blender or food processor. Set aside.

Melt butter in a large heavy-bottom soup pot, then add onions and celery and sauté for about 5 minutes. Stir in cayenne, pureed lima beans and remaining whole lima beans, tomatoes, corn, and soy sauce and simmer for 8 to 10 minutes. Add milk and

stir until heated through. (Do not boil.) When ready to serve, garnish individual servings with cheese. Serve immediately.

10 to 12 servings

Vegetable Soups

Borscht

This traditional Russian beef soup improves with overnight aging. It can be served hot or cold.

3 to 4 medium-size beets, peeled and shredded*
4 cups Vegetable Stock (page 111) or Beef Stock (page 110)
2 tablespoons honey
¼ cup vinegar
 soy sauce, to taste
¼ medium-size head cabbage, shredded (about ½ pound)
½ cup tomato puree or tomato juice
 yogurt or sour cream

Combine beets and stock in a large soup pot and cook, covered, over medium heat until beets are tender, 20 to 25 minutes.

Add honey, vinegar, and soy sauce to taste. Add cabbage, cover, and cook until cabbage begins to soften, 7 to 10 minutes. Stir in tomato puree or juice and cook an additional 10 to 15 minutes. Place a dollop of yogurt or sour cream on top of individual servings of soup.

4 to 6 servings

*Cooked or home-canned beets may be substituted. If this is done, use beet water to replace part of the stock.

Corn Chowder

2½ cups water
1 large potato, cubed
1 bay leaf
¼ teaspoon ground sage
1 teaspoon cumin seeds
1 medium-size onion, finely chopped
3 tablespoons butter, melted

3 tablespoons whole wheat flour
1 cup heavy cream, scalded
2 cups fresh corn (cut from 2 to 4 ears)
1 tablespoon minced fresh chives
1 tablespoon minced fresh parsley
1 teaspoon ground nutmeg
   pepper, to taste
¼ cup lemon juice

In a 4-quart soup pot place water, potato, bay leaf, sage, and cumin seeds. Bring to a boil, cover, and simmer until potato is tender, about 15 minutes. Strain out potato water into a separate bowl and reserve.

In a medium-size skillet, sauté onions in butter until translucent. Add flour and mix well. Stirring with a wire whisk, add cream and cook over low heat for 1 minute.

Combine sauce with potatoes in pot. Measure 2 cups reserved potato water and add to pot along with corn, chives, parsley, nutmeg, and pepper. Simmer soup for about 10 minutes. Stir in lemon juice, remove bay leaf, and serve.

4 to 6 servings

Variation:

Corn Chowder with Cheese: Along with lemon juice, stir in 1½ cups grated sharp cheddar cheese and heat until melted.

Leek and Potato Soup

4 cups coarsely chopped potatoes
6 cups Poultry Stock (page 110)
3 cups thinly sliced leeks
½ cup nonfat dry milk
1 cup water
   kelp powder, to taste
   soy sauce, to taste
1 tablespoon vegetable oil
   chopped fresh parsley

Place potatoes in a 4-quart saucepan. Add stock and bring to a boil. Stir in 2 cups leeks and simmer mixture 7 to 10 minutes, or until potatoes are tender. Puree potatoes, leeks, and liquid in a blender or food processor, then return mixture to pan.

Combine dry milk and water with a wire whisk and add to soup. Reheat soup and season with kelp powder and soy sauce.

Sauté remaining leeks in oil until tender. Add to soup just before serving. Garnish with parsley.

6 to 8 servings

Fresh Tomato Soup

½ cup finely diced onions
¼ cup finely diced celery
¼ cup finely diced carrots
2 cloves garlic, minced
2 tablespoons butter or vegetable oil
4 large tomatoes (about 2 pounds), peeled,
   seeded, and finely diced
1 bay leaf
¼ cup minced fresh parsley
1 teaspoon minced fresh thyme or ½ teaspoon
   dried thyme
1 teaspoon minced fresh marjoram or ½
   teaspoon dried marjoram
1 tablespoon minced fresh basil
4 cups Poultry Stock (page 110) or tomato juice
   whipped cream, sour cream, or yogurt
   minced fresh herbs (parsley, chives, basil,
   or chervil)

In a 4-quart soup pot sauté onions, celery, carrots, and garlic in butter or oil until onions are translucent. Add tomatoes, bay leaf, parsley, thyme, marjoram, and basil. Cover and cook over low heat for 10 to 15 minutes, or until mixture is soft and thick.

Gradually stir in stock or juice, cover, and bring to a boil. Reduce heat and simmer gently for 15 to 20 minutes, or until vegetables are soft. Remove bay leaf. Serve garnished with whipped cream, sour cream, or yogurt and minced fresh herbs.

6 servings

Variations:

▪ Garnish with croutons, grated cheese, cooked rice, or cooked tiny soup pasta instead of dairy produce.

▪ Reduce stock to 1 cup and stir into vegetables. Heat 3 cups milk or light cream and stir into soup just before serving. Omit dairy garnish, if desired.

▪ Use 1 teaspoon minced fresh sage instead of basil.

▪ Puree the soup after cooking, then return to heat and warm thoroughly.

▪ Add 1 teaspoon honey with tomatoes and herbs.

Eight-Vegetable Soup with Millet

This recipe makes enough to serve half and freeze half. It is a light whole meal in a soup bowl.

   3 tablespoons butter
   2 medium-size onions, chopped
   4 carrots, chopped
   3 stalks celery, with leaves, chopped
   1 large potato, chopped
   2 small zucchini, chopped
   ½ pound fresh string beans, sliced (about
       2 cups)
   6 cups Poultry Stock (page 110)
   2 medium-size tomatoes, chopped
   1 bay leaf
   ½ teaspoon dried thyme
   3 leaves fresh basil or ½ teaspoon dried basil
   ¼ teaspoon pepper
6 to 8 leaves spinach or Swiss chard, finely
       shredded
   1 cup cooked millet
   1 cup skim milk

Melt butter in a large soup pot. Add onions and sauté until translucent. Then add carrots, celery, potatoes, zucchini, and beans. Stir in stock and tomatoes and bring to a boil. Reduce heat, add herbs and pepper, cover, and simmer for 45 minutes.

Let soup cool, then remove bay leaf and puree using a sieve or food mill. Return to same pot and stir in shredded spinach or chard, millet, and milk. Adjust seasoning, if desired. Simmer for 5 minutes, or until heated through. (Do not allow to boil.)

   12 servings

Minestrone Genovese

Minestrone is what the Italians call a mixed vegetable soup. It is unusual to see a version that calls for eggplant, as this one does.

   ¼ cup olive oil
   2 large eggplants, peeled and diced
   1 medium-size head cabbage, coarsely shredded
       and then chopped
   2 small acorn squashes, peeled and cubed
   1 cup cauliflower florets
   1 cup fresh or frozen lima beans

   ½ pound mushrooms, quartered or sliced
   6 cups Beef Stock (page 110)
   2 medium-size tomatoes, peeled, seeded, and
       coarsely chopped
   pepper, to taste
   chopped fresh parsley
   grated Parmesan cheese

In a large skillet, heat oil and sauté eggplants, cabbage, acorn squash, cauliflower, and lima beans until slightly softened. Transfer to a separate bowl. Add mushrooms to same skillet and sauté lightly. Set aside.

In a large soup pot, heat stock, then add sautéed vegetables, except mushrooms. Cook slowly until tender but not mushy, 7 to 10 minutes.

Add tomatoes and mushrooms during last 5 minutes of cooking, just long enough to heat through but not lose color and texture. Add pepper. Garnish with parsley and serve with bowl of Parmesan cheese.

   8 to 10 servings

Miso-*Wakame* Soup

   3½ ounces dried *wakame*
   2 medium-size onions, quartered and thinly
       sliced lengthwise
   3 tablespoons sesame oil
   3 cloves garlic, minced
   3 stalks celery, thinly sliced on the diagonal
   3 carrots, thinly sliced on the diagonal
   2 cups finely chopped cabbage
   8 cups Vegetable Stock (page 111)
   ¾ teaspoon cayenne pepper
   ½ teaspoon dried rosemary
   3 tablespoons miso
   1 cup finely chopped scallions
   ½ cup thinly sliced radishes

Wash *wakame* under cold running water. Cover with fresh water and soak for 10 minutes. Drain and reserve soaking water. Remove the center vein, then chop *wakame* into ½-inch pieces. Set aside.

In a 4-quart soup pot, sauté onions in oil until translucent. Add garlic, celery, and carrots and sauté for 2 minutes. Toss cabbage and *wakame* in mixture until coated with oil.

Pour stock over vegetables. Add cayenne and rosemary. Bring to a boil and then simmer until all ingredients, including *wakame,* are tender, about 30 minutes.

Dissolve miso in enough reserved soaking water to form a thin paste. Remove soup from heat and stir miso paste into it. Ladle soup into bowls and garnish each bowl with scallions and radishes.

6 to 8 servings

Tomato, Leek, and Onion Soup

¼ cup olive oil
2 medium-size onions, diced
2 leeks, thinly sliced (2 medium-size onions may be substituted)
1 clove garlic, minced
2 tablespoons chopped fresh parsley
1 teaspoon minced fresh thyme
1 bay leaf
2 cups diced peeled tomatoes
3 cups Poultry Stock (page 110) or Beef Stock (page 110)
  soy sauce, to taste
1 to 2 teaspoons honey
  chopped fresh parsley
  chopped scallion tops

In a large skillet heat oil and sauté onions, leeks, and garlic until translucent, but not brown.

Combine sautéed vegetables, parsley, thyme, bay leaf, tomatoes, and stock in a 2-quart saucepan. Cover and simmer until tomatoes are cooked and flavors are well combined, 20 to 30 minutes. Remove bay leaf.

Season with soy sauce and honey. Garnish with parsley and scallions before serving.

4 to 6 servings

Soupe au Pistou

This hearty French vegetable soup is named after the pungent sauce that is added to provide undeniable character.

1 cup dried navy beans
8 cups water
1 large onion, thinly sliced
1 clove garlic, minced
1 large leek, finely sliced
3 medium-size carrots, sliced
3 large potatoes, cubed
1 bouquet garni (celery, parsley, thyme, bay leaf, and 2-inch piece orange rind)
1 cup uncooked whole wheat elbow macaroni
1½ cups sliced fresh green beans (1-inch lengths)
2 small zucchini, sliced
1 medium-size pattypan squash, cubed
  Pistou (see below)

Soak navy beans (see page 261 for soaking directions). Drain, then place in a large heavy-bottom soup pot. Add water and bring to a boil. Add onions, garlic, leek, carrots, potatoes, and bouquet garni to boiling water. Cover and simmer for about 45 minutes, or until beans are soft but still hold their shape.

Add pasta and cook for 5 minutes. Then add green beans, zucchini, and pattypan squash and cook for another 12 minutes, or until pasta is tender. Remove bouquet garni and discard. If soup is too thick, add about 1 cup hot water.

When ready to serve, place *pistou* in a separate bowl so that each diner can stir a portion into his soup before eating.

8 to 10 servings

Pistou

4 large cloves garlic
  pinch of cayenne pepper
⅓ cup packed fresh basil
1 medium-size tomato, peeled, seeded, and chopped
1 cup grated Parmesan cheese
¾ cup olive oil

Mince garlic in a blender or food processor. Add cayenne, basil, tomatoes, and ½ of the cheese. Puree mixture. Slowly add oil—drop by drop—continuing to blend. Add remaining cheese and blend until a coarse sauce is formed. Serve at room temperature.

Pistou will keep 7 to 10 days in the refrigerator in a tightly covered container.

Yields about 2½ cups

NOTE: The *pistou* will naturally separate as it sits, so stir it occasionally.

Whole Garden Soup with Rice and Pesto

This northern Italian soup is thick with lots of vegetables and beans, wholesome, and fragrant with pesto.

2 tablespoons olive oil
1 large onion, coarsely chopped
1 medium-size leek, coarsely chopped
2 cups shredded cabbage
1 small potato, cubed
6 cups cold water
2 large tomatoes (about 1 pound), peeled and
  cut into chunks
¼ pound sliced fresh string beans (about 1 cup)
1 cup cooked cannellini, white kidney, or
  other small white beans, drained
1 cup cooked short grain brown rice
3 leaves Swiss chard, with stems removed,
  shredded
  pinch of crushed red pepper
3 tablespoons Pesto Sauce (page 329)
  grated Parmesan cheese

Heat oil in a heavy 6-quart soup pot. Add onions, leeks, and cabbage and cook, stirring frequently, for 5 minutes. Add potatoes and toss, then add water and tomatoes. Bring to a boil, then reduce heat and cook for 25 minutes, partially covered.

Add string beans, cooked beans, and rice and cook 10 minutes longer. Stir in shredded chard, red pepper, and pesto sauce. Serve hot with grated Parmesan.

6 to 8 servings

Cream Soups

Buttermilk Soup

1 tablespoon whole wheat flour
½ cup water
½ cup raisins
3 tablespoons honey
4 cups buttermilk
2 egg yolks, lightly beaten
  ground cinnamon

In a medium-size saucepan, combine flour, water, raisins, and honey. Place over medium heat, bring to

a boil, then reduce heat to low and simmer for 5 minutes. Gradually add buttermilk and heat to just below boiling point.

Stir a few tablespoons of hot soup into egg yolks, then slowly stir egg yolk mixture into soup and simmer for 2 minutes. (Do not boil.) Garnish with cinnamon and serve immediately.

4 servings

Country Tomato-Carrot Soup

¼ cup olive oil
2 scallions, with tops, chopped
2 cloves garlic, minced
2 stalks celery, with leaves, coarsely chopped
4 cups diced carrots
2 cups chopped Italian-style tomatoes
4 cups Poultry Stock (page 110)
1 tablespoon dried oregano
  milk, for thinning
2 cups yogurt
  thin carrot slices

In a large heavy-bottom soup pot, heat oil. Add scallions and stir. Stir in garlic and remaining vegetables, one at a time. Add stock and oregano. Bring to a boil, then reduce heat, cover, and simmer 10 to 12 minutes, or until vegetables are tender. Stir occasionally.

Remove from heat and cool. Puree vegetables and liquid until smooth, using a food mill or sieve. Return to pot and add milk if a thinner consistency is desired. Reheat if necessary, but do not boil if milk has been added. Just before serving, stir in yogurt and garnish with carrot slices.

6 to 8 servings

Cream of Asparagus Soup

3 cups water
1 pound asparagus
¼ cup finely chopped onions
¼ cup finely chopped celery
1 clove garlic, minced
2 tablespoons butter or vegetable oil
2 tablespoons whole wheat flour
1 cup light cream or milk
1 tablespoon lemon juice
  ground coriander

Bring water to a boil in a medium-size saucepan. Cut 2-inch tips from asparagus spears (reserve remainder) and add to boiling water. Cook about 3 minutes, or until tender. Remove tips from water, cut into ½-inch pieces, and set aside. (Do not discard cooking water.)

Remove woody ends from remainder of spears and pare tough outer fibers, if necessary. Cut into small pieces and place in same cooking water along with onions, celery, and garlic. Cover and bring to a boil again. Reduce heat and simmer for 30 minutes.

Puree mixture using a sieve or food mill. Set puree aside.

Heat butter or oil in a 3-quart saucepan. Stir in flour and cook for a few minutes, but do not brown. Gradually add cream or milk, stirring constantly until smooth. Cook over medium heat for 5 minutes, or until thickened. Add asparagus puree and lemon juice, stirring constantly. Heat through, but do not boil. Serve garnished with reserved asparagus tips and a sprinkling of coriander.

4 to 6 servings

Variations:

Creamy Asparagus-Cheese Soup: Before adding asparagus puree, add ½ cup grated Swiss, cheddar, or Parmesan cheese to thickened white sauce and stir until cheese is melted and sauce is smooth.

Zesty Cream of Asparagus Soup: Add 1 teaspoon each French-style mustard and grated horseradish to thickened white sauce.

Cream of Cauliflower Soup

2 tablespoons butter
1 small onion, chopped
1 cup Beef Stock (page 110) or Poultry Stock (page 110)
2 large potatoes, diced
1 small head cauliflower (about 1 pound), broken into florets
½ cup boiling water
⅛ teaspoon ground coriander
⅛ teaspoon ground nutmeg
½ teaspoon white pepper
2 cups half-and-half
chopped fresh chives, watercress, or parsley

In a large saucepan, melt butter. Add onions, and sauté until soft. Add stock and potatoes, cover, and cook for 7 to 10 minutes, or until potatoes are tender. Puree potato mixture using a blender or food processor, then return it to saucepan.

Meanwhile, in another saucepan, cook cauliflower in the water for about 7 minutes, or until barely tender. (Do not drain.) Remove 1 cup florets with a slotted spoon and reserve. Puree remaining cauliflower with its cooking water, then add this to potato mixture.

Cut reserved florets into very small pieces (½-inch lengths) and set aside.

Add coriander, nutmeg, and pepper to soup and simmer for 3 minutes. Stir in half-and-half, then add reserved florets. Heat through but do not boil the soup. Garnish each serving with chives, watercress, or parsley.

4 to 6 servings

Cream of Chicken Soup

½ cup diced onions
½ cup diced carrots
½ cup diced celery
⅔ cup diced mushrooms
1 cup diced cooked chicken
1 tablespoon minced fresh parsley
1 teaspoon minced fresh rosemary
3 cups Poultry Stock (page 110)
3 tablespoons butter or vegetable oil
3 tablespoons whole wheat flour
1 cup light cream or milk
1 egg, beaten
½ cup cooked fresh peas
chopped fresh parsley

Combine onions, carrots, celery, mushrooms, chicken, minced parsley, rosemary, and stock in a large saucepan. Cover and bring to a boil, then reduce heat and simmer for 30 minutes.

Puree mixture using a sieve or food mill. Return to saucepan.

Heat butter or oil in a small saucepan. Stir in flour, then heat for several minutes longer, but do not brown. Gradually add cream or milk, stirring constantly. Cook until slightly thickened.

Stir a little hot sauce into egg, then add egg mixture to remaining sauce. Add to pureed soup, along with peas. Heat through but do not boil. Serve garnished with chopped parsley.

4 to 6 servings

Cream of Broccoli Soup

1 small head broccoli (about 1½ pounds)
1 cup minced onions
½ cup sliced celery
1 leek, sliced
1 clove garlic, minced
2 tablespoons butter
6 cups Poultry Stock (page 110)
2 cups light cream
  pepper, to taste

Coarsely chop broccoli stems and set florets aside.
In a 3-quart saucepan, sauté onions, celery, leeks, and garlic in butter over low heat for 20 minutes. Add chopped broccoli stems and stock. Bring to a boil, then reduce heat, cover, and simmer for 15 minutes. Add florets and simmer 15 minutes longer.

Puree mixture, using a food mill or sieve, and return to pan. Add cream and bring soup to a simmer. (Do not boil.) Season with pepper and serve.

6 servings

Cream of Carrot Soup

2 tablespoons butter
4 medium-size carrots, thinly sliced
1 small onion, sliced
1 teaspoon chopped fresh tarragon or ½
    teaspoon dried tarragon
1 teaspoon lemon juice
1½ cups water
1 cup heavy cream, scalded
2 egg yolks, lightly beaten
1 scallion, minced

Melt butter in a large saucepan. Add carrots and onions and sauté over medium heat for 1 to 2 minutes, or until onions are translucent. Add tarragon, lemon juice, and water. Bring to a boil, then reduce heat, cover, and simmer for 10 minutes.

Place carrot mixture in a blender or food processor and add cream. Process on low speed until smooth. (Do not remove soup from container yet.) Stir a little pureed soup into yolks, then add yolk mixture to rest of soup and process again on low speed. To serve, reheat soup if necessary (do not boil) and garnish with scallions.

4 servings

Cream of Endive Soup

2 tablespoons butter
6 scallions, finely chopped
4 cups finely chopped endive
1 pound carrots, diced
¼ teaspoon pepper
1 tablespoon plus 1 teaspoon minced fresh mint
1½ teaspoons minced fresh marjoram
2 cups Poultry Stock (page 110)
1 cup light cream
1½ cups milk
2 tablespoons cornstarch
  mint sprigs or chopped scallions

Melt butter in a 2- to 3-quart saucepan. Add finely chopped scallions, endive, and carrots. Cover and sauté, stirring occasionally, for 10 minutes. Add pepper, minced mint and marjoram, and stock. Bring to a boil, then reduce heat, cover, and simmer for 10 minutes.

Puree mixture in two batches, using a blender or food processor. Return puree to saucepan. Add cream and all but 2 tablespoons milk. Heat over medium heat until soup begins to simmer.

Dissolve cornstarch in remaining 2 tablespoons milk and slowly stir into soup. Bring to just below a boil, then reduce heat and simmer, stirring occasionally, for 5 minutes. Serve garnished with mint sprigs or chopped scallions.

4 servings

Cream of Fresh Green Pea Soup

4 cups fresh peas
6 cups milk
4 sprigs marjoram, minced, or ¼ teaspoon dried
    marjoram
1 sprig thyme
2 leaves fresh mint (optional)
  pepper, to taste

Place a small amount of water in a 2-quart saucepan and bring to a boil; reduce heat and add peas. Simmer for 5 to 10 minutes (do not allow to boil), then drain.

Place 1 cup peas in a blender or food processor. Add 1½ cups milk and herbs and process on low speed until smooth. Pass mixture through a sieve into the top of a double boiler. Repeat process with remaining peas and milk.

Heat soup through, but do not boil. Season with pepper and serve.

8 servings

Cream of Leek Soup

1 cup Poultry Stock (page 110)
4 cups milk
4 leeks
4 scallions
2 medium-size onions, diced
1 teaspoon dried rosemary
1 teaspoon dried thyme
    white pepper, to taste
1 cup cubed sharp cheddar cheese

In a large soup pot, gently heat stock and milk. (Do not boil.)

Cut green portions of leeks and scallions into ½-inch pieces and cut white bulbs into ¼-inch pieces. Add to soup pot. Stir in onions, rosemary, thyme, pepper, and cheese. Cook over low heat, stirring constantly, until cheese melts.

4 servings

Cream of Mushroom Soup

2 tablespoons butter or vegetable oil
½ pound mushrooms, finely chopped
¼ cup finely chopped onions
1 clove garlic, minced
1 tablespoon minced fresh parsley
⅛ teaspoon ground nutmeg
    dash of cayenne pepper or hot pepper sauce
1 tablespoon whole wheat flour
2 cups Beef Stock (page 110), Poultry
    Stock (page 110), or Vegetable
    Stock (page 111)
1 cup light cream, sour cream, yogurt, or milk
    chopped fresh parsley

In a 2-quart saucepan heat butter or oil. Add mushrooms, onions, garlic, parsley, nutmeg, and cayenne or pepper sauce and sauté until mushrooms soften and lose their liquid. Sprinkle flour over mixture and continue cooking for several minutes. Gradually add stock, stirring constantly. Bring to a boil, then reduce heat, cover, and simmer for 15 minutes.

Puree mixture using a blender or food processor, then return to saucepan. Stir in cream, sour cream, yogurt, or milk and heat thoroughly, but do not boil. Serve garnished with chopped parsley.

4 servings

Sunshine Soup

This sun-colored soup is an appetizing answer to the annual squash deluge. The peanut butter garnish is delightful.

1 medium-size onion, halved
⅓ stalk celery, chopped
1 sprig thyme or ½ teaspoon dried thyme
1 sprig savory or ½ teaspoon dried savory
1 cup chopped tomatoes
2 cups Poultry Stock (page 110)
3 to 4 cups cubed peeled acorn, pumpkin,
    butternut, or hubbard squash
1 medium-size potato, cubed
½ cup nonfat dry milk
½ cup milk
1 tablespoon peanut butter

Place onion, celery, thyme, savory, tomatoes, and stock in the bottom of a 2-quart steamer. Place squash and potato cubes in top container of steamer. Cover and steam for 15 to 20 minutes, or until vegetables are very tender.

Remove squash and potato cubes and puree through a sieve or food mill until perfectly smooth. Place puree in a large saucepan. Pour stock mixture through sieve into pureed vegetables (discard residue). Simmer until slightly thickened.

Stir dry milk and milk together until smooth. Use several tablespoons of it to thin peanut butter to a smooth consistency. (The mixture should be as thick as heavy cream.) Add remaining milk to pureed soup and heat through but do not boil. Just before serving, garnish by swirling peanut butter mixture on top of soup.

4 to 6 servings

Cream of Sorrel Soup

¾ to 1 pound fresh sorrel
    ¼ cup butter or vegetable oil
    ¼ cup minced scallions
    ¼ cup whole wheat flour
    4 cups Poultry Stock (page 110)
    1 cup light cream or milk, or more if needed
        minced fresh chives
        minced fresh sorrel

Remove stems from sorrel and cut leaves into thin strips.

In a large saucepan, heat butter or oil. Add scallions and sauté until soft. Stir in sorrel, cover, and cook over low heat for 3 to 5 minutes, or until leaves have thoroughly wilted. Sprinkle flour over sorrel mixture and stir over medium heat for 2 to 3 minutes (do not brown). Gradually add stock, stirring constantly. Bring to a boil, then reduce heat and simmer for 5 minutes.

Puree mixture using a blender or food processor, then return to saucepan over low heat.

In a small saucepan, thoroughly heat cream or milk (do not boil). Gradually stir this into soup. Serve hot or chilled. (Thin if necessary, with additional cream or milk.) Garnish with minced chives and sorrel before serving.

4 to 6 servings

Variation:

Enriched Cream of Sorrel Soup: Beat 2 egg yolks into cream or milk before heating.

Cream of Watercress Soup

    1 tablespoon safflower oil
    1 tablespoon butter
    4 scallions, chopped
    1 large bunch watercress, with stems, coarsely
        chopped
        dash of ground nutmeg
    1½ cups Poultry Stock (page 110)
    1 cup light cream
        parsley sprigs

Heat oil and butter in a large saucepan. Add scallions and sauté over low heat. Add watercress and stir over medium heat until wilted. Stir in nutmeg and

stock. Bring to a boil, then reduce heat, cover, and simmer for 8 to 10 minutes.

Puree mixture using a blender or food processor, then return to saucepan. Add cream and heat through (do not boil). Serve garnished with parsley.

4 servings

Sour Cream-Potato Soup

    2 cups grated potatoes
    3 cups Beef Stock (page 110), Poultry Stock
        (page 110), or water
    1 medium-size onion, sliced or diced
    ½ teaspoon pepper
    1 cup sour cream
    ¼ cup chopped fresh parsley

Place potatoes, stock or water, onions, and pepper in a 2-quart saucepan. Bring to a boil, then reduce heat, cover, and simmer for 15 minutes, or until vegetables are tender. Stir in sour cream and heat to just below the boiling point. Serve hot, topped with parsley.

6 servings

Panades (Bread Soups)

Onion Soup Gratiné

    ½ cup butter
    3½ pounds Bermuda onions, thinly sliced
    1 teaspoon honey
    1 tablespoon whole wheat flour
    1 clove garlic, minced
    7 cups Beef Stock (page 110)
    ½ bay leaf
    ¼ teaspoon pepper

    Topping
    6 slices stale whole grain or French bread
    2 tablespoons butter, melted
    1 tablespoon olive oil
    ¼ cup grated Gruyère cheese
    ¼ cup grated Parmesan cheese

Melt butter in a 4-quart soup pot. Add onions. Stir and cook over low heat until onions are translucent, about 20 minutes. Add honey. Increase heat to medium and continue cooking until onions are a rich golden color, about 20 minutes more. Sprinkle with flour, add garlic, and stir for a few minutes. Add stock, bay leaf, and pepper and bring to a boil. Then reduce heat, partially cover, and simmer 45 minutes longer. Remove bay leaf.

To make topping: Place bread on a baking sheet. Combine melted butter with oil and spread over bread. Mix cheeses together and sprinkle bread evenly with ¼ cup of mixture. Place under broiler for a few minutes until cheese melts.

Preheat oven to 350°F.

Pour soup into an 8- or 10-cup ovenproof casserole, float bread on top, and sprinkle remaining cheese over bread. Bake for 20 minutes, or until a melted crust of cheese has formed on top of soup.

6 servings

Provincial Bread Soup

> 3 tablespoons butter or vegetable oil
> ¾ cup diced onions
> ¼ cup diced celery
> 4 cups Poultry Stock (page 110) or Vegetable
>   Stock (page 111)
> ¼ cup minced fresh parsley
> 1 teaspoon minced fresh thyme
> 1 bay leaf
> 4 cups diced stale whole wheat bread
> 1 tablespoon whole wheat flour
> 1 cup light cream or milk
> 1 egg, beaten
>   chopped fresh parsley
>   grated nutmeg

In a large soup pot, heat 2 tablespoons butter or oil and sauté onions and celery until soft and golden. Add stock, parsley, thyme, bay leaf, and bread. Cover and bring to a boil, then reduce heat and simmer for 30 minutes. Remove bay leaf.

Puree mixture using a sieve or food mill. Return puree to soup pot.

Heat remaining 1 tablespoon butter or oil in a small saucepan. Stir in flour and heat for several minutes longer, but do not brown. Gradually add cream or milk, stirring constantly. Cook until slightly thickened.

Stir a little hot sauce into egg, then add egg mixture to remaining sauce. Add to pureed soup and blend thoroughly. Heat through, but do not boil. Serve garnished with chopped parsley and nutmeg.

4 to 6 servings

Variation:

Vegetable-Bread Soup: Before pureeing add ½ cup cooked greens (such as sorrel, watercress, spinach, lettuce, or chard) or cooked mixed vegetables to bread mixture.

Chilled Soups

Chilled Broccoli Soup

> 2 tablespoons butter or vegetable oil
> ½ cup diced onions
> 1 clove garlic, minced
> 1 small head broccoli (about 1 pound), coarsely
>   chopped
> 4 cups Poultry Stock (page 110) or Vegetable
>   Stock (page 111)
> 1 tablespoon minced fresh parsley
> ½ teaspoon minced fresh rosemary
> 1 tablespoon lemon juice
> ¾ cup light cream, sour cream, yogurt, or milk
>   chopped fresh parsley

In a 3-quart saucepan, heat butter or oil and sauté onions and garlic until translucent. Add broccoli, stock, and minced herbs. Cover and bring to a boil, then reduce heat and simmer for 15 minutes, or until broccoli is tender.

Puree mixture using a strainer or food mill. Place puree in a bowl and add lemon juice. Cover and refrigerate until chilled.

Just before serving, stir in cream, sour cream, yogurt, or milk and blend thoroughly. Or, if using sour cream or yogurt, place a dollop on top of each serving instead. Garnish with chopped parsley.

4 to 6 servings

Variation:

Chilled Broccoli Soup, Indian Style: While onions and garlic are sautéing, sprinkle over them ¼ teaspoon each ground cumin, turmeric, coriander, cloves, cardamom, and cayenne pepper. Garnish chilled soup with minced scallions.

Chilled Carrot Soup

1 pound carrots, thinly sliced (about 2½ cups)
½ cup diced onions
1 clove garlic, minced
½ cup uncooked brown rice
3 cups cold water
2 cups apple juice
1 tablespoon lemon juice
1 cup light cream, sour cream, yogurt, or milk
   minced fresh herbs (parsley, dill, chives,
   or chervil)

Place carrots, onions, garlic, rice, water, and apple juice in a 3-quart saucepan. Cover and bring to a boil, then reduce heat and simmer until carrots and rice are tender, about 45 minutes.

Puree mixture using a blender or food processor. Place pureed soup in a bowl, then add lemon juice, cover, and chill.

Before serving, stir in cream, sour cream, yogurt, or milk and blend thoroughly. Or, add a dollop of sour cream or yogurt to top of individual servings. Garnish with minced herbs.

4 to 6 servings

Variations:

Cold and Zesty Carrot Soup: Stir in 1 teaspoon each grated horseradish and French-style mustard during cooking.

Cold Orange-Carrot Soup: Omit garlic. Substitute 2 cups orange juice for apple juice, and add ½ teaspoon ground ginger before cooking. Garnish with grated nutmeg.

Chilled Mint-Pea Soup

3 cups fresh peas
1½ cups shredded lettuce
½ cup sliced scallions
3 tablespoons minced fresh mint
2 cups water
⅓ cup light cream, sour cream, or yogurt
   chopped fresh mint

Place peas, lettuce, scallions, minced mint, and water in a 3-quart saucepan, cover, and bring to a boil. Reduce heat and simmer until peas are very tender, about 20 minutes.

Puree mixture through a strainer or food mill. Place puree in a covered container and refrigerate until chilled.

Just before serving, stir in cream, sour cream, or yogurt and blend thoroughly. Or, place a dollop of sour cream or yogurt on individual servings of soup. Garnish with chopped mint.

4 to 6 servings

Cold Melon Soup

1 large ripe cantaloupe
¼ teaspoon ground cinnamon (optional)
2½ cups orange juice
3 tablespoons lime juice
   mint sprigs

Remove seeds and membrane from melon. Peel and cut pulp into cubes.

Place cantaloupe, cinnamon (if used), and ½ cup orange juice in a blender or food processor and puree.

Combine remaining orange juice with lime juice and then stir into puree. Pour mixture into a bowl, cover, and refrigerate at least 1 hour before serving.

When ready to serve, stir mixture and pour into soup tureen or individual soup bowls. Garnish with mint.

4 to 6 servings

Gazpacho

6 medium-size tomatoes, peeled and chopped
   (3 cups)
½ cup finely chopped onions
1 cucumber, peeled, seeded, and diced
½ cup finely chopped green peppers
1 small clove garlic, minced
3 tablespoons chopped fresh parsley
2 tablespoons chopped fresh chives
2 cups tomato juice
⅓ cup red wine vinegar
¼ cup olive oil
¼ teaspoon cayenne pepper
   thin cucumber slices

In a large bowl, combine tomatoes, onions, cucumbers, green peppers, garlic, parsley, and chives. Add tomato juice, vinegar, oil, and cayenne and mix well.

Cover bowl and refrigerate for at least 2 hours to chill and blend flavors. Serve soup "ice cold." Garnish with cucumber.

4 to 6 servings

Strawberry Soup

3¾ cups sliced fresh strawberries
5 tablespoons honey
2½ tablespoons cornstarch, dissolved in ½ cup orange juice
½ cup sour cream or yogurt

Place strawberries in a medium-size bowl. Add 3 tablespoons honey and stir well to coat berries evenly. Set aside for 1 hour or so.

Drain berries. You should have about 1½ cups strawberry juice and 2¼ cups berries. Pour juice into blender or food processor and add ½ of the berries. Process to a very liquid puree.

Place puree in a 2-quart saucepan and heat to the boiling point. Stir cornstarch mixture into boiling puree. Cook 1 to 2 minutes, or until clear and thickened. Cool slightly. Add remaining honey and strawberries. Chill thoroughly.

Serve with a dollop of sour cream or yogurt on top of each bowl. Or, if desired, make a creamy soup by first stirring a little soup into sour cream or yogurt, to thin it, and then add this mixture to remaining soup. Chill completely before serving.

4 to 6 servings

Swiss Cherry Soup

½ cup raisins
¼ cup lemon juice
1 stick of cinnamon, 2 inches long
6 thin slices navel orange
5 thin slices lemon
3 cups water
2 cups pitted fresh sweet cherries
2 cups sliced peeled peaches
⅓ cup honey
2 tablespoons cornstarch, dissolved in ¼ cup cold water
yogurt

In a medium-size saucepan, combine raisins, lemon juice, cinnamon stick, orange slices, and lemon slices. Add water. Place over medium heat and bring to a boil. Reduce heat, cover, and simmer for 15 minutes. Remove cinnamon stick.

Add cherries, peaches, and honey to soup mixture and bring to a boil. Slowly add cornstarch mixture to hot soup. Cook, stirring constantly, until soup is clear, about 2 to 3 minutes. Remove saucepan from heat, immediately pour soup into a bowl, and cool.

Cover and place in refrigerator for several hours or overnight. Serve chilled soup accompanied by yogurt.

6 to 8 servings

Frosty Tomato Soup

2 cups tomato juice
1 small onion, stuck with 3 cloves
1 bay leaf
1 envelope unflavored gelatin
¼ cup lemon juice
1½ tablespoons honey
dash of cayenne pepper
2 egg whites
yogurt
radish roses

Place 1 cup tomato juice in a 1-quart saucepan. Add onion and bay leaf, cover, and simmer gently for 10 minutes.

Pour remaining tomato juice into a small bowl and sprinkle gelatin on top. Set aside for 5 minutes to soften. Then add to hot juice in saucepan along with lemon juice, honey, and cayenne. Stir until gelatin is completely dissolved. Strain mixture through a sieve into a shallow pan (discard residue) and place pan in freezer for about 1 hour.

Beat egg whites until stiff but not dry. Remove mixture from freezer and place in a deep bowl. Beat well until smooth. Fold beaten egg whites into tomato mixture and return to freezer until serving time.

To serve, scoop frappé into stemmed glasses, garnish each with a dollop of yogurt and a radish rose. Serve immediately.

4 to 6 servings

Vichyssoise

2 tablespoons butter or vegetable oil
3 cups thinly sliced leeks (green tops only)
1/3 cup diced celery
1 tablespoon minced fresh parsley
1½ cups diced potatoes
3 cups Poultry Stock (page 110) or Vegetable
    Stock (page 111)
1 cup light cream, sour cream, or yogurt
    chopped fresh chives and parsley
    ground nutmeg

Heat butter or oil in a 3-quart saucepan. Add leeks, celery, and minced parsley. Cover and cook over low heat for 10 to 15 minutes, or until vegetables are limp and golden. Stir in potatoes and stock, then cover and bring to a boil. Reduce heat and simmer until potatoes are very tender, about 30 minutes.

Puree mixture using a strainer or food mill. Pour puree into a bowl, then cover and chill thoroughly. Before serving, stir in cream, sour cream, or yogurt. (Or, if desired, heat soup, then stir a little of it into cream, sour cream or yogurt before adding this to pot of soup; serve hot.) Garnish with chopped herbs and nutmeg.

4 to 6 servings

Seafood Soups

Bourride

2 pounds cod, flounder, bass, or haddock fillets,
    or a combination of these
1 medium-size onion, sliced
1 bay leaf
1 teaspoon dried fennel
1 teaspoon dried thyme
2 cloves garlic, minced
1 piece orange rind, 3 inches long
4 medium-size tomatoes, peeled, seeded, and
    quartered
8 cups water or Fish Stock (page 111)
    pepper, to taste
    Aïoli Sauce (page 144)
12 slices French bread

Cut fish in pieces. Place in a large soup pot with all other ingredients except aïoli sauce and bread.

Cover and simmer over medium-high heat for 10 to 15 minutes, or until fish is tender.

Pour soup through a strainer into a pot or bowl. Remove fish from strainer and discard residue. Slowly stir 1/3 of the aïoli sauce into broth. Serve soup over slices of French bread placed in individual soup crocks. Fish may be served separately or with soup, along with rest of aïoli.

12 servings

Bouillabaisse

This is an all-shellfish version of the famous fish stew of Marseilles. The original is a melange of fin fish and shellfish based on the bounty at hand.

1/3 cup olive oil
½ medium-size onion, chopped
½ cup chopped leeks
1 tablespoon minced garlic
3 medium-size tomatoes, peeled, seeded, and
    finely chopped
¼ cup plus 1 tablespoon tomato paste
2 bay leaves
½ teaspoon saffron
6 fennel seeds
5 cups Fish Stock (page 111) or clam juice
    pepper, to taste
1 tablespoon lemon juice
1 pound uncooked lobster (either whole or
    tails), cut into 4 sections*
1 pound uncooked medium-size shrimp, peeled
    and deveined*
1 pound fresh or frozen crab meat, cartilage
    removed*

Topping
1 tablespoon finely chopped pimiento
1 to 2 red chili peppers, steamed until tender
    (dried chili peppers may be substituted)
3 cloves garlic, minced
1/3 cup olive oil
1 tablespoon minced fresh parsley
½ cup whole grain bread crumbs

Heat oil in a large soup pot. Add onions and leeks and sauté until soft. Add garlic and sauté 1 minute longer. Stir in tomatoes, tomato paste, bay leaves, saffron, and fennel seeds. Add stock or clam juice and pepper. Cover and simmer over moderate heat for 25 minutes.

Add lemon juice and lobster and cook for 10 minutes. Stir in shrimp and crab meat and simmer 10 minutes longer. Remove from heat and discard bay leaves.

Remove shell from lobster. Cut meat into chunks and return to pot.

To make the topping: Place pimientos in a small bowl and crush with a fork. Finely chop chili peppers, then add to bowl along with garlic, oil, and parsley. Soak bread crumbs in water to cover for a minute or so, then squeeze out excess moisture and add to bowl. Blend entire mixture into a paste.

To serve, pass bread crumb mixture at the table for diners to spoon into individual bowls of hot bouillabaisse.

6 to 8 servings

*Clams, mussels, or other shellfish may be substituted for the ones listed above, depending on preference and availability.

Clam Chowder, New England Style

3 dozen clams
4 cups water
2 tablespoons plus 1 teaspoon butter
1 medium-size onion, chopped
1 stalk celery, finely chopped
3 medium-size potatoes, diced
1 bay leaf
2 cups heavy cream
    pepper, to taste
    parsley sprigs

Wash clams and place in a large pot. Add water and 1 teaspoon butter, then cover pot and steam until shells open, about 8 to 10 minutes. Remove clams from shells and chop. Strain broth into a bowl through a double layer of cheesecloth set in a large sieve. Reserve both clams and broth.

Melt remaining 2 tablespoons butter in a large saucepan. Add onions and celery and sauté until soft. Stir in reserved clam broth, then add potatoes and bay leaf. Bring to a boil, then reduce heat and cook until potatoes are tender, 7 to 10 minutes. Remove

from heat and take out bay leaf. Add cream, chopped clams, and pepper. Heat through but do not boil. Garnish each serving with a sprig of parsley.

6 to 8 servings

Lobster Bisque

¼ cup plus 1 tablespoon olive oil
½ cup chopped carrots
½ cup chopped celery
½ cup chopped onions
2 uncooked lobsters or lobster tails, each cut
    into 3 sections
2 cups Fish Stock (page 111)
1 tablespoon lemon juice
1 bay leaf
1 teaspoon dry mustard
2 tablespoons butter
2 tablespoons whole wheat flour
1 cup milk
1 teaspoon soy sauce
1 cup heavy cream
    several dashes of ground nutmeg
    pepper, to taste

In a large soup pot heat oil and sauté vegetables for 5 minutes. Add lobster sections and toss for several minutes. Stir in stock, lemon juice, bay leaf, and mustard, cover, and simmer over low heat for 5 minutes. Remove lobster from pot and allow to cool so that lobster meat may be extracted from shells. Continue cooking vegetable and stock mixture.

Break shells into pieces or pound with a mortar, then put shell fragments through a food grinder or fine sieve. Dice lobster meat and set aside.

Remove bay leaf from stock. Mix ground shells with vegetables and stock and puree mixture through a sieve or food mill.

In a medium-size saucepan, melt butter. Stir in flour, then slowly add milk and continue stirring until mixture has thickened, about 5 minutes. This should be done over moderate heat, making sure it does not boil. Add puree and soy sauce. Stir and cook over low heat for 10 minutes. (Do not allow to boil or soup may curdle.) Add cream, nutmeg, and diced lobster. Stir and cook for 5 minutes. Serve garnished with pepper.

4 to 6 servings

Fish Chowder

  1 pound haddock, cod, perch, or other firm-
    fleshed white fish, gutted
  3 cups water
  ½ cup apple juice
  2 tablespoons butter or vegetable oil
  ¾ cup diced onions
  ¼ cup diced celery
  ¼ cup diced green peppers
  ¼ cup diced carrots
  2 cups diced potatoes
  2 cups light cream or milk
  2 tablespoon minced fresh parsley
  2 tablespoons minced fresh fennel
  1 teaspoon minced lemon rind
    butter
    paprika
    chopped scallions and fresh parsley

Place fish in a large saucepan. Add water and apple juice and bring to a boil. Then reduce heat, cover, and simmer until fish is tender and flakes easily with a fork, about 10 to 15 minutes. Remove fish from stock and set both aside.

In a large soup pot, heat butter or oil and sauté onions, celery, green peppers, and carrots until soft, about 5 minutes. Add potatoes and reserved stock, cover, and bring to a boil. Reduce heat and simmer for 30 to 45 minutes, or until potatoes are tender.

Remove any skin or bones from cooked fish, then cut fish into 1-inch pieces and add to soup. Stir in cream or milk and minced parsley, fennel, and lemon rind. Heat thoroughly but do not boil. To serve, garnish each bowl of hot chowder with a pat of butter, paprika, and chopped scallions and parsley.

  6 servings

Variation:
  Fish Chowder, Manhattan Style: Add ½ cup tomato sauce or ¼ cup tomato paste with potatoes and stock.

Shrimp Bisque

  3 tablespoons butter
  1 carrot, sliced
  2 scallions, chopped, or 2 leeks (white part
    only), sliced
  1 pound uncooked medium-size shrimp, peeled
    and deveined
  ¼ cup uncooked brown rice
  1 bay leaf
  1 teaspoon dried thyme
  3 sprigs parsley
    pepper, to taste
    dash of cayenne pepper
    dash of paprika
  2 medium-size tomatoes, chopped
  8 cups water
  ¾ cup heavy cream or half-and-half

Melt butter in a 4-quart soup pot. Add carrots, scallions or leeks, and shrimp and sauté lightly. Add rice, herbs, seasonings, tomatoes, and water and simmer, uncovered, for about 40 minutes.

Remove bay leaf and parsley, then puree mixture through a strainer or food mill. Return to pot, add cream, and cook over low heat just until heated through. Do not boil.

  10 servings

Sauces

Well-conceived sauces—simple and delicate, or rich and spicy—can elevate even the most routine dishes. Today's versions of the classics are much more simplified, free from most of the tedium once associated with fine saucery. True, some cooks still fancy the time-honored methods that take so long and require so much care, but there are accepted new ways to turn out first-class sauces quickly and with minimal effort. For example, you can use a food processor or a blender to speed up the preparation of numerous sauces that once required extended, cautious beating or whipping by hand.

Although many of the best-known sauces originated in France, the cuisine of virtually every country includes several sauces which exalt its favorite dishes. French cuisine frequently weds the flavors of meat, fish, fowl, or vegetable dishes with a gentle steeping of sauce; for Italian pasta, a wide range of sauces, from delicate Alfredo to a hearty tomato, may grace the occasion. Asian cooking, distinguished by its restraint, has its own techniques of saucing food with basic and healthful ingredients. Sauces also play some totally functional roles, as in thickening cream soups or binding casseroles and croquettes.

Though often elementary in composition, sauces tend to border on the extravagant and require a certain amount of discretion in their preparation and use. Sauces based on cream, butter, and eggs are likely to be very rich (high in calories and fats) but such ingredients can be blended in wise proportions to produce sauces that enhance the nutrition and taste of a dish without overpowering it. The trick is to make the most of sauce, accenting the right flavors yet achieving a balance between the sauce and the food it will dress. When it is right, the sauce will complement a good dish, but it cannot be expected to mask all the deficiencies of a really poor one. It is a good rule to omit a sauce if you are doubtful about its final effect on a dish.

Always use a sauce lightly, remembering that the sauce is only a seasoning. If a dish is delicate or bland tasting it may be accented by a rich sauce, but one whose ultimate effect will be to highlight the basic flavor of the food it dresses. Sole with white sauce, or flounder with hot butter and parsley, reflects such subtle treatment. Stronger-tasting fish, meat, or vegetables need not be handled so timidly. Assertive sauces, such as those flavored with pungent cheeses, aromatic herbs, or with lemon juice or tomatoes, work splendidly with these foods. Sometimes a sauce may be used for a dish that stands quite well on its own, to add piquancy or to provide a desirable contrast of flavors. Pork, very tasty when unadorned, is sometimes bathed in a zesty sweet and sour pineapple sauce, popular in oriental cooking. Salmon, usually dressed with tangy hollandaise sauce, may also be prepared this way.

Some sauces add to foods and make them more nourishing. A white sauce based on milk or cream and sometimes eggs introduces more calcium, vitamins, and minerals to any meal, and when used with grain or legume dishes, it raises the protein value as well. Sauces made from nut or seed milk or butter also enhance the overall nutrition of a meal. Sauces and dressings made from soymilk and other soy products are both tasty and nourishing.

If you are concerned about calories that come from the rich ingredients often used in sauces, consider yogurt made from low-fat milk, buttermilk, or sour cream as a replacement for heavy cream. These foods cut down on calories, and lower cholesterol intake as well. Some slight adjustments will have to be made, and the flavors may be slightly altered, but you will find there are many dishes that are greatly flattered by these sauces. These ingredients are suitable for most hot sauces and they make very refreshing cold sauces. Cold yogurt sauces are a traditional accompaniment to many Middle Eastern and Caucasian dishes, such as lamb and cooked vegetables. In Finland, hot yogurt sauces, served with seafood or eggs, are a favorite.

Whether you opt for the traditional recipes or some of their newer versions, an acquaintance with the "matriarch sauces" can supply some fundamental precepts in the art of sauce making. The matriarch—or mother—sauces comprise the core from which all the classic variations flow. These sauces include béchamel and velouté—two basic white sauces; espagnole, or brown sauce—which includes tomato-based sauces; hollandaise and mayonnaise—emulsion sauces; hot and cold butter sauces; and oil and vinegar dressings.

White and Brown Sauces

A roux, a flour and butter (or oil) combination, usually of equal parts, is the most popular way to thicken a white or brown sauce. About one tablespoon each of flour and butter added to two cups of liquid will produce a thin sauce. For a thicker sauce you may double or triple the amount of flour and butter. This carefully cooked mixture may be *blanc, blond,* or *brun*—white,

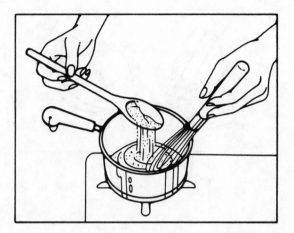

golden, or brown—depending on the type of sauce desired. Only white refined flour will produce the stark white color often associated with cream sauces. But whole grain flour—pastry or regular—may be used quite successfully for either white or brown sauces, with only pleasant variations in taste, texture, and color.

For a white sauce made from a white roux, the flour is added to the butter as soon as the butter is melted. This heating and blending period is most important. It is best done in the top of a double boiler or in a heavy skillet over a low flame, to protect the mixture from burning. The roux should be constantly stirred with a wire whisk and cooked long enough to remove the raw flour taste—about five to seven minutes. The stirring will also help distribute the heat and allow the starch granules of the flour to swell evenly so they will absorb the liquid that will be used for the body of the sauce.

A brown sauce is derived from the same procedure, but the butter is sometimes first browned slightly to a golden color. Care must be taken that the heat not be too high, or the butter will turn black and become bitter.

Liquids

Milk, cream, or a flavored stock are the most common liquids used for sauces. The liquid that will form the body of the sauce is slowly added

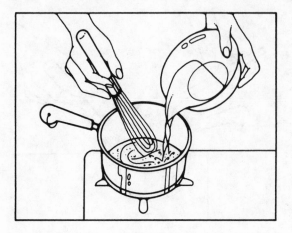

to the cooked roux. Béchamel, one of the two basic white or cream sauces, is derived from a white roux with milk and cream or cream alone. To velouté, the other leading white sauce, either poultry, veal, or fish stock is added. A fish velouté is derived from a *fumet*—an essence of rich fish stock or court bouillon in which fish has been cooked. The same hearty stocks or *fonds de cuisine* used in soup making (see page 100) may also be used for flavoring sauces.

Béchamel and velouté—their elegant names reflect their origins in haute cuisine—are two basics from which several more sophisticated sauces are composed: *aurore, mornay,* and *soubise.*

A béchamel sauce may grace many vegetables and creamed dishes, including mild-flavored fish, poultry, dairy foods, and pasta. A velouté sauce most often adorns the food from which the flavor of its liquid is derived. A vegetable casserole lavished with a generous serving of a white sauce, then crowned with toasted, buttered bread crumbs and grated cheese is transformed into a simple but tasty au gratin dish.

The most common liquid used for a brown sauce is a meat stock. While sauces made with milk, cream, or white stock mingle well with delicate and light-colored foods, the darker brown sauce is better suited for darker meats and richer foods. There are exceptions. For example, most game meats demand a dark and pungent sauce; however, some more delicate game animals or birds may take a light cream sauce.

Unlike white sauces, brown sauces are not enriched with cream or cheese. A *mirepoix*—a mixture of finely diced carrots, onions, and celery sautéed in butter—may be used as a foundation contributing its robust seasoning.

Sautéing, roasting, braising, or browning meat or poultry creates juices that can also add more savor to a brown sauce. These pan gravies, as well as fat-free stocks reduced to a glaze, are quite effective in flavoring sauce and normally reflect the flavor of the food they will garnish. (See Gravy for Meat and Poultry, page 141).

Thickeners

Although it is not always the case, a sauce is commonly thought of as a thickened liquid. In French cuisine a properly thickened sauce has *"du corps,"* or body. This texture may also be described as *à la nappe,* meaning the sauce will coat a spoon. Flour or egg yolk is the agent most commonly used to give a sauce its necessary thickness. However, there are occasions when another type of thickener may be more desirable.

Sauces native to Chinese cooking most often use cornstarch to thicken, resulting in a desired

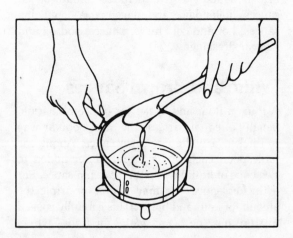

translucent quality. The cornstarch is mixed with a little cold water, then added to the hot liquid. One tablespoon of cornstarch will thicken 1½ to 2 cups of liquid.

A delicate, almost fragile texture results when arrowroot, a starch derived from the root of a tropical plant, is used to thicken a sauce. It thickens well at low heat and so is good for sauces containing egg yolks. However, arrowroot will neither hold nor reheat well, so sauce thickened with it should be served within 15 minutes of preparation. Its flavor is unobtrusive and, unlike wheat flour, it need not be cooked to remove rawness. Use one level tablespoon to thicken one cup of liquid.

Kudzu is a high-quality, imported, white cooking starch that may be used interchangeably with arrowroot and cornstarch. It has the same properties for thickening sauces and may be used in the same proportion as arrowroot. Kudzu tends to form clumps or crystals in storage, so it may be necessary to pound it to a more powdery state before measuring. It is usually available in natural foods stores and is considerably more expensive than arrowroot or cornstarch.

Potato flour or starch, like cornstarch, will result in a semitransparent sauce. Only a short simmering period is required. If the sauce is heated beyond 176°F it will lose its body and thin out again. Sauces thickened with potato flour should be served soon after preparation. One tablespoon of potato starch may be used to thicken 1½ cups of liquid.

Some brown sauces and gravies may be thickened with the blood from the animal whose meat the sauce will accompany. Blood contributes flavor as well as body. You may add it to the sauce just before it is to be served, blending it in the same manner as you do butter swirls (see Enrichment and Flavoring, opposite). The sauce may be simmered, but do not permit it to boil after the blood has been added or it will curdle. Fresh blood may be refrigerated for up to two days. If you plan to store it, mix the blood with one or two tablespoons of vinegar to prevent clotting.

Reduction—the slow evaporation of liquid to thicken a sauce—may be used to bring brown or white sauces to the desired texture. Low simmering leads to a sauce rich with essential flavors. Sauces thickened by reduction are best seasoned right before being served. To thicken a sauce by means of reduction, simply simmer it, uncovered, until the desired thickness is attained. Stir constantly to avoid burning or sticking.

Enrichment and Flavoring

Spices and fresh or dried herbs should be added just before a sauce has reached completion, so their flavors are released but not diminished with cooking. This is especially true for black pepper, which may become bitter if cooked too long.

Sometimes it is the very enrichment that defines a sauce. A primary béchamel enriched with cream or egg yolk and cheese becomes a classic mornay sauce. Heavy cream and egg yolk transform a velouté into sauce supreme. These and many sauces may be sufficiently rich and sumptuous, but further enrichment may be desired for a sauce that is to complement a particular simple or subtle dish. There are several classic methods for doing this.

Beurre manié (kneaded butter) and butter swirls are two classic enrichment methods for brown and white sauces. White sauces may also be enriched with cream or egg yolk, depending on the result desired.

Beurre manié is made by cutting softened butter into an equal amount of flour and manipulating the mixture with your fingers or a pastry blender until little balls form. The *beurre manié* is stirred in to the sauce until it is sufficiently thickened and should be added near the end of the sauce's cooking. About two tablespoons of the mixture will thicken one cup of sauce.

A sauce may also be *finie au beurre* (finished with butter swirls) by depositing bits of

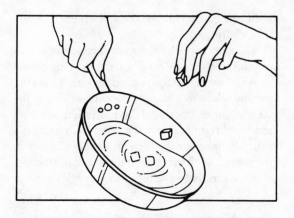

unmelted butter on top of the finished sauce just after it is removed from the heat. The pan is then rotated slowly, allowing the melting butter to form a spiraling swirl in the hot sauce. Do not use a spoon to stir and do not reheat the sauce. Use about 1 to 1½ tablespoons of butter for finishing two cups of sauce this way.

Another way to improve the color and texture of a sauce, increase its flavor, and bind it together is with a liaison. This is a mixture of cream and beaten egg yolk—added to the sauce at the last minute. To avoid any curdling, the liaison is usually blended with a small amount of the hot sauce before being totally incorporated.

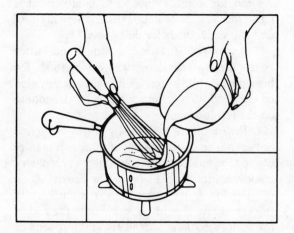

A meat glaze, or *glace de viande,* is a meat stock that has been strained and reduced until it is very thick and syrupy. This highly concen-

trated essence can be used to flavor a brown sauce or gravy. (See Stocks, page 100.) Just one-half teaspoon of this condensed liquid can enrich and flavor sauces.

Emulsion Sauces

Though not based on any primary sauce, hollandaise is sometimes considered part of the white sauce group. For dressing fish and boiled vegetables, a well-made hollandaise has no peer. Béarnaise, fragrant with the sweetness of tarragon, is a sister sauce that is savored on broiled and grilled dishes. Mayonnaise is the cold counterpart of these characteristically thick emulsion sauces. The quick blender recipes given here will yield smooth sauces. However, their ideal satiny texture can only be achieved if the melted butter or the oil is stirred into the egg yolks very gradually and mixed in thoroughly. For hollandaise or béarnaise, a double boiler or heavy-bottom saucepan is used and the cooking temperature kept low. If the sauce begins to curdle, you can save it by putting a fresh egg yolk in another pan and gradually whipping the curdled mixture into it. Another method is to add some cold water to the mixture and blend it well.

Mayonnaise may appear with many cold appetizers, entrées, and salads and is often appropriate wherever most oil and vinegar dressings are used. A smooth delicacy and a pronounced tanginess make it a perfect condiment for cold fish and shellfish. Its flavor complements many foods and it serves as the foundation for other sauces, including creamy salad dressings and tartar sauce. Compounded with crushed garlic, a mayonnaise recipe yields a lavishly piquant *aïoli* sauce.

When making this cold emulsion sauce, always start with both the egg yolks and the oil at room temperature. Add the first few drops of oil slowly and then pour a thin stream continuously, whipping the mixture constantly. Add a little vinegar whenever the mixture gets too thick. Two egg yolks will hold about one cup of oil.

Light Sauces

Several internationally famous chefs have devised simple techniques for adding a host of lighter, but equally flavorful sauces to augment the classic repertoire of sauces. These sauces are not really new since the basics of classic sauce making have been retained in their preparation. However, these sauces provide alternatives for lessening the caloric content (particularly that from fat) of sauces—without diminishing the body and flavor. This is especially significant for those striving to control their weight or reduce their fat intake.

The following are the most important guidelines applied to making light sauces:

Reduction and meat glaze: The success of light sauces derives from an attempt to create rich flavor as opposed to rich body. Reducing stocks to a concentrate of their native flavor is one of the most effective ways to do this. A meat glaze, or *glace de viande,* a highly reduced stock, is commonly used to bolster the flavor of all sauces and soups and is particularly useful to light sauces.

Nonfat and low-fat dairy products: These products are used almost solely as a liaison to finish or enrich a light sauce (rather than as the body of the sauce).

Vegetables and fruits: Pureed, cooked vegetables and fruits have long been popular accompaniments to meat, fish, and fowl in French cuisine. It is only natural to extend their role to that of delicate, light sauces. Such low-calorie, high-nutrition foods are important elements in making light sauces. Some vegetables and fruits when cooked and pureed are rich enough in texture and flavor to form the entire body of a sauce. Few additions, if any, may be needed.

Aromatic ingredients: Although aromatic ingredients such as mushrooms, onions, garlic, tomatoes, lemon, parsley, and fresh herbs can be important additions to any sauce, they are especially handy in bringing light sauces to life. These and other highly flavored ingredients add zest and fragrance to sauces that might otherwise seem bland. They go a long way in seasoning, so they need be used only in small amounts. In classic sauce making most of these ingredients are sautéed in butter or oil at the start of the sauce's cooking. In light sauce making there is little sautéing, so these ingredients are often added as a cooked puree to finish the sauce; or they may be cooked and pureed along with the sauce. Cooks who make light sauces regularly find it useful to keep flavoring agents such as mushroom and tomato purees on hand for quick use.

Enrichment with a liaison: Classic sauce making methods generally rely on the thickening power of the roux; a liaison may be used to further enrich the sauce. Light sauces often forgo the roux for body, texture, and sometimes flavor in favor of the liaison only. The classic egg, or egg and cream liaison may be used but only in small proportions. Instead, the following ingredients are more commonly used to bind a light sauce:

yogurt, buttermilk, nonfat milk, or small amounts of cream or crème fraîche

pureed vegetables, alone or blended with small amounts of the above dairy products.

Butter Sauces

Grilled or fried fish and hearty vegetables, such as cauliflower or broccoli, fare well when lightly flavored with butter sauce. Simple butter sauces, creamed or browned and then enlivened with parsley, lemon juice, or other herbs and flavorings, produce classic variations.

The *beurres composés,* or the compounded butters, are highly flavored combinations, with ingredients such as shellfish, mustard, shallots, or chives contributing to their potency. Besides being used with fish, meat, and vegetables, they may be used for finishing other hot sauces. When melting butter to be used as sauce, avoid heating it to oiliness. A creamy appearance marks the desired consistency.

Clarified butter may be used in making brown or white sauces, or it may be served as a sauce for lobster and other shellfish. Clarified butter, also known as drawn butter or ghee, can be made by melting butter slowly over low heat. When the butter is removed from the heat and allowed to stand several minutes the milk solids—which cause butter to burn—will sink to the bottom. The butterfat, clear and yellow, can then be skimmed off and strained into a container. Clarified butter may also be used for making brown or black butter. Simply cook the clarified butter over very low heat, stirring constantly, until it is golden or dark brown. Season each cup of butter with 1½ teaspoons of lemon juice. Serve over cooked vegetables or fish.

Marinades

A marinade is a seasoned cooked or uncooked liquid in which meat, fish, or vegetables may be steeped. It is sometimes added to a finished sauce for richer flavor. Some oil and vinegar dressings may serve as a marinade for raw vegetables. A marinade, aromatic and tenderizing, impregnates the soaking food with its blend of flavors and brings out the native flavor of the food. Vinegar or lemon juice is usually part of the marinade, along with oil, herbs, garlic, or onion. The acid ingredient helps to tenderize meat and fish, and to cut down on the cooking time. Marinated vegetables need not be cooked at all.

Size and texture determine how long meat or fish should be marinated. Food left to marinate longer than one hour should be refrigerated. Each pound of food usually requires about one-half to three-quarters cup of marinade. Food should not be marinated so long that its original flavor is lessened. (For more information and specific recipes for marinating meat, fish, poultry, and vegetables, see Index.)

Storing Sauces

Most sauces are at their peak taste and texture immediately after preparation and should be served then. However, if this is not possible, any basic white or brown sauce may be held in a container covered with a thin layer of melted butter or fat for up to a week. Refrigerated tomato sauces will keep for a few days longer than white or brown sauces. All three—or the roux alone for brown and white sauces—may be frozen for as long as several months. Freeze in small quantities, then thaw and reheat as needed in the top of a double boiler, stirring often to lessen the tendency to separate.

Store mayonnaise in the warmest part of the refrigerator, since extreme cold will cause separation. Never freeze it. Though hollandaise and béarnaise may be stored for a day or two at most, it is advisable to make only what is needed for the meal. These emulsion sauces are highly subject to bacterial activity, so care should be taken to store them properly.

Tips for Making Successful Sauces

• In general, the amount of sauce to make for a dish should equal about one-third the amount of solid food it dresses. Allow a little more than this for light sauces, and a little less for rich sauces.

• When making sauces, temper cold ingredients by combining them separately with a small amount of the heated liquid before adding them to the saucepan.

• When adding the liquid to a roux, remove the pan from the heat. Return it after incorporating the roux with the liquid.

• Be especially careful not to boil sauces made with egg yolk or yogurt, or they will curdle.

• Do not overheat a cornstarch-thickened sauce or it may thin out.

• Do not cover a hot sauce, or the steam created may cause thinning out and separation.

Hot butter sauces should be refrigerated for no more than one day and should not be frozen. Dairy-free sauces, with a fruit or vegetable base will keep well in the refrigerator for four or five days.

Gravy for Meat and Poultry

Pan juices that result from sautéing, roasting, braising, or browning meat are highly desirable ingredients for meat and poultry gravies. Gravies are usually made with these degreased juices just before the meat is to be served. Most cooks make the gravy in the same pan used to cook the meat. First, place the meat on a platter. Then remove as much fat as possible from the pan juices (use a syringe, if necessary). Now reheat the juice and scrape into it any solidified particles from the pan's sides and bottom. Then transfer this liquid into another container. If more liquid is needed, use stock flavored by the same type of meat you plan to serve with the gravy. Use the following method to make gravy for any meat or poultry:

1. Make a roux (see White and Brown Sauces, page 135) in the same pan. Use two to three tablespoons each of flour and butter. If you prefer, you may substitute fat skimmed from the pan juice for the butter.

2. To the cooked roux, slowly add the reserved pan juice (and stock or water, if you are adding more liquid), stirring constantly. You may add about 1½ to 2 cups of liquid, depending on how much roux you have and how thin you would like the gravy to be.

3. Cook the gravy until smooth, stirring frequently.

4. Allow gravy to simmer about five minutes. Season with fresh or dried herbs and freshly ground pepper, if desired. The gravy should be sufficiently rich and flavorful from the pan juice, but if you want to enrich it further, add about one-quarter cup of milk or cream and cook a few minutes longer. Serve in a gravy boat.

White Sauces

Béchamel Sauce
(Basic White Sauce)

This is the "cream sauce" cooks often use for vegetables and casseroles. It is also the basis for other popular sauces.

> 2 tablespoons butter
> 2 tablespoons whole wheat pastry flour
> 1½ cups milk
> ¼ teaspoon white pepper
> ⅛ teaspoon ground nutmeg
> 1 teaspoon grated onions (optional)

Melt butter in a heavy-bottom saucepan. Add flour and cook over low heat for 5 to 7 minutes, stirring constantly. Add the milk slowly and continue to cook, stirring with a wire whisk, until thickened, about 10 minutes. Stir in pepper, nutmeg, and onions (if used).

Yields 1¼ cups

NOTE: This yields a medium white sauce. For a *thin* white sauce, use only 1 tablespoon each of butter and flour. For a *thick* white sauce, use 3 tablespoons each of butter and flour.

Basic Duxelles
(Chopped Mushroom Sauce Base)

Add to stuffings, or combine with other sauces and gravies to impart the flavor of mushrooms to meat and fish dishes.

> 1 cup sliced mushrooms
> 2 tablespoons butter
> 1 small onion, minced
> ⅛ teaspoon ground nutmeg
> ¼ teaspoon pepper

Use a food processor or blender to finely chop mushrooms. Remove and put in a piece of cheesecloth or a man's large linen handkerchief, twist, and squeeze out the moisture.

Melt butter in a small skillet. Add the onions and cook over low heat until translucent. Add mushrooms, nutmeg, and pepper. Raise the heat, stir, and cook until the moisture evaporates. Cool, then store in refrigerator.

Yields ½ cup

Velouté Sauce
(White Sauce with Stock)

A creamy sauce to serve with poultry, veal, fish, and vegetable dishes.

2 tablespoons butter
2 tablespoons whole wheat pastry flour
1 cup Poultry Stock (page 110) or Fish Stock
   (page 111)
¼ teaspoon white pepper

Melt butter in a heavy-bottom saucepan. Blend in flour and cook over low heat for 5 to 7 minutes, stirring constantly. Gradually add stock and continue cooking, stirring with a wire whisk, until thickened, 10 to 15 minutes. Add pepper. Serve hot.

Yields 1 cup

Variations:
Enriched Velouté Sauce (Sauce Supreme): Beat 1 cup heavy cream and 3 egg yolks together. Gradually add this mixture to 1 cup Velouté Sauce and cook over low heat, stirring constantly, until thickened. Do not allow sauce to boil, or it will curdle.

***Aurore* Sauce:** Add 1 cup Enriched Velouté Sauce to ½ cup tomato sauce.

Soubise Sauce: Sauté ⅓ cup finely chopped onions in 1 tablespoon butter. Then add onions and ½ teaspoon lemon juice to 1 cup Velouté Sauce.

Mornay Sauce

A delicious cheese sauce—excellent for seafood, egg, and vegetable dishes.

¼ cup butter
¼ cup whole wheat pastry flour
1 cup Poultry Stock (page 110)
1 cup light cream
2 tablespoons grated Parmesan cheese
2 tablespoons grated cheddar or Swiss cheese
¼ teaspoon paprika
½ teaspoon grated onions

Melt butter in a heavy-bottom saucepan. Stir in flour. Add stock and milk, stirring with a wire whisk to avoid lumps. Add cheeses, paprika, and onions and cook until cheese has melted.
Serve with seafood, poultry, or vegetables.

Yields about 2½ cups

Duxelles Velouté
(Mushroom Sauce)

Serve hot over chicken, veal, or fish.

¾ cup Velouté Sauce (see opposite)
3 tablespoons Basic Duxelles (page 141)
¼ cup tomato paste
1 teaspoon lemon juice

Heat velouté sauce in the top of a double boiler. Add remaining ingredients and cook until hot.

Yields about 1 cup

Soymilk Cream Sauce

A tasty alternative to traditional white sauces.

2 tablespoons butter
¾ cup pureed cooked white beans
1½ cups soymilk
1 teaspoon soy sauce

In a heavy-bottom saucepan, brown butter over medium heat. Watch carefully so butter does not burn. Add puree and mix well. Gradually add soymilk and stir with a wire whisk until milk is heated thoroughly and mixture starts to thicken. Add soy sauce and continue to stir until sauce is thick and smooth.

Yields 2 cups

Variations:
Soymilk Cheese Sauce: Add 1 cup grated sharp cheddar cheese.
Soymilk Curry Sauce: Add 1 teaspoon curry powder.

Brown Sauces

Sour Cream Gravy

Good with veal cutlets, veal kidneys, pork chops, wild game, and venison.

2 tablespoons butter
2 tablespoons minced onions
1 tablespoon finely chopped fresh parsley
1½ tablespoons whole wheat pastry flour
   dash of cayenne pepper
1½ cups sour cream

In a small skillet, melt butter over medium heat. Add onions and parsley and sauté for about 2 minutes. Do not allow to brown. Blend in flour and cayenne. Gradually add sour cream, stirring constantly. Bring to a boil, then reduce heat, and allow to cook very slowly until thickened.

Yields 1¾ cups

Variation:

Brown Sour Cream Gravy: Make this delicious gravy right in the roasting pan after removing roasted meat. Use 2 tablespoons meat fat and drippings in place of butter. If meat is highly seasoned, omit onions and parsley.

Mirepoix

This is a blend of vegetables that may be used as a base for poaching. Or use to cover roasts of meat or poultry and shellfish. Mirepoix is an essential ingredient in Sauce Espagnole (see opposite).

2 tablespoons vegetable oil or butter
2 carrots, finely chopped
1 medium-size onion, finely chopped
2 stalks celery, finely chopped

Heat oil or butter in a large skillet. Add vegetables and cook until soft, about 10 minutes.

Yields about 1¼ cups

Meat or Vegetable Herb Sauce

This sauce makes an excellent substitute for gravy.

2 tablespoons butter
2 tablespoons whole wheat pastry flour
1 cup Beef Stock (page 110), Poultry Stock (page 110), or Vegetable Stock (page 111)
¼ teaspoon dried basil
1¼ teaspoons dried chives
¼ teaspoon dried thyme
dash of cayenne pepper

In a heavy-bottom saucepan, melt butter. Cook over low heat until butter is a golden brown, about 7 minutes. Add flour and stir until smooth and bubbly. Remove from heat and slowly add stock, stirring with a wire whisk to avoid lumps. Add basil, chives, thyme, and cayenne and cook over high heat, stirring constantly, until sauce boils. Reduce heat and simmer for a few minutes, or until sauce has thickened.

Yields 1 cup

Variation:

Sauce Espagnole (Brown Sauce): Add ¼ cup heavy cream and 2 tablespoons tomato puree to sauce. Blend well and add ½ cup *Mirepoix* (see opposite). Cook sauce over low heat until heated through, about 5 minutes.

Emulsion Sauces

Hollandaise Sauce

Dress up the simplest vegetable, egg, or meat dish with this elegant sauce.

3 egg yolks
2 teaspoons water
½ cup butter, softened
¼ teaspoon cayenne pepper
2 tablespoons lemon juice

In the top of a double boiler, over 2 inches of hot but not boiling water, beat egg yolks and water together with a wire whisk until slightly thickened. Cut butter into 3 or 4 pieces. Add one piece at a time, beating constantly after each addition until blended, smooth, and thickened. Add cayenne and lemon juice. Serve warm.

Yields ¾ cup

NOTE: If sauce begins to curdle, reconstitute by putting a fresh egg yolk in another pan and gradually whipping the curdled mixture into it. Or place sauce in a blender, add a small amount of water, and blend well.

Variations:

Sauce Maltaise: Add 1 tablespoon orange juice and ½ teaspoon grated orange rind. Especially good with asparagus.

Yogurt Hollandaise Sauce: Substitute yogurt for water and omit lemon juice.

Aïoli Sauce
(Garlic Mayonnaise)

Serve over fish or boiled beef, or use as a dipping sauce for artichokes or other chilled vegetables.

      3 large cloves garlic, minced
      ¼ cup plus 2 tablespoons lemon juice
      2 eggs
      ½ teaspoon white pepper
      1½ cups olive oil
      1 whole clove garlic

In a blender, process garlic and lemon juice. Add eggs and pepper and process again at high speed, stopping frequently to scrape down sides of container.

Add oil, a few drops at a time at first, while blender is going. Then gradually add oil in a steady stream.

When mixture has thickened, spoon into a bowl and refrigerate. Stir before serving and top with whole garlic clove to identify the sauce, since it resembles mayonnaise.

Yields about 2 cups

Sauce Béarnaise

A flavorful herb sauce especially good served over broiled meat and fish.

      2 tablespoons water
      2 teaspoons minced fresh tarragon or ½
         teaspoon dried tarragon
      2 tablespoons minced scallions
      1 tablespoon minced fresh parsley
      ¼ cup plus 2 tablespoons wine vinegar
      ¾ cup butter
      4 egg yolks
      1 tablespoon lemon juice
      ¼ teaspoon cayenne pepper

In a small, heavy-bottom saucepan, mix water, tarragon, scallions, parsley, and vinegar. Cook slowly until it is almost a glaze. Set aside.

Melt butter and keep it hot.

In a blender, place egg yolks, lemon juice, and cayenne. Blend and add hot butter slowly but steadily until thickened. Add herb mixture and beat well. Serve warm.

Yields 1 cup

Mayonnaise

      2 egg yolks, at room temperature, lightly beaten
      2 tablespoons lemon juice or vinegar, at room
         temperature
      ½ teaspoon dry mustard
      1⅓ cups vegetable oil, at room temperature
      2 teaspoons boiling water

Warm a glass or stainless steel bowl and a wire whisk in hot water. Dry thoroughly.

Place egg yolks in the bowl and add 1 tablespoon lemon juice and the mustard. Beat well. Continue beating constantly as you add the oil, one drop at a time. Be sure the yolks are absorbing the oil. This may require that you stop adding the oil and just beat the yolks for a few seconds. After about 1/3 cup oil has been incorporated into the yolks, add remaining oil by the tablespoon. Beat well after each addition.

When mayonnaise is thick and stiff, beat in remaining lemon juice to thin. To prevent mayonnaise from separating, blend in the boiling water.

Store in a covered glass jar in the refrigerator.

Yields about 1¼ cups

Variation:

Blender Mayonnaise: Warm a blender container in hot water, then dry thoroughly.

Combine egg yolks, lemon juice, and mustard in the container. Blend at medium speed about 1 minute.

Add oil a few drops at a time, continuing to blend at medium speed, until ⅓ cup oil has been incorporated into the yolks. At this point remaining oil may be added by the tablespoon, until all the oil has been used.

To ensure against mayonnaise separating, blend in boiling water.

Tofu Mayonnaise

This mayonnaise is perfect for those wishing to limit or avoid eggs in their diets.

      10 ounces soft tofu, drained (1 cup)
      1 to 2 teaspoons French-style mustard
      3 tablespoons lemon juice
      ½ cup vegetable oil
         dash of pepper (optional)

Place tofu and mustard in a blender and add 1 tablespoon lemon juice. Blend at high speed, stopping frequently to scrape down sides of the container.

Add oil a few drops at a time while blender is going. Then gradually add oil in a steady stream. When about 1/3 of the oil has been added, slowly add another tablespoon lemon juice while blending. Dribble in another 1/3 of the oil and then the remaining lemon juice. Add a bit of pepper if desired. Continue adding oil until it is gone. Store in covered container. Mayonnaise will keep in refrigerator for several weeks.

Yields 1½ cups

Avgolemono
(Greek Egg and Lemon Sauce)

If you are on a diet, try this sauce instead of mayonnaise, since it contains no butter or oil.

    3 eggs
      juice of 1 large lemon
    1 cup Poultry Stock (page 110) or Fish Stock
      (page 111)
    1 tablespoon cornstarch, dissolved in ½ cup
      cold water
    ¼ teaspoon white pepper

In a small bowl, beat eggs with a wire whisk until foamy. Slowly add lemon juice.

In a saucepan, bring stock to a boil. Add cornstarch to boiling stock, and add pepper. With a whisk, beat stock very slowly into the egg-lemon mixture. Return mixture to pot and cook over medium heat, beating constantly, until thickened.

Serve hot or cold.

Yields 1 cup

NOTE: Substitute Beef Stock (page 110) if sauce is to be used with meat, or Vegetable Stock (page 111) if using sauce with vegetables.

Light Sauces

Enhance your most elegant meal with one of the following low-calorie, high-nutrition sauces— flavorful alternatives to the rich classic sauces.

Carrot Sauce

    2 cups cooked carrots
    2 tablespoons chopped celery

    ¾ cup Beef Stock (page 110)
    ¼ cup tomato paste
      pepper, to taste

Puree all ingredients in a food processor or blender. Heat and serve with meat loaf, liver, or green vegetables.

Yields about 1½ cups

Hot Apple Meat Sauce

    3 cups unsweetened applesauce
    2 tablespoons minced onions
    1 tablespoon honey
    ¼ teaspoon French-style mustard
    2 tablespoons vinegar
      pepper, to taste
    1 teaspoon horseradish (optional)

Combine all ingredients. If using horseradish, omit pepper. Simmer, stirring occasionally until onions cook. Serve hot over meat.

Yields about 2 cups

Light Brown Sauce with Herbs

    2 cups Beef Stock (page 110)
    2 tablespoons cornstarch
    ½ cup white grape juice
    1 tablespoon minced fresh tarragon or 1
      teaspoon dried tarragon
    1 tablespoon chopped fresh chives
    1 clove garlic, halved
    1 teaspoon lemon juice
      pepper, to taste

Shake ½ cup stock and cornstarch in a jar with a tight-fitting lid. Heat remaining stock to a boil and then reduce heat to medium. Add cornstarch mixture and simmer for 5 minutes, stirring constantly.

In a small saucepan, boil grape juice, tarragon, chives, and garlic over medium heat until reduced by half. Strain, and add to thickened stock. Heat, adding lemon juice and pepper. Serve with beef or potatoes.

Yields about 2 cups

Light Cream Sauce

2 cups water
1 cup nonfat dry milk
3 tablespoons cornstarch

Mix all ingredients in a food processor or blender.
In a small saucepan, simmer sauce until thickened, about 2 minutes. Serve with poultry, veal, fish, and vegetable dishes.

Yields about 2 cups

Variations:
Light Cheese Sauce: Add ½ cup grated cheddar cheese or ¾ cup Swiss cheese and 1 teaspoon dry mustard to thickened sauce. Heat just until cheese has melted.
Light Dill Cream Sauce: Add 1 tablespoon fresh dill to thickened sauce.
Light Egg Cream Sauce: Add chopped hard-cooked eggs and pepper to thickened sauce.

Light Curry Pear Whip

1 cup chopped peeled pears
1 cup part-skim ricotta cheese
2 teaspoons curry powder
½ teaspoon ground allspice

Blend all ingredients in a food processor or blender. Chill. Serve as a dip for assorted raw vegetables.

Yields about 2 cups

Light Curry Sauce

1 tablespoon cornstarch
2 cups yogurt
3 to 4 teaspoons curry powder
4 teaspoons honey
1 teaspoon lemon juice
½ teaspoon ground ginger
pepper, to taste

In a medium-size saucepan thoroughly blend cornstarch and yogurt. Add remaining ingredients, mixing well, and cook over medium heat, stirring constantly, just until sauce simmers. Remove from heat and serve at once over rice or vegetables.

Yields about 2 cups

Light Mayonnaise Sauce

2 eggs
⅛ teaspoon white pepper
1 tablespoon honey
1 teaspoon dry mustard
2 teaspoons cornstarch
1 cup skim milk
2 tablespoons lemon juice
1 tablespoon vegetable oil

Blend all ingredients together in a food processor or blender. Pour into a small saucepan and cook over medium heat, stirring constantly, until mixture thickens. Do not boil.

Yields about 1½ cups

NOTE: This sauce will thicken in the refrigerator to a mayonnaise consistency.

Light Tomato Sauce

10 to 12 medium-size tomatoes, peeled and finely
chopped (about 4 cups)
1 tablespoon minced dried basil
1½ teaspoons minced dried oregano
⅛ teaspoon garlic powder
⅛ teaspoon pepper
2 tablespoons olive oil

Combine all ingredients. Toss with cooked pasta.

Yields about 4 cups

Sauce Florentine

2 to 3 tablespoons olive oil
1 small onion, chopped
¼ teaspoon garlic powder (optional)
¼ pound spinach, chopped
½ cup cooked white beans, drained
2 tablespoons tomato paste

In a large skillet, heat 2 tablespoons olive oil. Add onions and sauté, adding garlic powder (if used). Add spinach and lightly sauté, adding more oil if necessary.
In a food processor or blender puree spinach, onions, beans, and tomato paste, adding water to thin if necessary.
Heat in a medium-size saucepan and serve over chicken, veal, vegetables, or pasta.

Yields about 1½ cups

Parsley Sauce

3 soft-cooked eggs, cooled
½ cup chopped fresh parsley
¼ cup freshly squeezed lemon juice
⅛ teaspoon pepper

In a food processor or blender combine eggs and remaining ingredients and process until smooth. Strain. Warm and serve over cooked vegetables.

Yields about 1 cup

Oriental Peach Sauce

2 tablespoons soy sauce
2 tablespoons peanut oil
2 tablespoons honey
1 cup pureed peaches
¼ teaspoon ground ginger
1 tablespoon minced scallions
2 tablespoons sesame seeds, toasted

Mix together all ingredients and serve over cold sliced or diced chicken or cold pork.

Yields about 1 cup

Sorrel Sauce

1 tablespoon butter
½ cup chopped sorrel
1 cup Poultry Stock (page 110)
1 teaspoon minced fresh tarragon
2 teaspoons cornstarch
2 egg yolks
1 tablespoon cold water

In a medium-size saucepan, melt butter and sauté sorrel until wilted. Add ½ cup stock and tarragon, and simmer for 3 minutes.

Shake remaining stock and cornstarch in a jar with a tight-fitting lid.

Whisk egg yolks, adding cold water. Spoon a little of the hot mixture into egg yolks, return to pan and whisk over low heat for 2 minutes. Gradually add cornstarch mixture, whisking until thickened. Serve with fish or veal.

Yields about 1 cup

Ruby Raspberry Sauce

¼ cup orange or apricot preserves
½ cup white grape juice
½ cup Poultry Stock (page 110)
1 tablespoon grated orange rind
1 teaspoon honey
2 egg yolks, lightly beaten
1 teaspoon cornstarch
1 cup fresh raspberries

In a medium-size saucepan, combine preserves, grape juice, stock, orange rind, and honey. Simmer, stirring constantly, until preserves melt.

Put a little of the hot mixture into egg yolks. Return to pan whisking well. Remove from heat.

In a jar with a tight-fitting lid, shake cornstarch with a little of the sauce. Slowly stir back into saucepan. Cook over medium heat, stirring constantly, until sauce has thickened. Add berries and heat through.

Serve over chicken or pork.

Yields about 2½ cups

Sauce Piquant

½ cup tomato sauce
½ cup Light Mayonnaise Sauce (page 146)
3 tablespoons lemon juice
½ teaspoon grated lemon rind
5 or 6 drops hot pepper sauce, or to taste

Combine all ingredients. Chill. Serve with cold fish.

Yields about 1 cup

Sauce Verde

1 head broccoli (about 1 pound)
¾ cup Poultry Stock (page 110)
⅛ teaspoon pepper
2 tablespoons crème fraîche (page 450)

Cook broccoli in a small amount of water for 10 to 15 minutes. Drain. When cool, coarsely chop.

Combine broccoli and remaining ingredients in a food processor or blender and process until smooth. Heat and serve over vegetables.

Yields about 2½ cups

Purple Plum Sauce

½ cup grape juice
1 tablespoon cornstarch
1 cup Poultry Stock (page 110)
1 teaspoon ground cinnamon
¼ teaspoon ground nutmeg
1 tablespoon lemon juice
10 purple plums, pitted and halved

In a jar with a tight-fitting lid, shake grape juice with cornstarch.

Heat stock, cinnamon, and nutmeg. Slowly add lemon juice and simmer, stirring constantly, until sauce has thickened. Add plums and heat through.

Serve with pork.

Yields about 2 cups

Sweet Mustard Sauce

1 tablespoon French-style mustard
¼ cup honey
2 teaspoons minced fresh dill
1 cup buttermilk

In a small saucepan, heat mustard and honey just until blended. Remove from heat and stir in dill and buttermilk. Serve over cold fish or pork.

Yields about 1 cup

NOTE: For a thicker sauce, replace half of the buttermilk with ½ cup of low-fat cottage cheese.

Butter Sauces

Clarified Butter

Clarified or drawn butter is simply melted butter with the sediment removed. It is often used for sautéing chicken, veal, or fish because it doesn't burn as easily. Nice also as a dipping sauce for shellfish.

1 cup butter
½ teaspoon lemon juice

Combine butter and lemon juice in a small saucepan and melt over low heat. Transfer mixture to a container and refrigerate until butter solidifies. The solid yellow top is clarified butter. The milky whey on the bottom

may be discarded or added to a cream sauce. Store clarified butter in refrigerator or freezer.

Yields about ¾ cup

Basil Butter

Spread lightly over steaks, hamburgers, or roast beef for a delicious, buttery flavor.

⅓ cup butter, at room temperature
1 tablespoon tomato paste
1 teaspoon dried basil

In a small bowl, combine all ingredients and beat with a wooden spoon until smooth and creamy. Cover tightly and store in refrigerator until ready to use.

Yields about ½ cup

Herb Butter

Slice pieces of this butter, as needed, and place on top of hot sliced meats, poultry, fish, or vegetables just before serving.

¼ cup butter, at room temperature
½ teaspoon lemon juice
dash of cayenne pepper
½ teaspoon prepared mustard
¼ teaspoon soy sauce
2 teaspoons chopped fresh parsley
1 teaspoon minced fresh thyme
1 teaspoon minced fresh tarragon

With a fork, wire whisk, or wooden spoon, blend all ingredients until well mixed and smooth.

Put mixture on wax paper, and shape into roll about 1 inch in diameter. Chill.

Yields about ¼ cup

Tarragon Butter

Serve over fillets of sole or other white fish.

3 tablespoons butter
1½ cups chopped mushrooms
3 tablespoons chopped shallots or scallions
2 teaspoons dried tarragon
1 tablespoon lemon juice

In a medium-size skillet, melt butter over medium heat. Add mushrooms and shallots or scallions, and sauté until soft, about 5 minutes. Add tarragon and lemon juice. Use at once.

Yields about 1½ cups

Quick Sauces

Avocado Sauce

Delicious mixed with hot or cold cooked chicken, or served over fresh fruit.

> 1 cup mashed avocado
> 2 tablespoons lemon juice
> 2 teaspoons honey
> ¼ cup buttermilk
> dash of ground cinnamon (optional)

Combine all ingredients in a small bowl and beat until smooth. Serve immediately.

Yields 1¼ cups

Basic Barbecue Sauce

This sauce is excellent for basting or marinating chicken breasts or flank steak.

> 1 tablespoon butter
> ¼ cup chopped onions
> 1 cup tomato sauce
> 1 tablespoon honey
> 1 tablespoon soy sauce
> 1 tablespoon prepared mustard

In a medium-size skillet, melt butter over medium heat. Add onions and sauté about 5 minutes. Blend in remaining ingredients and cook until heated through, about 10 minutes. Cool slightly, and then place sauce in a jar. Cover tightly and store in refrigerator.

Yields ¾ cup

Variations:

Herb Barbecue Sauce: Add ½ teaspoon dried rosemary and 1 tablespoon chopped fresh parsley. Simmer for 1 minute longer.

Tangy Barbecue Sauce: Add a dash of cayenne pepper, 1 clove minced garlic, and 1 teaspoon celery seeds. Simmer for 1 minute longer.

Blue Cheese Sauce

Use over hot or cold grains, pasta, or cooked or raw vegetables.

> 1 cup cottage cheese
> 1 tablespoon lemon juice
> 1 ounce blue cheese, crumbled (Roquefort, Stilton, or Gorgonzola cheese may be substituted)

In a food processor or blender, combine cottage cheese and lemon juice and process until smooth and creamy. Then fold in cheese. Store in a tightly covered container in refrigerator.

Yields about 1¼ cups

Cardamom-Yogurt Sauce

Try spooning this sauce over chilled, mixed citrus fruit for a light dessert.

> 1 egg, lightly beaten
> ¼ cup orange juice
> 1 tablespoon honey
> ½ teaspoon ground cardamom
> 1 cup yogurt

In a small saucepan, combine egg, orange juice, honey, and cardamom. Cook and stir over medium-low heat until mixture thickens, about 5 minutes. Cook and stir for 2 minutes longer. Cool.

Fold yogurt into cooled egg mixture. Cover and chill thoroughly.

Yields 1⅓ cups

Cool Yogurt-Cucumber Sauce

A nice sauce to use over cold cooked fish or over chilled raw vegetables as a salad alternative.

> 1 cup yogurt
> 1 medium-size cucumber, peeled and shredded
> 2 teaspoons chopped fresh dill or ½ teaspoon dried dillweed
> dash of cayenne pepper
> ½ teaspoon soy sauce

Mix all ingredients in a small bowl and chill well.

Yields 1½ to 2 cups

Chinese Sweet and Sour Sauce

¾ cup pineapple juice
¼ cup vinegar
1 tablespoon soy sauce
2 tablespoons honey
1 small sweet red pepper, shredded
½ cup Poultry Stock (page 110)
2 teaspoons minced peeled ginger root or 2
　　teaspoons ground ginger
2 tablespoons cornstarch, dissolved in ⅓
　　cup water

In a medium-size saucepan, mix pineapple juice with vinegar, soy sauce, and honey. Add pepper, stock, and ginger and bring to a boil.

Add cornstarch to boiling sauce, stirring constantly with a wooden spoon. Cook for 1 minute or until sauce is thick and clear. Pour over fish, poultry, or cooked vegetables.

Yields 2 cups

Creamy Peanut-Yogurt Sauce

Use as a topping for hot or cold chicken or as a dip for fresh fruit.

½ cup yogurt
½ cup creamy peanut butter
¼ cup chopped banana

Place all ingredients in a food processor or blender and process until smooth.

Yields 1 cup

Variation:
　Coconut-Peanut-Yogurt Sauce: Substitute ¼ cup freshly grated coconut for banana.

Curried Yogurt Sauce

Good over hot cooked beef, chicken, or cooked green vegetables.

⅓ cup Beef Stock (page 110)
½ cup yogurt
½ teaspoon curry powder

In a small saucepan, bring stock to a boil. Remove from heat and stir in remaining ingredients. Reheat, but do not boil. Serve immediately.

Yields about ¾ cup

Enchilada Sauce

A spicy sauce for serving over enchiladas, tacos, or other Mexican dishes.

1 teaspoon olive oil
½ cup chopped onions
2 cups tomato sauce
2 cups chopped canned tomatoes
1 can (4 ounces) green chilies, drained
　　and chopped
1 teaspoon minced, peeled, seeded jalapeño
　　pepper or ⅛ teaspoon cayenne pepper
½ teaspoon dried oregano
½ teaspoon dried basil

In a medium-size saucepan, heat oil and sauté onions for about 1 minute. Stir in remaining ingredients and bring to a boil, then reduce heat and simmer for 10 minutes.

Yields about 4 cups

Variation:
　Cheese Enchilada Sauce: Add ⅔ cup grated cheddar cheese. Serve over hot cooked pasta or grains.

Fluffy Horseradish Sauce

2 egg yolks
2 tablespoons cider vinegar
3 tablespoons horseradish
2 teaspoons honey
1 tablespoon prepared mustard
1 tablespoon water
½ cup heavy cream

Place egg yolks in the top of a double boiler and beat lightly. Stir in vinegar, horseradish, honey, mustard, and water. Place over hot water and cook, stirring constantly, until mixture thickens, about 7 minutes. Remove from heat, cover, and chill.

Whip cream until it holds soft peaks. Stir cooled horseradish mixture until smooth and then fold into cream. Cover and chill until ready to use. Sauce will keep for 4 days in refrigerator.

Yields 1½ cups

Variation:
　Yogurt-Horseradish Sauce: For a tangy, low-calorie sauce, substitute yogurt for cream.

Coriander Sauce

An easy way to spice up baked or poached fish. Garnish with lime for extra zest.

1½ tablespoons vegetable oil
1 large onion, thinly sliced
1 teaspoon minced fresh garlic
2 cups chopped canned tomatoes
⅛ teaspoon cayenne pepper
1½ tablespoons ground coriander
1 teaspoon ground cumin
1 small bay leaf

In a medium-size saucepan heat oil over medium heat. Add onion slices and sauté until soft. Add garlic and continue to cook for 1 minute longer. Add remaining ingredients and bring to a boil. Then reduce heat and simmer, uncovered, for 10 minutes. Remove bay leaf.

Yields 1¾ cups

Onion Sauce

A simple sauce to give added zip to broiled hamburgers, steaks, or vegetarian entrées.

1 medium-size sweet onion
2 teaspoons vegetable oil
1 tablespoon lemon juice
1 tablespoon prepared mustard
¼ cup catsup

Slice onion into ¼-inch slices, then separate into rings. (This will yield about 2 cups of onion rings.)

In a medium-size saucepan, sauté onion rings in oil for 3 to 5 minutes, or until tender. Stir in remaining ingredients, reduce heat to low, cover, and simmer for 5 to 7 minutes longer. Serve hot.

Yields about 1 cup

Peanut Sauce

Serve over hot cooked grains or use as a dip for crisp raw vegetables.

¼ cup Poultry Stock (page 110)
¼ cup creamy peanut butter
2 tablespoons soy sauce
dash of cayenne pepper
1 teaspoon minced garlic

In a small saucepan, heat stock. Add remaining ingredients and mix well. Store in a tightly covered jar in refrigerator.

Yields about ⅔ cup

Remoulade Sauce
(Pungent Mayonnaise Sauce)

Especially good with shellfish, cold meat, and poultry.

1 cup mayonnaise
1 tablespoon finely chopped scallions
2 teaspoons dry mustard
1 hard-cooked egg, finely chopped
2 teaspoons minced fresh tarragon or ½ teaspoon dried tarragon
1 teaspoon lemon juice

Blend all ingredients together and chill for 1 hour or more to develop flavor.

Yields 1 cup

Rosy Sauce Louis

Serve with cold seafood or stuffed artichokes.

1 cup mayonnaise
¼ cup tomato sauce
1 tablespoon lemon juice
2 tablespoons chopped fresh parsley or chives
1 teaspoon horseradish
1 teaspoon soy sauce
2 tablespoons yogurt

Combine all ingredients and mix well. Store in a tightly covered jar in refrigerator.

Yields 1½ to 1¾ cups

Sesame-Ginger Sauce

Pour over poached or baked fish.

2 tablespoons dark sesame oil
2 tablespoons grated peeled ginger root
1 tablespoon soy sauce
1 tablespoon lemon juice
1 tablespoon water
½ cup chopped scallions

Combine all ingredients in a small saucepan and bring to a boil. Serve immediately.

Yields about ½ cup

Sauce *Rouille*

This sweet pepper and garlic sauce is served over broiled fish or with poultry or fish soups.

2 thick slices whole grain bread
¼ cup Poultry Stock (page 110)
1 hot chili pepper
2 large sweet red peppers
2 large cloves garlic
¼ cup olive oil
1 teaspoon lemon juice

Soak bread in stock. Squeeze out excess moisture and reserve. Bread should be mushy and not too dry. Roast, peel, and seed chili (see page 54).

Place red peppers, garlic, chili pepper, and bread in a food processor or blender and process for 2 minutes. With the machine still running, trickle the oil slowly into the mixture. Then add 2 tablespoons of the reserved stock and the lemon juice. Let stand for 1 hour to develop flavor.

Yields about 1½ cups

Tomato-Yogurt Sauce

A colorful sauce to serve over hot or cold cooked trout or other delicate fish.

1 cup yogurt
½ cup tomato sauce
2 tablespoons lemon juice
1 teaspoon grated lemon rind
dash of cayenne pepper

Combine all ingredients and mix well.

Yields 1½ cups

Sweet-Sour Barbecue Sauce

1 cup sesame oil
¼ cup vinegar
½ to 1 teaspoon dry mustard, or to taste
1 clove garlic, minced
dash of cayenne pepper
¼ cup honey
1 egg yolk, lightly beaten

In a medium-size saucepan, combine oil, vinegar, mustard, garlic, cayenne, and honey. Simmer for 4 minutes.

Mix 2 tablespoons hot sauce with egg yolk and blend into sauce. Cook for 1 minute longer.

Yields 1¼ cups

Variation:
Creamy Barbecue Sauce: Reduce oil to ½ cup and add ½ cup yogurt to sauce just before serving.

Zesty Cucumber Sauce

½ cup mayonnaise
½ cup coarsely shredded peeled cucumber
1 teaspoon grated lemon rind
2 teaspoons lemon juice
¼ teaspoon dillweed
dash of cayenne pepper

Combine all ingredients in a small bowl and mix well.

Serve immediately over broiled or poached fish.

Yields 1 cup

Salads

Salads bring color, crunch, and light coolness to meals. What better way to set off hearty meats, casseroles, sandwiches, and thick soups than with a lush salad of mixed greens? Of course, salads built around meat, poultry, fish, fruit, or vegetable combinations can be substantial enough to stand on their own as a main dish.

There are no rules for composing salads, only a few generalizations and lots of room for experimentation. As you plan a salad, let the occasion and its use—appetizer, side dish, salad course, main dish, or dessert—dictate the ingredients and the size.

A small salad of tart fruit stimulates the appetite, so it makes a good appetizer. Create a satisfying main dish with a substantial salad of whole grains, fish, and greens married with a delicate homemade mayonnaise and garnished with chopped nuts. To soothe the palate after a spicy meal, serve a bland salad. For a satisfying dessert dress sliced strawberries and citrus sections with a cream thinned and sweetened with fruit juice.

In putting together a salad from the myriad combinations of foods and seasonings at hand, try to balance the textures, colors, and flavors. A mild base of romaine lettuce accepts assertive complements such as cucumbers, onions, pineapple, or a nippy Roquefort dressing. Soft cubes of turkey benefit from crisp celery slices, crunchy carrot rounds, and chewy pecan bits. Avoid using colors and flavors that compete. A salad of just carrots, beets, red peppers, tomatoes, and red radishes, for example, would fall short in terms of eye appeal and flavor interest. And, keep garnishes simple and edible. Often a dash of paprika or a sprig of watercress is sufficient. The best arrangements have a natural look, not one that seems artificially composed.

Salads beg for originality in the way they are served. Arrange a lovely antipasto with all kinds of raw and cooked vegetables, eggs, fish, poultry, and fruit on a large platter for a family help-yourself. Or, set up a salad bar presentation and

---

Salad Bowls

In selecting a bowl for preparing salads, consider the size of the bowl as well as its composition. A salad bowl should be large enough to accommodate bulky ingredients as they are tossed. Look for a bowl made from ceramic, glass, or wood; a plastic bowl is serviceable but hardly elegant. Some connoisseurs prefer wooden bowls, which can be seasoned with garlic and oil. Others like glass or ceramic ones which are easy to clean though these bowls cannot be seasoned.

If you choose a wooden bowl, season and care for it in the following manner. Rub the interior with a cut garlic clove. After using, simply wipe the bowl clean with dry paper towels. Continual soaking and washing of a wooden bowl strips the delicate seasoning and eventually ruins the wood itself. If, after a period of time, the oils and seasonings absorbed by the wood become rancid and impart off-flavors instead of pleasant ones, then wash the bowl and reseason it. If washing does not remove the flavor, the bowl must be refinished or replaced.

154

let each person make his own antipasto. On another occasion compose individual molded salads and serve them bedded on lettuce. Use a large molded salad as the focal point for a festive birthday dinner. Or, present platter salads — foods grouped attractively on a platter instead of tossed together in a bowl. Hollowed-out avocado halves, tomato cases, and green pepper shells make fancy, edible serving dishes for picnics and buffets.

Salad Greens

The freshest of greens is essential for making attractive-looking salads with optimum flavor and nutrition. Farmers' markets usually have the best greens, but supermarkets with a high turnover are also good places to buy. Generally, greens displayed in chilled cases are the crispest.

Whenever possible, look for unpackaged greens; then, closely inspect the leaves. Check for bright green color and crisp appearance. Avoid lettuce with rust since the spots often go through the entire head. Lettuce and cabbage should have compact, firm heads and should be heavy for their size. Whenever possible, buy the dark greens—spinach, kale, collard, beet, and turnip greens. Dark greens are high in iron and calcium as well as vitamins A and C. (The ever-present iceberg lettuce offers little in terms of nutrition.) Some greens such as Swiss chard and spinach may be high in these nutrients but they also contain oxalates which restrict the absorption of their calcium. That means these particular greens are not a prime source of calcium. (See Popular Greens table, page 156.)

Preparing Greens

Expert cooks have differing opinions about the best time for washing greens. Some like to wash greens as soon as they are brought in from the garden or the store. Others prefer to wash them right before use. Either method is fine, so long as you thoroughly dry the greens after rinsing. Too

much moisture will cause the greens to rot, but a touch of it will help crisp them. Dressings cling best to dry greens.

Before washing loose greens remove and discard any damaged or wilted leaves. Rinse the greens under cold running water or quickly swish them in sinkful of icy water. Never soak loose greens since vitamins that are water soluble easily leach into the wash water.

To clean head lettuce first rap the core sharply on a counter to loosen it, then remove it; or, cut out the core with the point of a sharp knife. (If you plan to store lettuce for several days, though, leave the core intact.) Next, hold the head under cold running water. The force of the water will separate the leaves and flush out dirt, sand, and insects. Drain, then pat the leaves dry.

Heads of cabbage with their compact, tight leaves are more difficult to wash. First, discard the outermost tough leaves which are usually damaged during the trip to the market. Then, slice through the core to cut the cabbage into quarters. Soak the pieces for 10 to 15 minutes in cool water (some vitamin C will be lost). Soaking encourages any dirt and insects lodged in the cabbage to float to the surface. Rinse and thoroughly drain.

Most greens will crisp nicely if loosely wrapped in dry toweling, slipped into a plastic bag, and stored in the refrigerator for two or more hours. Watercress and parsley keep best

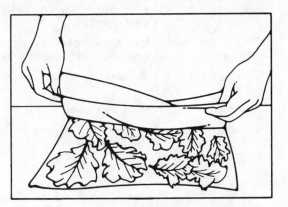

when stood in a glass of cold water, covered with a plastic bag, and placed in the refrigerator. All will stay at peak quality for up to three days.

Once washed, greens are easy to prepare for eating. Break away coarse stems and tear large leaves into bite-size pieces. With a sharp chef's knife, coarsely shred cabbage. Kitchen shears simplify snipping parsley and watercress. As a rule, one to two cups of greens will serve one person.

Salads based on greens are most appealing when well chilled and crisp. Prepare these salads shortly before serving so that the weight of other ingredients does not crush the greens. To keep greens crisp, add dressings (and juicy tomato wedges and cucumber slices) at the last possible minute. With salads destined for picnics, keep the greens crisp by carrying them undressed in a plastic bag. When ready to serve, pour the dressing into the bag and gently shake it until all the greens are coated.

Salads made with only mixed greens benefit from the simplicity of an oil and vinegar dressing. First, moisten the greens with a small amount of the oil. Toss the greens until all leaves glisten; then toss again with a little flavorful herb vinegar (or lemon juice for mild flavor).

Freshly minced herbs are another nice addition to a tossed green salad. As a rule, two tablespoons of herbs are enough for one quart of greens. Sprinkle the herbs directly on the greens or mix them with the vinegar.

Popular Greens

Green	Description	Dressings and Serving Suggestions
Arugula	dark green; bitter	vinegar and olive oil dressings; good with mixed greens
Beet greens	reddish stems; tender leaves; mild cabbage flavor	yogurt dressings, vinaigrettes
Belgian endive (sometimes called witloof chicory)	slender, long, bleached leaves; slightly bitter flavor	mayonnaise dressings, vinaigrettes; good with beets
Cabbage		
Chinese	long, tight head; pale green; mild flavor	cooked or creamy dressings, mayonnaise dressings; good with mixed greens
White, green, red, or savoy	round, compact head; color depends on variety; coarse leaves (ruffled on savoy); distinctive flavor	cooked or creamy dressings, mayonnaise dressings; good with mixed greens
Chicory (often called curly endive)	frilly, sprawling heads; coarse leaves with dark-green edges, white center; bitter flavor	onion dressings, strong-flavored cheese dressings; good with mixed greens
Collard greens	dark green; large leaves; spinachlike flavor	cheese dressings, creamy dressings, vinaigrettes; good with mixed greens
Dandelion	small, dark leaves; slightly bitter flavor	cooked dressings; good with mixed greens
Escarole	broad, coarse, flat leaves; distinctive rib; slightly bitter flavor	garlic dressings, vinaigrettes; good with mixed greens

Popular Greens—*Continued*

Green	*Description*	*Dressings and Serving Suggestions*
Garden cress	small leaves; spicy hot flavor	cooked dressings, herb dressings, vinaigrettes; good with mixed greens
Kale	dark bluish green; medium to large leaves with curly edges; crunchy; cabbagelike flavor	mild-flavored cheese dressings, vinaigrettes; good with mixed greens
Lamb's-quarters	small, dark, spoon-shaped leaves; loosely clustered; biting, radishlike flavor	mild-flavored cooked dressings; good with mixed greens
Lettuce		
Bibb	small head; pale to medium green; tender leaves; delicate, mellow flavor	herb dressings, vinaigrettes; good as a bed for main dish and molded salads
Boston (butterhead)	loose head; deep green; large, soft leaves; delicate flavor	herb dressings, yogurt dressings, light vinaigrettes; good as a bed for main dish and molded salads
Iceberg (head)	large head; crisp leaves; little flavor	cooked dressings, mayonnaise dressings; good as a bed for fruit, main dish, and molded salads
Loose-leaf (garden)	curly, loose, coarse leaves; mild flavor	herb dressings, lemon juice, mild-flavored vinaigrettes
Red-leaf	red-tinged, large, loose leaves; tender texture; delicate flavor	mild-flavored cheese dressings, yogurt dressings, vinaigrettes; good with mixed greens and as a bed for vegetable, main dish, and molded salads
Romaine (cos)	medium green; large, long, crisp leaves; mild flavor	strong-flavored cheese dressings
Mustard greens	dark green; rough-textured leaves; peppery flavor	yogurt dressings, vinaigrettes; good with mixed greens
Parsley	dark green; small, frilly leaves; distinctive flavor	strong-flavored cheese dressings, creamy dressings, herb dressings; good with mixed greens
Sorrel	bright green; crisp, tongue-shaped leaves; sour flavor	cooked dressings, vinegar and oil dressings; good with mixed greens
Spinach	dark green; tender leaves; mild but distinctive musky flavor	creamy dressings, vinaigrettes; good with mixed greens or with mushrooms and hard-cooked eggs
Turnip greens	dark green; large, tender leaves; mild cabbage flavor	yogurt dressings, vinaigrettes; good with mixed greens
Watercress	dark green; dime-size, glossy leaves; spicy, peppery flavor	cooked dressings, mayonnaise dressings; good with mixed greens

Vegetable Salads

All types of raw and cooked vegetables make appetizing, nutrient-packed salads that nicely round out any meal (see Salad Vegetables table, below). Served on Bibb lettuce, a salad of sliced beets and onions brightens a dinner of meat and potatoes, and it is quick and simple to make. Potato salad is always welcome at picnics or for buffets, and marinated legumes make an intriguing side dish alone or tossed with greens.

Of course, the simplest preparation of vegetables for salads is to use them raw. You only need to scrub and cut them into bite-size pieces. More elaborate preparation might involve steaming and marinating root vegetables and wilting delicate ones. Some vegetables, such as green peppers and tomatoes, make excellent casings (edible bowls) for other salad ingredients.

Traditional Salad Vegetables

Vegetable	Ways to Use in Salads
Beans	
Dry	cooked; whole; marinated mixed bean salads, tossed salads
Green	cooked or raw; julienne strips, whole; marinated bean salads, molded salads
Beets	cooked or raw; grated, sliced, whole; garnishes; marinated beet salads
Broccoli	cooked or raw; florets, sliced stalks; antipasto, marinated salads, molded salads, tossed salads
Carrots	cooked or raw; curls, diced, grated, julienne strips, sliced; antipasto, marinated salads, molded salads, slaws, tossed salads
Cauliflower	cooked or raw; florets, sliced stalks; marinated salads, molded salads, tossed salads
Celery	raw; diced, julienne strips, sliced; meat and poultry salads, molded salads, slaws, tossed salads
Corn	cooked; whole kernel; molded salads, relish-type salads
Cucumbers	raw; diced, shredded, sliced; antipasto, molded salads, tossed salads
Mushrooms	cooked or raw; diced, sliced, whole caps; marinated salads, molded salads, spinach salads, tossed salads
Onions	cooked or raw; diced, sliced, whole; marinated salads, meat and poultry salads, molded salads, tossed salads
Peas	cooked or raw; whole; marinated salads, molded salads, tossed salads
Peppers, red and green	cooked or raw; diced, rings, sliced, as edible bowls; antipasto, meat and poultry salads, molded salads, stuffed with salads, tossed salads
Potatoes, waxy	cooked or raw; diced, sliced, whole; antipasto, potato salads
Radishes	raw; diced, roses, sliced, whole; molded salads, tossed salads
Scallions	raw; snipped, whole; antipasto, meat and poultry salads, molded salads, pasta salads, tossed salads
Squashes, summer	cooked or raw; cubed, grated, julienne strips, sliced; molded salads, tossed salads
Tomatoes	raw; cubed, sliced, wedges, whole, as edible bowls; antipasto, aspics, marinated salads, molded salads, stuffed with salads, tossed salads

Fruit Salads

Fruit salads lend color and refreshment to a meal. Chilled melon balls garnished with fragrant sprigs of mint make a subdued, sweet appetizer or dessert. Smothered in yogurt, blueberries are a perfect finale for a dinner. When several fresh fruits are arranged with a scoop of cottage cheese and nestled on a bed of red-leaf lettuce, the result is an ideal luncheon dish for a hot summer's day.

Preparing fruits for salads is easy (see Preparing Fruits, page 608). Generally, pieces for salads are cut into halves, cubes, balls, or wedges. Whenever you can, divide the fruit in such a way that a portion of the skin remains on each cut piece. Preserving the skin maximizes taste, texture, fiber, and nutrients. When left on pears and apples, it also lends an attractive touch of color. For a few salads you will need to peel the fruit. On those occasions pare as thinly as possible.

As you cut fruit, keep the pieces somewhat large (about bite-size or slightly bigger). Large pieces are less susceptible to loss of nutrients from overexposure to light and air. They also maintain the character of the fruit you are eating.

Cut fruit pieces must remain colorful and bright to be appetizing in a salad. To slow the browning of bananas, apples, peaches, and pears, sprinkle lemon juice over the fruit immediately after cutting. (Cortland apples, unlike other types, remain white and fresh looking for hours after they have been cut, and therefore may not need lemon juice.)

Make the most of fruit salads by presenting them in attractive ways. Make boats of pineapple shells or baskets from cantaloupes. Grapefruit and orange rinds turn into colorful cups. Bananas become canoes or stick men.

High-Protein Main Dish Salads

Any cooked meat, poultry, or fish lightly coated with a mayonnaise or French dressing makes a substantial salad that is worthy of service as a main dish. These salads also make excellent fillings for sandwiches.

In making meat, poultry, or fish salads, you can use leftovers or freshly cooked foods. Simply slice or cube leftover meats and poultry, then add the dressing. Fish should be gently flaked. If you are cooking meat or poultry expressly for use in a salad, boil it for a soft, tender texture. Other methods of cooking tend to dry meat. After boiling, marinate the meat to make up for the flavor lost to the cooking water. Either braising or poaching is an appropriate way to cook fish destined for salads.

Eggs are yet another excellent protein source for salads. They are usually hard-cooked, then sliced for an antipasto, chopped for use as a garnish on a spinach salad, or grated and added to the dressing on potatoes. With a little dressing and minced onion, chopped eggs by themselves make a tasty salad or sandwich filling.

Whole grains, too, make satisfying salads either by themselves or in combination with meat, fish, poultry, fruits, or vegetables. The grains—rice, bulgur—and pastas that retain their shape and some firmness after being cooked and dressed result in the best-looking salads. Bulgur, for instance, makes a hearty traditional Middle Eastern salad, tabbouleh.

Several of the natural cheeses work well as protein sources for salads. Cottage cheese is often the primary ingredient in fruit and molded salads. And, blue, Roquefort, and cheddar cheeses turn bland dressings into rich nippy ones. Use strong cheeses like Parmesan and Romano sparingly. Mild, firm cheeses look attractive when sliced, cubed, or shredded and then arranged as a garnish on the salad.

Seeds, nuts, and sprouts make other wholesome, tasty garnishes on salads. Try adding sesame, sunflower, pumpkin, or caraway seeds; or, use almonds, cashews, peanuts, walnuts, or pecans for a crunchy surprise in soft meat or grain salads. For garden freshness add a sprinkling of alfalfa, radish, lentil, chick-pea, wheat, rye, sunflower, or mung bean sprouts.

Since the flavor of main dish salads will mellow and improve with time, chill meat, poultry, fish, egg, and whole grain salads for an hour or so before serving. To savor the full flavor of a delicate fish salad, first chill and then allow it to return to room temperature for serving. On picnics always keep fish, poultry, egg, and potato salads safe by packing them in ice so they stay well chilled.

Molded Salads

Molded salads add shimmer and grace to formal dinners, buffets, and even picnics. A cranberry ring, set on a bed of lettuce and filled with cottage cheese, looks beautiful next to a large roasted turkey. And, a savory aspic in a fish-shaped mold makes an attractive centerpiece for a special buffet.

Molds for Shaping Salads

When selecting a mold, let your imagination take over. To create individual circular salads, use small fish cans or muffin tins. Or, try deeper cans and slice the gel once it is firmly set. You can mold gels in large, shallow (one to two inches deep) pans; then cut your own designs. (Cookie cutters are great for cutting stars, hearts, and other common shapes.) If you are less adventurous, you will find a ready solution in very attractive commercially shaped molds. For a sturdy gel select a ring mold with the supportive center wall instead of a large, deep, bowl mold.

Molded salads are also ideal for disguising leftovers. Team leftover grains and fruits in a gel based on pineapple juice, or pair up leftover roast beef and vegetables and marry the flavors with a gelatinous beef or vegetable stock.

Either agar (a vegetable gelatin made from sea moss, an algae) or unflavored, unsweetened gelatin gives structure to fruit and vegetable salads. (Flavored gels work, too, but they are loaded with sugar and artificial flavorings and colorings.) Gelatinous stock holds vegetables, meat, poultry, or fish together to form appealing, nutritious aspics. About two tablespoons of agar

flakes or gelatin (two envelopes) thicken three to four cups of liquid nicely. (The same proportions of gelatin to liquid can be used to set a non-gelatinous or watery stock.)

To use gelatin or agar, soak the recommended amount in one-quarter cup of cold water. Let it sit for five minutes, stirring occasionally. When softened, stir in hot liquid. Chill until the liquid is the consistency of raw egg whites. Next, quickly rinse a mold with cold water and pour the mixture into it. (Rinsing the mold makes it easy to unmold the salad later.)

Add other ingredients which have been pureed, shredded, or diced into smaller-than-bite-size pieces. (Fresh pineapple, figs, papaya, and kiwi fruit all contain an enzyme that interferes with the jelling property of gelatin. Heat destroys that enzyme, so use a canned variety of those fruits or cook the fresh fruits before mixing them with the gelatin.) The timing for adding ingredients to gelatin is critical. If added too soon, fruit, vegetable, and meat pieces will sink to the bottom; if added too late, they will perch on the top. Finally, chill the gelatin until firm.

Ideally, you should make gelatin salads early in the day (or the day before) since they take three to four hours to set. But sometimes it is desirable to set the gel in one or two hours. At those times use only half the amount of hot liquid, then stir in ice cubes instead of the remaining liquid. When the mixture reaches the raw egg white stage, remove any undissolved cubes and proceed as usual to complete the salad.

If you are using a gelatinous stock to make an aspic, heat—but do not boil—the stock until it becomes liquid. Once fluid, the stock should be cooled until, like other gelatin mixtures, it reaches the consistency of raw egg whites. Then add desired ingredients and chill until set.

Layered molded salads are time-consuming but fun and easy to make. First, set the top layer (which is on the bottom of the mold until the salad is turned out); then, pour in the gelatin mixture for the second layer. Proceed in this manner until all the desired layers have been added and set. Remove the salad from the mold and you have a truly impressive presentation.

When it is time to unmold, fill a sink or a large bowl with warm water that is deep enough to cover the sides of the mold. Carefully dip the mold into the water. Do not let any water run over the top edge! In about 30 seconds the warm water will soften the gelatin around the sides. (Of course, the entire gel will soften if left in the heat too long.) After taking the mold from the water, gently shake it to be sure the gelatin is loose. Then, invert a wet plate over the mold (the wetness helps in centering the mold on the plate) and deftly flip both plate and mold over to turn out the gelatin. If it does not drop to the plate, loosen it with an abrupt, firm shake. Refrigerate the gel for 15 minutes to reset the sides.

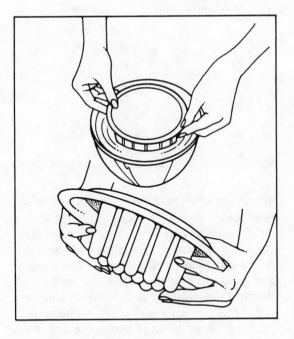

If dipping the mold into warm water makes you uneasy, try this method. Invert the mold on a serving plate. Immerse a dish towel in hot water, then wring it out. Quickly wrap the hot towel around the inverted mold. Remove the towel and the mold the moment the salad drops down.

Gelatin salads keep well in the refrigerator for several days. After that they tend to become rubbery from a gradual loss of water. Never freeze gelatin dishes.

Molded salads benefit from judiciously applied garnishes. A few mint leaves or sprigs of parsley or several lemon wedges work nicely with both side and main dish salads. Nestle individual salads on cups of Bibb lettuce. To softly finish a dessert salad, spoon on a dollop of yogurt or a fluffy dressing of whipped cream. Chopped nuts scattered on a cranberry mold lend a delightful crunch, and raisins give just the right touch of sweetness and color contrast to a peach-yogurt gel.

Salad Dressings

It takes a flavorful dressing to marry the various vegetables, fruits, or meats in a salad perfectly. The dressing can be thick or thin, sweet or tart, traditional or experimental, but it should always suit your taste and the dish. Choose a light, tart dressing for appetizer, side dish, and main course salads. Sweet and rich dressings sate the appetite, so they are best reserved for dessert salads.

Most dressings originate from one of three basic types: vinaigrette, mayonnaise, or cooked. Sweet cream and yogurt-based dressings do not belong to any of these categories, yet they are popular and easy to make.

Vinaigrette—often called French, oil and vinegar, or Italian—is the simplest of the dressings. It is based on an oil and vinegar combination, and often includes herbs. Vinaigrettes must be shaken vigorously before each use because they separate readily.

For easy preparation and serving, make a vinaigrette in a jar. Mix two or three parts oil to one part vinegar. Any one of the light oils makes a pleasing dressing (see Salad Oils table, page 162). Wine vinegar, cider vinegar, or one of the herb vinegars (see Herb Vinegars, page 50) lends a good flavor. But white distilled vinegar is too harsh, tending to overpower the other salad

Salad Oils

Oil	Flavor	Suitability for Salads	Fatty Acids Saturated	Polyunsaturated
Safflower	minimal	unsuitable (unless blended with olive or aromatic nut oils)	very low (has lowest ratio)	very high
Corn	light	suitable	low	high
Sunflower	mild	suitable (especially for raw vegetable salads)	low	very high
Olive	fruity, rich, delicate	suitable	low	high
Sesame	nutty	suitable	low	high
Peanut	mild	suitable	low (slightly higher than corn or olive oil)	high (slightly lower than corn oil)
Soy	mild to slightly beany	suitable	low	high (about the same as corn oil)
Avocado	light, slightly nutty, sharp	suitable	low	high
Almond	mildly sweet, barely nutty	suitable	low	high
Hazelnut	nutty (toasted flavor)	suitable	low	high
Walnut	nutty	suitable	low	high

ingredients (see Vinegars table, page 164). If vinegars in general are sharper than you like, try the subtler lemon or lime juice.

When using herbs, add them to the vinegar before the oil. To awaken the fragrance of dried herbs, crush them in your fingers, then soak them in the vinegar for at least 25 minutes before adding the oil. Basil, borage, burnet, chervil, chives, coriander, dill, fennel, marjoram, mint, oregano, parsley, rosemary, summer savory, tarragon, thyme, and fines herbes (a mix of chervil, chives, parsley, and tarragon) complement salad ingredients.

With the addition of chopped foods, a vinaigrette becomes a chiffonade. Tasty companions are parsley, sweet red pepper, green pepper, celery, onion, and hard-cooked egg.

Mayonnaise is a fairly stable emulsion of oil, egg yolk, and lemon juice. Rich and creamy, it goes exceptionally well with meat, fish, poultry, and potato salads. It is also the base for such flavorful preparations as Russian dressing and tartar sauce. (See Emulsion Sauces, page 138.)

A thick white sauce makes the base for a cooked salad dressing. Lemon juice or vinegar, seasonings, and a fat transform the sauce into a rich dressing such as a blue cheese or a savory sour cream.

Both mayonnaise and cooked dressings benefit from the addition of fresh or dried herbs,

Can Be Interchanged with Other Oils for Salad Dressings	Comments
yes	Recommended for those who must watch cholesterol levels. Very high in essential nutrients. Texture unpleasant; greasy in salad dressings.
yes	Most popular, versatile oil.
yes	Suitable for salad dressings; less so for cooking.
yes	Pleasant, but definite flavor. Popular for salad dressings.
yes	Brown sesame oil is highly flavored and best added to other oils for salad dressings. The lighter sesame oil can be used full strength.
yes	Peanut oil imported from France is preferred for salads.
yes	Best-tasting varieties are found in oriental grocery stores.
no	Experts consider it primarily a novelty.
no	Best for special effect.
no	Best for special effect.
no	Best for special effect.

yogurt, sour cream, chili sauce, catsup, crumbled Roquefort, grated hard-cooked eggs, grated onions, finely diced cucumbers, minced bell peppers, or chopped nuts. Fruit and vegetable juices also blend well into dressings. Three tablespoons of freshly crumbled herbs or one tablespoon of dried herbs to one cup of dressing works well. Use about three tablespoons of eggs, onions, cucumbers, peppers, or nuts and one-half to one cup of yogurt, juice, catsup, cream, cheese, or chili sauce to one cup of dressing.

Many dressings, such as vinaigrettes, develop the most flavor about 30 minutes after they have been made. From there taste quality slowly goes downhill, so prepare minimal amounts, no more than you will use in a day or two. Store leftover dressings, covered, in the refrigerator.

The best time to apply the dressing depends on the salad. Add vinaigrettes to crisp vegetables, greens, and fresh fruits just before serving to prevent wilting. But apply mayonnaise and cooked dressings to meat, poultry, potato, fish, pasta, beet, and cabbage salads one to two hours ahead of serving. Those salads improve by marinating. And, for outstanding flavor in meats and poultry destined for tossed salads, marinate those protein foods in a French dressing for an hour or so before tossing them with the greens. Use the same dressing on the entire salad. Keep the salad

Using Garlic in Salads

Garlic adds a delightful assertive snap to salads—tossed, potato, meat, poultry. Too much, though, overpowers all other ingredients. Here are four easy ways to keep garlic flavor subtle.

- Before adding the greens rub the bowl with a cut garlic clove.
- Toss a chapon with the salad, then remove it before serving. A chapon is a dry crust of bread that had been rubbed on all sides with the cut edge of a garlic clove.
- Place two or three crushed cloves in the bottom of the salad bowl, add the dressing, and allow the flavors to mellow for ten minutes. Remove the cloves before serving the salad.
- Slice garlic into the salad oil, then warm it briefly over low heat. Cool the oil and remove the garlic before serving. Avoid letting the garlic stand long in the oil; it will become bitter.

ingredients well chilled until serving time but warm all vinaigrette dressings to room temperature.

Avoid overdressing salads since the delicate flavors of other ingredients are easily masked. Generally speaking, three to four tablespoons of dressing are ample for one quart of prepared

greens. One-quarter to one-half cup mayonnaise readily coats three to four cups of potatoes, meat, or poultry. Use a dressing that is thin enough to blend easily with the salad but not so thin that it immediately drains to the bottom of the bowl.

Trickle or spoon the dressing over the salad and gently toss until all ingredients glisten with a light coating. For salads dressed at the last minute, you can add the dressing to the salad in a large serving bowl or pass it for each person to apply his own. Occasionally, you may prefer to put the dressing on first instead of last. If so, place several sturdy greens over the dressing in the bottom of the bowl to protect the more tender greens from the moisture. Toss the salad at serving time.

Making Your Own Croutons

It is easy to make croutons at home. Simply cut crusts and pieces of dry bread into small cubes. Then, sprinkle the cubes with garlic powder and toast them in the broiler, or sauté them in one to two tablespoons butter in a moderately hot skillet. Toasted croutons have fewer calories and less fat than sautéed ones.

Vinegars

Vinegar	Source	Characteristics
Cider	apple cider	Apple-acid flavor is strong, but good for oil and vinegar dressings—especially highly seasoned ones.
Herb	cider vinegar or red or white wine vinegar with herbs added	Flavor is characteristic of the herb added. Good in salads.
Malt	barley malt or other cereal grains	Flavor is too strong for salads.
Rice	rice	Flavor has about half the sharpness of cider vinegar with a touch of sweetness. Tasty in salads—especially in those made with oriental vegetables.
White or distilled	alcohol	Strong, acidic flavor is too sharp for salad dressings.
Wine	red, rosé, or white wine	Red or rosé wine vinegars are robust and go well with pungent greens, meat, and cheese salads. White wine vinegar is more delicate and excellent with tender lettuces.

Green Salads

Caesar Salad

The traditional anchovies are eliminated in this recipe because of their high salt content.

    1 large head romaine lettuce, torn into bite-size
        pieces
    2 cloves garlic
    2 eggs
    ¼ teaspoon dry mustard
    ¼ cup olive oil
        juice of ½ lemon, at room temperature
    1 tablespoon wine vinegar
    ½ teaspoon soy sauce
    ¼ cup grated Parmesan cheese
        freshly ground pepper
    ½ cup croutons

Dry lettuce thoroughly. Cut garlic cloves in half and rub them all over the inside of a large wooden salad bowl, then discard.

Cook eggs gently in simmering water for 1 minute. When cool enough to handle, break eggs into salad bowl and mix rapidly with a wooden spoon until well blended and lightened in color. Stirring constantly, add dry mustard, then slowly pour oil into egg mixture. Add lemon juice, vinegar, and soy sauce. Mix well.

Toss lettuce in mixture. Sprinkle cheese and a generous amount of pepper into salad. Toss again, add croutons, and serve immediately.

    4 servings

Cool Coleslaw

    2 cups shredded cabbage
    1 cup diced celery or 1 teaspoon celery seeds
    1 carrot, shredded
    1 to 2 young stalks dill, chopped
    2 tablespoons chopped fresh basil
    1 teaspoon poppy seeds
    3 tablespoons mayonnaise
    1 to 2 tablespoons wine vinegar
        pepper, to taste

Combine all ingredients in a large bowl and chill for at least 1 hour before serving, to allow flavors to blend.

    4 servings

Romaine and Fennel Salad

    2 cloves garlic
    ¾ cup vegetable oil
    3 tablespoons lemon juice
    3 egg yolks
        freshly ground pepper, to taste
    2 heads romaine lettuce, torn into bite-size pieces
    2 bulbs fennel, finely slivered
    1½ cups diced tofu, drained, or ¾ cup diced
        tofu and ¾ cup ricotta cheese
    1½ cups chopped walnuts
        grated Parmesan cheese, to taste

Cut garlic cloves in half and rub them all over bottom of a very large wooden salad bowl, then discard.

In a small bowl whisk together oil, lemon juice, egg yolks, and pepper until well blended. Pour into salad bowl and stir well. Place lettuce, fennel, tofu, and ricotta (if used) in salad bowl and toss lightly until coated with dressing. Garnish with Parmesan cheese.

    6 to 8 servings

Stuffed Lettuce, Country Style

    1 whole, large, firm head lettuce
    1 tablespoon crumbled Roquefort cheese
    3 tablespoons grated carrots
    1 tablespoon chopped pimientos
    2 tablespoons chopped green peppers
    1½ tablespoons grated onions
    1 teaspoon lemon juice
    ¼ cup tomato puree

Remove core of lettuce and hold head under cold running water. Drain well. Using your fingers and a serrated knife, hollow out center of lettuce, leaving a shell about 1 inch thick. Place shell upside down on paper toweling and drain well.

Finely chop scooped-out heart of lettuce and combine with remaining ingredients. Pack mixture firmly into lettuce shell. Wrap stuffed lettuce head in wax paper or cheesecloth and chill thoroughly.

Slice into wedges and serve with Herb Dressing (page 182), Vinaigrette (page 184), or any favorite dressing.

    6 to 8 servings

Spinach-Mushroom Salad with Sweet-Sour Mustard Dressing

1 tablespoon vegetable oil
1 pound mushrooms, sliced
1 small onion, chopped
  pepper, to taste
1 tablespoon lemon juice
1 pound spinach, torn into bite-size pieces
  Sweet-Sour Mustard Dressing (see below)
3 hard-cooked eggs, sliced or coarsely grated
½ cup croutons (optional)

Heat oil in a medium-size skillet. Add mushrooms and brown quickly over high heat, stirring often. Add onions during last 30 seconds of cooking. (Do not overcook.) Transfer mixture to a bowl. Sprinkle with pepper and lemon juice, toss lightly, and set aside to cool.

Combine spinach with cooled mushrooms and onions in a large salad bowl. Add dressing and toss. Top with eggs and croutons (if used).

6 servings

Sweet-Sour Mustard Dressing

2 tablespoons vinegar
1 tablespoon honey
¼ cup vegetable oil
1 teaspoon French-style mustard
  pepper, to taste

Heat vinegar and honey in a small saucepan, stirring until honey is dissolved. Let cool. Combine with remaining ingredients in a jar with a tight-fitting lid. Shake well.

Yields about ½ cup

Tossed Green Salad

½ head iceberg lettuce
¼ head curly endive
¼ pound fresh spinach
½ bunch radishes, sliced or cut into wedges
½ medium-size cucumber, sliced
1 cup croutons
  Herbal Vinaigrette (page 185)
3 medium-size tomatoes, cut into wedges

Tear lettuce, endive, and spinach into bite-size pieces. Combine with radishes and cucumbers in a large salad bowl. Toss with croutons and vinaigrette, then decorate with tomatoes. Or, serve vinaigrette in a separate bowl.

6 to 8 servings

Variations:
Replace spinach and radishes with any of the following:
  watercress
  grated carrots
  grated turnips
  cauliflower florets
  shredded red or green cabbage

Stuffed Head Lettuce

This salad is especially nice for a picnic since each serving will have its own "dressing" when carved into wedges.

½ cup minced unpeeled cucumber
¼ cup minced onions
2 tablespoons minced green peppers
3 tablespoons vinegar
2 tablespoons honey
  dash each of ground allspice, turmeric, ground cloves, and celery seeds
1 whole, medium-size, firm head lettuce
8 ounces cream cheese, softened
2 teaspoons tomato paste
2 hard-cooked eggs, finely chopped

Combine cucumbers, onions, and peppers and drain well. Place in a small saucepan with vinegar, honey, spices, and celery seeds. Cook over moderately high heat for 5 to 10 minutes, or until vegetables are tender and mixture has reduced to ½ to ⅓ cup. Set aside to cool.

Meanwhile, prepare lettuce by removing core and holding under cold running water. Allow to drain well. Using a serrated grapefruit knife and your fingers, hollow out lettuce until cavity will hold about 1 cup filling, leaving wall of ½ to 1 inch in thickness. Shred scooped-out lettuce and set aside. Place lettuce head, hole-side down, on paper towels and allow to drain again until almost dry.

Mix cream cheese and tomato paste in a small bowl until well blended. Stir in cooled vegetable mixture and hard-cooked eggs, then pack into hollowed-out lettuce head, shaking well so that mixture reaches bottom of hole. Place lettuce in a small bowl, filled-side up, cover, and refrigerate for several hours until center is firm.

When ready to serve, place lettuce head, filled-side down, on bed of reserved shredded lettuce. Carve into wedges with a sharp knife.

6 to 8 servings

Spinach Salad

1 pound spinach, torn into bite-size pieces
¼ cup chopped leeks or fresh chives
2 white radishes, sliced (optional)
10 mushrooms, thinly sliced
1 carrot, cut into julienne strips

Combine all ingredients in a salad bowl and toss with dressing. Goes especially well with Creamy Cucumber Salad Dressing (page 181), Green Garden Dressing (page 182), or Mushroom Dressing (page 183).

4 to 6 servings

Tossed Sesame Salad with Tarragon Dressing

2 heads Boston lettuce, torn into bite-size pieces
¼ cup sesame seeds
¼ cup thinly sliced water chestnuts
¼ cup grated Parmesan cheese
Tarragon Dressing (see below)

Place lettuce, sesame seeds, water chestnuts, and cheese in a large salad bowl. Toss lightly with enough dressing to coat (reserve remainder for another salad). Serve immediately.

6 to 8 servings

Tarragon Dressing

⅔ cup vegetable oil
⅓ cup vinegar
1½ teaspoons dried tarragon
1 teaspoon honey

½ teaspoon dry mustard
½ clove garlic, crushed

Combine all ingredients in a jar with a tight-fitting lid. Shake well.

Yields about 1 cup

Vegetable Salads

Carrot Salad

½ cup walnuts
½ pound unpeeled carrots, cut into chunks (4 to 5 medium size)
½ cup raisins
¼ cup mayonnaise

Chop walnuts coarsely in a blender at low speed, then scrape into a serving bowl.

Place carrots in blender, then add raisins and enough water to cover. Process briefly, at low speed, until carrots are coarsely chopped. Drain well in a colander or strainer. Add carrot mixture to nuts, stir in mayonnaise, chill and serve.

2 to 4 servings

Cucumber Salad

1 medium-size cucumber, thinly sliced
pepper, to taste
dillweed, to taste
1 medium-size onion, thinly sliced
¼ teaspoon light honey
2 tablespoons corn oil
2 tablespoons cider vinegar

Place cucumber slices in a shallow bowl and lightly sprinkle with pepper and dillweed.

Separate onion slices into rings and add to cucumbers. Add honey and gently toss with a fork. Add oil and toss until each slice is coated. Add vinegar and toss again. Chill for 1 hour. Lightly toss with a fork before serving.

4 servings

Eggplant Salad

1 medium-size eggplant, cubed (about 3 cups)
2 tablespoons minced onions
½ cup chopped pecans
½ cup chopped celery
½ cup chopped green peppers
¼ cup plus 2 tablespoons vegetable oil
3 tablespoons vinegar
  pepper, to taste
1 teaspoon dried basil
  salad greens
2 tablespoons chopped fresh parsley

Cook eggplant in as little water as possible, or steam, until tender. Combine with other ingredients and chill in refrigerator. Serve on salad greens, garnished with chopped parsley.

4 to 6 servings

Fresh Raw Vegetables with Vinaigrette Sauce

  Bibb lettuce, chicory, or other salad greens
1 cup shredded peeled beets
1 cup shredded carrots
1 cup slivered celery
½ cup shredded black radishes
¾ cup shredded peeled turnips
12 cherry tomatoes
1 small cucumber, seeded and shredded
  Vinaigrette Sauce (see below)

Line a platter with greens and arrange vegetables on top in a decorative manner. Pour vinaigrette over all and serve immediately.

6 servings

Vinaigrette Sauce

1 egg yolk
1 tablespoon French-style mustard
2 tablespoons tarragon or wine vinegar
1 tablespoon chopped scallions
½ teaspoon freshly ground white pepper
¾ cup olive oil

Combine egg yolk, mustard, vinegar, scallions, and pepper in a bowl. Beat with a wire whisk for 1 minute. Add oil very slowly, beating constantly with whisk until sauce is consistency of thin mayonnaise.

Yields about 1¼ cups

Fresh Mushroom Salad

1 pound mushrooms
¼ cup plus 1 tablespoon olive oil
2 tablespoons wine vinegar
¼ cup chopped fresh parsley
1½ tablespoons chopped fresh tarragon or 1
  teaspoon dried tarragon
⅛ teaspoon freshly ground pepper
  watercress

Remove stems from mushrooms and reserve for another use. Slice large mushroom caps about ¼ inch thick; cut small caps in half. Place sliced mushrooms in a mixing bowl. Add oil, vinegar, parsley, tarragon, and pepper. Toss salad well, then cover and chill in refrigerator for 1 hour, to blend flavors.

To serve, spoon salad into serving dish lined with watercress.

6 servings

Variation:

Mushroom and Dill Salad: Omit tarragon and substitute 1½ tablespoons chopped fresh dill.

Kefir Potato Salad

6 medium-size potatoes
1½ cups chopped cooked carrots
1 cup diced, cooked, fresh green beans
1 cup cooked fresh or frozen peas
½ cup chopped scallions
¼ cup chopped celery
⅛ teaspoon pepper
⅛ teaspoon garlic powder
2 cups kefir (page 448)
  salad greens
  thin tomato wedges
  chopped fresh parsley

Cook potatoes in enough water to cover until tender, 30 to 40 minutes. Drain, cool, then dice them into a large bowl. Add carrots, beans, peas, scallions, celery, pepper, garlic powder, and kefir. Toss gently until well combined. Cover and chill for several hours.

When ready to serve, spoon into a bowl lined with crisp salad greens and garnish with tomato wedges and parsley.

4 to 6 servings

Lalap
(Indonesian Salad)

2 teaspoons vegetable oil
1 teaspoon paprika
¼ cup vinegar
   dash of crushed red pepper, or to taste
2½ tablespoons honey
   dash of soy sauce
1 cup bean sprouts
1 leek, thinly sliced
1 cucumber, thinly sliced
½ cup roasted cashews

Heat oil in a small saucepan. Add paprika and sauté for several minutes until color becomes brighter. Add vinegar, red pepper, honey, and soy sauce and bring to a boil. Remove from heat and set aside to cool to room temperature.

In a salad bowl, toss together sprouts, leeks, and cucumbers. Pour cooled dressing over vegetables and toss until well coated. Sprinkle cashews on top and serve.

4 to 6 servings

Three-Bean Salad

The beans in this salad are marinated the night before to allow flavor to develop fully.

¼ cup plus 2 tablespoons olive oil
3 tablespoons red wine vinegar
2 cloves garlic, minced
¼ teaspoon dried oregano
½ teaspoon pepper
1 cup fresh green beans, cut into 1-inch pieces
1 cup hot, cooked, white marrow beans, drained
1 cup hot cooked kidney beans, drained
1 large Bermuda or red onion
2 stalks celery
2 ounces sharp cheddar cheese, cubed
2 tablespoons minced fresh parsley
   romaine lettuce or other salad greens

Combine oil, vinegar, garlic, oregano, and pepper in a small bowl or jar and mix together well. Set marinade aside.

Steam green beans for 5 minutes. Then place hot green beans in a medium-size bowl along with hot marrow and kidney beans. Pour marinade over combined beans and toss lightly until all are well coated. Cover bowl and chill overnight in refrigerator.

Next day, thinly slice onion and separate into rings. Thinly slice celery stalks. Cut cheese into ½-inch cubes. Combine onion rings, celery, cheese, and parsley with marinated beans and toss together until well mixed. Serve in a bowl lined with romaine or other salad greens.

4 to 6 servings

Potato–Wax Bean Salad

8 medium-size unpeeled red potatoes
2½ pounds fresh wax beans
½ to 1 cup olive oil
2 teaspoons vinegar
   pepper, to taste
1 tablespoon chopped fresh basil
4 scallions, chopped

Cook potatoes in enough water to cover until tender, 30 to 40 minutes. Cook beans in a small amount of boiling water, or steam, until just tender, about 20 minutes. Drain potatoes and beans and cut into bite-size pieces. While still warm, toss with enough oil to lightly coat vegetables. Add vinegar, pepper, basil, and scallions and toss again. Marinate for at least 1 hour before serving at room temperature.

8 servings

Raw Vegetable Salad

2 cups coarsely grated carrots
2 cups finely shredded cabbage
2 cups peeled, seeded, and coarsely grated
   cucumbers
1 to 2 cups bean sprouts (optional)
   salad greens

Arrange vegetables and sprouts (if used) in separate mounds on a platter lined with crisp salad greens. Serve a dressing in a separate container. Goes well with Curried Mayonnaise (page 182), Horseradish-Yogurt Dressing (page 182), or Rocky Roquefort Salad Dressing (page 183).

Or, lightly toss each vegetable in a dressing before arranging mounds on platter. Sprinkle sprouts over all.

6 to 8 servings

Tangy Potato Salad

4 medium-size unpeeled potatoes
2 hard-cooked eggs, chopped
2 stalks celery, diced
2 scallions or 1 small onion, finely chopped
1 small cucumber, chopped
2 tablespoons chopped fresh parsley
½ cup sunflower seeds (optional)
3 tablespoons yogurt
2 tablespoons lemon juice
1 teaspoon caraway seeds
½ teaspoon dry mustard
1 teaspoon chopped fresh dill or ½ teaspoon
    dillweed
paprika

Cook potatoes in enough water to cover until tender, 30 to 40 minutes. Drain, cool, then dice them into a large bowl. Add eggs, celery, scallions, or onions, cucumbers, parsley, and sunflower seeds (if used). Mix well.

In a small bowl combine yogurt, lemon juice, caraway seeds, mustard, and dill. Pour over potato mixture and toss gently. Garnish with paprika.

4 servings

Fruit Salads

Roquefort Apples

6 medium-size apples
3 tablespoons lemon juice
⅓ cup crumbled Roquefort cheese
¼ cup vegetable oil
⅓ cup chopped walnuts
3 tablespoons raisins

Cut slice off top of each apple and reserve. Remove core, then scoop out pulp in large pieces (do not discard), leaving shell ¼ inch thick. Brush insides of shells with lemon juice.

Dice scooped-out pulp into a small bowl. Add remaining ingredients and toss lightly. Fill apple shells with mixture and replace reserved tops. Chill first, or serve immediately.

4 to 6 servings

Curried Melon Salad

½ cup chopped onions
2 tablespoons Clarified Butter (page 148)
2 teaspoons curry powder, or to taste
¾ cup mayonnaise
    juice of ½ lime
1 cantaloupe
¼ cup diced celery
¼ cup diced tart apples
1 honeydew melon, cut into 4 to 6 wedges
    lettuce leaves
    lime wedges

In a small saucepan sauté onions in clarified butter until translucent. (Do not brown.) Add curry powder and continue to cook until foamy, about 2 minutes. Cool mixture, then add mayonnaise and lime juice and blend well.

Remove seeds and membrane from cantaloupe and scoop flesh into balls or cut into cubes (about 2 to 2½ cups). Drain well on paper toweling.

In a large bowl combine cantaloupe, celery, apples, and mayonnaise mixture. Toss lightly and serve immediately in wedges of honeydew melon set on lettuce leaves. Garnish with lime wedges.

4 to 6 servings

Orange, Fennel, and Watercress Salad

4 large oranges, separated into segments
2 tablespoons white wine vinegar
2 tablespoons vegetable oil
1 tablespoon honey
1 bulb fennel
¼ cup chopped dates
1 bunch watercress, with stems removed

Holding orange segments over a mixing bowl to collect any juice, remove white membranes and break segments into pieces. Place pieces in bowl along with vinegar, oil, and honey. Stir to coat all pieces well.

Separate fennel into stalks and slice into thin slivers. Stir into orange sections. Add chopped dates. Cover and marinate in refrigerator about 30 minutes.

Just before serving, drain liquid from orange sections into a separate container to serve as dressing. Toss watercress with orange sections and fennel. Serve immediately with reserved dressing.

4 to 6 servings

Pear and Roquefort Salad

4 ounces Roquefort cheese
¼ cup butter, softened
3 large pears
   lemon juice, for sprinkling
½ cup yogurt
   paprika
   salad greens

In a small bowl beat together cheese and butter until smooth.

Peel, halve, and core pears, then lightly sprinkle each half with lemon juice. Divide cheese mixture evenly over pear halves and press mixture down with a spoon. Divide yogurt among pear halves and spread lightly to coat. Garnish with paprika. Chill well before serving on a platter lined with salad greens.

6 servings

Waldorf Salad

4 medium-size unpeeled tart apples, cored
   and cubed
¼ cup chopped celery
¼ cup raisins
½ cup chopped walnuts
1 tablespoon lemon juice
2 tablespoons yogurt
2 tablespoons mayonnaise
2 teaspoons honey
   salad greens

In a large bowl combine apples, celery, raisins, and walnuts. In a separate bowl mix together lemon juice, yogurt, mayonnaise, and honey. Stir until well blended. Add dressing to apple mixture, toss together, and serve on a bed of salad greens.

4 to 6 servings

Rice and Dried Fruit Salad
with Sweet and Zesty Dressing

1 cup orange juice
1½ cups water
1 cardamom pod, crushed
1 stick of cinnamon, 1 inch long
1 tablespoon sliced peeled ginger root
6 dried apricots, cut in half
3 slices dried pineapple
1 cup uncooked brown rice

¼ cup raisins
   Sweet and Zesty Dressing (see below)
¼ cup chopped scallions
¼ cup chopped green or sweet red peppers

In a medium-size saucepan combine orange juice, water, cardamom, cinnamon, and ginger. Simmer gently for 10 minutes, tightly covered. Add apricots and pineapple and simmer about 5 minutes longer, or until fruits are just tender. Remove saucepan from heat. Pour mixture through a strainer. Reserve juice, discard spices, and set cooked fruit aside to cool.

Return strained juice to saucepan and stir in rice and raisins. Bring to a slow boil, then cover, reduce heat to a simmer, and cook until rice is tender and liquid is absorbed, about 30 minutes. (It may be necessary to add a small amount of water to prevent sticking.) Remove cooked rice and raisins from heat and allow to stand, still covered, for 20 minutes undisturbed.

Pour dressing over warm rice. Use 2 forks to fluff rice and coat thoroughly with dressing. Chop apricots and pineapple and add to rice. Cool to room temperature. Just before serving, toss in scallions and peppers.

4 to 6 servings

Sweet and Zesty Dressing

¼ cup fruit juice (apple, pineapple, or
   white grape)
2 tablespoons cider vinegar
½ cup vegetable oil
¼ teaspoon white pepper

Place ingredients in a jar with a tight-fitting lid and shake vigorously.

Yields about ¾ cup

Apple and Orange Salad

4 oranges
1 apple, cored and diced
1 cup sour cream
¼ cup chopped pecans or walnuts
   pinch of ground nutmeg

Separate oranges into segments and remove skins. Combine with remaining ingredients. Chill before serving.

6 to 8 servings

Pear Crunch Salad

Try this salad as a main dish for a light, nutritious lunch.

    1 cup chopped celery
    ½ cup chopped walnuts
    1 cup raisins
    ½ cup mayonnaise
    1½ cups cottage cheese
    6 pears
        lemon juice, for sprinkling
        salad greens

In a small bowl combine celery, walnuts, raisins, mayonnaise, and cottage cheese. Set aside.

Halve and core pears. Lightly sprinkle each half with lemon juice and top with a spoonful of cottage cheese mixture. Serve on a platter lined with salad greens.

    6 servings

Main Dish Salads

Bavarian Meatball Salad

Black bread and sweet butter are a nice accompaniment to this salad.

    Dressing
    1 cup sour cream
    ½ cup chopped onions
    ½ teaspoon chopped fresh dill

    Meatballs
    1½ pounds lean ground beef, or ¾ pound lean
        ground beef and ¾ pound lean ground pork
    ½ cup whole grain bread crumbs
    ½ teaspoon ground ginger
    ¼ teaspoon ground cloves
    1 teaspoon ground cinnamon
    ½ teaspoon ground allspice
    2 tablespoons dried currants
    1 egg
    3 tablespoons wine vinegar

    Poaching Broth
    1 cup rich Beef Stock (page 110)
    ¼ cup chopped onions

        lettuce leaves

To make the dressing: Combine sour cream, onions, and dill and stir until well blended. Set aside for 1 hour to allow flavors to mellow.

To make the meatballs: Combine ground meat, bread crumbs, ginger, cloves, cinnamon, allspice, currants, egg, and vinegar. Mix with moistened hands until well blended. Roll into small balls, using 1 tablespoon of the mixture for each.

To poach the meatballs: In a large skillet bring stock and onions to a low simmer. Add meatballs to simmering broth, not more than 2 deep. Cover and allow to steam over high heat for 5 to 10 minutes, or until meat is no longer pink. Uncover and allow liquid to evaporate until only rendered fat from the meat remains. Remove meatballs with a slotted spoon and allow to cool.

To serve, place spoonful of meatballs onto a serving plate lined with lettuce leaves. Top with a dollop of sour cream dressing.

    4 to 6 servings

Basic Fish Salad

    2 cups flaked cooked haddock, flounder,
        shrimp, crab meat, tuna, salmon, or fillet
        of sole
    1 small onion, minced
    ½ stalk celery, minced, or ½ teaspoon celery
        seeds
    ½ teaspoon lemon juice
    1½ tablespoons chopped fresh parsley
    ⅓ cup yogurt
    ⅓ cup mayonnaise
        salad greens
        lemon wedges

In a medium-size bowl combine fish, onions, celery, lemon juice and parsley. Add yogurt and mayonnaise and gently mix until all ingredients are moist. Chill for 1 hour.

Serve on a bed of salad greens and garnish with lemon wedges. Or, make sandwiches with whole grain bread and lettuce.

    4 servings

Broccoli, Mushroom, and Pasta Salad

2 cups rich Poultry Stock (page 110) or
    Vegetable Stock (page 111), or more
    if needed
2 to 2½ cups small mushrooms
2 to 2½ cups broccoli florets
2 cloves garlic, minced
⅓ cup vegetable oil
1 teaspoon dried oregano
1 tablespoon grated Parmesan cheese
¼ cup wine vinegar
    dash of cayenne pepper
1 cup uncooked tiny whole wheat pasta (orzo,
    marina, or shells)
2 to 3 tablespoons chopped roasted sweet red
    peppers or pimientos

Bring stock to a boil in a 1-quart saucepan. Reduce heat, add mushrooms and cook for 5 minutes. Remove mushrooms with a slotted spoon and set aside in a large bowl. Add broccoli to simmering liquid and cook for 2 to 4 minutes. Remove broccoli with slotted spoon and set aside with mushrooms.

In a blender or jar with a tight-fitting lid, place garlic, oil, oregano, cheese, vinegar, and cayenne. Blend several seconds or shake vigorously. Pour dressing over mushrooms and broccoli and allow to cool.

Bring stock to a boil again. Stir in pasta, reduce heat to a simmer, and cook, uncovered, until pasta is tender and liquid has been absorbed. Stir from time to time and add more liquid as necessary to prevent sticking. When pasta is tender, remove from heat, cover, and allow to cool. Just before serving, use forks to fluff up pasta. Toss with broccoli mixture and serve.

4 to 6 servings

Chicken and Rice Salad

2 cups cubed cooked chicken (turkey may be
    substituted)
1 cup cooked brown rice
½ cup pecans or walnuts, coarsely chopped
1 small onion, chopped
1 stalk celery, chopped
    pepper, to taste
¼ cup yogurt

¼ cup mayonnaise
    lettuce leaves
2 sprigs parsley, chopped

Toss together all ingredients except lettuce and parsley. Chill for 1 to 2 hours. Spoon onto a serving plate lined with lettuce leaves and garnish with parsley.

4 to 6 servings

Chick-pea and Savoy Cabbage Salad

2 cups chopped savoy cabbage
1 cup dried chick-peas, cooked and drained
½ cup chopped or thinly sliced red onions
¼ cup chopped pimientos
½ teaspoon dried basil
½ cup cider vinegar
⅓ cup olive oil
1 tablespoon honey
1 tablespoon mayonnaise

Combine cabbage, chick-peas, onions, pimientos, and basil in a medium-size bowl.

In a small bowl mix together vinegar, oil, honey, and mayonnaise. Add to cabbage mixture and toss. Refrigerate until thoroughly chilled before serving.

4 to 6 servings

Chick-pea and Tuna Salad

1 medium-size Bermuda onion
2 cloves garlic, crushed
½ cup vegetable oil
    juice of ½ lemon
1 can (6 to 7 ounces) water-packed tuna, flaked
1½ tablespoons wine vinegar
2 cups cooked chick-peas, drained
¼ cup chopped fresh parsley
½ teaspoon freshly ground pepper

Sliver onion by cutting from top to bottom and separating into petals. Measure 1 cup onion slivers and place in a 2-quart bowl. (Reserve any remaining slivers for use in other dishes.) Add garlic and oil and toss gently. Set aside to marinate for 1 hour. Toss in remaining ingredients and serve at room temperature.

6 to 8 servings

Chili con Carne Salad

    1 cup tomato sauce
    ¼ teaspoon ground cumin
    ¼ teaspoon ground coriander
      dash of crushed red pepper, or to taste
    1 clove garlic, minced
    ½ teaspoon dried basil
    ¼ teaspoon dried oregano
    2 teaspoons vinegar
    1 teaspoon honey
1½ to 2 cups cooked kidney beans, drained
    ½ cup diced celery
    ¼ cup diced green or sweet red peppers
    ½ cup chopped onions
    1 pound lean ground beef
      shredded lettuce

Combine tomato sauce, cumin, coriander, red pepper, garlic, basil, oregano, vinegar, and honey in a small saucepan and simmer for 5 minutes.

Place beans in a large bowl and pour hot tomato mixture over beans. Toss gently to combine, then refrigerate for several hours or overnight.

Add diced celery, peppers, and onions to marinated bean mixture and toss to combine. Set aside.

Sauté beef until cooked but not overbrowned. Try to keep beef in chunks. Drain off fat and cool slightly. Toss meat with bean and vegetable mixture. To serve, use a slotted spoon to place salad in a serving dish lined with shredded lettuce. Any marinade remaining in the bowl may be strained and passed at the table as extra dressing.

    4 to 6 servings

Chinese Hot Chicken Salad in Rolled Lettuce Leaves

Use this salad as a main course or serve as an unusual, delectable finger food for a party.

  6 to 8 Chinese dried mushrooms
    ¼ cup vegetable oil
    ¾ cup finely chopped onions
10 to 12 water chestnuts, finely chopped
    2 cups cooked chicken, shredded
    ¾ cup rich Poultry Stock (page 110), or more
      if needed
    1 tablespoon cornstarch, or more if needed
    1 tablespoon soy sauce

    ½ teaspoon honey
    ½ cup coarsely chopped roasted cashews
    1 large head lettuce, separated into leaves

Soak mushrooms in hot water for 15 minutes. Drain, then finely chop them.

In a large skillet heat oil and sauté onions. Add mushrooms, water chestnuts, and chicken. Toss and heat thoroughly.

Combine stock, cornstarch, soy sauce, and honey. Pour over chicken mixture and stir lightly over high heat until thickened. (Add more stock if mixture is too thick or more cornstarch mixed with cool stock if too thin.)

To serve, place hot chicken salad in a warm bowl and sprinkle with cashews. Place a platter of icy cold lettuce leaves beside salad. Each person spoons a generous portion of chicken mixture onto a lettuce leaf and rolls it with his fingers "cigar" style.

    4 to 6 servings

Curried Chicken and Corn Salad

    ⅓ cup Curried Mayonnaise (page 182)*
2½ to 3 cups cubed cooked chicken
    1½ cups cooked corn
    3 tablespoons chopped green peppers
      lettuce leaves
      tomato wedges
      onion rings

Combine mayonnaise, chicken, corn, and peppers. Chill 1 hour to mellow flavors.

To serve, bring almost to room temperature. Then place scoops of salad on individual plates lined with lettuce leaves and garnish with tomato wedges and onion rings.

    4 to 6 servings

*If Curried Mayonnaise is not available, sauté ¾ teaspoon curry powder in 2 tablespoons Clarified Butter (page 148). Add to ⅓ cup mayonnaise.

Egg Salad

    5 hard-cooked eggs, chopped
    1 small onion, chopped
    ½ cup chopped celery, with leaves
    3 tablespoons finely chopped green peppers
    2 teaspoons minced fresh parsley

¾ cup mayonnaise, or to taste
   dash of ground cumin
   paprika

In a medium-size bowl toss together eggs, onions, celery, green peppers, and parsley. Add mayonnaise and blend well. Stir in cumin and chill. When ready to serve, garnish with paprika.

4 servings

Leftover-Roast Salad with Pan Juice Dressing

Pan drippings and meat left over from Sunday's roast combine to form a salad perfect for a picnic, potluck, or quick supper.

  1½ pounds cold roasted beef, lamb, or pork
6 to 8 small new potatoes (about 1 pound)
   3 scallions, diagonally sliced
   Pan Juice Dressing (see below)
   freshly ground pepper
  ¼ cup minced fresh parsley

Cut meat into thin slices or slivers and place in a large mixing bowl.

Boil potatoes in enough water to cover until tender, about 25 minutes. Drain, cool, and cut into ½-inch cubes. Add to meat along with scallions and combine.

Pour dressing over meat mixture and gently toss. Sprinkle with pepper and parsley. Serve at room temperature.

6 servings

Pan Juice Dressing

  ¼ cup cider vinegar
  ½ teaspoon soy sauce
  1 clove garlic, minced
  ⅓ cup sesame oil
  ¼ cup degreased leftover pan juices

In a small bowl combine vinegar, soy sauce, and garlic. Add oil in a thin stream, beating constantly, then beat in pan juices.

Yields about ¾ cup

Mint and Lamb Salad

  ¾ cup olive oil
  ¼ cup plus 2 tablespoons lemon juice
  ¾ cup chopped fresh mint

  1½ cups cubed cooked lamb
  ½ pound mushrooms, thinly sliced
  ¼ cup chopped pimientos
  1½ pints cherry tomatoes, halved
  1 head Bibb lettuce, torn into bite-size pieces
  ½ bunch watercress, with stems removed

In a small mixing bowl combine oil, lemon juice, and mint. Mix well, then set dressing aside.

In a large mixing bowl combine lamb, mushrooms, pimientos, and tomatoes. Pour ½ of the dressing over all and toss to mix. Cover and chill.

When ready to serve, combine lettuce and watercress in a salad bowl, then toss with remaining dressing. Arrange lamb salad over the dressed greens.

6 servings

Summer Rice Salad

  3 cups hot cooked brown rice
  ¼ cup plus 1 tablespoon olive oil
  ¼ cup plus 3 tablespoons wine vinegar, or to taste
  1 teaspoon chopped fresh tarragon or ½
    teaspoon dried tarragon
  ½ cup chopped green peppers
  ½ cup finely chopped celery
  ¼ cup chopped fresh parsley
  ¼ cup finely chopped scallions
  3 tablespoons chopped fresh chives
  ½ cup diced cucumbers
  3 tablespoons chopped pimientos
    iceberg or romaine lettuce leaves
    hard-cooked eggs, quartered
    tomatoes, quartered

Place rice in a large mixing bowl. Add oil, ¼ cup vinegar, and tarragon. Toss together lightly. Set aside to cool at room temperature.

Add peppers, celery, parsley, scallions, chives, and cucumbers to marinated rice. Add remaining vinegar 1 tablespoon at a time. (Reduce amount of vinegar if a less-tart salad is desired.)

Cover and refrigerate salad until ready to serve; or, if desired, serve at room temperature. To serve, heap rice salad onto the center of a serving platter, surround it with lettuce leaves, and garnish with egg and tomato quarters.

6 servings

Peas and Cheese Salad

2 cups fresh peas, or 1 package (10 ounces)
   frozen peas, thawed
6 ounces colby or Monterey Jack cheese,
   shredded
¼ cup thinly sliced scallions
2 tablespoons chopped fresh parsley
½ cup mayonnaise
   freshly ground pepper
   lettuce leaves

Blanch peas for 1 minute in boiling water. Drain and chill quickly in cold water. Drain well.

Set ¼ cup cheese aside. In a medium-size bowl toss peas with remaining cheese. Fold in all other ingredients until blended, then chill mixture until serving time. Serve on a platter lined with lettuce leaves and garnish with reserved cheese.

4 to 6 servings

South Seas Chicken Salad

2 to 2½ cups diced cooked chicken
   1/3 cup chopped celery
   ¼ cup chopped green or sweet red peppers
   2 tablespoons chopped scallions
   2 tablespoons chopped chutney
   1 tablespoon lemon juice
   ½ teaspoon grated lemon rind
   ½ cup mayonnaise
   2/3 cup nuts (peanuts, macadamia nuts, or
      cashews), toasted
   1 can (8 ounces) unsweetened pineapple
      chunks, drained
      salad greens
      unsweetened shredded coconut, toasted

Combine chicken, celery, peppers, scallions, chutney, and lemon juice in a large bowl. Toss to mix well. Stir lemon rind into mayonnaise and then fold into chicken mixture. Cover and chill for several hours.

Just before serving fold in nuts and pineapple. Spoon into a serving bowl lined with salad greens and sprinkle with toasted coconut.

4 servings

Variation:

South Seas Shrimp Salad: Replace chicken with 2 to 2½ cups diced cooked shrimp.

Three-Fruit Fish Salad with Ginger Sauce

½ large ripe pineapple
1 large orange
1½ cups cooked halibut, scrod, or other firm-
   fleshed fish, broken into bite-size pieces
12 green seedless grapes, halved
10 large purple grapes, halved
10 large red grapes, halved
   salad greens
   Ginger Sauce (see below)
½ cup sliced or slivered almonds, toasted

Slice pineapple in half lengthwise. Cut away rind and tough center core. Cut pineapple into small cubes and place in a large bowl. Holding rind over bowl, scrape inner side to extract all fruit and juice.

Separate orange into segments, remove skins, and break flesh into small pieces. Add to bowl of pineapple, along with fish and grapes.

Toss salad gently with enough ginger sauce to moisten well. Mound in the center of a serving platter, surround with salad greens, and sprinkle top with almonds.

4 servings

Ginger Sauce

½ cup mayonnaise
½ cup sour cream
1 teaspoon minced peeled ginger root
1 tablespoon lime or lemon juice
1 teaspoon mild honey

Combine all ingredients and blend well.

Yields about 1 cup

Norwegian Fish Salad

3 cups flaked cooked fish
2 red apples, cored and diced
1 tablespoon minced onions
1 cup sour cream
2 tablespoons wine vinegar
¼ teaspoon white pepper
2 teaspoons chopped fresh dill
   salad greens
4 small cooked beets, peeled and sliced
2 hard-cooked eggs, quartered
3 sprigs dill

In a large bowl toss fish with apples and onions. Mix sour cream with vinegar, pepper, and chopped dill and add to fish, stirring carefully. Mound mixture in center of platter lined with salad greens. Chill for 30 minutes, then surround outside of platter with beets on one side and eggs on the other. Garnish with dill.

6 to 8 servings

Red Lentils and Red Onion Salad with Tangy Mustard Dressing

1 carrot
1 small onion
½ stalk celery
1 bay leaf
2 cups water
2 cups dried red lentils
1 medium-size red onion
Tangy Mustard Dressing (see below)

Place carrot, small onion, celery, and bay leaf in a medium-size saucepan and cover with water. Bring to a boil, then cover and cook until carrot is tender, 20 to 30 minutes.

Remove carrot, slice into coins, and set aside. Strain hot cooking liquid (discarding onion, celery, and bay leaf) and pour over lentils in a bowl. Set aside to cool, at room temperature, until lukewarm.

Drain and rinse soaked lentils. Cover lentils with fresh water and boil for several minutes until just tender. (Do not overcook.) Drain, then rinse with cool water and drain again.

Cut 2 or 3 thin slices from red onion and reserve; chop remainder. Combine chopped onions, carrots, and lentils in a serving bowl. Toss with dressing and garnish with reserved onion slices separated into rings.

4 to 6 servings

Tangy Mustard Dressing

1 tablespoon dry mustard
1 teaspoon whole wheat flour
¼ cup cold water
3 tablespoons vinegar
½ teaspoon turmeric
1 tablespoon honey

¼ cup vegetable oil
½ teaspoon garlic powder
2 teaspoons soy sauce
dash of cayenne pepper

In a small saucepan blend dry mustard, flour, and water to the consistency of a paste. Add remaining ingredients and mix well. Cook for several minutes over moderate heat, stirring constantly, until thickened. Cool before adding to salad.

Yields about ¾ cup

Tropical Beet and Tuna Salad

¼ cup cider vinegar
¼ cup pineapple juice
2 tablespoons honey
2 whole cloves
1 stick of cinnamon, ½ inch long
1 clove garlic
2 cups sliced, peeled, cooked beets
²/₃ cup mayonnaise
1 small head lettuce, torn into bite-size pieces
¾ cup unsweetened pineapple chunks, broken into smaller pieces
1 can (6 to 7 ounces) water-packed tuna, flaked
1 medium-size red onion, sliced and separated into rings
2 hard-cooked eggs, cut into wedges

Combine vinegar, pineapple juice, honey, cloves, cinnamon, and garlic in a small saucepan. Bring to a boil, then reduce heat, cover, and simmer for 10 minutes. Pour hot marinade over beet slices and refrigerate for several hours or overnight.

Drain beets, discarding spices and garlic clove but reserving marinade. Combine mayonnaise with enough marinade to thin it to a pouring consistency. Set aside to use as dressing.

To serve, arrange lettuce to cover bottom of a large salad bowl. Place beets on top of lettuce, overlapping slices like petals. Leave a border so lettuce shows around edge. Place pineapple on beets, tuna on pineapple, onion rings on tuna, and, finally, egg wedges on top, always allowing a border of each ingredient to show, making concentric circles. Serve with marinade-mayonnaise dressing.

4 to 6 servings

Trout Salad with Mediterranean Dressing

This main dish salad, which is marinated overnight, can also be served as a seafood cocktail with lemon wedges and salad greens or as a spread for crackers or toast points.

     4 peppercorns
     1 bay leaf
     1 slice onion, stuck with 2 cloves
     1 sprig tarragon or ¼ teaspoon dried tarragon
2 or 3 slices lemon
     2 tablespoons lemon juice
       pinch of crushed red pepper
     ½ cup water
2 or 3 medium-size whole trout
       Mediterranean Dressing (see below)
       lemon wedges

In a large saucepan combine all ingredients except trout, dressing, and lemon wedges. Bring to a simmer, then add trout and gently poach until fish flakes easily with fork, about 5 to 7 minutes. Allow fish to cool in liquid.

When fish is cool, remove all skin and bones and flake flesh into a bowl. (Discard cooking liquid.) Pour dressing over fish, then cover and marinate in refrigerator overnight. Serve with lemon wedges.

     4 to 6 servings

Mediterranean Dressing

     ½ cup vegetable oil
     ¼ teaspoon grated peeled ginger root
       juice of 1 lemon
     2 cloves garlic, minced
     1½ teaspoons dried oregano

Combine all ingredients and mix well.

Yields about ¾ cup

Molded Salads

Avocado Mold

     ½ cup cold water
     2 envelopes unflavored gelatin
     3 avocados, mashed (about 4 cups)

     1 cup yogurt
     2 tablespoons lemon juice
     1 clove garlic, crushed
     ½ cup chopped cucumbers
     1 large tomato, chopped

Pour water into a small Pyrex bowl and sprinkle gelatin on top. Let stand 5 minutes to soften, then place bowl in a pan of very hot water and stir until gelatin has dissolved.

In a large mixing bowl combine dissolved gelatin with mashed avocados, yogurt, lemon juice, and garlic. Beat thoroughly.

Chill until slightly thickened and mixture forms a mound when dropped from a spoon. Then fold in cucumbers and tomatoes and turn into a 6-cup mold. Chill overnight or until firm. Unmold and serve.

     6 servings

Black Cherry–Almond Mousse Molded Salad

       1½ cups red grape juice
       2 envelopes unflavored gelatin
2½ to 3 cups fresh sweet cherries (1 pound), pitted
       1 tablespoon lemon juice
       1 whole chicken breast
       2 cups rich Poultry Stock (page 110)
       ¼ cup cold water
       ½ teaspoon dried thyme
       ½ teaspoon freshly grated nutmeg
         pinch of ground rosemary
         dash of white pepper
       ⅔ cup blanched almonds, toasted
       3 ounces cream cheese, softened
       ½ cup mayonnaise

       Dressing
       ½ cup sour cream or yogurt
       ½ cup mayonnaise

Place ½ cup grape juice in a small saucepan. Sprinkle 1 envelope gelatin on top and set aside for a few minutes to soften. Then set saucepan over moderate heat and stir constantly until gelatin has completely dissolved. Stir in remaining grape juice, cherries, and lemon juice. Pour into a 4 × 8-inch loaf pan or a 6-cup mold and refrigerate until firm, 1 to 2 hours.

Poach chicken breast in stock until tender, about 20 minutes. Lift chicken out of stock, then remove skin and bones and set aside. Reserve stock.

Sprinkle second envelope of gelatin over water and set aside.

Add thyme, nutmeg, rosemary, and pepper to reserved stock. Boil stock, uncovered, until reduced to 1 cup. Add softened gelatin to reduced stock, return to heat, and simmer gently until gelatin has completely dissolved. Set aside to cool to room temperature.

Chop toasted almonds coarsely. Chop reserved chicken finely, or process in a blender or food processor. Combine cream cheese, mayonnaise, and cooled stock-gelatin mixture in a 1-quart bowl and beat until very smooth. Add chicken and almonds. Pour mixture over cherry layer in mold. Chill for several hours until firm. Unmold and slice into serving pieces.

To make the dressing: Combine sour cream or yogurt with mayonnaise and mix well. Serve with molded salad.

10 servings

Blue Cheese Mousse in Cantaloupe Rings

    1 medium-size cantaloupe (honeydew melon
        may be substituted)
    ¼ cup cold water
    1 envelope unflavored gelatin
    2 tablespoons lemon juice
    8 ounces blue cheese, softened
    3 ounces cream cheese, softened
        dash of cayenne pepper
        dash of white pepper
    ½ cup heavy cream, whipped
        salad greens

Pare outside rind of cantaloupe with a sharp paring knife. Slice off stem end to point where seed cavity just begins. Use a spoon or serrated grapefruit knife to hollow out seed cavity (as if making a jack-o'-lantern). Stuff cavity with paper towels and allow to drain, open-end down, while preparing mousse.

Pour water into a small saucepan and sprinkle gelatin on top. Set aside for several minutes until gelatin has softened. Add lemon juice and stir mixture over moderate heat until gelatin has completely dissolved. Remove from heat and allow to cool.

In a blender combine blue cheese, cream cheese, cayenne, white pepper, and gelatin mixture and process until perfectly smooth. Carefully fold in whipped cream.

Remove the paper towels from cavity of melon. Blot any remaining liquid with additional paper towels.

Pour cheese mixture into cavity, then place melon in a small bowl, open-end up, so it will not fall over. Chill for several hours until center is firm. Use a long sharp knife to slice melon into rings. Place each ring on a bed of salad greens and serve.

6 to 8 servings

Cranberry Mold

    4 cups fresh cranberries
    3½ cups boiling water
    ¾ cup honey
    ¾ cup cold water
    3 envelopes unflavored gelatin
    1 cup chopped pecans
    1 cup unsweetened pineapple chunks
    1 cup green seedless grapes
        lettuce leaves

In a large saucepan cook cranberries in boiling water until berries burst. Stir in honey.

Pour water into a small bowl and sprinkle gelatin on top. Set aside for several minutes to soften, then add to hot cranberry mixture. Cool. Add pecans, pineapple, and grapes.

Turn into an 8-cup mold and chill for several hours until firm. To serve, invert onto a platter lined with crisp lettuce leaves.

6 to 8 servings

Tuna Mold

    2 cans (6 to 7 ounces each) water-packed tuna
    2 hard-cooked eggs, chopped
    2 tablespoons chopped fresh chives or onions
    ¼ cup cold water
    3 envelopes unflavored gelatin
    1 cup mayonnaise

In a medium-size bowl combine tuna, eggs, and chives or onions.

Pour water into a small bowl and sprinkle gelatin on top. Set aside for several minutes to soften, then stir in mayonnaise. Fold into tuna mixture until well blended.

Pour into a 3-cup mold and chill for several hours until firm. To serve, unmold onto a bed of watercress.

6 to 8 servings

Orange and Tomato Aspic

This aspic makes a nice accompaniment to seafood or vegetable salads.

>   2 cups strained orange juice
>   2 cups tomato juice
>   1 tablespoon white wine vinegar
>   juice of 1 lemon
>   1 teaspoon honey
>   dash of cayenne pepper
>   2 envelopes unflavored gelatin
>   salad greens

Combine orange juice, tomato juice, vinegar, lemon juice, honey, and cayenne in a 2-quart saucepan. Sprinkle gelatin over mixture and set aside for 5 minutes until gelatin has softened. Then bring to a simmer over moderately high heat, stirring constantly, until gelatin has completely dissolved.

Pour mixture into a 4½-cup mold and place in refrigerator for several hours until firm. To serve, unmold onto a serving plate and garnish with salad greens.

4 to 6 servings

Salmon in Fish Aspic

>   2½ cups Fish Stock (page 111)
>   1 envelope unflavored gelatin
>   ¾ pound salmon fillet, skinned
>   1 hard-cooked egg, cut into 4 slices
>   lettuce leaves
>   Green Mayonnaise (page 181)
>   lemon slices

Clarify stock if it is very cloudy (see page 105 for directions).

Place ½ cup stock in a small bowl. Sprinkle gelatin on top and set aside for 5 minutes to soften.

Heat 1½ cups stock in a small saucepan. Add softened gelatin mixture and bring to a simmer, stirring to dissolve gelatin. Set this fish aspic mixture aside at room temperature while preparing salmon.

Poach salmon in remaining ½ cup stock until fish flakes easily with fork, about 10 minutes. Drain off excess liquid and chill fish in refrigerator.

Into each of 4 ½-cup molds, place 2 tablespoons fish aspic. Center a slice of egg in each one, yolk-side down. Place molds on level rack in freezer for 10 to 15 minutes, or until gelatin is set.

Cut salmon into 4 neat blocks of equal size to fit molds. After thin layer of aspic in molds has jelled, place salmon portion in each one. Fill remaining space in molds with additional fish aspic. Pour remaining aspic into a separate small container to form a thin layer. Place molds and container on level refrigerator rack and chill until gelatin is set.

To serve, unmold onto individual serving plates lined with lettuce leaves. Use a fork to break up aspic in extra container and arrange pieces around molds. Serve with Green Mayonnaise and lemon slices.

4 servings

Tomato Aspic

>   3 cups tomato juice
>   1 stalk celery, with leaves, cut into 3-inch pieces
>   1 small onion, quartered
>   3 sprigs parsley
>   ¼ teaspoon crushed bay leaf
>   dash of cayenne pepper
>   4 teaspoons unflavored gelatin
>   1 teaspoon honey
>   ½ teaspoon soy sauce
>   2 tablespoons lemon juice
>   ½ teaspoon horseradish, drained
>   salad greens or watercress

In a 1-quart saucepan combine 2 cups tomato juice, celery, onion, parsley, bay leaf, and cayenne. Place saucepan over medium heat and bring to a boil. Reduce heat and simmer, uncovered, for 15 minutes. Remove from heat and strain mixture, discarding residue and returning liquid to saucepan. Set aside.

Meanwhile, place remaining 1 cup tomato juice in a small bowl. Sprinkle gelatin over top and allow to stand until softened, about 5 minutes. Add softened gelatin to hot tomato mixture and stir until gelatin has dissolved. Stir in honey, soy sauce, lemon juice, and horseradish. Cool slightly.

Pour cooled tomato mixture into a 1-quart ring mold and place in refrigerator for several hours until firm.

Unmold aspic onto a serving platter and surround with salad greens or watercress. Center may be filled with coleslaw, cottage cheese, or chicken, potato, or egg salad, as desired.

6 servings

White Grape-Mint Mold

3½ cups white grape juice
2 envelopes unflavored gelatin
¼ cup lemon juice
¼ cup honey
¼ cup minced fresh mint
1 to 1½ cups white seedless grapes
   salad greens

Place ½ cup grape juice in a small saucepan and sprinkle gelatin on top. Set aside for several minutes to soften. Heat mixture over moderate heat, stirring constantly, until gelatin has completely dissolved. Remove from heat and add remaining grape juice, lemon juice, and honey. Stir until well blended, then set aside to cool to room temperature.

Stir in mint leaves and refrigerate until slightly thickened and mixture forms a mound when dropped from a spoon. Fold in grapes.

Pour into a 4-cup mold and refrigerate for several hours or overnight. Unmold onto a bed of salad greens. Garnish with additional grapes, if desired.

6 to 8 servings

Dressings

Almost a Miracle Dressing

1 teaspoon dry mustard
2 tablespoons cornstarch
½ cup cold water
⅓ cup cider vinegar
2 tablespoons plus ½ teaspoon honey
2 egg yolks
3 tablespoons lemon juice
1 cup vegetable oil

In a small saucepan combine dry mustard and cornstarch, then gradually whisk in cold water. Add vinegar and 2 tablespoons honey and cook over moderate heat, stirring constantly, until mixture comes to a boil and thickens. Set aside to cool to room temperature.

Combine egg yolks, remaining ½ teaspoon honey, and lemon juice in a blender. Process at high speed while adding oil in thin, steady stream until sauce is consistency of mayonnaise. Turn blender to low setting and add cooled thickened mixture by the tablespoon.

Store in a covered jar in refrigerator. Dressing keeps up to 2 weeks. Use in pasta, meat, poultry, or fish salads. Also very tasty in coleslaw.

Yields 2 cups

Creamy Cucumber Salad Dressing

½ cup low-fat cottage cheese
1 tablespoon yogurt
½ teaspoon honey
1 teaspoon vinegar
½ cup finely chopped cucumbers
2 tablespoons minced scallions
   dash of white pepper

Sieve cottage cheese, or process in a blender, until very smooth. Blend in yogurt, honey, and vinegar. Drain chopped cucumbers very well, squeezing in paper towel to remove excess moisture. Fold cucumbers and scallions into cottage cheese mixture. Season with pepper. Serve over mixed green salads.

Yields 1½ cups

Green Mayonnaise

1 egg
2 tablespoons lemon juice
1 cup vegetable oil
2 tablespoons chopped fresh chives
2 tablespoons minced, mixed, fresh herbs
   (parsley, marjoram, tarragon, thyme, sorrel,
   basil, or savory)
1 clove garlic, minced

Combine egg and lemon juice in a blender. Process at high speed while adding oil in thin, steady stream until mayonnaise forms and all oil is incorporated. Add chives, herbs, and garlic. Scrape down mayonnaise with a rubber spatula, then process at high speed until herbs are pureed and mayonnaise turns light green.

Stored in a tightly covered jar in refrigerator, mayonnaise keeps up to 3 days. Serve over mixed green salads.

Yields about 1½ cups

Curried Mayonnaise

2 teaspoons curry powder
1 cup plus 2 tablespoons vegetable oil
2 egg yolks
2 tablespoons vinegar

In a small saucepan sauté curry powder in 2 tablespoons oil until foamy, about 2 minutes. Set aside to cool.

Place egg yolks and vinegar in a blender. Process at high speed while adding 1 cup oil in thin, steady stream. Continue until mayonnaise forms and all oil is incorporated. Stir in cooled curry mixture. Allow to mellow several hours in a tightly covered container in refrigerator (will keep up to 1 week).

Serve over mixed greens and other vegetable salads.

Yields 1 cup

Green Garden Dressing

½ cup chopped fresh parsley
¼ cup mayonnaise
¼ cup yogurt or buttermilk
½ teaspoon dried thyme
1 tablespoon prepared mustard or ½ teaspoon dry mustard

Process all ingredients in a blender until smooth. Serve over mixed green salads.

Yields 1 cup

Herb Dressing

½ cup vegetable oil
3 tablespoons wine vinegar
¼ teaspoon dried thyme
¼ teaspoon dried marjoram
1 teaspoon chopped fresh tarragon or ¼ teaspoon dried tarragon
1 tablespoon chopped fresh basil or ½ teaspoon dried basil
1 tablespoon chopped fresh parsley

Combine all ingredients in a jar with a tight-fitting lid and shake vigorously. Allow to stand for 15 minutes before serving. Shake well before adding to crisp salad greens.

Yields ⅔ cup

Horseradish-Yogurt Dressing

1 cup yogurt
1 tablespoon lemon juice
3 tablespoons grated horseradish (rinsed and drained prepared horseradish may be substituted)
½ teaspoon honey
½ teaspoon prepared mustard

Combine all ingredients and mix well. Serve with green salads or with cold meats.

Yields 1½ cups

Kefir-Fruit Dressing

1 cup kefir (page 448)
2 teaspoons honey
½ teaspoon finely grated lemon rind
¼ teaspoon ground nutmeg
¼ teaspoon ground cinnamon
¼ teaspoon ground ginger
¼ cup unsweetened shredded coconut
¼ cup unsweetened crushed pineapple, drained (optional)

Combine all ingredients and mix well. Chill. Serve over mixed fresh fruits and berries.

Yields 1½ cups

Low-Calorie All-Purpose Dressing

1 medium-size cucumber
½ teaspoon honey
1 scant teaspoon dry mustard
¼ teaspoon dried tarragon
1 teaspoon minced fresh parsley
2 tablespoons lemon juice
1 tablespoon olive oil
3 tablespoons safflower oil
1 egg white
1 teaspoon minced garlic

Peel cucumber and cut into large chunks. Puree cucumber pieces in a food processor or blender. Add remaining ingredients and blend thoroughly.

May be stored in an airtight jar in refrigerator, but flavor is best when used fresh. Shake before using. Serve over crisp salad greens.

Yields about 1 cup

Kefir-Tomato Dressing

2 medium-size tomatoes
1 teaspoon dried basil or dillweed
1 clove garlic, minced, or 1 teaspoon chopped
    fresh chives
1 cup kefir (page 448)

Peel, seed, chop, and drain tomatoes. (You should have about 2 cups.)

In a blender combine tomatoes, basil or dillweed, and garlic or chives. Process until smooth. Fold in kefir and stir gently until smooth. Serve with crisp fresh vegetables or whole grain crackers.

Yields 3 cups

Mushroom Dressing

½ cup plus 1 tablespoon vegetable oil
1½ cups mushrooms, minced
2 cloves garlic, minced
2½ tablespoons lemon juice
1 hard-cooked egg yolk, sieved
¼ teaspoon dry mustard
½ teaspoon dried oregano
1 tablespoon grated Parmesan cheese

Heat 1 tablespoon oil in a medium-size skillet and sauté mushrooms and garlic over high heat, stirring constantly, until mushrooms are cooked and excess liquid has evaporated. Place in a pint jar with a tight-fitting lid and add remaining ingredients. Shake vigorously until well blended. Allow dressing to marinate overnight in refrigerator for maximum flavor. Good with all green salads.

Yields ¾ to 1 cup

Orange-Yogurt Dressing

1 large orange
¼ teaspoon ground cinnamon
1½ tablespoons honey
1 cup yogurt

Grate rind from orange (about 1 tablespoon) and squeeze out juice (¼ to ⅓ cup). Blend together rind, juice, cinnamon, honey, and yogurt and allow to chill for 1 hour to blend flavors. Use dressing with fruit salads.

Yields about 1½ cups

Rocky Roquefort Salad Dressing

1 cup mayonnaise
1 cup sour cream
4 ounces Roquefort cheese, coarsely crumbled

Combine ingredients and refrigerate overnight in a covered container to allow flavors to mellow. Good with fresh garden tomatoes and green salads. Keeps 1 week, refrigerated.

Yields 2 to 2½ cups

Russian Dressing

½ cup yogurt
1 cup mayonnaise
½ cup catsup
1 teaspoon horseradish, drained

Combine yogurt and mayonnaise with a wire whisk, then mix in catsup and horseradish. Serve with green salads.

Yields 2 cups

Sesame Seed Dressing

½ cup vegetable oil
1 tablespoon sesame seeds
1 clove garlic
2 tablespoons cider vinegar or rice vinegar
2 teaspoons soy sauce
    few drops of dark sesame oil (optional)

Combine vegetable oil and sesame seeds in a small saucepan. Peel garlic clove, drop into oil, and crush slightly using back of a spoon. Place saucepan over moderate heat and stir until seeds and garlic have become a toasted color, about 2 minutes. Do not overbrown seeds or garlic. Remove from heat immediately. Set aside to cool to room temperature. Remove garlic clove.

Place cooled oil and seeds in a jar with a tight-fitting lid. Add remaining ingredients and shake vigorously to blend. This delicately flavored dressing is good with salads of sprouts and soft-leaved lettuces.

Yields ¾ cup

Sour Cream and Vinegar Dressing

1 egg yolk
1/3 cup sour cream
1 tablespoon lemon juice
1 tablespoon white wine vinegar
1/2 teaspoon honey
1/2 cup vegetable oil
1 clove garlic, minced
1 teaspoon minced fresh parsley
1/2 teaspoon celery seeds
    pinch of minced fresh oregano
    pinch of minced fresh thyme

Place all ingredients in a pint jar with a tight-fitting lid. Shake vigorously until well blended. Allow to chill in refrigerator at least 1 hour so flavors can mellow. Goes well with sliced tomatoes, cucumbers, watercress, and green salads.

Yields 1 cup

Sour Cream Salad Dressing

1 cup sour cream
2 teaspoons prepared mustard
1 teaspoon honey (optional)
1 1/2 tablespoons lemon juice
1 teaspoon chopped fresh chives

Combine all ingredients and mix well. Use immediately or store in a tightly covered container in refrigerator. Dressing will keep for 3 to 4 days without separating.

Excellent when served over crisp greens and other vegetable salads. Also delicious with cabbage salads.

Yields 1 1/2 cups

Variations:
Sour Cream Fruit Salad Dressing: Omit mustard and chives and add 1 tablespoon grated orange rind.
Sour Cream-Garlic Dressing: Omit chives and add 1/2 teaspoon minced garlic.
Sour Cream-Shallot Dressing: Add 1 tablespoon finely chopped shallots or scallions.

Spicy Yogurt Dressing

1 cup yogurt
1/2 teaspoon onion powder
1 clove garlic, minced
1/4 teaspoon paprika

1 teaspoon wine vinegar
1 tablespoon honey
2 tablespoons lime juice
    pinch of crushed red pepper, or to taste
    dash of ground cinnamon
    dash of ground coriander
    dash of ground cumin

Combine ingredients and blend well. Allow to chill at least 1 hour to blend flavors. Very good with legume salads.

Yields about 1 1/4 cups

Sweet and Sour Dressing

1 egg
3 tablespoons cider vinegar
1/3 cup honey
1 teaspoon cornstarch
1/4 cup plus 1 tablespoon water
    dash of freshly ground pepper

Combine egg, vinegar, and honey in a small saucepan and whisk until frothy. Mix cornstarch and water together until smooth. Add to ingredients in saucepan. Cook over moderate heat, stirring constantly, until mixture reaches a boil and thickens. Remove from heat and stir in pepper. Serve warm over strong-flavored greens or potato salad.

Yields about 1 cup

Tangy Soy Dressing

1 medium-size tomato, halved
2 tablespoons soy sauce
2 tablespoons cider vinegar
1/3 cup sunflower or sesame oil
1 clove garlic, halved (optional)
1 teaspoon dried thyme

Process all ingredients in a blender until smooth. Serve over mixed green salads.

Yields 1 to 1 1/4 cups

Vinaigrette

3 tablespoons cider vinegar
1 teaspoon honey
1/2 cup olive oil

In a screw-top jar shake vinegar and honey together until blended. Add oil and shake until thoroughly mixed. Serve over any salad of crisp greens and other vegetables. Flavor is best when used fresh.

Variations:

Curried Vinaigrette: Add ½ teaspoon curry powder and 1 minced shallot to vinegar and honey. Shake well before adding oil.

Garlic Vinaigrette: In a small bowl crush 1 clove garlic with ¼ teaspoon white pepper to a paste. Stir in vinegar and honey. Transfer mixture to a screw-top jar. Add oil and shake well. Prepare at least 2 hours before serving.

Herbal Vinaigrette: Add 2 teaspoons each minced fresh chives, parsley, basil, and tarragon to Vinaigrette, Curried Vinaigrette, or Garlic Vinaigrette.

Mustard Vinaigrette: Shake 1 teaspoon dry mustard together with vinegar and honey. Add oil and shake well.

Tomato Vinaigrette: Add 1 tablespoon tomato paste to Mustard Vinaigrette or Garlic Vinaigrette.

Yields ¾ cup

Yogurt, Lime, and Ginger Dressing

½ cup yogurt
½ cup sour cream
1 tablespoon lime juice
1 teaspoon grated lime rind
¼ teaspoon grated peeled ginger root
¼ teaspoon ground mace
¼ teaspoon freshly grated nutmeg

Combine ingredients and blend well. Chill several hours or overnight. Especially good with seafood.

Yields 1 cup

Yogurt-Tahini Dressing

½ cup yogurt
¼ cup tahini (sesame butter)
juice of ½ lemon
1 tablespoon soy sauce
1 small clove garlic, halved

Process all ingredients in a blender until smooth. If too thick, add a small amount of hot water. Serve over salads of mixed crisp greens.

Yields about ¾ cup

Zesty Italian Herb Dressing

1½ cups vegetable oil
½ cup wine vinegar
2 cloves garlic, crushed
½ teaspoon dried basil
½ teaspoon dried oregano
¼ to ½ cup grated Parmesan cheese (optional)
    freshly ground pepper, to taste

Combine ingredients in a quart jar and shake well. Refrigerate overnight before serving. Use with mixed green salads.

Yields 2 cups

Vegetables

Vegetables are the edible parts of plants often served as part of a meal—roots, bulbs, stems, blossoms, seeds, and fruits. Custom and starch content usually dictate when you call a fruit a vegetable or a seed a vegetable. Most people think of tomatoes as a vegetable and serve them that way, though they are a fruit by botanical definition. Peas are true seeds, but they are prepared and served as a vegetable too.

Loaded with vitamins, minerals, and fiber, yet low in calories and fat, vegetables are the perfect answer for dieters. Most bring fewer than 50 calories per serving to a meal when served either raw or steamed. The calorie reading climbs when a pat of butter or a dollop of sour cream tops a serving.

When you select vegetables for a menu, consider your choice in the context of the whole meal. You want flavors, colors, shapes, and textures to balance and enhance the other dishes, not compete with them. Never plan several purees, all white foods, or all highly spiced foods for a single meal. Instead, dramatize bland-colored grain dishes by serving them with slices of juicy red tomatoes and shiny green pepper rings. Add crunch to meals featuring meat or poultry dishes with crisp green salads, firm carrot sticks, and red radishes.

Buying Vegetables

Fresh: For top-quality, tasty vegetables at the best price, buy them fresh and in season when the supply is plentiful. If you can, buy directly from a farm producing its own vegetables. If that is not convenient, shop in a market that keeps the vegetables cold or where the turnover is high. Always buy vegetables as close to the time you plan to eat them as you can, since some (peas and corn, for example) become starchy quickly and others (such as salad greens) wilt rapidly. Look for vegetables that are without defects and are of moderate size. Oversized or undersized ones are rarely a bargain. Fresh vegetables should have a bright color and should be ripe yet feel firm. If you want to avoid chemical residues that are difficult, or impossible, to remove (see Removing Waxes and Pesticides, page 188), seek out vegetables grown without sprays (usually more expensive). Even better, grow your own if time and space permit.

Frozen: Select packages of frozen vegetables from a freezer case where the temperature registers 0°F or below. Look to see that the package you want is below the freezer line and that it is clean and firm. Dirty or soggy packages indicate mishandling. Shake the package. The food within should rattle around if the food has remained completely frozen while in storage. If it does not, the food has probably thawed and become refrozen as a solid block. Taste, texture, color, and nutrients suffer each time vegetables thaw and refreeze.

Canned: When buying canned vegetables, you have to rely on the package labels for information. The labels should tell you something about the quality of the vegetables when they were packed. Quality is often indicated by these grades:

Fancy or U.S. Grade A—the most flavorful, best-looking vegetables available. This grade frequently appears on labels.

Extra Standard or U.S. Grade B—not as nice looking as Grade A. Vegetables with this grade are often unmarked.

Standard or U.S. Grade C—overmature vegetables that lack uniform shape. This grade is rarely indicated on the label probably because manufacturers prefer no label to one showing the contents as only standard. (Since nutrients are the same for all three grades, standard is often a good buy for use in casseroles and purees.)

Labels also state whether the vegetables are whole, sliced, or diced, and if seasonings such as salt and sugar have been added. Occasionally a color preservative is added to a vegetable such as potatoes. Never buy rusted, dented, or bulging cans; the contents are suspect and could have dangerous levels of bacteria or toxins.

Canned vegetables are characterized by diminished crispness, color, flavor, and nutritional content. You may find their best use in casseroles, purees, and soups.

Dried: Other than legumes, most dried vegetables are available as instant soups and other processed foods. Read the label carefully so you know what additives have been used. If you are lucky enough to shop at a market that carries plain, dried vegetables, look for those with bright colors and with no evidence of insect damage or mold.

Storing Vegetables

Keeping vegetables in top condition at home is easy if you follow a few basic rules. Never wash fresh vegetables before storing them, since moisture encourages rot and tends to reduce the amount of water-soluble nutrients in the vegetables. To maintain crispness, refrigerate most fresh vegetables in the crisper bin or in plastic bags to maintain proper humidity. Store hard-rind winter squashes, sweet potatoes, white potatoes, and dry onions in a cool (45 to 50°F), dry, dark area instead of in the refrigerator. (Don't put onions and potatoes together in a container because onions will pick up moisture from the potatoes and spoil quickly as a result.)

Frozen vegetables should be kept solidly frozen and canned ones stored in a cool, dry area. Use tightly covered containers or plastic bags for dried vegetables and put them in a cool, dry place. Always refrigerate leftover vegetables in covered containers and use them within two days.

Preparing Vegetables

Good preparation techniques can make the difference between great-looking vegetables and those that are simply passable. Wash vegetables thoroughly, but never soak them. (Exceptions are sandy spinach and cauliflower, broccoli, and cabbage that can have bugs. Soak those vegetables only long enough to remove the unwanted extras.) While washing, inspect the vegetables for damaged spots, and remove them before cooking. Damaged parts tend to discolor during cooking and often impart off-flavors. Pare hard-skinned vegetables such as rutabagas and winter squash. Others—potatoes, carrots, parsnips, young beets, and immature turnips—need only scrubbing. Leave skins intact, since they are a source of fiber and valuable nutrients.

Avoid cutting vegetables when you can, since small pieces with many exposed surfaces lose nutrients to the cooking water. Cook young, tender, succulent vegetables whole. But to reduce cooking times and avoid uneven cooking of roots, tubers, and large vegetables with tough, woody portions, cut them into quarters or one-inch pieces. Since exposure to light and air begins the destruction of nutrients, cut just before you are ready to cook. (Never soak cut potatoes to stop them from darkening; they will lose water-soluble vitamin C. Besides, the color change is reversed during cooking.) To lessen bruising, use a sharp knife to cut firm vegetables, but simply tear sensitive greens.

Removing Waxes and Pesticides

In the market, some vegetables such as rutabagas, potatoes, tomatoes, cucumbers, and green peppers often feel waxy because producers have applied a coating to make the vegetable look brighter and to prevent shriveling from moisture loss. Although the U.S. Food and Drug Administration has approved the wax coatings for consumption, you may find them unappealing, as many health-conscious people do, and feel concern about eating them.

The best and most certain way to remove the coatings is to peel off the outer layer of the vegetable. Some authorities suggest scrubbing with warm water and a mild detergent if you want to retain the vegetable's peel and yet eliminate the wax. Unfortunately, the wax does not always dissolve entirely, and sometimes detergent residues remain on the vegetable.

Pesticides applied correctly become harmless in a number of days and, though still covered with pesticide residues, sprayed vegetables harvested after a recommended waiting period are safe to eat according to current information from the U.S. Department of Agriculture. Unfortunately, there is no sure way to know if the growers do apply the sprays correctly or wait the required number of days to ensure the safety of the produce.

The best way to remove the surface residues of pesticides is to scrub the produce thoroughly under running water. There is no way to get rid of the residues of pesticides absorbed through a vegetable's root system.

Basic Handling of Vegetables

Vegetables are crisp, colorful, and flavorful when handled properly. The procedure is simple.

Select the method of cooking—baking, boiling, steaming, stir-frying—that best enhances the vegetable's natural attributes. For example, sweet potatoes with their high moisture content make excellent bakers, and delicate, green sweet peas that are small and tender make great steamers. Use herbs to bring out a vegetable's flavor, not to mask poor cooking techniques.

Do not use baking soda to heighten the color of green vegetables. Baking soda destroys vitamin C and thiamine, a B vitamin; it imparts a bitter taste and leaves vegetables mushy. On the other hand, a tablespoon of vinegar or lemon juice added to red cabbage will help it stay red. (The old German custom of adding a tart apple to red cabbage will achieve the same result.) If you forget to put the acid in during cooking, add some later. The color change in red vegetables, unlike that of green vegetables, is reversible. Leave the skins and two inches of the tops on red beets to keep them from leaching their color. Add vinegar to their cooking water to help them stay bright red as well.

Top vegetables with acidic sauces (such as tomato sauce) only after cooking is complete since acids slow softening.

Cooking times should always be minimal. Lengthy cooking of any vegetable works against its flavor, nutrients, and color. Strong vegetables—brussels sprouts, broccoli, cauliflower, and turnips—become stronger when overcooked because they release offensive sulfur compounds. Overcooked cauliflower turns from a pleasing white to an unappealing brownish gray; green beans and other green vegetables take on a dull olive color.

Save nutrients and shorten cooking time as well by cooking vegetables in tightly covered saucepans. The strong-flavored vegetables will stay mild, though, if you cook them uncovered.

To determine whether vegetables are done, either taste them or pierce them with a sharp pronged fork or the point of a small, sharp knife. When properly done, vegetables are crisp-tender (slightly crunchy) with the flavor characteristics of the raw vegetable. When in doubt about the cooking time for a vegetable, aim to undercook it.

Reheating a vegetable lowers its nutritional content and mushes its texture. The best way to use leftover vegetables is by adding them to soufflés, salads, timbales, omelets, and other dishes that call for vegetables that are already cooked.

Frozen: In recipes frozen vegetables may often be used interchangeably with fresh ones. All are easy to get ready and add year-round variety to cooked vegetable dishes.

To prepare both commercially and home-frozen vegetables, cook all except greens, such as spinach and kale, and corn on the cob without thawing. Thaw corn on the cob thoroughly but greens only slightly.

To boil commercially frozen vegetables, follow the package directions. Boil or steam home-frozen vegetables the same as you would fresh ones, but separate the frozen pieces with a fork and you will shorten the cooking time by several minutes. Vegetables are partially cooked in preparation for freezing, so they need slightly less cooking before serving than fresh ones do.

To bake frozen vegetables, separate vegetable pieces and spread them in an oiled or buttered ovenproof casserole. Cover the dish and bake at 350°F until the vegetables are tender. Baking may take as long as 45 minutes.

If you want to pressure-cook frozen vegetables, reduce the cooking time by one-half of that for fresh. Watch the time closely since the vegetables will be done almost before you can look at the clock—some will take less than 15 seconds.

Canned: Commercially canned vegetables need only reheating. To avoid cooking them until they disintegrate totally (vegetables are already overcooked by the canning process), drain the liquid into a saucepan and bring it to a boil. Then add the vegetables only long enough to heat them through.

Heat home-canned vegetables the same way as commercially canned ones if you are absolutely sure they have been processed correctly at the recommended temperature (see Canning, page 766). If you have any doubt, cook most varieties at a full rolling boil for at least 10 minutes. Boil corn and spinach for 20 minutes.

Dried: There is nothing mysterious or difficult about using dried vegetables. They must be rehydrated when used in dishes low in liquids (see Using Dried Foods, page 786). Otherwise, simply add them as they are to soups, stews, sauces, and other dishes high in liquids and increase the cooking liquid accordingly. You can also make instant cream soups by grinding dried vegetables to a powder and adding them to hot white sauce.

Steeping is the simplest and most reliable method for rehydrating vegetables other than beans and peas (see Legumes chapter). Put the vegetables in a warm saucepan, and pour enough boiling water over the vegetables to cover them. Immediately put a tight-fitting lid on the pan and keep the water hot but not boiling, or rehydrating will be uneven. Stop the process when most of the vegetables are reconstituted. After removing the newly plumped vegetables, save any unabsorbed liquid—it is flavorful and contains water-soluble nutrients—for making soup stocks.

When adding dried vegetables to stews, use an extra cup of water for every cup of dried vegetables. For soups, increase the liquid by two or more cups for every cup of dried vegetables. The vegetables will absorb the extra water as they rehydrate so that the finished soup or stew will have the consistency called for in the recipe. After combining the vegetables and the liquid, bring everything to a boil, cover the pot, and reduce the heat. Simmer the vegetables for 10 to 20 minutes.

Dried vegetables are excellent sources of nutrients, but their texture and color are different from those of fresh vegetables. Dried vegetables are best used in such dishes as casseroles, omelets, stews, and souffles.

Popular Ways of Cooking Vegetables

Vegetables are delightful when served raw and crunchy or cooked in any one of several basic ways described below. You can add variety by dressing up plain vegetables with freshly snipped herbs, grated cheese, or toasted bread crumbs, and by mixing several vegetables together. Making simple vegetable salads, timbales, or cream soups are other popular ways for including vegetables in your diet.

Baking and Broiling

Baking brings out a full, pleasant flavor in vegetables, especially in those with a high-moisture content: potatoes, squash, sweet potatoes, tomatoes, onions, and eggplant. Whether you bake the vegetables by themselves or roast them with meat, leave the skins on so that the vegetables retain their nutrients and moisture. (Steam that forms inside the jackets actually cooks the vegetables.)

If you want to bake sliced vegetables (and those with a low-moisture content), smother them in a tasty sauce or broth, and cover the baking dish to keep them moist. Serve the sauce with the vegetables since it contains a lot of flavor and valuable nutrients that leached out during cooking.

A moderately hot oven (350°F) is good for baking most vegetables, but a hot one (400°F) is fine for potatoes and sweet potatoes if you want to speed up the cooking. (See Vegetables table, page 192.)

The same vegetables that make good bakers make good broilers. To prevent scorching, place them about six inches below the heat source. Check them frequently and baste with a light butter sauce to keep them moist.

Boiling

Keep vegetables whole to preserve nutrients or cut into quarters for faster cooking when boiling them. Use water sparingly; usually one-half to one cup is plenty for most vegetables. The exceptions are summer squash, which contains a lot of water and so requires much less, and greens which need only the water clinging to the leaves after washing.

For most vegetables, bring the water to a boil; then add the vegetable. As the water returns to a boil, cover, lower the heat to simmer, and time the cooking. When the food is almost done according to the clock, check the tenderness; it is easy to overcook boiled vegetables. With greens, place them in the pot; cover and heat over medium heat until the water boils. Reduce the heat and cook briefly. Drain the vegetables before serving and save the nutrient-rich cooking water for soup stocks. (See Vegetables table, page 192.)

Steaming

Steaming is an excellent way to cook vegetables and yet retain nutrients, shape, and distinctive flavor. Adjustable baskets for steaming are inexpensive and easy to find. Put the steamer filled with one or more vegetables in a saucepan that has about an inch of boiling water. Cover with a tight-fitting lid and leave the pan on moderately high heat so that the vegetables cook in the steam. Remove the vegetables when they are still brightly colored and just fork-tender. (See Vegetables table, page 192.)

Pressure-cooking

If properly timed, vegetables cooked in a pressure saucepan (often called a pressure cooker) retain about the same nutritional value and texture as those that are boiled. But, for best results, use this saucepan to cook longer-cooking vegetables such as potatoes. Tender vegetables such as peas can become overcooked extremely easily.

Always follow the manufacturer's directions for filling the saucepan, regulating the pressure, and venting the steam. For nicely cooked vegetables, bring the pressure up to 10 or 15 pounds quickly. Since you cannot readily take the lid off to check the progress, time the cooking exactly. As little as half a minute in such intense heat can make the difference between vegetables that are just tender and vegetables that are mushy. (See Vegetables table, page 192.) When done, reduce pressure and cool cooker according to manufacturer's directions or as directed in individual recipe.

Stir-Frying

This method (sometimes called panning or braising in older cookbooks) of preparing vegetables originated in China where fuel supplies were short, so cooking foods rapidly was particularly desirable. Cut vegetables into small pieces or thin slices, or shred them so they take only three to five minutes to cook. Then, heat one to two tablespoons of oil in a large, heavy skillet or wok over medium-high heat. The pan is ready for cooking when droplets of water dance as they are sprinkled in it. (The hot oil will seal in fresh vegetable flavor, valuable nutrients, and juices and keep the vegetables from sticking to the pan.) Add vegetables and cook, tossing them quickly and constantly until they are crisp-tender. If you are cooking a mixture of vegetables, partially stir-fry the extra-firm vegetables, then add the tender, quick-cooking ones. If you prefer vegetables slightly softer than crisp-tender, finish the cooking by covering the pan. For some extra-firm vegetables, steam them adding one to two tablespoons of boiling water before covering the pan. Serve the hot vegetables immediately.

Deep Frying

Potatoes are probably the best known of the deep-fried vegetables. Tasty as they are, these and other fried vegetables acquire extra fat absorbed during cooking. If you choose to fry vegetables despite the fat, here is the procedure.

Allow the vegetables to warm to room temperature if they have been refrigerated. Wash and slice the vegetables; then, pat dry to reduce foaming when they come into contact with the hot fat. Before frying squash rounds, eggplant slices, onion rings, cauliflower pieces, or broccoli florets, bread them or dip them in batter (they become fritters when dipped). Let the coating dry for ten minutes while the fat is heating. Be certain you use a fat that has a high smoking point such as corn or peanut oil. When the fat reaches 350 to 385°F (less fat is absorbed when it is hot and the cooked vegetables will be crisp, not soggy), fry several vegetable pieces at a time until they are golden brown; then remove them with a slotted spoon and drain on a paper towel. Repeat until you have cooked all the vegetable pieces.

Selecting, Storing, and Using Vegetables

Vegetable	Quantity for 4	Peak Season	Look For	Storage	
Artichokes Globe	2 pounds	April-May	Plump heavy globe; tight fleshy leaves of uniform green color.	Refrigerate in plastic bags; will keep 3-4 days.	
Jerusalem	1 pound	October-March	Not true artichoke; firm unscarred tuber with tender beige to brown skin.	Refrigerate in perforated plastic bags; will keep 2 days.	
Asparagus	1 pound	April-June	Firm, smooth, round spears; closed compact tips; rich green color.	Wrap stems in moist toweling. Refrigerate in plastic bags or in covered container; will keep 2-3 days.	
Beans Snap (green, string, wax)	¾-1 pound	May-October	Crisp, long, slender pods; velvety feel; seeds less than half grown; should snap when broken. Green beans—bright green color; wax beans—pale yellow color.	Refrigerate in plastic bags; will keep 2-5 days.	
Lima (butter)	2½ pounds (unshelled) or 1 pound (shelled)	April-August	Well-filled, clean, shiny green pods.	Refrigerate in shells; will keep 2-5 days.	

*Cooking time will be longer at higher altitudes.

Preparation	Boil	Steam	Pressure-cook	Bake	Popular Uses	Complementary Herbs
			Cooking Time (minutes)			
Rinse. Remove loose leaves and thorny leaf tips. Cut off 1 inch of top. Cook, covered, in enough boiling water to cover. Simmer until a leaf pulls out easily.	25-40	30-45	10-12	...	Cooked or raw: appetizers, salads. May top with butter or hollandaise sauce. Available: canned, fresh, frozen.	bay leaves, marjoram, thyme
Under running water, scrub with vegetable brush. Pare thinly, if desired. Cook, covered, in a small amount of simmering water. Or, bake at 350°F.	15-35	35	15	30-60	Cooked or raw: creamed, hors d'oeuvres, plain, salads, soups. May sprinkle with lemon juice. Available: fresh.	parsley, pepper
Break off woody stem where it snaps easiest; remove scales. Rinse. Tie spears together and cook standing. Place stalk-end-down in small amount of boiling water. Cover pan.	5-15	10-20	1-1½	...	Cooked or raw: creamed, custards, plain, quiches, salads, soups. May top with almonds, buttered bread crumbs, grated cheese, hollandaise sauce, or lemon juice. Available: canned, fresh, frozen.	caraway seed, mustard seed, nutmeg, parsley, pepper, sesame seed, tarragon
Rinse. Snap off ends. Cook whole beans, lengthwise strips, or 1-inch pieces in small amount of simmering water. Leave pot uncovered for first 2 minutes. Finish cooking with lid on.	15-25	15-30	1-3	...	Cooked or raw: casseroles, cream soups, plain, salads. May mix with almonds, corn, mushrooms, pimientos, or tomato sauce. Available: canned, fresh, frozen.	basil, bay leaves, dill, marjoram, mint, mustard seed, nutmeg, oregano, parsley, pepper, savory, tarragon, thyme
Rinse. Shell by snapping or cutting pod open and squeezing out beans. Cook, covered, in small amount of simmering water.	20-30	25-40	2-3	...	Cooked: casseroles, plain, vegetable soups. May combine with corn. Available: canned, dried, fresh, frozen.	celery seed, chili powder, curry powder, marjoram, oregano, parsley, pepper, sage, savory, tarragon, thyme

[continued]

Selecting, Storing, and Using Vegetables—*Continued*

Vegetable	Quantity for 4	Peak Season	Look For	Storage	
Beets	1½ pounds	June–October	Smooth, firm, round root with slender tap; rich, deep-red color; small to medium size.	Cut off tops 2 inches above root; refrigerate in plastic bags; will keep 1-2 weeks.	
Broccoli (Italian asparagus)	1½–2 pounds	October–May	Small, closed buds with no trace of yellow; moderate size; firm yet tender stems and branches; dark almost purplish green head.	Refrigerate in plastic bags; will keep 3-5 days.	
Brussels sprouts (Tom Thumb cabbage)	1½ pounds	October–November	Miniature cabbage; hard heads with tight-fitting leaves; bright green color.	Refrigerate in plastic bags; will keep 2-4 days.	
Cabbage White (green) Red Savoy	1 pound	year-round	White—hard, tight-leaved, compact head; heavy for size; greenish white color. Red—hard, tight-leaved, compact head; reddish purple color. Savoy—crumpled leaves; dark green color.	Refrigerate in plastic bags; will keep 1-2 weeks.	
Chinese (celery)	1 pound	June–November	Elongated, crisp, green leaves.	Same as white cabbage.	

*Cooking time will be longer at higher altitudes.

Preparation	Boil	Steam	Pressure-cook	Bake	Popular Uses	Complementary Herbs
Scrub under running water. Leave 1-2 inches of tops attached. Cook, covered, in enough simmering water to cover. Cool; slip off skins when beets are tender. Or, bake at 350°F.	30-45	40-75	12-18	40-60	Cooked: pickled, plain, salads, soups. Vary with orange glaze. Available: canned, fresh.	allspice, bay leaves, caraway seed, cloves, dill, ginger, mustard seed, nutmeg, parsley, pepper, savory, thyme
Remove insects by soaking in cold water for 10 minutes. Rinse. Remove tough outer leaves and ends of stalks. Split stalks in 3-4 places for quick cooking. Cook standing up in 1-inch of simmering water. Leave cover off for first 2-3 minutes. Finish cooking with lid on.	9-15	15-18	1½-2	...	Cooked or raw: plain, salads. Vary with grated cheese, hollandaise sauce, or lemon juice. May use florets in salads. May cut stalks into sticks for using with dips or into penny-size slices for salads. Available: fresh, frozen.	caraway seed, dill, mustard seed, parsley, pepper, oregano, tarragon
Remove insects by soaking in cold water for 10 minutes. Rinse. Cut off stem ends and peel away discolored leaves. Cook, covered, in small amount of simmering water.	8-10	15-20	1-2	...	Cooked or raw: creamed, plain, salads. May sprinkle with grated cheese or toasted bread crumbs. May mix with celery. Available: canned, fresh, frozen.	basil, caraway seed, dill, garlic, mustard seed, parsley, pepper, sage, thyme
Remove and discard outer leaves. Wash thoroughly. Cook in small amount of simmering water. Leave uncovered for first 1-2 minutes. Finish cooking with lid on.	6-10	9-12	½-1	...	Cooked or raw: creamed, pickled, plain, salads, scalloped. May top with cheese sauce, grated cheese, hollandaise sauce, or toasted bread crumbs. Available: fresh.	allspice, basil, caraway seed, celery seed, dill, mint, mustard seed, nutmeg, oregano, parsley, pepper, savory, tarragon
Cut off root end; discard wilted outer leaves.	4-5	...	½-1	...	Same as white cabbage. Available: fresh.	Same as white cabbage.

[continued]

Selecting, Storing, and Using Vegetables—*Continued*

Vegetable	Quantity for 4	Peak Season	Look For	Storage	
Carrots	1-2 pounds	year-round	Crisp, smooth, tapering roots; yellow to orange red color.	Cut off tops; discard. Refrigerate in plastic bags; will keep at least 1-2 weeks.	
Cauliflower	3-3½ pounds	September-January	Firm, clean head with compact florets; white to creamy white color; tender green leaves.	Refrigerate in plastic bags; will keep 3-5 days.	
Celery Green (pascal) White (bleached)	1 stalk	year-round	Rigid, crisp, tightly packed stalks with good heart formation; glossy surface.	Refrigerate in plastic bags; will keep at least 1 week.	
Celery root (celeriac)	1½ pounds	August-May	Three-inch diameter or less; rough, brownish skin; crisp.	Refrigerate in plastic bags; will keep 1 week.	

*Cooking time will be longer at higher altitudes.

Preparation	Cooking Time* (minutes) Boil	Steam	Pressure-cook	Bake	Popular Uses	Complementary Herbs
Scrub under cold running water. Scrape thinly, if desired. Cook, covered, in small amount of simmering water. Or, bake at 350°F.	10-25	15-40	3-15	30-60	Cooked or raw: creamed, plain, salads, scalloped. May combine with onions or peas. Or, sprinkle with lemon juice. Available: canned, fresh, frozen.	allspice, aniseed, bay leaves, caraway seed, chili powder, chives, curry powder, dill, fennel, ginger, mace, marjoram, mint, nutmeg, parsley, pepper, thyme
Remove leaves and woody core. Wash thoroughly. Cook in small amount of simmering water. Leave pan uncovered for first 2-3 minutes. Cover for remaining cooking time. Or, bake at 350°F.	8-20	10-25	3-10	60	Cooked or raw: creamed, plain, salads, scalloped. May top with cheese sauce, grated cheese, hollandaise sauce, or toasted bread crumbs. May slice leaves and add to salads. Available: fresh, frozen.	caraway seed, celery seed, curry powder, dill, mace, mustard seed, nutmeg, paprika, parsley, pepper
Trim roots; scrub thoroughly. Cut into desired lengths. Cook, covered, in small amount of simmering water.	10-15	25-30	2-3	...	Cooked or raw: appetizers, casseroles, cream soups, plain, salads, stews. May cut stalks for using with dips or fill stalks with cheese or nut spreads. Available: fresh.	basil, bay leaves, chervil, chives, cumin seed, dill, fennel, mace, marjoram, mint, oregano, paprika, parsley, pepper, savory, tarragon, thyme
Remove leaves and root fibers. Rinse. Cook, covered, in enough simmering water to cover. Peel thinly, if desired, after cooking.	40-60	...	...	...	Cooked or raw: appetizers, creamed, plain, salads. Available: fresh.	basil, bay leaves, chervil, chives, cumin seed, dill, fennel, mace, marjoram, mint, oregano, paprika, parsley, pepper, savory, tarragon, thyme

[continued]

Selecting, Storing, and Using Vegetables—*Continued*

Vegetable	Quantity for 4	Peak Season	Look For	Storage	
Corn	8 ears	May-September	Moist, green husks; bright, plump, yellow or white kernels.	Refrigerate in husks; will keep 1-2 days. Best if used within 1-2 hours after harvest.	
Cucumbers	2 medium	May-July	Tender, dark green skins; crisp and firm; slender.	Refrigerate in plastic bags; will keep 3-5 days.	
Eggplant	1 medium (about 1½ pounds)	August-September	Firm, heavy body; 4-6 inches in diameter; small blossom end scar; rich purple color; shiny, tight, smooth skin.	Store in cool place or in refrigerator; put in plastic bag to retain moisture; will keep 2-4 days.	
Fennel *(Finocchio)*	2 bulbs	October-January	Compact, greenish white bulb; crisp green stalks with green feathery shoots.	Refrigerate in perforated plastic bags; will keep 5-7 days.	

*Cooking time will be longer at higher altitudes.

Preparation	Cooking Time* (minutes)				Popular Uses	Complementary Herbs
	Boil	Steam	Pressure-cook	Bake		
Remove silk and husks. Cook, covered, in small amount of simmering water. Or, leave in husk and moisten husk with water. Bake at 350°F, turning each cob once.	4-5	10-15	½-1½	20-30	Cooked: creamed, fritters, puddings, salads, soups. May mix with lima beans. Available: canned, dried, fresh, frozen.	celery seed, chili powder, chives, curry powder, parsley, pepper
Rinse. Peel if waxed. Cook, covered, in small amount of simmering water.	5-10	15-20	1½-3	30	Cooked or raw: creamed, dips, plain, salads, sandwiches, soups, stuffed. May sprinkle with lemon juice. Available: fresh.	basil, chili powder, chives, dill, garlic, mint, parsley, pepper, tarragon
Rinse. Peel if skin is tough. Cook whole or thickly sliced in small amount of simmering water. Or, bake at 350°F.	5-15	15-20	...	25-30	Cooked: casseroles, marinated, plain, salads, sautéed, scalloped, stews, stuffed. May top with grated cheese or toasted bread crumbs. Available: fresh.	allspice, basil, bay leaves, chili powder, chives, garlic, marjoram, oregano, parsley, pepper, sage, sesame seed, thyme
Discard coarse outer stalks. Trim off feathery tops and save to use as an herb. Scrub bulb thoroughly. Cook, covered, in small amount of simmering water.	7-15	25-30	2-3	...	Cooked or raw: casseroles, plain, salads, soups, stews, stuffings. May top with finely ground nuts, grated cheese, or toasted bread crumbs. Available: fresh.	basil, bay leaves, chervil, chives, cumin seed, dill, mace, marjoram, mint, oregano, paprika, parsley, pepper, savory, tarragon, thyme

[continued]

Selecting, Storing, and Using Vegetables—*Continued*

Vegetable	Quantity for 4	Peak Season	Look For	Storage	

Greens†
   Amaranth
   Beet greens
   Chicory
   Collards
   Dandelion
   Endive
   Escarole
   Kale
   Lettuce
   Mustard greens
   Sorrel
   Spinach
   Turnip greens
   Watercress
	1½-2 pounds	varies	Crisp, tender leaves; bright green color typical of variety; fine veins and stems.	Refrigerate in perforated plastic bags; will keep 3-5 days.	

Kohlrabi (cabbage turnip)	6-8 bulbs	June-July	Firm, crisp bulbs 2-3 inches in diameter; crisp green tops; light green bulb.	Refrigerate. Green tops will keep 2-3 days. Bulbs will keep 1-2 weeks in plastic bags.	
Mushrooms	1 pound	year-round	Small to medium, clean, creamy white or light brown caps; pink or light tan gills, if showing; caps closed around stem.	Refrigerate in closed paper bag; will keep 1 week.	
Okra	1 pound	May-October	White or bright green color; pods tender enough to bend under light pressure and less than 4½ inches long.	Store in cool, damp place or refrigerate in perforated plastic bags; will keep 3-4 days.	

*Cooking time will be longer at higher altitudes.
†For information on using greens in salads, see Salad Greens, page 155.

Preparation	Cooking Time* (minutes)				Popular Uses	Complementary Herbs
	Boil	Steam	Pressure-cook	Bake		
Rinse thoroughly (but do not soak) in cold water. Drain. Remove thick stems, if desired. Cook in tightly covered pot with no added water. Moisture from washing is enough for cooking.	5-15	5-20	0-1½	...	Cooked or raw: cream soups, plain, pureed, salads. Available: canned (spinach only), fresh, frozen.	allspice, basil, chives, cinnamon, dill, garlic, mace, marjoram, nutmeg, oregano, parsley, pepper, rosemary, tarragon
Wash and peel. Save crisp, tender greens for salads.† Cook bulbs, covered, in small amount of simmering water.	25-30	30-35	...	...	Cooked or raw: creamed, plain, relish tray, salads. Vary with French dressing. Available: fresh.	marjoram, parsley, pepper
Wipe clean with damp cloth or soft mushroom brush. Trim away end of stems. Sauté over low heat. Use only small amount of butter or oil. Or, bake at 350°F.	...	15-20	...	15	Cooked or raw: casseroles, creamed, hors d'oeuvres, marinated, plain, quiches, salads, soups, stews, stuffed. May combine with other vegetables. Available: canned, dried, fresh, frozen.	parsley, pepper, rosemary, tarragon, thyme
Rinse. Cut off stems. Cook, covered, in small amount of simmering water.	8-15	20	3-4	...	Cooked: soups, stews. May use in cheese and mushroom sauces. May combine with tomatoes, corn, or green pepper. Vary with grated cheese, lemon juice, or yogurt. Available: canned, fresh, frozen.	basil, bay leaves, chervil, chives, dill, fennel, parsley, pepper, savory, thyme

[continued]

Selecting, Storing, and Using Vegetables—*Continued*

Vegetable	Quantity for 4	Peak Season	Look For	Storage	

Onions
  Dry onions
    Bermuda
    Red
    Shallots
    Small white
    Spanish
    Yellow
	1½ pounds	year-round	Clean, hard, well-shaped globes with dry, papery skins; color varies with type.	Store in net bags in cool, dry, dark place; will keep at least 1 month.	

Green onions
  Leeks
  Scallions
	2 bunches	May-August	Crisp, straight stems; white, tender bulbs; bright green tops.	Refrigerate in plastic bags; will keep 3-4 days.	

Parsnips	1 pound	October-March	White; smooth, firm, clean, tapered root of small to medium size.	Refrigerate in plastic bags; will keep 2 weeks.	
Peas Sweet green	2-3 pounds (unshelled) or 1 pound (shelled)	February-July	Crisp, bright green pods filled but not bulging with peas.	Best when used quickly after harvesting. Refrigerate, uncovered, in pods; will keep 2-4 days.	

Snow (sugar)
  Sugar snap
  (edible pods)
	1 pound	May-September	Crisp, slender, bright green pods with immature peas.	Best when used quickly after harvesting. Refrigerate in plastic bags; will keep 1-2 days.	

*Cooking time will be longer at higher altitudes.

Preparation	Cooking Time* (minutes)				Popular Uses	Complementary Herbs
	Boil	Steam	Pressure-cook	Bake		
Peel under cold water to reduce tearing. Cook, covered, in enough simmering water to cover. Or, bake at 350°F.	15-30	25-40	3	50-60	Cooked or raw: baked, casseroles, creamed, garnishes, salads, sauces, sautéed, soups, stuffed, stuffings. May sprinkle with grated cheese or toasted bread crumbs. Available: canned, dried, dry (aged to prevent spoilage), frozen.	basil, caraway seed, chili powder, curry powder, ginger, mustard seed, nutmeg, oregano, parsley, pepper, sage, thyme
Cut off roots; wash; remove loose skin. Cook, covered, in small amount of simmering water.	2-10	10-30	...	...	Same as dry onions. Available: fresh.	Same as dry onions.
Scrub thoroughly under running water. Scrape thinly, if desired. Cut off ends. Cook, covered, in small amount of simmering water. Or, bake at 350°F.	10-30	35-40	4-10	35-40	Cooked: mashed, plain, soups, stews. May top with herbed white sauce, horseradish, lemon juice, or orange glaze. Available: fresh.	caraway seed, cardamom, celery seed, chervil, chives, cinnamon, coriander, cumin, dill, fennel, ginger, mace, mint, nutmeg, parsley, savory, tarragon, thyme
Shell peas. Cook, covered, in small amount of simmering water.	5-10	10-20	0-1	...	Cooked or raw: casseroles, creamed, plain, pureed, salads, soups, stews. May serve with carrots. Vary with lemon or lime juice. Available: canned, dried, fresh, frozen.	basil, chili powder, dill, marjoram, mint, mustard seed, oregano, parsley, pepper, poppy seed, rosemary, sage, savory, tarragon
Rinse briefly; pat dry. Cook, covered, in small amount of simmering water.	5-10	10-20	...	...	Same as sweet green peas. Vary with sautéed mushrooms or toasted almonds. Available: fresh, frozen.	Same as sweet green peas.

[*continued*]

Selecting, Storing, and Using Vegetables—*Continued*

Vegetable	Quantity for 4	Peak Season	Look For	Storage	

Peppers
   Green or red sweet
   Hot‡
	4 peppers	June–September	Glossy, medium to dark green or red color; relatively heavy; firm walls and sides.	Refrigerate in plastic bags; will keep 3-5 days.	

Potatoes
   All-purpose
   Mealy (baking, Idaho, russet)
   New (immature, red,)
   Waxy (Maine)
	1-1½ pounds	year-round	Well-shaped, firm, with no green discoloration under skin.
			New—small; thin, feathery skin.
			Waxy—well-shaped, firm, with no green discoloration under skin.
				Store in cool, dry, well-ventilated, dark place; will keep 2 months. Use before they sprout.	

Radishes
   Black
   Red
   White (icicle)
	½ pound	April-June	Black: firm, smooth, round roots; black exterior.
			Red: firm, smooth, round roots ¾-1⅛ inches in diameter; good red color.
			White: firm, slender tap root 3-4 inches long; white color.
				Refrigerate in plastic bags; will keep 2 weeks.	

*Cooking time will be longer at higher altitudes.
‡For information on using hot peppers, see Chilies, page 53.

Preparation	Cooking Time* (minutes)				Popular Uses	Complementary Herbs
	Boil	Steam	Pressure-cook	Bake		
Wash; pat dry. If waxed, char skin under broiler. Let cool; peel. To roast: char skin under broiler; let cool; peel; then, parboil in water to cover, with lid on pan. Drain, then bake at 350°F.	5	...	...	25-30	Cooked or raw: casseroles, dips, garnishes, salads, sauces, soups, stuffed. Available: canned (as pimientos only), fresh, frozen.	basil, bay leaves, garlic, oregano, thyme
Scrub under running water; remove any sprouts. Cook, covered, in enough simmering water to cover. Or, prick skin in several places (to prevent bursting) and bake at 400°F.	20-35	20-45	3-11	45-60	Cooked or raw: baked, casseroles, mashed, pancakes, plain, salads, scalloped, soups, stews. Vary with herbed butter sauce. All-purpose—fine for baking or boiling. Mealy—ideal for baking, frying, mashing. New—ideal for creamed potatoes, stews. Waxy—ideal for boiling and slicing in salads and scalloped potatoes. Available: canned, dried, fresh, frozen.	basil, bay leaves, caraway seed, celery seed, chives, dill, garlic, mustard seed, oregano, paprika, parsley, pepper, poppy seed, thyme
Black: Scrub and peel thinly; then, cook or use raw. Red: Wash; drain; trim off root. Cook, covered, in small amount of simmering water. May also cook green tops in small amount of simmering water. Use lid on pan. White: Scrub and cut off ends. Use raw.	5-15	5-20	0-1½	...	Cooked or raw: garnishes, plain, salads. Available: fresh.	parsley, pepper

[continued]

Selecting, Storing, and Using Vegetables—*Continued*

Vegetable	Quantity for 4	Peak Season	Look For	Storage	
Rutabaga (Swedish turnip)	1-2 pounds	October–December	Not true turnip; medium size; smooth; heavy for size; thick, yellow to buff skin; few leaf scars.	Store in cool, dry place; will keep several weeks.	
Salsify (oyster plant)	1-1½ pounds	October–November	Firm, tapered roots with black or white skin.	Refrigerate in plastic bags; will keep 2-3 weeks.	

Squashes
  Summer
    Patty pan (cymling, scalloped, white)
    Yellow (crookneck, straight)
    Zucchini (cocozelle, courgette, Italian)
	2-3 pounds	April–August	Firm, glossy, tender skin; fairly heavy for size. Patty-pan 4 inches or less in diameter; others slender; 6-8 inches long. Patty-pan—white skin; yellow—light yellow skin; zucchini—dark green skin.	Refrigerate in plastic bags; will keep 3-5 days.	

Winter
    Acorn
    Buttercup
    Butternut
    Chayote
    Hubbard
    Pumpkin
    Spaghetti
	2-3 pounds	October–February	Hard rind (chayote with soft rind is exception); heavy for size. Acorn, buttercup, and hubbard—dark green rind; butternut—beige rind; chayote—pale green rind; pumpkin—warm orange rind; spaghetti—yellow rind.	Store in cool, dry place; will keep several months.	

*Cooking time will be longer at higher altitudes.
§For information on roasting seeds, see Roasting or Toasting Nuts and Seeds, page 401.

Preparation	Cooking Time* (minutes)				Popular Uses	Complementary Herbs
	Boil	Steam	Pressure-cook	Bake		
Scrub; pare if waxed. Cut into 1-inch cubes or strips. Cook, uncovered, in enough simmering water to cover.	20-40	35-40	4-8	...	Cooked or raw: casseroles, mashed, plain, soups. May top with cheese sauce or parsley white sauce. May combine with potatoes. Available: fresh.	cardamom, chervil, cinnamon, cumin, dill, fennel, ginger, mace, nutmeg, paprika, parsley, pepper, savory, tarragon
Cut off tops; pare thinly, if desired. To slow browning, drop in cold water that contains small amount of lemon juice or vinegar. Leave whole or cut in julienne strips. Cook, covered, in small amount of simmering water.	10-20	...	...	...	Cooked: creamed, mashed, plain, sautéed, stews. May top with butter or buttered bread crumbs. Available: fresh.	chives, nutmeg, parsley, pepper
Wash, pat dry. Cut off stem and blossom end. Cook, covered, in very small amount of simmering water. Or, bake at 350°F.	8-30	15-20	1½-3	30-60	Cooked or raw: casseroles, garnishes, mashed, plain, salads, soups, stews, stuffed. All are interchangeable in recipes. May top with grated cheese; minced, sautéed onions; or toasted bread crumbs. Available: fresh, frozen.	basil, bay leaves, chives, garlic, mace, marjoram, mustard seed, paprika, parsley, pepper, rosemary
Scrub and cut in half lengthwise. Remove seeds and stringy pulp. Wash and save seeds for roasting.§ Cut flesh with rind still attached into 3-4-inch cubes. Cook, covered, in enough simmering water to cover. Drain; scrape flesh from rind and mash flesh. Or, bake halves at 400°F.	15-30	25-30	6-8	60	Cooked: mashed, pie fillings, plain, soups. May combine with yams. May mash with cream or sprinkle with grated ginger root or orange rind. Available: canned, fresh, frozen.	allspice, basil, cinnamon, cloves, fennel, ginger, mustard seed, nutmeg, parsley, pepper, rosemary

[*continued*]

Selecting, Storing, and Using Vegetables—*Continued*

Vegetable	Quantity for 4	Peak Season	Look For	Storage	
Sweet potatoes Dry-meated (sweet potatoes) Moist-meated (yams)	1-2 pounds	September-December	Smooth, well-shaped, firm tubers; medium size. Dry-meated—pale, golden brown skin; moist-meated—pale, brownish to reddish skin.	Store in cool, dry place; will keep 1-2 days.	
Tomatoes	1-2 pounds	May-September	Firm, plump bodies with uniform red or yellow color; small blossom end scar; shape varies with type.	Keep unripe tomatoes at room temperature but out of sun. Refrigerate ripe tomatoes; will keep 1 week.	
Turnips	1-2 pounds	October-March	Small to medium size, 2-3 inches in diameter; round shape with flat top; uniformly tender white skin with purple tinge; heavy for size; few leaf scars or roots.	Refrigerate in plastic bags; will keep at least 1 week.	

*Cooking time will be longer at higher altitudes.
†For information on using greens in salads, see Salad Greens, page 155.

Preparation	Cooking Time* (minutes)				Popular Uses	Complementary Herbs
	Boil	Steam	Pressure- cook	Bake		
Scrub. Cook, covered, in enough simmering water to cover. When tender, drain and slip off skins. Or, bake at 400°F.	30-35	35-40	6-10	30-50	Cooked: candied, mashed, plain, souffléed. May use in biscuits, breads, cakes, cookies, custards, muffins, pies. May combine with pumpkin. Available: canned, dried, fresh, frozen.	allspice, cardamom, cinnamon, cloves, ginger, mace, nutmeg, parsley, pepper, poppy seed
Wash; cut out stem. Cook in covered pan with no added water. Or, bake at 350°F. May be peeled: Dip in boiling water for 30-60 seconds. Cool; remove skin. May remove seeds: Cut tomato in half and gently squeeze out seeds. Cut slices vertically (top to bottom) to retain the most juice.	3-8	10	1-1½	15-30	Cooked or raw: baked, broiled, catsup, chili sauce, juice, paste, plain, relishes, salads, sandwiches, soups, stuffed. May sauté green tomatoes. Available: canned, fresh.	basil, bay leaves, celery seed, chervil, chili powder, chives, cumin, dill, fennel, marjoram, mint, mustard seed, oregano, paprika, parsley, pepper, sage, sesame seed, tarragon
Cut off roots and greens; save greens.† Scrub; peel thinly, if desired. Cook, covered, in a moderate amount of simmering water.	15-30	20-25	1½-8	...	Cooked or raw: casseroles, creamed, dips, glazed, mashed, salads, stews. May top with grated cheese or grated lemon or orange zest. Vary with minced onions. Available: fresh.	allspice, caraway seed, celery seed, chives, dill, oregano, parsley, pepper, poppy seed

Basic Vegetable Recipes

Stuffed Vegetables

    4 large green peppers, cucumbers, onions,
        potatoes, summer or winter squash, sweet
        potatoes, or tomatoes
    2 cups cooked brown rice or bulgur, or whole
        grain bread crumbs
    1 teaspoon minced fresh parsley
    1 teaspoon dried thyme
    ⅛ teaspoon pepper
    1 cup tomato sauce or Poultry Stock (page 110)

Parboil and hollow out vegetables.

In a medium-size bowl, combine brown rice,
bulgur, or bread crumbs with parsley, thyme, pepper,
and ¾ cup sauce or stock. Mix thoroughly.

Preheat oven to 350°F.

Place vegetables in a lightly oiled 2-quart ovenproof casserole. Fill each vegetable with the rice or
other mixture and top with remaining sauce or stock.
Cover and bake until the vegetables are tender, about
45 minutes.

    4 servings

Creamed Vegetables

    3 cups coarsely chopped assorted vegetables
    1 cup medium Béchamel Sauce (page 141)
    ½ teaspoon curry powder (optional)
    ¼ teaspoon nutmeg or paprika, or 1 tablespoon
        minced fresh parsley

Cook vegetables, covered, in a small amount of
simmering water for 15 to 20 minutes, or until tender.
Drain.

While vegetables are cooking, prepare sauce.

Add vegetables and curry powder (if used) to
warm sauce and mix thoroughly. Cook until mixture is
just heated through. Serve garnished with nutmeg,
paprika, or parsley.

    4 to 6 servings

Glazed Vegetables

    1 cup Poultry Stock (page 110) or water
    2 teaspoons honey
    2 teaspoons butter
    1 pound carrots, onions, sweet potatoes, or
        turnips, sliced into 1-inch pieces or cubes

Place stock or water, honey, butter, and vegetables
in a medium-size saucepan and cook, covered, for 10
to 15 minutes or until almost tender. Uncover and
continue cooking until tender, basting to coat vegetables evenly with glaze, about 10 minutes. Shake
the pan to keep vegetables from sticking.

    4 servings

Scalloped Vegetables

    3 cups coarsely chopped mixed vegetables
    1½ cups medium Béchamel Sauce (page 141)
    3 tablespoons fine whole grain bread crumbs

Cook vegetables, covered, in a small amount of
simmering water for 15 to 20 minutes, or until tender.
Drain.

While vegetables are cooking, prepare sauce.

Preheat oven to 350°F.

Place vegetables and sauce in a lightly buttered
1-quart ovenproof casserole in alternating layers. Start
with vegetables and end with the sauce. Sprinkle with
bread crumbs and bake until crumbs are lightly
browned, about 25 minutes.

    6 servings

Variation:

    Easy au Gratin Vegetables: Add ½ cup grated
cheddar cheese to Béchamel Sauce before pouring
over vegetables.

Vegetable Marinade

    ½ cup vegetable oil
  ⅓ to ½ cup cider vinegar
    ¼ cup finely chopped fresh parsley
    2 cloves garlic, pressed
    1 tablespoon prepared mustard
    1 teaspoon honey
    ½ teaspoon dried oregano
    ½ teaspoon dried basil
    ½ teaspoon dried tarragon
    ⅛ teaspoon cayenne pepper

Combine all ingredients and mix well.

Pour marinade over raw or lightly steamed,
mixed vegetables. Chill for at least 2 hours, stirring
occasionally.

    Yields 1 cup

Vegetables Tempura

This style of light-batter deep frying is favored by the Japanese. With vegetables it allows for quick cooking that maintains firmness.

1 cup rye or whole wheat flour
½ teaspoon baking powder
1 egg, beaten
1 cup milk
1 pound assorted vegetables (broccoli or cauliflower florets, ½-inch-thick onion rings, whole or sliced mushrooms)
vegetable oil, for frying

Combine flour and baking powder in a small bowl. Add egg and milk and stir until well mixed. Let stand for 30 minutes.

Meanwhile prepare vegetables. Then heat oil in a deep fryer (oil should reach 375°F). Dip vegetables into batter and then lower coated vegetables into hot oil. Cook until batter is browned to your liking. Drain on paper towels.

Serve with your favorite dipping sauce, or a variety of sauces such as Sesame-Ginger Sauce (page 151), Peanut Sauce (page 151), or Sweet-Sour Barbecue Sauce (page 152).

6 to 8 servings

Vegetable Pie

Crust
1¼ cups cornmeal
3 tablespoons vegetable oil
½ cup hot water, or more as needed

Filling
1 medium-size onion, chopped
1 medium-size green pepper, chopped
1 stalk celery, chopped
2 tablespoons vegetable oil
1 large tomato, chopped
1 teaspoon chili powder
½ teaspoon ground cumin
¼ teaspoon pepper
2 teaspoons cornstarch, dissolved in ¼ cup cold water
1½ cups vegetables (any of the following, alone or in combination: corn, green beans, peas, or zucchini; cooked carrots, chick-peas, kidney beans, pinto beans, or spinach)
2 ounces Monterey Jack cheese, grated

To make the crust: In a medium-size bowl, mix cornmeal, oil, and enough hot water to make a pliable dough. Press dough into a well-oiled 8-inch pie plate. Preheat oven to 350°F.

To make the filling: In a large skillet, sauté onions, green peppers, and celery in oil until soft. Add tomato, chili powder, cumin, and pepper and cook for 3 minutes longer. Add cornstarch mixture, stirring constantly until mixture thickens. Fold in vegetables. Spoon filling into piecrust, sprinkle with cheese, and bake for 35 minutes.

4 servings

Artichokes

There are two vegetables known as artichokes, the globe type—the "true" artichoke—and the Jerusalem.

Globe artichokes are relished as a gourmet treat. The cooked leaves may be eaten hot accompanied by a butter or hollandaise sauce, cold with a vinaigrette dressing, or stuffed as in the recipe on page 212.

Jerusalem artichokes are crisp tubers with a sweet and nutty taste. They are especially rich in vitamin B_1 and are a good source of iron.

Artichokes in Cream

2 cups thinly sliced peeled Jerusalem artichokes
½ cup lentil sprouts
½ cup shredded zucchini
1 cup thinly sliced green peppers
1 cup sour cream or ricotta cheese
2 teaspoons soy sauce
parsley sprigs

Combine artichokes, sprouts, zucchini, and peppers in a salad bowl.

In a cup, mix sour cream or ricotta cheese and soy sauce. Pour dressing over vegetables and toss thoroughly. Garnish with parsley.

4 to 6 servings

Jerusalem Artichokes with Stir-Fry Vegetables

2 tablespoons safflower oil
2 cloves garlic, pressed
1 piece ginger root, 1 inch long, peeled and
finely grated
1 medium-size onion, cut into 6 slices and
separated into rings
2 cups coarsely chopped broccoli
4 cups sliced Chinese cabbage, bok choy, or
cabbage
2 cups cubed zucchini
4 teaspoons cornstarch
¼ cup soy sauce
1 cup Vegetable Stock (page 111)
pepper, to taste
2 cups thinly sliced peeled Jerusalem artichokes
8 scallions, chopped

Preheat a wok or heavy skillet. Add oil, garlic, ginger, onion, broccoli, and cabbage. Stir-fry about 4 minutes. Add zucchini and stir-fry another 2 minutes.

Mix cornstarch with soy sauce and stock and then add to vegetables. Stir until liquid thickens. Add pepper and stir in artichokes. Remove from heat and turn into serving dish. Garnish with scallions and serve with cooked brown rice.

4 servings

Stuffed Artichokes

12 small to medium-size or 8 large globe artichokes

Stuffing
1½ cups whole grain bread crumbs
½ cup grated Parmesan cheese
1 teaspoon dried basil
1 teaspoon dried parsley
1 teaspoon dried oregano
1 teaspoon dried thyme
2 cloves garlic, minced
2 tablespoons olive oil
1 tablespoon soy sauce

Cut off artichoke stems and trim ½ inch from tops of artichoke leaves.

To make the stuffing: In a large bowl mix together the bread crumbs, Parmesan, dried herbs, garlic, oil,

and soy sauce. Holding each artichoke over the bowl, stuff breading into spaces between leaves with hands or with a spoon.

Place artichokes on a rack above boiling water in a large pot and steam for 30 to 45 minutes over medium heat, or until leaves pull away easily.

6 to 8 servings

Asparagus

Malaysian Asparagus

1 tablespoon soy sauce
1½ teaspoons minced peeled ginger root
1 clove garlic, crushed
2 tablespoons vegetable oil
1 pound asparagus, cut into 2-inch pieces

Sauce
½ cup half-and-half or light cream
2 teaspoons cornstarch

Combine soy sauce, ginger, and garlic. Mix well and let stand for 30 minutes.

In a skillet or wok, heat oil over high heat. Add soy sauce mixture and asparagus. Stir-fry about 2 minutes. Then cover and steam until asparagus is just tender.

To make the sauce: In a small saucepan, blend together half-and-half or cream and cornstarch. Heat until sauce thickens, stirring constantly.

When asparagus is done, pour cream sauce over it and serve immediately.

4 servings

Asparagus Casserole with Sesame Seeds

1 pound asparagus, cut into 1-inch pieces
2 hard-cooked eggs, sliced
¼ cup shredded cheddar cheese
1 tablespoon sesame seeds
3 tablespoons whole grain bread crumbs
1 cup Poultry Stock (page 110)

Steam asparagus until tender, about 10 minutes.

Arrange half the asparagus on the bottom of a buttered ovenproof casserole. Cover with egg slices, and then add remaining asparagus.

Combine cheese, sesame seeds, and bread crumbs. Spread evenly over asparagus. Pour stock over all and place under broiler until cheese is melted.

3 servings

Asparagus Soufflé

3 tablespoons whole wheat pastry flour
1 cup milk
4 eggs, separated
1 cup cooked asparagus, finely chopped
  pepper, to taste
  dash of nutmeg or pinch of dried tarragon

Preheat oven to 375°F.

In a medium-size saucepan blend flour with 1/3 cup milk until smooth. Add remaining milk. Bring to a boil and cook, stirring constantly, until thickened. Continue stirring and add egg yolks, one at a time. Bring mixture to a boil again, and stir in asparagus and seasonings. Set aside to cool.

Beat egg whites until stiff but not dry, and then fold into asparagus mixture. Pour into a buttered ovenproof casserole. Bake on lowest rack in oven for 30 to 40 minutes.

6 servings

Variation:

Vegetable Soufflé: Use almost any cooked vegetable in place of the asparagus. Choose seasonings that will enhance the vegetable you are substituting: aniseed or thyme on carrots, for instance; marjoram on mushrooms, zucchini, or peas; basil with eggplant or tomatoes. Grated Parmesan or Romano cheese may be sprinkled on top.

Basil Asparagus with Pasta

1 medium-size onion, chopped
2 tablespoons vegetable oil
2 cups chopped tomatoes
½ teaspoon dried basil
¼ teaspoon pepper
1 pound asparagus, cut into 1-inch pieces
8 ounces uncooked whole wheat noodles

In a large skillet, sauté onions in oil until soft. Add tomatoes, basil, pepper, and asparagus. Simmer, with the cover ajar, until asparagus is tender, about 10 minutes.

Meanwhile, cook noodles until tender, then drain. Serve asparagus and sauce over noodles.

4 servings

Beans

Dill Vegetables in a Rice Ring

2 cups cooked brown rice
¼ cup minced fresh parsley
1 sweet red pepper, finely chopped (optional)
1 cup fresh green beans, cut into 1-inch pieces
1 medium-size summer squash, quartered
  lengthwise and sliced
1 stalk celery with leaves, sliced
¾ cup water
3 tablespoons butter
1 tablespoon dillweed
  pepper, to taste

Combine rice, parsley, and red pepper, if used. Form mixture into the shape of a ring on a serving plate.

Combine beans, squash, celery, and water in a large saucepan and cook, covered, until vegetables are tender, about 10 minutes. Drain well. Cut butter into pieces and add it to vegetables along with dillweed and pepper. Stir to mix. Spoon vegetables into the center of the rice ring.

6 servings

Herb Green Beans with Sunflower Seeds

1 pound fresh green beans, cut into 1-inch pieces
½ teaspoon dried basil
½ teaspoon dried marjoram
½ teaspoon dried chervil
1 tablespoon chopped fresh parsley
2 teaspoons chopped fresh chives
⅛ teaspoon dried savory
⅛ teaspoon dried thyme
1 small onion, chopped
1 clove garlic, minced
2 tablespoons vegetable oil
½ cup sunflower seeds
¼ teaspoon pepper

Cook beans in a small amount of water for 10 to 12 minutes or until crisp-tender. Drain.

Meanwhile, combine herbs in a small bowl. Then sauté onions and garlic in oil until soft. Add herbs and sunflower seeds.

Add cooked beans to herb mixture, season with pepper, toss lightly, and serve immediately.

4 to 6 servings

Polynesian Vegetable Medley

2 tablespoons vegetable oil
1 small onion, chopped
1 green pepper, chopped
1 stalk celery, chopped
2 large carrots, thinly sliced
1 cup fresh green beans, cut into 1-inch pieces
¼ cup Poultry Stock (page 110) or water
1 cup pea pods
¾ cup unsweetened crushed pineapple
1 tablespoon soy sauce
4 ounces water chestnuts, sliced
2 teaspoons cornstarch, dissolved in 2 tablespoons water

Heat oil in a medium-size skillet. Add onions, peppers, and celery and sauté for 3 to 5 minutes. Do not brown. Add carrots, beans, and stock or water. Simmer, covered, until vegetables are tender, 10 to 12 minutes. Add pea pods, pineapple, and soy sauce, and simmer for 2 minutes longer. Add water chestnuts and cornstarch mixture, stirring constantly until thickened.

4 servings

NOTE: Two cups fresh green beans may be substituted for 1 cup green beans and 1 cup pea pods.

Chilled Green Beans

1 pound fresh green beans, cut into 1-inch pieces
½ medium-size onion, minced
1 small clove garlic, minced
¼ cup plus 2 tablespoons olive oil
2 tablespoons wine vinegar
pepper, to taste
grated Parmesan cheese

Cook beans in a small amount of water for 10 to 15 minutes or just until tender. Drain.

Combine beans with remaining ingredients, except for cheese. Chill. Top with cheese just before serving.

4 to 6 servings

Green Bean Casserole with Corn Bread Topping

1½ pounds fresh green beans, cut into 1-inch pieces
1½ to 2 cups milk
2 tablespoons butter
dash of white pepper
2 tablespoons whole wheat flour

Corn Bread
1 cup cornmeal
½ cup whole wheat flour
1 tablespoon baking powder
1 egg
⅔ cup milk
2 tablespoons honey
3 tablespoons butter, melted and cooled

Cook beans in a small amount of water for 10 to 12 minutes or until crisp-tender. Drain, reserving liquid. Place beans in a buttered 9-inch-square baking dish. Add enough milk to the reserved liquid to equal 2 cups.

In a small saucepan, heat 1½ cups of the liquid with butter and pepper.

Pour remaining ½ cup liquid into a jar. Add flour, cover, and shake until smooth. Pour flour mixture into the hot milk, stirring constantly, and cook until sauce bubbles and thickens. Pour over beans.

Preheat oven to 400°F.

To make the corn bread topping: Mix cornmeal, flour, and baking powder with a fork until well blended. In a bowl, beat together egg, milk, honey, and butter. Pour all at once into dry ingredients. Stir until just mixed.

Spoon batter over beans and sauce. Bake for 20 to 22 minutes, or until corn bread has risen and is brown on top.

6 servings

Green Beans Vinaigrette

A cool side dish or an easy take-along food for a picnic.

1 cup vegetable oil
⅓ cup red wine vinegar
1 tablespoon chopped pimientos
1 tablespoon chopped fresh chives or scallions
1 tablespoon chopped green peppers
½ teaspoon soy sauce
2½ cups fresh whole green beans

Combine all ingredients, except green beans, in a bottle or jar. Cover and shake well.

Place beans in a large bowl and pour dressing over them. Cover and refrigerate for at least 3 hours, stirring occasionally. Drain before serving.

4 servings

Swiss Green Beans

1½ pounds fresh green beans, cut into 1-inch pieces
2 tablespoons butter
2 tablespoons whole wheat flour
¼ teaspoon pepper
½ teaspoon grated onions
1 cup yogurt
½ pound Swiss cheese, grated

Topping
1 cup whole wheat flour
½ cup rolled oats
1 tablespoon minced fresh parsley
pepper
3 tablespoons butter, softened

Cook beans in a small amount of water for 10 to 15 minutes or just until tender. Drain.

Melt butter in a medium-size saucepan. Stir in flour, pepper, and onions and cook for 2 minutes. Reduce heat, add yogurt, and stir until smooth. Fold

in beans and heat gently. Turn into a buttered oven-proof casserole and sprinkle with cheese.

Preheat oven to 400°F.

To make the topping: Combine flour, oats, parsley, and pepper. Work in butter until evenly blended. Sprinkle topping over cheese. Bake for 20 minutes, or until bubbly and crumbs are browned.

8 servings

Quick Bean Dish

4½ cups fresh green beans
¾ cup finely chopped walnuts, almonds, or peanuts
1½ cups yogurt
¾ cup mayonnaise
2 cloves garlic, crushed

Mix beans and nuts together. In a separate bowl, combine yogurt, mayonnaise, and garlic. Pour dressing over mixture. Toss lightly and serve.

6 servings

Lima Bean Goulash

1 tablespoon butter
½ pound lean ground beef
1 cup chopped onions
1 cup chopped celery
1½ cups quartered tomatoes
1 teaspoon paprika
2 cups cooked lima beans, drained with liquid reserved
1 teaspoon grated lemon rind
1 tablespoon lemon juice
1 cup sliced mushrooms

Heat butter in a large skillet with a tight-fitting lid over medium-high heat. When it starts to sizzle, add ground beef. Stir and fry until browned. Add onions and celery and cook for 3 to 4 minutes longer. Stir in tomatoes and paprika. Add 2 cups reserved bean liquid, adding water if necessary to make the full amount. Stir in lemon rind, lemon juice, and beans. Cover, lower heat, and simmer for 30 minutes. Add mushrooms and cook, covered, for 15 minutes more.

4 to 6 servings

Lima-Stuffed Tomatoes

2 cups pureed cooked lima beans
¼ teaspoon onion powder
½ cup cottage cheese
4 to 6 medium-size tomatoes
1 tablespoon sesame seeds, toasted, or finely
    chopped walnuts
lettuce leaves

Combine puree, onion powder, and cottage cheese.
Cut tops off tomatoes and hollow out centers. Fill
centers with bean mixture and decorate with sesame
seeds or walnuts. Chill. When ready to serve, arrange
tomatoes on crisp lettuce leaves.

4 to 6 servings

Lima-Tuna Casserole

*This main-dish meal may be prepared a day
ahead or frozen and saved for that busy, no-
time-to-cook day.*

3 eggs, beaten
1 cup milk
2 cups cooked lima beans, chopped
1 cup finely chopped celery
1 can (6 to 7-ounces) water-packed tuna, flaked
2 tablespoons grated onions
½ teaspoon dillweed
¼ cup chopped fresh parsley

Preheat oven to 350°F.
In a small bowl, combine eggs and milk.
In another larger bowl, mix beans, celery, tuna,
onions, dillweed, and parsley. Then add egg mixture
and stir lightly. Spoon mixture into a buttered loaf pan
and bake for 35 minutes.

4 to 6 servings

Hot and Spicy Lima Beans

3 pounds unshelled lima beans
3 tablespoons corn oil
1 large onion, chopped
2 cloves garlic, finely chopped
1 medium-size tomato, chopped
1 tablespoon chopped peeled ginger root
1 teaspoon ground coriander
½ teaspoon turmeric
¼ to ½ teaspoon cayenne pepper
¼ teaspoon paprika
1 green chili pepper, sliced

Steam beans until tender, about 15 minutes. Cool.
Heat oil in a medium-size skillet. Add onions and
garlic and sauté for 3 minutes. Stir in tomato, ginger,
coriander, turmeric, cayenne, paprika, chili pepper,
and lima beans. Cover and cook for 5 minutes over
medium heat.

8 servings

Succotash

3 tablespoons butter
1 medium-size onion, chopped
1 cup fresh baby lima beans
1 cup corn
½ cup water
½ teaspoon pepper
½ cup heavy cream

Heat butter in a large skillet. Add onions and
sauté until wilted. Add beans, corn, water, and pepper
and cook, covered, over medium heat for 10 to 15
minutes, or until vegetables are crisp-tender. Stir in
cream and cook for 5 to 8 minutes, or until vegetables
are tender.

4 servings

Mellow Wax Beans and Mushrooms

1½ pounds fresh wax beans, cut into 1-inch pieces
½ pound mushrooms, sliced
1 teaspoon dried basil
½ cup Beef Stock (page 110) or Poultry Stock
    (page 110)

In a medium-size saucepan, cook beans until partially done, about 5 minutes. Drain. Then add mushroom slices, basil, and stock and bring to a boil.
Reduce heat and simmer for about 5 minutes, or
until tender.

8 servings

Beets

Dutch Vegetable Salad

1 cup diced peeled cooked beets
2 cups diced cooked potatoes
1 cup cooked green beans or peas
2 tart apples, diced
3 tablespoons vegetable oil
3 tablespoons cider vinegar·
  lettuce leaves
  mayonnaise
2 hard-cooked eggs, sliced

In a large bowl, combine beets, potatoes, beans or peas, apples, oil, and vinegar. Toss gently to mix. Chill. Spoon mixture onto a bed of lettuce on a platter. Cover with a thin layer of mayonnaise and garnish with slices of egg.

4 to 6 servings

Harvard Beets

6 medium-size beets
2 teaspoons cornstarch
¼ cup vinegar
¼ cup honey

Place beets in a large saucepan. Add enough water to cover and cook, covered, for 30 minutes, or until tender. Let beets cool slightly and then drain, saving ¼ cup of the liquid for the sauce. Peel and slice beets.

In a large saucepan, add the beet cooking liquid, cornstarch, vinegar, and honey. Stir and cook over medium heat until sauce clears and thickens. Add cooked beets to the sauce, stirring to coat. Warm the mixture until beets are heated through.

4 servings

Molded Beet Salad with Sour Cream Dressing

3 large beets
1 small celery heart with leaves, chopped
2 scallions with tops, chopped
1 envelope unflavored gelatin
1 tablespoon honey
  juice of ½ lemon

1 cup sour cream or yogurt
½ medium-size cucumber, finely chopped

Place beets in a medium-size saucepan. Add enough water to cover and cook, covered, for 30 minutes, or until tender. Let beets cool slightly and then drain, saving 1¾ cups of the beet juice for the gelatin mixture. Peel and dice beets.

Sprinkle celery and scallions in a 1½-quart ring mold. Add beets.

In a small saucepan, combine reserved beet juice, gelatin, and honey, and cook over low heat, stirring constantly, until gelatin and honey are dissolved. Stir in lemon juice and then pour mixture gently over vegetables. Chill in the refrigerator until set.

When ready to serve, run a table knife around the edges of the mold, dip mold briefly in hot water, then place a serving plate on top, and invert to unmold.

Mix together sour cream or yogurt and cucumber, and then spoon into center of mold.

6 to 8 servings

Broccoli

Near Eastern Broccoli

2¼ cups Poultry Stock (page 110)
1 cup bulgur
1 tablespoon lemon juice
1 clove garlic, minced
1 small onion, minced
½ teaspoon dried oregano
½ head medium-size broccoli, coarsely chopped

In a medium-size saucepan, bring stock to a boil. Stir in remaining ingredients. Cover and simmer for 15 to 20 minutes, or until broccoli is tender.

4 to 6 servings

Broccoli Puff

1 head broccoli
1 small onion, chopped
2 eggs
½ cup heavy cream
¼ teaspoon pepper
¼ teaspoon ground nutmeg
¼ cup whole grain bread cubes
½ cup shredded sharp cheddar cheese

Preheat oven to 350°F.

Cut florets from broccoli. Steam broccoli until tender, about 8 minutes. Cool slightly and puree in a blender with onions, eggs, and cream. Pour into a medium-size mixing bowl and stir in pepper, nutmeg, bread cubes, and cheese.

Pour into a buttered 8-inch-square baking pan and bake for 30 to 40 minutes.

4 to 6 servings

Vegetable Nut Pie

A satisfying meatless main course dish in which the nuts provide a nice surprise in texture and flavor. Choose the basic pastry or try the nut pastry for an extra nutty taste.

Whole Wheat Pastry
¼ cup plus 2 tablespoons butter
1¼ cups whole wheat flour
3 tablespoons ice water

Preheat oven to 400°F.

In a medium-size bowl cut butter into flour until mixture resembles coarse crumbs. Stir in ice water until pastry holds together and forms a ball.

Roll dough on a lightly floured cloth to make a 12-inch round. Fit into a 9-inch pie plate. Trim and flute to make a stand-up edge. Prick dough generously with a fork.

Bake for 10 minutes. Remove pastry from oven.

OR

Whole Wheat and Nut Pastry
¼ cup plus 2 tablespoons butter
1 cup whole wheat flour
⅓ cup ground pecans

Preheat oven to 350°F.

In a medium-size bowl cut butter into flour until mixture resembles coarse crumbs. Stir in nuts. Press over bottom and sides of a 9-inch pie plate.

Bake for 8 minutes. Remove pastry from oven.

Vegetable Nut Filling
3 slender carrots, sliced (about 1 cup)
½ head broccoli, cut into florets
¼ cup chopped scallions
1 cup chopped pecans, peanuts, or cashews
1 tablespoon butter
¾ cup shredded Gruyère cheese
3 eggs
1 cup milk
½ teaspoon dillweed

Preheat oven to 350°F.

Cook carrots in a small amount of boiling water for 5 minutes. Add broccoli and cook for 5 minutes longer. Drain. Chop broccoli to make 1½ cups.

Sauté scallions and nuts in butter in a small skillet for 3 to 5 minutes.

Sprinkle ¼ cup of cheese over bottom of baked crust, spoon vegetables and sautéed nuts over cheese, and sprinkle ¼ cup of cheese over vegetables.

Beat eggs with milk in a small bowl. Stir in dillweed. Pour mixture over vegetables, sprinkle with remaining cheese, and bake for 30 minutes, or until knife inserted in center comes out clean. Remove from oven and let stand for 10 minutes before serving.

4 to 6 servings

Brussels Sprouts

Vary your vegetable menu with brussels sprouts, a member of the cabbage family. Brussels sprouts are a good source of vitamins A and C.

Brussels Sprouts and Carrots in a Potato Ring

1 pint brussels sprouts
6 carrots, cut into 1-inch pieces
¼ cup plus 2 tablespoons butter

¾ cup Poultry Stock (page 110)
1 tablespoon honey
1 tablespoon cornstarch
2 tablespoons cider vinegar
6 medium-size potatoes, cut into 1-inch pieces
2 tablespoons butter
1 egg
2 tablespoons milk
   white pepper, to taste

Combine brussels sprouts, carrots, ¼ cup butter, and stock in a large saucepan. Cover and cook until vegetables are tender, about 20 minutes. Add honey. Mix cornstarch and vinegar together, and then add mixture to the saucepan. Simmer for 1 minute, stirring constantly.

Cook potatoes in enough water to cover. When tender, drain potatoes. Steam potatoes dry over low heat, shaking the pan, for 2 to 3 minutes. Mash potatoes with remaining butter, egg, and milk. Add pepper and form potatoes into the shape of a ring on a serving plate. Fill the center with the brussels sprouts and carrots.

6 servings

Brussels Sprouts with Yogurt

2 to 2½ pounds brussels sprouts
   1 medium-size tomato, chopped
   2 teaspoons chopped fresh chives
   ½ teaspoon ground nutmeg
   ¼ teaspoon pepper
   1 cup yogurt, whisked
   ¼ cup grated Parmesan cheese
   ¼ cup toasted blanched almonds

Steam brussels sprouts until tender when pierced with the tip of a knife, about 7 minutes.

Preheat oven to 350°F.

Place cooked sprouts in a buttered ovenproof casserole. Sprinkle tomatoes and chives over top, add nutmeg and pepper, and then pour yogurt over all. Sprinkle with cheese and almonds and bake for 15 minutes.

6 to 8 servings

Brussels Sprouts Kabobs

1 pint brussels sprouts
2 tablespoons soy sauce
2 tablespoons corn or other vegetable oil
2 tablespoons lemon juice
2 tablespoons chopped fresh parsley
1 pint cherry tomatoes
½ pound mushrooms

Steam brussels sprouts until tender when pierced with the tip of a knife, about 7 minutes. Cool.

To make the marinade, combine soy sauce, oil, lemon juice, and parsley and mix well. Add tomatoes and mushrooms and marinate at room temperature for 30 minutes, stirring occasionally.

Alternate sprouts, tomatoes, and mushrooms on skewers, leaving a small space between each one. Broil kabobs for 5 minutes, turning once and basting with the marinade.

4 servings

Brussels Sprouts in Walnut-Brown Butter Sauce

1 pint brussels sprouts
¼ cup butter
1 cup coarsely chopped walnuts

Steam brussels sprouts until tender when pierced with the tip of a knife, about 7 minutes.

Place butter and walnuts in a heavy iron skillet and heat, while stirring, over moderately high heat until butter foams and turns deep tan and nuts are toasted.

Place brussels sprouts in a serving dish, pour butter evenly over sprouts, and serve immediately.

4 to 6 servings

Variation:

Vegetables in Walnut–Brown Butter Sauce: Substitute 2 cups cubed cooked potatoes, carrots, or rutabagas for brussels sprouts.

Cabbage

Chinese Cabbage-Sour Cream Roll

This strudellike roll is a tempting side dish—perfect for a company meal.

¼ cup butter
1 medium-size head Chinese cabbage, finely chopped
1 cup finely chopped walnuts
1 cup golden raisins
2 cups whole grain bread crumbs
1 teaspoon ground cinnamon
pastry for Sour Cream Piecrust (page 719)

In a large skillet, melt butter. Add cabbage and simmer until cabbage turns light brown, stirring occasionally. With a slotted spoon, remove cabbage from skillet and place in a medium-size bowl. When cabbage is cool, stir in walnuts, raisins, bread crumbs, and cinnamon. Set aside.

Preheat oven to 375°F.

Roll out pastry into a 14 × 16-inch rectangle, about ⅛ inch thick. Spread the cooled cabbage filling evenly over the pastry, leaving a 1-inch-wide border all around the pastry. Roll pastry up carefully, with long edge toward you. Place jelly-roll style in a jelly-roll pan, seam-side down, and bake for 30 minutes, or until pastry is golden brown.

8 to 10 servings

Shrimp-Cabbage Stir-Fry

Marinade
2 tablespoons rice vinegar
2 teaspoons soy sauce
2 teaspoons cornstarch
2 teaspoons tomato paste
2 tablespoons water

1 pound uncooked medium-size shrimp, peeled and deveined
2 large heads Chinese cabbage

Sauce
½ cup Poultry Stock (page 110) or Fish Stock (page 111)
2 teaspoons cornstarch
2 teaspoons soy sauce
2 teaspoons honey

¼ cup safflower or peanut oil
4 cloves garlic, minced
1 piece ginger root, ¼ inch long, peeled and minced
6 mushrooms, quartered
4 scallions, white parts thinly sliced (reserve green parts)
4 cups coarsely chopped spinach

To make the marinade: In a medium-size bowl mix together vinegar, soy sauce, cornstarch, tomato paste, and water. Add shrimp, turning to coat pieces well, and refrigerate for 2 to 3 hours.

Trim cabbage leaves from the ribs. Slice ribs diagonally into ½-inch pieces. Cut leaves into 2-inch squares.

To make the sauce: Mix together stock, cornstarch, soy sauce, and honey. Then drain marinade from the shrimp into this sauce.

Heat 1 tablespoon of oil in a wok or heavy skillet. When a small piece of scallion dropped in the oil dances around, the oil is ready. Sauté half of the shrimp until they turn pink. Remove to a bowl. Repeat with remaining shrimp. Remove shrimp and any liquid to the bowl.

Heat remaining oil. Sauté garlic and ginger briefly in the oil. Then add mushrooms, white parts of scallions, and cabbage ribs. Stir for 1 minute and add cabbage leaves and spinach. Add sauce and cook, stirring constantly, until thickened. Return shrimp to the wok or skillet and cook until warmed, about 1 minute. Garnish with reserved scallions and serve with hot cooked brown rice.

4 servings

Winter Vegetable Quiche

A complete meal in itself for those seeking a vegetarian alternative.

Pastry
½ cup cold butter, cut into small pieces
1¾ cups whole wheat pastry flour
1 egg yolk
3 tablespoons sour cream

Filling
2 small heads Chinese cabbage
1 tablespoon butter
1 onion, thinly sliced
4 eggs

1 cup milk
½ cup light cream
¼ teaspoon chopped fresh thyme
⅛ teaspoon freshly grated nutmeg
⅛ teaspoon freshly ground pepper
    dash of cayenne pepper

½ cup grated Swiss cheese

To make the pastry: Keep butter, yolk, and sour cream cold and work as fast as possible.

Cut butter into flour until mixture is in small, even crumbs.

Beat egg yolk slightly with a fork. Reserve ½ teaspoon. Mix with sour cream and add this liquid to flour mixture. Quickly form into a ball and, on a floured surface, roll pastry out to fit a 10-inch pie plate.

Line pie plate with pastry and slightly crimp the edges of the dough over the rim of the plate. Refrigerate until baking time.

To make the filling: Trim ribs from cabbage leaves and reserve. Steam cabbage leaves for 4 to 5 minutes, or until they become just limp. Remove from heat and chop coarsely. Set aside.

Cut reserved ribs into ¼-inch slices. In a medium-size skillet, melt butter and sauté ribs with onion slices until both are tender, about 5 minutes. Set aside to cool.

In a medium-size bowl, beat together eggs, milk, cream, thyme, nutmeg, black pepper, and cayenne. Stir in onion mixture and cabbage leaves.

Preheat oven to 425°F.

Prick empty piecrust generously with a fork and bake for 10 minutes. Then, brush bottom of crust with reserved egg yolk. Return to oven for 2 more minutes.

Reduce oven temperature to 375°F. Pour egg and vegetable mixture into crust, sprinkle with cheese, and bake for 35 minutes, or until top begins to brown and knife inserted in center comes out clean. Allow to cool at room temperature for about 10 minutes before slicing.

6 servings

Snappy Savoy Cabbage

1 small head savoy cabbage, shredded
3 tablespoons butter, melted

1 teaspoon lemon juice
1 teaspoon horseradish, drained
¼ teaspoon pepper
1 teaspoon honey

Steam cabbage for about 10 minutes, or until crisp-tender. Drain and spoon into a serving dish.

Combine butter, lemon juice, horseradish, pepper, and honey. Add to cabbage, toss, and serve.

6 to 8 servings

Sweet and Sour Red Cabbage

1 small head red cabbage, coarsely chopped*
1 cup water
¼ teaspoon pepper
2 tablespoons butter
2 tart apples, sliced
2 tablespoons cider vinegar
1 tablespoon honey
½ teaspoon caraway seeds
1 tablespoon cornstarch, dissolved in ¼ cup
    cold water

In a large saucepan, combine cabbage, water, pepper, and butter. Cook, covered, until cabbage is crisp-tender, about 10 minutes. Add apples and cook for 3 to 5 minutes, or until soft. Stir in vinegar, honey, and caraway seeds. Pour in cornstarch mixture, stirring gently over low heat until sauce bubbles and thickens. Simmer for 1 minute.

6 servings

*Green cabbage may be substituted for red cabbage.

Dutch Cabbage in Milk

2 cups milk
5 cups shredded cabbage
2 tablespoons grated fresh horseradish root or
    prepared horseradish, drained
⅛ teaspoon pepper

In the top of a double boiler, heat milk over direct heat. Add cabbage, horseradish, and pepper, and stir thoroughly. Cover tightly, place over boiling water, and cook for 15 to 20 minutes, stirring occasionally.

6 servings

Stuffed Cabbage

Plan on serving this dish often. The flavors of rice and mint combine with cabbage leaves— accented by tomato sauce.

¼ cup uncooked brown rice
⅓ cup water
3 tablespoons olive oil
1 medium-size onion, finely chopped
½ medium-size green pepper, finely chopped
1½ cups thinly sliced mushrooms
2 cloves garlic, minced
1½ teaspoons minced fresh mint or ½ teaspoon
    dried mint
1 medium-size tomato, finely chopped
1 teaspoon dried oregano
½ teaspoon soy sauce
¼ cup sunflower seeds or pine nuts
    cayenne pepper, to taste
12 large cabbage leaves
1½ cups thin tomato sauce
½ lemon, thinly sliced
    chopped fresh mint

Bring rice and water to a boil in a 2-quart saucepan. Cover, reduce heat to low, and cook until water has been almost completely absorbed, about 10 minutes.

Add 2 tablespoons of oil, the onions, and green peppers to the rice. Cook over low heat, stirring frequently, until vegetables are limp. Then stir in mushrooms, garlic, mint, tomato, oregano, and soy sauce, and cook gently, uncovered, until liquid from the tomato has been absorbed. Add sunflower seeds or pine nuts and sprinkle with cayenne. Remove pan from heat and set aside.

If cabbage leaves have thick ribs, trim backs of the ribs even with the leaves, keeping leaves intact. Steam just until color deepens.

Gently place leaves in a single layer on a clean surface. Place a tablespoon of stuffing at base of each leaf. Fold leaf end over stuffing, then fold in sides, and roll. The finished roll should look like a short, fat cigar.

Place a thin layer of remaining oil over the bottom of a heavy saucepan large enough to hold all the rolls in a single layer. Pour ¾ cup of the tomato sauce into the pan, add cabbage rolls, seam-side down, cover with remaining tomato sauce, and simmer, covered, for 45 minutes.

Place lemon slices over cabbage rolls and simmer an additional 20 minutes. Before serving, garnish with chopped mint.

4 servings

Carrots

Baked Carrot and Apple Casserole

2 cups sliced carrots
5 apples, cut into ¼-inch slices
2 tablespoons whole wheat flour
4 tablespoons honey
4 tablespoons butter
¾ cup orange juice

Steam carrots for 12 minutes.
Preheat oven to 350°F.

Put half the apples in a shallow 1-quart baking dish and cover them with half of the carrots. Sprinkle 1 tablespoon of the flour over carrots and apples; then drizzle 2 tablespoons of the honey over the flour. Dot with 2 tablespoons of butter. Repeat the layers.

Pour orange juice over entire casserole, and bake for 40 to 45 minutes. Serve hot.

6 servings

Ginger Carrots in Orange Cups

2 large oranges
6 carrots, thinly sliced
¼ cup butter
1 tablespoon honey
½ teaspoon ground ginger
    parsley sprigs

Using a zig-zag pattern, cut oranges in half crosswise to form 4 cups. Press out juice and scoop out pulp. Reserve 3 tablespoons of juice. Dip cups in boiling water and drain.

Steam carrots for 15 to 20 minutes, or until tender. Drain.

In a medium-size skillet, combine butter, reserved orange juice, honey, and ginger. Cook over low heat, stirring, until bubbly. Add carrots and stir to glaze evenly, about 5 to 7 minutes. Spoon carrots into orange cups and garnish with parsley. Serve immediately.

4 servings

Carrot Celebration

1 pound carrots
3 tablespoons butter
3 tablespoons concentrated orange juice
1 to 2 tablespoons honey
  chopped walnuts

Cut carrots into halves, then cut into quarters lengthwise. Steam carrots for 20 to 25 minutes, or until tender.

In a small saucepan, heat together butter, orange juice, and honey. Then toss with carrots in a serving dish and garnish with chopped walnuts.

6 to 8 servings

Parslied Carrots and Zucchini Julienne

1 pound carrots
3 medium-size zucchini
½ cup butter, melted
¼ teaspoon pepper
½ cup chopped fresh parsley

Cut carrots into sticks lengthwise, then into julienne strips, 2 to 3 inches long. Cut zucchini in half lengthwise and remove seeds. Cut halves into sticks, then julienne strips.

In 2 separate saucepans steam vegetables for 20 to 25 minutes, or until crisp-tender. Drain. Then combine vegetables in a heated serving dish and toss gently with butter, pepper, and parsley.

6 to 8 servings

Vegetable Sunburgers

These tasty burgers are easy to prepare and will be favorites with your family. Served with a salad, they are a nutritious alternative to the popular hamburger.

½ cup grated carrots
½ cup finely chopped celery
2 tablespoons chopped onions
1 tablespoon chopped fresh parsley
1 tablespoon chopped green peppers
1 egg, beaten
1 tablespoon vegetable oil

¼ cup tomato juice
1 cup ground sunflower seeds
2 tablespoons wheat germ
⅛ teaspoon dried basil

Preheat oven to 350°F.

In a medium-size bowl combine all ingredients, and shape into patties.

Arrange in an oiled shallow baking dish. Bake until brown on top, about 15 minutes. Turn patties and bake until reverse sides are brown, 10 to 15 minutes.

4 servings

Cauliflower

Baked Cauliflower and Broccoli au Gratin

1 small head broccoli
1 small head cauliflower
2 cups milk
¼ teaspoon white pepper
3 tablespoons butter
¼ cup plus 1 tablespoon whole wheat flour
½ pound cheddar cheese, coarsely grated
½ cup whole grain bread crumbs
2 tablespoons wheat germ
  paprika

Cut broccoli into 1-inch lengths. Break cauliflower into small florets. In two separate saucepans steam vegetables for 12 to 15 minutes, or until just tender. Drain. Place vegetables in an 8½ × 11-inch baking dish, and mix gently.

Preheat oven to 350°F.

Scald 1½ cups milk in a small saucepan. Add pepper and 2 tablespoons butter. Stir until butter is melted. Pour remaining ½ cup milk into a jar. Add flour, cover, and shake until smooth. Pour flour mixture into hot milk, stirring constantly, and cook until mixture thickens and bubbles. Add cheese and stir until melted. Pour sauce over vegetables, top with bread crumbs and wheat germ, dot with remaining butter, sprinkle with paprika, and bake for 30 minutes.

6 to 8 servings

Rosy Cauliflower with Onions

2 large white onions, cut into ⅛-inch slices
3 tablespoons vegetable oil
1 tablespoon mild honey
1 large head cauliflower, broken into florets
1 cup tomato juice
1 tablespoon chopped fresh parsley

In a large skillet sauté onions in oil until tender. Add honey and cook until lightly browned, about 3 minutes. Stir in cauliflower and tomato juice, cover, and cook over medium heat until cauliflower is crisp-tender. Sprinkle with parsley just before serving.

6 servings

Celery

Spiced Celery and Fruit

1 tablespoon butter
1 medium-size onion, chopped
6 stalks celery, cut into ½-inch slices
1 tablespoon curry powder
1 tablespoon whole wheat flour
1¼ cups water
1 piece fresh ginger root, 1 inch long, peeled and finely chopped
3 tablespoons lemon juice
½ cup dried apricots
2 apples, coarsely sliced
1 banana, cut into ½-inch slices
½ cup raisins
½ cup sour cream

In a large skillet melt butter. Add onions and celery and sauté until golden. Combine curry powder and flour and then stir into celery-onion mixture. Cook for 2 to 3 minutes over medium heat, stirring constantly. Stir in water, ginger, lemon juice, apricots, apples, banana, and raisins and cook, covered, over low heat until apples and apricots are tender, about 20 minutes. Just before serving, fold in sour cream.

8 servings

Celery Root Remoulade

3 to 4 celery roots (celeriac)
½ cup cottage cheese
¼ cup mayonnaise
¼ cup sour cream or yogurt
1 tablespoon French-style mustard
1 tablespoon soy sauce
¼ cucumber, cut into small pieces
¼ green pepper, cut into small pieces
¼ stalk celery, cut into small pieces
4 radishes, cut into small pieces

Cut off leaves and root fibers of celery roots, peel, and cut into very thin julienne strips. Place in a serving dish or on individual plates.

In a blender, place cottage cheese, mayonnaise, sour cream or yogurt, mustard, and soy sauce and blend on low speed until well mixed. Gradually add pieces of cucumber, pepper, celery, and radish, blending until vegetables are finely chopped. Pour or spoon over celery root and serve cold.

6 servings

Celery Root Timbales

An elegant company vegetable dish—well worth the extra preparation time.

2 to 3 celery roots (celeriac)
3 to 4 medium-size potatoes, cubed
2 teaspoons butter
1 leek, cut into ½-inch slices
1¼ cups light cream
1 egg plus 2 egg yolks, beaten
dash of nutmeg
dash of dried thyme
10 ounces fresh spinach, chopped
2 teaspoons vegetable oil
½ cup sliced mushrooms
¼ cup diced onions
2 tablespoons whole wheat flour

Cut off leaves and root fibers of celery roots, peel, and cube. Cook celery roots and potatoes in a small amount of water until very tender. Drain well and puree.

In a small skillet melt butter, and sauté leeks until tender (be careful not to brown). Puree leeks and then mix with pureed vegetables.

Preheat oven to 375°F.

Add ¼ cup cream, beaten egg and egg yolks, nutmeg, and thyme to pureed mixture. Blend well. Pack into 6 ½-cup-size timbale molds or custard cups that have been well buttered and lined with small rounds of wax paper on the bottom. Place molds in a 9 × 13-inch baking pan, and pour hot water into bottom of pan until water reaches a depth of ⅔ the way up sides of molds. Cover with a piece of buttered wax paper and bake for 30 minutes, or until set.

Fifteen minutes before timbales are to be finished, sauté spinach in oil for 5 minutes, or until wilted. Remove spinach and cook mushrooms and onions in remaining pan juices until tender. Sprinkle flour over ingredients in skillet and blend thoroughly. Gradually whisk in 1 cup cream. Set ½ of this creamed mixture aside and blend remaining half into the wilted spinach.

Pack creamed spinach mixture into bottom of ovenproof serving dish. Unmold celery root timbales onto spinach-lined serving dish. Top with reserved mushroom sauce and, just before serving, place under broiler until lightly browned. Serve immediately.

6 servings

Hearts of Celery

4 celery hearts
1 large tomato, peeled and cut into wedges
⅓ cup olive oil
2 tablespoons lemon juice
½ teaspoon minced fresh basil
   soy sauce, to taste
3 tablespoons chopped fresh parsley

Split each celery heart in half lengthwise. Cut out the root. Trim leaves, leaving only the smallest. Cut into 1½-inch pieces, wipe dry, and place in a salad bowl. Add tomato wedges.

Combine oil, lemon juice, basil, and soy sauce; pour over celery and tomatoes. Mix well. Top with parsley for garnish.

6 servings

Corn

New England Corn Pudding

3 tablespoons butter, melted and cooled slightly
2 eggs
1⅓ cups milk
3 tablespoons whole wheat flour
¼ teaspoon white pepper
1 teaspoon honey
2 cups fresh corn, cut from 4 to 6 ears
   dash of nutmeg

Preheat oven to 325°F.

In a blender, combine butter, eggs, milk, flour, pepper, and honey and blend until well mixed. Pour into a buttered 1½-quart ovenproof casserole. Stir in corn and sprinkle with nutmeg. Set casserole in a square baking pan and pour hot water into bottom of pan until water reaches a depth ⅓ the way up sides of casserole. Bake for 45 minutes, or until knife inserted in center comes out clean.

4 to 6 servings

Pennsylvania Dutch Corn Pie

pastry for 2 Basic Rolled Piecrusts (page 718)
2 tablespoons whole wheat flour
2 cups fresh corn, cut from 4 to 6 ears
   dash of white pepper
1 tablespoon chopped fresh parsley
2 hard-cooked eggs, sliced
1 tablespoon butter
½ cup milk

Preheat oven to 375°F.

Roll out ½ of the pastry and line a 9-inch pie plate. Sprinkle bottom with flour, and add corn. Add remaining ingredients in order listed. Roll out remaining pastry for top crust, cover filling, and crimp edges to seal. Cut vents in top crust and bake for about 45 minutes. Serve in soup plates. If desired, heat additional milk with a little butter to pour over each portion.

4 to 6 servings

Sautéed Corn with Sour Cream

2 tablespoons butter
2 cups fresh corn, cut from 4 to 6 ears
¼ cup chopped red and green peppers
1 tablespoon chopped onions
    dash of cayenne pepper, to taste
¾ cup sour cream

In a medium-size skillet, heat 1 tablespoon butter and sauté corn for 5 minutes. Add remaining butter, peppers, onions, and cayenne and cook for 5 minutes longer, or until onions and peppers are tender.

Add sour cream and cook, stirring constantly, until cream is heated through.

4 servings

Welshkorn Puffers

2 egg whites
2 cups fresh corn, cut from 4 to 6 ears
3 tablespoons whole wheat pastry flour
2 teaspoons chopped fresh parsley
¼ teaspoon pepper

Beat egg whites until stiff, but not dry. Set aside. Chop corn finely with sharp knife on cutting board, or use a food processor or blender until coarsely chopped and slightly creamy, but not pureed. Fold into egg whites, along with flour, parsley, and pepper. Drop by the teaspoon onto hot, lightly oiled griddle in silver dollar-size dollops and cook until dry and golden underneath, about 7 minutes. Carefully turn and cook about 7 minutes on reverse side. Serve immediately.

4 to 6 servings

Eggplant

Baked Eggplant Parmigiana

¼ cup plus 1 tablespoon olive oil
2 medium-size eggplants, cut into thin slices
    whole wheat flour
1 teaspoon minced garlic
1 can (28 ounces) Italian-style tomatoes, drained
¼ cup tomato paste
¼ teaspoon pepper

2 tablespoons minced fresh basil or 1 teaspoon dried basil
2 tablespoons minced fresh parsley
½ cup grated Parmesan cheese
½ pound mozzarella cheese, sliced

Heat ¼ cup oil in a large skillet. Dredge eggplant slices in flour and sauté in hot oil until lightly browned on both sides. (During cooking, add more oil if needed.)

While eggplant is cooking, heat the tablespoon of oil in a medium-size skillet. Add garlic and sauté for 2 minutes. Add tomatoes, paste, pepper, basil, and parsley and simmer, uncovered, for 20 minutes. Stir occasionally.

Preheat oven to 350°F.

Layer eggplant, sauce, and grated Parmesan cheese in an 8½ × 11-inch baking pan, beginning and ending with sauce and Parmesan cheese. Arrange mozzarella slices on top. Bake casserole for 35 minutes, or until brown and bubbly.

6 to 8 servings

Sesame-Eggplant Bake

¼ cup olive oil
2 small or 1 large eggplant
2 eggs
1 cup milk
    pepper, to taste
1 cup tomato sauce
½ cup sesame seeds, ground
½ cup grated Parmesan cheese

Coat a baking sheet with olive oil. Slice eggplant about ¼ inch thick, arrange on the baking sheet, and brush with oil and place under broiler until lightly browned. Turn over, brush with oil, and brown. Place slices in an oiled 9 × 13-inch baking pan.

Preheat oven to 375°F.

Beat eggs and milk together. Season with pepper. Pour over eggplant and bake for 20 minutes, or until knife inserted in center comes out clean.

Pour tomato sauce over top and sprinkle with sesame seeds and cheese. Place under broiler or in very hot oven until top is lightly browned. Serve at once.

4 to 6 servings

Roasted Eggplant

1 large eggplant
5 cloves garlic
  pepper, to taste
3 tablespoons olive oil
  wine vinegar, to taste

Preheat oven to 375°F.

Cut 5 slits in whole eggplant lengthwise. Cut garlic cloves into halves. Place 2 halves of garlic in each "pocket" of eggplant. Sprinkle pepper in "pockets."

Place eggplant in an oiled baking dish and sprinkle top with 1 tablespoon olive oil. Bake about 50 minutes, or until fork tender. Cool.

Remove skin and garlic, and place eggplant in a serving dish. Season with remaining olive oil, vinegar, and pepper, to taste. Serve with whole grain toast.

6 servings

Ratatouille

Seasoned eggplant mixed with several other vegetables.

2 tablespoons olive oil
2 cloves garlic, crushed
1 large onion, halved and thinly sliced
1 small eggplant, cubed
2 medium-size green peppers, coarsely chopped
4 large tomatoes, coarsely chopped
3 small to medium-size zucchini, cut into ¼-inch
  slices
1 teaspoon dried basil
½ teaspoon dried oregano
½ teaspoon dried thyme
2 tablespoons chopped fresh parsley

In a 4-quart pot, heat oil. Add garlic and onions and cook until soft, about 7 minutes. Add eggplant and stir until coated with oil. Add peppers and stir in well. Cover pot and cook over medium heat for 10 minutes, stirring occasionally to avoid sticking.

Add tomatoes, zucchini, and herbs and mix well. Cover and cook over low heat about 15 to 20 minutes, or until eggplant is tender, but not mushy. Serve hot or, if desired, chill and use as a savory condiment.

4 servings

Fennel
Celery Parmesan and Fennel

The slightly anise flavor of fennel combines with the celery for a pleasing and unusual dish.

3 medium-size fennel bulbs (about 1½ pounds)
⅓ cup vegetable oil
2 cups sliced celery
½ cup Poultry Stock (page 110)
¼ cup grated Parmesan cheese

Separate fennel into "leaves" and slice thinly. (Use only bottom bulb of fennel; discard any stems or feathery leaves.)

Place oil in a deep saucepan. Add vegetables and toss in oil until well coated. Sauté carefully, stirring for 5 minutes. Be careful that vegetables do not brown. Add stock, cover tightly, and bring to a boil. Reduce heat to simmer, and cook about 10 to 15 minutes, or until crisp-tender. With a slotted spoon remove vegetables to a serving dish and keep warm.

Bring liquid in saucepan to a boil until volume is reduced by ½. Pour over vegetables in serving dish, sprinkle with cheese, and serve immediately.

4 to 6 servings

Greens
Sautéed Spinach and Pignoli

3 tablespoons olive oil
2 large cloves garlic, bruised
1 dried chili pepper or ⅛ to ¼ teaspoon crushed
  red pepper
¼ cup pine nuts
2 tablespoons sesame seeds
1 pound spinach
2 tablespoons Poultry Stock (page 110) or water
  lemon wedges

Heat oil in a large deep skillet or a Dutch oven. Add garlic and pepper to brown. Remove garlic. Add pine nuts and sesame seeds and cook, stirring constantly, until lightly toasted, 1 to 2 minutes. Add spinach and stock or water, cover, and cook over high heat for 4 to 5 minutes, tossing with a fork once or twice, just until wilted and tender. Serve hot with lemon wedges.

4 servings

Spanakopeta
(Greek Spinach Pie)

Crust

1⅓ cups whole wheat pastry flour
2 tablespoons vegetable oil
¼ cup cold milk

Filling

2 pounds spinach
⅓ cup olive oil
2 bunches scallions with tops, chopped
    pepper, to taste
2 tablespoons dillweed
2 cups crumbled feta cheese

Preheat oven to 350°F.

To make the crust: Mix together flour, oil, and milk. Roll dough between 2 sheets of lightly floured wax paper to fit an 8-inch pie plate. Trim edges and make a fluted rim. Reserve trimmings for lattice. Prick crust generously with a fork and bake for 7 minutes. Set aside.

To make the filling: Steam spinach over low heat in just the water that clings to the leaves after washing. When wilted, drain spinach, then squeeze dry, and chop.

In a medium-size skillet, heat oil and sauté scallions until soft. Add spinach, pepper, dillweed, and cheese. Stir to mix.

Spoon filling into pie crust. Roll out pastry trimmings and cut lattice strips for the top. Bake pie for 20 to 25 minutes, or until crust is brown.

4 to 6 servings

Spinach-Stuffed Tomatoes

6 large tomatoes
⅓ cup butter
¼ cup chopped onions
1 clove garlic, minced
1 tablespoon minced fresh parsley
½ cup whole grain bread crumbs
2 tablespoons wheat germ
⅓ cup grated Parmesan cheese
1½ cups cooked chopped spinach, well drained

Preheat oven to 350°F.

Cut off tomato tops. Scoop out centers, leaving fleshy shells intact.

Melt butter in a small saucepan. Add onions and garlic and sauté until onions are translucent. Add parsley.

In a small bowl, combine bread crumbs, wheat germ, and cheese.

Place tomato shells in an ovenproof casserole small enough to hold them upright. Spoon spinach into the shells, top each with some of the bread crumb mixture, spoon butter mixture over crumbs, and bake for 30 minutes, or until tender.

6 servings

Endive-Stuffed Tomatoes

2 tablespoons olive oil
4 cloves garlic, minced
1 onion, chopped
3 cups finely chopped endive
4 large firm tomatoes
⅛ teaspoon pepper
1 tablespoon wine vinegar
1 cup soft whole grain bread crumbs
½ cup shredded cheddar cheese
¼ cup grated Parmesan cheese
½ cup ground walnuts

Heat oil in a large skillet and sauté garlic, onions, and endive until onions are tender and endive turns a dull green color.

Hollow out tomatoes by scraping out seeds, pulp, and juice with a spoon. Add pulp mixture to the sautéing endive along with pepper and vinegar. Break up any large pieces of pulp with a spoon. Simmer until juice from tomato evaporates. Remove from heat and stir in bread crumbs, ¼ cup cheddar, Parmesan, and nuts.

Preheat oven to 350°F.

Fill tomatoes with warm stuffing, top with remaining cheddar, and bake in a buttered baking pan on upper rack for 15 to 20 minutes.

4 servings

Italian Winter Greens Soup

1 small onion, coarsely chopped
1 clove garlic, minced
1 tablespoon butter
1 tablespoon minced fresh parsley
1½ teaspoons dried basil

3 cups Poultry Stock (page 110)
2 medium-size tomatoes, finely chopped
½ pound spinach or chard-type greens, chopped
    into large pieces
½ teaspoon soy sauce
    juice of ½ lemon
¼ to ½ teaspoon freshly ground black pepper
    grated Parmesan cheese

In a 3-quart saucepan sauté onions and garlic in butter until soft. Add parsley and basil and cook for 2 more minutes.

Add stock and tomatoes to vegetables and bring liquid to a slow boil. Then add greens to the hot stock and simmer, covered, for 15 minutes. Stir in soy sauce, lemon juice, and pepper and serve hot with Parmesan cheese sprinkled on top.

4 servings

Swiss Chard-Cottage Cheese Puff

2 teaspoons vegetable oil
1 clove garlic, minced
½ cup sliced leeks
1 stalk celery, sliced
3 to 4 cups chopped Swiss chard
1 cup cottage cheese, well sieved
3 tablespoons whole wheat flour
2 eggs
¼ cup finely grated sharp cheddar cheese
4 tablespoons grated Parmesan cheese

Heat oil in a large skillet. Add garlic, leeks, and celery and sauté until very tender but not browned. Add Swiss chard and steam, tightly covered, until wilted and tender. Remove mixture from heat and then puree in a blender. Combine mixture with cottage cheese, flour, eggs, and cheddar and beat until light and fluffy.

Preheat oven to 350°F.

Sprinkle 2 tablespoons Parmesan over bottom of a buttered 1-quart baking dish, pour in mixture, and sprinkle top with remaining Parmesan. Place baking dish in a pan and pour hot water into bottom of pan until water reaches halfway up the sides of the baking dish. Bake for 1 hour or until puffed and golden brown. Serve immediately.

4 to 6 servings

Vegetables with Oriental Sauce

½ cup walnuts
1 cup thinly sliced celery
1 cup thinly sliced onions
1 sweet red pepper, cut into thin strips (optional)
2 to 3 tablespoons vegetable oil
½ pound spinach
2 cups bean sprouts

Sauce
3 tablespoons soy sauce
½ cup Poultry Stock (page 110) or water
    pinch of ground ginger
⅛ teaspoon garlic powder
2 teaspoons cornstarch
1 tablespoon honey

Place the walnuts in a small saucepan with enough water to cover. Bring to a boil. Drain.

In a large skillet stir-fry celery, onions, and red pepper, if used, in 1 tablespoon oil until crisp-tender. Remove with a slotted spoon. Then sauté walnuts until lightly brown, adding more oil to the pan as needed. Remove walnuts. Stir-fry spinach and sprouts until spinach has just wilted and then return celery, onions, red pepper, and walnuts to skillet.

In a small saucepan, combine all the sauce ingredients, except the honey, and bring to a boil, stirring constantly. Add honey and stir until dissolved. Pour sauce over vegetables, heat through, and serve.

4 to 6 servings

Kale in Sour Cream

2 cups cooked kale, drained
1 teaspoon butter
½ teaspoon honey
    dash of pepper
1 teaspoon lemon juice
¾ cup sour cream

In a medium-size saucepan, heat kale, butter, honey, pepper, and lemon juice. When very hot, reduce heat and slowly stir in sour cream. As soon as cream is hot, remove from heat and serve.

4 servings

Stir-Fried Kale with Chinese Mushrooms

Serve over hot cooked brown rice or whole wheat noodles for a quick and different entrée or side dish.

> 10 dried shiitake mushrooms*
> 2 cups hot water
> 6 scallions with tops
> 2 medium-size tomatoes, chopped
> 1½ tablespoons soy sauce
> 1½ teaspoons red wine vinegar
> 1½ teaspoons honey
> 2 tablespoons vegetable oil
> 4 ounces firm tofu, drained and cut into ½-inch cubes
> 2 teaspoons minced fresh hot red chili pepper or 1 teaspoon dried hot red pepper
> 2 cloves garlic, minced
> ½ pound kale, coarsely chopped
> 2 tablespoons cornstarch, dissolved in 2 tablespoons water

Soak mushrooms in hot water until spongy, about 30 minutes. Drain, reserving half the soaking water. Remove and discard tough stems.

Quarter half of the mushrooms; slice remaining mushrooms into ¼-inch strips.

Slice white part of scallions thinly on the diagonal. Chop tender green part of scallions finely (keep separate).

Combine reserved water, tomatoes, soy sauce, vinegar, and honey in a small bowl.

Heat 2 teaspoons oil in a large wok or large heavy skillet. When oil is very hot, add tofu and stir-fry until golden. Remove tofu and add remaining oil to the wok or skillet. When oil is hot, stir in red pepper and garlic. Then add scallion bottoms. Add half the kale and all the mushrooms, tossing continuously. When wilted, stir in remaining kale. Continue to stir-fry until kale becomes bright green. Pour in tomato mixture, stir once, and cover. Reduce heat to medium and simmer for 5 minutes. Stir in cornstarch paste and cook, stirring slowly until sauce thickens. Add tofu to kale mixture. Sprinkle with scallion greens and serve immediately.

4 to 6 servings

*Shiitake mushrooms are commonly available in oriental grocery stores.

Mustard Greens with Dill, Lemon, and Soy Sauce

> 3 cups Beef Stock (page 110), Poultry Stock (page 110), Vegetable Stock (page 111), or boiling water
> 4 tablespoons soy sauce
> 1 cup barley
> 1 medium-size onion, chopped
> 2 tablespoons safflower oil
> 1 pound fresh mustard greens, chopped, or 2 packages (10 ounces each) frozen mustard greens, thawed and chopped
> ½ teaspoon dillweed
> ¼ cup lemon juice
> freshly ground pepper, to taste

Combine stock or water and 2 tablespoons soy sauce in a medium-size saucepan. Add barley and bring to a boil. Lower heat, cover, and simmer for 45 to 60 minutes, or until tender.

In a large skillet, sauté onions in oil until translucent, stirring occasionally. Add mustard greens, stir to mix, cover, and gently steam for 15 minutes. Add dillweed, lemon juice, remaining soy sauce, and pepper, and steam for another 10 minutes. Serve greens over barley, spooning juice proportionally over each serving.

4 to 6 servings

Sorrel-Stuffed Eggs

> 8 hard-cooked eggs
> ½ pound sorrel, chopped
> 1/3 cup cottage cheese, well drained
> 2 tablespoons freshly grated Parmesan cheese
> 1 tablespoon chopped fresh parsley
> dash of white pepper
> few grindings of freshly ground nutmeg, to taste
> salad greens
> cherry tomatoes, tomato wedges, or other sliced salad vegetables

Slice eggs in half lengthwise, remove yolks, and set white halves aside.

Place egg yolks, sorrel, cottage cheese, Parmesan, parsley, and pepper in a food processor or blender. Process with short on-off bursts until a smooth paste of mayonnaise consistency is formed. If necessary, thin slightly with small amount of milk or mayonnaise. Pile mixture high into egg white halves. Sprinkle with nutmeg. Serve on fresh greens garnished with cherry tomatoes, tomato wedges, or other sliced salad vegetables.

4 to 6 servings

Kohlrabi

Golden Kohlrabi Patties

    4 to 6 medium-size kohlrabi
    1 egg, beaten
    3 tablespoons whole wheat flour
    ¼ cup butter
    1 small onion, finely chopped
    ⅛ teaspoon pepper

Trim kohlrabi of stems, peel, and then shred. Place in a medium-size saucepan with enough water to cover. Bring to a boil, lower heat, and simmer, covered, for 10 minutes. Drain and cool. Mix kohlrabi, egg, and flour in a large bowl.

Melt butter in a large skillet, add onions, and sauté until translucent. Add kohlrabi mixture, sprinkle with pepper, and cook over medium heat until bottom is golden brown and crusty. Divide into quarters and turn each quarter over with a spatula and brown on the other side. Serve hot.

4 servings

Mushrooms

Mandarin Mushrooms

    ½ cup chopped onions
    ½ cup sliced green peppers
    ½ cup thinly sliced celery
    1 pound mushrooms, cut into chunks

    Sauce
    1 tablespoon grated orange rind
    2 tablespoons honey

    1 tablespoon vinegar
    ½ cup orange juice
    ½ cup Poultry Stock (page 110) or Vegetable
        Stock (page 111)
    ½ teaspoon grated peeled ginger root
        (½-inch piece)
    1 tablespoon soy sauce
        dash of cayenne pepper, or to taste
    1 tablespoon cornstarch, dissolved in 1
        tablespoon water
    1 cup skinned orange segments

Preheat oven to 350°F.

Place onions, peppers, celery, and mushrooms in an 8-inch-square baking dish.

To make the sauce: In a medium-size saucepan, combine orange rind, honey, vinegar, orange juice, stock, ginger root, soy sauce, and cayenne. Bring to a boil and simmer, covered, for 5 minutes.

Add cornstarch mixture to sauce, stirring until mixture thickens. Remove from heat. Stir in orange segments, pour sauce over vegetables, and bake, uncovered, for 25 minutes. Serve with brown rice or whole wheat noodles.

4 servings

Marinated Mushrooms

    1 pound mushrooms
    ½ cup soy sauce
    1 tablespoon honey
    3 tablespoons butter
    1 tablespoon whole wheat flour
    ½ cup water

Slice mushrooms into thirds parallel to the stem. Place in a medium-size bowl and cover with soy sauce and honey. (Marinade will not cover mushrooms completely so stir occasionally.) Marinate for 30 minutes at room temperature. Drain, reserving marinade.

In a medium-size skillet, melt butter. Stir in mushrooms. Sprinkle flour over mushrooms and stir gently until mushrooms are coated. Add water and 1 tablespoon reserved marinade. Simmer, uncovered, for 5 minutes. Serve hot.

4 to 6 servings

Skewered Vegetable Antipasto

2 large green peppers
8 large mushrooms
4 tablespoons olive oil
1 tablespoon wine vinegar
1 clove garlic, sliced
½ teaspoon dried basil
    pepper, to taste
2 medium-size onions, quartered
    fresh or dried oregano, to taste
2 large tomatoes, quartered
4 ounces provolone cheese, cut into 1-inch cubes

Cut each pepper into 8 chunks. Remove mushroom stems, leaving caps whole.

In a large skillet, heat 2 tablespoons oil. Add mushroom caps and sauté until lightly brown. Remove mushrooms and then sauté peppers until softened slightly.

Place mushrooms and peppers in a large bowl. Add remaining 2 tablespoons oil, vinegar, garlic, basil, and pepper. Marinate for several hours in refrigerator, stirring once or twice.

Place onions in a small saucepan with enough water to cover and simmer, covered, until tender.

Sprinkle oregano over tomatoes.

Using 4 metal skewers, pass each skewer through alternating chunks of green pepper, mushroom, onion, and tomato. Broil for about 5 minutes, or until hot and brown.

Serve with cheese cubes.

4 servings

Stuffed Mushrooms
with Ricotta, Spinach, and Dill

½ to ¾ pound fresh spinach or 1 package (10
    ounces) frozen chopped spinach
½ cup finely chopped onions
1 tablespoon olive oil
1 pound extra large mushrooms (about 15 to
    a pound)
1 cup ricotta cheese
½ cup grated Parmesan cheese (optional)
1 teaspoon dillweed
1 tablespoon soy sauce

freshly ground pepper, to taste
2 tablespoons grated Parmesan cheese

Steam fresh spinach over low heat in just the water that clings to the leaves after washing, about 5 minutes, or just until tender. If using frozen spinach, cook according to package directions. Drain and chop finely.

Sauté onions in oil slowly until soft.

Carefully remove mushroom stems from the caps and reserve. Then place caps in an oiled baking dish. Preheat oven to 400°F.

Finely chop reserved stems and add to sautéed onions. Sauté another 3 minutes and remove from heat. Stir in spinach, ricotta, the ½ cup Parmesan, if used, dillweed, soy sauce, and pepper. Spoon mixture into mushroom caps, piling high. Sprinkle each one with a little grated Parmesan and bake for 20 minutes, or until mushrooms release their juices and tops are lightly browned.

Makes about 15

Okra

Mixed Vegetables, Delta Style

1 tablespoon vegetable oil
2 tablespoons butter
1 green pepper, coarsely chopped
1 medium-size onion, chopped
1 clove garlic, minced
¾ cup Poultry Stock (page 110) or water
1 cup sliced okra
2 cups chopped peeled tomatoes
1½ cups lima beans
1 cup corn
½ teaspoon dried marjoram
¼ teaspoon crushed red pepper (optional)
1 tablespoon cornstarch, dissolved in ¼ cup water

Heat oil and butter in a large skillet. Add green peppers, onions, and garlic and sauté until soft. Stir in stock or water, okra, tomatoes, and lima beans and simmer, covered, until vegetables are almost tender, about 20 minutes. Add corn and cook for 5 minutes. Stir in marjoram, red pepper, if using, and cornstarch mixture, and cook, stirring constantly, until thickened. Simmer for 1 minute longer.

6 servings

Onions

Nut-Stuffed Baked Onions

6 large onions
2 tablespoons butter
1 cup cooked brown rice
1½ cups chopped pecans
2 eggs, beaten
¼ teaspoon pepper
6 pecan halves

Cut ½-inch slices off top end of onions and reserve. In a medium-size saucepan boil onions and tops in a small amount of water for 30 minutes. Drain and cool. Scoop out center of onions, leaving shells with ½-inch walls. Chop scooped-out onion centers and top ends.

Preheat oven to 350°F.

In a small skillet, melt butter. Add chopped onions and simmer until liquid evaporates. In a small bowl, mix cooked onions, rice, chopped pecans, eggs, and pepper. Stuff onions with the mixture and garnish with a pecan half. Place stuffed onions in an ungreased 9 × 13-inch baking pan. Pour ¼ inch of hot water into bottom of pan, cover with foil, and bake for 40 to 45 minutes. Any extra filling may be baked separately.

6 servings

Spicy Onion Fritters

1 cup whole wheat flour
½ teaspoon cayenne pepper
½ teaspoon baking soda
1 tablespoon lemon juice
½ cup water
1 clove garlic, finely chopped
⅔ cup chopped onions
vegetable oil, for deep frying

In a medium-size bowl mix flour, cayenne, baking soda, lemon juice, water, garlic, and onions.

Heat oil to 350 to 360°F.

Drop batter from a large spoon into the hot oil and cook for 2 to 3 minutes, or until golden. Drain well on paper towels. Keep warm until serving.

Makes about 1 dozen

Parsnips

Cinnamon Parsnips à l'Orange

1½ cups orange juice
1 tablespoon slivered orange rind
1 stick of cinnamon, broken into pieces
1 tablespoon honey
1 pound parsnips, peeled and cut into chunks
1 tablespoon whole wheat flour, mixed with 1 tablespoon butter
2 oranges, sliced

Combine juice, rind, cinnamon, honey, and parsnips in a medium-size saucepan. Cover tightly and cook until parsnips are tender, about 15 minutes. Remove parsnips and cinnamon with slotted spoon. Add butter and flour mixture to liquid in saucepan and cook rapidly until sauce has thickened. Pour sauce over parsnips and garnish with orange slices.

4 to 6 servings

Shredded Parsnips

2 cups shredded peeled parsnips
½ cup chopped green peppers
1 cup grated or finely chopped carrots
1 medium-size apple, cored and diced
2 tablespoons sour cream
3 tablespoons corn oil
1 tablespoon cider vinegar
soy sauce, to taste
1 small head leafy lettuce (optional)

Combine parsnips, peppers, carrots, and apples in a medium-size bowl.

Mix together sour cream, oil, vinegar, and soy sauce. Add to vegetables and toss. Serve over lettuce leaves, if desired.

6 servings

Peas

Steamed Peas Piquant

   2 cups fresh or frozen peas
   ¼ cup chopped scallions
   ¼ cup diced celery
   ¼ cup diced sweet red pepper
   4 large spinach leaves
   4 large romaine lettuce leaves
   1 tablespoon lemon juice, heated, or 1
      tablespoon grated lemon rind

Steam peas, scallions, celery, and red peppers for 3 to 4 minutes.

Arrange 1 spinach leaf and 1 lettuce leaf on each plate. Top with steamed pea mixture. Sprinkle with the warm lemon juice or grated rind and serve immediately.

   4 servings

Peas and Shrimp Salad

This is a fine salad that satisfies as a one-dish meal. A perfect contribution to a neighborhood picnic.

   ¼ cup yogurt
   ¼ cup mayonnaise
   1½ teaspoons minced onions
   1½ teaspoons minced fresh parsley
   ⅛ teaspoon white pepper
   ⅔ cup cooked whole wheat macaroni
   2 cups fresh or frozen peas
   ¼ cup diced carrots
   ½ cup cooked small shrimp
      lemon wedges

In a small bowl mix yogurt, mayonnaise, onions, parsley, and pepper. Chill, covered, for 1 hour.

In a large bowl gently toss macaroni, peas, carrots, and shrimp. Add chilled yogurt mixture and carefully mix. Chill for 1 hour. Serve garnished with lemon wedges.

   4 to 6 servings

Braised Peas and Lettuce, French Style

   2 leeks (white part only) or 1 medium-size
      onion, chopped

   2 tablespoons olive oil
   2 cups shredded iceberg lettuce
   2 pounds fresh peas or 2 packages (10 ounces
      each) frozen peas
   2 tablespoons water
   ¼ teaspoon pepper
   ⅛ teaspoon dried mint
   ½ teaspoon dried basil
   1 cup whole grain bread cubes
   ¼ cup butter

In a medium-size skillet sauté leeks or onions in oil until soft. Add lettuce, peas, and water. (If using frozen peas, omit water.) Cover and simmer until peas are tender, 10 to 15 minutes (5 minutes for frozen). Stir in pepper, mint, and basil and simmer for 1 minute longer.

In a small skillet sauté bread cubes in butter until toasted and golden, about 5 minutes. Serve peas topped with the croutons.

   6 servings

Peppers

Green Peppers and Pineapple en Brochette

   1 can (20 ounces) unsweetened pineapple
      chunks, drained with juice reserved
   3 large green peppers, cut into 2-inch squares
   3 tablespoons tomato paste
   3 tablespoons honey
   2 tablespoons cider vinegar
      dash of ground cloves
      dash of ground cinnamon
      dash of ground allspice

Place reserved pineapple juice into a medium-size saucepan and bring to a boil. Reduce heat, add green pepper squares, and simmer for about 5 minutes, or until crisp-tender. Remove pepper squares immediately with slotted spoon and thread alternately on 4 skewers with pineapple chunks.

Add remaining ingredients to juice in pan and heat. Place skewers on broiler tray and brush with heated sauce. Broil several inches from heat, turning and brushing frequently with sauce. Serve immediately.

   4 servings

Green Peppers Stuffed with Spinach

6 slices whole grain bread, torn into small pieces
¼ cup milk
4 large green peppers
1 pound spinach
2 tablespoons butter
1 medium-size onion, chopped
¼ teaspoon pepper
1 egg, beaten
3 ounces cream cheese
½ cup grated Parmesan cheese
½ cup grated Swiss cheese

Preheat oven to 350°F.

In a small bowl soak bread pieces in milk.

Parboil peppers in a small amount of water for 5 minutes. Cool and then cut into halves lengthwise and remove seeds.

Steam spinach over low heat in just the water that clings to the leaves after washing. When tender, drain spinach, then squeeze dry.

In a large skillet melt butter. Add onions and sauté until translucent. Remove from heat, add spinach, and mix.

In a medium-size bowl mix together bread and milk mixture, pepper, egg, and cheeses. Add spinach and onion mixture and mix well. Then stuff peppers with mixture and place in a buttered 8-inch-square pan and bake for 20 minutes.

4 servings

Roasted Peppers with Peanut Butter Sauce

6 large green peppers
3 tablespoons peanut butter
½ cup Poultry Stock (page 110) or Vegetable Stock (page 111)
1 teaspoon grated onions
1 teaspoon lemon juice

Preheat oven to 450°F.

Roast peppers on aluminum-foil-lined baking sheet until skins are blackened and peppers are tender, about 25 minutes. Cool. Slip off skins and discard stems and seeds. Cut peppers into 1-inch-wide strips and place in a serving dish.

Place a medium-size saucepan over medium-low heat, add peanut butter, and slowly whisk in stock.

Add grated onions and lemon juice and simmer for about 5 minutes, stirring constantly. Pour over pepper strips and mix. Serve warm.

6 servings

Pickled Green Peppers

4 large green peppers
¼ cup lemon juice or wine vinegar
¼ cup olive oil
freshly ground pepper, to taste

Broil green peppers, turning often, until they blister. Cool slightly and then peel. Remove cores and seeds. Cut peppers into ½-inch-wide strips and place in a medium-size bowl.

In another small bowl mix together lemon juice or wine vinegar, oil, and pepper. Pour over green peppers, cover, and refrigerate for at least 2 hours before serving.

6 to 8 servings

NOTE: Peppers will keep in the refrigerator, covered, for up to 1 month.

Potatoes

Hash-Brown Potatoes

3 medium-size potatoes
¼ cup minced onions
¼ teaspoon pepper
3 to 4 tablespoons butter

Place potatoes in a medium-size saucepan, and add enough water to cover. Bring water to a boil, lower heat, and simmer, covered, for about 15 minutes. Drain and cool.

Shred potatoes and mix with onions and pepper in a medium-size bowl.

Melt 3 tablespoons butter in a 10-inch skillet over low heat. Add potato mixture and spread into pan.

Cover and cook over low heat for 15 to 20 minutes, or until bottom is brown and slightly crusty. Cut with spatula into quarters and turn. Continue cooking until potatoes are fully cooked, adding additional tablespoon of butter, if necessary.

4 servings

Mashed Potatoes

5 or 6 medium-size potatoes
¼ cup butter
¼ teaspoon pepper
½ teaspoon soy sauce (optional)
1 cup warm milk

Peel and quarter potatoes. Place in a 6-quart saucepan, and add enough water to cover. Bring water to a boil, reduce heat, and simmer for 20 to 25 minutes, or until potatoes are tender. Drain.

Mash potatoes with a masher or electric mixer. Add butter, pepper, and soy sauce, if using. Gradually add warm milk until potatoes are light and fluffy.

6 to 8 servings

Scalloped Potatoes

5 medium-size potatoes, thinly sliced
¼ teaspoon pepper
¼ cup whole wheat flour
3 tablespoons butter
1 small onion, thinly sliced (optional)
2 cups milk, or more as needed

Preheat oven to 350°F.

Place ⅓ of the potatoes on bottom of a buttered 1½- or 2-quart ovenproof casserole. Sprinkle with ⅓ of the pepper and flour. Dot with 1 tablespoon butter. Top with onion slices, if desired. Repeat process until all potatoes, pepper, flour, butter, and onions are used.

Pour milk over top and bake, covered, for 60 to 70 minutes, or until potatoes are tender and casserole is bubbly.

6 servings

Twice-Baked Potatoes

4 medium-size to large baking potatoes
1 egg
2 tablespoons milk
2 tablespoons grated Parmesan cheese
1 tablespoon butter
1 tablespoon finely chopped onions
1 teaspoon crushed dried thyme
⅛ teaspoon pepper
paprika, to taste

Preheat oven to 400°F.
Bake potatoes for 45 to 60 minutes, or until they are easily pierced with a fork.

Cut about ¾ inch off top of each potato. Scoop out cooked potato and place in a large bowl. Reserve shells. Add egg, milk, cheese, butter, onions, thyme, and pepper and beat until smooth. Spoon the potato mixture back into the potato shells, sprinkle with paprika, and bake at 350°F for about 30 minutes, or until thoroughly heated.

4 servings

Lefse
(Potato Pancakes)

The traditional Norwegian lefse were wrapped around a piece of food such as a meatball. Today, however, many Norwegian-Americans butter their lefse and roll it up to eat as a type of bread.

3 large potatoes, cooked and mashed
½ teaspoon pepper
3 tablespoons butter, melted
3 tablespoons heavy cream
2 teaspoons mild honey
1½ cups whole wheat flour

While potatoes are still hot, add pepper, butter, cream, and honey. Gradually add flour. When cool to the touch, turn out onto a well-floured surface (dough will be sticky). Knead with floured hands for 5 minutes. Then chill for 1 hour.

Divide dough into 12 balls, about the size of golf balls. On a floured surface, roll each ball paper thin. Keep balls chilled while working. Drape and roll pancake over a rolling pin and carefully unroll onto a well-seasoned, medium-hot griddle. Cook until bottom is dappled brown. Turn carefully and cook reverse side. Keep warm until all are made. Serve with extra melted butter, cinnamon, and honey, if desired.

4 to 6 servings

Cheese and Nut-Stuffed Potatoes

These potatoes may be prepared ahead, several hours before serving–a plus for the busy host or hostess.

6 medium-size to large baking potatoes
½ cup butter
¾ cup hot milk
1 cup shredded Gruyère or Swiss cheese
¾ to 1 teaspoon freshly ground pepper

½ teaspoon grated nutmeg
⅓ cup finely chopped slivered almonds, toasted, or cashews, roasted
⅓ cup sliced almonds

Preheat oven to 400°F.

Bake potatoes for 45 to 60 minutes, or until they are easily pierced with a fork.

Cut about ¾ inch off top of each potato. Scoop out cooked potato and place in a large bowl. Reserve shells. Mash potatoes in bowl or press through a ricer. While hot, add butter and gradually beat in hot milk until potatoes are light and fluffy. Add cheese, pepper, nutmeg, and chopped almonds or cashews. Spoon mixture into reserved potato shells. Top with sliced almonds. (Potatoes may be refrigerated at this point.)

About 25 to 35 minutes before you plan to serve them, bake at 350°F until heated through and browned on top.

6 servings

Herb-Roasted Potatoes and Onions

6 large potatoes, quartered
6 medium-size onions, quartered
⅓ cup vegetable oil
½ teaspoon pepper
1 tablespoon dried parsley
1 teaspoon dried basil
½ teaspoon dried marjoram

Preheat oven to 375°F.

Place potatoes and onions in a shallow roasting pan. Pour oil over vegetables and sprinkle with pepper, parsley, basil, and marjoram. Stir vegetables to coat all sides with oil and seasonings and bake, uncovered, for about 1 hour, or until fork-tender, turning occasionally to keep from sticking to the bottom of the pan. Serve immediately.

6 servings

Cheese, Potato, and Carrot Casserole

3 to 4 medium-size potatoes, thinly sliced
2 large carrots, thinly sliced
4 ounces Swiss, Jarlsberg, or Gruyère cheese, shredded
pepper, to taste
¼ teaspoon ground nutmeg
1 tablespoon butter
¾ to 1 cup Poultry Stock (page 110) or Beef Stock (page 111)

Preheat oven to 350°F.

Place ⅓ of the potatoes and carrots into an 8-inch-square baking dish. Sprinkle with ⅓ of the cheese, pepper, and nutmeg. Dot with ⅓ of the butter. Arrange 2 more layers the same way.

Bring stock to a boil. Add enough hot stock to the baking dish to come up to the level of the vegetables.

Bake casserole for 1 hour, or until vegetables are tender and top is brown. Add more stock during baking if mixture seems too dry.

4 servings

Radishes

Sautéed Radishes and Cucumbers

3 medium-size cucumbers
1 large bunch red radishes
2 tablespoons cider vinegar
2 tablespoons butter
1 tablespoon lemon juice
sprigs fresh mint

Quarter cucumbers lengthwise, remove seeds, and cut into 1½-inch pieces. Place cucumbers in a medium-size bowl with whole radishes. Add vinegar and toss. Allow to stand for 30 minutes and then drain well.

Sauté cucumbers and radishes in butter for 5 minutes, or until tender but still very crisp. Sprinkle with lemon juice and serve immediately. Garnish with sprigs of fresh mint.

4 to 6 servings

Radishes Baked in Mustard Sauce

1 pound radishes, thinly sliced
½ cup vegetable oil
¼ cup lemon juice
1 teaspoon prepared mustard
¼ teaspoon dry mustard
¼ teaspoon pepper
1 teaspoon dried parsley

Preheat oven to 350°F.

Place radishes in a 1½-quart baking dish.

Beat together oil, lemon juice, prepared mustard, dry mustard, pepper, and parsley until well blended. Pour this mixture over radishes and bake, covered, for 30 minutes, or until radishes are pink and soft.

4 servings

Rutabagas

Golden Puree in Orange Cups

   3 pounds rutabagas, carrots, or sweet potatoes,
     peeled and sliced
   ¼ cup butter
    dash of ground nutmeg
   6 orange shell halves
   3 tablespoons maple syrup

Cook vegetables in a small amount of water until very tender, about 35 minutes. Drain well and puree in a blender. Beat in butter and season with nutmeg. Pile into orange shells. Drizzle with maple syrup and serve immediately.

   6 servings

Rutabaga Ring

  2½ tablespoons butter
   2 tablespoons honey
   3 tablespoons whole wheat flour
   1 cup milk
   4 egg yolks, lightly beaten
   2 cups cooked mashed rutabaga
   2 tablespoons chopped fresh parsley
   ¼ teaspoon pepper
   4 egg whites

Preheat oven to 375°F.

Melt butter in a 1½-quart saucepan over low heat. Stir in honey and then flour, stirring until smooth. Gradually stir in milk and cook, while stirring, until thickened and smooth. Remove from heat.

Place beaten egg yolks in a medium-size bowl. Gradually stir in white sauce. Add rutabaga, parsley, and pepper and mix.

Beat egg whites until stiff, but not dry. Fold in ¼ of the egg whites. Then gently fold in remaining egg whites. Turn into a well-buttered 1-quart ring mold and bake for 30 to 35 minutes.

Remove from oven, cover with a towel, and let rest for 5 minutes before unmolding onto a heated serving platter.

   4 to 6 servings

Squashes

Candied Butternut Squash

   1 large butternut squash
   ¼ cup butter, melted
   ¼ cup honey
   ½ cup ground walnuts
   ¼ teaspoon ground nutmeg

Preheat oven to 350°F.

Quarter squash lengthwise and scoop out seeds. Arrange pieces, cut-side down, in an 11 × 15-inch baking dish. Add ¼ inch of hot water to the pan and bake for 1 hour, or until tender. Cool and then peel squash.

Cut squash into ½-inch slices, and place in a 9 × 13-inch baking dish. Pour butter and honey over squash, sprinkle with walnuts and nutmeg, and bake for 20 minutes, or until squash is hot and topping is crusty.

   6 to 8 servings

Twice-Baked Squash

   2 medium-size baking potatoes
   1 medium-size acorn squash
   2 tablespoons butter
    white pepper, to taste
    milk
    ground nutmeg

Preheat oven to 400°F.

Bake potatoes for 20 minutes.

While potatoes are baking, cut squash into quarters and scoop out seeds. Place squash in oven with potatoes and bake until potatoes and squash are fork-tender, about 25 minutes.

Carefully scoop squash and potato from their shells and place in a large bowl. (Reserve squash shells.) Mash with butter and pepper, and add enough milk to make a smooth consistency. Fluff with a wire whisk or fork, and then gently spoon mixture into reserved squash shells. Garnish with nutmeg and bake for another 15 minutes. Serve in the shells.

   4 servings

Baked Acorn Squash with Nuts

3 medium-size acorn squashes
¼ cup plus 2 tablespoons butter
½ teaspoon ground cinnamon
½ teaspoon ground ginger
⅓ cup honey or maple syrup
⅓ cup apple cider
1 cup chopped nuts (combination of pecans,
    walnuts, and hazelnuts or almonds)

Preheat oven to 375°F.

Cut squashes in half lengthwise and scoop out seeds. Arrange squashes, cut-side down, in an 11 × 15-inch shallow baking pan. Add ¼ inch of hot water to the pan and bake squashes for 30 minutes.

While squashes bake, prepare nut filling. Melt butter in a small saucepan. Add cinnamon, ginger, honey or maple syrup, and cider. Bring to a boil, lower heat, and simmer, uncovered, for 4 to 5 minutes. Then stir in nuts.

Remove squashes from oven. Pour out liquid from baking pan and turn squashes cut-side up. Spoon nut mixture into cavities and bake for 20 minutes more, basting occasionally with sauce.

6 servings

Batter-Sautéed Summer Squash

4 eggs
2 tablespoons wheat germ
¼ cup whole wheat flour
¼ teaspoon pepper
    vegetable oil, for frying
2 medium-size summer squashes, cut into
    ½-inch slices

Mix together eggs, wheat germ, flour, and pepper until smooth.

In a large skillet, heat enough oil to coat the pan. Dip squash slices into batter and sauté in the hot oil on both sides until golden brown and tender inside. If batter seems too thick, add 1 to 2 teaspoons water. Add more oil to pan, if needed. Keep squash warm until all slices are cooked.

4 servings

Baked Stuffed Summer Squash

1¼ cups whole grain bread crumbs
2 tablespoons wheat germ
¼ teaspoon ground thyme
1 tablespoon minced fresh parsley or ½
    teaspoon dried parsley
⅛ teaspoon pepper
½ small onion, minced
½ medium-size green pepper, finely chopped
2 tablespoons butter, melted
1 egg, beaten
⅓ to ½ cup Beef Stock (page 110)
1 large summer squash

Preheat oven to 350°F.

In a medium-size bowl, mix bread crumbs, wheat germ, thyme, parsley, pepper, onions, and green peppers. Add butter and toss to mix. Add egg and toss to mix again. Stir in enough stock to just moisten mixture.

Cut summer squash in half lengthwise and scoop out seeds. Stuff squash with bread mixture and place in an 11 × 15-inch shallow baking pan. Add ½-inch of hot water to the pan and place a piece of aluminum foil loosely over the top.

Bake squash for 45 minutes. Add more water to the pan as necessary. Remove foil and bake for 15 minutes longer. Squash should be tender when pierced with the tip of a sharp knife.

4 servings

Pattypan Squash with Sesame Seeds

1 medium-size pattypan squash, cubed
1 tablespoon chopped fresh chives
¼ cup butter, browned
1 tablespoon sesame seeds, toasted

Cook squash in a small amount of water or steam until tender, about 35 minutes. Drain.

Place squash in a serving dish, add chives and butter, and toss. Garnish with sesame seeds before serving.

4 servings

Spaghetti Squash Special

1 large spaghetti squash
1 pound mozzarella cheese, sliced
1 to 1½ cups tomato sauce
½ cup grated Parmesan cheese

Place whole squash in a large pot with enough water to cover. Bring to a boil and then simmer, covered, for 30 minutes, or until skin is tender. Remove from water and allow to cool until squash can be handled. Preheat oven to 350°F.

Cut squash in half and remove seeds. Using a fork, scrape pulp from shell and pull apart into spaghettilike strands. Arrange squash, mozzarella cheese, and sauce in layers in a buttered ovenproof casserole. Sprinkle with Parmesan, and bake for 30 minutes. Serve hot.

6 servings

Spaghetti Squash with Vegetarian Sauce

1 large spaghetti squash

Sauce
2 teaspoons vegetable oil
1 large stalk celery, finely minced
1 large carrot, grated
1 clove garlic, pressed
1 teaspoon dried basil
1 teaspoon dried oregano
1½ cups pureed tomatoes
¼ cup grated Parmesan cheese

Place whole squash in a large pot with enough water to cover. Bring to a boil and then simmer, covered, for 30 minutes, or until skin is tender. Remove from water and allow to cool until squash can be handled.

Cut squash in half and remove seeds. Using a fork, scrape pulp from shell and pull apart into spaghettilike strands. Keep warm until serving time. While squash is cooking, prepare the sauce.

To make the sauce: Place oil in a deep saucepan and heat over medium temperature. Add celery and carrots and allow steam to form. Cover vegetables tightly, do not stir, and allow to steam in their own juices until tender, about 20 minutes. Add seasonings and cook for 5 minutes. Stir in tomato puree and cheese and cook, uncovered, until thickened, about 15 minutes.

To serve, place drained squash on large, deep platter. Top with vegetable sauce and sprinkle with grated Parmesan.

4 to 6 servings

Zucchini-Beef Bake

3 medium-size zucchini, sliced
¼ cup olive oil
1 pound lean ground beef
1 medium-size onion, chopped
3 eggs
1 tablespoon chopped fresh parsley
⅛ teaspoon garlic powder
pepper, to taste
1 cup whole grain bread crumbs
2 cups milk
2 tablespoons cornstarch
1 cup shredded mild cheddar cheese

In a large skillet, lightly brown zucchini slices in oil. Remove from pan and set aside.

In the same skillet, brown beef and onions. Drain off fat and allow beef to cool.

Beat together eggs, parsley, garlic powder, and pepper. Combine egg mixture, bread crumbs, and beef. Preheat oven to 350°F.

Heat 1¾ cups milk in a medium-size saucepan. Dissolve cornstarch in remaining ¼ cup cold milk. Add this mixture to the hot milk, stirring constantly, and cook until mixture thickens and bubbles. Add cheese and cook, stirring, until it is just melted.

Layer sauce, zucchini, and beef in a 2-quart ovenproof casserole, beginning and ending with the sauce. Bake, covered, for 30 minutes.

4 servings

Zucchini Italiano

1 teaspoon minced fresh garlic
¼ cup vegetable oil
1 can (28 ounces) Italian-style tomatoes, drained
¼ cup tomato paste
¼ teaspoon pepper
1 teaspoon dried oregano
2 tablespoons minced fresh parsley
3 medium-size zucchini, sliced
8 ounces mozzarella cheese, coarsely grated

In a medium-size skillet, sauté garlic in oil until translucent. Add tomatoes, tomato paste, pepper, oregano, and parsley, and simmer, uncovered, for 20 minutes, or until thickened. Stir occasionally.

Preheat oven to 350°F.

Pat zucchini slices dry. Arrange slices in an oiled jelly-roll pan. Top with sauce, sprinkle with cheese, and bake for 30 minutes, or until zucchini is just tender.

4 servings

Zucchini Pancakes

2 cups coarsely grated zucchini
½ medium-size onion, grated
1 cup grated Jarlsberg or Gruyère cheese
½ cup whole wheat flour
¼ teaspoon pepper
2 eggs

In a medium-size bowl, mix all ingredients together until well blended. Spoon batter onto a lightly oiled medium-hot griddle, and cook until cakes are brown on both sides, 5 to 10 minutes.

Makes about 10

Sweet Potatoes

Most cooks use sweet potatoes and yams interchangeably and with predictable success. Yams are generally the larger of the two and the more fibrous.

Sweet Potato Custard Pie

6 medium-size sweet potatoes
    pastry for 1 Basic Rolled Piecrust (page 718)
2 eggs, beaten
½ cup milk
1 cup grated cheddar cheese
1 tablespoon whole wheat flour
1 tablespoon soy sauce
⅛ teaspoon ground ginger
    freshly ground pepper, to taste

Place potatoes in a 6-quart saucepan, and add enough water to cover. Bring water to a boil, lower heat, and simmer, covered, for 20 to 30 minutes, or until fork-tender. Cool in a colander and then peel and mash with a fork.

While potatoes are cooking, roll out pastry and line a 9-inch pie plate. Set aside.

Preheat oven to 375°F.

Combine eggs and milk and add to sweet potatoes, mixing well. Mix cheese with flour and stir into sweet potato mixture. Season with soy sauce, ginger, and pepper. Spread into piecrust and bake for 45 to 50 minutes, or until knife comes out clean when inserted in the center. Serve hot.

6 to 8 servings

Sweet Potato Munchies

These crunchy slices may be served as a side dish or as an afternoon or late-evening snack.

sweet potatoes
vegetable oil
cheddar cheese, sliced

Peel and slice sweet potatoes crosswise. Sauté in a small amount of oil and drain quickly on paper towels. While still hot, place a slice of cheddar cheese between 2 slices of sweet potato. (Hot potato slices melt cheese.)

Sweet Potato Pone

4 cups peeled and grated sweet potatoes
1½ cups molasses
2 tablespoons mild honey
½ cup butter, melted
1 cup light cream
1 teaspoon ground cinnamon
¼ cup raisins
1 teaspoon ground ginger or grated peeled
    ginger root
    grated rind of 1 orange
    grated rind of 1 lemon
2 tablespoons coarsely chopped peanuts or
    pecans
1 cup heavy cream, whipped

Preheat oven to 325°F.

In a large bowl, mix sweet potatoes with molasses, honey, butter, cream, cinnamon, raisins, ginger, and grated rinds. Turn out into a well-buttered 1½-quart baking dish and bake for 1 hour.

Sprinkle with chopped nuts and return to oven for 15 to 20 minutes, or until top is crusty and brown. Serve warm with whipped cream.

4 servings

Jamaican Sweet Potatoes

    5 small sweet potatoes
    3 tablespoons butter
    ¾ teaspoon curry powder
    ⅔ cup walnuts, pecans, or cashews
    ¼ cup chopped onions
    ¼ teaspoon grated lime rind
    1 tablespoon lime juice
    ½ cup apple cider or Poultry Stock (page 110)

In a medium-size saucepan cook sweet potatoes in enough boiling water to cover until just tender, about 30 minutes. Drain. When cool enough to handle, remove jackets.

While potatoes cook, heat 1 tablespoon butter with curry in a large skillet. Add nuts and sauté for 6 to 8 minutes. Remove nuts with a slotted spoon and reserve.

Add remaining butter to skillet and sauté onions until soft. Stir in lime rind, lime juice, and cider or stock.

Cut potatoes in half lengthwise and then into ¾-inch slices. Add to skillet, cover, and cook over low heat for 5 minutes. Stir in reserved nuts.

    6 servings

Candied Sweet Potatoes

    4 medium-size sweet potatoes, peeled and sliced
    4 small tart apples, quartered
    ½ cup raisins
    2 tablespoons honey
    3 tablespoons pineapple juice
    3 tablespoons butter, melted

Preheat oven to 350°F.

Arrange potatoes, apples, and raisins in alternate layers in a buttered 2-quart ovenproof casserole.

Mix together honey, juice, and butter. Pour over vegetable and fruit mixture, cover, and bake for 30 minutes. Serve hot.

    6 to 8 servings

Tomatoes

Fresh Tomato and Mushroom Flan

A flan in Spain could be a quiche in France—both custard-based dishes. This one is a no-meat main course attraction.

    pastry for 1 Basic Rolled Piecrust (page 718)
    3 medium-size tomatoes, peeled
    2 tablespoons butter
    1 small onion, minced
    1 cup sliced mushrooms plus 1 whole mushroom
    ¼ teaspoon dried savory
    2 large eggs, beaten
    2 tablespoons light cream
    2 tablespoons grated Gruyère cheese

Preheat oven to 425°F.

Roll out pastry and line a 7-inch flan pan. Prick dough generously with a fork. Bake crust for 10 minutes.

While piecrust is baking, cut 1 tomato into 8 wedges and set aside. Chop remaining tomatoes finely.

Melt butter in a large skillet. Add onions and sauté until tender. Add sliced mushrooms and sauté lightly. Remove from heat. Stir in chopped tomatoes and savory. Add eggs and cream, and blend well. Pour mixture into prebaked shell, and top with cheese. Reduce oven temperature to 350°F and bake for 30 minutes.

Remove flan from oven and arrange reserved tomato wedges around edge and whole mushroom in center. Bake for 10 minutes longer. Cool slightly before serving.

    4 servings

Hoosier Fried Green Tomatoes

    1 cup whole wheat flour or cornmeal
    1½ teaspoons pepper
    6 large green tomatoes, cut into ½-inch slices
    ¼ cup plus 2 tablespoons butter
    ½ cup heavy cream
    1 tablespoon minced fresh basil or ¼ teaspoon
        dried basil

Combine flour or cornmeal and pepper. Dip tomato slices into flour mixture.

Melt butter in a large heavy skillet. When hot, add tomato slices, one layer at a time. Reduce heat, and cook slowly until brown on one side. Turn carefully and cook until inside is tender and second side is brown. Remove to a warm serving dish.

Add cream to pan drippings and stir. Cook, stirring constantly, until slightly thickened. Pour over tomatoes, sprinkle with basil, and serve.

4 to 6 servings

Mexican Tomatoes

    8 medium-size tomatoes, peeled
    1 scallion, sliced
    1 clove garlic, pressed
    1 tablespoon fresh chopped coriander (optional)
    1 teaspoon chopped fresh basil
    1 tablespoon chopped fresh parsley
    2 tablespoons red wine vinegar
      dash of cayenne pepper, or to taste

Push 2 tomatoes through a sieve or process in a blender or food processor and strain. Place remaining tomatoes in a large glass or ceramic bowl. In a small bowl, combine scallions, garlic, coriander, if used, basil, parsley, vinegar, and cayenne with sieved tomato puree. Blend well, and pour over tomatoes in bowl. Cover and allow to marinate in refrigerator for several hours. Serve cool or at room temperature.

4 to 6 servings

Stewed Tomatoes

    6 large tomatoes, peeled
    2 tablespoons minced onions
    2 tablespoons minced green peppers
    2 tablespoons butter or vegetable oil
    ½ teaspoon honey

Cut tomatoes into wedges.

In a medium saucepan, sauté onions and green peppers in butter or oil until slightly soft. Add tomatoes and honey, cover, and cook over medium heat for 10 to 20 minutes.

4 to 6 servings

Stuffed Tomatoes

    ½ tablespoon butter
    1 small onion, minced
    ⅔ cup uncooked brown rice, bulgur, or barley
    ⅔ cup Poultry Stock (page 110)
    1 tablespoon lemon juice
    ¼ cup minced fresh parsley
    4 large tomatoes
    ½ cup shredded cheddar or Swiss cheese
    ¼ cup coarsely chopped walnuts

Melt butter in a medium-size skillet. Add onions and sauté until golden. Stir in rice, bulgur, or barley, stock, and lemon juice. Bring mixture to a boil, cover skillet, and cook for 45 minutes, or until grain is tender and stock has been absorbed. Remove from heat, fluff mixture with a fork, and stir in parsley.

Remove loose pulp from center of tomatoes. Stuff tomatoes with grain mixture, top with cheese, and garnish with walnuts. Place under broiler until cheese is melted and bubbly. Serve hot.

4 servings

Turnips

Carrots and Turnips in Vinegar Sauce

    4 cups thinly sliced peeled turnips
    1 cup thinly sliced carrots
    1 teaspoon soy sauce
    ½ cup vinegar
    1 tablespoon honey
    ½ to 1 teaspoon freshly grated peeled ginger
        root (optional)

Place turnips and carrots in a large bowl.

In a small jar, mix soy sauce, vinegar, and honey and pour over vegetables. Mix thoroughly and chill. Before serving, add ginger, if desired.

6 servings

Spiced Turnip with Apple Rings

4 apples
1 medium-size turnip, peeled and diced
¾ cup water
4 tablespoons butter
¼ teaspoon pepper
¼ teaspoon ground nutmeg
½ teaspoon ground cinnamon

Peel and dice 2 apples. Combine turnip and diced apples in a medium-size saucepan. Add water and simmer, covered, until turnip and apples are tender enough to mash, about 25 minutes. Drain and mash with 2 tablespoons butter, pepper, and nutmeg.

Slice remaining apples into rings. (Do not peel.) Sauté apple rings in remaining 2 tablespoons butter until they are tender and lightly browned on both sides. Sprinkle rings with cinnamon.

To serve, mound mashed turnip and apples in a serving dish and garnish with overlapping apple rings.

6 servings

Turnip-Cheese Bake

2 cups diced peeled turnips
1 cup cottage cheese
1 cup yogurt or buttermilk
1 cup grated cheddar cheese
1 tablespoon minced fresh parsley
½ cup chopped onions
2 eggs, beaten
1 clove garlic, minced
1 tablespoon fresh marjoram

Cook turnips in a small amount of water for 20 to 30 minutes, or until tender. Drain.

Preheat oven to 350°F.

Combine cottage cheese, yogurt or buttermilk, cheddar, parsley, onions, eggs, garlic, and marjoram. Add turnips and mix together.

Pour mixture into a buttered baking dish and bake, covered, for 40 minutes.

4 to 6 servings

Turnips with Apples en Casserole

4 to 6 cups finely chopped peeled turnips
1 cup minced apples
2 tablespoons dried currants
¼ cup chopped dates
2 tablespoons crumbled whole grain bread crumbs
¼ teaspoon ground cinnamon
pinch of ground mace
pinch of ground ginger
1 tablespoon butter

Preheat oven to 350°F.

Mix turnips, apples, currants, and dates together. Place in a 1½-quart buttered ovenproof casserole. Cover and bake for 45 to 60 minutes, or until tender. Uncover. Combine bread crumbs, cinnamon, mace, ginger, and butter and then sprinkle over top of casserole. Bake, uncovered, for 15 minutes longer.

4 to 6 servings

Sea Vegetables

The cultures of the Far East have long honored sea vegetables as a source of delicious, readily available nourishment. Cooks there commonly use them to enfold rice or fish, flavor soup, or accompany other vegetables. But sea vegetables are not confined to the cuisines of China and Japan. They appear in the native diets of regions throughout the world where sea vegetables are easily harvested right from the ocean. The beautiful purple seaweed *Porphyra* (also called nori, laver, or amanori) grows as abundantly off the rocky European shores as it does off the Japanese coast. In parts of France and Britain, cooks boil it for hours to get a dark-brown, viscous mass called marine sauce, or "sloke," which they serve with lemon juice or vinegar. The Welsh make a bread out of seaweed, and the English, Irish, and French all make use of its gelatinous quality for cooking. Hawaiian dishes frequently include seaweed.

Dulse has long been popular in parts of New England where it is most commonly harvested, but many other types of seaweed are finding their way into American cuisine. Westerners find that the taste and texture of sea vegetables differ considerably from the foods most commonly used in this part of the world. But anyone who likes the flavor of other foods from the sea is likely to enjoy sea vegetables.

The nutritional treasures of seaweed, including a small amount of protein and 1 to 9 percent fat, enhance its value as a food source. Most vitamins are also present in sea vegetables in varying proportions. The greatest nutritional attribute that sea vegetables have is their minerals. They usually contain iodine in abundance and have traces of many other minerals, including the interdependent elements calcium, phosphorus, and magnesium. Like other plants, sea plants contain carbohydrates in the form of starches and sugars.

Popular Types of Sea Vegetables

The bulk of the edible sea vegetables sold commercially in the United States comes from Japan. They are packaged in dried form and sold under generic Japanese names—*nori* or *laver, kombu, hijiki, wakame, arame.* Once you have some experience with the different sea vegetables, their broad differences in taste will soon become apparent. Though the flavors vary considerably, you can successfully substitute one type of seaweed for another in most recipes.

Nori, which grows at the water's edge as a thin leaf about a foot long, tastes like briny corn when fresh. A popular Japanese dish called sushi consists of vinegar-rice wrapped in nori.

Kombu, like nori, may be used as a wrapping for other foods—rice, tofu, vegetables, ground meat, or seafood.

Hijiki has a mild, almost beany flavor that blends well with sharper-tasting foods, but it is

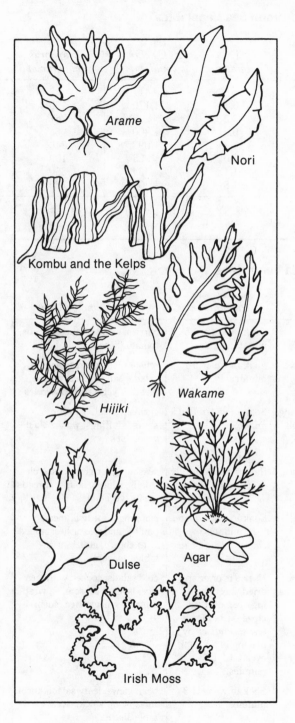

Arame

Nori

Kombu and the Kelps

Hijiki

Wakame

Dulse

Agar

Irish Moss

often served alone with a sprinkling of vinegar or lemon juice. Like all sea vegetables, its low-calorie content makes *hijiki* a perfect snack food for diet-conscious persons.

Wakame, a sea vegetable somewhat akin to leafy land vegetables, makes a tasty cold salad. Its nutritional goodness includes a good dose of the mineral calcium.

Arame is closely related to *wakame* and can be used in the same way, or its rich seafood flavoring can make a welcome addition to spicy sauces and condiments as well as to soups and salads.

Dulse is the most prolific of edible American seaweeds. Its thin fronds resemble a waving hand. When freshened (reconstituted from the dried state by soaking in water), it is often used as one would use spinach. Its flavor also enhances relishes and salad dressings.

Kelp, which flourishes on the Pacific coast, is the seaweed most revered by nutritionists—due largely to its abundant stores of calcium and iodine. Its high sodium content, however, warrants its use in moderation. Granular kelp can improve the food value of soups, sauces, and spreads, as well as thicken and flavor these mixtures. Kelp powder is most often used as an alternative to table salt. If you decide to use it in this way, use about one-half as much kelp as you would table salt.

Sea Gelatin

Agar and *Irish moss* are two sea vegetables famed for their jelling qualities. The use of agar as a jelly in Japan dates back to the 16th century. Kanten, agar, and agar-agar are names used interchangeably on packaging and in recipes calling for this natural gelatin.

Irish moss, or sea moss, yields the extract carrageenin, named after the Irish town Carragheen. Irish moss is used interchangeably with agar, but unlike agar, it will not gel and retain

Nutrients in Some Common Sea Vegetables

Sea Vegetable—Dried (100 grams)	Calories	Protein (grams)	Fat (grams)	Calcium (milligrams)	Phosphorus (milligrams)
Agar	323	6.2	---	417	52
Arame	235	6.0	0.1	1,170	150
Dulse	---	20	3.2	296	267
Hijiki	173	4.5	0.8	1,400	56
Kelp	---	---	1.1	1,093	240
Kombu	219	5.6	1.0	955	199
Nori (laver)	235	22.2	1.1	434	350
Wakame	276	12.7	1.5	1,300	260

Guide to Sea Vegetables

Sea Vegetable	Primary Sources	Appearance (dried form)	Preparation	Most Common Uses
Arame	southern coastal regions of Japan	charcoal black, wavy fronds	Soak in water 3-5 minutes.	curries, salads, sauces, soups, tomato dishes
Dulse	Atlantic and Pacific coastal waters	thin, glove-shaped fronds	Soak in water 5-7 minutes.	relishes, salad dressings, salads, sandwiches; grain, meat, or vegetable casseroles
Hijiki	rocky, low waters of northern and southern coasts of Japan	short, thin, curling strands; blackish color	Soak in water 12-15 minutes.	garnishes, salads, soups, stews, stuffings, wok-cooked vegetables
Kelp	Pacific coast from Mexico to Canada	powdered, granular, or tablet form	Sun or mechanically dry; then pulverized.	seasoning for grain casseroles, salads, sauces, soups, spreads, meats, vegetables
Kombu	Pacific coastal waters	strands or wide, flat sheets	Soak in warm water 7-10 minutes.	condiment for fish, meat, poultry, and rice dishes; stuffed with cheese, grains, vegetables; toasted
Nori (laver)	rocky coastal waters of southernmost islands of Japan and both coasts of United States	ruffled-fan-shaped, thin, parchmentlike sheets	Use as is or crisp dried sheets by holding open over hot stove burner for a few seconds or by placing in a 250°F oven for 2 to 3 minutes.	cold salads; cooked with meat, rice; layered casseroles; wrapping for vinegar-rice (sushi)
Wakame	waters near southernmost islands of Japan	olive green to brownish strands	Soak in water 2-3 minutes.	bean stews, leafy salads, meat, miso, soup stock, rice, vegetable dishes

248

Iron (milligrams)	Sodium (milligrams)	Potassium (milligrams)	Thiamine (B_1) (milligrams)	Riboflavin (B_2) (milligrams)	Vitamin C (milligrams)	Vitamin A (international units)
21	102	1,125	---	---	---	---
12	---	---	0.02	0.20	---	---
150	2,100	8,060	0.63	0.50	24	---
29	---	---	0.01	0.02	---	555
---	3,007	5,273	---	---	---	---
11.2	2,500	---	0.07	0.26	11	430
28.3	1,294	3,503	0.24	1.34	10	960
---	1,100	---	0.01	0.02	15	140

its firmness without refrigeration. Like the other sea vegetables, agar and Irish moss add nutrition to food as well as bulk that appeases the appetite, yet they contain fewer calories than does animal gelatin. Agar and Irish moss can be used to make bouillons, aspics, vegetable salads and dessert molds (see Molded Salads, page 160), and sauces and jellies.

Cooking with Sea Vegetables

Sea vegetables in dry and fresh form can be incorporated into your daily diet easily. Fresh or freshened, if they have been dried, their uses are as limitless as those of land vegetables. Like many vegetables they require no special cooking and may be eaten raw. Cooking helps their pungent flavors and aromas mingle with those of the other ingredients. Also, like land vegetables, they lend themselves to preparations with many types of foods. Dishes in just about every category of food can be made more distinctive with sea vegetables. Grains, pasta, and legumes are all enlivened in a tasty, nutritious way when a sea vegetable is added to the recipe; the same is true of meat, fish, and poultry. Nuts and seeds also mix well with sea vegetables and are especially good toasted together.

Prepare sea vegetables just as you do other vegetables. They may be sautéed, fried, or parboiled, and then seasoned and spiced to be served alone or added to other dishes. Try lightly sprinkling sea vegetables with sesame oil or safflower oil and toasting them on a baking sheet in a moderate oven (325 to 350°F) for 5 to 7 minutes, or until crispy. Add the toasted vegetables to salads or other cooked vegetables for another dimension in flavor. Or you may serve the toasted sea vegetables as is, lightly seasoned, or with a dip. Grinding the crisped vegetables in a blender or with a mortar and pestle yields a powder that may then be used as a tangy seasoning for many foods.

Storing Sea Vegetables

If you are able to harvest sea vegetables directly from their source, you need only rinse them well in fresh water; then drain and prepare them for a meal. Like other fresh vegetables, fresh sea plants should be stored in the refrigerator. Once dried, they may be stored in plastic bags or containers, or in glass jars, and kept in a cool, dry place (heat and moisture may affect their vitamin C content) for up to two years. Cooked sea vegetables should be stored in glass or ceramic containers since plastic containers may affect the taste.

Drying Fresh Sea Vegetables

Freshly foraged sea vegetables may be dried to preserve them for future use. Simply rinse them well in fresh water before laying them on a clean cloth in the sun. (Setting them to dry on paper, plastic, or rubber may affect their flavor.) Turn the plants over periodically—at least every 45 to 50 minutes, more often if possible—so they dry evenly. The drying process takes about 12 hours. When the plants are dried, they may be used immediately or stored for future use.

Freshening Dried Sea Vegetables

Most types of sea vegetables mentioned here are available in dried form at natural foods stores or in shops where oriental food products are sold.

To freshen dried sea vegetables, immerse them in a bath of water—about four to five times their dried volume. They will increase their volume two to five times as they freshen. The water used to freshen them may be at room temperature, but for the firmer sea plants, such as kombu and *hijiki,* warmer water will do the job faster. Once freshened, sea vegetables may be refrigerated, either drained or in the soak water, for up to a week. The soak water may be used to make soup or stock or to cook other vegetables.

Sometimes, even after a long soaking, part of the sea vegetable remains tough. Just trim this firm midrib away and add it to soups or stocks for flavoring.

When cooking sea vegetables, choose cookware that is of flameproof enamel or ceramic. Woks and heavy iron skillets are also suitable for preparing them.

Arame

Nippy *Arame* Sandwich

½ cup loosely packed dried *arame*
1½ cups water
1 tablespoon soy sauce
1 tablespoon sesame oil
mayonnaise
2 slices sourdough, whole wheat, or rye bread
lemon juice

Soak *arame* in the water for 15 minutes. Lift out with a slotted spoon and place in a small saucepan. Allow soaking water to settle, then pour over *arame,* discarding the gritty residue. Simmer, covered, for 25 minutes. Add soy sauce and oil and simmer, uncovered, for another 5 minutes. Cool.

Spread mayonnaise thinly on both slices of bread. Place 2 or 3 tablespoons *arame* on 1 side of 1 slice, sprinkle with lemon juice, and close up sandwich. Serve with vegetable soup and/or salad.

Makes 1

Arame with Tempeh

Fragrant with garlic and ginger, this combination is a filling dinner entree, accompanied with cooked brown rice.

2¼ cups water
½ cup soy sauce
¼ cup lemon juice
1 tablespoon minced garlic
1 tablespoon grated peeled ginger root
8 ounces tempeh, cut into 12 pieces
½ cup loosely packed dried *arame*
2 to 3 tablespoons vegetable oil
1 tablespoon sesame oil
1 medium-size onion, chopped
1 carrot, diced

In a medium-size bowl combine ¼ cup water, soy sauce, lemon juice, garlic, and ginger. Add tempeh and marinate for 1 to 5 hours, turning pieces over once.

Soak *arame* in 2 cups water for 20 minutes.

Heat vegetable oil in a medium-size skillet. Then remove tempeh, reserving marinade, and sauté in hot oil. Drain on paper towels.

In a separate skillet heat sesame oil and sauté onions and carrots for 5 to 7 minutes, or until onions are soft. Lift *arame* from soaking water with a slotted spoon and add to vegetables. Allow soaking water to settle, then add ¼ cup to vegetable mixture. Stir in tempeh and ¼ cup of the reserved marinade and mix well. Cook, covered, over low heat, for 20 minutes.

4 to 6 servings

Steamed Sesame String Beans

The tofu and arame *transform this favorite into an entirely new taste experience.*

> ¾ pound fresh string beans, cut into julienne strips (about 2 cups)
> 8 ounces soft tofu, drained
> 1 to 2 tablespoons soy sauce
> ½ cup water
> 3 tablespoons loosely packed dried *arame*
> ¼ cup sesame seeds, toasted

Place string beans in a steamer basket.

In a small bowl or on a plate, mash tofu and soy sauce with a fork until well mixed and crumbly. Sprinkle over beans.

Soak *arame* in ½ cup water for 15 minutes. Drain *arame,* chop coarsely, and sprinkle over tofu. Steam all for 15 minutes. Transfer to a bowl.

Grind sesame seeds using a mortar and pestle or a blender. Add to bean mixture, and mix well.

Serve as an accompaniment to grains and other vegetables.

4 to 6 servings

Zucchini, *Arame,* and Mushroom Stir-Fry

Serve this colorful mixture as a side dish with other oriental preparations.

> ¼ cup loosely packed dried *arame*
> 1 cup water
> 1 tablespoon sesame oil
> 1 sweet red pepper, cut into ½-inch pieces
> ½ pound mushrooms, sliced
> 2 small zucchini (about 1 pound), sliced
> 1 large clove garlic, minced
> 2 tablespoons soy sauce

Soak *arame* in water for 15 to 20 minutes.

Heat oil in a large skillet. Add pepper, stir a few seconds, and then add mushrooms. Cook over medium-high heat, stirring often, until mushrooms start to shrink and release liquid. Pour off about 1½ to 2 tablespoons mushroom liquid into a small bowl or cup. Return vegetables to heat, add zucchini, and cook over high heat for 3 to 4 minutes, stirring continuously. Add garlic.

Drain *arame,* coarsely chop, and add to skillet. Add soy sauce to mushroom water and sprinkle over vegetables. Stir well and cook, covered, over low heat for 4 minutes. Remove cover, cook for another 3 to 4 minutes, or until some of the liquid evaporates.

4 to 6 servings

Dulse

Oat-Dulse Scones

These savory scones with a seaside character have a chewy and dense texture that makes them a filling snack item or accompaniment to a light luncheon.

> 1 cup loosely packed dried dulse
> 2½ cups rolled oats
> 1 cup whole wheat flour
> 1 cup chopped onions
> 2 teaspoons dried thyme
> ¼ cup corn oil
> ¾ cup water

Soak dulse in enough water to cover for 10 to 15 minutes. Rinse, drain, and chop into small bits.

Combine dulse and remaining ingredients in a large bowl and mix well. The result should look like thick tuna salad.

Preheat oven to 325°F. Shape into patties about 3 inches in diameter and ½ inch in height. Place on oiled baking sheet and bake for about 25 minutes.

Makes 1 dozen

Roasted Pumpkin Seeds with Dulse

An unusual flavoring is added to a favorite snack food. These seeds may also be mixed into an appetizer spread.

> ½ teaspoon corn or sesame oil
> 1 cup pumpkin seeds
> ½ teaspoon powdered dulse

Place oil and seeds in a 1-quart stainless steel saucepan. Place pan over medium-high heat and, stirring constantly, roast seeds for about 8 minutes, or until they puff up slightly and begin to change color. Sprinkle dulse over seeds and mix. Remove from heat. Cool before serving.

Yields 1 cup

NOTE: Use only a metal saucepan since the high heat and lack of water may cause enameled saucepans to crack.

Hijiki

Ginger-Dressed Seaweed Salad

> ½ cup crumbled dried *hijiki* or *arame*
> 2 cups water
> 2 tablespoons soy sauce
> ¼ cup rice vinegar
> 1 head Boston lettuce, torn into bite-size pieces
> ½ bunch of watercress
> 2 red radishes, sliced
> 1 cup alfalfa sprouts
> Ginger Dressing (see below)

Soak *hijiki* or *arame* in the water for 20 minutes. Lift out with a slotted spoon and place in a small saucepan. Allow soaking water to settle, then pour 1 cup soaking water over *hijiki* or *arame,* discarding the gritty residue. Add soy sauce and vinegar, and simmer, covered, for 15 minutes. Drain and cool.

Mix lettuce and watercress in a large salad bowl with radishes and sprouts. Chop the *hijiki* or *arame* coarsely a few times and sprinkle over top of salad. Serve with the dressing.

4 to 6 servings

Ginger Dressing

> ¼ cup tahini (sesame butter)
> 1 tablespoon soy sauce

> 3 tablespoons water
> 2 tablespoons lemon juice
> 1 teaspoon grated peeled ginger root
> 1 clove garlic, minced

Mix tahini and soy sauce until smooth. Then beat in water and lemon juice, 1 tablespoon at a time, until creamy. Blend in ginger and garlic. Serve 1 to 2 tablespoons over each serving of salad.

Yields about 1 cup

Hijiki with Mushrooms and Carrots

> ½ cup loosely packed dried *hijiki*
> 5 dried shiitake mushrooms*
> 2 cups water
> 1 to 3 carrots, cut into julienne strips (about ½ cup)
> 1 small turnip, peeled and cut into julienne strips (about ½ cup), or ¼ cup slivered burdock
> 1 tablespoon sesame oil
> 1½ tablespoons soy sauce

Soak *hijiki* and mushrooms in the water for 20 minutes. Remove mushrooms with a fork and place on chopping board. Lift out *hijiki* with a slotted spoon and place in a 2- or 3-quart saucepan. Allow soaking water to settle, then pour over *hijiki,* discarding the gritty residue. Place over moderate heat.

Remove stems from mushrooms, slice caps into strips, and add to *hijiki.* Simmer, with cover ajar, for 10 minutes.

Sauté carrots and turnip in oil for 5 to 6 minutes, or until they begin to brown. Add to *hijiki* along with soy sauce and simmer, covered, for another 20 minutes, stirring occasionally. Serve with brown rice and steamed green vegetables.

4 to 6 servings

*Shiitake mushrooms are commonly available in oriental grocery stores.

Kakiage (Tempura Vegetables) with Oriental Dipping Sauce

Serve these Japanese treats as an appetizer, as a side dish to a light dinner meal, or as a main course. They are very filling.

> 2 tablespoons loosely packed dried *hijiki*
> ½ cup water
> 1 cup whole wheat pastry flour
> 1 tablespoon arrowroot

½ cup slivered carrots
½ cup slivered zucchini
½ cup slivered turnips
½ green pepper, thinly sliced
3 cups sesame or safflower oil
Oriental Dipping Sauce (see below)

Soak *hijiki* in the water for 15 minutes. Lift out with a slotted spoon and set aside.

Allow soaking water to settle, then pour into a large bowl, discarding the gritty residue. Add flour and arrowroot, and mix to make a medium-thick batter. Add *hijiki* and then carrots, zucchini, turnips, and pepper slices. Mix well.

In a large heavy skillet or wok heat oil to 350°F. (Do not allow it to smoke.) With a slotted spoon, gently lower vegetables into hot oil. (Batter should just hold them together and the clusters of vegetables should float on the oil.) Cook until lightly browned and firm. Drain well on paper towels and then keep warm in a 200°F oven.

Serve with small individual bowls of dipping sauce.

4 to 6 main-course servings

Oriental Dipping Sauce

¼ cup soy sauce
¼ cup water
1 tablespoon grated peeled ginger root or 2 tablespoons grated white radishes

Combine all ingredients in a small bowl and mix well.

Yields ½ cup

Kombu

Chick-pea Stew

2 pieces dried kombu, 3 inches long
2 cups dried chick-peas
6 cups hot water
2 small carrots, cubed
1 medium-size onion, cubed
1 stalk celery, chopped
2 bay leaves
¼ cup olive oil
4 slices peeled ginger root
2 to 3 tablespoons soy sauce

Place kombu on bottom of a slow cooker, then add all other ingredients. Cover and cook for 8 hours on low setting. If you do not have a slow cooker, place ingredients in a large heavy-bottom saucepan, bring to a boil, reduce heat, and then simmer, covered, for 2 to 3 hours, or until chick-peas are tender.

6 to 8 servings

Fried Kombu Chips

Serve these chips as a light snack instead of nuts, or mix into nut snacks.

3 pieces dried kombu, 3 inches long
1 cup vegetable oil

Rinse kombu quickly under cold water and pat dry with a paper towel. Allow to rest wrapped in paper towel for 10 minutes to soften. Cut lengthwise into 3 thin strips with scissors. Tie each strip into a knot.

In a large heavy skillet or wok heat oil until it begins to move. Gently slide kombu knots into oil, cook for several seconds until they puff up, and then remove with a slotted spoon as soon as they have stopped expanding. Drain well on paper towels.

Makes 8 to 10

Watercress and Carrot Soup

1 piece dried kombu, 3 inches long
1 to 3 carrots, cut into julienne strips (about ½ cup)
4 cups water
4 ounces firm tofu, drained and cut into ½-inch cubes
2 tablespoons miso, or to taste
⅔ cup loosely packed watercress, with thick stems removed

In a large saucepan combine kombu, carrots, and water, and bring to a boil. Reduce heat and simmer, covered, for 5 minutes. Remove kombu with a slotted spoon and keep to use one more time in a broth or soup. Add tofu and simmer, covered, for another 10 minutes. Place miso in a small bowl and dissolve with a few spoonfuls of soup. Add miso to soup and turn off heat.

Just before serving, add watercress.

4 servings

Poached Sea Trout

6 cups water
1 carrot, coarsely chopped
1 stalk celery, coarsely chopped
1 medium-size onion, coarsely chopped
1 shallot, chopped (optional)
10 peppercorns
¼ teaspoon dried thyme
3 large sprigs parsley
1 large bay leaf
1 piece dried kombu, 3 inches long
2 tablespoons soy sauce
2 pounds sea trout or other firm-fleshed
    fish fillets
1 cup mayonnaise
  lemon wedges
  watercress
  cherry tomatoes

In a large pot combine water, carrots, celery, onions, shallot (if used), and peppercorns. Then add thyme, parsley, bay leaf, kombu, and soy sauce, and bring to a boil. Reduce heat and simmer, covered, for 30 minutes.

Using a strainer, pour vegetable liquid into a medium-size bowl.

Place fish in a single layer in a large oiled baking pan. Pour hot, strained vegetable stock over fish and cover pan with foil. Place pan on 2 burners and let liquid simmer for 5 minutes. Do not boil.

Transfer fish to a serving platter, reserving fish stock. Keep platter warm while preparing sauce.

Mix mayonnaise with reserved fish stock, adding 2 tablespoons at a time, until it reaches desired consistency. Garnish fish with lemon wedges, watercress, and cherry tomatoes and serve with the sauce.

4 servings

Nori

Brown Rice and Sesame Balls

This unusual dish may be served as an appetizer or as a side dish with Japanese entrées.

6 sheets dried nori
3 cups cooked short grain brown rice

2 teaspoons *umeboshi* plum paste*
½ cup sesame seeds, toasted

Toast each nori sheet by holding open over a hot stove burner for a few seconds or by placing in a 250°F oven for 2 to 3 minutes. With scissors, cut nori sheets down the middle at right angles with the fold and set aside.

With moistened hands pick up ¼ cup of cooked rice and squeeze firmly into a patty. Place about ⅛ teaspoon plum paste in center and close up again. Roll in sesame seeds and place on a plate. Repeat until all rice balls are made.

Moisten nori sheets with wet hands to soften them. Place 1 rice ball in middle of each nori sheet and wrap sheet around it, as if it were a package. Squeeze tightly all around to make nori stick together. Serve as a snack, or pack for a lunch or picnic.

Makes 1 dozen

*Umeboshi plum paste is available in natural foods stores or oriental grocery stores.

Brown Rice Sushi

These tidbits provide the perfect introduction to the special qualities of sea vegetables. Sushi bars, quite common in America's larger cities, offer an endless variety of fillings in these vegetable wraps.

1 large carrot
1 egg
1 tablespoon water
4 sheets dried nori
3 cups cooked brown rice
1 cucumber, cut into 4 long thin strips
4 tablespoons rice vinegar, cider vinegar, or
    lemon juice

Cut carrot into 4 long thin strips (as long as nori sheets are wide). Steam carrot strips until just soft, about 6 minutes.

Beat egg with water. Heat a 9-inch, lightly oiled skillet, and spoon egg mixture into skillet. Tilt and turn to make an egg pancake, and cook for about 1 minute or until set. Turn out of skillet onto a plate, and cut 4 ½-inch strips along the widest part.

Toast each nori sheet by holding open over a hot stove burner for a few seconds or by placing in a 250°F oven for 2 to 3 minutes.

Place a damp paper towel on a working surface or on a sushi mat.* Moisten hands and smooth 1 nori sheet over the damp paper towel. Working with moist hands, take ¾ cup rice and pat down firmly all over the lower three-quarters of the nori sheet, making an even thickness and leaving an uncovered edge about 1½ inches wide along the top (the part farthest away from you).

Place 1 carrot, cucumber, and egg strip across center of rice, and sprinkle all with 1 tablespoon vinegar or lemon juice. Starting at edge nearest you, roll up gently, using paper towel (and mat, if you're using one), rolling toward the uncovered edge of nori. Moisten uncovered edge lightly, and finish rolling as if rolling a cigar. (Make sure paper towel is not in the roll.) Squeeze gently with your whole hand all along the roll to firm. Slice across roll with a thin, sharp, wet knife to make 5 pieces. Serve pieces standing up. The orange, green, and yellow of the vegetables and egg should form a cluster in center of rice. Repeat with each nori sheet.

4 to 6 servings

*Sushi mats are available at cooking supply stores or Japanese specialty shops.

Japanese *Soba* Noodles with Sauce

A delicious side dish to serve in place of rice or potatoes.

2 tablespoons kudzu* or arrowroot
2 tablespoons peanut butter
1½ tablespoons soy sauce
1⅓ cups water
1 sheet dried nori
8 ounces uncooked *soba* noodles

Place kudzu or arrowroot, peanut butter, soy sauce, and water in a blender and process for a few seconds, or mix thoroughly by hand. Pour into a small saucepan and heat, stirring constantly with a wooden spoon, until mixture thickens and begins to simmer. Allow to simmer for 2 minutes.

Toast each nori sheet by holding open over a hot stove burner for a few seconds or by placing in a 250°F oven for 2 to 3 minutes. With scissors, cut each nori sheet once lengthwise and then across in ½-inch widths to make strips.

Cook noodles. Drain, rinse, and serve with the hot sauce topped with nori strips.

4 to 6 servings

*Kudzu is available in natural foods stores or oriental grocery stores.

Tofu-Nori Sandwiches with Ginger-Lemon Dipping Sauce

8 slices firm tofu, ¼ inch thick and 3 inches long, drained
vegetable oil, for sautéing
soy sauce, to taste
2 sheets dried nori
8 long scallion greens, trimmed
8 thin slices white radish or daikon
¼ cup shredded carrots or red cabbage
Ginger-Lemon Dipping Sauce (see below)

Sauté tofu in oil until crisp on both sides. Just before removing from skillet, sprinkle with soy sauce. Place on a paper towel to drain.

Toast each nori sheet by holding open over a hot stove burner for a few seconds or by placing in a 250°F oven for 2 to 3 minutes. With scissors, cut each nori sheet along fold, then in half crosswise so that you have 4 pieces for each sheet. Moisten each piece with wet hands to soften. Place 1 tofu slice in a nori piece and wrap up like a package. Repeat process.

Drop scallions in boiling water for 30 seconds, then drain. Use them to tie nori packets.

Arrange packets around the edge of a serving plate alternating with radish or daikon slices. Pile shredded carrots or red cabbage in middle and serve with the sauce.

Makes 8

Ginger-Lemon Dipping Sauce

2 tablespoons water
2 tablespoons soy sauce
1 teaspoon lemon juice
½ teaspoon grated peeled ginger root

Combine all ingredients in a small bowl and blend well.

Yields ¼ cup

Wakame

Fish Poached in Seaweed Broth

1 ounce dried *wakame*
2 cups water
1 medium-size onion, finely chopped
1 tablespoon vegetable oil
2 cloves garlic, minced
5 teaspoons soy sauce
¼ teaspoon ground ginger
1 bay leaf
2 small zucchini, sliced
2 small yellow summer squashes, sliced
1 whole sea trout, red snapper, mackerel, or
     other fresh fish (1½ to 2 pounds), gutted
6 scallions, chopped
1½ tablespoons kudzu* or arrowroot, dissolved in
     ¼ cup water
2 tablespoons chopped fresh parsley

Soak *wakame* in the water for 15 minutes, or until quite soft. Lift out *wakame* with a slotted spoon and set aside. Reserve soaking water.

To prepare the poaching liquid: In a small saucepan sauté onions in oil until very brown, then add garlic. Add 1½ cups reserved *wakame* soaking water, soy sauce, ginger, and bay leaf and simmer, covered, for 15 minutes.

Meanwhile, arrange zucchini and summer squash slices in a shallow baking pan. Unravel the long strands of *wakame* and lay them over vegetables across the pan from top to bottom, letting them overhang.

Preheat oven to 400°F.

Wash and dry fish, place lengthwise on *wakame,* and stuff with scallions. Pour poaching liquid over fish. Fold overhanging seaweed strands gently over fish so that fish is wrapped from head to tail and lies lengthwise over vegetables. Cover pan with foil and bake for 20 to 30 minutes.

Remove from oven. Unwrap fish and, with 2 spatulas, transfer gently and quickly onto an oven-proof serving platter. Place *wakame* in a bowl and reserve. Remove vegetables with a slotted spoon and arrange around fish. (Do not discard pan liquid.) Cover platter with the foil and return to the turned-off oven while you make sauce.

To prepare the sauce: Pour liquid from fish pan into a small saucepan and bring to a boil. Reduce liquid to 1¾ cups. Chop 2 tablespoons reserved *wakame* and add to liquid. Stir kudzu or arrowroot mixture well and add to liquid. Stir continuously until thickened. Continue to simmer for 1 more minute. Add parsley, pour into a warmed sauceboat, and serve with fish.

4 to 6 servings

*Kudzu is available in natural foods stores or oriental grocery stores.

Scrambled Eggs with *Wakame*

1 piece dried *wakame,* 2 inches long
½ cup water
1 scallion, chopped
2 eggs
1 teaspoon sesame oil

Soak *wakame* in water for 15 minutes. Drain. Then remove tough center rib and chop *wakame* finely. Place 1 tablespoon in a small bowl. Add scallions and eggs, and beat well with a fork.

In a skillet warm oil over low heat. Add eggs and stir with a spoon until just set, about 3 to 4 minutes. Serve immediately. Good with whole wheat toast and salad.

1 serving

Rainbow Stir-Fried Vegetables

6 large stalks bok choy
1 piece dried *wakame,* 4 inches long
½ cup water
2 tablespoons kudzu* or arrowroot
2 tablespoons water or Vegetable Stock
     (page 111)
2 tablespoons safflower oil
1 medium-size onion, sliced
1 teaspoon minced garlic
½ teaspoon minced peeled ginger root
1 large carrot, sliced
¼ pound mushrooms, sliced
½ large sweet red pepper, cut into diamonds
     or squares
1 medium-size zucchini, cut into julienne strips

1 medium-size yellow summer squash, sliced
2 tablespoons soy sauce
20 snow pea pods

Separate leafy greens from white stalks of bok choy. Cut leaves 2 to 3 inches around and reserve. Cut stalks in half lengthwise if they are wide (over 1½ inches across), then cut into 1½-inch lengths and reserve.

Soak *wakame* in the water for 15 minutes. Drain, reserving soaking water. Remove tough center rib and chop *wakame*. Set aside.

Mix kudzu or arrowroot with water or stock and reserve.

Heat a large heavy skillet or wok over high heat for 5 to 10 seconds. Then add oil. Rotate wok to coat cooking surface with oil. Add onions and stir-fry for 1 minute. Then add garlic and ginger and stir-fry for 1 minute. Add chopped *wakame,* carrots, and mushrooms and stir-fry for 2 minutes. Add pepper pieces and bok choy stalks and stir-fry for 2 more minutes. Add zucchini and yellow squash and stir-fry for 1 minute. Stir in ½ cup reserved *wakame* soaking water and soy sauce. Cover skillet or wok and cook for 2 minutes. Add snow peas and bok choy leaves, cover, and cook for 1 minute longer.

Push vegetables to side of skillet or wok and slowly pour in well-mixed kudzu or arrowroot mixture, stirring liquid in skillet or wok as you pour. When liquid is thick enough to coat vegetables nicely without being either overly thick or watery, turn off heat and mix vegetables quickly with sauce. Remove to a serving platter or bowl and serve immediately.

4 to 6 servings

*Kudzu is available in natural foods stores or oriental grocery stores.

Wakame-Sesame Condiment

This tasty combination is an excellent flavor enhancer–a good substitute for salt.

6 pieces dried *wakame,* 3 to 4 inches long*
½ cup sesame seeds, toasted

Roast *wakame* in a 350°F oven for 10 minutes, or until very crisp. Pulverize *wakame* with a mortar and pestle or in a blender and measure 1 tablespoon. Add sesame seeds to *wakame* and grind together thoroughly. Store in a tightly sealed jar. Serve as a condiment.

Yields about ½ cup

*The *wakame* may be replaced with granulated kelp or powdered dulse, available in natural foods stores or oriental grocery stores.

Sea Gelatin (Agar)

Broccoli Aspic

Serve this as part of an elegant buffet spread, as an appetizer, or as a special luncheon salad.

2 bars kanten (agar) or 5 tablespoons agar flakes
4 cups water or Vegetable Stock (page 111)
1½ tablespoons soy sauce, or to taste
1 teaspoon grated peeled ginger root
2 cups broccoli florets
lettuce
parsley sprigs
radishes

If using kanten bars, rinse under cold water until soft. Place bars or flakes in a large saucepan with water or stock. Add soy sauce and ginger, bring to a boil, reduce heat, and simmer for 3 to 5 minutes, stirring constantly until kanten or agar has dissolved. Pour into a bowl or mold, and refrigerate until mixture thickens to consistency of egg whites, 15 to 20 minutes.

Steam broccoli for 3 to 4 minutes, or until broccoli turns bright green. Drain and then place into aspic in an appealing pattern. Chill until well set, about 3 to 4 hours. Garnish unmolded aspic with lettuce, parsley sprigs, and radishes.

4 to 6 servings

Apricot-Almond Custard

    3 cups apricot juice or apricot-apple juice
    1 cup water
    2 bars kanten (agar) or 5 tablespoons agar flakes
    1 teaspoon vanilla extract
    ¼ teaspoon almond extract
    ½ cup roasted almond butter
    1 cup almonds, toasted and chopped

Place juice and water in a 1½-quart saucepan. If using kanten bars, rinse briefly under cold water to soften, then tear into pieces, and drop into saucepan. If using flakes, sprinkle over juice. Bring mixture to a boil, reduce heat, and simmer for 5 minutes, stirring constantly until kanten or agar is well dissolved. Add vanilla and almond extracts and simmer for another minute. Pour into a shallow baking pan and chill. When thoroughly set, cut up jelled juice with a spatula and place in a blender with almond butter. Process at low speed until creamy. (Add more juice if necessary.) Serve dessert in bowls with toasted almonds sprinkled on top.

    4 to 6 servings

Kiwi Fruit Tart

    1 cup almonds
    ¼ cup maple syrup
    ⅛ teaspoon almond extract
    2 egg whites
    2 cups sliced fruit (1 kiwi, 1 orange, 1 apple, and strawberries)
    ¼ cup orange juice
    1½ tablespoons agar flakes
    1½ cups apple juice
    ½ teaspoon vanilla extract

Line a 9-inch pie plate with buttered parchment paper.

Grind almonds finely in a blender or food processor. Combine maple syrup and almond extract, and add to almonds.

Beat egg whites until stiff but not dry, then fold gently into almond mixture. Pour mixture into pie plate, and bake at 300°F for 35 to 40 minutes, or until set and lightly browned. Remove from oven and cool.

While tart base bakes, toss sliced fruit with orange juice and allow to marinate.

Sprinkle agar over apple juice in a small saucepan. Add vanilla, and simmer for 5 minutes, stirring until agar dissolves. Cool slightly, at room temperature or in refrigerator, until glaze thickens to consistency of egg whites. Do not allow to set.

Arrange fruit attractively over tart base, with kiwi fruit on top. Pour thickened agar glaze over fruit. Chill until firmly set.

    6 to 8 servings

Bulgur Pudding with Raisin Sauce

This lightly sweet dish makes a satisfying dessert; it may also be served as a breakfast food.

    1 cup bulgur
    2 cups apple juice
    1 cup water
    ½ cup chopped almonds
    1½ teaspoons vanilla extract
    grated rind of 1 lemon
    2 tablespoons lemon juice
    Raisin Sauce (see below)

Combine bulgur, apple juice, water, almonds, vanilla, lemon rind and juice in a medium-size saucepan, and simmer, covered, for 10 to 15 minutes, or until all liquid has been absorbed. Pour into individual dessert bowls, or into a 9-inch-square shallow baking pan, and chill. Serve with the sauce.

    4 to 6 servings

Raisin Sauce

    1 cup raisins
    1 stick of cinnamon
    1¼ cups water
    1 tablespoon agar flakes

Combine all ingredients in a small saucepan and simmer for 5 minutes, stirring constantly to dissolve agar flakes. Remove cinnamon stick and cool sauce in refrigerator until set. When set, process in a blender or food processor until creamy.

    Yields about 1¼ cups

NOTE: This sauce may also be made with chopped prunes, but use less of them since they absorb more water than raisins.

Legumes
Dried Beans, Peas, and Lentils

In spite of their centuries-old reputation as poor man's food, the stunning variety of textures and flavors among beans ensures that everybody will have a few favorites. And for vegetarians, dried beans, or legumes, are a vital staple. Legumes also star in dishes favored by those anxious to limit their meat intake for health reasons.

By themselves, dried beans, peas, and lentils have most of meat's protein values, but not all—a lack easily remedied by serving them with grains or dairy foods. And, contrary to their reputation, legumes are not fattening—a four-ounce serving of cooked beans contains about 135 calories. In fact, they are an ideal food for weight control because these carbohydrate foods are very satisfying.

Add low cost to the many other attractions of legumes. They provide more protein for the money than do many other foods. Easily grown, dried, and stored, beans, peas, and lentils are a versatile resource that provides new opportunities to stretch a tight budget, enhance the family's nutrition, and break away from monotonous menus. Their newfound popularity is well deserved.

Legumes dominate the cuisine of many cultures that consider meat a luxury. The result is a legacy of imaginative, savory dishes featuring those foods—Mexican *frijoles refritos,* Italian *pasta e fagioli,* and Indian *dal,* to name a few.

The legume family is a colorful and varied clan that can add depth and zest to both main courses and side dishes. Crunchy, nutlike chickpeas (garbanzos), fleshy lima beans, and grainy split peas—they and their cousins all promise eating pleasure. And they are most accommodating, mixing well as a part of or as an accompaniment to many dishes.

Buying Tips

American supermarket shelves only hint at the variety of legumes that are commonly available in other countries. Split peas, lentils, and several of the more common varieties of beans are usually displayed in our markets. However, if a Hispanic community is nearby, demand requires that the choice be more varied. When you cannot find the type of bean you want where you usually shop, it may prove fruitful to canvas the specialty shops—food co-ops, natural foods stores, and various ethnic groceries—to fill your requirements.

Mail-order sources (see Appendix 4) provide an excellent means of getting beans that might not be available at ordinary shopping outlets.

Whether buying the one-pound cellophane-wrapped supermarket beans or loose beans in bulk, check the color and the size. Beans, peas, and lentils should have a fairly clear uniform color. A faded look suggests too-long storage.

260

Also, the size of the beans in the package should be uniform; mixed sizes will result in uneven cooking. Look for any visible defects. Cracked or shriveled seed coats, foreign material, and pinholes caused by insects are signs of low quality.

Preparing Dried Beans

The proper preparation of dried beans is neither mysterious nor complicated. Though beans do require time to cook, they need little attention during the process. In fact, beans should not even be stirred very often as they cook, since too much disturbance will break the skins.

Before cooking, sort through the beans and remove any little stones or other debris that might remain after the initial cleansing.

Beans are a dried food so they must be rehydrated. A simple, no-fuss presoaking method is used for all legumes, except for split peas and lentils, which need no presoaking. Soaking begins the process of increasing the dried bean's volume, which cooking then completes.

Overnight Soak

Soak the beans in cold water that is three to four times their volume for six to eight hours, or overnight. If you choose to soak the beans overnight, they should be refrigerated; otherwise, they might ferment and become spoiled. Before proceeding with cooking, remove any beans that float. (Beans that float indicate premature harvesting. The bean will shrink within its seed coat and may become moldy or contain trapped dirt.)

Quick Soak

An alternate method is to boil the amount of water you would normally use to soak the beans. Drop the beans in slowly so as not to interrupt the boil. Let the pot boil for two minutes more, then remove it from the heat and let the beans sit for an hour or more. Boiling ruptures the hard shells of the beans so the beans swell. Then they cook the same as they would after an overnight soak. The overnight soak is slightly preferred because fewer nutrients are lost in that process.

Cooking Beans

Cook soaked beans in the soaking water—it preserves food value. (Soybeans are an exception; the water gets bitter so it must be drained and replaced.) Add water if the beans have absorbed most of it, then cover the pot and simmer the beans over low heat for the appropriate time (see Cooking Legumes table, page 264, for approximate cooking times).

If you must stir the beans to ensure even cooking, do so as little as possible, and use a wooden spoon to avoid breaking the beans' skins. Otherwise, no stirring is necessary.

The cooking time for dried beans is subject to several variables—where they were grown, their age, the altitude of the cooking place, and the hardness of the water in which they are cooked—so it is difficult to be exact about it. Generally speaking, most beans will cook in 1½ to 2½ hours, with lentils and peas requiring less time, and chick-peas and soybeans requiring more. The times given in this chapter should therefore be regarded as approximate. Test the beans, either with a fork or by tasting them, after an appropriate amount of time has passed. When ready, they should be firm but tender, and not mealy. Another simple test is to spoon out a few beans and blow on them; if the skins burst, the beans are sufficiently cooked.

Beans cook best by themselves. Molasses, fats, salt, and acids such as tomato or vinegar all harden the bean's skin and lengthen cooking time, so they should not be added until after the beans are cooked. Do not add baking soda to the water to hasten the cooking process—it tends to destroy the thiamine (vitamin B_1) and can have an adverse effect on the taste of the beans.

Tips for Storing, Cooking, and Using Legumes

• Store uncooked dried beans in tightly covered glass jars. Stored in a cool dry place, beans will keep for months. Adding a couple of bay leaves to each container discourages insects and other unwanted creatures.

• Beans cook best in cast-iron enamelware, unglazed pottery, or a heavy-bottom stainless steel pot.

• Since preparing dried beans is a lengthy procedure, cook the beans you want now and for some future meals all at once. Beans freeze well and keep for as long as five months. Freeze the extra beans in several separate containers that you can thaw as needed. Remember to date the containers. Most beans keep their shape and texture nicely, though lentils tend to become mushy.

• Keep a jar of marinated cooked beans in the refrigerator, and use them to add texture and zest to a green salad.

• Preparing cooked beans with molasses increases their calcium value.

• Use leftover bean dishes as a stuffing base for peppers or cabbage, or mix with fresh vegetables in casseroles.

• If the flatulence that sometimes follows eating dried beans concerns you, try this: Soak the dried beans in water for at least three hours. Throw away the soaking water and cook the beans in fresh water for at least 30 minutes. Discard the cooking water, add fresh water, and continue cooking until the beans are done. This process does lose some nutrients, but it rids the beans of oligosaccharides, the culprits of the gas problem.

Pressure-Cooker Method

Pressure-cooking greatly reduces the time it takes to cook beans. Soak the beans, using either the overnight or the quick-soak method, and place them in the cooker with the water. To avoid possible clogging of the vent pipe by foam, do not fill the cooker more than one-third full of soaked beans and liquid. (One tablespoon of vegetable oil added to the pot will prevent the contents from foaming up and keep any loose seed coats from clogging the steam escape valve.) Next, place the cover on securely and put the pressure regulator on the vent pipe. Follow the manufacturer's directions for bringing the cooker to the desired pressure. Start to monitor the cooking time as soon as the pressure is reached (see Cooking Legumes table, page 264).

Cook the beans as directed. At the end of the cooking period (or any time before that, if you want to check the contents), reduce the interior pressure by removing the cooker from the heat and letting it stand for about five minutes, until the pressure drops. The skins are less likely to break if the pressure is allowed to rise and fall gradually.

Bean Puree

Bean puree can be used to boost the nutritional value of many foods. It retains moisture in baked goods, lends a creamy texture to casseroles, moistens stuffings, and can be used to thicken soups. Puree cooked beans in a blender, about one cup at a time, on medium to high speeds until a smooth consistency is reached. The puree can be used immediately or refrigerated for three to six days. It will thicken as it cools. Frozen, it keeps up to six weeks.

To enrich baked goods, add two to three tablespoons of thick bean puree to yeast bread mixtures along with the liquid ingredients. For quick bread recipes, replace one tablespoon of each cup of liquid with one tablespoon of bean puree. The resulting baked goods will be slightly denser and very moist.

For casseroles, stuffings, and soups, add approximately one tablespoon of bean puree for every cup of ingredients per recipe. Blend the puree in with either the liquid or the dry ingredients before cooking or baking.

Bean Flour

Bean flour can be added to baked goods as a nutritional booster. It is made by grinding any type of *dried* beans to a fine consistency. Grind about one-quarter cup of beans at a time, and make only as much as you need for the recipe being used; bean flour's shelf life is short term. To use bean flour in baked goods, substitute it for two to three tablespoons of every cup of wheat flour called for. Expect a slight but pleasant change in taste, texture, and color.

Soybeans

Whole books have been devoted exclusively to the soybean and its many derivatives. Like other beans, soybeans and soybean products are a familiar part of the culinary scene in oriental cultures, and have been so for many centuries.

Dried soybeans can be purchased the year round and are prepared for eating in the same way as other dried beans (see Cooking Legumes table, page 264). The following list of soyfood products commonly used today suggests the scope of the soybean world. Most of these products can be found in natural foods stores, co-ops, and usually in supermarkets serving an Asian community. Some, such as tofu and soymilk, can be made right in your kitchen.

Soy Products

Tofu, bean curd, or soy cheese: The pulpy, custardlike product derived from soymilk is called by any of these names. The liquid should be drained off before use, but some water should be

---

Tofu Equivalent Measurements
(1 pound firm tofu)

Form	Amount (cups)
1-inch cubes	2⅔
Crumbled or mashed	2
Pressed or squeezed, then crumbled	1¼
Beaten with electric mixer	1¾
Pureed	1¾

---

restored to cover leftover tofu before refrigerating it in a tightly covered container. It will remain fresh that way for about a week.

In this country tofu can be purchased as either "firm" or "soft." Firm tofu is the Chinese style and soft tofu (also called *kinugoshi*) is Japanese-style tofu. Flavor-wise, there is very little difference between firm and soft tofu. Firm tofu simply has more water pressed from it and therefore has a firmer consistency. Firm tofu is more suitable for use in recipes where you would like the tofu to keep its shape. For recipes where the tofu will be crumbled, mashed, or creamed, either type may be used. Soft tofu may be specified for use in recipes where its high water content makes it more easily blended or creamed.

Tofu is one of the most versatile soyfoods. It can be served in a number of ways in both hot and cold dishes. Because its own flavor is on the bland side, it blends readily with strong-flavored foods and with any kind of seasoning. It can be stir-fried with onions and garlic or any mixed vegetables. It can be cubed and added to soups for flavor, texture, and nutrition. In cold salads it will absorb the flavor of the dressing and become very tasty.

Tofu can be mashed and mixed with eggs, cheese, and seasonings in much the same way ground meat is, then baked as a savory loaf or fried like meatballs.

When frozen for several hours the texture of tofu becomes pleasantly chewy and meatlike, and its color changes to yellow. It will change back to white when thawed, and the tofu can be used in exactly the same way as fresh tofu. One of the quickest, most delicious ways to prepare frozen tofu is to soak slices of it for an hour or two in a marinade of vinegar, soy sauce, ginger, and garlic, and then to coat the slices with bread crumbs or cornmeal and brown them in oil. The "tofu cutlets" can be enjoyed as is or made into a Parmesan dish, with cheese and tomato sauce.

Fresh slices of tofu go well on cold sandwiches, especially in pita bread pockets with garnishes of sprouts, tomatoes, and onions.

Guide to Cooking Legumes

Dried Beans (1 cup)	Appearance	Approximate Cooking Time Regular	Pressure-cook
Adzuki	tiny, deep red, cylindrical	45-50 minutes	15-20 minutes
Black (Turtle)	small ovals with black skins and white interiors	45-60 minutes	10 minutes
Black-eyed pea	tiny, creamy, white ovals with a distinctive small black eye	1 hour	10 minutes
Chick-pea (Garbanzo)	beige, irregular, rumpled-looking exterior; firm texture	2 hours	15-20 minutes
Fava	flat and kidney-shaped (resembles lima)	45-60 minutes	not recommended
Kidney	light and dark red varieties, kidney-shaped	1½ hours	10 minutes
Lentil	small, grayish brown or brownish orange disks	30 minutes	6-8 minutes
Lima	flat and kidney-shaped; large and small varieties	45-60 minutes	not recommended
Baby lima	flat and kidney-shaped	45-50 minutes	not recommended
Mung	olive green, lozenge-shaped	1½ hours	8-10 minutes
Pea, split	green or yellow, small half spheres	35-40 minutes	not recommended
Pinto	pale pink, brown-speckled oblongs	1½ hours	10 minutes
Soybean	small, round, of various shades; smooth texture	3 hours	15 minutes
White (Great Northern, Marrow, Navy, Pea)	various sizes	45-60 minutes	4-5 minutes

Tofu dishes can appear as main courses, as side dishes, or as hors d'oeuvres. Tofu may even be whipped in the blender as a base for mayonnaise, dips, or salad dressings. It can also be used as the base for sweet dishes, such as cheesecake and other desserts (see Index).

Tempeh: This Indonesian soyfood is made by inoculating cooked soybeans with a special culture and then incubating them for 24 hours. The result is a fragrant, firm, white cake with a chewy texture and a mild, meaty flavor. Tempeh can be fried, baked, broiled, or simmered. It works well as a burger, or in tempura, soups, or casseroles.

Okara, **or soy pulp:** This solid material, left after soymilk has been prepared, has a bland flavor and coarse texture, but retains some protein. When used in combination with other foods *okara* adds nutritive value, and in ground meat dishes it serves well as an extender. *Okara* should be heated thoroughly before being used, to eliminate the beany flavor.

Cooking Water (cups)	Cooked Volume (cups)	Most Common Uses	Suggested Substitutes
4	2½	baked goods, salads, sprouts	mung, soybean
4	2½	casseroles, soups, stews	pinto
4	2½	casseroles, rice dishes, soups	white
4	3¼	purees, salads, stews	fava
4	2½	casseroles, pasta dishes, soups	lima
3	2½	casseroles, chili, mashed into cakes and fried, pasta dishes, soups, stews	pinto
4	2¾	casseroles, *dal,* soups	split pea
4	2½	casseroles, soups, stews	fava
4	2¼	casseroles, soups, stews	fava
4	2½	Chinese stir-fry dishes, salads, sprouts	adzuki, soybean
3	2¼	*dal,* soups	lentil
3	2	casseroles, Mexican refried beans	black, kidney
5	2¾	baked goods, casseroles, salads, tofu and tempeh making, vegetarian pâtés	adzuki, mung
4	2½-3	casseroles, pasta dishes, soups, stews	kidney, lima

Soy flakes: Whole soybeans are toasted for about 30 seconds, then flaked in a roller mill to make this product. The flakes have all the qualities of whole soybeans with the advantage of being easier and faster to cook. They can be used in a variety of ways, much the same as soybeans — with rice dishes, in casseroles, in baking.

Soy flour: This flour made of ground soybeans has a high protein (35 percent) and high fat (20 percent) content. To modify a recipe with soy flour, substitute two tablespoons from every cup of wheat flour with soy flour. Soy flour cannot completely replace wheat flour because it lacks the gluten necessary for texture. Because products containing soy flour brown more quickly, baking time or temperature may need to be reduced slightly. Soy flour should be stored in a cool dry place to keep it from turning rancid.

Soy grits: These are coarsely ground soybeans. (Sometimes the oil is removed for even quicker cooking.) They differ from soy flakes in that they are neither cooked nor treated with heat, but simply mechanically ground. Grits can be cooked with rice pilaf or added to any grain dish. They also add a nutritional boost to baked foods.

Soymilk: This milk, prepared from soybeans, can substitute for cow's milk in many recipes, or it can be used as a beverage on its own. Those who have allergies to other milks find soymilk a particularly valuable resource. It serves as the base for soymilk desserts, such as ice cream and sherbets, and for soymilk yogurts, cream cheese, cottage cheese, sour cream, kefir, buttermilk, and other cultured drinks.

Soy oil: This product is rich in polyunsaturated fats. Unrefined soy oil is dark brown, strong flavored, and aromatic. Though it can be used in the same way as other oils, it may alter the taste of a dish unfavorably. Be wary of this one. Before using it full strength, try blending it (one-to-one ratio) with another oil—peanut, sesame, or safflower.

Soy sauce, shoyu, tamari, and miso: These related by-products of soybeans are rich-flavored seasonings that add a meatlike taste to many dishes. All are relatively high in sodium and are best added to foods in small amounts because their seasoning power is highly concentrated. Shoyu is a naturally fermented soy sauce introduced thousands of years ago by the Chinese. It is made over a period of a year from soybeans and cracked, roasted wheat in equal portions of water, salt, and mold starter.

The original Japanese version, tamari (meaning "liquid drip"), is a fermented soy sauce made from soybeans, salt, water, and inoculated grain (koji), but no wheat. Tamari has a slightly deeper flavor, darker brown color, and richer consistency than shoyu. The product sold in this country as tamari is actually shoyu.

Miso is a fermented seasoning that can take from two months to three years to make from a mixture of soybeans, grain (either rice or barley), salt, water, and mold starter. Miso has the consistency of peanut butter and is used as a

condiment, soup starter, or spread. Miso-tamari is the delicious liquid that accumulates at the top of miso during its aging process.

How to Make Soymilk and Tofu

This recipe will yield enough soymilk to make one pound of tofu—fine for a first try, but time consuming considering the modest-size brick you get for your effort. You may want to double or triple the recipe the next time.

Soymilk

   1 cup dried soybeans
     water

Soak soybeans in 4 cups water overnight, using a deep container so the beans are well covered to allow for expansion. In the morning, drain beans. Puree them for 2 minutes in a blender, using 1 cup soaked beans to 1½ cups water at a time. In a large heavy-bottom pot, combine pureed beans with 4½ cups water. Bring mixture to a slow rolling boil, stirring frequently to minimize sticking. After it has reached the boiling point (when foam suddenly rises, threatening to overflow), reduce the temperature and simmer soy mixture for 10 to 15 minutes.

Ladle mixture into a colander that has been lined with cheesecloth and positioned over a large bowl to catch the liquid. Strain out as much of the milk as possible, leaving the residue in the cheesecloth. This residue is *okara*. Lift cheesecloth out of colander, place wrapped *okara* into a separate container full of cold water, and stir the water through the *okara*. Lift cheesecloth, place wrapped *okara* back into colander, and again strain out the moisture into the bowl holding liquid obtained from first pressing. Pour 2 cups water through *okara*, again straining this through the cloth, twisting, squeezing, and pressing it to drain all water into the bowl. What you now have gathered is soymilk. It may be used as is, or you may go on to make tofu out of it. The *okara* may be used for other recipes.

   Yields about 1½ quarts

Tofu is curdled from soymilk in much the same way that cheese is curdled from dairy milk. In cheese making, rennet is commonly used, but in tofu making the easiest solidifier to obtain is magnesium sulfate—Epsom salts—a perfectly natural, safe ingredient.

Tofu

    Soymilk (see preceding recipe)
2¼ teaspoons Epsom salts, dissolved in 1 cup
    water

Pour soymilk into a 4-quart saucepan and heat to the boiling point. Add ⅓ of the Epsom salt solution to soymilk, stirring well. Wait for milk to settle, then sprinkle another ⅓ of the solution over it, and stir gently. Cover and let stand for 7 to 8 minutes. Gently sprinkle remaining solution over milk, cover, and again let soymilk stand, this time about 4 minutes. Gently stir top 2 or 3 inches of mixture while curdled milk gathers together into soft curds. The yellow, clear liquid left between curds is the whey.

Line a colander or tofu forming box* with a quadrupled layer of cheesecloth. Place the colander or forming box over a large bowl or pan, and gently ladle curds and whey into the cheesecloth. The whey will slowly drain out. (Save this whey, as it is a good soup or sauce stock, high in protein and the B-complex vitamins.)

Fold the cloth over top of drained curds and place a flat object weighing 3 to 5 pounds (such as a water-filled jar) on top of wrapped curds. Try to distribute the weight as evenly as possible over draining curds. Whey will continue to drip out under the pressure, allowing curds to solidify into a block of tofu. The more whey that is allowed to drain out, the firmer your tofu will be. Depending on the weight used to press whey from curds, a usable block of tofu will result in 1½ to 2 hours. When tofu has cooled well, unwrap it. Tofu may be covered with water in a well-sealed container and stored in the refrigerator for a week, or slightly longer if you change the water occasionally.

    Yields about 1 pound

*Forming boxes are available in some natural foods stores.

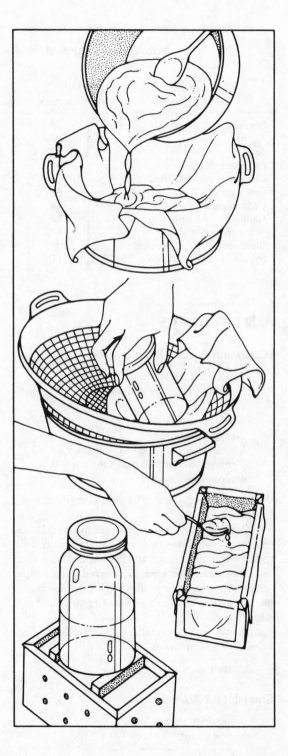

Nutritional Values of Soyfoods and Other Selected Foods

Food (100 grams)	Calories	Protein (grams)	Fat (grams)	Carbohydrates (grams)	Fiber (grams)	Calcium (milligrams)
Soymilk	33	3.4	1.5	2.2	...	21
Tempeh	157	19.5	7.5	9.9	1.4	142
Tofu	72	7.8	4.2	2.4	0.1	128
American cheese	398	25.0	32.2	2.1	...	750
Chicken drumstick, fried	235	32.6	10.2	1.0	...	15
Cow's milk	65	3.5	3.5	4.9	...	118
Ham, roasted	374	23.0	30.6	...	...	10
Hamburger, cooked	286	24.2	20.3	...	...	11
Potato, baked in skin	93	2.6	0.1	12.1	0.6	9
Rice, white enriched, cooked	109	2.0	0.1	24.2	0.1	10
Spaghetti, white enriched, cooked	111	3.4	0.4	23.0	0.1	8

Adzuki Beans

Potato and Adzuki Bean Patties

1 cup dried adzuki beans
5 medium-size unpeeled potatoes
1 egg
2 tablespoons butter
pepper, to taste
3 tablespoons chopped fresh parsley
1 cup grated Parmesan cheese
¼ cup vegetable oil

Soak beans (see page 261 for soaking directions). Drain.

Cook potatoes in enough water to cover. Drain, reserving 1 cup water. Peel potatoes, then mash them together with egg, butter, and pepper, and set aside.

Cook beans, covered, in reserved potato water until tender and water is absorbed. Combine beans, parsley, and potatoes. Shape into 12 patties and coat with cheese.

Heat oil in a large skillet and fry patties on both sides until golden brown.

Makes 1 dozen

Squash and Adzuki Beans

1 cup dried adzuki beans
3½ cups water
1 piece dried kombu*

1 cup diced butternut squash
½ teaspoon grated peeled ginger root
1 tablespoon chopped fresh parsley

Place beans, water, and kombu in a medium-size saucepan. Bring to a boil, then reduce heat and simmer, covered, for 1 hour. Stir in squash and ginger root, then cover and simmer 30 minutes longer. Mix gently with a wooden spoon, and break up the kombu which has softened. Serve garnished with parsley.

4 to 6 servings

*Kombu may be purchased in natural foods stores or oriental grocery stores.

Black Beans

Beef, Black Beans, and Rice

This is a good, cold weather entrée, inexpensive and filling.

2 tablespoons vegetable oil
½ pound lean ground beef
1 cup chopped onions
1 cup chopped green peppers
1 clove garlic, minced
1 tablespoon lemon juice
1 tablespoon prepared mustard
1 teaspoon chili powder
2 tablespoons soy sauce
dash of cayenne pepper

Phosphorus (milligrams)	Iron (milligrams)	Sodium (milligrams)	Potassium (milligrams)	Vitamin A (international units)	Thiamine (milligrams)	Riboflavin (milligrams)	Niacin (milligrams)	Vitamin C (milligrams)
48	0.8	...	...	40	0.08	0.03	0.2	...
240	5.0	...	...	...	0.28	0.65	2.52	...
126	1.9	7	42	...	0.06	0.03	0.1	...
478	1.0	700	82	1,310	0.03	0.46	0.1	...
236	2.3	...	...	140	0.07	0.40	7.1	...
93	...	50	144	140	0.03	0.17	0.1	1
236	3.0	...	...	...	0.51	0.23	4.6	...
194	3.2	47	450	40	0.09	0.21	5.4	...
65	0.7	4	503	...	0.10	0.04	1.7	20
28	0.9	374	28	...	0.11	...	1.0	...
50	0.9	1	61	...	0.14	0.08	1.1	...

1 cup tomato sauce
2 cups cooked black beans, drained
3 cups hot cooked brown rice

Heat oil in a large skillet over medium heat. Add beef, onions, green peppers, and garlic and sauté until tender, stirring frequently.

In a small bowl combine lemon juice, mustard, chili powder, soy sauce, and cayenne with a small amount of tomato sauce and whisk until thoroughly blended. Stir in remaining tomato sauce, then add to meat mixture. Add beans and cook for 20 minutes, or until flavors are well blended.

To serve, spoon over rice.

6 servings

Black Bean Burger Loaf

1 small onion, halved
3 slices whole grain bread
2 cups cooked black beans, drained
1 pound lean ground beef
1 cup canned tomatoes, drained
2 eggs
⅛ teaspoon garlic powder

Preheat oven to 375°F.
Mince onion in a food processor. Add bread and process to fine crumbs. Then add beans and puree the mixture. Add beef, tomatoes, eggs, and garlic powder and process until well blended. Turn into loaf pan and bake for 50 minutes.

4 servings

Sweet Bean-Stuffed Squash

3 large acorn squash
1½ cups hot cooked brown rice
3 tablespoons butter
1½ cups cooked black beans, drained
¼ cup honey
1 cup unsweetened applesauce
ground cinnamon, to taste

Preheat oven to 350°F.
Cut squashes in half lengthwise and scoop out seeds and membranes. Place each half, cut-side down, in a shallow baking dish. Pour in about 1 inch of hot water and bake for 30 minutes. Remove from oven. Drain off water and put squash back into baking dish, cut-side up.

While squash is baking, combine rice and 2 tablespoons butter in a medium-size bowl, and stir with a wooden spoon until butter melts. Stir in beans, honey, and applesauce. Spoon mixture into squash hollows, sprinkle with cinnamon, and dot with remaining 1 tablespoon butter. Continue to bake until squash is tender and heated through, about 30 minutes.

6 servings

Vegetarian Sloppy Joes

¼ cup olive oil
1 cup chopped onions
1 cup chopped sweet red or green peppers
3 cups cooked black beans, drained
2 tablespoons wine vinegar
⅛ teaspoon dried oregano
1 teaspoon honey
⅛ teaspoon cayenne pepper
1 cup tomato sauce
4 to 6 whole grain burger buns or pita bread pockets, warmed

In a large skillet, heat oil. Add onions and peppers and sauté for 2 to 3 minutes. Add beans, vinegar, oregano, honey, cayenne, and tomato sauce. Simmer for 10 to 15 minutes, or until flavors are well blended.

Serve on burger buns or in pita bread pockets.

4 to 6 servings

Black-eyed Peas

Chilled Black-eyed Pea Salad

2 cups cooked black-eyed peas, drained
1 cup peeled, seeded, and chopped tomatoes
1 cup shredded carrots
½ cup chopped yellow squash or zucchini
1 small onion, chopped
½ cup vegetable oil
¼ cup cider vinegar
1 teaspoon honey
4 drops hot pepper sauce

Combine peas, tomatoes, carrots, squash, and onions in a large bowl.

In a jar with a tight-fitting lid, shake together remaining ingredients. Pour over vegetables and toss to coat. Refrigerate salad until well chilled before serving.

4 servings

Hopping John
(Black-eyed Peas, Rice, and Pig's Feet)

2 cups dried black-eyed peas
6 cups water
¾ cup chopped onions
¼ cup chopped celery
1 pair pig's feet (1½ to 2 pounds)
1 cup uncooked brown rice
¼ teaspoon pepper

Soak peas in the 6 cups water (see page 261 for soaking directions).

Transfer soaked peas and soaking liquid to a large pot and add onions, celery, and pig's feet. Cover and cook over medium heat until peas are almost tender but still whole, about 45 minutes. Add rice and pepper, cover, and simmer for about 1 hour, or until rice is tender.

Remove meat from pig's feet and discard bones and fat. Mix meat into peas and rice. Serve hot.

6 to 8 servings

Pineapple Baked Beans

1½ cups dried black-eyed peas
3 cups pineapple juice
1 cup water
1 medium-size onion, minced
1 tablespoon light molasses
⅛ teaspoon ground ginger
1 tablespoon honey
1 cup shredded fresh pineapple

Preheat oven to 300°F.

In a large saucepan, combine peas, juice, and water. Bring to a boil and continue to boil for 2 minutes. Remove from heat and let stand for 1 hour. Then cover and simmer until peas are tender, about 1 hour. Drain, reserving liquid.

In a large ovenproof casserole or bean pot, combine peas, onions, molasses, ginger, honey, and pineapple. Add 1½ cups reserved liquid, cover, and bake for 3 hours. Uncover and bake 1 hour longer, adding a little more reserved liquid if peas appear to be drying out.

4 to 6 servings

Vegetarian Taco Stacks

½ cup vegetable oil
1 medium-size onion, chopped
1 clove garlic, minced
1½ cups cooked black-eyed peas, drained
1 cup cooked black beans, drained

4 cups canned tomatoes
¼ cup chopped green or red chili peppers
  (optional)
1 tablespoon chili powder, or more to taste
½ teaspoon ground cumin
⅛ teaspoon pepper
12 Corn Tortillas (page 392)
1½ cups shredded cheddar cheese
½ head lettuce, shredded
2 large tomatoes, finely chopped
1 medium-size onion, finely chopped

Heat 3 tablespoons oil in a Dutch oven. Add chopped onions and garlic and sauté until onion is translucent. Add peas, beans, canned tomatoes, chilies (if used), chili powder, cumin, and pepper. Simmer for 15 minutes.

In a large skillet, heat remaining 5 tablespoons oil and lightly sauté tortillas on both sides, one at a time, placing each in a warm oven as completed.

Stack cooked tortillas in 4 piles of 3 each. Spread bean filling and cheese between layers and on top of each stack. Garnish with lettuce and chopped tomatoes and onions.

4 servings

Chick-peas

Mixed Beans with Rice and Sour Cream

1 tablespoon vegetable oil
1 clove garlic, minced
1½ cups cooked chick-peas, drained
1½ cups cooked white beans, drained
1 cup cooked brown rice
½ cup sour cream
½ cup rich Poultry Stock (page 110)
1 egg, beaten

Heat oil in a medium-size saucepan. Add garlic and sauté over low heat for 3 minutes. Add chick-peas, beans, and rice. Toss gently until mixture is hot.

Gently blend sour cream and stock together, then slowly stir mixture into beans and rice. Heat gently, then stir in egg. As soon as sauce has thickened slightly, remove from heat. (Do not allow to boil.) Serve hot or cold.

4 to 6 servings

Falafel with Tahini Sauce

2 cups dried chick-peas
1 large onion, quartered
½ cup minced fresh parsley
2 cloves garlic, crushed
1 tablespoon ground cumin
1 tablespoon ground coriander
1 teaspoon pepper or ¼ teaspoon cayenne pepper
  vegetable oil, for frying
12 pita bread pockets, warmed
  shredded lettuce
  tomato slices
  sweet or hot pepper slices (optional)
  Tahini Sauce (see below)

Soak chick-peas (see page 261 for soaking directions). Drain.

Process soaked chick-peas, onion, and parsley through medium-fine blade of a food or meat grinder. Add garlic, cumin, coriander, and pepper. Blend well and allow mixture, which should be a light shade of green, to stand 1 or more hours to enhance flavor. (Or, mixture may be stored in refrigerator for as long as 4 days.)

When ready to cook, shape mixture into small balls about 1 inch in diameter. Heat oil in a large skillet and sauté balls until crisp. (Do one test ball first, and taste for seasoning before forming the rest. Correct seasoning in mixture if necessary.)

Cut off one edge, about 4 inches long, of each pita bread pocket to form an opening. Into this, layer sideways a bed of lettuce topped with 6 or 7 *falafel* balls, tomato slices, and, pepper slices (if used). Sprinkle tahini sauce over all.

4 to 6 servings

Tahini Sauce

¼ cup yogurt
¼ cup tahini (sesame butter)
2 tablespoons lemon juice
2 tablespoons hot water, or more as needed

In a small bowl, mix together yogurt and tahini. Blend in lemon juice and water. If consistency seems too thick, add a little more hot water to thin out.

Yields about ½ cup

Mexi-Bean Salad

2 cups cooked chick-peas, drained
2 cups cooked kidney beans, drained
1 cup cubed cheddar or Monterey Jack cheese
1 cup chopped peeled tomatoes
2 tablespoons finely chopped onions
1 cup yogurt
1 teaspoon chili powder
2 teaspoons prepared mustard
2 teaspoons dillweed
6 cups shredded cabbage

In a large bowl, stir together chick-peas, kidney beans, cheese, tomatoes, and onions. Cover and chill about 1 hour.

In a small bowl, stir together yogurt, chili powder, mustard, and dillweed. Cover and chill.

To serve, place 1 cup cabbage on each of 6 salad plates. Spoon salad mixture over cabbage and top with dressing.

6 servings

Bean and Rice Balls

2 cups cooked brown rice
1 cup pureed cooked chick-peas
½ cup chopped fresh parsley
1 tablespoon soy sauce
½ teaspoon curry powder
½ teaspoon garlic powder
½ cup sesame seeds, toasted

In a medium-size bowl combine all ingredients except sesame seeds. Mix well, then form into 1-inch balls and roll in sesame seeds.

Serve well chilled. Or, place balls on greased baking sheet, bake at 350°F for 10 minutes, and serve hot.

4 to 6 servings

Fava Beans

Bean and Rice Ring with Tuna Sauce

¼ cup plus 2 tablespoons butter
1 small onion, minced
2 tablespoons whole wheat flour
1 cup milk
¼ teaspoon ground ginger
1 can (6 to 7 ounces) water-packed tuna, flaked
3 cups hot cooked brown rice
½ cup chopped seeded tomatoes
2 cups hot cooked fava beans, drained

Melt 2 tablespoons butter in a medium-size saucepan. Add onions and sauté until soft.

In a jar with a tight-fitting lid, shake together flour and ¼ cup milk. Add to onions in saucepan. Gradually add remaining milk and cook, stirring constantly, until thickened. Stir in ginger and tuna. Keep hot.

In a 2-quart bowl combine rice, tomatoes, beans, and remaining butter. Stir with a wooden spoon until butter is melted, then pack mixture in a buttered 2-quart ring mold.

To serve, unmold onto a platter and pour warm sauce over ring.

4 servings

Fava Bean Casserole

6 tablespoons grated Parmesan cheese
2 tablespoons chopped fresh parsley
1 teaspoon chopped fresh chives
1 teaspoon dried basil
2 cups cooked fava beans, drained with liquid reserved
1 large onion, sliced
3 medium-size tomatoes, peeled and sliced
1¼ cups reserved bean liquid, Beef Stock (page 110), or Poultry Stock (page 110)

Preheat oven to 350°F. Butter an 8-inch ovenproof casserole.

In a small bowl, combine 3 tablespoons cheese, parsley, chives, and basil.

Place ½ of the beans into casserole, arrange ½ of the onions and tomatoes over the beans, then sprinkle cheese-herb mixture over all. Make another layer with remaining beans and top with remaining onions and tomatoes. Pour reserved bean liquid or stock over all and sprinkle with remaining cheese. Cover casserole and bake for 45 minutes. Then uncover and bake 15 minutes longer, or until top is golden brown.

4 servings

Curried Fava Bean Salad

⅔ cup sour cream or mayonnaise
¼ cup lemon juice
1½ teaspoons curry powder
4 cups cooked fava beans, drained
2 cups coarsely shredded cabbage
1 cup grated carrots
½ cup chopped sweet red peppers
   salad greens

In a large bowl, mix sour cream or mayonnaise with lemon juice and curry powder. Add beans, cabbage, carrots, and peppers and toss lightly. Cover and chill overnight.

When ready to serve, warm to room temperature and arrange on a bed of greens.

4 to 6 servings

Bean-Stuffed Peppers

1 cup bulgur
2 cups boiling water
8 green peppers
2 cups cooked fava beans, drained and mashed
   slightly
5 medium-size tomatoes, peeled, seeded, and
   chopped
1 medium-size onion, chopped
½ cup chopped almonds
¼ cup plus 2 tablespoons olive oil
2 tablespoons lemon juice
¼ teaspoon garlic powder

In a medium-size bowl combine bulgur and water and let stand for 20 minutes.

Preheat oven to 350°F. Oil a 9 × 13-inch baking dish.

Cut peppers in half lengthwise, removing seeds and pith. Drain bulgur thoroughly, pressing out moisture. Mix bulgur together with beans, tomatoes, onions, almonds, ¼ cup oil, lemon juice, and garlic powder. Spoon mixture into pepper halves and place in baking dish. Drizzle remaining 2 tablespoons oil over tops and bake until peppers are tender, about 40 minutes.

4 servings

Kidney Beans

Mexican Kidney Beans

2 tablespoons corn oil
1½ cups sliced onions
2 large cloves garlic, minced
2 teaspoons chili powder
¼ teaspoon ground cumin
1 large green pepper, cut into strips
1 jalapeño pepper, diced
2 cups chopped tomatoes
2 cups cooked kidney beans, drained with liquid
   reserved
½ cup coarsely chopped peanuts

Heat oil in a large skillet which has a tight-fitting lid. Add onions and garlic and sauté for 3 minutes, stirring frequently. Add chili powder, cumin, green peppers, and jalapeño peppers and cook 1 minute longer. Add tomatoes and beans, then stir in 2 cups of the reserved bean liquid, adding water if necessary to make the full amount. Bring to a boil, stirring occasionally. Cover pan, reduce heat, and simmer for 30 minutes. Stir in peanuts and cook 10 minutes longer.

4 to 6 servings

Kidney Bean and Salmon Salad

1 can (7¾ ounces) red or pink salmon
1½ cups cooked kidney beans, drained
2 tablespoons chopped onions
¼ cup chopped celery
2 tablespoons lemon juice
1 teaspoon prepared mustard
¼ cup chopped fresh parsley
   salad greens

Drain salmon and remove bones and skin. Break into bite-size pieces.

In a small bowl, lightly toss salmon with beans, onions, celery, lemon juice, mustard, and parsley. Chill. When ready to serve, arrange on a bed of salad greens.

4 to 6 servings

Cucumber-Kidney Bean Salad

This is a good luncheon salad or accompaniment to a hot meal. It keeps well, so it can be prepared in advance.

>   2 cups cooked kidney beans, drained
>   ¾ cup chopped green peppers
>   ½ cup chopped onions
>   1 clove garlic, minced
>   1 cup chopped cucumbers
>   ½ cup chopped celery
>   ½ cup vegetable oil
>   ¼ cup cider vinegar
>   1 teaspoon honey
>   1 teaspoon soy sauce
>   1 tablespoon prepared mustard
>   1 teaspoon curry powder
>   ⅛ teaspoon paprika
>   dash of cayenne pepper
>   2 tablespoons chopped fresh parsley
>   salad greens
>   1 cup yogurt or sour cream

In a large bowl, combine beans, green peppers, onions, garlic, cucumbers, and celery.

In a small bowl, mix together oil, vinegar, honey, soy sauce, mustard, curry powder, paprika, cayenne, and parsley. Stir until well blended.

Pour dressing over bean mixture and toss gently. Chill for at least 1 hour. When ready to serve, arrange on a bed of salad greens and top with yogurt or sour cream.

   6 servings

Lentils

Indian Lentils
(Dal)

>   1 cup dried lentils
>   3 cups water
>   1 tablespoon vegetable oil
>   1 clove garlic, minced
>   1 medium-size onion, sliced
>   ½ teaspoon turmeric
>   ½ teaspoon ground ginger
>   ¼ teaspoon chili powder
>   ¼ cup tomato juice

Combine lentils and water in a medium-size saucepan, partially cover pan with a lid, and bring to a boil. Watch carefully to prevent lentils from boiling over. Reduce heat and simmer for 45 to 60 minutes, or until lentils are tender.

Meanwhile, heat oil in a small skillet and sauté garlic and onions. Add spices and then tomato juice. Cook until onions are soft and mixture is well blended.

Combine onion mixture with lentils and puree in a blender. Serve with brown rice.

   4 to 6 servings

Lentil Casserole with Pork Chops

>   4 lean pork chops
>   3 cups cooked lentils, drained with liquid
>   reserved (lima beans or white beans may
>   be substituted)
>   1 cup chopped onions
>   2 cups coarsely chopped tart apples
>   dash of ground cloves
>   1 tablespoon prepared mustard

In a large hot skillet brown pork chops, using only their own fat, until golden brown on both sides.

Preheat oven to 350°F. Butter an 8-inch-square or 9-inch-round ovenproof casserole.

Spoon lentils into casserole, cover with onions, add apples, and sprinkle with ground cloves. Arrange chops on top of apples and lightly spread each chop with mustard. Pour 1 cup reserved lentil liquid over all. Bake for 40 minutes.

   6 servings

Lentil Loaf

>   1 medium-size onion, minced
>   2 cloves garlic, minced
>   ¼ pound mushrooms, minced
>   2 tablespoons butter
>   1 cup dried lentils, ground
>   1 tablespoon fresh thyme or ½ teaspoon
>   dried thyme
>   1 pinch each of ground cloves, pepper, ground
>   nutmeg, and cayenne pepper
>   2 eggs, beaten
>   1 cup tomato juice
>   2 tablespoons slivered almonds

Preheat oven to 350°F. Butter a 9 × 5-inch loaf pan.

In a large skillet sauté onions, garlic, and mushrooms in butter until very soft. Remove from heat and stir in remaining ingredients. Pour into loaf pan and bake for 30 minutes, or until top is lightly browned and loaf is dry.

6 servings

Lentil-Nut Rolls

These nutritious, savory rolls are an excellent and filling main dish for meatless meals.

2 cups cooked lentils, pureed
½ cup cottage cheese
1 cup minced onions
1 cup soft whole grain bread crumbs
2 tablespoons chopped fresh parsley
1 teaspoon soy sauce
½ cup finely chopped almonds

Preheat oven to 400°F. Grease a baking sheet.

In a large bowl, combine lentil puree, cottage cheese, onions, bread crumbs, parsley, and soy sauce. Mix thoroughly.

Divide mixture into 8 parts. Shape each portion into a roll, then coat each roll evenly with almonds. Place rolls on baking sheet and bake for 30 minutes, or until golden brown. Serve hot or cold.

4 to 6 servings

Lentil Tabbouleh

1½ cups cooked lentils, drained
1½ cups cooked bulgur
2 tablespoons vegetable oil
2 tablespoons vinegar
½ cup chopped fresh mint or parsley
½ cup finely chopped onions
1 teaspoon minced garlic
1 tablespoon prepared mustard
1 teaspoon dried oregano
½ cup thinly sliced scallions

In a large bowl, combine lentils and bulgur.

In a small bowl, whisk together oil, vinegar, mint or parsley, onions, garlic, mustard, and oregano until well blended. Pour over lentils and bulgur and toss gently until mixture is well coated with dressing. Chill. When ready to serve, top with scallions.

4 to 6 servings

Lima Beans

Sausage-Three Bean Casserole

1 cup cooked lima beans, drained
1 cup cooked black-eyed peas, drained
1 cup cooked kidney beans, drained
1½ pounds fresh sausage links
1 large onion, chopped
1½ cups tomato sauce
1 tablespoon honey
¼ teaspoon pepper
¼ teaspoon dry mustard

Preheat oven to 375°F.

Combine lima beans, peas, and kidney beans in a large ovenproof casserole.

In a large skillet, cook sausage until almost done. Drain, cut into 1-inch pieces, and add to beans.

Combine onions, tomato sauce, honey, pepper, and mustard and stir into beans and sausage. Bake, covered, for 1 hour.

4 servings

Lima Bean-Cheese Loaf

1 cup fine whole grain bread crumbs
2 cups cooked lima beans, drained and pureed
1½ cups grated cheddar cheese
¼ cup minced onions
¼ teaspoon garlic powder
1 cup milk
3 eggs, beaten
1 cup tomato sauce

Preheat oven to 350°F. Butter a 9 × 5-inch loaf pan.

In a large bowl mix together bread crumbs, pureed beans, cheese, onions, and garlic powder. Gradually stir in milk, then mix in eggs, one at a time. Turn into loaf pan. Place loaf pan in a larger pan and add 1 inch of hot water to outer pan. Bake for about 1 hour, or until knife inserted in center of loaf comes out clean.

Heat tomato sauce and serve on the side.

4 servings

Bread and Butter Bean Pickled Medley

4 cups cooked lima beans, drained
1 carrot, sliced into ¼-inch rounds
½ small head cauliflower, broken into florets
1 sweet red pepper, cut into 1-inch strips
1 large onion, coarsely chopped
5 cloves garlic, slightly crushed
5 bay leaves
2½ teaspoons celery seeds
3 cups white vinegar
1½ cups water
¾ cup honey
1½ teaspoons dry mustard
½ teaspoon turmeric

In a large bowl toss beans, carrots, cauliflower, peppers, and onions together. Place 1 clove garlic and 1 bay leaf in each of 5 pint jars, then fill them to 1 inch from the top with vegetable mixture. (Try to evenly distribute all vegetables among the jars.) Sprinkle ½ teaspoon celery seeds into each jar.

Combine vinegar, water, honey, mustard, and turmeric in a 2-quart saucepan and bring to a boil. Pour liquid over vegetables to ½ inch from the top and seal tightly. Cool, then store in refrigerator. Let vegetables marinate at least 1 week before opening, to allow flavors to develop.

Makes 5 pints

NOTE: These pickles must be refrigerated.

Curried Bean Pot

3 tablespoons vegetable oil
1 medium-size onion, chopped
1 large green pepper, chopped
1 clove garlic, minced
1½ cups sliced carrots
1½ cups sliced fresh green beans
1 cup cauliflower florets
2 cups cooked lima beans, drained
1 cup water
1 teaspoon cornstarch, dissolved in ½ cup cold water
1 medium-size apple, peeled, cored, and chopped
1 tablespoon tomato paste

2 teaspoons curry powder
¼ teaspoon pepper
4 cups hot cooked brown rice
½ cup chopped raisins
½ cup chopped peanuts

In a large saucepan, heat oil and sauté onions, green peppers, and garlic. Add carrots, green beans, cauliflower, lima beans, and water. Simmer, covered, for 15 to 20 minutes, or until vegetables are fork-tender.

Add cornstarch mixture to vegetables, then stir in apples, tomato paste, curry powder, and pepper. Cook, stirring constantly, until thickened. Serve with rice on the side and with raisins and peanuts as garnish.

4 servings

Vegetable-Lima Aspic

pastry for 1½ Basic Rolled Piecrusts (page 718)
1½ cups cold water
2 envelopes unflavored gelatin
2 cups Beef Stock (page 110)
1 tablespoon lemon juice
2 cups cooked lima beans, drained
1 cup chopped seeded tomatoes
2 hard-cooked eggs, sliced
½ cup sour cream
½ cup mayonnaise

Preheat oven to 400°F.

Roll out pastry dough and line an 11-inch flan pan with removable bottom. Cut wax paper circle and place over dough so that paper comes up and over sides of pan. Weight crust down by filling completely with dried beans. Bake for 10 minutes, then reduce heat to 350°F and continue to bake for 15 minutes. Remove paper and beans and continue to bake crust until golden, about 10 minutes more. Remove from oven and carefully take crust out of pan.

Place ½ cup water in a small bowl. Sprinkle gelatin over water and set aside for several minutes to soften.

In a medium-size saucepan, bring stock and remaining 1 cup water to a boil. Add gelatin and stir to dissolve. Remove from heat and add lemon juice. Refrigerate until thickened but not set, stirring often.

In a small bowl, mix together lima beans and tomatoes. Add ¾ of the gelatin, then turn mixture into baked piecrust. Arrange egg slices attractively on top, smooth on remaining gelatin, and refrigerate until set.

Mix together sour cream and mayonnaise and serve with aspic.

6 servings

Pennsylvania Dutch-Style Beans and Corn Custard

  1 tablespoon butter
  4 eggs, separated
  1 cup cooked lima beans, drained
  ½ cup cooked corn
  ½ cup heavy cream
  ½ teaspoon soy sauce
  ⅛ teaspoon pepper or dash of cayenne pepper
  ¼ cup finely chopped mild onions
  3 tablespoons finely chopped green peppers
  1 tablespoon minced fresh parsley, or 2
       teaspoons minced fresh parsley and 1
       teaspoon minced fresh dill

Preheat oven to 400°F.

Place butter in a 9-inch-round baking dish and put baking dish in the preheating oven while you prepare the rest of the ingredients.

In a medium-size bowl, beat egg yolks well. Stir in beans, corn, cream, soy sauce, pepper, onions, green peppers, parsley, and dill (if used).

Beat egg whites in a separate bowl until soft peaks form. Fold whites into vegetable mixture and pour mixture into the hot baking dish. Bake for 10 minutes. Reduce heat to 350°F and bake 15 minutes more, or until top is browned and center of custard is just set.

4 servings

Succotash Pie Mornay

  ¼ cup plus 2 tablespoons butter
  ¼ cup whole wheat flour
  2 cups milk
    white pepper, to taste
  1 cup grated Parmesan cheese
  1 cup cooked corn
  1 cup cooked lima beans, drained
    pastry for 1 Basic Rolled Piecrust (page 718)

In a medium-size saucepan melt ¼ cup butter. With a wire whisk mix in flour to form a paste. Slowly stir in milk. Simmer until mixture thickens, stirring constantly, and continue to cook for 3 minutes. Remove from heat and add remaining 2 tablespoons butter, pepper, and cheese, stirring until butter melts. Add corn and beans to sauce.

Preheat oven to 425°F.

Line a 9-inch pie plate with rolled-out pastry dough. Prick dough with a fork, then add a handful of dried beans to weight down crust. Bake until lightly browned, about 15 minutes.

While piecrust is baking, heat corn mixture, stirring frequently with a wooden spoon. Turn succotash into piecrust and serve.

6 servings

Mung Beans

Creamy Mung Beans

  3 tablespoons vegetable oil
  ½ cup chopped onions
  ½ cup chopped sweet red peppers
  1 cup chopped tomatoes
  2 cups cooked mung beans, drained
  1 teaspoon soy sauce
  ½ teaspoon dried basil
  1 teaspoon chopped fresh chives
  ½ cup sour cream
  ½ cup yogurt
  2 tablespoons chopped fresh parsley

Heat oil in a medium-size skillet. Add onions and peppers and sauté for 5 minutes. Add tomatoes, beans, soy sauce, basil, and chives. Cook, stirring frequently, for 15 minutes. Remove from heat, stir in sour cream and yogurt, top with parsley, and serve immediately.

4 to 6 servings

Mung Bean-Vegetable Stew

    2 tablespoons butter or vegetable oil
    ½ cup chopped onions
    1 clove garlic, minced
    ½ cup chopped celery
    1 cup sliced carrots
    1 cup Poultry Stock (page 110) or Vegetable
        Stock (page 111)
    1 large unpeeled potato, cubed
    1 teaspoon dried tarragon (optional)
    1 tablespoon soy sauce
    2 cups cooked mung beans, drained
    ½ cup chopped fresh parsley

In a large skillet or saucepan which has a tight-fitting lid, heat butter or oil, add onions and garlic, and sauté for 5 minutes. Add celery, carrots, and stock. Cover and simmer for 30 minutes. Add potatoes, tarragon (if used), and soy sauce and cook 15 minutes longer. Stir in mung beans and parsley and continue to cook until just heated through, 8 to 10 minutes.

    4 to 6 servings

Pinto Beans

Burritos

    6 Flour Tortillas (page 392)
    2 tablespoons vegetable oil
    ⅔ cup chopped onions
    2 cups cooked pinto beans, drained and mashed
        (lentils, chick-peas, or kidney beans may
        be substituted)
    1 large tomato, peeled, seeded, and chopped
    1 cup shredded cheddar cheese
    ½ cup shredded lettuce or spinach
    1 avocado, peeled, pitted, and coarsely chopped
    2 cups tomato sauce, warmed

Preheat oven to 350°F.

Place tortillas in a large covered ovenproof casserole and put casserole in oven while preparing filling.

Heat oil in a large skillet and sauté onions until tender but not brown. Add beans, then cook until heated through, stirring frequently.

Remove tortillas from oven and spoon about ⅓ cup beans onto center of each. Top with tomatoes, cheese, lettuce, and avocado. Fold bottom edge of tortilla (nearest you) up and over filling, then fold in the 2 sides (envelope fashion) and fold top edge down.

Arrange tortillas on an ungreased baking sheet and bake for 15 minutes, or until just heated through. Serve with tomato sauce on the side.

    4 to 6 servings

Frijoles Refritos

    2 cups dried pinto beans
    4 cups water
    ⅔ cup pureed tomatoes
    2 tablespoons olive oil
    1 cup coarsely chopped onions
    1½ teaspoons minced garlic
    1 green chili pepper, seeded and minced (about
        ⅓ cup)
    1 teaspoon soy sauce
    ½ teaspoon cayenne pepper

Soak beans in the 4 cups water (see page 261 for soaking directions). Transfer soaked beans and soaking liquid to a large pot and bring to a boil. Reduce heat, cover, and simmer for 20 minutes. Remove lid, stir in pureed tomatoes, and simmer until beans have absorbed most of the cooking liquid, stirring occasionally.

Heat oil in a large skillet. Add onions, garlic, and chilies and sauté until soft. Stir in soy sauce and cayenne. Gradually add beans to skillet, mashing them in the pan with a potato masher. Stir frequently to prevent scorching. When all beans have been added to skillet, fry to taste.

    4 to 6 servings

Vegetable-Bean Patties

1½ cups pureed cooked pinto beans or any
    other beans
1½ cups whole grain bread crumbs, or more
    as needed
¼ cup wheat germ
 1 egg
¼ cup bran
¼ cup sesame seeds
 1 large carrot, grated
½ medium-size onion, chopped
 1 clove garlic, minced
 2 tablespoons chopped fresh parsley
¼ cup soy sauce
¼ cup cider vinegar
 1 teaspoon dried basil
¼ cup vegetable oil
8 to 10 slices cheddar cheese

In a large bowl combine all ingredients except oil
and cheese. Mix well, then form into 8 to 10 patties. If
mixture is too loose to hold its shape when formed,
add more bread crumbs.

Heat oil in a large skillet and brown patties well
on both sides. Place 1 slice cheese on top of each patty
during last 3 minutes of browning, and cover pan to
melt cheese.

Serve on whole grain or pita bread topped with
shredded lettuce, sprouts, and tomatoes. Or, serve
with a fresh green vegetable and cooked brown rice.

Makes 8 to 10

Split Peas

Carrot, Potato, and Split Pea Patties

*These patties are an excellent entrée and
satisfy as a flavorful meat substitute.*

4 to 6 tablespoons butter
 2 tablespoons chopped onions
 1 teaspoon minced garlic
 2 cups cooked split peas

 1 medium-size potato, cooked until crisp-tender,
    then grated
 2 carrots, cooked until crisp-tender, then grated
 1 cup whole grain bread crumbs
 2 eggs, beaten
    dash of cayenne pepper
 1 tablespoon soy sauce

Heat 2 tablespoons butter in a small skillet. Add
onions and garlic and sauté until tender, about
7 minutes.

In a large bowl, mash split peas lightly with a
fork. Add potatoes, carrots, onion-garlic mixture, ½
cup bread crumbs, and eggs. Mix well, then add
cayenne and soy sauce. Shape into patties, then coat
with remaining bread crumbs.

Melt 2 tablespoons butter in a large skillet and fry
patties on both sides over medium heat until lightly
browned, adding more butter as needed. Do not
overcook. Serve hot, with tomato sauce on the side if
desired.

Makes 8 to 10

Split Pea Stuffing

*Makes an excellent poultry or vegetable
stuffing. Or serve by itself as a tasty addition to
any meal.*

 2 tablespoons vegetable oil
¼ cup chopped leeks or onions
¼ cup chopped celery
¼ cup chopped sweet red peppers
 1 cup whole grain bread crumbs
 2 cups cooked split peas

Heat oil in a large skillet. Add leeks or onions,
celery, and peppers and sauté for about 7 minutes.
Add bread crumbs and stir until crumbs are slightly
toasted. Stir in split peas.

Use as a filling for poultry or any large, scooped-out
vegetables, such as eggplants, tomatoes, or sweet
peppers. Or, bake in a lightly buttered 1-quart ovenproof casserole at 350°F for 25 minutes.

Makes 3½ cups

White Beans

Double Bean-Double Cheese Bake

> 3 tablespoons olive oil
> 1 small onion, chopped
> 1 clove garlic, minced
> 1 pound lean ground beef
> 2 cups tomato sauce
> ½ cup ricotta cheese
> 4 ounces cream cheese, softened
> ¼ cup sour cream
> 4 ounces whole wheat noodles, cooked
> ¾ cup cooked navy beans, drained
> ¾ cup cooked black beans, drained

Preheat oven to 350°F.

In a large skillet, heat oil and sauté onions and garlic until limp but not brown. Add beef and cook until browned. Drain off grease, then add tomato sauce and simmer for 5 minutes. Add ricotta cheese, cream cheese, and sour cream and stir until well blended.

Fold noodles into meat mixture. Stir in beans with a wooden spoon. Turn mixture into a large ovenproof casserole and bake until heated through, about 30 minutes.

6 servings

Nested Cabbage Rolls

> 8 large leaves cabbage
> 1 pound cooked ground beef, drained
> 1 cup cooked navy beans, drained
> 1½ cups cooked brown rice
>   pepper, to taste
> 1 egg, beaten
> 1 medium-size onion, chopped
> 5 tablespoons butter
> 2 cups Beef Stock (page 110)
> 2 tablespoons cornstarch
> 1 pound uncooked spinach whole wheat noodles
>   paprika

Cover cabbage leaves with boiling water and let stand until leaves are soft and pliable. Cut hard spine off back of each leaf.

Mix together beef, beans, rice, pepper, and egg. Divide between cabbage leaves. Roll up, tucking in ends so that no filling is exposed. Place rolls, seam-side down, on a wire rack in a steamer and steam for 30 minutes.

In a large skillet, sauté onions in 2 tablespoons butter. Add 1¾ cups stock. Shake remaining stock and cornstarch together in a jar with a tight-fitting lid. Add to skillet, stirring constantly over medium heat until mixture thickens.

Cook noodles until tender. Drain and toss with remaining butter. Spread noodles on a large platter, then place cabbage rolls on top. Sprinkle with paprika and spoon some sauce over all. Serve immediately with remaining sauce on the side.

4 to 6 servings

New England Baked Beans

> 2 cups dried navy beans or other white beans
> 8 cups water
> 2 medium-size onions
> ¾ cup dark molasses
> 1½ teaspoons dry mustard

Soak beans in the 8 cups water (see page 261 for soaking directions). Transfer soaked beans and soaking liquid to a large pot and bring to a boil. Reduce heat and simmer gently until beans are tender. Drain, reserving liquid.

Preheat oven to 350°F.

Place whole onions in a 4-quart ovenproof casserole. Combine reserved bean liquid with molasses and mustard and add to casserole. Add beans. If there is not enough liquid to come to 1 inch from top of casserole, add water.

Cover casserole and bake for 2 hours. Remove cover and continue to bake 2 hours longer. Add boiling water if necessary to keep beans moist during baking.

4 to 6 servings

Sweet and Sour Beans

> 1 tablespoon butter
> ½ pound lean ground beef
> 1 cup chopped onions
> 1 cup thinly sliced carrots
> 1 cup sliced tart apples
> ⅔ cup raisins
> 2½ cups cooked white beans, drained with liquid
>   reserved

1 tablespoon honey
2 tablespoons vinegar
2 cups shredded cabbage

In a large skillet with a tight-fitting lid, melt butter over medium-high heat. When it has started to turn golden in color, add beef and onions. Stir and fry until lightly browned. Then add carrots, apples, raisins, beans, honey, vinegar, and 1½ cups reserved bean liquid. Cover and simmer for 20 minutes.

Add cabbage and continue to simmer 10 minutes longer, or until cabbage is crisp-tender.

4 to 6 servings

Sweet Cheddar-Meringue Pie

This pie may be served with vinaigrette vegetables as an entrée or, since it is mildly sweet, as a dessert.

pastry for 1 unbaked Basic Rolled Piecrust
(page 718)
2 cups pureed cooked white beans
1 cup milk
3 egg yolks, lightly beaten
½ teaspoon ground nutmeg
½ teaspoon ground cinnamon
⅓ cup honey
⅔ cup grated cheddar cheese
3 egg whites

Preheat oven to 450°F.
Line a 9-inch pie plate with rolled-out pastry dough.

Combine pureed beans and milk in a large bowl. Add egg yolks, nutmeg, cinnamon, and honey. Stir in cheese. Pour into piecrust and bake for 10 minutes. Then reduce heat to 350°F and bake 25 minutes longer, or until set.

Just before pie is finished baking, beat egg whites until stiff but not dry. When pie is removed from oven, top with beaten egg whites. Return to oven and bake for another 10 minutes, or until golden brown.

6 servings

White Beans in Tomato Sauce on Pasta

3 tablespoons olive oil
1 medium-size onion, chopped
1 clove garlic, minced

3 cups canned tomatoes
1 can (6 ounces) tomato paste
1 teaspoon dried oregano
¼ teaspoon dried basil
2 cups cooked navy beans, drained
1 pound uncooked spinach or whole wheat
noodles or other pasta

In a Dutch oven, heat oil. Add onions and garlic and sauté until soft but not brown. Add tomatoes and simmer for 15 minutes. Add tomato paste, oregano, and basil and simmer for 20 minutes, stirring occasionally. With a wooden spoon, stir in beans and cook until heated through.

Cook pasta until tender. Drain, toss with hot bean sauce, and serve.

4 to 6 servings

White Bean-Meat Casserole

1 pound fresh sausage
3 cups cooked navy beans, drained
1 cup chopped onions
1 cup diced carrots
1 cup chopped peeled tomatoes
¼ teaspoon garlic powder
1 bay leaf
½ teaspoon dried oregano
⅛ teaspoon pepper
2 cups Poultry Stock (page 110)
2 cups diced cooked chicken
1 cup diced cooked pork
1 cup soft whole grain bread crumbs
¼ cup grated Parmesan cheese

In a Dutch oven, cook sausage, then drain well. Add beans, onions, carrots, tomatoes, garlic powder, bay leaf, oregano, and pepper. Mix well. Add stock and bring to a boil. Then reduce heat and simmer for 30 minutes.

Preheat oven to 325°F.
Remove bay leaf. Add chicken and pork, stirring with a wooden spoon. Turn into a 2-quart ovenproof casserole.

In a small bowl, mix bread crumbs with Parmesan cheese. Spread on top of casserole and bake until heated through, about 30 minutes.

6 servings

White Bean Bake

2 tablespoons chopped onions
2 tablespoons chopped green peppers
2 tablespoons butter or vegetable oil
1½ cups tomato sauce
2 teaspoons honey
2 teaspoons cider vinegar
1 teaspoon prepared mustard
3 cups cooked white beans, drained

Preheat oven to 375°F. Butter a 1-quart ovenproof casserole.

In a large skillet, sauté onions and peppers in butter or oil for about 7 minutes. Add remaining ingredients and mix well. Pour into casserole and bake for 35 to 45 minutes.

4 to 6 servings

Soybeans

Dry-Roasted Soybeans

1 cup dried soybeans
½ teaspoon ground thyme
½ teaspoon dried basil, ground

Soak soybeans (see page 261 for soaking directions).

Preheat oven to 350°F.

Drain soybeans and pat dry on paper towels. Place on baking sheet and bake for 35 to 45 minutes, or until beans are dry and golden brown.

Place beans in a small bowl, sprinkle thyme and basil over them, and toss until all beans are coated evenly. Serve immediately while still warm. Or, store in an airtight container, then heat briefly at 325°F for 10 minutes before serving.

Makes 2½ cups

Variation:

Sunflower-Soy Roast: Substitute 1 cup soy flakes for soybeans and add 1 cup sunflower seeds to beans 10 minutes before removing from oven.

Poulet au Jardin
(Chicken with Beans and Vegetables)

2 tablespoons vegetable oil
2 tablespoons butter
1 chicken (broiler-fryer, about 3 pounds), cut into serving pieces
2 cups chopped leeks or onions
¼ cup chopped fresh parsley
1 large clove garlic, minced
1 cup sliced carrots
1½ cups water or Poultry Stock (page 110)
4½ teaspoons soy sauce
3 cups cooked soybeans, drained

In a large heavy skillet or Dutch oven with a tight-fitting lid, heat oil and butter over medium heat. Add chicken pieces and brown evenly on all sides. Add leeks or onions, parsley, garlic, carrots, water or stock, and soy sauce. Cover and cook for about 1 hour, or until chicken is tender. Add soybeans and continue to cook until beans are heated through.

To serve, spoon beans and vegetables onto a heated serving platter and arrange chicken on top.

4 to 6 servings

Soybean Croquettes

2 tablespoons butter
1 cup chopped onions
2 cloves garlic, minced
2 cups cooked soybeans, drained (chick-peas, pinto beans, or white beans may be substituted)
2 eggs, beaten
1 cup chopped peeled tomatoes
¼ cup lemon juice
½ cup chopped peanuts
½ cup chopped walnuts
2 cups whole grain bread crumbs
2 tablespoons vegetable oil

In a small skillet, melt butter and sauté onions and garlic until slightly golden.

Combine onion mixture, soybeans, eggs, tomatoes, lemon juice, peanuts, walnuts, and 1 cup bread crumbs in a large bowl. Mix well. Form into 8 to 10 croquettes, then coat with remaining bread crumbs.

Heat oil in a large skillet and gently fry croquettes until golden brown. Serve plain or with tomato sauce.

4 to 6 servings

Soybean-Wheat Casserole

½ cup cooked soybeans, drained
2 cups corn
2 cups stewed tomatoes, drained

1 cup chopped onions
1 clove garlic, crushed
½ teaspoon dried thyme
    pinch of cayenne pepper
¼ cup tomato paste
½ cup Poultry Stock (page 110) or Beef Stock
    (page 110)
2½ cups cooked wheat berries
1/3 cup grated Parmesan cheese

Preheat oven to 350°F. Oil a 4-quart ovenproof casserole.

In a large bowl combine soybeans, corn, tomatoes, onions, garlic, thyme, and cayenne. Set aside.

In a small bowl combine tomato paste and stock. Set aside.

Place ½ of the wheat berries on bottom of casserole. Cover wheat with vegetable mixture, then spread stock mixture over vegetables. Cover this layer with remaining wheat, sprinkle with cheese, and bake, uncovered, for 30 minutes.

6 to 8 servings

Corn Bread and Bean Stuffing

5 cups crumbled Corn Bread (page 301)
1/3 to ½ cup milk
¼ cup butter
2 tablespoons sesame seeds, toasted
2 medium-size onions, finely chopped
1 stalk celery, finely chopped
1 tablespoon minced fresh parsley
1 cup fresh green soybeans or lima beans
1 teaspoon dried basil
¼ teaspoon dried marjoram
½ teaspoon ground sage
¼ teaspoon pepper
2 eggs, beaten

In a large bowl combine bread and enough milk to moisten it without it becoming mushy.

In a small skillet, melt butter and add sesame seeds, onions, and celery. Sauté until celery softens. Stir in parsley, beans, basil, marjoram, sage, and pepper and sauté for 1 minute longer. Add mixture to corn bread along with eggs and stir well.

Serve as stuffing for chicken breasts or pork chops.

Makes 4 cups

Beans Italiano

2 tablespoons olive oil
2 large cloves garlic, minced
2 cups sliced mushrooms
2 cups fresh green soybeans or lima beans
1 tablespoon dried basil
½ teaspoon dried oregano
    pinch of dried tarragon
2 tablespoons wine vinegar
2 cups stewed tomatoes, crushed
1 pound uncooked whole wheat spaghetti or
    other pasta
½ cup grated Romano cheese

Heat oil in a large saucepan. Add garlic and mushrooms and sauté for 2 minutes. Add beans, basil, oregano, tarragon, vinegar, and tomatoes. Cover and simmer for 10 minutes, then remove lid and simmer 10 minutes more.

Cook pasta until tender. Drain.

Stir ½ of the cheese into sauce, then spoon over hot pasta and sprinkle with remaining cheese.

4 servings

Sweet-Pungent Stir-Fried Beans

1 tablespoon cornstarch
1 can (8 ounces) unsweetened pineapple chunks,
    drained with juice reserved
1 tablespoon sesame oil
1 large onion, halved, then sliced lengthwise
    from top to bottom
1 clove garlic, minced
3 cups fresh green soybeans or lima beans
¼ teaspoon grated peeled ginger root
1/8 teaspoon pepper
3 tablespoons rice vinegar
2 teaspoons brown soy sauce
3 cups hot cooked brown rice

Dissolve cornstarch in reserved pineapple juice and set aside.

Heat oil in a wok. Add onions and garlic and stir-fry for 30 seconds. Add beans, ginger, and pepper and stir-fry for 3 minutes. Stir in pineapple chunks, vinegar, and soy sauce. Then add cornstarch mixture and stir for 2 minutes longer. Serve over rice.

4 servings

Tempeh

Bean-Tempeh Stew

8 ounces tempeh
  whole wheat flour
1 tablespoon vegetable oil
4 cups Beef Stock (page 110)
1 cup tiny white onions
1 cup coarsely sliced celery (1-inch lengths)
1 cup coarsely sliced carrots (½-inch rounds)
2 cups cooked lima beans, drained
1 teaspoon dried basil
¼ teaspoon pepper
1 cup buttermilk or yogurt (optional)
  chopped fresh parsley

Cut tempeh into 1-inch cubes and dust with flour.
Heat oil in a large heavy skillet and brown tempeh on all sides. (This step is important for flavor and texture.) Remove from skillet and set aside.

In the same skillet, heat stock. Add onions, celery, and carrots and simmer for 35 minutes. Then add beans, tempeh, basil, and pepper and cook 15 minutes longer. Remove from heat, stir in buttermilk or yogurt (if used), top with parsley, and serve immediately.

4 to 6 servings

Tempeh Burgers

2 eggs, beaten
¼ cup chopped onions
1 clove garlic, minced
½ cup chopped tomatoes
½ cup whole grain bread crumbs
8 ounces tempeh, crumbled
2 teaspoons vegetable oil
4 to 6 whole grain burger buns

Combine eggs, onions, garlic, tomatoes, bread crumbs, and tempeh in a large bowl and mix well. Form into 4 to 6 patties.

Heat oil in a large skillet and fry patties until golden brown on both sides. Serve on whole grain burger buns. May be topped like a hamburger with mustard, mayonnaise, and chopped lettuce.

Makes 4 to 6

Tempeh Chili

3 tablespoons vegetable oil
1 large onion, coarsely chopped
2 green peppers, coarsely chopped
4 cups coarsely chopped tomatoes
5 teaspoons chili powder
1 pound tempeh, crumbled
1¼ cups tomato juice, or to taste
  cayenne pepper, to taste
¼ cup grated cheddar cheese (optional)

In a large skillet, heat oil and sauté onions until translucent. Add green peppers, tomatoes, chili powder, and tempeh. Thin with tomato juice. Add cayenne and simmer for 20 to 30 minutes. Serve with grated cheese on top, if desired.

6 to 8 servings

Vegetables and Tempeh au Gratin

1 cup coarsely chopped broccoli
1 cup chopped carrots
1 cup chopped leeks
2 tablespoons butter or vegetable oil
2 cups cubed tempeh
1 teaspoon soy sauce
2 cups cooked brown rice
1½ cups Mornay Sauce (page 142)
3 tablespoons buttered whole grain bread crumbs

Preheat oven to 350°F. Oil an 8-inch-square ovenproof casserole.

Steam broccoli, carrots, and leeks until crisp-tender.

In a large heavy skillet, heat butter or oil and sauté tempeh cubes for about 15 minutes. Add soy sauce and cook 1 minute longer, stirring frequently.

Spoon rice into casserole, and then cover with vegetables. Add tempeh, spoon sauce over all, and sprinkle with buttered crumbs. Bake for 20 minutes, or until mixture is well heated and sauce is bubbly and golden brown.

4 to 6 servings

Tofu

Cheese-Tofu Rarebit

½ cup soymilk
1 teaspoon soy sauce

10 ounces firm tofu, drained
2 cups grated sharp cheddar cheese
1 tablespoon whole wheat flour

In a blender, combine soymilk, soy sauce, and tofu and process until smooth. Transfer mixture to a 2-quart saucepan and heat over medium heat.

Combine cheese and flour. Add to hot tofu mixture and cook over low heat, stirring constantly, until mixture is very smooth and cheese is melted.

Serve over whole wheat crackers or toast.

4 servings

Marinated Tofu Cutlets

1 pound frozen tofu, thawed
¼ cup wine vinegar
¼ cup soy sauce
¼ cup water
2 cloves garlic, crushed
1 teaspoon dried basil
1 tablespoon chopped fresh parsley
1 teaspoon pepper
½ teaspoon ground ginger
1 egg, beaten with 2 tablespoons water
   cornmeal, for dredging
   vegetable oil, for frying

Drain tofu well, squeezing out excess moisture with a towel. Cut into slices about 2 inches square and ½ inch thick.

Combine vinegar, soy sauce, water, garlic, basil, parsley, pepper, and ginger in a medium-size bowl. Toss in tofu pieces and mix until marinade is completely absorbed. Dip one piece at a time in egg mixture, then coat with cornmeal.

In a large heavy skillet heat about ¼ inch oil. Fry breaded tofu until golden brown on both sides, adding more oil as needed. Drain on paper toweling.

Serve hot with rice, steamed vegetables, and a sauce or gravy. Or, serve cold as an appetizer, pairing each piece of tofu with a piece of pimiento.

4 servings

Cassoulet with Tofu

¼ cup sunflower oil
1 medium-size onion, chopped
2 cloves garlic, minced

1 pound firm tofu, drained and cut into 1-inch cubes
2 teaspoons dried thyme
1 bay leaf
¼ teaspoon pepper
1 tablespoon soy sauce
4 cups cooked navy beans, drained with liquid reserved
1 cup reserved bean liquid or Vegetable Stock (page 111)
2 tablespoons chopped fresh parsley
½ cup corn germ*

Preheat oven to 300°F.

In a large skillet, heat oil and sauté onions and garlic until soft. Add tofu and sauté lightly. Add thyme, bay leaf, pepper, and soy sauce and sauté 3 minutes longer. Stir in beans and bean liquid or stock.

Pour mixture into a 1-quart ovenproof casserole, sprinkle top with parsley and ¼ cup corn germ and bake for 45 minutes. Remove from oven, stir contents down gently, and sprinkle on remaining corn germ. Bake 30 minutes longer, or until topping is crisp.

6 servings

*Corn germ is available in natural foods stores.

Tofu and Beans with Chinese Vegetables

3 tablespoons olive oil
3 cups cooked lima, kidney, or fava beans, drained
1¼ pounds firm tofu, drained and cut into ½-inch cubes
1 cup bean sprouts
½ pound pea pods, cut into thirds
⅓ cup sliced water chestnuts
2 tablespoons vinegar
1 tablespoon soy sauce

In a large skillet or wok, heat oil. Add beans and stir-fry for 2 minutes. Then add tofu and stir-fry 2 minutes longer. Add sprouts, pea pods, and water chestnuts. Toss and fry only until all vegetables are heated through. Quickly stir in vinegar and soy sauce and toss 1 minute longer. Serve immediately.

4 to 6 servings

Tofu-Guacamole Deviled Eggs

12 hard-cooked eggs, halved lengthwise
½ cup soft tofu, drained
3 scallions, finely chopped
½ teaspoon soy sauce
    dash of cayenne pepper
1 medium-size ripe avocado
    paprika
    lettuce leaves

Remove yolks from eggs and mash in a small bowl together with tofu. Add scallions, soy sauce, and cayenne and mix well.

In another bowl, mash avocado. Add egg yolk mixture and stir until thoroughly blended. Mound mixture into egg white hollows, sprinkle with paprika, and serve on crisp lettuce leaves.

Makes 1 dozen

Tofu Lasagna

10 ounces tofu, drained
¼ cup grated Parmesan cheese
2 cloves garlic, crushed
½ pound mushrooms, sliced and sautéed
¼ cup chopped fresh parsley
2 to 2½ cups tomato sauce
2 cups grated mozzarella, Swiss, or Monterey
    Jack cheese
1 pound whole wheat lasagna noodles, cooked

Mash tofu, or slice it for a layer effect. Mix together with Parmesan cheese and garlic. Have mushrooms, parsley, sauce, and grated cheese ready for assembly.

Preheat oven to 350°F. Oil an 8½ × 11-inch baking pan. Line bottom of baking pan with a layer of noodles. (Save those noodles in the best shape for top layer.) Dot with ½ of the tofu mixture, then ½ of the mushrooms, ½ of the parsley, about ½ cup sauce, and 1/3 of the grated cheese.

Now add another layer of noodles, then repeat procedure with each filling. Place noodles on top, sprinkle with remaining grated cheese, and top with remaining tomato sauce. Bake for about 45 minutes, or until nicely browned.

6 to 8 servings

Tofu Stroganoff

2 pounds firm tofu
1 tablespoon butter
3 tablespoons vegetable oil
    dash of soy sauce
½ cup thinly sliced scallions
½ pound mushrooms, thinly sliced
1 tablespoon whole wheat flour
½ cup lemon juice
½ cup sour cream
1 tablespoon tomato puree
    pepper, to taste
2 tablespoons finely chopped fresh parsley

Drain, press, and cut tofu into slices 2 inches square and ½ inch thick. In a heavy 12-inch skillet, heat butter and 2 tablespoons oil over medium heat until butter foams. Add tofu. Sprinkle with soy sauce and fry tofu until lightly browned on both sides. With a slotted spoon, transfer to a plate.

Pour remaining oil into skillet, add scallions and mushrooms, and sauté for 3 to 4 minutes, stirring often, until lightly browned. Gradually mix in flour, lemon juice, and sour cream, stirring constantly. Blend in tomato puree and pepper. Add tofu, coating thoroughly with the sauce. Cover and simmer for 2 to 3 minutes, or until heated through. Sprinkle with parsley and serve with noodles or brown rice.

4 to 6 servings

Tofu-Tuna Bake

1 can (6 to 7 ounces) water-packed tuna, flaked
¾ cup mayonnaise
2 tablespoons grated onions
1 tablespoon chopped sweet red peppers or
    pimientos
2 tablespoons lemon juice
½ cup grated cheddar cheese
½ package (about 5 ounces) frozen peas
1¼ cups cubed firm tofu, drained
½ cup chopped almonds
¼ cup wheat germ

Preheat oven to 350°F. Oil a 2-quart baking dish.

Combine tuna, mayonnaise, onions, peppers or pimientos, lemon juice, cheese, and peas in a medium-size bowl. Mix well, then stir in tofu.

Spoon mixture into baking dish, sprinkle with almonds and wheat germ, and bake for about 45 minutes, or until lightly browned. Serve immediately, or chill and slice for sandwiches.

4 to 6 servings

Tofu-Zucchini Custard

4 to 5 small zucchini (about 1½ pounds)
 2 tablespoons butter
 ¾ cup chopped onions
 ½ cup chopped sweet red peppers
 10 ounces firm tofu, drained and cut into ½-inch cubes
 1 cup shredded sharp cheddar cheese
 2 eggs, beaten

Preheat oven to 350°F. Butter a 1-quart baking dish.

Cook whole zucchini in a small amount of water until crisp-tender. Cool.

In a large skillet melt butter and sauté onions and peppers until golden. Remove from heat. Cut zucchini into cubes or slices and add to onion mixture. Stir in tofu and ¾ cup cheese, then add eggs.

Spoon mixture into baking dish, top with remaining cheese, and bake for 30 minutes.

4 to 6 servings

Tofu Meat Loaf

 1 pound lean ground beef
1 to 1½ pounds tofu, drained (1⅔ to 2½ cups)
 1 medium-size onion, finely chopped
 ½ cup chopped celery
 ¼ cup chopped fresh parsley
 ¼ teaspoon ground cloves (optional)
 2 eggs
 ½ cup wheat germ
 ¼ cup soymilk or water
 ⅓ cup sunflower seeds

Preheat oven to 350°F.
Combine all ingredients except sunflower seeds in a large bowl and beat with an electric mixer until smooth.

Spoon mixture, which will be quite moist, into a loaf pan and top with sunflower seeds. Bake for 1 to 1½ hours. Serve hot with a sauce, or slice cold for sandwiches.

8 to 10 servings

Tofu-Spinach Balls

 1 package (10 ounces) frozen spinach
 1½ cups whole grain cracker crumbs or bread crumbs
 1 pound tofu, drained and mashed
 ½ cup finely chopped onions
 3 eggs, beaten
 ⅓ cup butter, melted
 ¼ cup grated Parmesan cheese
 ½ teaspoon pepper
 ½ teaspoon garlic powder
 ¼ teaspoon dried thyme

Preheat oven to 325°F. Grease a baking sheet.
Cook spinach and drain well.

In a large bowl combine spinach with remaining ingredients and mix well. Then shape into 1-inch balls, place on baking sheet, and bake for 15 to 20 minutes.

6 to 8 servings

NOTE: Balls may be prepared in advance and frozen unbaked. When ready to use, thaw for 10 to 15 minutes and then bake as indicated.

Vegetarian Tofu Burgers

 2 eggs, beaten
 1½ cups soft tofu, drained
 ½ cup finely chopped onions
 1 clove garlic, minced
 ½ teaspoon dried basil
 ½ teaspoon dried oregano
 ⅛ teaspoon pepper
 2 tablespoons grated Parmesan cheese
 1½ cups cooked brown rice or bulgur
 ½ cup whole grain bread crumbs, or more as needed
4 to 6 whole grain burger buns

In a large bowl, combine eggs and tofu, using a fork to mash them together. Add onions, garlic, basil oregano, pepper, and cheese. Mix well, then stir in rice or bulgur. Stir in bread crumbs, adding more if necessary to make a mixture that holds together.

Form into 4 to 6 patties. Fry patties in a lightly oiled large skillet until golden brown, about 2 to 3 minutes on each side. Serve on burger buns.

Makes 4 to 6

Grains

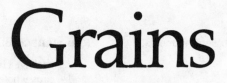

Whole grains present a limitless source of low-cost, nutrition-rich eating pleasure. When you replace some of the meat on the menu with grains, you serve less fat (particularly less saturated fat) and fewer calories; you provide more trace minerals and more fiber.

To bring this variety of whole grains into your own diet, you might take inspiration from some world-famous dishes — the oatmeal porridge of Scotland, the polenta (cornmeal) of Italy, the kasha (buckwheat) of Russia, the couscous (wheat) of northern Africa, to name a few. You will find that grains work well as a fundamental base for all other foods. Serving just a little milk and fruit or vegetable with any of the staple grains will give you a dish that provides both variety and sustenance. Adding a dairy product to any grain raises the grain's protein value.

Grains are best when processed in the simplest way — sprouted or stone ground into meal or flour — rather than milled in factories where the germ and the bran are usually removed. Many of the commercially prepared grain cereals are lacking in some food value because they have been refined to increase their shelf life and shorten preparation time. "Enriched" or "restored" on the label or list of ingredients simply means some of the nutritive value lost in processing has been put back, but this hardly approximates the original quality of the whole grain. The same wholesome, delicious, health-giving grain foods that have pleasured and nourished the world for thousands of years are still available, so why settle for anything less?

How to Cook Grains

Grains are easy to prepare; they need only be cooked in liquid until swollen and tender. The same basic cooking method works with all the cereal grains. Just remember that they do expand in cooking. Millet and barley grow to between three and four times their original volume, while other grains more than double — even triple — in volume. Plan to serve one-half cup of cooked grain per person for breakfast or as a side dish, and one cup of cooked grain for main dish servings.

Basic Cooking Method

Refer to the Cooking Grains table, page 290, to find the appropriate amount of cooking liquid and length of cooking time. Then:

1. If surface grit is present, rinse the raw grain in cold water and drain well. This will help remove both grit and excess starch and start the swelling process as well. If no dirt is present, do not rinse since some of the B vitamins, which are water soluble, may be washed away, too.

2. Bring the correct amount of cooking liquid to a boil in a pot large enough to accommodate the increase in volume after cooking. Meat or vegetable stock, juice, milk, or water may be used. The more flavorful the cooking liquid, the more flavorful the cooked grain will be.

3. Add the grain to the boiling liquid. Stir once.

4. Allow the liquid to return to a boil, then reduce heat to the lowest possible setting. Cover and let the grain cook slowly until it is soft and the cooking liquid has been absorbed. This will take anywhere from 15 minutes for bulgur to two hours for wheat berries and the harder grains.

To determine if the grain is cooked, use the taste test: Well-cooked grain will be chewy but not pasty, and not tough or hard either. If not quite done, add a little more liquid, cover, and continue cooking.

Other Cooking Methods

For the time and attention required, the basic cooking method is the most efficient. However, there may be times when one of the following cooking methods better suits your needs.

Thermos Method

All grains may be cooked by the thermos method. Place 1 cup of grain in a quart thermos (preferably widemouthed) and add boiling water almost to the top, leaving a one-inch headspace between water and stopper of thermos. Using a long wooden spoon handle, stir the grain to distribute the water evenly. Close the thermos and let it stand for 8 to 12 hours. (For brown rice add only 1½ cups of boiling water and let stand for only 8 hours.)

Pilaf Method

Cooking time for the pilaf method is about the same as for the basic method. Brown rice, bulgur, barley, millet, and wild rice are especially good when cooked this way. Sauté the grain, usually mixed with minced onion, in oil and then add stock or water—approximately twice as much liquid as grain. Cook the grain, covered, over medium-low heat until the liquid has been absorbed and the grain is tender.

Egg Method

Buckwheat is traditionally prepared by this method, which involves stirring a raw egg into the dry grain before adding stock or water and cooking until tender. This replaces the need for sautéing the buckwheat in oil and is done to keep the grains separate throughout the cooking process. For one cup of buckwheat groats, the required amount of water is two cups for the "egg method"

of cooking buckwheat and five cups when cooking it without egg, to be eaten as a cereal.

Oven Method

Grains can be cooked in a preheated oven to bring out their subtle nut flavor. If you are already using the oven to bake something else, you may consider this method so as to conserve energy. At 400°F the grain will cook about the same length of time in the oven as with the basic method. Before putting it in the oven, sauté one cup grain in one tablespoon butter in an ovenproof casserole for about a minute. Add the correct amount of water, then cover and bake until the grain is tender and all the water has been absorbed.

Tips for Cooking Grains

- Cook grain in a large, heavy pan to avoid possible scorching.
- Too much stirring makes the grain gummy, so stir only as suggested—and use a fork.
- To attain distinct, separate cooked grains, add a tablespoon of vegetable oil or butter to the cooking water.
- For a creamier grain for porridge or pudding, do not heat the cooking liquid initially; instead, first combine it with the uncooked grain, then bring the mixture to a boil, cover, and cook.
- Cooked grain can be held in a covered pot off the heat until needed. It will hold its heat for quite a while.
- To enhance the flavor and shorten the cooking time, toast grain in a dry, medium-hot iron skillet, stirring constantly, until it has a pleasant fragrance and takes on a darker color. This also enables the grain to be "cracked" by briefly grinding it in an electric blender.
- You may shorten the cooking time of hard grains such as wheat, rye, and triticale by bringing them to a boil in the required amount of water, letting them boil for 10 minutes, then soaking them for 8 to 12 hours in this same water. After soaking they may be cooked in the same water for 15 to 20 minutes and will be tender enough to eat.

Guide to Cooking Grains

Grain (1 cup dry measure)	Appearance	Approximate Cooking Time	Cooking Water (cups)	
Amaranth	Seeds about the size of millet, ranging in color from purple black to buff yellow.	20-25 minutes	3	
Barley	Short, stubby kernels with a hard, outer shell. Pearled barley (outer layer removed) is white translucent.	55 minutes*	3	
Buckwheat groats	Groat contained inside dark-brown, 3-cornered seeds that resemble beechnuts.	15 minutes	2 or 5†	
Cornmeal	Grainy white or yellow meal ground from plump, round kernels. Texture ranging from coarse to fine.	25 minutes	4	
Millet	Tiny, round, yellow; resembles seeds more than grains.	45 minutes	3	
Oats	Long, light brown. Grain is seldom seen in its whole form. Rolled or cut oats are flat, papery, tan flakes with brownish flecks.	30-40 minutes	3	
Rice, brown	Long, medium, or short kernels covered with a green-brown husk. Brown rice has husk removed. White rice has lost its germ and several outer layers.	35-45 minutes	2	
Rice, wild	Long, dark, almost black kernels slightly longer and thinner than long grain brown rice.	1 hour or more	3	
Rye berries	Long, dark-brown kernels longer and thinner than those of wheat.	1 hour or more‡	4	
Sorghum	Roundish seeds (slightly smaller than peppercorns). Brown with mixed yellow and red coloration.	45 minutes	3	

*If whole grain (pot or Scotch) barley is used, it must be soaked overnight in 4 cups water (and then drained) before cooking.

†Buckwheat is traditionally cooked by first stirring a raw egg into the dry grain (to keep grains separate) and then adding 2 cups of liquid for a dry, fluffy, cooked grain. Or, it can be cooked without the egg, in 5 cups of liquid, to yield a creamy consistency for eating as a cereal.

‡To shorten the cooking time, bring grain to a boil in the required amount of water and let boil for 10 minutes. Next, soak grain in the same water for 8 to 12 hours, then cook—again in the same water—for 15 to 20 minutes, or until tender.

Cooked Volume (cups)	Most Common Uses	Suggested Grain Substitutes
2½	Toasted seeds can be milled into flour or boiled in fruit juice as cereal, also popped like corn or used as thickening agent.	millet, sorghum
3	Flavors and thickens soups, stews. Flakes or whole grains make chewy breakfast cereal. Sprouts are used to make malt and caffeine-free beverage.	brown rice, wheat
2½ or 4	Used most often as flour, in pancakes, biscuits, muffins. Groats are used for kasha, *varnishkas,* blini.	oats, bulgur
3	Used in hasty and Indian puddings, mush, unleavened breads, pones, muffins, polenta, griddle cakes, tortillas.	amaranth, millet
3½	Boiled like rice for breakfast and main dishes. Thickens and flavors soups, stews. Used in Indian chapati or added to wheat bread. Used as bird feed.	amaranth, cornmeal, sorghum
3½	Thickens and enriches soups. Stretches meat dishes. Used in stuffings, pilaf, breads, cakes, pancakes, granola, Swiss *muesli.*	buckwheat groats, brown rice
3	Boiled as basic food, served alone or with meat, vegetables, in casseroles, soups, stews, stuffings, puddings, pilaf, paella.	barley, wheat
4	Used in stuffings, casseroles, as a side dish for fish or fowl— especially duck and Cornish game hen.	long grain brown rice
2⅔	Boiled and mixed with other grains, legumes, vegetables as a side dish. Added to casseroles, soups, stews. Ground to make flour. Groats can be cooked by the egg method, like buckwheat groats.	triticale, wheat
3½	Boiled seeds can be eaten whole, like boiled rice. Ground into meal for cereal, or milled into flour.	amaranth, millet

[continued]

Guide to Cooking Grains—*Continued*

Grain (1 cup dry measure)	Appearance	Approximate Cooking Time	Cooking Water (cups)
Triticale	Gray-brown, oval-shaped kernels. Larger than wheat grains and plumper than rye grains.	1 hour‡	4
Wheat Berries	Short, rounded kernels of varying shades of brown.	2 hours‡	3
Cracked	Brownish. Coarsely cracked wheat berries, unevenly shaped.	25 minutes	2
Bulgur	Resembles cracked wheat in appearance. Grains have been parboiled.	15-20 minutes	2

‡To shorten the cooking time, bring grain to a boil in the required amount of water and let boil for 10 minutes. Next, soak grain in the same water for 8 to 12 hours, then cook—again in the same water—for 15 to 20 minutes, or until tender.

Storing Grains

Unhulled grain with its germ still intact has a higher oil content than refined grain, so it must be protected against rancidity by proper storage. Sealed in a tightly covered container and stored in a cool, dry place, most grains will keep for about a year. Because they are especially quick to spoil, buckwheat groats and oatmeal should be refrigerated or stored in the freezer. If that is not possible, try to use them within a month. Bulgur—the parcooked grain—stores very well because is has a good resistance to rancidity.

Insects thrive on healthy grain, so you need a tightly closed container to protect your supply against infestation.

Types of Grains

Most natural foods stores carry a wide selection of whole grains and their flours. However, grains such as amaranth, sorghum, and triticale are sometimes harder to find. You can often order these from mail-order sources that carry whole grains (see Appendix 4).

Amaranth

Amaranth, a significant crop in scattered areas of the world, is only now being introduced to American cooks. It is especially valued for its nutritious leaves and its high-protein seeds containing protein that is of a higher quality than that of any other grain. Boiled in water and then chilled, amaranth seeds can be used to replace cornstarch as a thickening agent.

Barley

Barley is most often associated in American minds with beer brewing, but its best use is in the kitchen where one can make, among many possibilities, a delicious pilaf of barley cooked in chicken broth with onions and mushrooms.

Pearled barley, with its nutritious outer husk removed by abrasion, is the most readily available form of this grain. Whole grain brown barley

Cooked Volume (cups)	Most Common Uses	Suggested Grain Substitutes
2½	Cooked whole or cracked to make breakfast cereal. Milled to make flour for yeast breads with ryelike flavor.	rye, wheat
2⅔	Boiled grains can be added to rice and burgers for a chewy texture, or blended into casseroles, meatloaf, stuffings.	rye, triticale
2⅓	Can be used much the same as wheat berries or bulgur.	buckwheat groats, short grain brown rice, rye, triticale
2½	Used as breakfast cereal or as a side dish. Can replace rice in most recipes. Used in casseroles, tabbouleh. Sautéed with vegetables.	buckwheat groats, short grain brown rice, rye, triticale

(also known as *pot* or *Scotch barley*) is more nutritious because only a single outer layer has been removed, but it is harder to find. This form of barley must be soaked overnight before cooking.

Buckwheat

Botanically speaking, buckwheat is a fruit (related to the rhubarb plant), but its three-cornered seed is treated as a grain. The nutty, appealing flavor of *buckwheat groats* receives the most serious attention in Russian cuisine—*varnishkas,* blini, and kasha, for example—but the cooks in America are fast learning that *buckwheat flour* can be used for more than pancakes.

Corn

Cornmeal may be ground from either white or yellow corn. White cornmeal, when cooked, has a slightly rougher texture than the yellow, but there is so little difference in flavor that they are virtually interchangeable in recipes. Most cooks use the color specified in a recipe only to get the texture intended. Whichever you choose, try to buy stone-ground cornmeal. *Bolted* and *degermed cornmeal* have had much of the germ-bearing hull removed with sieves, thus losing large portions of the nutrients present in whole cornmeal. Whole meal is more perishable, but better all around.

Masa harina is a special corn flour popular throughout Mexico and Latin America. This fine cornmeal soaked in limewater gives tortillas their characteristic nutty-sweet flavor. It can be purchased in Mexican or Spanish grocery stores and from many suppliers that carry whole grains.

Cornstarch, made from the heart or endosperm of the corn, is a silken powder with little nutritive value, but it is quite suitable as a thickening agent (see Thickeners, page 136).

Hominy and *hominy grits* are highly refined products of corn. Corn that has been hulled and degermed is called by the Algonquin name, hominy. Hominy grits are dried hominy ground to a meal to give uniform granular particles. The precious corn germ and bran are almost completely absent in both of these products, and they contain only one-half to one-third of the B vitamins found in whole corn.

Millet

Millet has a texture and taste somewhere between egg-rich pasta and cornmeal. It swells tremendously when cooked, and makes a delicious breakfast cereal when topped with fruit and maple syrup. It is the major staple grain in Africa.

Oats

Oats is the only one of all the grains that emerges from the rigors of processing still clinging to its nutrients. Only the fibrous hull which has little nutritional value is removed in milling, leaving the groat which contains the bulk of the bran, endosperm, and germ. *Steel-cut oats* are made by cutting the groats into pieces with steel rollers. *Rolled oats,* the most familar form, are made by flaking the groats, a process that cracks the kernel and makes the nutrients in it more available to the digestive system. At the same time it permits the oats to absorb liquid faster, and so reduces cooking time. Steel-cut or rolled oats is the product grandma added to boiling water, simmered for 40 minutes, and served with milk, cinnamon, fruit, or maple syrup.

Rice

Brown rice has always taken a backseat, in terms of popularity, to the less nutritious white product in the United States. White rice is "enriched" just as white bread is, meaning a few nutrients are returned to it after processing, but much of the fiber, fat, and several other nutrients contained in the discarded bran and germ are lost forever. White rice has a rather bland flavor when compared with the brown; it cooks up in 12 to 14 minutes. Brown rice has a rich, nutty, definite taste and requires more cooking time, but no more fuss,

than the white. *Long grain brown rice,* used in Chinese, Indian, Indonesian, and Middle Eastern cooking, is dry and fluffy and the grains remain separate when cooked. *Short grain brown rice,* starchier and stickier than long grain rice when cooked, is used primarily in Japanese cooking. *Sweet brown rice,* a short grain brown rice with high sugar and starch content, is a sweet-tasting, sticky grain suited to oriental rice cakes and puddings.

Nutritious Rice Supplements

Consider adding these nutritious and tasty rice products to your pantry stock. Two to three tablespoons mixed into food dishes will notably increase the amount of B vitamins without altering flavor. They are available in natural foods stores.

Rice bran, the nutty-tasting outer bran layer that is a by-product of processed brown rice, can be added to baked goods or cereals and used in much the same way as wheat bran.

Rice grits, coarsely cracked brown rice, add taste and chewy texture to soups, stews, and casseroles. Use rice grits cup for cup to replace regular rice, following the same cooking directions.

Brown rice flour, made from ground short grain brown rice, can replace up to 15 percent of the wheat flour used in baking, yielding a drier, crispier texture.

Parboiled or *converted rice* falls midway between brown rice and white rice in terms of nutrition. This rice is steamed before being dried, and then polished to make it white. The steaming forces 70 percent or more of the B vitamins and some minerals in the bran and germ into the rice kernel.

Wild rice is not a grain but the seed of an aquatic grass related to the rice family. Its unique flavor is akin to that of grains, however, and it is used in much the same way. As its name implies, it is a wild crop, growing in northern Minnesota, Wisconsin lake country, and southern Canada. The system of harvesting, carefully controlled by law and custom, makes it rare and, consequently, expensive.

Rye

Rye flour is the most common form of that grain. It is most popular in Scandinavian countries where people eat a lot of *knäckebröd,* a rye crisp bread baked from unsifted whole rye flour. Rye grain is quite hardy and can be used much the same as whole wheat or triticale grain. Whole rye grains, called *rye berries,* will cook faster if allowed to soak for several hours (see Tips for Cooking Grains, page 289).

Sorghum

Sorghum, also known as *milo,* is another grain that has a much better image in other parts of the world than it does in the United States. Here it is used mainly by industry as a sweetener in the form of syrup boiled down from the sap of sweet sorghum stalks. In Africa and parts of India, sorghum is a major cereal grain; the Chinese and Japanese savor it boiled, as they boil rice.

Triticale

Triticale, the youngest of all grains, is a crossbreed of wheat and rye. Its name derives from *triticum* and *secale,* the Latin for wheat and rye. The new grain successfully combines the best in flavor, nutrition, and cooking possibilities of wheat and rye.

Wheat

Wheat berries (as the whole wheat grain is usually called) are sometimes sprouted to make a sweeter flour or to make diastatic malt (see Sprouts chapter). Like rye and triticale they are slow cooking and so are particularly suited to the thermos method. Wheat berries can also be heated and pressed flat and sold as *wheat flakes.* Wheat flakes resemble oatmeal in appearance and can be used similarly.

Cracked wheat is produced by cracking the whole wheat grain between rollers. *Bulgur* is actually cracked wheat that has been hulled and parboiled. The parboiling conserves most of the nutrients by leaching them from the outer layer to the center of the grain.

Farina is a wheat product prepared by grinding and sifting the wheat grain to a granular form. Made from wheat other than durum, it has the bran and most of the germ removed. Enriched farina has some of the B vitamins and minerals returned.

Bran and Germ

The bran and germ portions of grains are generally discarded in modern processing, leaving only the starchy endosperm as the end product. Bran, the brown husk of the grain that gives whole wheat flour its characteristic color, fell victim to the whiter-is-better philosophy. Wheat germ spoils very quickly because the fat it naturally contains tends toward rancidity; also, its nutrients attract insects and rodents. Manufacturers remove the germ to increase the shelf life of flour.

Bran is a concentrated source of B vitamins and minerals, but fiber is its greatest asset. Now that the role of fibrous foods in the prevention of many modern-day diseases has been defined and upheld by medical research, bran is finding its way into more diets as a supplement. It can be found in most natural foods stores and is easy to add to all types of dishes—sprinkle it on top of breakfast cereals, include it in the mix for homemade bread, muffins, and cookies, or add a few tablespoons to casseroles and meat loaves. Bran has a nutty, wholesome flavor when toasted.

Many health-minded people take wheat germ more seriously than commercial millers do. They are not willing to sacrifice important vitamins and minerals for a lighter, fluffier bread with a longer shelf life. The tiny embryo of the grain contains a nutritional powerhouse—the entire B complex, except B_{12}, plus protein, iron, and other minerals.

Because the germ is perishable, it should be stored carefully—tightly sealed and refrigerated. Toasting is the best way to preserve wheat germ, though it reduces the nutrient content slightly. You can toast wheat germ by spreading it evenly on a baking sheet and baking it for 15 to 20 minutes at 325°F until lightly browned. Stir occasionally to avoid burning. (Toast bran the same way.) Toasted germ will keep from two to six months if refrigerated or stored in the freezer. Of course, if it smells rancid or tastes bitter, discard it. Frozen wheat germ can be used directly from the freezer.

Wheat germ is easily incorporated into anybody's diet. It can be eaten by itself as a cold or hot cereal, or added to any dish. Athletes and health-conscious people take wheat germ as a nutritional supplement, blended with yogurt, fruit, and nuts to make a health shake, or sprinkled on fruit or vegetable salads, ice cream, and pudding. It can be added to pancakes and any baked goods. Wheat germ blends well with ground meat and can also be used to make a superb coating mix for fish or chicken.

Corn germ, another nutritious by-product of milling, is usually processed for its oil. Like wheat germ, corn germ is a good source of protein, vitamins, and minerals, and can be used interchangeably with wheat germ.

Amaranth

Baked Amaranth Pudding

This lemony, fragrant custard is enhanced with the taste and texture of amaranth grains.

    3 eggs
    1 cup milk
    ½ cup honey
    1 teaspoon vanilla extract
    1 teaspoon grated lemon rind
    1 teaspoon lemon juice

    ½ cup raisins
    2 cups cooked amaranth

Preheat oven to 350°F. Butter 8 to 12 individual custard cups.

In a large bowl beat eggs, then add milk and honey and mix well. Add remaining ingredients and blend together thoroughly.

Pour mixture into custard cups and set cups inside a large shallow baking pan containing 1 inch boiling water. Bake for about 1 hour, or until custards are firm. (Point of a knife inserted near edge of custard should come out clean.) Serve warm or cold. May be accompanied by fresh cream, if desired.

    8 to 12 servings

Vegetable, Amaranth, and Bulgur Pilaf

    1 large onion, chopped
    1 carrot, halved lengthwise, then thickly sliced
    1 stalk celery, finely chopped
    2 tablespoons butter
    2 cloves garlic, minced
    ¼ cup brown amaranth
    ½ cup bulgur
    1 teaspoon crumbled dried sage
    1¼ cups water
    2 tablespoons minced, fresh, mixed herbs
        (chervil, dill, and parsley, or other herbs)
    ⅓ cup grated Parmesan cheese
    ¼ cup slivered almonds

In a 1½- to 2-quart heavy-bottom saucepan sauté onions, carrots, and celery in 1 tablespoon butter over medium heat for a few minutes, or until onion separates. Add garlic and amaranth and cook for 5 more minutes, stirring occasionally.

Add remaining butter and bulgur. Cook and stir a few minutes, until bulgur becomes more golden. Stir in sage and then water. Cover and bring to a boil. Stir thoroughly, scraping bottom of pan, then cover again and reduce heat to a slow simmer. Cook for about 30 minutes, or until bulgur is tender and fluffy.

Season with fresh herbs and stir in cheese just before serving. Top with almonds.

    4 servings

Barley

Beef, Whole Barley, and Dried Lima Bean Stew (Cholent)

Cholent is a traditional lunch for Jews on Saturday upon returning from synagogue (shul). Some say the word is derived from the German Shule ende (meaning, synagogue services have ended—time to eat). Preparation of this stew begins the night before serving.

2 or 3 cloves garlic
  1 teaspoon paprika
  ½ teaspoon pepper
  2½ pounds lean, boneless, first-cut brisket of beef
  1½ cups dried large lima beans
  3 tablespoons chicken fat
  4 medium-size onions, thinly sliced
  7 cups hot Poultry Stock (page 110), or more as needed
  1 cup whole barley
  2 bay leaves

Using a mortar and pestle, mash garlic with paprika and pepper until a paste is formed. Smear paste on both sides of meat, cover loosely, and refrigerate overnight.

Soak lima beans overnight (see page 261 for soaking directions).

Next day, heat 2 tablespoons chicken fat in a large skillet until very hot. Add meat and brown on both sides. Transfer to a large heavy ovenproof casserole with a cover.

In same skillet heat remaining chicken fat. Add onions and sauté until well browned. Add 2 cups stock and stir and scrape bottom of pan to deglaze. Pour over meat in casserole.

Preheat oven to 400°F.

Drain lima beans and add to casserole along with barley, remaining 5 cups stock, and bay leaves. Cover and bake for 30 minutes, then check to see that liquid still covers ingredients. Add more stock if necessary. Reduce heat to 225°F and bake for 2½ hours longer.

To serve, lift out meat and remove bay leaves. Cut meat into equal portions and replace on top of casserole. Serve hot.

6 to 8 servings

Three-Bean, Barley, and Greens Casserole

A budget-aware meal-in-a-dish, this colorful bean and grain casserole is flavored with diced lamb, spinach, and herbs and topped with a cool mint-yogurt sauce.

  ½ cup dried lentils
  2 tablespoons olive oil
  1 large clove garlic, minced
  1 large onion, finely chopped
  ½ pound boneless lamb, trimmed of fat and cubed
  ½ teaspoon pepper
  pinch of crushed red pepper
  1 teaspoon turmeric
  ¼ cup uncooked long grain brown rice
  ½ cup barley
  3 cups Beef Stock (page 110)
  1 cup cooked chick-peas, drained
  1 cup cooked kidney beans, drained
  4 cups shredded spinach
  2 scallions, thinly sliced
  ½ cup minced fresh parsley
  ¼ cup minced fresh dill

  Sauce
  1 cup yogurt
  2 tablespoons minced fresh mint

Soak lentils (see page 261 for soaking directions). Drain and set aside.

Heat oil in a 5-quart heavy-bottom pot. Add garlic and onions and sauté over medium heat until softened. Add lamb, both kinds of pepper, and turmeric and cook, stirring, until meat loses pink color. Add rice and barley and stir for 2 minutes longer. Add stock and bring to a boil, then reduce heat, stir once, and cover pot. Simmer over low heat for 20 minutes.

Add lentils and cook for 15 minutes more. Stir in chick-peas and kidney beans and cook for another 5 to 10 minutes, or until all liquid has been absorbed.

Mix spinach, scallions, parsley, and dill together in a bowl and then add to pot. Stir gently over low heat until greens wilt. Transfer mixture to a warmed casserole to serve.

To make the sauce: Mix yogurt and mint together and serve separately in a sauce boat.

6 to 8 servings

Whole Barley and Mixed Fruit Pudding

The barley is soaked for 24 hours in preparing this delicate, fruity pudding.

1 cup whole barley
4 cups water
½ cup dried apples, cut into small pieces
¼ cup raisins
1 cup mixed dried fruits, cut into halves
(apricots, pears, and pitted prunes, or other fruits)
1 teaspoon shredded orange or tangerine rind
¼ teaspoon ground cloves
1 teaspoon ground cinnamon
3 to 4 tablespoons mild honey
2 tablespoons frozen orange juice concentrate
1 tablespoon butter

Combine barley with water and set aside to soak for 24 hours. Drain soaking water into a 1-quart measuring cup and add enough additional water to equal 4 cups. Pour into a large saucepan and bring to a boil. Add barley, cover pot, reduce heat, and simmer for 10 minutes.

Preheat oven to 350°F. Butter bottom and sides of a 2-quart soufflé dish.

Mix remaining ingredients together, except butter, and add to barley and liquid. Spoon into soufflé dish and bake for 40 minutes. Remove from oven, stir once, and dot with butter. Return to oven to bake for 15 minutes more. Serve warm, accompanied by cold milk poured from a pitcher at the table.

6 to 8 servings

Baked Barley-Prune Custard

4 cups milk
¼ cup barley
2 eggs
2 tablespoons honey
½ teaspoon vanilla extract
¼ cup chopped dried prunes
ground cinnamon

Place milk in a large saucepan. Add barley, cover, and cook slowly for 45 to 55 minutes, or until barley is tender.

Preheat oven to 350°F.

In a small bowl beat eggs. Add honey, vanilla, and prunes.

Slowly stir egg mixture into barley and cook over very low heat for 5 minutes, stirring constantly. Spoon mixture into 4 to 6 individual custard cups and sprinkle lightly with cinnamon.

Bake for 10 to 15 minutes, or until custard is set. Cool, then refrigerate. Serve cold.

4 to 6 servings

Barley-Rice Pilaf

This is a superior side dish with lamb or poultry. With the suggested variations it becomes a satisfying meatless main course.

1 tablespoon butter
1 medium-size onion, chopped
2 cloves garlic, minced
½ cup barley
½ cup uncooked brown rice
2 cups Beef Stock (page 110) or Poultry Stock (page 110)
1 tablespoon lemon juice

Melt butter in a medium-size skillet. Add onions, garlic, barley, and rice. Stirring constantly, sauté until onions are translucent and rice and barley are slightly browned. Let cool for 1 to 2 minutes.

Add stock and lemon juice and stir briefly with a fork. Bring pilaf quickly to a boil over high heat, then reduce heat to low, cover with a tight-fitting lid, and cook until liquid has been absorbed, 45 to 55 minutes.

4 to 6 servings

Variations:

Add ½ cup of one or more of the following to pilaf before serving:
coarsely chopped almonds, cashews, peanuts, pecans, or walnuts
hot, sautéed, coarsely chopped green peppers
hot, sautéed, sliced mushrooms

Barley with Grapes and Sweet-Sour Cabbage

1 tablespoon butter
1 medium-size onion, finely chopped (about ¾ cup)
4 cups shredded cabbage
3 tablespoons white wine vinegar
1 tablespoon honey
1½ cups white grape juice
2 cups cooked barley
½ teaspoon pepper
3 tablespoons minced fresh parsley
18 blue and red grapes

Melt butter in a large heavy skillet. Add onions and sauté until lightly browned. Add cabbage and stir and cook over low heat for 3 minutes.

Mix vinegar, honey, and grape juice together, then add to cabbage and onions and continue to cook for 20 minutes.

Stir in barley and pepper and simmer, covered, for 10 more minutes, or until cabbage is tender and most liquid has been absorbed. Before serving, sprinkle with parsley and dot with grapes.

6 servings

Barley with Peas, Shredded Carrots, and Mint

This side dish is quick to prepare and is especially good with chicken.

    3 tablespoons butter
    1 medium-size onion, finely chopped
    3 cups cooked barley
    ½ cup rich Poultry Stock (page 110)
    1 cup shredded carrots
    1 package (10 ounces) frozen green peas, partially thawed
    ¼ teaspoon pepper
    1 tablespoon minced fresh mint or 1 teaspoon dried mint

In a medium-size skillet melt butter. Add onions and sauté until lightly browned. Stir in barley and cook for 5 minutes. Stir in remaining ingredients, except mint. Cover skillet and cook over medium heat for 5 minutes. Spoon into a warmed serving dish and sprinkle with mint.

6 servings

Buckwheat

Eggplant and Buckwheat Patties

Crisp on the outside, this side dish is nutty and flavorful and can also be used as a no-meat main dish.

    1 medium-size eggplant, peeled and cubed (2½ cups)
    2 cloves garlic, minced
    juice of 1 lemon
    grated rind of 1 lemon
    2 tablespoons olive oil
    1 tablespoon butter

    1 large onion, minced
    2 cups cooked fine buckwheat groats
    2 tablespoons minced celery leaves or fresh lovage
    ¼ teaspoon pepper
    1 tablespoon minced fresh parsley
    1 egg, beaten
    3 tablespoons light buckwheat flour, or more if needed
    corn oil, for frying

Steam eggplant in a vegetable steamer for 8 to 10 minutes, or until tender. Transfer to a glass or ceramic bowl and toss with garlic, lemon juice, lemon rind, and olive oil. Set aside to marinate for 1 hour. Then finely chop in a food processor or blender, along with marinating liquid.

Meanwhile, heat butter and brown onions in a large skillet. Cool, then add remaining ingredients, except corn oil. Stir in chopped eggplant. Mixture should be fairly stiff; add a little more flour if necessary.

Heat corn oil in another large skillet. Drop mixture by the tablespoon into hot oil and fry until golden brown on each side. Drain on paper towels. Serve hot.

Makes about 1½ dozen

Kasha

This traditional buckwheat dish from eastern Europe is an excellent alternative to potatoes or rice as part of a meal. It goes especially well with brisket of beef and gravy.

    1 egg, beaten
    1½ cups coarse buckwheat groats
    3 to 4 cups boiling water
    1 medium-size onion, diced
    ½ cup sliced mushrooms (optional)
    2 tablespoons chicken fat or vegetable oil

Add egg to groats and mix well with a fork. Heat a large heavy skillet and add groats mixture. Stir constantly over moderate heat until groats are dry and toasty. Add 3 cups boiling water gradually, while stirring. Cover pan, reduce heat, and cook for 15 minutes, or until grains fluff up and are tender. If kasha begins to dry out, add more boiling water, a little at a time.

While groats are cooking, brown onions and mushrooms (if used) in fat or oil and then add them to groats. Stir and serve.

6 servings

Liver, Buckwheat, and Onions in Potato Nests

Prepare in advance and bake just before dinner, to serve as a side dish—or make very tiny ones for party hors d'oeuvres.

> 3 tablespoons chicken fat or butter
> 6 to 7 medium-size onions, coarsely chopped
> ¼ pound mushrooms, coarsely chopped
> ½ pound calf's liver
> 1 cup cooked coarse or medium buckwheat groats
> 1 tablespoon minced fresh parsley
> 3 tablespoons sour cream
> ⅛ teaspoon white pepper
> 6 to 7 medium-size potatoes, cooked until tender
> 2 eggs
> 1 teaspoon baking powder
> ⅛ teaspoon cayenne pepper
> ½ cup light buckwheat flour

Melt chicken fat or butter in a large heavy skillet. Add onions and sauté over medium-high heat until browned, about 15 to 20 minutes. Stir constantly to prevent burning. Transfer ¾ cup browned onions to a large bowl and place remainder (about ¼ cup) in a medium-size bowl. Let cool.

In same skillet sauté mushrooms for 1 to 2 minutes, then add to bowl containing ¼ cup onions.

Sauté liver in same skillet for 1 to 2 minutes on each side over medium-high heat. (The center should be slightly pink.) Remove liver, cut into small pieces, and add to mushroom mixture. Place in a food processor along with buckwheat and parsley and chop finely. Remove filling from processor and combine with sour cream and white pepper. Set aside.

Mash potatoes together with reserved ¾ cup onions, eggs, baking powder, and cayenne. Add flour last.

Flour hands well and divide potato mixture into 20 equal portions. Form into balls and place on a greased baking sheet. With the back of a round soup-spoon, press a well in each ball to form a "nest." Evenly distribute liver filling among potato nests, forming a mound in each one. Cover and refrigerate until cooking time.

Preheat oven to 350°F.

Bake for about 25 minutes, or until potatoes are lightly golden. Serve hot.

Makes 20

Sunflower Seed-Buckwheat Patties

> 1 cup buckwheat groats
> 3 eggs
> 2 cups boiling water
> 2 small onions, thinly sliced
> ½ pound mushrooms, chopped
> 1 teaspoon vegetable oil
> 1 tablespoon chopped fresh parsley
> 1 tablespoon chopped sunflower seeds

In a large heavy saucepan combine buckwheat with 1 egg and sauté, stirring constantly, until groats are dry and toasty. Add boiling water, cover, and simmer for 15 to 20 minutes, or until water has been absorbed.

While groats are cooking, sauté onions and mushrooms in oil for about 5 minutes, then add to cooked groats. Beat parsley, remaining 2 eggs, and sunflower seeds together and combine with groats.

Form mixture into 3-inch patties or drop by the tablespoon into a hot oiled skillet. Sauté on both sides until browned. Serve hot.

Makes 8

Corn

Baked Indian Pudding

> 4 cups milk
> ¼ cup butter
> ⅔ cup molasses
> 3 tablespoons honey
> ⅔ cup cornmeal
> ¾ teaspoon ground cinnamon
> ¾ teaspoon ground nutmeg

Heat 3 cups milk in a 2-quart saucepan. Stir in butter, molasses, and honey. Combine cornmeal with spices and stir gradually into warm milk mixture, using a wire whisk to avoid lumps. Cook over low heat, stirring constantly, for about 10 minutes, or until thick.

Preheat oven to 300°F.

Turn pudding into an oiled 2-quart ovenproof casserole, pour remaining 1 cup milk over top (do not stir), and bake for 3 hours. Serve warm.

6 to 8 servings

Corn Bread

1 cup stone-ground cornmeal
1 cup whole wheat flour
½ cup nonfat dry milk
2 teaspoons baking powder
2 eggs, beaten
1 cup buttermilk
3 tablespoons vegetable oil

Preheat oven to 350°F.

In a large bowl stir together cornmeal, flour, dry milk, and baking powder. Make a well in center of dry mixture and into this place eggs, buttermilk, and oil. Mix lightly, only until ingredients are moistened.

Pour batter into a well-buttered 8-inch-square baking pan. Bake for 30 minutes, or until browned and wooden pick inserted into center of bread comes out clean. Cool slightly, then cut into 2-inch squares. Serve warm or cold.

Makes 16 squares

Paprika Corn Wafers

Delicate, fragile, and paper thin, here is an inexpensive snack food that can be served as a change from potato chips.

⅔ cup Quaker cornmeal*
2 tablespoons butter, cut into small pieces
¾ cup boiling water
⅛ teaspoon chili powder
paprika

Preheat oven to 400°F. Line a large baking sheet with foil. Butter the foil generously and set aside.

Place cornmeal in a medium-size bowl. Put butter pieces into a small bowl or jar and pour boiling water over them, stirring to melt. Then add to cornmeal and stir. Add chili powder, mix, and let stand for 5 minutes. Batter will be very thin.

Stirring after each spoonful, drop batter by the teaspoon onto baking sheet. Spoon only 3 to a row and no more than 9 on a sheet, since they spread. Bake for 7 to 10 minutes, or until dry and very lightly browned at the edges. Lift off carefully with a wide spatula, place on a wire rack to cool, and dust with paprika.

Makes 2 to 2½ dozen

*Use Quaker cornmeal for best results.

Peppered Corn Nuts

Try this crunchy snack as an inexpensive alternative to nuts.

1 cup dried corn
2 tablespoons corn oil
pepper, to taste

Soak corn overnight in water to cover. Drain, rinse, and dry thoroughly on paper towels.

Heat oil in a medium-size heavy skillet until very hot. Add corn and, shaking pan or stirring constantly, toast for about 5 minutes, until corn begins to turn a light golden brown. Drain on paper towels and sprinkle with pepper. Serve warm.

Makes 1 cup

Variation:

Peppered Hominy Nuts: Replace soaked dried corn with 1 cup cooked whole hominy and toast as directed.

Spoon Bread

Spoon bread makes a fine accompaniment to a meat course, or it may be served as a luncheon dish with sour cream, cottage cheese, or a tomato or mushroom sauce.

1½ cups milk
¾ cup cornmeal
3 eggs, separated
3 tablespoons vegetable oil

Preheat oven to 375°F.

Scald milk in a 1-quart saucepan. With a wire whisk stir in cornmeal and cook for 15 minutes, or until thickened. Add egg yolks and oil and mix well. Remove from heat and cool slightly.

Beat egg whites until stiff but not dry, then fold into cornmeal mixture. Transfer batter to a well-buttered 8-inch-square baking pan and bake for 35 to 40 minutes. Serve hot.

8 servings

Variation:

Spoon Bread, Italian Style: After adding egg yolks and oil, stir in ¾ cup shredded sharp cheddar cheese and 1 tablespoon each chopped green peppers and chopped scallions.

Polenta Cheese Squares

This traditional Italian favorite appears in many regions in place of pasta and, like pasta, can be served with a variety of sauces to vary the importance of its role in the meal.

    5 cups water
1½ cups white or yellow cornmeal
    1 cup grated sharp cheddar cheese
⅓ cup grated Parmesan cheese
1½ cups tomato sauce, warmed

In a large heavy saucepan bring water to a boil. Add cornmeal very slowly, stirring constantly with a wire whisk or long wooden spoon until mixture is thick and free from lumps. Transfer mixture to top of a double boiler, cover, and cook for 30 minutes, stirring occasionally. Cornmeal is ready when it leaves sides of pan.

Remove cornmeal from heat and turn into a lightly oiled 9-inch-square baking pan. Cool and refrigerate for 3 to 4 hours, until stiff enough to cut. (Or, refrigerate overnight.)

Preheat oven to 400°F.

Cut polenta into 16 squares and arrange these in an oiled 9 × 13-inch baking dish. Sprinkle with cheddar and Parmesan cheeses and bake for 15 minutes, or until cheese has melted and browned. Serve immediately, topped with tomato sauce.

6 to 8 servings

NOTE: Polenta may also be prepared by adding cheddar cheese to cornmeal mixture just before removing from heat. Sprinkle with Parmesan cheese before placing in oven.

Rhode Island Jonnycakes

The name is said to be a corruption of "journey cakes," since these cornmeal breads were commonly carried by travelers in earlier times for convenient nourishment on the road. Today, they are a popular accompaniment to seafood or poultry.

    1 cup stone-ground white cornmeal
1¼ cups boiling water
¼ cup milk, or more to taste
    1 tablespoon honey
    1 tablespoon butter, melted

Place cornmeal in a 2-quart bowl. Stir in water, milk, honey, and butter. Mix thoroughly. For thinner and crisper cakes add a little more milk.

Drop batter by the tablespoon onto a hot well-buttered griddle and cook for 6 to 8 minutes, or until browned and crisp on bottom. (For best results, do not turn cakes prematurely.) Then turn cake over and cook reverse side for 4 to 5 minutes, or until browned. Serve hot with butter or maple syrup.

Makes about 15

Millet

Chinese Stir-Fried Vegetables with Tofu and Millet

Sauce
½ cup Poultry Stock (page 110) or Vegetable Stock (page 111)
    2 tablespoons soy sauce
½ teaspoon crushed aniseed or Chinese Five-Spice Powder (page 62)*
    1 teaspoon mild honey
    2 teaspoons cider vinegar
½ teaspoon grated peeled ginger root
    1 tablespoon plus 1 teaspoon cornstarch

Vegetables
    2 tablespoons peanut oil
    1 small hot chili pepper (optional)
    1 large onion, cut in half vertically and thinly sliced
    1 clove garlic, minced
    1 teaspoon grated peeled ginger root
1½ cups tiny cauliflower florets
1½ cups thinly sliced mushrooms
1½ cups cubed zucchini
    2 small sweet red peppers, cut into ¾-inch squares
    2 tablespoons Poultry Stock (page 110), mixed with 1 tablespoon soy sauce
    1 cup bean sprouts
    1 cup fresh or frozen peas
    2 cups shredded Swiss chard or spinach
    12 ounces firm tofu, drained and cubed

3 to 4 cups hot cooked millet
⅓ cup roasted cashews
    1 tablespoon minced fresh coriander

To make the sauce: Blend all sauce ingredients together and set aside.

To make the vegetables: Have all ingredients cut, measured, and assembled in separate piles, in order of use, before beginning to stir-fry.

Heat a wok or a large skillet over high heat and add peanut oil. When oil is very hot, add chili (if used), onions, garlic, and ginger. Stir constantly, keeping ingredients moving at all times, until onions are translucent. Remove chili and discard. Add cauliflower and stir and cook for 2 minutes. Then add mushrooms and stir and cook for 1 minute. Add zucchini and sweet peppers and stir-fry for 2 minutes. Stir in stock and soy sauce and cook for 1 minute more. Add bean sprouts, peas, and Swiss chard or spinach and stir-fry for 2 minutes. Then stir in tofu and reserved sauce. Sauce should glaze vegetables and thicken in 2 minutes' time. Keep vegetables moving constantly throughout cooking. When crisp-tender and glazed, pile on top of hot millet, sprinkle with cashews and coriander, and serve at once.

6 servings

*Five-spice powder is also available in oriental grocery stores.

Marinated Millet Salad with Layered Vegetables and Bean Sprouts

This piquant salad must be prepared several hours in advance. It can be kept in the refrigerator for 3 to 4 days, and will then become red from the beet juice.

Marinade

½ cup red wine vinegar
¼ cup water
2 teaspoons mixed pickling spices
2 tablespoons safflower oil
2 or 3 drops sesame oil
2 teaspoons soy sauce

Salad

2 cups soy or mung bean sprouts
1 cup cooked millet
1½ cups shredded carrots
1 large green pepper, cut into julienne strips
1 medium-size beet, peeled and shredded
2 tablespoons minced fresh chives

lettuce leaves

To make the marinade: Combine all marinade ingredients in a small saucepan. Bring to a boil, then reduce heat and simmer for 5 minutes. Remove from heat and cool to room temperature.

To assemble the salad: First, place bean sprouts in a small bowl and add boiling water to cover. Let stand for 10 to 15 seconds to blanch, then drain and set aside.

In a clear glass bowl with deep sides, arrange millet, carrots (reserve ½ cup for garnish), blanched sprouts, peppers, and beets in layers in the order given. Pour marinade through a strainer across top of salad. Arrange reserved carrots in a ring on top of beet layer and sprinkle with chives. Cover and refrigerate for several hours or overnight.

To serve, use a slotted spoon to lift out vegetables and grain. Place salad on individual plates lined with lettuce leaves.

6 servings

Millet-Stuffed Peppers

4 green peppers, halved lengthwise and cored
1 tablespoon vegetable oil
1 medium-size onion, minced
½ pound lean ground beef
½ cup millet, cooked
2 tablespoons chopped fresh parsley
1 teaspoon dried oregano
1 tablespoon soy sauce
2 tablespoons wheat germ
2 tablespoons grated Parmesan cheese
1½ cups tomato sauce, warmed

Place pepper halves in a vegetable steamer and steam for 5 minutes. Set aside.

Heat oil in a large skillet. Add onions and beef and sauté for about 5 minutes, stirring to brown meat evenly.

Preheat oven to 350°F.

Combine meat mixture with cooked millet, parsley, oregano, and soy sauce and mound into pepper halves. Sprinkle tops with wheat germ and cheese. Place stuffed peppers in a large shallow baking pan and bake for 20 minutes. Serve hot, topped with tomato sauce.

4 to 6 servings

Millet, Ricotta, and Pineapple Pie with Pecan Crust

Easy and delicious, this is the ideal pie for people who are intimidated by the thought of making pastry crusts.

Crust

1½ cups plus 2 tablespoons ground pecans
   (7 to 8 ounces)
2 tablespoons butter, cut into small pieces and
   softened

Filling

1½ cups ricotta cheese
2 tablespoons frozen pineapple-orange juice
   concentrate
1 can (8 ounces) unsweetened crushed
   pineapple, drained
1 tablespoon honey
¾ cup cooked millet
1 teaspoon grated orange rind
1 teaspoon vanilla extract

⅛ teaspoon ground cinnamon

To make the crust: First, preheat oven to 350°F. Place pecans (reserve 2 tablespoons for garnish) and butter in a small bowl. Crush butter with your fingertips to incorporate it into ground nuts. When a mass is formed, press into a 9-inch pie plate, covering sides as well as bottom of plate. (Press thin to cover evenly.) Bake for 10 minutes, then remove from oven and let crust cool before adding filling.

To make the filling: Combine remaining ingredients, except cinnamon, in a bowl and beat with a wooden spoon until smooth.

Spoon filling into cooled crust. Mix reserved ground pecans with cinnamon and sprinkle over top of pie. Chill for 30 minutes before serving.

6 servings

Millet Soufflé

5 cups water
2 tablespoons vegetable oil
1 cup millet meal (whole millet coarsely ground
   in blender)
4 eggs, separated
¼ cup nonfat dry milk
½ teaspoon crushed dill seeds (optional)
3 tablespoons minced fresh chives or grated
   onions
1 cup grated or shredded sharp cheese

In a 2-quart saucepan bring 4 cups water and oil to a boil. Gradually add millet meal, stirring constantly with a wire whisk until smooth. Transfer mixture to top of a double boiler, cover, and cook for 20 to 30 minutes, or until all water has been absorbed. Stir mixture occasionally. Remove from heat and cool slightly.

Preheat oven to 350°F. Butter bottom and sides of a 2-quart soufflé dish.

In a large mixing bowl beat egg yolks with an electric mixer until foamy and thickened. Using a wire whisk combine dry milk with remaining 1 cup water, then beat mixture gradually into yolks.

With mixer set at medium speed, blend cooked millet into yolk mixture until thoroughly combined. Stir in dill seeds (if used) and chives or onions. Add cheese.

In a separate bowl beat egg whites until soft peaks form, then gently fold into millet mixture. Pour into soufflé dish and bake for 35 to 45 minutes. Serve immediately.

6 servings

Millet and Cheese Cocktail Snack

1 cup grated soft sharp cheddar cheese
1⅔ cups cooked millet
2 teaspoons prepared mustard
2 teaspoons horseradish, drained

In a small bowl combine cheese with ⅔ cup millet, mustard, and horseradish. Spread remaining millet onto a sheet of wax paper or across bottom of a pie plate.

Form cheese mixture into 20 balls, about ½ inch in diameter, then roll each ball in millet, pressing with your fingers so grains will adhere. Place balls on a plate lined with wax paper and chill for 45 minutes.

Preheat broiler.

Transfer balls to a shallow baking pan and place under broiler. Broil just until tops start to brown. Then remove from oven and use a spatula to turn them over carefully (they are fragile). Broil again for 1 to 2 minutes, or until reverse side is lightly browned. Serve at once, accompanied by whole grain crackers.

Makes 20

Sweet and Sour Meatballs, Middle Eastern Style

Meatballs

1 pound lean ground chuck
1 small onion, grated
2 tablespoons minced fresh parsley
½ cup cooked millet
¼ teaspoon ground cumin
⅛ teaspoon pepper
2 tablespoons tomato juice
1 egg, beaten
2 tablespoons olive oil

Sauce

3 tablespoons olive oil
6 medium-size onions, thinly sliced
1 cup tomato juice
1½ cups water
1 small butternut squash (about 1 pound), peeled, seeded, and cubed
⅓ cup raisins
10 pitted dried prunes
½ cup blanched almonds
1 teaspoon grated lemon rind
¼ cup lemon juice
¼ cup mild honey
1 teaspoon Syrian mixed spices* or ground allspice

4 cups hot cooked millet
1 tablespoon minced fresh parsley

To make the meatballs: Place all meatball ingredients, except oil, in a large bowl and knead until smooth. Add oil and knead again until incorporated. Wet hands and shape mixture into about 20 small balls, using 1 tablespoon mixture for each. Place meatballs on a plate lined with wax paper and refrigerate.

To make the sauce: Heat oil in a large skillet. Add onions and sauté over high heat, stirring occasionally, until browned. Add tomato juice and water and bring to a boil, then reduce heat and simmer for 5 minutes. Place meatballs in simmering liquid and cook until no longer pink. Remove meatballs with a slotted spoon and set aside.

To same skillet add remaining ingredients, except millet and parsley. Cover and simmer for 25 minutes, stirring gently once or twice during cooking. Then return meatballs to skillet, baste with cooking liquid (most of it should have been absorbed), and cook 5 minutes longer.

To serve, place hot millet in a mound on a large serving dish. With a slotted spoon lift fruit, vegetables, and meatballs out of skillet and arrange around base of millet. Spoon any remaining sauce over top of millet and sprinkle with parsley.

6 to 8 servings

*Syrian mixed spices is available in Middle Eastern grocery stores.

Oats

Almond Crunch Cereal

3 cups rolled oats
1½ cups unsweetened shredded coconut
½ cup wheat germ or soy grits
1 cup sunflower seeds
¼ cup sesame seeds
½ cup honey
¼ cup vegetable oil
½ cup cold water
1 cup slivered blanched almonds
½ cup raisins (optional)

Preheat oven to 225°F. Lightly oil a large shallow baking pan.

In a large mixing bowl combine oats, coconut, wheat germ or soy grits, sunflower seeds, and sesame seeds. Toss ingredients together thoroughly.

Combine honey and oil in a separate bowl. Add to dry ingredients, stirring until well mixed. Add water, a little at a time, mixing until crumbly. Pour mixture into baking pan and spread evenly to edges of pan.

Place pan on middle rack of oven and bake for 1½ hours, stirring every 15 minutes. Add almonds and continue to bake for 30 minutes longer, or until mixture is thoroughly dry and light brown in color. Cereal should feel crisp to the touch.

Turn oven off and allow cereal to cool in oven. Add raisins to cereal at this point (if used). When cool, remove cereal from oven and place in a tightly covered container. Store in a cool dry place. Serve with cold milk and fresh fruit.

Makes 8 cups

Cinnamon Oatmeal with Raisins and Seeds

Eating this hot breakfast cereal is like eating an oatmeal cookie!

2 cups water
½ cup raisins
1 cup rolled oats
½ teaspoon vanilla extract
1 teaspoon ground cinnamon
¼ cup sunflower or sesame seeds

In a 1-quart saucepan combine water and raisins and bring to a boil. Gradually stir in oats, vanilla, and cinnamon. Reduce heat and cook for 10 minutes.

Pour hot cereal into bowls and top with seeds. Serve with milk or yogurt.

4 servings

Meat Loaf with Oats

2 pounds ground chuck or round
⅓ cup wheat germ
½ cup rolled oats
2 tablespoons chopped fresh parsley
½ teaspoon freshly ground pepper
2 tablespoons soy sauce
½ cup chopped onions
2 tablespoons vegetable oil
2 eggs, beaten
¼ cup sour cream or yogurt
½ cup tomato juice
vegetable oil, for glazing

Preheat oven to 350°F. Oil a 9 × 5-inch loaf pan.

In a large mixing bowl combine ground beef, wheat germ, oats, parsley, pepper, and soy sauce. Set aside.

Sauté onions in 2 tablespoons oil until soft but not brown. Add to meat mixture.

Blend eggs together with sour cream or yogurt. Add to meat mixture. Then add tomato juice and mix thoroughly. Turn out meat mixture into loaf pan, packing down well. Allow to rest for 10 to 15 minutes in refrigerator.

Run a spatula around edge of meat loaf to loosen. Carefully turn out into a lightly oiled, large, shallow baking pan, keeping original shape as much as possible. Brush all sides of loaf with oil, then place on middle rack of oven and bake for 1¼ hours. Remove from oven and allow to rest for 10 minutes before serving.

6 to 8 servings

Oat Groats with Toasted Almonds and Soy Sauce

Soaked overnight, this may be served as a simple, hearty side dish with dinner—or omit the soy sauce and almonds and enjoy it as a basic hot cereal for breakfast.

1 cup oat groats
3 cups water
soy sauce, to taste
½ cup sliced or slivered almonds, toasted

Place oats in a 2-quart heavy-bottom saucepan, cover with the water, and allow to soak overnight in refrigerator.

Next day, bring mixture to a boil, then reduce heat to low and cook, uncovered, for 25 minutes, or until groats are soft. Stir often.

Serve hot, sprinkled with soy sauce and almonds.

6 servings

Scottish Oat Cakes

These cookielike crackers make an enjoyable snack or teatime treat. Serve them accompanied by jams or spreadable cheeses.

¼ teaspoon baking soda
¼ cup boiling water
½ cup date sugar
1 cup rolled oats
1 cup whole wheat flour
½ cup bran
¾ cup butter, softened
1 teaspoon soy sauce

Preheat oven to 350°F. Grease 2 baking sheets.

Add baking soda to boiling water and set aside to cool.

Mix all dry ingredients together in a large bowl. Using a pastry blender or 2 knives, cut in butter until mixture is crumbly. Add cooled baking soda water and soy sauce and knead mixture 4 or 5 times to make a fairly firm dough.

Place dough between 2 sheets of wax paper and roll out until quite thin, about ⅛ inch thick. Remove 1 sheet of wax paper and use a sharp knife to cut rolled dough into 2-inch squares. Transfer squares carefully onto baking sheets with a wide spatula. (Squares may be placed close together since they can be broken apart easily when baked and cooled.)

Gather any leftover dough together, roll out again, and cut more 2-inch squares, placing them on baking sheets as before. Bake for 10 to 12 minutes, or until edges are lightly browned.

Makes about 4 dozen

Tropical Fruit and Oat Bars

    1 cup pitted dates
    ¾ cup unsweetened crushed pineapple
    ¼ cup pineapple juice
    1½ cups whole wheat flour
    1 cup rolled oats
    ¼ cup date sugar
    ½ cup unsweetened flaked coconut
    ¼ teaspoon baking soda
    ½ cup butter
    1 egg, beaten

In a 1-quart saucepan combine dates, pineapple, and pineapple juice. Bring to a boil, then reduce heat to low and cook for about 5 minutes, stirring occasionally, until mixture has thickened.

Preheat oven to 375°F. Butter an 8-inch-square baking pan.

In a large mixing bowl combine flour, oats, date sugar, coconut, and baking soda. Cut in butter with a pastry blender or 2 knives, or put mixture into a food processor and blend until crumbly.

Take ½ of the crumb mixture and press it firmly across bottom of baking pan with your fingers. Then spoon and evenly spread pineapple-date mixture on top.

Add egg to remaining crumb mixture, then spread this evenly over layer of filling. Bake for 25 to 30 minutes, or until lightly browned. Cool in pan on a wire rack. When cold, cut into 2-inch squares.

Makes 16

Granola

Granola has become a popular cereal or snack food. It can be made even more delicious by adding several of the suggested variation ingredients.

    6 cups rolled oats
    ½ cup wheat germ
    ¼ cup honey
    ¼ cup vegetable oil
    1 cup raisins

Preheat oven to 300°F. Grease 3 large baking sheets with rims.

In a large bowl mix oats together with wheat germ.

In a small saucepan heat honey and oil until honey is thin and runny. Add mixture to oats and blend well.

Spread granola thinly and evenly on baking sheets and bake about 15 minutes, or until lightly browned. Cool. Spoon into a large bowl, add raisins, and mix thoroughly. Store in a tightly covered container and keep in a cool dry place.

Makes 7 cups

Variations:

■ Add ¼ cup of any one or combination of the following to oats along with wheat germ:

    coarsely chopped almonds, cashews, peanuts,
        or walnuts
    bran
    unsweetened shredded coconut
    sesame or sunflower seeds
    nonfat dry milk

■ Replace raisins with 1 cup of chopped dried apples, apricots, figs, peaches, pears, pineapple, prunes, or mixed dried fruits.

Rice

Brown Rice and Eggplant with Cheese Custard

This meatless version of Greek moussaka can be assembled a day ahead, and the cheese custard added before baking and serving. It is a festive and satisfying lunch or supper dish and is attractive enough for a party buffet.

1 large eggplant (about 1 pound), peeled and
   cut into ½-inch slices
5 tablespoons olive oil
1 large onion, finely chopped
1 large clove garlic, minced
4 large tomatoes, chopped
1 small carrot, shredded
1 teaspoon minced fresh basil or ½ teaspoon
   dried basil
¼ teaspoon pepper
½ teaspoon ground cinnamon
¼ cup minced fresh parsley
1 cup frozen peas
2 cups cooked long grain brown rice
½ cup coarsely chopped walnuts

   Custard
2 tablespoons butter
2 tablespoons whole wheat pastry flour
1½ cups low-fat milk
¼ teaspoon white pepper
⅛ teaspoon ground nutmeg
1 cup ricotta cheese
2 eggs, beaten
¼ cup grated Parmesan cheese

Preheat oven to 400°F.

Place eggplant slices in a lightly oiled 9 × 13-inch baking pan and drizzle 3 tablespoons olive oil over them. Bake on lowest rack in oven for 15 minutes.

While eggplant is baking, heat remaining oil in a large skillet. Add onions and garlic and stir and cook over medium heat until onions have wilted. Add tomatoes, carrots, basil, pepper, and cinnamon. Stir in parsley and peas and set aside.

Spread rice in a layer over eggplant slices and evenly spoon tomato mixture over it. Sprinkle with walnuts. At this point the dish may be refrigerated for several hours or overnight.

To make the custard: First, preheat oven to 350°F.

Melt butter in a 1-quart saucepan and then stir in flour. Add milk gradually, stirring constantly with a wire whisk, and cook over low heat for about 10 minutes, or until sauce is slightly thickened. Remove from heat and add pepper, nutmeg, and ricotta cheese, stirring with whisk. Add eggs, beating well with whisk, and then add Parmesan cheese. Pour custard over casserole and bake for 45 minutes. Let stand for 15 minutes before cutting into squares to serve.

   6 to 8 servings

Brown Rice Salad with Radishes and Snow Pea Pods

2 cups cooked long grain brown rice
3 or 4 scallions, chopped (about ¾ cup)
¼ pound snow pea pods (about 1 cup), blanched
¾ cup finely chopped celery, with leaves
1 medium-size cucumber, diced (about 1 cup)
8 to 10 large radishes, thinly sliced
1 small sweet red pepper, finely chopped
   (about ½ cup)
⅓ cup minced fresh parsley
2 tablespoons rice vinegar
2 tablespoons lemon juice
1 tablespoon soy sauce
¼ teaspoon pepper
½ teaspoon paprika
⅓ cup safflower oil

Combine rice, scallions, pea pods, celery, cucumbers, radishes, red peppers, and parsley in a large bowl.

Place vinegar, lemon juice, soy sauce, pepper, and paprika in a small bowl. Add oil gradually, beating constantly with a wire whisk, until well blended. Pour dressing over rice and vegetables and toss to combine. Cover and chill for 2 hours before serving.

   6 servings

Cashew-Rice Casserole

¼ cup butter
3 tablespoons olive or vegetable oil
½ cup chopped onions
½ cup chopped celery
2 cups sliced mushrooms
1 cup uncooked brown rice
¼ cup chopped fresh parsley
¼ cup chopped fresh dill
¼ teaspoon dried thyme

¼ teaspoon pepper
2½ to 3 cups hot Beef Stock (page 110)
    2 cups diced zucchini
    2 cups loosely packed spinach
    1 cup roasted cashews (pecans, almonds, or
        chopped Brazil nuts may be substituted)
    1 cup shredded Gruyère or Swiss cheese

Preheat oven to 325°F.

Heat butter and 2 tablespoons oil in a large skillet. Add onions, celery, and mushrooms and sauté over medium-high heat until onions are light golden in color. Add rice and continue to cook, stirring often, until rice is golden. Stir in parsley, dill, thyme, and pepper. Add 2½ cups stock and bring to a boil. Carefully pour mixture into a buttered 2-quart baking dish. Cover and bake for 1 hour, stirring once after 30 minutes of baking.

While rice bakes, heat remaining oil in skillet. Add zucchini and sauté for 2 minutes, or just until it changes color. Add spinach and cook just until wilted. Remove from heat.

After rice is removed from oven, stir in ¾ cup nuts and then sautéed vegetables. Return casserole to oven and bake 30 minutes longer, or until rice is tender, adding more stock if necessary. Then sprinkle remaining nuts and cheese over top and place under broiler just long enough to melt cheese.

6 servings

East Indian *Dosa* with Onion-Potato Filling
(Brown Rice and Lentil Flatbread)

The rice and lentils used in this wheat-free, pancakelike bread are soaked overnight and then fermented for 24 hours to enhance flavor and lightness. The basic dosa recipe makes 10 flatbreads. They are then stuffed with spiced vegetables and topped with yogurt for a complete meal.

    Dosa
    1 cup uncooked short grain brown rice
3½ cups water
    ½ cup dried green lentils
1 to 2 tablespoons milk
      pinch of baking soda
    1 tablespoon butter, melted
  ⅛ teaspoon cayenne pepper

    Filling
    2 tablespoons butter
  ½ teaspoon mustard seeds
    1 medium-size onion, chopped (about ¾ cup)
    1 large tomato, coarsely chopped
    2 medium-size potatoes (about ¾ pound),
      cooked and diced
  ¼ teaspoon cayenne pepper
  ¼ teaspoon turmeric
  ⅛ teaspoon pepper
    1 tablespoon minced fresh coriander

    yogurt, for topping

To make the *dosa:* Place rice in a bowl with 2 cups water and soak overnight. In a separate bowl soak lentils in 1½ cups water overnight. Next morning drain liquid from both, combine, and reserve.

In a blender puree rice plus ¼ cup reserved soaking water. Transfer puree to a bowl. Repeat process with lentils and same amount of water. Mix purees together, cover, and allow to ferment in a warm place for 24 hours.

To make the filling: Next day, before completing *dosa,* prepare filling. Melt butter in a medium-size skillet and add mustard seeds. Cook and stir for 1 minute. Add onions and sauté for 5 minutes, then add tomatoes and cook for 2 minutes more. Add potatoes, cayenne, turmeric, and pepper. Stir and cook until liquid has been absorbed and mixture is dry. Stir in coriander. Keep warm while *dosa* are cooked.

When ready to prepare *dosa,* add just enough milk to fermented mixture to make a batter the consistency of heavy cream. Stir in baking soda, melted butter, and cayenne.

Heat a 9-inch skillet. When hot, add ½ cup batter, turning pan quickly to distribute batter into a thin layer about 6 inches in diameter. Cook until surface is dry and small bubbles form on top, then invert onto a sheet of wax paper. Place another piece of wax paper on top and invert again. Peel surface piece of wax paper off and invert uncooked side of bread back into pan to cook for 1 to 2 minutes more. Slide bread carefully out of pan and keep in a warm oven until all batter is used up.

To serve, place several spoonfuls of onion-potato filling in the middle of each bread and top with a spoonful of yogurt. Fold 2 edges of bread over filling, as you would for a stuffed crepe, and eat with fingers or a fork.

4 servings

Herb, Tomato, and Rice Soup with Orange Rind and Nutmeg

The surprise of orange rind and nutmeg turns this simple soup into a gourmet treat. It is best made when fresh tomatoes are at their peak.

      2 tablespoons butter
      1 large onion, finely chopped
  7 to 8 medium-size tomatoes (2½ pounds),
          peeled and quartered
      4 cups Poultry Stock (page 110)
      4 sprigs thyme, tied together with string
      1 bay leaf
      4 leaves basil, minced
      1 strip of orange rind, 2 inches long
      1 cup cooked long grain brown rice
      ¼ cup heavy cream
      2 teaspoons honey, or to taste (optional)
      2 tablespoons minced fresh parsley
          few gratings of nutmeg

Melt butter in a large heavy-bottom saucepan. Add onions and sauté until wilted but not browned. Stir in tomatoes and stock and bring to a boil. Add thyme, bay leaf, basil, and orange rind, then cover pot and simmer for 20 minutes.

Remove thyme, bay leaf, and orange rind. Puree soup in a food processor or blender and return to pot. Add cooked rice and simmer for 10 minutes more. Then add cream. Stir in honey if a sweeter taste is desired. Before serving, sprinkle with parsley and nutmeg.

   6 servings

Green Rice Ring Mold Filled with Carrots

      7 tablespoons butter
      3 scallions, finely chopped (about ½ cup)
      1 large clove garlic, minced
      1 hot green chili pepper, seeded and chopped,
          or pinch of crushed red pepper
      ¼ cup minced fresh parsley
      ½ cup chopped celery leaves or fresh lovage
      1 cup shredded fresh sorrel, with ribs and
          stems removed
      ½ cup broccoli florets, finely chopped
      1 cup shredded Swiss chard (leaves only)
   2½ cups cooked short grain brown rice
      ¼ cup grated Gruyère cheese
  3 to 4 carrots, cut into 1-inch lengths

      1 teaspoon honey
      ⅛ teaspoon ground nutmeg

Preheat oven to 325°F. Generously butter a 6-cup ring mold.

Heat 3 tablespoons butter in a large skillet and sauté scallions, garlic, and chili or red pepper until soft. Process in a blender or food processor to a very fine puree. Set aside in a bowl. Then process parsley, celery leaves or lovage, sorrel, broccoli, and Swiss chard until very fine. Stir into scallion mixture. (This should be done in several batches.)

Melt 3 tablespoons butter and add to pureed mixture along with rice and cheese. Stir well.

Press rice mixture firmly into ring mold. Cover with foil and set mold in a larger pan. Pour boiling water into pan until it reaches ¾ of the way up the outside of the mold. Bake for 30 minutes.

Meanwhile, steam carrots for about 15 minutes, or until crisp-tender. Toss with honey, remaining 1 tablespoon butter, and nutmeg. Keep hot.

When mold is removed from oven, allow to rest for 5 minutes, then invert onto a serving platter. Spoon hot carrots into center of mold and serve.

   6 servings

Rice Mountain with Walnut Chicken and Vegetables

      2 cups hot, cooked, short grain brown rice
      ¼ cup peanut oil
      2 large whole chicken breasts, boned, skinned,
          and cut into 2-inch pieces
      1 slice peeled ginger root, ½ inch thick, minced
      2 large cloves garlic, minced
      1 large onion, cut into 8 pieces
      2 carrots, sliced paper thin on the diagonal
          (1 cup)
      1 cup tiny broccoli florets
      2 tablespoons soy sauce
      ¾ cup Poultry Stock (page 110)
      1 tablespoon cornstarch, dissolved in
          2 tablespoons water
      ¾ cup walnuts, roasted
      1 small bunch watercress or several sprigs
          fresh coriander (optional)

Press rice into a deep buttered bowl and keep warm in oven.

Heat oil in a wok until very hot. (Test for temperature by sprinkling a drop or two of water into pan.

If water "pops," temperature is correct.) Add chicken, ginger, and garlic and stir-fry for 2 minutes. Add onions, carrots, and broccoli and stir-fry for 1 minute. Remove vegetables with a slotted spoon and set aside.

Add soy sauce and stock to wok and bring to a boil. Cover and continue cooking for 3 minutes. Remove cover and add cornstarch and water mixture. Stir and wok over high heat for 1 minute, or until sauce thickens. Add vegetables, cover wok, and cook for 2 minutes more.

To serve, invert rice from bowl onto a large serving platter. Spoon chicken and vegetables on top and around sides of rice. Sprinkle with walnuts and garnish with watercress or coriander (if used). Serve immediately.

6 servings

Old-fashioned Rice Pudding

½ cup uncooked brown rice
1 cup nonfat dry milk
3½ cups water
⅓ cup honey
¼ teaspoon ground or grated nutmeg
⅓ cup raisins

In top of a double boiler, combine rice, dry milk, water, honey, and nutmeg. Cook, covered, for 2½ hours, or until rice is tender. Stir mixture occasionally. During last 30 minutes of cooking, stir in raisins. Serve warm or cold.

5 to 6 servings

Risotto

This Milanese rice dish requires constant attention during cooking—and the delicious result is well worth it.

2 tablespoons butter
2 tablespoons corn oil
1 cup uncooked short grain brown rice
1 cup chopped onions
1 clove garlic, minced
1 cup sliced mushrooms
4 cups hot Poultry Stock (page 110)
½ cup grated Parmesan cheese (optional)

Heat butter and oil in a 3-quart saucepan. Add rice and stir to coat with oil, then add onions, garlic, and mushrooms. Sauté until onions are golden and rice

is browned. Add 1 cup hot stock and cook slowly, uncovered, until stock is almost absorbed, stirring occasionally. (Do not let rice dry out.) Then add 1 cup more stock. Continue to cook, stir, and add stock gradually as it is absorbed, until all stock has been used and rice is tender but firm—about 1 hour in all. When done, sprinkle with cheese (if used) and serve immediately.

4 servings

Onions Stuffed with Wild Rice, Mushrooms, and Herbs

Steaming the onions first, as called for in this side dish, gives them a more delicate flavor.

6 large onions
¼ cup plus 2 tablespoons butter
1 cup chopped mushrooms (about ¼ pound)
2 tablespoons minced fresh parsley
1 teaspoon crushed dried sage
¼ teaspoon paprika
¼ teaspoon pepper
1 teaspoon lemon juice
2 cups cooked wild rice
Poultry Stock (page 110), for poaching

Steam onions in a vegetable steamer for 10 minutes. Drain and cool.

Using a small sharp knife, hollow out each onion at stem end, leaving a ½-inch-thick shell. Reserve centers of onions. Set shells in a buttered oven-to-table flat casserole with deep sides. Chop reserved onion centers and measure out ¾ cup. (Use remainder in another recipe.)

Preheat oven to 450°F.

In a medium-size skillet, melt butter. Add mushrooms and add ¾ cup chopped onions and sauté over medium heat for 5 minutes. Stir in parsley, sage, paprika, pepper, and lemon juice, then toss this mixture with rice.

Fill each onion shell to the top with stuffing. (If any remains, use to fill green or red peppers for a colorful accompaniment.) Pour enough stock in bottom of casserole to reach halfway up the sides of the onions. Bake for 20 minutes, spooning some stock gently over rice while baking. Spoon any remaining juices over onions when serving.

6 servings

Saffron Rice

The delicate flavor saffron brings to this rice makes it an ideal foil for spicy dishes, such as Indian curries.

1½ teaspoons saffron threads
3½ cups plus 3 tablespoons boiling water
¼ cup plus 2 tablespoons butter
1 stick of cinnamon, 2 inches long
4 whole cloves
2 cups uncooked brown rice
¼ teaspoon cardamom seeds, finely crushed
1 cup raisins
½ cup slivered almonds, toasted

Soak saffron in 3 tablespoons boiling water for about 10 minutes.

Meanwhile, melt butter in a large heavy skillet. Add cinnamon and cloves and stir to coat. Sauté lightly over low heat for about 5 minutes, being careful not to burn spices.

Add rice to skillet and stir until coated evenly with butter mixture. Cook over low heat for about 5 minutes. Add remaining 3½ cups water and cardamom and bring to a boil over high heat. Add saffron and its soaking water and stir gently. Then cover, reduce heat, and simmer for 20 to 25 minutes, or until rice is tender. Drain off any remaining liquid. Remove cloves and cinnamon stick, stir in raisins and almonds, and serve immediately.

8 servings

Southern Brown Rice Pancakes

Totally wheat-free, these crisp little pancakes need not be limited to breakfast. Try them for dessert, snack, or lunch.

1½ cups cooked short grain brown rice
6 tablespoons butter
¼ cup honey
1½ cups milk
2 eggs, separated
1½ cups brown rice flour
2 teaspoons baking powder
½ teaspoon ground cinnamon
⅛ teaspoon ground nutmeg

In a large saucepan combine rice, 3 tablespoons butter, honey, and milk and heat until butter melts. Beat egg yolks until frothy with a wire whisk and add to rice mixture. In a small bowl mix together flour, baking powder, cinnamon, and nutmeg and add to rice mixture. Beat egg whites until stiff and then fold into rice mixture.

Heat 1 tablespoon butter in a large heavy skillet. Drop batter by the tablespoon to form pancakes, and cook over medium heat until brown and crisp on both sides, turning once. Use 1 tablespoon butter for cooking each batch of pancakes. Keep warm and serve with maple syrup or fruit.

Makes about 2 dozen

Spinach, Mushrooms, and Brown Rice with Cheese

Here is a fast, filling, and nutritious hot luncheon dish, or a side dish that goes beautifully with broiled fish.

1 tablespoon olive oil
3 tablespoons butter
1 large clove garlic, minced
1 cup sliced mushrooms
1½ pounds spinach, shredded (about 5 cups)
¼ teaspoon pepper
1¼ cups shredded cheddar cheese (about 4 ounces)
½ cup small-curd cottage cheese
3 cups cooked short grain brown rice
6 thin slices mozzarella cheese
paprika

Preheat oven to 400°F. Oil an 8-inch-square baking dish.

Heat oil and butter in a 10-inch skillet. Add garlic and mushrooms and cook, stirring, for 1 minute. Add spinach and stir and cook about 2 minutes, or until spinach wilts. Stir in pepper, cheddar cheese, and cottage cheese and set aside.

Make a layer of rice on bottom of baking dish. Spoon spinach-cheese mixture evenly over rice. Top with mozzarella cheese and sprinkle with paprika. Bake for 8 to 10 minutes and then broil for about 1 minute, or until cheese is bubbly and brown. Cut into squares and serve very hot.

6 servings

Rye

Lentil-Rye Pilaf

1 tablespoon vegetable oil
1 small onion, minced
½ cup diced carrots
½ cup diced celery
½ cup rye berries, cooked
½ cup dried lentils, cooked
1 teaspoon caraway seeds (optional)
¼ teaspoon dried thyme
¼ teaspoon crumbled dried sage
1 tablespoon soy sauce
    pepper, to taste
3 cups Poultry Stock (page 110)
1 cup fresh peas, cooked until tender (optional)

Heat oil in a large skillet and sauté onions, carrots, and celery until tender. Add cooked rye and lentils, caraway seeds (if used), thyme, sage, soy sauce, pepper, and stock. Stir to combine, then cover and cook over low heat for 10 minutes. Lightly toss with hot cooked peas (if used) and serve.

4 servings

Rye Berries with Sweet-Sour Red Cabbage, Apples, and Caraway Seeds

This crunchy-textured, sweet-sour side dish tastes best when made a day ahead, to allow flavors to develop. It is excellent served with poultry or pork.

2 cups Poultry Stock (page 110)
1 cup rye berries
2 tablespoons chicken fat or butter
1 large onion, chopped (about 1 cup)
1 large head red cabbage (2 pounds), coarsely
    chopped (about 8 cups)
²/₃ cup apple cider
¹/₃ cup red wine vinegar
2 tablespoons mild honey
½ teaspoon ground allspice
¼ teaspoon ground cloves
¼ teaspoon pepper
2 small red delicious apples, cored and shredded
½ teaspoon caraway seeds
2 tablespoons minced fresh parsley

Bring stock to a boil in a 4-quart saucepan. Add rye, then reduce heat, cover, and simmer for 1 hour.

Meanwhile, heat chicken fat or butter in a large heavy skillet. Add onions and sauté for 2 minutes. Add cabbage and continue to cook over high heat for 5 minutes, stirring frequently.

Mix cider, vinegar, and honey together and add to skillet. Add remaining ingredients, except parsley, then cover pan, reduce heat, and cook for 40 minutes.

When rye is done, stir into cabbage mixture, cover, and cook for 10 minutes more. Serve hot, sprinkled with parsley.

6 to 8 servings

Triticale

Cheese, Nut, and Triticale Casserole

1 tablespoon vegetable oil
1 tablespoon butter
1 medium-size onion, chopped
3 large stalks celery, with leaves, chopped
½ cup chopped cashews
½ cup chopped walnuts
½ cup sunflower seeds
1 cup cooked triticale
1 cup ricotta cheese
2 teaspoons chopped fresh chives
2 tablespoons chopped fresh parsley
1 tablespoon chopped fresh thyme or
    1½ teaspoons dried thyme
2 eggs, beaten
¼ cup wheat germ
¼ cup sesame seeds

In a large skillet heat oil and butter. Add onions and sauté until wilted. Add celery, then cover and cook for 5 minutes.

In a mixing bowl combine nuts, sunflower seeds, triticale, cheese, chives, parsley, thyme, and eggs. Add onion-celery mixture and mix thoroughly.

Preheat oven to 350°F. Butter a 1½-quart oven-proof casserole.

Sprinkle ½ of the wheat germ on bottom and sides of casserole, then spoon triticale mixture over it. Sprinkle remaining wheat germ and sesame seeds on top and bake for 1 hour.

6 to 8 servings

Triticale-Sesame Seed Wafers

These paper-thin crackers have the crunchy, nutty taste of freshly roasted sesame seeds.

⅔ cup triticale flour
⅓ cup whole wheat pastry flour
2 tablespoons butter, cut into small pieces and softened
1 tablespoon tahini (sesame butter)
 pinch of cayenne pepper
1 egg yolk
¼ cup sesame seeds, roasted
1 to 2 tablespoons ice water

Preheat oven to 350°F. Cover 2 rimless baking sheets with foil and set aside.

Mix flours together in a bowl. Using a food processor or 2 knives, cut butter, tahini, and cayenne into flour until crumbly. Lightly stir in egg yolk, sesame seeds, and just enough ice water to form a stiff dough.

Divide dough evenly into 18 pieces and roll into circles between sheets of lightly floured wax paper until about ¼ inch thick. Place circles on baking sheet, widely spaced, and cover with a sheet of wax paper. Continue to roll out as thinly as possible (about ⅛ inch thick) right on baking sheet. Circles should not touch after rolling. Bake for 10 to 15 minutes, or until light golden in color. Carefully lift off with a wide spatula and cool on a wire rack.

Makes 1½ dozen

Wheat

Bulgur Confetti Salad with Sesame Seed Dressing

2 cups cooked medium bulgur
1 cup finely shredded red cabbage
1 cup shredded carrots
1 cup soy sprouts
½ cup diced sweet red peppers
½ cup minced scallions
½ cup minced fresh parsley
24 small seedless grapes
½ small avocado, cut into ½-inch cubes
3 to 4 tablespoons Sesame Seed Dressing (see opposite)
 curly leaf lettuce

Allow bulgur to cool to room temperature. Then, in a large bowl mix together bulgur, cabbage, carrots, sprouts, peppers, scallions, parsley, and grapes. Add avocado cubes and dressing and toss lightly, being careful not to mash avocado. Pile onto a platter lined with lettuce and serve.

6 servings

Sesame Seed Dressing

¼ cup lemon juice or rice vinegar
1 teaspoon French-style mustard
¼ teaspoon pepper
¼ cup plus 2 tablespoons safflower oil
1 teaspoon sesame oil
1 teaspoon soy sauce
1 teaspoon sesame seeds, toasted

Place lemon juice or vinegar in a small bowl. In a separate bowl, using a wire whisk, combine mustard, pepper, both oils, and soy sauce. Whisk mixture into lemon juice or vinegar, then add sesame seeds.

Yields ¾ cup

Baked Zucchini Boats Stuffed with Bulgur and Ground Lamb

Here is a colorful and satisfying main course that uses only one-half pound of meat for six servings.

3 medium-size zucchini (about 2 pounds)
2 scallions
½ green pepper
3 sprigs parsley
1 cup canned tomatoes, drained with liquid reserved
½ pound lean ground lamb
¼ teaspoon pepper
⅛ teaspoon cayenne pepper
½ teaspoon ground allspice
¾ cup coarse bulgur
 tomato paste, to taste
 lemon wedges

Place zucchini in a large deep skillet and add enough boiling water to cover. Cook for 10 to 12 minutes, then chill quickly under cold water. Cut off stem end of each zucchini and split lengthwise. Starting from wide end of vegetable, scoop out pulp with a spoon, leaving a ½-inch-thick shell; reserve pulp. Place shells in a 9 × 13-inch oven-to-table baking dish.

Preheat oven to 350°F.

In a food processor mince scallions, green peppers, and parsley. Add drained tomatoes, reserved zucchini pulp, lamb, spices, and bulgur and process until well mixed.

Generously spoon mixture into scooped zucchini shells. Add enough water to reserved tomato liquid to make 1 cup, stir in a little tomato paste, and pour around bottom of baking dish. Cover pan with foil and bake for 35 minutes, removing foil every 10 minutes to baste with liquid. Remove foil completely for last 5 minutes of baking. Serve hot, with lemon wedges.

6 servings

Bulgur, Fresh Beans, and Chick-peas in Basil-Tomato Puree

2 tablespoons olive oil
1 medium-size onion, finely chopped
2 cups pureed tomatoes, or 2 cans (8 ounces each) Italian-style tomatoes, pureed
1 cup fresh fava beans or broad beans (about 2 pounds unshelled)
1 cup cooked chick-peas, drained
1 cup cooked bulgur
½ teaspoon dried oregano
2 tablespoons minced fresh basil
¼ teaspoon pepper
2 thin scallions, minced

Heat olive oil in a large skillet. Add onions and sauté until wilted. Add tomato puree and bring to a boil, then reduce heat and add beans. Cover skillet and cook for 5 minutes. Add chick-peas, bulgur, oregano, basil, and pepper. Cover and simmer for 15 to 20 minutes, or until beans are tender. Remove from heat and let stand for a few minutes to absorb any remaining liquid. Spoon into a warmed serving dish and sprinkle with scallions.

6 servings

Bulgur Pilaf with Shallots and Parsley

2½ tablespoons butter
6 shallots, finely chopped
1½ cups coarse or whole bulgur
3 cups Poultry Stock (page 110)
¼ teaspoon pepper
½ cup minced fresh parsley

Melt butter in a large skillet. Add shallots and cook over medium heat until wilted. Stir in bulgur and stock and bring to a boil. Turn off heat, cover tightly, and let stand for 45 minutes.

Before serving, toss with 2 forks and warm over low heat for 5 to 10 minutes. Stir in pepper and parsley and serve.

6 servings

Orange-Nut Bulgur

1 orange
1 cup cold water
¼ cup butter
½ cup chopped onions
½ cup chopped celery
1 cup coarsely shredded carrots
1 cup bulgur
2 tablespoons chopped fresh flat-leaf parsley
⅛ teaspoon dried rosemary
½ to ¾ cup almonds, pecans, coarsely chopped cashews, or pine nuts, toasted
2 cups hot Poultry Stock (page 110)
chopped pistachios
celery leaves

Pare rind from orange with a vegetable peeler; reserve orange segments. Cut rind into ⅛ × 1-inch slivers, place in a small saucepan with 1 cup cold water, and bring to a boil. Drain and reserve rind.

Preheat oven to 325°F.

In a large skillet melt butter and sauté onions, celery, and carrots over medium-high heat for 5 to 7 minutes, or until onions begin to brown. Add bulgur and continue cooking and stirring until bulgur is lightly browned. Stir in reserved orange rind, parsley, rosemary, and nuts. Turn out mixture into a 5-cup oven-to-table baking dish.

Add stock to skillet and stir over low heat to deglaze any browned bits. Pour over bulgur, cover, and bake for 40 to 45 minutes, or until all liquid has been absorbed. Stir once or twice during baking.

To serve, slice reserved orange segments and arrange slices on top of baked bulgur. Sprinkle with pistachios and garnish with crisp pale celery leaves. Serve hot or slightly cooled.

6 servings

Bulgur Couscous with Lamb Stew

Stew

2 tablespoons vegetable oil
2 pounds boneless lamb, cut into 2-inch cubes
1 clove garlic, minced
3 medium-size onions, quartered
3 carrots, cut into 1-inch chunks
¼ teaspoon ground ginger
¼ teaspoon ground cumin
⅛ teaspoon ground cloves
½ teaspoon ground coriander

Couscous

2 cups bulgur, finely ground
2 cups water, or as needed
¾ cup dried chick-peas, cooked and drained
2 small zucchini, cut into 1-inch slices and
    lightly steamed

To make the stew: Heat oil in a deep soup pot and brown lamb on all sides. Add garlic, onions, carrots, seasonings, and just enough water to cover. Bring to a boil, then reduce heat and simmer, covered, for about 1 hour.

To make the couscous: While stew is cooking, place ground bulgur in a bowl and, with your hands, work about 1 cup water into it, or enough to moisten each grain. Place bulgur in a cheesecloth-lined strainer which is small enough to fit into pot in which stew is cooking. Place strainer over stew above level of liquid so bulgur will steam, not boil. Replace cover and cook for 30 minutes.

Remove strainer and turn out bulgur into a bowl. With your fingers, separate grains and add about 1 cup water to moisten all particles again. Place bulgur back into strainer, replace over stew, and continue to steam for another 15 minutes.

Lift out bulgur and add cooked chick-peas and zucchini to stew. Replace bulgur over stew and continue to cook just long enough to heat chick-peas and zucchini through.

Serve bulgur couscous immediately, topped with lamb stew.

6 servings

Bulgur with Cauliflower, Lemon, and Tarragon

3 tablespoons butter
1½ cups coarse bulgur
2½ cups Poultry Stock (page 110)
½ cup minced scallions
3 cups cauliflower florets, lightly steamed
1 carrot, shredded
1 tablespoon minced lemon rind
1 tablespoon minced fresh tarragon or ½
    teaspoon dried tarragon
juice of ½ lemon
¼ teaspoon pepper

Melt 2 tablespoons butter in a large skillet. Add bulgur and sauté until lightly browned, stirring occasionally. Pour stock over bulgur and bring to a boil. Then reduce heat, cover skillet, and simmer for 15 minutes, or until stock has been absorbed.

In another large skillet, melt remaining butter. Add scallions and cook for 1 minute, stirring continuously. Add remaining ingredients, toss to combine, and cook for 1 minute. Add to bulgur, fluff with 2 forks, and serve.

6 servings

Bulgur-Nut Casserole

¼ cup chopped onions
¼ cup chopped celery
2 tablespoons butter
1 cup bulgur
2 cups water, Poultry Stock (page 110), or Beef
    Stock (page 110)
1 egg
¼ cup pine nuts
¼ cup Brazil nuts
¼ cup chopped fresh parsley
½ teaspoon dried marjoram
½ teaspoon dried basil
2 tablespoons soy sauce

In a large skillet sauté onions and celery in butter until translucent. Add bulgur and cook and stir thoroughly for about 3 minutes. Add water or stock slowly, stirring grains. Cover and allow to simmer for 20 minutes, or until liquid has been absorbed.

Preheat oven to 325°F.

Add egg, pine nuts, Brazil nuts, parsley, marjoram, basil, and soy sauce to bulgur mixture and blend together well. Turn out mixture into an oiled 2-quart ovenproof casserole, cover, and bake for 15 minutes.

4 to 6 servings

Wheat Berry, Spiced Cauliflower, and Onion Salad

Prepare this salad a day ahead to allow the flavors to blend well—but serve it at room temperature to bring out the taste of the spices.

    1 head cauliflower (2½ pounds), separated into
        small florets
    2 teaspoons sesame seeds
    ½ teaspoon cumin seeds
    ¼ teaspoon coriander seeds
    ¾ teaspoon mustard seeds
      seeds from 4 cardamom pods
    ¼ cup plus 2 tablespoons butter
    2 large onions (about 1 pound), thinly sliced
    ½ teaspoon caraway seeds
    1½ cups yogurt
    ¼ teaspoon pepper
    2 cups cooked wheat berries
    1 large bunch fresh parsley

Steam cauliflower in a small amount of water about 5 to 6 minutes, or until crisp-tender. Rinse under cold water, drain, and set aside.

Combine sesame, cumin, coriander, mustard, and cardamom seeds in a small heavy skillet, cover with a splatter guard, and place over medium heat until mustard seeds begin to pop. Transfer to a spice or coffee grinder, blender, or mortar and pestle and pulverize until fine. Set aside.

Melt butter in a large skillet over low heat and then stir in onions. Cover pan and cook, stirring frequently, about 10 minutes, or until soft. Remove cover, raise heat to high, and continue to stir and cook onions about 10 to 12 minutes more, or until lightly browned. Add caraway seeds and reserved ground spices and cook for 1 to 2 minutes, stirring constantly. Add cauliflower and stir and cook for 1 to 2 minutes. Remove from heat. Stir in yogurt and pepper, blend well, and refrigerate overnight.

Next day, combine cauliflower mixture with cooked wheat berries and set aside to bring salad to room temperature. To serve, mince 2 tablespoons parsley for garnish and arrange remaining parsley sprigs in a ring on a serving platter. Spoon salad onto center of platter and sprinkle with minced parsley. Do not chill before serving.

6 servings

Tabbouleh Salad

    4 cups boiling water
    1¼ cups bulgur
    ¼ cup dried navy beans, cooked and drained
    ¾ cup chopped scallions or onions
    3 medium-size tomatoes, chopped
    1½ cups chopped fresh mint or parsley
    1 cucumber, chopped
    ½ cup lemon juice
    ¼ cup vegetable oil
    ¼ teaspoon pepper
      salad greens

Pour boiling water over bulgur and let stand for 1 hour, or until light and fluffy. Drain and press out excess water.

In a large bowl combine bulgur with cooked beans and remaining ingredients, except salad greens, and chill for about 1 hour. Serve on plates lined with salad greens.

8 servings

Wheat Germ Breading Mix

Use this mix instead of bread crumbs or flour to coat chops, fish, chicken, or vegetables that will be baked or fried. Or, add it to stuffings for meat, poultry, and fish.

⅓ cup cornmeal
⅓ cup rye flour
⅓ cup wheat germ

Combine all ingredients in a small jar. May be stored in refrigerator for up to 6 months.

Makes 1 cup

Mixed Grains

Mixed Grain, Black Bean, and Mushroom Loaf

For a meatless main course, try this tasty, nutritious loaf complete with grains, legumes, vegetables, cheese, and eggs.

3 cups Poultry Stock (page 110)
¼ cup millet
¼ cup barley meal (whole barley coarsely ground in blender)
¼ cup fine bulgur
¼ cup rolled oats
2 tablespoons corn germ*
3 tablespoons olive oil
½ cup thinly sliced leeks
½ cup thinly sliced scallions
1 clove garlic, minced
⅔ cup chopped celery
5 large mushrooms, coarsely chopped
¼ teaspoon dried oregano
⅛ teaspoon dried rosemary
¼ teaspoon ground cumin
½ teaspoon chili powder

1 cup cooked black beans, drained
1 cup shredded sharp cheddar cheese
2 eggs, beaten
butter
minced fresh parsley

Preheat oven to 350°F. Butter and flour a 9 × 5-inch loaf pan.

Bring stock to a boil in a 5-quart pot. Mix together millet, barley, and bulgur and slowly add them to boiling stock. Cover pot, reduce heat, and simmer for 15 minutes, stirring occasionally. Stir in oats and corn germ and set aside to cool.

In a medium-size skillet heat oil and add leeks, scallions, garlic, and celery. Stir and cook over medium heat for 5 minutes. Stir in mushrooms, herbs, and spices.

Add vegetable mixture, beans, and cheese to cooked grains, then stir in eggs. Pack into loaf pan, dot surface with butter, and bake for 1 hour. Remove from oven and cool in pan for 5 minutes before inverting onto a serving dish. Garnish with parsley and serve.

6 servings

*Corn germ is available in natural foods stores.

Basic Mixed-Grains Breakfast Cereal

3 cups cooked mixed grains (any combination)
1½ cups milk or light cream
½ cup chopped walnuts or pecans
¼ cup raisins
1 teaspoon vanilla extract
1 teaspoon ground cinnamon or nutmeg
¼ cup maple syrup .

Mix all ingredients in a 2-quart heavy-bottom saucepan and warm over low heat for about 10 minutes, stirring occasionally. If desired, serve with extra milk or cream and sliced fresh fruit.

4 to 6 servings

Pasta

The history of pasta is as colorful and varied as its numerous shapes and sizes and the many sauces that flavor it. The most popular legend has it traveling from China to Italy with Marco Polo. However, drawings of pasta cookware in Etruscan caves show that pasta existed in Italy long before that famed voyage. Another theory holds that pasta was actually introduced to Italy by Arabs who had easy access to Venice during the Middle Ages. At that time both the Arabs and the Indians were already eating noodles, calling them *rishta* and *sevika,* the Persian and Indian words for thread. Italians eventually called their version *spaghetti*—from the word *spago,* or string.

In the Western world Italian versions may dominate the pasta scene, but Asian cuisine has created a unique variety of noodles—Chinese cellophane noodles and rice noodles and Japanese *soba* noodles, to name but a few. The Chinese are generally accepted as the first to develop the noodle.

Making your own pasta at home is so easy that, once you try it, you may never go back to commercial brands again. It is less expensive, tastes better, and is more nutritious. Traditionally, commercial pasta has been made from semolina, the starchy endosperm of the hard durum wheat. This golden grain gives store-bought pasta its yellow color and an exceptionally high amount of gluten, which produces a hard-textured pasta that stands up well to cooking and to sauces. Unfortunately, the flour used in this type of noodle is nutritionally depleted in milling. Commercial "enriched" pasta has some B vitamins returned, but the small yet significant amounts

of fiber and minerals are not replaced. In terms of nutrition, whole grain pasta is far superior, and the calorie content is about the same as the processed product (200 calories per two-ounce serving). Whatever type of pasta you choose, the protein in it is complemented well by matching it with beans and cheese, such as in lasagna, ravioli, and *pasta e fagioli* (pasta with beans).

When shopping for pasta, it may help you to know that federal food-labeling regulations permit products labeled "macaroni" to be prepared from just flour and water. However, "noodles" must contain fresh, dried, or frozen whole eggs or egg yolks.

Types of Pasta

You may want to experiment with some of the newer versions of pasta now sold in natural foods stores and gourmet shops. To the familiar egg, whole wheat, and spinach pastas are added tomato, carrot, hot pepper, artichoke, and others.

The shapes and styles of pasta are of basically four types:

Strings and cords: *capellini, fusilli,* spaghetti, *spaghettini,* vermicelli.

Tubular: *cavatelli, ditalini,* macaroni, *mostaccioli,* rigatoni, *tubetti, ziti.*

Flat ribbons: fettuccine, lasagna, linguine, *tagliatelle.*

Forms to be stuffed: cannelloni, cappelletti, *conchiglie* (large shells), manicotti, ravioli, tortellini.

In addition to the above, there is soup pasta and an endless variety of fancy shapes—*conchigliette, farfalle, ruote, stellette.*

Oriental pasta can be found as chow mein noodles, cellophane noodles (also called bean thread), *harusame* (Japanese soy noodles), *soba* (Japanese buckwheat noodles), rice stick or rice flour noodles, and wonton.

How to Make Pasta

Unlike making bread, which can be time-consuming and is sometimes tricky, making pasta is fairly quick and almost foolproof. Very little can go wrong. The equipment required is basic—a rolling pin and a large knife are usually all you need. (However, if you intend to make pasta regularly you might want to invest in a pasta crimper or, on a larger scale, a pasta machine.) Traditionally, the dough is made on a large, wooden pastry board and rolled out with a long, thin, "broomstick" type of rolling pin. But any smooth, hard surface—Formica, plastic, marble —will suffice.

The Dough

Pasta making, like most cooking, is not an exact science, so the proportions of flour and egg used in a dough recipe may need to be changed slightly

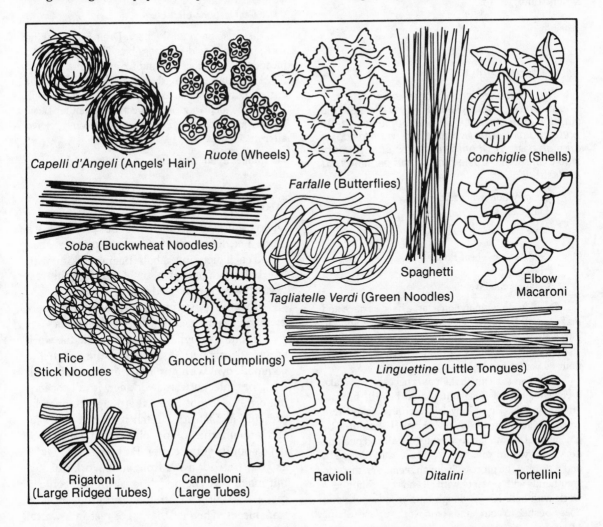

Capelli d'Angeli (Angels' Hair)

Ruote (Wheels)

Farfalle (Butterflies)

Conchiglie (Shells)

Soba (Buckwheat Noodles)

Tagliatelle Verdi (Green Noodles)

Spaghetti

Elbow Macaroni

Rice Stick Noodles

Gnocchi (Dumplings)

Linguettine (Little Tongues)

Rigatoni (Large Ridged Tubes)

Cannelloni (Large Tubes)

Ravioli

Ditalini

Tortellini

each time, depending on the size of the eggs, type of flour, humidity, temperature of the kitchen, and other uncontrollable variables. The recipes that follow are basic formulas. You should not hesitate to alter the amounts of ingredients to make the dough "feel right."

Ideally, pasta should be made, cut, and cooked on the same day. If you cannot use all the dough immediately, you can wrap it in plastic wrap and keep it in the refrigerator overnight or for a couple of days. (Tightly wrapped dough can be kept in the freezer indefinitely.) When you want to use the dough, be sure to bring it to room temperature and to add more flour as needed when rolling it out.

Basic Pasta Dough

Two choices of ingredients are listed here. The second grouping yields a bit less pasta but the addition of oil makes for a more-supple dough. Try both, and pick your favorite. Each will provide enough pasta for about four main course or eight side dish servings. The recipes can be increased as desired.

1½ cups whole wheat flour
2 large eggs

OR

1 cup whole wheat flour
1 large egg
2 teaspoons olive oil

Pile flour in a mound on a large hard surface and make a well in the center. Drop eggs, or egg and oil, into well, then gently blend them together with flour. Use a fork or your fingers, gradually bringing in more flour as you mix.

Incorporate as much flour as is necessary to make a cohesive ball of dough. It should be stiff but not unmanageable. Brush any leftover flour away from work surface. Knead dough for 5 to 10 minutes by placing heel of your hand on center of ball and pushing dough away from you, then folding it over, turning it, and repeating the process. If dough seems dry, moisten your hands with water or with oil and then continue to work with ball. Knead dough until it is smooth and does not stick to your hands or to work surface. Shape

dough as described in Forming the Pasta, below, or in individual recipes in this chapter.

Makes ¾ to 1 pound

Spinach Pasta Dough

Pasta verdi–green pasta–has shown a steady increase in popularity over recent years and can now be found on many a supermarket shelf. Making your own is more satisfying, and the product is reliably fresh and nutritious. This recipe yields enough pasta for eight to ten main course portions.

1 pound fresh spinach
3 cups whole wheat flour
3 extra-large eggs
1 tablespoon olive oil

Steam spinach until tender. Drain well, making sure spinach is as dry as possible. Then puree it in a blender or food processor and set aside until cool.

Place flour in a large bowl and make a well in the center. Drop spinach, eggs, and oil into the well. Proceed by following same directions given for Basic Pasta Dough (opposite). Dough should be evenly colored after kneading.

Makes about 2 pounds

Forming the Pasta

Divide your ball of dough into four pieces with a knife. Let dough rest for several minutes, then knead each piece into a ball. Begin working with one ball of dough at a time, keeping the rest covered with an inverted bowl.

If using a pasta machine, proceed from here by following the manufacturer's directions.

If rolling dough by hand, sprinkle the work surface lightly with flour. Flatten the dough into a smooth oval with a rolling pin, then stretch it from the center outward, working with all portions uniformly. Do not make the dough thinner by pressing it. Instead, stretch it by wrapping an end around the rolling pin and moving both hands out from the center. Pull the dough wider as you stretch it away from you. Work quickly, but make sure the dough is as thin as you can make it. Roll and stretch until the sheet is translucent. Then let that piece rest in a warm,

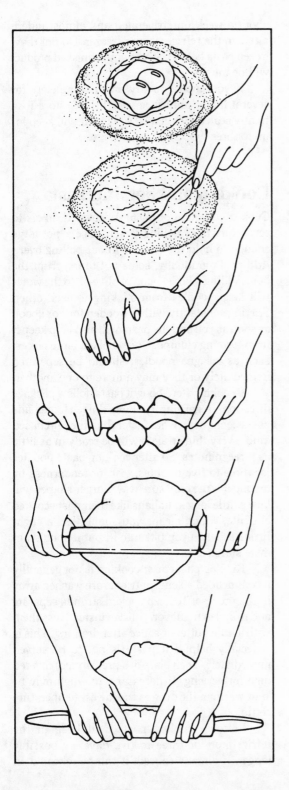

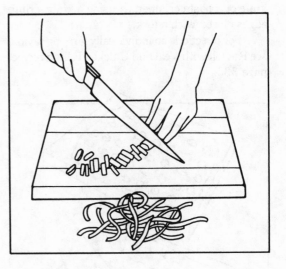

dry place while you repeat the process with the remaining balls of dough.

When the rolled-out dough is dry and supple (in 45 to 60 minutes) but before it becomes brittle, it is ready to cut to form pasta. The size may vary to your liking, of course, but general shapes are created as follows:

For noodles: Loosely roll each sheet of dough like a jellyroll, then cut noodles to the desired width with a large knife. Carefully unroll strips one at a time.

For lasagna noodles: Cut sheets into long, narrow strips—about 2 by 11½ inches for use in a 9 × 13-inch pan.

For cannelloni or manicotti: Cut rolled-out dough into large rectangles—about four by five inches is typical. (Store-bought versions of these are preformed into a tubular shell, then cooked and stuffed. If homemade, the pasta is first cooked, as a rectangle, then rolled around a filling to form a tube shape.)

For tortellini: A pasta machine works best for making these small, stuffed rings. See Tortellini recipe, page 334, for shaping instructions.

For ravioli: Use two large sheets of dough. Spoon filling mixture onto one sheet at regular intervals, then cover all with the second sheet of dough. Gently press down the spaces between the lumps of filling and cut out squares with a knife or a pasta crimper. (If using a knife, crimp edges closed with a fork.)

For directions on individually forming ravioli, see Ravioli with Veal and Chicken Filling recipe, page 333.

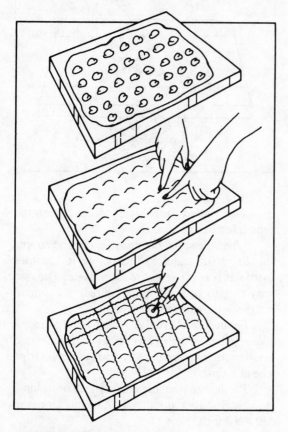

Drying Pasta

Allow pasta noodles and other shapes to dry in the open air for at least an hour before cooking or storing them. (This brief drying helps pasta to stay firm and not become soggy when cooked.) Lay pieces flat on wax paper or a towel, or drape them, as the Italians do, over the backs of kitchen chairs or on a horizontal broomstick.

Storing Pasta

Store uncooked homemade pasta in tightly sealed plastic bags or shallow plastic containers with airtight tops. Add a handful of cornmeal to keep pasta from sticking together. It will keep for about a week unrefrigerated and almost indefinitely in the refrigerator or freezer. Do not thaw frozen pasta before cooking or the finished product will be mushy.

If you choose to dry pasta completely for several hours until it is very brittle, store it in tightly sealed jars in a cool place. It will keep for up to three weeks.

Cooking and Serving Pasta

Cook each pound of pasta, uncovered, in six to seven quarts of boiling water. (Use a pot large enough to hold the water without boiling over.) Add pasta gradually, so as not to interrupt the boil. Adding a tablespoon of olive oil to the water will keep noodles from sticking to each other. Stirring constantly with a wooden fork or spoon as soon as you add the pasta will also help keep it from forming clumps. Once cooked, large pieces, such as lasagna noodles, should be separated immediately or they may adhere to one another.

If cooking store-bought pasta, follow package directions regarding cooking time. Homemade pasta cooks somewhat faster than the purchased kind—very thin strands will be ready in as little as three minutes. So after cooking pasta noodles for three to five minutes, test for tenderness by tasting it—the only sure way. Larger shapes will take a little longer. Italians like their pasta cooked al dente, which means you should feel a slight firmness when you bite into it, but it should not taste starchy.

Rinsing pasta after cooking is not generally recommended—some nutrients are washed away in the process. To keep cooked strands separate and to add extra flavor, you can instead toss them with a little butter or sauce after draining. This is especially helpful if pasta is not to be served immediately. Then place in a prewarmed, covered dish for serving. If necessary, the dish may be kept warm in the oven at the lowest temperature setting.

Leftover cooked pasta will keep in the refrigerator for three to five days, or possibly longer. If already sauced, it can be reheated on top of the stove, or covered and warmed in the oven. If unsauced, cover the pasta with boiling water for about two minutes, then drain well.

The Sauce

Italians do not overwhelm the delicate flavor of pasta with large quantities of sauce. They use sauce on pasta to add aroma, flavor, and color, and to keep pieces from sticking together. Some sauces are lightly tossed with hot pasta before serving, while others are traditionally poured on top of the pasta and tossed at the table. Cream sauces should always be mixed with pasta until each strand is well coated. Serve extra sauce in a pitcher to be added by the diners as desired.

Dumplings

Dumplings, bound together by eggs and then steamed to a light, spongy texture, add substance and variety to soups and stews. They can be simple or enhanced with spices and herbs. Middle Eastern nockerln, derived from a butter-egg base, and German spaetzle are traditional dumplings served with stews or meat dishes. Some dumplings owe their flavor to a base of pureed vegetable. Gnocchi, Italian potato dumplings, are plumped up in simmering water, then drained and accompanied by any of the diverse pasta sauces.

Most dumplings are made from an amply thick batter, dropped by spoonfuls on top of a liquid that can be water, a soup, or a stew. The secret to light-textured dumplings is to steam them on top of simmering liquid for 10 to 15 minutes without crowding each other, or they will stick together. (Do not allow the liquid to boil, or the egg protein will toughen.) Cover the pot as soon as the batter starts to float in the liquid; the steam will cook the dumplings. They are done when all have risen to the surface. When cooked in water, dumplings can be drained and held for several hours in a covered container before being served.

Quenelles are a special type of French dumpling, delicate and flavorful. Made from a smooth paste of meat or fish mixed with cream and whole eggs or egg whites, they are poached just like dumplings. Quenelles are best complemented with a light, velvety sauce or herb butter.

Pasta Sauces

With the exception of Basic Tomato Sauce and Tomato-Beef Sauce (which yield larger quantities), all recipes in this section will make enough sauce for one pound of pasta, or four to six main course servings.

Basic Tomato Sauce

Lasagna, spaghetti, and other forms of pasta are well complemented by this basic, meatless sauce—but its versatility extends to other foods as well. Try it with meat loaf, patties, or any course that calls for a topping of tomato sauce. Or, use it in place of the purchased variety of sauces for a more-flavorful recipe ingredient. This recipe provides enough sauce for 1½ pounds of pasta.

    3 tablespoons olive oil
3 or 4 cloves garlic, chopped
    4 medium-size tomatoes, peeled
    1 cup tomato puree
    ¼ cup plus 2 tablespoons tomato paste
    1 cup water, Beef Stock (page 110), or Vegetable
        Stock (page 111)
 1½ teaspoons dried oregano
    ½ teaspoon dried basil
    ½ teaspoon dried thyme
    2 tablespoons soy sauce
        pepper, to taste

Heat oil in a 2-quart saucepan and sauté garlic until lightly browned. Process tomatoes in a blender until smooth, or pass them through a strainer and discard seed residue. Add tomatoes, tomato puree, and tomato paste to pan. Gradually stir in water or stock, then cook sauce for about 45 minutes over medium heat, stirring occasionally. Add herbs and seasonings and cook for 15 to 20 minutes longer. Sauce keeps well for 7 to 10 days, refrigerated.

Yields 3 cups

Variation:
Tomato-Chicken Sauce: Add 2 cups diced cooked chicken when sauce has finished cooking. Simmer sauce 5 minutes longer, or until chicken is heated through.

Tomato-Beef Sauce

This sauce freezes well and can be thawed as needed for lasagna or a quick pasta dinner.

¼ cup olive oil
1¼ cups chopped onions
1 large clove garlic, minced
1 carrot, grated
1 pound lean ground beef
2½ pounds fresh plum tomatoes (10 to 12), peeled and chopped, or 1 can (2 pounds, 3 ounces) Italian-style tomatoes
3 tablespoons tomato paste
pinch of crushed red pepper
1 teaspoon chopped fresh oregano or ½ teaspoon dried oregano
¼ teaspoon pepper
2 tablespoons minced fresh parsley

Heat oil in a large heavy pot. Add onions and sauté for 5 minutes. Add garlic and carrots and continue to cook for 2 minutes, then add beef. Stir and cook until meat begins to lose pink color.

Place tomatoes in pot and crush them with a wooden spoon. Stir in tomato paste, red pepper, oregano, and pepper. Cover and simmer for 45 minutes, stirring occasionally. Add parsley, then correct seasonings to taste.

Yields about 7 cups

Alfredo Sauce

Fettuccine is the pasta traditionally used with this flavored white sauce. Its origin is attributed to the chef of a modest trattoria in Rome, which grew into one of the most elegant and fashionable restaurants in the city on the strength of this sauce.

¼ cup butter
2 cloves garlic, minced
2 cups heavy cream
4 to 6 ounces Parmesan cheese, grated
freshly ground pepper, to taste
minced fresh parsley

Melt butter in top of a double boiler or in a 1-quart saucepan over very low heat. Add garlic and cook for 3 to 5 minutes. (Do not allow garlic to brown.) Slowly add cream, stirring continuously with a wire whisk. Heat slowly for 15 to 20 minutes, or until sauce is thick enough to coat a spoon. Remove from heat.

Just before serving add Parmesan and pepper and toss with hot pasta. Garnish with parsley.

Yields 2¾ cups

Variations:
■ Before adding cream, add any of the following to garlic butter and cook until soft:
1 cup chopped mushrooms
½ cup minced onions
½ cup chopped green peppers
■ Add either of the following to cooked sauce and heat briefly before adding Parmesan and pepper:
1 cup small cooked shrimp
1 can (6 to 7 ounces) water-packed tuna, flaked

Blue Cheese and Almond Sauce

3 tablespoons butter
1 small onion, minced
3 cups heavy cream
8 ounces blue cheese, crumbled
½ teaspoon white pepper
½ cup slivered almonds

In a large saucepan melt butter and sauté onions until translucent. Add cream and bring to a slow boil. Cook, stirring constantly, for about 12 minutes, or until mixture has reduced in volume by 1/3. Add cheese and pepper and continue to cook until cheese has melted. Add almonds, then toss with hot pasta.

Yields about 3½ cups

Chicken Liver and Tomato Sauce

¼ cup olive oil
1 pound chicken livers
½ cup finely chopped onions
½ cup finely chopped celery
1 cup sliced mushrooms

1 cup Poultry Stock (page 110)
1½ cups Basic Tomato Sauce (page 325)
1 tablespoon chopped fresh parsley
¼ teaspoon dried marjoram
¼ teaspoon crumbled dried sage
¼ teaspoon dried rosemary
  freshly ground pepper, to taste

Heat oil in a large skillet, then add chicken livers. Stir and sauté livers for about 2 minutes on each side, or until lightly browned. Remove from heat and set aside.

Add onions and celery to same skillet. Stir and cook for 2 minutes, then add mushrooms and sauté until golden. Stir in remaining ingredients, except sautéed livers, and simmer for 30 minutes.

Coarsely chop chicken livers and return to skillet. Simmer for an additional 15 minutes, stirring often. Spoon over hot pasta.

Yields about 4 cups

Classic Cream and Egg Sauce

¼ cup butter
1 large onion, chopped (about 1 cup)
2 egg yolks, lightly beaten
1 cup light cream or milk
  dash of ground nutmeg, or to taste
  dash of cayenne pepper, or to taste
¼ cup grated Parmesan cheese

Melt butter in a small saucepan. Add onions and sauté until soft. Remove pan from heat.

Combine yolks with cream or milk. Stir into butter-onion mixture and return pan to heat. Cook over low heat, stirring often, until sauce will coat a spoon, about 8 minutes. (Do not boil.) Add nutmeg and cayenne and blend well. Pour over hot pasta and sprinkle with cheese.

Yields 1¾ cups

Variation:
Tangy Cream and Egg Sauce: Substitute ½ cup yogurt for ½ cup cream or milk.

Fennel Sauce

Try this quick-to-make sauce with its mildly licorice taste over spinach spaghetti for an appealing accompaniment to a meal.

⅓ cup olive oil
1 tablespoon fennel seeds
⅓ cup ground pine nuts
½ cup butter
⅛ teaspoon garlic powder
2 tablespoons chopped fresh parsley
⅛ teaspoon pepper
½ cup grated Parmesan cheese

In a small saucepan combine oil, fennel seeds, nuts, butter, garlic powder, parsley, and pepper. Heat until butter has melted, then toss with hot pasta. Sprinkle with cheese and toss again.

Yields about ¾ cup

Fish Sauce with Lemon, Parsley, and Tomato

Loaded with chunks of white fish, this sauce is a good choice when your time is limited. Goes well with linguine.

¼ cup olive oil
¼ cup finely chopped shallots
½ cup Fish Stock (page 111)
1 cup chopped tomatoes
½ teaspoon chopped fresh thyme or ¼ teaspoon dried thyme
1 teaspoon minced fresh basil or ½ teaspoon dried basil
1 pound turbot, halibut, or whiting fillets, cut into 1-inch cubes
1 teaspoon grated lemon rind
2 tablespoons lemon juice
¼ cup minced fresh parsley

Heat oil in a large saucepan, then add shallots and sauté, stirring constantly, until wilted. Add stock, then cook for 1 minute. Stir in tomatoes, thyme, basil, and fish and cook over medium heat for 7 to 8 minutes, or until fish is opaque. Add lemon rind, lemon juice, and parsley. Toss with hot pasta.

Yields 3 cups

Fresh Tomato, Zucchini, Pepper, and Fennel Sauce

Flavored with just a touch of sausage, this licoricelike quick sauce is chunky with vegetables. Serve with short, tubular pasta or those designed to hold sauces.

    1 tablespoon olive oil
    ¼ pound fresh pork sausage, with casings removed
    1 medium-size onion, chopped
    2 small, dried, hot chili peppers
    2 stalks fennel, thinly sliced
    2 sweet red peppers, cut into thin strips
    1 medium-size thin zucchini, sliced into ¼-inch rounds
    3 medium-size tomatoes, peeled and diced
    ¼ teaspoon fennel seeds
    1 teaspoon chopped fresh oregano or ½ teaspoon dried oregano
    ¼ teaspoon pepper
    2 tablespoons minced fresh parsley
    grated Parmesan cheese

Heat oil in a large heavy skillet. Crumble sausage into skillet and cook for 5 minutes, stirring often. Add onions and chili peppers. Cook and stir for 2 minutes, then add sliced fennel, red peppers, zucchini, and tomatoes. Bring to a boil, then reduce heat. Stir in fennel seeds, oregano, and pepper and simmer, uncovered, for 10 to 12 minutes.

Remove chili peppers from sauce. Spoon over hot pasta and garnish with parsley and Parmesan cheese.

Yields 3 cups

Oil and Garlic (*Olio e Aglio*) Sauce

Garlic-flavored olive oil makes up this classic Italian sauce. A mere half cup is sufficient to coat one pound of pasta, for about eight side dish servings. With the addition of sliced vegetables, it becomes a trifolati sauce—some form of which appears on almost every Italian menu.

    ½ cup olive oil (butter may be substituted for part of oil)
    4 or 5 cloves garlic, or more to taste
    1 small, dried, hot chili pepper
    1 tablespoon minced fresh parsley
    grated Parmesan cheese
    freshly ground pepper

Heat oil slowly in a small saucepan. When hot, add garlic cloves and chili. Cook until garlic is lightly browned, then remove garlic and chili with a slotted spoon. Remove pan from heat and allow oil to cool for a few minutes (or it will make pasta gummy).

Toss with hot pasta. Add parsley and toss again. Parmesan and pepper may be sprinkled on top or passed at the table.

Yields ½ cup

Variations:

Oil, Garlic, and Rosemary Sauce: Add 2 sprigs rosemary to hot oil along with garlic and chili. Remove and discard before tossing with pasta.

Trifolati Sauce: Heat oil in a larger saucepan. After removing garlic and chili from oil, add ½ cup Poultry Stock (page 110) and any one of the following vegetables.

    3 cups thinly sliced broccoli florets
    3 cups shredded fresh spinach
    2 cups thinly sliced mushrooms
    2 cups coarsely shredded carrots
    1 cup pureed cooked artichoke hearts, thinned with 2 tablespoons light cream

Cover pan and simmer for 2 to 4 minutes before proceeding with recipe.

Marinara Sauce

A pureed tomato topping frequently served over spaghetti, marinara can be prepared in several ways—often with seafood added.

    2 tablespoons olive oil
    2 small onions, chopped (about ½ cup)
    2 small carrots, minced (about ¼ cup)
    1 large clove garlic, minced
    ¼ teaspoon pepper, or more to taste
    2 pounds fresh plum tomatoes (8 to 10), peeled and diced, or 1 can (1 pound, 12 ounces) Italian-style tomatoes
    1 small bay leaf, crushed
    ¼ teaspoon dried thyme
    1 tablespoon butter
    ⅛ teaspoon crushed red pepper
    1 teaspoon grated lemon rind
    2 tablespoons minced fresh parsley

Heat oil in a large skillet. Add onions, carrots, and garlic and sauté for about 5 minutes, or until soft. Add pepper, tomatoes, bay leaf, and thyme. Cook, uncovered, over low heat for 15 to 20 minutes, stirring often.

Puree mixture in a food mill or pass it through a strainer; discard seed residue. Stir in butter, red pepper, and lemon rind. Spoon over hot pasta and garnish with parsley.

Yields 3 cups

Pesto Sauce

This flavorful and very aromatic sauce is a lusty, no-meat pasta topping that does not even need to be cooked. An easy favorite for a novice to make. A little goes far—about two tablespoons per serving.

    2 cloves garlic, quartered
    1½ cups fresh basil (about 36 leaves)
    ½ cup pine nuts
    ½ cup grated Parmesan cheese
    ¾ cup olive oil

Using a large mortar and pestle pound garlic and basil to a rough paste. Add pine nuts and continue pounding until nuts are ground. Transfer to a bowl.

Gradually blend in Parmesan. (Mixture will be fairly thick.) Then slowly stir in oil and mix until well blended. Thoroughly toss with hot pasta. Covered and refrigerated, it keeps well up to 1 week.

Yields 2 cups

Variation:

Parsley Pesto Sauce: Substitute fresh parsley for ½ or all of the basil.

Red and Green Tomato Sauce with Yellow Peppers

If you have a garden, or a friend who does, try this colorful sauce of both green and ripe tomatoes. Use with medium-size, tubular pasta or other shapes best suited to holding sauce.

    3 cloves garlic
    ½ cup olive oil
    2 large onions, thinly sliced
    4 medium-size green tomatoes, sliced
    3 sweet yellow peppers, cut into ½-inch strips

    5 large ripe tomatoes, peeled and cubed
    ¼ teaspoon crushed red pepper
    ¼ teaspoon dried rosemary
      pinch of dried oregano
    ¼ teaspoon pepper
    2 tablespoons minced fresh parsley

Place garlic cloves and oil in a large heavy skillet and sauté over medium heat. When garlic begins to sizzle and brown, remove from skillet and discard. Quickly add onions and cook, while stirring, for about 8 minutes. Add green tomatoes and yellow peppers and cook for 5 minutes longer. Stir in ripe tomatoes, red pepper, rosemary, and oregano and cook for another 5 minutes. Add pepper and 1 tablespoon parsley. Serve hot or at room temperature, spooned over hot buttered pasta and garnished with remaining parsley.

Yields 3½ cups

Red Clam Sauce

Vongole (clams) and pasta are a popular combination in Italian cuisine—and deservedly so. Serve this tasty tomato-based sauce over spaghetti.

    2 dozen cherrystone clams in shells
    2 cups water
    3 tablespoons olive oil
    1 clove garlic, minced
    1 small onion, chopped
    3 cups canned tomatoes, drained and chopped
    ⅛ teaspoon pepper
    ½ teaspoon dried oregano
    2 tablespoons minced fresh parsley
    ¼ cup tomato paste

Scrub clams thoroughly. Place 2 cups water in a large steamer or pot and steam clams until they open. Drain, reserving ½ cup clam juice. Set clams aside to cool.

In a large skillet heat oil. Add garlic and onions and sauté until onions are translucent. Add tomatoes, reserved clam juice, pepper, oregano, and parsley. Simmer for 5 minutes. Stir in tomato paste and simmer for 5 minutes longer.

While sauce is cooking, remove clams from shells and chop them. Add to sauce and cook until heated thoroughly. Spoon over hot pasta.

Yields about 4 cups

Ricotta-Nut Sauce

½ cup ricotta cheese (cottage cheese may be
    substituted)
¼ cup olive oil
¼ cup light cream
1 small clove garlic, minced
2 tablespoons chopped, fresh, flat-leaf parsley
    dash of cayenne pepper
1 tablespoon chopped fresh basil or 1 teaspoon
    dried basil
1/3 cup walnuts or pistachios

Combine all ingredients in a blender and process
until smooth. Spoon over hot pasta.

Yields 1 cup

Tuna Sauce

½ cup olive oil
½ cup butter
3 cloves garlic, minced
½ cup raisins
3 tablespoons chopped fresh parsley
1 teaspoon dried basil
1 teaspoon dried oregano
⅛ teaspoon pepper
1 can (6 to 7 ounces) water-packed tuna, flaked
½ cup coarsely chopped pine nuts
    crushed red pepper, to taste (optional)

Heat oil and butter in a Dutch oven. Add garlic
and sauté for about 3 minutes. Stir in raisins, parsley,
basil, oregano, and pepper. Continue to cook until
raisins are plumped, stirring constantly. Add tuna and
nuts and cook until heated through. Toss with hot
pasta and sprinkle with red pepper (if used).

Yields 1¾ cups

Walnut Cream Sauce

*A quick, uncooked sauce, this works best with
cavatelli or any small pasta that holds sauce well.*

1½ cups walnuts, toasted
1 clove garlic, quartered
2 tablespoons chopped fresh parsley

1 tablespoon chopped fresh marjoram or ½
    teaspoon dried marjoram
3 tablespoons olive oil
½ cup milk, or more as needed
1 cup ricotta cheese
⅛ teaspoon cayenne pepper

In a blender chop nuts, garlic, and herbs together.
Add oil and blend until incorporated, then add milk,
cheese, and cayenne and process again until smooth.
(Thin with additional milk if sauce is too thick.) Toss
with hot pasta.

Yields about 2½ cups

White Clam Sauce

*The reward in added flavor is well worth any
extra effort it takes to get fresh clams for this classic
sauce, often served with spaghetti or vermicelli.*

2 dozen cherrystone clams in shells
8 tablespoons olive oil
1 clove garlic, quartered
⅛ teaspoon pepper
2 tablespoons chopped fresh parsley
1 teaspoon chopped fresh basil or ½ teaspoon
    dried basil
¼ teaspoon crushed red pepper (optional)

Scrub clams thoroughly. Heat 2 tablespoons oil
in a large skillet. Add clams and push them around
with a wooden spoon as they cook over medium heat
until all have opened. Remove clams and set aside.

Pour oil and juice from skillet through a fine
strainer and reserve. When cool enough to handle,
remove clams from shells and chop them.

Heat remaining 6 tablespoons oil in same skillet
over medium heat. Add garlic, pepper, strained juice
and oil from cooking clams, parsley, basil, chopped
clams, and red pepper (if used). Simmer for 15 minutes,
then discard garlic. Toss with hot pasta.

Yields 2¼ cups

White Fish Sauce

½ cup Fish Stock (page 111)
1 tablespoon lemon juice
½ teaspoon minced garlic

¼ cup chopped fresh parsley
¼ teaspoon dried basil
¼ teaspoon dried oregano
   dash of cayenne pepper
1 cup flaked poached haddock fillet

Heat stock in a small saucepan. Add lemon juice, garlic, parsley, basil, oregano, and cayenne. Bring to a boil and cook for 1 minute. Stir in fish and continue to cook until heated through. Spoon over hot pasta.

Yields 1½ cups

Zucchini Sauce

There is a fresh and earthy character to this sauce—a nice idea for using abundant zucchini. Try it over fettuccine or spaghetti.

4 cups chopped peeled zucchini
¼ cup butter, at room temperature
2 teaspoons lemon juice
   dash of pepper
1 teaspoon soy sauce

Steam zucchini for 5 minutes. Then drain thoroughly, place in a blender, and process to a coarse puree. Transfer puree to a small saucepan and place over medium heat until heated thoroughly.

Whisk in butter, a little at a time. Add lemon juice, pepper, and soy sauce and stir to blend. Spoon over hot pasta.

Yields 3 cups

Variation:

Garden Vegetable Sauce: Add 2 large tomatoes, peeled and finely chopped, and ¼ cup chopped fresh chives to puree just before heating. Omit butter.

Filled Pasta

Just as pasta can be served with any sauce of your choice, fillings for stuffed pasta are equally variable. A basic cheese filling is given below. For other types, you may want to "mix and match" pasta shapes with any of the fillings in the recipes that follow.

Cheese Filling for Pasta

A simple, basic filling for lasagna, manicotti, ravioli, tortellini, or other stuffed pasta.

1 pound ricotta cheese
2 large eggs
¼ cup chopped fresh parsley or basil
1/3 cup grated Parmesan cheese
1 tablespoon chopped fresh thyme, basil, oregano, or a combination of these
½ teaspoon pepper

In a large bowl mix all ingredients together with a wooden spoon until well blended.

Yields 2½ cups

Lasagna

4 cups Basic Tomato Sauce (page 325) or Tomato-Beef Sauce (page 326), warmed
1 pound whole wheat lasagna noodles, cooked until al dente
   Cheese Filling for Pasta (see above), at room temperature
1 pound mozzarella cheese, grated
4 ounces Parmesan cheese, grated

Preheat oven to 325°F.

Spread ½ cup sauce over bottom of a 7 × 11-inch baking pan or ovenproof casserole. Cover with one layer of lasagna noodles. Layer 1/3 of the filling over noodles, spoon about 1 cup sauce over this, and top with 1/3 of the mozzarella. Continue in this way, ending with layer of noodles, until all filling, mozzarella, and noodles are used. (Or, reserve some mozzarella to melt on top, if desired.) Spread remaining sauce on top and sprinkle with Parmesan cheese. Bake, uncovered, for 25 to 30 minutes, or until heated through. Allow to stand for several minutes before serving, to set layers (or lasagna will be runny when you cut it).

8 servings

NOTE: This recipe makes a 3-layered lasagna (4 layers of noodles). If you prefer 2 thicker layers, or use a larger baking pan, use fewer noodles and increase the toppings between them proportionately.

Spinach Lasagna

Spinach Filling
1 pound fresh spinach or 2 packages (10 ounces each) frozen spinach
2 cloves garlic, minced
1 tablespoon chopped fresh parsley
1 tablespoon chopped fresh basil
1 teaspoon dried oregano
½ cup wheat germ
2 cups tomato sauce
1 can (6 ounces) tomato paste

Cheese Filling
1 pound ricotta cheese
pinch of pepper
2 tablespoons chopped fresh parsley

9 whole wheat lasagna noodles, cooked
½ cup grated Parmesan cheese
8 ounces mozzarella cheese, sliced
1 cup tomato sauce

To make the spinach filling: Cook or steam spinach until tender. Drain well, then place in a blender. Add garlic, parsley, basil, and oregano and process until mixed but not liquified. Combine wheat germ, tomato sauce, and tomato paste in a medium-size bowl. Add spinach mixture and stir to blend.

To make the cheese filling: Mix ricotta, pepper, and parsley together in a small bowl.

Preheat oven to 375°F. Butter bottom of a 9 × 13-inch baking pan.

Arrange 3 lasagna noodles side by side in baking pan. Using ⅓ of each amount, add a layer of spinach filling, ricotta filling, Parmesan, and mozzarella, in that order. Place 3 more noodles on top and repeat process until all ingredients are used, ending with mozzarella. Pour remaining 1 cup tomato sauce over all. Bake for 30 minutes, or until heated through. Allow to stand for several minutes before serving, to set layers.

8 servings

Creamy Seafood Manicotti

Filling
3 tablespoons butter
1 cup sliced mushrooms
¾ pound uncooked large shrimp, peeled, deveined, and quartered
¾ pound sea scallops, quartered, or bay scallops
1 large tomato, peeled, seeded, and chopped
⅛ teaspoon white pepper
3 hard-cooked eggs, finely chopped

Sauce
¼ cup plus 1 tablespoon butter
¼ cup plus 2 tablespoons cornstarch
4 cups milk
1 cup grated mild cheddar cheese

12 whole wheat manicotti shells, cooked
¼ cup grated Parmesan cheese

To make the filling: Melt butter in a Dutch oven. Add mushrooms, shrimp, and scallops and sauté only until seafood is opaque. (Do not overcook or shrimp will toughen.) Add tomatoes and pepper and cook just until tomato is heated. Drain well. Lightly toss with chopped eggs and set aside.

Preheat oven to 350°F.

To make the sauce: In a large saucepan melt butter. Stir in cornstarch to make a paste. Add milk gradually, stirring constantly, and cook for 3 minutes, or until sauce thickens. Add cheddar cheese and continue to cook until cheese melts.

Combine ½ of the cheese sauce with seafood filling. Stuff manicotti shells with mixture.

Spread thin layer of remaining cheese sauce over bottom of a large shallow baking pan. Arrange filled manicotti in single layer over sauce, top with remaining sauce, and sprinkle with Parmesan. Bake about 20 minutes, or until heated through.

4 to 6 servings

Meat and Mushroom Manicotti

Sauce
¼ cup olive oil
1 clove garlic, minced
1 small onion, chopped
1 cup sliced mushrooms
4 cups canned tomatoes, chopped
1 teaspoon dried basil
2 teaspoons dried oregano
1 can (6 ounces) tomato paste

Filling
2 tablespoons butter
1 large onion, chopped
½ cup chopped mushrooms

1 clove garlic, minced
1 pound lean ground beef
1 cup sour cream

12 whole wheat manicotti shells, cooked

To make the sauce: Heat oil in a large skillet. Add garlic, onions, and mushrooms and sauté until onions are translucent. Add tomatoes, basil, and oregano, then stir in tomato paste and simmer for 10 to 15 minutes.

Preheat oven to 350°F.

To make the filling: Melt butter in another large skillet. Add onions, mushrooms, and garlic and sauté until onions are translucent. Add beef and cook until browned.

Place mixture in a strainer to drain off grease, pushing with back of a spoon to eliminate as much as possible. Transfer to a small bowl and mix with sour cream. Fill manicotti shells with meat mixture.

Spread thin layer of sauce over bottom of a 9 × 13-inch shallow baking pan. Arrange stuffed manicotti in single layer over sauce and pour remaining sauce over them. Bake for 40 minutes, or until sauce is bubbly and manicotti are heated through.

4 to 6 servings

NOTE: Manicotti may be made ahead and stored, covered, in the refrigerator. Allow 1 hour for baking.

Variation:

Cheese-Stuffed Manicotti: Omit meat filling and substitute Cheese Filling for Pasta (page 331).

Ravioli with Veal and Chicken Filling

If you have a pasta machine, or prefer to form ravioli individually, try this method of making them. Otherwise, see page 323 for directions on rolling out and forming the pasta from entire sheets of dough.

Filling
2 tablespoons butter
1 pound boneless veal, cooked and cubed (about 2¾ cups)
½ pound boneless chicken, cooked and cubed (about 1½ cups)
1 clove garlic, quartered
⅛ teaspoon pepper
½ pound spinach, cooked and drained

1 teaspoon dried basil
½ teaspoon dried oregano
¼ teaspoon dried thyme
⅓ cup grated Romano cheese

Pasta
Basic Pasta Dough (page 322) or Spinach Pasta Dough (page 322)
6 quarts water
2 tablespoons vegetable oil

Sauce
½ cup butter
¼ cup olive oil
1 clove garlic, halved

grated Romano cheese

To make the filling: Melt butter in a large skillet. Add cooked veal, cooked chicken, and garlic and sauté for a few minutes. Transfer to a food processor or food mill and add pepper, spinach, basil, oregano, thyme, and cheese. Process until smooth and well blended. Set aside.

To make the pasta: Divide dough into 4 pieces. (Keep pieces not being worked under an inverted bowl until ready to use.) Pass 1 piece of dough through a pasta machine to form a rectangle about 1/16 inch thick. Cut into 4 × 2-inch strips.

Place rounded teaspoon of filling at one end of each strip, leaving room to seal edges. Wet edges with a bit of water, fold dough in half lengthwise over filling, and pinch together to seal well. Repeat with remainder of dough until all filling has been used.

Place water and oil in a large pot and bring to a boil. Cook about ½ of the ravioli at a time, uncovered, in rapidly boiling water for 8 minutes, or until tender. Remove carefully with a slotted spoon and allow to drain.

To make the sauce: While ravioli are cooking, heat butter, oil, and garlic in a small saucepan for several minutes. Discard garlic.

Pour sauce over cooked ravioli and serve immediately. Accompany with a bowl of extra Romano cheese to be added at the table.

4 to 6 servings

Variation:

Ravioli with Cheese Filling: Omit meat filling and substitute Cheese Filling for Pasta (page 331). Use garlic sauce as noted, or top with a tomato-based sauce.

Sea Shells with Avocado or Chili Sauce

Go mild or zesty in your choice of sauce to accompany this creamy crab-stuffed pasta.

Filling

1 pound fresh or frozen crab meat, cartilage removed
2 tablespoons minced onions
1 teaspoon dried tarragon
½ cup sour cream
½ cup mayonnaise

12 jumbo whole wheat pasta shells, cooked and chilled
Creamy Avocado Sauce or Tangy Chili Sauce (see below)

To make the filling: In a small bowl mix together crab meat, onions, and tarragon. Combine sour cream and mayonnaise and fold into crab mixture.

Blot pasta dry with paper towels, then stuff shells with crab mixture and set them on a plate. Cover and refrigerate until thoroughly chilled.

Prepare sauce. Serve with chilled stuffed shells.

4 to 6 servings

Creamy Avocado Sauce

1 small onion
¾ cup mayonnaise
1 very ripe avocado, peeled, pitted, and cut into chunks
1 teaspoon lemon juice

Mince onion in a blender or food processor. Add remaining ingredients and process until blended.

Yields about 1 cup

Tangy Chili Sauce

½ cup sour cream
½ cup chili sauce
1 tablespoon horseradish, drained

Combine all ingredients and mix well.

Yields 1 cup

Tortellini

Tortellini can be formed from circles or squares of rolled-out dough, but they should be almost paper thin—so use a pasta machine for best results. As with manicotti and ravioli, this tiny stuffed pasta may be served with a variety of fillings and sauces. This basic recipe makes about 200.

Filling

2 tablespoons vegetable oil
1 small onion, chopped
1 pound lean ground pork
1 pound lean ground beef
¼ teaspoon garlic powder
2 eggs
8 ounces Parmesan cheese, grated
pepper, to taste

Pasta

Basic Pasta Dough (page 322) or Spinach Pasta Dough (page 322)
3 quarts Poultry Stock (page 110)

grated Parmesan cheese

To make the filling: Heat oil in a large skillet. Add onions and lightly sauté. Add pork, beef, and garlic powder and cook until well browned. Drain off fat and allow meat to cool. Then place in a food processor or food mill and add eggs, cheese, and pepper. Process briefly until smooth. Cover and set aside in refrigerator while dough is being formed.

To make the pasta: Divide pasta dough into 4 pieces. (Keep pieces not being worked in a bowl covered with a damp tea towel until ready to use.) Pass 1 piece of dough through a pasta machine until it is as thin as possible. (From this point on, work quickly, for the dough will soon dry and be difficult to shape.) Cut into strips 1½ inches wide, then cut strips into 1½-inch squares.

Place about ¼ teaspoon filling in middle of each square of dough. Fold each into a triangle, wet edges with a bit of water, and press to seal firmly. Carefully bend triangle in half so that side points join. Wet mating tips and twist them together so that pasta forms a ring. Repeat process until all dough has been used.

In a large pot bring stock to a boil. Add as many tortellini as will fit in pot without crowding. Reduce heat and simmer, uncovered, for 15 minutes. Repeat process until all tortellini are cooked. Serve hot with Parmesan cheese.

8 to 10 servings

Shells Florentine

Sauce
¼ cup olive oil
1 medium-size onion, chopped
1 clove garlic, minced
¾ pound lean ground beef
2½ cups canned tomatoes, chopped
1 can (6 ounces) tomato paste
1 teaspoon dried basil
1 teaspoon dried oregano

Filling
2 tablespoons butter
1 small onion, finely chopped
1 pound spinach, steamed, drained, and finely chopped
1½ cups ricotta cheese
¼ cup milk
1 cup grated Jarlsberg cheese

24 jumbo whole wheat pasta shells, cooked

To make the sauce: Heat oil in a large skillet. Add onions and garlic and sauté until golden. Add ground beef and stir and cook until browned. Drain off grease, then add tomatoes with their juice. Stir in tomato paste, basil, and oregano and simmer for 15 minutes.

Preheat oven to 350°F.

To make the filling: While sauce is cooking, melt butter in a medium-size saucepan. Add onions and sauté until translucent. Add spinach and heat through. Remove from heat. In a small bowl blend ricotta, milk, and Jarlsberg cheese together, then stir mixture into spinach. Fill shells with spinach mixture.

Spread layer of sauce over bottom of a large shallow baking pan. Arrange stuffed shells in single layer over sauce, then pour remaining sauce over them. Cover with foil and bake about 45 minutes, or until heated through and sauce is bubbly.

4 to 6 servings

Pasta Casseroles and Salads

Cheese and Pasta Casserole with Tuna Cakes

Sauce
3 tablespoons butter
1 tablespoon cornstarch
2 cups milk
4 ounces Monterey Jack cheese, grated
1 teaspoon French-style mustard

Tuna Cakes
1 can (12½ ounces) water-packed tuna, flaked
1 cup soft whole grain bread crumbs
2 eggs, beaten
1 tablespoon minced onions
1 teaspoon chopped fresh parsley

8 ounces whole wheat pasta twists, cooked
1 pound asparagus, cooked until tender, then cut into thirds
½ cup soft whole grain bread crumbs
butter, for topping

To make the sauce: Melt butter in a medium-size saucepan. Stir in cornstarch to make a paste, then gradually stir in milk. Bring mixture to a boil over medium heat and, stirring constantly, boil for 3 minutes, or until thickened. Add cheese and mustard and continue to cook until cheese melts. Remove from heat.

To make the tuna cakes: In a medium-size bowl combine tuna, 1 cup bread crumbs, eggs, onions, and parsley. Mix until well blended (mixture will be wet), then form into 6 cakes.

Preheat oven to 325°F.

Gently mix together pasta, sauce, and asparagus. Turn mixture into a large baking dish. Sprinkle with ½ cup bread crumbs, dot with butter, and arrange tuna cakes on top. Bake for about 30 minutes.

6 servings

Artichoke, Cauliflower, and Pasta Casserole

6 tablespoons butter
3 tablespoons cornstarch
2 cups milk
½ cup grated cheddar cheese
1 cup sliced mushrooms
1 cup cauliflower florets
10 frozen artichoke hearts, cooked and cut into halves
2 cups whole wheat noodles or other small pasta, cooked

In a large saucepan melt 3 tablespoons butter. Stir in cornstarch to make a paste. Slowly stir in milk and bring to a boil. Stirring constantly, boil for 3 minutes. Add cheese and continue to cook just until cheese melts. Remove from heat.

In a large skillet melt remaining 3 tablespoons butter and sauté mushrooms and cauliflower. Add artichoke hearts and lightly sauté. Stir in vegetables and pasta.

Preheat oven to 350°F. Lightly butter a 2-quart ovenproof casserole.

Turn pasta mixture into casserole and bake for about 20 minutes, or until bubbly.

4 servings

Baked Salmon Cream

4 tablespoons butter
1 small green pepper, chopped
1 small onion, chopped
½ cup sliced mushrooms
1 pound salmon fillets, poached and then broken into chunks
8 ounces whole wheat elbow macaroni, cooked
2 tablespoons chopped pimientos
1½ cups sour cream
¼ cup milk
1 tablespoon French-style mustard

½ teaspoon Worcestershire sauce
½ cup whole grain bread crumbs

Preheat oven to 325°F.

In a small skillet melt 3 tablespoons butter. Add green peppers, onions, and mushrooms and sauté until onions are softened and golden.

In a 2-quart ovenproof casserole mix together all ingredients except bread crumbs and remaining 1 tablespoon butter. Top with bread crumbs, dot with butter, and bake for 30 minutes, or until bubbly.

4 servings

Chicken, Tomato, and Pasta Salad

Salad
8 ounces whole wheat *ditalini* or other pasta, cooked and chilled
1 cup cooked cannellini or other white beans, drained
4 hard-cooked eggs, chopped
1 small Bermuda onion, chopped
4 medium-size tomatoes, chopped
2 cups chopped cooked chicken

Dressing
½ cup olive oil
¼ cup vinegar
½ teaspoon dried oregano
⅛ teaspoon garlic powder
⅛ teaspoon pepper

lettuce leaves

To make the salad: In a large bowl combine pasta, beans, eggs, onions, tomatoes, and chicken.

To make the dressing: Shake together oil, vinegar, oregano, garlic powder, and pepper in a jar with a tight-fitting lid.

Pour dressing over salad and toss to coat. Serve on a platter lined with lettuce leaves.

4 servings

Chilled Pasta Salad with Basil and Cheese Dressing

1 pound small whole wheat pasta shells or
    elbow macaroni, cooked and chilled
1 small onion, chopped
2 medium-size tomatoes, seeded and chopped
½ cup sliced mushrooms
¾ cup cooked fresh or frozen peas
    Basil and Cheese Dressing (see below)

Combine all ingredients in a large bowl and mix together gently. Cover and chill thoroughly before serving.

6 servings

Basil and Cheese Dressing

1 cup fresh basil (about 24 leaves)
1 clove garlic, halved
1 cup mayonnaise
¼ cup grated Romano cheese
⅛ teaspoon pepper

Puree basil and garlic in a food processor or blender. Add mayonnaise, cheese, and pepper and process until smooth.

Yields about 1¾ cups

Variation:
    Parsley, Basil, and Cheese Dressing: Omit fresh basil. Substitute 1 cup chopped fresh parsley and 2 tablespoons dried basil.

Dieters' *Ditalini* and Vegetable Salad

This is a first-class picnic dish–inexpensive, easy to make, and can be done ahead of time without sacrificing texture.

2 cups creamed cottage cheese
2 tablespoons mayonnaise
½ teaspoon French-style mustard
8 ounces whole wheat *ditalini* or small pasta
    shells, cooked and chilled
1 small zucchini, peeled, seeded, and chopped

4 radishes, chopped
¾ cup chopped celery
2 teaspoons minced onions
1 large tomato, seeded and chopped
    lettuce leaves

Combine cottage cheese, mayonnaise, and mustard and stir to blend.

Place pasta and all vegetables, except lettuce, in a large bowl. Add cottage cheese mixture and toss to coat. To serve, mound salad on lettuce leaves.

4 servings

Fettuccine and Vegetable Salad

This eye-catching salad, crunchy with vegetables, is marinated overnight to fully develop its flavor.

Salad
1 pound spinach whole wheat fettuccine, cooked
    and chilled
1 sweet red pepper, chopped
1 small onion, chopped
2 cups cauliflower florets
1 pound mozzarella cheese, cubed

Dressing
¼ cup plus 2 tablespoons lemon juice
¼ cup French-style mustard
4 cloves garlic, minced
⅛ teaspoon pepper
1 cup olive oil

¼ cup pine nuts

To make the salad: Mix pasta, red peppers, onions, cauliflower, and cheese together in a large bowl.

To make the dressing: In a jar with a tight-fitting lid, shake together lemon juice, mustard, garlic, pepper, and oil.

Pour ½ of the dressing over salad and toss to coat. Cover and refrigerate overnight. Just before serving, toss with remaining dressing and top with pine nuts.

4 to 6 servings

Macaroni and Cheese

1 cup thin Béchamel Sauce (page 141)
½ teaspoon dry mustard (optional)
2 cups shredded mild or sharp cheddar cheese
8 ounces whole wheat elbow macaroni, cooked
    paprika
    minced fresh chives or parsley (optional)

Preheat oven to 350°F. Lightly butter a 2-quart ovenproof casserole.

In a large saucepan combine sauce, dry mustard (if used), and cheese. Place over low heat and stir constantly until cheese melts.

Place macaroni in casserole, add cheese sauce, and mix until macaroni is evenly coated with sauce. Sprinkle with paprika and top with chives or parsley, if desired. Bake for about 15 minutes, or until heated through.

4 servings

Variations:

Stir ½ cup of any of the following into macaroni when cheese sauce is added:
    diced cooked shrimp, meat, or poultry
    chopped tomatoes
    yogurt
    sautéed chopped onions, green peppers, or
        mushrooms

Macaroni Potpourri

3 tablespoons butter
1 clove garlic, minced
1 large onion, sliced
1 stalk celery, chopped
16 small mushroom caps
2 pounds boneless pork, trimmed of fat and cut
    into 1 × 2-inch strips
8 ounces whole wheat elbow macaroni or pasta
    twists, cooked
1 cup cooked brussels sprouts, cut into halves
3 cups canned tomatoes, chopped
1 cup grated mild cheddar cheese (optional)
1 teaspoon dried oregano

In a large skillet melt butter. Add garlic, onions, celery, and mushroom caps and sauté until onions are translucent. Remove from pan with a slotted spoon. Add pork strips to same skillet and stir-fry just until cooked through.

Preheat oven to 350°F.

In a 3-quart ovenproof casserole combine onion mixture, pork, and remaining ingredients and mix thoroughly. Cover and bake about 20 minutes, or until bubbly.

6 servings

Noodle-Crust Pizza

Sauce

3 tablespoons olive oil, or more as needed
1 medium-size onion, chopped
1 clove garlic, minced
1 pound lean ground beef
1 teaspoon dried oregano
½ teaspoon dried basil
⅛ teaspoon pepper
2 cups canned tomatoes, chopped and drained
3 tablespoons tomato paste

Crust

4 ounces uncooked spinach whole wheat noodles
4 ounces uncooked whole wheat noodles
½ cup milk
2 eggs

2 cups grated mozzarella cheese

To make the sauce: Heat oil in a large skillet. Add onions and garlic and sauté until onions are translucent. Add beef and brown well, adding more oil if needed. Stir in oregano, basil, pepper, and tomatoes and simmer for 5 minutes. Add tomato paste and simmer for 5 minutes longer.

Preheat oven to 350°F.

To make the crust: While sauce is simmering, cook noodles until tender. Drain thoroughly. Beat milk and eggs together, then mix with drained noodles. Spread mixture evenly on 2 oiled small pizza pans.

Spoon sauce over noodle crusts, sprinkle cheese over all, and bake about 20 minutes, or until bubbly. Allow to stand a few minutes before slicing.

4 to 6 servings

Noodles and Tomatoes au Gratin

4 ounces whole wheat egg noodles, cooked
2 cups soft whole grain bread crumbs
3 medium-size tomatoes, peeled, seeded, and chopped
1 small onion, minced
4 ounces Monterey Jack cheese, grated
½ teaspoon dried oregano
1 tablespoon minced fresh parsley
5 eggs
3 cups milk
¼ cup butter

Mix together noodles, bread crumbs, tomatoes, onions, cheese, oregano, and parsley. Turn mixture into a large shallow ovenproof casserole.

In a large bowl beat eggs well with a wire whisk. Preheat oven to 350°F.

Heat milk and butter in a 1-quart saucepan until milk is scalding and butter has melted. Gradually add scalded milk to eggs, beating continuously with whisk. Pour over noodles.

Set casserole inside a large roasting pan and place on top rack of oven. Pour hot water in roasting pan to reach level of food in casserole. Bake for 45 to 50 minutes, or until custard has set.

6 servings

Party Pasta Salad

Salad
½ pound frozen artichoke hearts (about 14), cooked and cut into halves
8 ounces whole wheat elbow macaroni, cooked and chilled
2 large tomatoes, each cut into 8 pieces
1 tablespoon chopped pimientos
1 pound cooked king crab meat, broken into chunks

Dressing
1 cup mayonnaise
1 teaspoon lemon juice
1 teaspoon milk
½ teaspoon paprika
½ teaspoon dry mustard
⅛ teaspoon white pepper

½ small onion, sliced into rings

To make the salad: Mix artichoke hearts, pasta, tomatoes, pimientos, and crab meat together in a large bowl.

To make the dressing: Combine mayonnaise, lemon juice, milk, paprika, dry mustard, and pepper.

Lightly toss salad with dressing. Chill thoroughly. Garnish with onion rings before serving.

4 servings

Pasta à la Caprese

4 large tomatoes, seeded and sliced into thin strips
4 cloves garlic, crushed
1 long, thin, green or yellow sweet pepper, sliced into strips
20 leaves basil, shredded
½ cup vegetable oil
1 tablespoon mild vinegar
freshly ground pepper, to taste
1 pound uncooked whole wheat pasta twists
8 ounces mozzarella cheese, shredded
grated Parmesan cheese

About 1 hour before serving time, combine tomatoes, garlic, pepper strips, basil, oil, vinegar, and pepper in a large bowl. Let stand at room temperature.

Shortly before serving, cook pasta until tender. Drain well, then toss with mozzarella until cheese begins to melt slightly. Add marinated tomato mixture and toss again. Serve slightly warm, garnished with Parmesan.

4 to 6 servings

Pasta Frittata

8 ounces uncooked whole wheat vermicelli or
   very thin *spaghettini*
2 tablespoons butter
3 tablespoons olive oil
4 eggs
1/3 cup grated Parmesan or Romano cheese
1/4 cup minced fresh parsley
1/2 cup coarsely shredded carrots
1/4 teaspoon pepper

Cook pasta until tender, then drain well and toss
with butter.

Heat oil in a 10-inch cast-iron skillet that can go
under broiler. Add pasta, flatten evenly across pan
with a spatula, and cook for 10 to 15 minutes over
medium-high heat, or until bottom is crisp and brown.

In a medium-size bowl beat eggs well, then stir in
remaining ingredients. (Mixture will be somewhat
thick.) Pour over pasta.

Place skillet in oven and broil for several minutes,
or until frittata is puffy and flecked with brown. Slide
frittata out of pan onto a heated serving dish and cut
into wedges. Serve hot.

6 servings

Sautéed Cabbage, Caraway, and Noodles

*This hearty and traditional combination from
middle Europe is made especially flavorful by the
caraway seeds coupled with the sweetness of
the cabbage.*

1/4 cup butter
1/2 large head cabbage, shredded
1 small onion, chopped
1/2 teaspoon caraway seeds
1/8 teaspoon pepper
1 pound uncooked whole wheat noodles or
   elbow macaroni
1/4 cup heavy cream
1/2 cup grated cheddar cheese

In a large skillet melt butter and sauté cabbage,
onions, and caraway seeds for 15 minutes, stirring
often. Add pepper.

Cook pasta until tender. Drain well, then toss
with cabbage. Add cream and cheese and toss again.
Serve immediately.

4 servings

Tortellini, Pimiento, and Sausage Salad

*Tortellini are usually available in the frozen
foods section of a supermarket, but your own
homemade version will be better. To make them,
see Tortellini recipe, page 334.*

8 ounces spinach whole wheat tortellini, cooked
8 ounces whole wheat egg tortellini, cooked
4 scallions, cut into 1/2-inch strips
2 large pimientos, cut into 1/2-inch strips
2 to 3 sausages (1 1/2 to 2 pounds), cooked and cubed
1 cup Pesto Sauce (page 329), mixed with 1/2
   cup water
3 tablespoons grated Parmesan cheese
2 tablespoons pine nuts, toasted
   freshly ground pepper, to taste

In a large bowl mix together tortellini, scallions,
pimientos, and sausage. Add diluted pesto sauce and
toss. Add Parmesan and toss again. Sprinkle with
nuts and pepper. Let stand at room temperature for 15
minutes before serving.

6 servings

South of the Border Casserole

2 tablespoons vegetable oil
1/2 cup chopped green peppers
1 large onion, chopped
1 clove garlic, minced
1 hot chili pepper, seeded and finely chopped
   (optional)
1 pound lean ground beef
2 cups canned tomatoes, chopped
1 cup cooked corn
2 teaspoons chili powder
1 teaspoon dried oregano
1/8 teaspoon ground cumin
8 ounces whole wheat elbow macaroni, cooked
1 cup sour cream
1/2 cup grated cheddar cheese

In a large skillet heat oil. Add green peppers,
onions, garlic, and chili (if used) and sauté until
onions are golden. Add beef and brown well. Add
tomatoes, corn, chili powder, oregano, and cumin.
Cook until heated through.

Preheat oven to 325°F.

Fold pasta and sour cream into beef mixture. Pour into a 3-quart casserole, sprinkle with cheese, and bake, uncovered, for 25 minutes.

4 servings

Oriental Pasta

Rice Stick Noodles with Pork

Ingredients for this Chinese dish should all be cut, assembled, and ready to use before beginning to stir-fry.

6 large Chinese dried mushrooms, soaked in ½ cup water for 2 hours
1 pound uncooked rice stick noodles, ½ inch wide
1 teaspoon sesame oil
1 tablespoon peanut oil
2 cloves garlic, minced
5 thin slices peeled ginger root, minced
1 pound boneless pork loin, trimmed of fat and cut into thin strips 1½ inches long
1 tablespoon soy sauce
dash of pepper
¼ pound snow pea pods
4 scallions, cut diagonally into 1½-inch strips
3 cups bean sprouts
1 cup Poultry Stock (page 110)
1 teaspoon cornstarch, dissolved in 3 tablespoons water

Drain mushrooms, reserving liquid. Cut into thin strips.

In a large pot cook noodles for 7 to 8 minutes, or until tender but not sticky. Drain well and place in a bowl. Toss with sesame oil and set aside.

Heat a wok or a large skillet. Add peanut oil. When oil is hot but not smoking, add garlic and ginger and stir-fry until golden. Add pork strips, soy sauce, and pepper and stir-fry for about 3 minutes, or until pork loses its pink color. Lift out pork with a slotted spoon and set aside.

To same wok or skillet add pea pods, sliced mushrooms, scallions, and bean sprouts and stir-fry for about 1 minute. Add about ½ of the stock and continue cooking until hot. Return pork to wok and stir together with vegetables. Add cooked noodles, remaining stock, and reserved soaking liquid from dried mushrooms. Stir and cook mixture just until hot. Then push vegetables and meat to one side and slowly pour cornstarch mixture into bottom of wok,

blending it thoroughly with revealed liquid. When the sauce begins to thicken, push vegetables and meat into sauce and stir to blend all ingredients. Transfer to a large serving platter and serve immediately.

6 servings

Soba Noodle Pancake with Scallions and Ginger

Crisp and flavorful, this baked oriental noodle pancake may accompany stir-fried vegetables and tofu, as a nice change from rice.

8 ounces uncooked *soba* noodles
1 teaspoon sesame oil
¼ cup minced scallions
1 teaspoon grated peeled ginger root
2 tablespoons soy sauce
3 or 4 drops hot pepper oil
2 tablespoons peanut oil

Preheat oven to 500°F.

Cook noodles for 5 minutes. Drain, then toss with all ingredients except peanut oil.

Heat peanut oil in a 10-inch cast-iron skillet. (Skillet must be able to go into the oven.) When hot, add noodle mixture, pressing down and spreading evenly across bottom of pan.

Place skillet on lowest rack of oven. Bake for 20 to 25 minutes, or until pancake is crisp and dark golden. Slide pancake out and cut into wedges. Serve hot.

6 servings

Soba Noodles with Sesame Seed Sauce

1 pound uncooked *soba* noodles (whole wheat noodles may be substituted)

Sauce
¼ cup butter, melted
2 tablespoons sesame oil
3 tablespoons sesame seeds

Cook noodles for 10 minutes. Then prepare sauce.

To make the sauce: Heat butter and oil in a 12-inch skillet. Add sesame seeds. When seeds begin to turn golden, which will be almost immediately, remove from heat.

Drain noodles and toss gently with sauce. Serve immediately as a side dish.

4 to 6 servings

Wonton

Wonton wrappers made from white flour may be purchased in oriental grocery stores or in many of the larger supermarkets. To make your own nutritious whole wheat wrappers, use the recipe included here.

36 Wonton Wrappers (see below)

Filling

1 pound lean ground pork, lamb, or beef; or
    ¼ pound lean ground pork, lamb, or beef
    and 1 to 1¼ pounds tofu (2 cups), drained
1 small onion, finely chopped
1½ to 2 teaspoons minced peeled ginger root or 1
    teaspoon ground ginger
¼ teaspoon crushed garlic, or ⅛ teaspoon garlic
    powder
2 tablespoons soy sauce
2½ teaspoons lemon juice
1 cup chopped bok choy, or 1 cup chopped
    mixed cabbage, celery, and celery leaves

4 quarts water

Prepare wonton wrappers.

To make the filling: Place all ingredients (except water) in a large bowl and mix together until well blended.

Place a tablespoon of filling near end of each wrapper, moisten edges with a bit of water, and fold in half lengthwise. Pinch edges firmly together to seal.

Bring water to a boil in a 6-quart pot. Cook wonton in 2 or 3 batches—do not crowd or they will not cook properly. Drop wonton, one at a time, into water. Allow them to boil until they rise to surface of water, then add about a cup of cold water and bring to a boil again. Remove dumplings with a slotted spoon and place on a tray covered with paper towels to drain.

Serve hot, as a side dish. Or, refrigerate for later use; reheat by sautéing in butter or vegetable oil. Wonton may also be used in place of noodles in soups.

6 to 8 servings

Wonton Wrappers

3½ cups whole wheat flour
¼ cup gluten flour
1 cup cold water
2 eggs

Sift flours together into a large bowl. In a separate small bowl beat water and eggs together. Make a well in center of flour and pour water-egg mixture into it.

Mix together until a soft ball of dough is formed. Knead on a floured surface until dough is satiny and smooth, 5 to 10 minutes. Divide into 4 or more portions.

(If you want to use only a small amount at this time, dough can be wrapped in plastic wrap and stored for later use. You might, however, prefer to roll out all of dough first, and then refrigerate or freeze it.)

On a floured surface roll out each portion of dough until ¹/₁₆ inch thick. With a knife cut dough into 2 × 4-inch rectangles.

Use immediately to make wonton. Or, store for later use by dusting each rectangle with cornstarch to prevent sticking, then stacking pieces together and wrapping tightly in plastic wrap to exclude air. Freeze or refrigerate. Return to room temperature before using.

Makes about 40

Dumplings

Basic Whole Wheat Dumplings

This recipe will make about eight large dumplings.

1¼ cups whole wheat flour
2 teaspoons baking powder
2 tablespoons chopped fresh parsley
⅔ cup milk
2 tablespoons vegetable oil

Combine flour, baking powder, and parsley in a small bowl. Add milk and oil and stir to blend. (The dough will be soft.)

Drop heaping tablespoons of dough into a pot of simmering soup or broth. Cover pot and allow to simmer for 15 to 20 minutes. When dumplings are fully cooked, they are breadlike inside and soft and mushy outside.

2 to 4 servings

Gnocchi

Gnocchi are small Italian potato dumplings with a soft, noodlelike texture.

2 small potatoes (½ pound)
1 small onion, finely chopped

2 tablespoons butter
1 egg yolk
¼ cup ricotta cheese
⅔ cup grated Parmesan cheese
¾ to 1 cup whole wheat pastry flour
4 quarts water
melted butter, for topping

Steam potatoes until tender. Peel, quarter, and set aside to dry a bit.

In a small skillet sauté onions in butter until tender. Remove from heat and cool.

While potatoes are still warm, rice or sieve them into a medium-size bowl. Stir in onions, egg yolk, ricotta, and ⅓ cup Parmesan cheese, then mix in ¾ cup flour. Knead into a soft smooth dough on floured surface, using only enough remaining flour as necessary to prevent sticking. Avoid overkneading—dough should be soft.

Shape dough into long finger-thick rolls and cut rolls into ½-inch pieces. Shape by using a lightly floured fork: With one finger press each piece against front of tines while pulling finger briefly along dough toward fork handle. Dough will roll into a shell shape with an indentation. Let dough fall onto a plate. Repeat until all pieces are formed.

Place water in a 6-quart pot and bring to a boil. Cook 2 dozen gnocchi at a time. Drop them into water and continue to boil for 15 seconds after dough rises to surface of water. (Taste at this point to see that gnocchi are cooked through but not soggy.)

Remove them with a slotted spoon and allow to drain. Top with butter and remaining Parmesan cheese. Serve immediately.

Or, place gnocchi in a buttered 1½-quart ovenproof casserole and top with a sauce of your choice (see Pasta Sauces, page 325). Bake at 375°F for 20 minutes, or until hot.

4 servings

Green Gnocchi

These spinach gnocchi are formed into simple ovals. Try them tossed with Pesto Sauce (page 329) for a colorful and tasty combination, or top or bake them with any sauce you prefer.

2 small potatoes (½ pound)
2 tablespoons butter

2 tablespoons finely chopped onions
5 cups finely chopped spinach, with stems removed (finely shredded cabbage, with ribs removed, may be substituted for ½ of this amount)
1¼ cups whole wheat flour
1 egg yolk
3 tablespoons dry ricotta cheese
3 quarts water
¼ cup melted butter
⅓ cup grated Parmesan cheese

Steam potatoes until tender. Peel, quarter, and set aside to dry a bit while preparing the greens.

In a Dutch oven melt butter and sauté onions over medium-high heat for 3 minutes. Add greens and cook, stirring occasionally, until liquid evaporates. Mixture must be quite dry. Cool quickly by transferring to a bowl set in cold water.

Place 1 cup whole wheat flour in a shallow medium-size bowl. Make a shallow well in center of flour, then rice or sieve potatoes into well. Top with cooled greens and mix lightly with a fork.

Add egg yolk and ricotta and stir until dough is smooth enough to knead. Knead lightly for 3 to 5 minutes, using as little of remaining flour as possible. Do not overwork dough—knead only until dough is well blended, soft, and smooth.

Shape dough into rolls ¾ inch thick and 12 inches long. Pinch off small piece from roll and quickly shape into marble-size oval between palms of your hands. Repeat until all dough is formed.

Bring water to a slow boil in a large pot. Drop in about ⅓ of the gnocchi at a time. As they float to surface of water, keep them from touching. Cook for 3 to 4 minutes after water returns to a boil. Test the first few; gnocchi should be slightly chewy, with no raw taste. If overcooked, they become waterlogged.

Remove them with a slotted spoon and drain in a sieve. Serve immediately, topped with melted butter and Parmesan cheese.

Or, place gnocchi in a buttered 2-quart baking dish and pour desired sauce over them. (A cream or tomato sauce goes well—see Pasta Sauces, page 325.) Top with Parmesan cheese and bake at 375°F about 25 minutes, or until hot and bubbly.

4 to 6 servings

Quenelles

½ pound boneless chicken breast or veal, ground
⅓ cup heavy or light cream
3 eggs
    freshly ground white pepper, to taste
    pinch each of ground mace, ground cloves,
      ground nutmeg, and dried thyme

Place all ingredients in a blender or food processor and process until smooth. Refrigerate for at least 1 hour.

Fill a large saucepan ¾ full of water and bring to a boil. Reduce heat to a simmer.

Form quenelles by using 2 teaspoons. (Or, for smaller dumplings, use 2 melon ball scoops.) Wetting utensils in hot water each time, scoop out a spoonful of meat mixture with one, and use the other to make a neat egg shape.

Drop quenelles into simmering water, taking care not to crowd them.Cook for 3 to 5 minutes, depending on size. Then remove pan from direct heat but leave quenelles in water until ready to serve. Cover pan to keep water warm.

Serve within 30 minutes, topped with Béchamel Sauce (page 141), Hollandaise Sauce (page 143), or Sauce Béarnaise (page 144).

4 to 6 servings

Pierogies with Cabbage, Potato-Cheese, or Spinach Filling

Three fillings are provided—try any one, or treble the dough recipe and try all three. Leftover dough may also be rolled out and cut to form noodles.

    Dough
1 cup mashed cooked potatoes
1 egg
¼ cup grated Parmesan cheese
1 to 1¼ cups whole wheat pastry flour

Cabbage Filling, Potato-Cheese Filling, or
    Spinach-Scallion Filling (see below)
butter and vegetable oil, for frying

To make the dough: Mix potatoes, egg, cheese, and ¾ cup flour in a medium-size bowl. Turn dough out onto floured surface, and knead until smooth, 5 to 7 minutes, adding only enough remaining flour as necessary. Do not overknead—dough should be soft and slightly sticky. Place in an oiled bowl to rest for 30 minutes.

Meanwhile, prepare filling. Set aside.

Divide dough into 15 pieces. Roll each piece into a 3½-inch circle, flouring work surface as needed. Place a rounded tablespoon of filling off to one side of circle, then moisten outside edges of dough with a bit of water. Fold dough over filling to form a half-moon shape. Press firmly to seal edges.

Cook pierogies, a few at a time, in gently boiling water, for 3 minutes on each side. Drain.

Heat enough butter and oil in a large skillet to form a thin layer. Brown pierogies over medium heat on both sides, adding more butter and oil as needed. Serve hot. Goes well with sour cream.

4 to 6 servings

Cabbage Filling

2 tablespoons corn oil
2½ cups shredded cabbage
1 small onion, finely chopped
1 teaspoon crushed caraway seeds
2 teaspoons cider vinegar
1 teaspoon soy sauce
⅓ cup shredded Swiss cheese

Heat oil in a large skillet. Add cabbage, onions, and caraway seeds and sauté until slightly wilted. Add vinegar and soy sauce and simmer about 10 minutes, or until tender and lightly browned. Cool. (You can cool filling quickly by placing it in a bowl set in cold water.) Stir in Swiss cheese.

Yields about 2¼ cups

Potato-Cheese Filling

¼ cup butter
½ cup chopped onions
1 cup creamed cottage cheese
1 cup mashed cooked potatoes
2 tablespoons grated Parmesan cheese
2 tablespoons chopped fresh parsley
1 teaspoon pepper

Melt butter in a small skillet. Add onions and sauté about 7 minutes, or until soft. Allow to cool slightly.

Combine cottage cheese, potatoes, Parmesan, parsley, and pepper in a medium-size bowl. Add cooled onions and mix well.

Yields about 2½ cups

Spinach-Scallion Filling

2 tablespoons butter
3 cloves garlic, minced
1 pound mixed fresh spinach and cabbage, chopped into ¾-inch squares (about 12 cups)
½ cup thinly sliced scallions, with tops
1 tablespoon chopped fresh dill
1 tablespoon minced fresh parsley
½ cup crumbled feta cheese

Melt butter in a Dutch oven. Add garlic and greens and sauté until very dry, stirring occasionally. Stir in scallions, dill, and parsley. Cool mixture quickly by placing in a bowl set in cold water. Add cheese and mix well.

Yields 2¼ cups

Spaetzle

Dough
1½ cups barley flour
1 cup soy flour
3 eggs
¾ cup cold water

3 quarts water
2 to 3 tablespoons vegetable oil
2 tablespoons minced onions (optional)
minced fresh parsley

To make the dough: Sift together barley and soy flours into a medium-size bowl. Make a well in center of flour and break eggs into it. Pour ½ cup cold water on top. Use a wooden spoon to beat until smooth. Gradually add remaining cold water and continue to beat mixture until well blended and smooth.

Bring water to a gentle boil in a 4-quart pot.

Rinse a spaetzle press with cold water, then add 2 to 3 tablespoons batter. Slowly press batter into water. Hold press 4 to 5 inches above water for long noodles, or 2 to 3 inches above for short noodles. If you do not have a spaetzle press, drop small bits of batter from a spoon into boiling water.

As soon as spaetzle rise to surface of water, remove them with a slotted spoon and place in a bowl of cold water (to prevent noodles from sticking together).

Rinse spaetzle press again, and repeat procedure until all batter has been used. Then drain noodles in a colander or strainer, rinse them with additional cold water, and allow to drain again for several minutes.

To reheat spaetzle: Heat oil in a large heavy skillet. Add onions (if used) and sauté for a few minutes. Add noodles and cook over medium heat until hot, turning noodles gently with a wide spatula to prevent them from breaking apart.

Serve immediately, garnished with parsley. Spaetzle go particularly well served with beef stew, beef Stroganoff, meatballs and gravy, or sauerbraten.

6 servings

Breads

Every land has its own version of an ideal life-sustaining bread. In France it is a crusty loaf as long and slim as your arm; in Scandinavia, a rounded, fragrant, moist loaf of rye; in India, a light disk called chapati—all cultural interpretations of a universal food concept.

When you make bread at home, you participate in this age-old creative process. There is nothing quite like the pleasure of working the warm dough with one's own hands, observing its mysterious rise, and sniffing the yeasty aroma as it bakes. When you eat bread that has been baked in your own oven, you know special pleasure.

The makings for a loaf of bread can be as elementary as flour, water, and yeast, or they can become more elaborate, enriched with such items as butter, milk, eggs, cheese, or yogurt. The bread can be a simple, traditionally shaped loaf, or it can be molded into small, scalloped rounds; long, rolled scrolls; or fancy braids. Some breads have flavored fillings, and some are slightly poached or griddled before they are baked. The world of bread making also encompasses quick breads and flatbreads, neither of which relies on yeast for rising and so are even simpler to make.

It is an added inducement to know that making your own bread is a way to make sure that it contains the highest food value possible. The mention of bread means wheat bread to most Americans, but a wide variety of other whole grains can be added to wheat to enhance flavor. A mixture of whole grain flours guarantees a better fiber content—something generally deficient in commercial breads.

Regrettably, white bread is made with flour whose bran and germ have been sifted out. The starchy endosperm, or heart of the grain, that remains is milled into white flour. Although this flour usually is enriched with some or all of the nutrients it lost with the bran and germ, the significant amounts of fiber are never recovered.

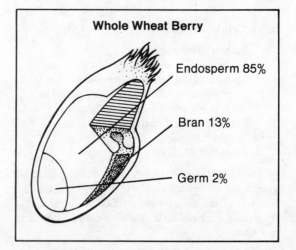

Whole Wheat Berry

Endosperm 85%

Bran 13%

Germ 2%

White flour is not used in the recipes given here. If you want to use it, for any reason, *unbleached* white flour is preferable because no chemical whiteners are added. If you should decide to use unbleached white flour, you can fortify its food value by using the following recipe, created by Dr. Clive McKay of Cornell University.

346

The Cornell Formula

> 1 tablespoon nonfat dry milk solids
> 1 tablespoon soy flour
> 1 teaspoon wheat germ

Combine all ingredients in a measuring cup, and fill out balance of cup with unbleached white flour. Do this for each cup of flour called for in recipe.

Baking Bread with Whole Grain Flours

Breads made with whole grains exclusively are denser and somewhat heavier than those made with refined flours, because the presence of the bran and wheat germ slightly inhibits the yeast's

Using Whole Grain and Other Flours in Bread Making

Flour or Meal	Portion of Each Cup of Whole Wheat Flour That Can Be Substituted with Other Flour or Meal (cups)	Taste Characteristics of Bread	Baked Characteristics of Bread
Amaranth	⅛	sweet	smooth, crisp crust; moist, fine crumb
Barley	¼	pleasant, malty aftertaste	firm, chewy crust; cakelike crumb
Brown Rice	¼	sweet	soft crust; dry, fine crumb
Buckwheat	¼	musty, robust flavor	soft crust; moist, fine crumb
Cornmeal	¼	bland, slightly sweet	unpronounced crust; grainy, slightly dry crumb
Gluten	½	tangy, earthy	crisp, thin crust; fine-grained, crumbly interior
Millet	¼	buttery, slightly sweet	smooth, thin crust; moist, dense crumb
Oat	⅓	sweet, nutty	firm crust; coarse, large crumb
Potato	¼	sweetly pungent	soft, dry crust; fine, springy crumb
Rye	½	tangy, slightly sour	smooth, hard crust; moist, supple crumb
Sorghum	⅛	sweet	crisp crust; fine crumb
Soy*	¼	slightly bitter	spongy crust; moist, fine crumb
Triticale	½	tangy	semifirm crust; dense-grained crumb
All whole wheat	. . .	sweet, nutty	supple crust; coarse, large crumb with stone-ground whole wheat flour; fine crumb with whole wheat pastry flour

*Soy (or soya) flour, made from soybeans, is actually a high-protein flour made from a legume, not a grain. It is often used to boost the nutritive value of many foods. Other legumes, including peas and lentils and the various types of dried beans, can be ground into flours to be used in making bread. Legume flours make bread especially nutritious because they are high in the very amino acids lacking in most grains. Therefore, the protein present in the accompanying grain becomes more efficient and is of a higher quality. The other legume flours will give bread about the same characteristics as soy flour and may be used in the same proportion as soy flour to wheat flour.

rising action. But the wholesomeness and flavor of these breads is truly superior to others, and you will find them filling and satisfying.

Experiment with combinations that appeal to you—try small amounts of cornmeal, rye, or buckwheat mixed with wheat flour, for example. Rye yields a moist, dense loaf, cornmeal adds a slightly dry, grainy texture. A little buckwheat flour gives whole wheat bread a pleasing, old-world taste. The opportunities for tasty discoveries are endless. The table Using Whole Grain and Other Flours on page 347 will give you an idea of what to expect when you combine whole grain and other types of flours with whole wheat flour in a recipe. Keep the pairings fairly simple so the flavor of each nonwheat flour retains its own identity in the final product.

Combinations of nonwheat flours and ground grains that complement each other well in nutrient value and final texture of bread include:

amaranth flour plus barley flour
brown rice flour plus ground millet
cornmeal plus brown rice flour
cornmeal plus buckwheat flour
gluten flour plus soy flour
oat flour plus soy flour
triticale flour plus cornmeal

These or any combinations, in any ratio of the two suggested flours, may be substituted for up to one-quarter of the amount of whole wheat flour called for in a recipe. For example, if a recipe calls for four cups of whole wheat flour, up to one cup may be replaced by any ratio of cornmeal to brown rice flour or of oat flour to soy flour, and so on.

Bear in mind, when combining whole grain flours, that at least one-half to three-quarters of the flour for each recipe must be wheat if you are to get a well-risen loaf. Wheat flour alone contains the proper amount of gluten-forming protein needed to take advantage of the yeast's rising action. Rye and triticale flours contain only small amounts of gluten—too little to provide a good rise on their own. But experience and individual taste will be the best guide to what combinations work well for you.

Gluten flour is made from wheat flour that has had some of its starch removed and its proteins concentrated so that it contains at least 70 percent pure gluten. It is sometimes added to a bread recipe to give the dough more resiliency.

In the United States we have both hard and soft varieties of wheat flour. Soft flour milled from winter wheat is not as high in protein and gluten as the hard spring wheat that is most often used for bread making. Graham flour is a coarse type of whole wheat flour ground from hard wheat. It may be used instead of whole wheat.

Buying Whole Grain Flours

Natural foods stores and specialty shops are good sources of whole grain flours for bread making, as are mail-order sources (see Appendix 4), especially if you intend to make bread quite often. Buy stone-ground flours whenever possible because less heat is involved in the milling process. That means fewer nutrients are destroyed. Most stone-ground flours are milled by stone rollers propelled by water power.

Storing Whole Grain Flours

All flours should be stored in airtight containers to protect them from loss of moisture. Be sure to label the container (and date it) if you remove the flour from its bag, or leave the label with the flour. Gluten flour can be kept at room temperature for up to six months. Whole grain flours with their germ and bran intact spoil easily, so they should be kept in the refrigerator (or the freezer, if you have space) and used within three months. Just remember that any flour must be allowed to warm to room temperature before use.

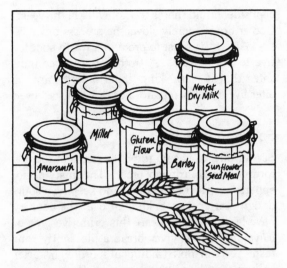

the machinery turn rancid and affect the taste of the next batch of whole grain you grind. These bits also attract insects.

Rice, buckwheat, millet, and rolled or steel-cut oats can be ground successfully in a regular kitchen blender if the blender has a strong motor. Grind one-quarter cup of grain at a time, making sure the appliance is not laboring too much.

Grinding Your Own Grains

Freshly milled grain is superior in taste to store-bought flour, and you can grind the amount of grain you need for each recipe. Finally, it permits a wider choice of flours to use in baking. Some grains, such as sorghum, amaranth, and millet, are not always available in flour form, so you may have to grind your own if you want to enjoy them.

Three types of grain mills are available—large electrical units, small hand units, and units that attach to appliances such as mixers. If you are considering the purchase of a grain mill, check your appliances to see if there are grain mill attachments available for them.

Electric mills are available with either stone or steel burr plates for grinding. Stone mills grind the flour finer, produce less heat at finer settings, and wear better. Steel-plate mills do not grind the flour as finely, but they can be cleaned easily and can be used for grinding foods other than grain—coffee beans, spices, nuts, beans, and peas, for example. Since stone grinders are not washable, only dry grain can be used in them.

Whether you choose an electric mill or a hand mill, be sure all the working parts are accessible for cleaning. Particles of grain left in

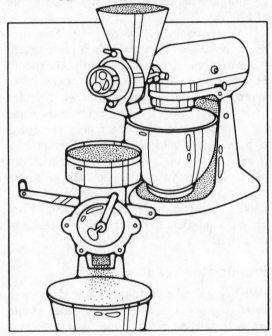

How Fine to Grind Grains

A fine flour is best for making so-called sandwich breads that are to be sliced thin and have to hold together. Bread made with coarse flour has more whole grain flavor and rises well but tends to fall apart easily. Coarse flour works particularly well in pancake recipes.

A fine grind exposes more surface area, and that allows for better assimilation of the grain's vitamins and minerals. But when the bran is ground too finely, its value as a fiber food is diminished. It makes sense to try for a mix of textures and uses for your home-ground grains.

Leavening

Yeast is crucial for raised bread. At work these living, single-celled fungi convert starches into carbon dioxide and alcohol. The carbon dioxide inflates the dough, and the alcohol bakes off. In the oven this action speeds up, and the bread is lightened more. Yeast cells thrive at 78 to 110°F, go into hibernation at 50°F, and begin to die at 120°F.

Commercially cultivated yeast (Saccharomyces cerevisiae) is available in a compressed, moist cake or in dry form. The fresh cake should be compact and of an even, creamy-beige color. Wrapped well and refrigerated, it will keep for about three weeks. Dry yeast is about the same color but doesn't change appearance when aging, so packages are marked with an expiration date. It will keep for up to six months in a cool, dry place. The dry yeast and the cake yeast are equally suitable and interchangeable for bread making: one tablespoon (or one envelope) dry yeast is equivalent to two-thirds of an ounce of cake yeast.

Proofing the Yeast

Both dry and cake yeast are dissolved and activated in a warm liquid—usually water, potato water, or milk. A small amount of sweetener may be added to provide food for the reproducing yeast, thereby speeding the process. One ounce of cake yeast or one tablespoon of dry yeast can be dissolved in about one-half cup of liquid, but this may vary with each recipe. The temperaure of the liquid can range from 78 to 110°F, but 90 to 100°F is most ideal. An exception to this is with the mixer method of mixing the dough, which some bakers feel is quicker. In this case the yeast, which has been blended first with part of the dry ingredients, is proofed with liquid that is 120 to 130°F. The hotter liquid is tempered by the dry ingredients. To test the liquid, sprinkle a few drops on the inside of your wrist. It should feel just warm but not hot. It is better to err on the cool side; liquid that is too hot will kill the yeast. Cooler liquid merely slows the process down.

Allow the yeast to proof in a warm spot for five to ten minutes. A frothy appearance indicates that it is working. If no bubbles appear after five minutes, discard the yeast and start over.

Sourdough Starter

San Francisco is said to be the home of today's formula for sourdough bread. The misty atmosphere is perfect for making and keeping a sourdough starter. But bakers all over the country have learned to duplicate this primitive type of leavening, which gives bread a pleasantly sour taste. You can mix a traditional sourdough starter at home with milk, honey, and flour, or you can use commercial yeast to produce a good bubbling batch.

Traditional Sourdough Starter

    2 cups sweet acidophilus low-fat milk (regular
       low-fat milk may be substituted)
    2 cups whole wheat flour
    1 teaspoon honey

Put milk into a small container, cover with cheesecloth, and leave at room temperature for 24 hours.

The next day add flour and honey, and stir well to blend mixture. Cover container with cheesecloth, and put in a warm place.

After 24 more hours, "captured" yeast should begin to activate. This may take 2 to 3 days. When starter becomes bubbly and begins to expand in size, it is ready for use.

The Handy Sourdough Starter recipe below takes a little less time than the Traditional Sourdough Starter and may be a little more reliable, especially if you live in a dry or very cold climate.

Handy Sourdough Starter

    1 tablespoon dry yeast
    2 cups warm water or potato water
    2 cups whole wheat flour

Combine ingredients in a glass or pottery (not metal) container. Cover with cheesecloth and let stand at room temperature for 48 hours. Stir down several times. A layer of bubbles and a fermentation smell indicate starter is ready for use. Stir down before using.

NOTE: All sourdough starters should be replenished with equal amounts of flour and water after each use. Starter should be stored in refrigerator, then taken out and brought to room temperature before being used.

Enrichment

Bread lends itself to all kinds of embellishments that can vary its taste, texture, nutritional value, and even its keeping quality. Eggs, butter, and milk, for example, are commonly used and add some special qualities to the final product.

Eggs and Butter

Eggs give bread a richer taste and supply protein that helps the loaf rise higher. Butter balances out the drying effect of egg whites, which coagulate during baking. Fats and oils flavor bread and enhance the gluten's elasticity by softening it, thereby producing a fuller risen loaf. Doughs high in fat usually require more yeast.

A soft crust and moist interior result from small amounts of egg and butter. Breads baked with eggs and butter or oil retain their moisture and stay fresh longer. Milk or beaten egg yolk brushed on top of the baking bread gives the crust a special crispness.

Liquids

The liquid used in bread can also influence its characteristics. Potato water—which is simply water in which potatoes have been boiled—adds its own sweet flavor and gives bread a rather delicate crumb. Plain water gives bread a dry, crunchy crust, while milk strengthens gluten and yields a smoother, moister crumb which will keep longer. Milk—including skim and nonfat dry—also adds to the bread's nutritional value by boosting its protein and calcium content.

Scalding milk that is to be used in bread making dates back to when milk was not pasteurized and its unwelcome bacteria could interfere with yeast fermentation. Although some cooks still recommend scalding milk, it is not necessary if the milk has been pasteurized. To scald milk, simply heat it until tiny bubbles appear around the edge of the pan.

Salt

A little salt may toughen the gluten in flour, giving it more elasticity, but too much salt affects yeast growth. Salt is not necessary in making bread and is not included as an ingredient in the bread recipes in this book. If you wish to add salt to your bread recipes for taste purposes, do so lightly—about one-half to one teaspoon per loaf is sufficient.

Sweeteners

A yeast bread can be sweetened with molasses, honey, or any of the grain syrups (see Grain Sweeteners, page 634) as well as sugar, of course. Sweeteners give bread a richer, darker color and act as a natural preservative. Too much sweetener, however, will inhibit the growth of yeast and cause the bread to burn.

Bulky Ingredients

Cheeses, herbs, pureed vegetables, dried fruits, and chopped nuts can be used to add something unusual to a plain loaf of bread. When you add a large quantity of dry, bulky ingredients, it is generally best to knead them in after the dough has risen once, so they will not hinder the yeast's leavening action.

Cracked wheat, sesame seeds, or rolled oats baked on top of a loaf of bread contribute flavor and crunch as well as an appetizing appearance.

Tips for a Lighter Loaf

Breads made with whole grain flours tend to be denser than those made with refined flours. Although the overall process of making bread with them differs very little, the dough may take longer to rise. This is especially so because bakers often add ingredients such as seed or nut meals, wheat or corn germ, bran, or nonfat dry milk to make their whole grain breads even more nutritious. The taste and food value are certainly enhanced, but the additions do make for a slightly heavier bread. As you become more confident with bread making, you will discover there are tricks you can use to make a lighter whole grain bread.

• Adding a teaspoon of baking powder or soda to the dry ingredients is a way to aid the yeast in raising the dough.

• Additional gluten flour may help the rising process and increase the fluffiness of the bread. (See Using Whole Grain and Other Flours table on page 347 for flour proportions.) Because it is high in protein, gluten flour gives the dough more elasticity.

• Lemon juice or vinegar added to the bread dough provides acid that helps soften the protein and increase the dough's elasticity. The result is a soft, light crumb and a higher risen loaf. Use 1 tablespoon of lemon juice or vinegar to every 2½ cups of flour. Don't add the acid ingredient until after some of the flour has been mixed with the activated yeast. Too much acid will interrupt the yeast fermentation, so be sure to keep the proportions correct.

• When eggs are called for in a bread recipe, try this formula for a lighter loaf: Separate the whites from the yolks. Beat the whites until stiff but not dry, and fold them into a small amount of the whole grain flour called for in the recipe before you add the rest of the flour and the other dry ingredients. Beat the yolks with oil or butter or, if no shortening is called for, any of the other liquid ingredients, then combine the two mixtures and proceed with the recipe directions.

Sponge Doughs

At one time sponge doughs were a popular method for bread making. To make a sponge dough, you proof the yeast in a large amount of liquid, then mix it with just a portion of the flour. This spongelike batter is allowed to rise for about an hour, then the remaining flour and ingredients are all added. The dough is allowed to rise one more time, then baked. The resulting breads are generally light, with a large crumb. Today most bread makers prefer the denser-textured but finer-grained breads that result from the conventional dough mixing method (see Mixing the Ingredients, below).

Equipment for Bread Making

The equipment you use for making bread can be as simple as a good pair of hands and a warm oven, or it can be much more elaborate and modern. If you use a large ceramic or glass bowl, 13 inches across the top, you can mix enough dough for two loaves of bread. The only other equipment you will need is:

large and small bowls
measuring cups
measuring spoons
wooden spoon for mixing
loaf pans (8½ × 4½-inch, medium, or
    9 × 5-inch, large)
wire rack for cooling the bread

Special pans such as muffin tins, brioche pans, cast-iron bread pans (for crustier loaves), Bundt pans, and two- or five-section loaf pans can be bought once you feel thoroughly committed to the art of bread making.

Mixing the Ingredients

Before you begin mixing the ingredients for a recipe, be sure to bring them all to room temperature first. The order in which you mix them does not matter, but either add all the wet ingredients (including oil or butter) to the dry, or add all the dry to the wet. You can proof the yeast directly in the mixing bowl and then add the dry ingredients, which you have combined in another bowl. Mix all the ingredients with a long wooden spoon until you have incorporated them into a formless, sticky mass that begins to resemble dough.

The amount of liquid absorbed by any type of flour depends on several variables, including weather and locale. On humid days the amount of liquid or flour may need to be altered slightly. Where and how the grain was grown, and its age, also will have an effect on a flour's absorbency. Freshly ground and stone-ground grain, in general, will take more liquid than older or steel-milled flour. As you become more familiar with bread making, you will become more proficient at judging how to adjust the liquid for each recipe.

When possible, mix nonwheat flours with the other ingredients first, then incorporate the wheat flour gradually until the proper consistency is reached. You will have to knead the dough for a while before you know if enough flour has been incorporated.

Kneading the Dough

When all the ingredients have been mixed and moistened in the bowl, you may use your hands for kneading. Food processors and electric mixers with proper attachments can knead bread dough with speed and efficiency, but many bakers find it relaxing to work the dough to its proper texture by hand.

Bear in mind as you knead the dough that the purpose is to distribute all the ingredients as uniformly as possible so that the yeast can raise the dough properly. Kneading also helps to develop the gluten network that traps the bubbles of carbon dioxide produced as the yeast digests the starches in the dough.

Choose a hard, smooth surface and dust it with flour. To knead the dough, begin by pulling the dough toward you, then push it away with the heels of your hands. Stretch and pull the dough slowly with both hands, then fold it over itself, give it a one-quarter turn, and repeat the process. Do not be afraid to add liberal amounts of flour as you knead, to keep the dough from sticking to your hands or the surface.

Most dough should be kneaded for 10 to 15 minutes. Underkneading or overkneading can have adverse effects on the gluten development and consequently on your bread. Dough has been kneaded enough when it no longer sticks to your hands or to the work surface. It should be firm and smooth but manageable.

The Rising

When the dough has been thoroughly kneaded, roll it into a smooth, even ball, and place it in a well-oiled bowl. Turn it over once to coat all sides of the dough with oil, which will keep a crust from forming as the dough rises. Cover the bowl with a damp cloth, and place it in a warm, draft-free spot. If necessary, heat the oven slightly for three minutes, turn it off, and place the bowl on the open oven door or nearby. Dough will rise well in a place where the temperature is 70 to 75°F. The warmer the spot, the faster will be the rise. For the best results in flavor and texture, dough should be allowed to rise slowly. You can hasten the rising if necessary, by exposing the dough to a temperature of 100°F. Rising can also be slowed down by putting the dough in a cool place or by refrigerating it. At any point the dough may be covered and refrigerated for up to four or five days. Before kneading and shaping refrigerated dough, allow it to warm to room temperature for about two hours.

Dough must be allowed to rise at least once, and usually twice or more. Dough that has risen

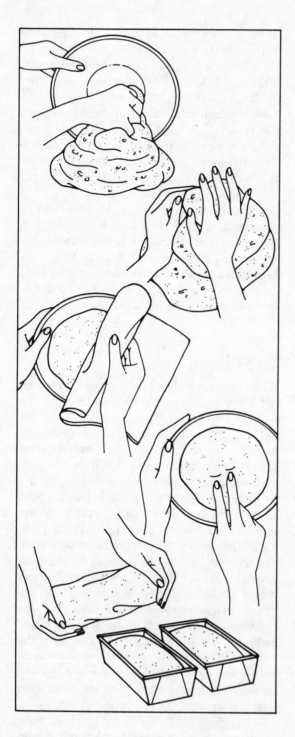

just once before baking will produce a coarse-textured loaf with large holes. For the first rise, dough should rise until it doubles in bulk, usually at least 1½ hours, even more for cooler places or heavier breads. (At high altitudes dough rises faster. No recipe adjustment is necessary, but do not allow dough to increase its volume more than is called for.)

Whenever you are in doubt about whether the dough has expanded to the proper volume, there is a foolproof test you can apply. Just poke two fingers into it. If the indentations remain, the dough is ready for you to punch it down with your fist, reshape it into a smooth ball, and allow it to rise for a second time. This lets carbon dioxide escape and mixes yeast cells more evenly throughout the dough, giving them access to fresh food and oxygen. The result is a more evenly grained bread and a lighter load. This second rising may be done after the loaves have been shaped and placed in the pans in which they will be baked. Be sure to allow room in the pan for the bread's expansion while baking. Individual recipes usually give instructions on how to prevent the baked bread from sticking. Generally, the pan or baking dish is buttered—generously—and a sprinkling of flour or cornmeal may or may not be required.

Baking Time and Temperature

You will find that the time and temperature for baking bread will vary with each recipe. A bread's actual baking time does not always coincide with the time specified in the recipe, and that can be due to altitude, ingredient freshness, or inconsistent oven temperature. It is wise to check the baking bread about 15 to 20 minutes before the end of its stated baking time, to make sure it is not cooking too fast. Often an oven is hotter in

Bake with Quarry Tiles for Crusty Breads

Breads baked on quarry tiles have a special crustiness to them. The porous tiles absorb moisture from the baking loaves and give an added crispness to the bottom crusts. To keep the crust from setting too quickly, humidity must be present during the cooking. This is supplied by a pan of hot water placed on the bottom shelf of an electric oven or the floor of a gas oven. During the baking, the oven should be sprayed periodically with water from an atomizer.

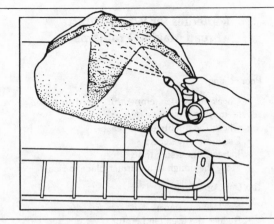

the back; if yours is, turn the bread around during baking. But do so only midway through the baking time. If part of the crust is browning too quickly, cover that part with foil.

The bread is done when its edges begin to pull away from the sides of the cooking vessel or when a light rap on the top or bottom crust produces a hollow sound. If the bread does not seem to be done, return it to the oven and test again in ten minutes. Freshly baked bread should be removed from the pan and cooled on a wire rack, to allow the air to circulate and to prevent steam from forming on its crisp crust. Allow the loaves to cool thoroughly before slicing them. This permits the flavor to develop fully and the loaf to set firmly enough to be sliced without crumbling.

Storing Freshly Baked Bread

When bread is thoroughly cooled, wrap it in plastic wrap or foil, and store it in a dry place or in a bread box. Home-baked bread will keep its fresh quality for about a week when stored this way. Wrapped and refrigerated, it will keep for at least two weeks. Bread securely wrapped in plastic wrap or foil, and then frozen, will be good for several months. Allow a frozen loaf to thaw for three to six hours, or heat it in the foil for 15 to 20 minutes at 400°F before serving.

Quick Breads

Sweetened, spiced, herbed, or filled, quick breads offer as many delicious variations as yeast breads, but they are simpler to make. You can vary them in any number of ways; a cupful of chopped nuts adds new appeal to a plain banana bread; a pureed vegetable adds moisture and flavor when it replaces some of the liquid in a recipe; yogurt instead of milk makes a heavier, moister product.

Quick bread refers to those breads in which the dough or batter is leavened with baking powder or soda or steam or beaten egg white, instead of yeast. Quick breads involve no proofing, kneading, or rising. Though they lack the fine texture and keeping qualities of yeast breads, you can incorporate nonwheat flours into their recipes more easily, since they do not rely on gluten.

Remedies for Whole Wheat Bread Making Problems

Poor Rising

• Check the water temperature used to proof yeast—may be too hot or too cold.
• Check the quality of the yeast.
• Use more sweetener.
• Increase the rising time.
• Move the dough to a warmer place to rise.

Too Dark or Crusty

• Use less sweetener.
• Reduce the oven temperature.
• Shorten the baking period.

Pale Color

• Use a higher oven temperature.
• Use more sweetener.
• Lengthen the baking period.

Dry

• Reduce the oven temperature.
• Shorten the baking period.
• Use less yeast.
• Use more sweetener.

Hard

• Reduce the oven temperature.
• Shorten the baking period.
• Use less yeast.
• Check the quantity or type of flour.
• Use more liquid.

Tough or Chewy

• Check the quantity or type of flour.
• Increase the rising time.
• Use less liquid.
• Shorten the baking period if tough.
• Lengthen the baking period if chewy.

Lacking Flavor

• Use more sweetener.
• Lengthen the baking period.

Uneven Loaves

• Check the oven temperature.

Still Damp after Baking

• Check the quantity of flour.
• Lengthen the baking period.
• Remove the bread from the pan and put it back in the oven for a few minutes with the oven turned off.

Filled with Air Bubbles

• Allow the dough to rise more slowly by moving it to a cooler place to rise.
• Use less yeast.
• Shorten the rising time.

Cracked Tops or Edges of Loaves

• Reduce the oven temperature.

Flat Rather Than Rounded Loaves

• Check the quantity of flour.
• Place the pans further apart in the oven while baking.

Leavenings for Quick Breads

Baking powder and baking soda are the most commonly used leavenings for quick breads.

In the presence of heat and moisture, baking soda releases carbon dioxide, and that causes the batter to expand. This alkaline ingredient must be neutralized by the addition of some acidic element such as sour milk, yogurt, or molasses, or it will give the bread a soapy taste.

Baking powder, which contains baking soda, includes its own acid—cream of tartar. Added cornstarch keeps the mixture dry enough so the soda and acid do not react in storage.

Generally speaking, recipes with acid ingredients specify baking soda; those with very little acid in the ingredients call for baking powder. A high proportion of acid ingredients in a recipe may require additional alkalinity, and in such a case, both baking powder and baking soda may be called for.

Double-acting baking powder is slower than old-fashioned single-acting. Double-acting means it begins to release carbon dioxide as soon as moistened, but a second rising action will take place in the oven.

Commercial double-acting baking powders often contain aluminum sulfate, a chemical (potentially harmful to the nervous system) that is not necessary in raising a quick bread. Commercial brands without this chemical are available, or you can mix your own baking powder as follows:

Baking Powder

½ teaspoon cream of tartar
¼ teaspoon sodium bicarbonate (baking soda)
¼ teaspoon cornstarch or arrowroot

NOTE: Mix only as much baking powder as you need per recipe, since it may lose its potency in storage.

Quick breads have some obvious advantages over yeast breads, particularly in terms of time and convenience. The quick bread batters can be mixed by hand with a wooden spoon or with an electric mixer. Dry ingredients can be mixed beforehand and set aside for a few hours or overnight, but once they have been combined with the liquid, the resulting batter should be baked immediately.

If the batter is mixed by hand with a spoon, the dry ingredients should be blended together first, then the liquid ones added. With an electric mixer the liquid ingredients are mixed first and the dry ingredients then added. Bulky whole foods such as nuts, seeds, and dried fruits should be gently blended into the batter last.

The consistency of the batter will vary, depending on the type of quick bread, but it will always be thinner and moister than a yeast dough. If it is too thick, add one-quarter cup of a liquid to the batter. If too thin, add more flour and adjust the sweetener.

Substitutes for Whole Milk

Sour milk, buttermilk, or yogurt may be substituted for whole milk in bread recipes. The result is a tarter-tasting product. Use one cup of sour milk or buttermilk to replace one cup of whole milk, but use only three-quarters cup of yogurt for one cup of milk.

To replace buttermilk or sour milk in a recipe, use one cup of whole milk mixed with one tablespoon of either vinegar or lemon juice, or with two teaspoons of cream of tartar. Let stand for five minutes before using.

For a crustier-textured bread, you may also substitute citrus or apple juice for milk. Use about half as much juice as milk, and fill out the balance of each cup with water.

Baking Quick Breads

The baking times and temperatures for quick breads may vary with each recipe as they do with yeast breads. It is wise to test the baking product about 15 minutes before the end of the specified baking time. A wooden pick or a very thin, pointed knife inserted gently into the center of the bread should come out clean when the bread is done. Most quick breads can be served immediately, while they are still warm. When thoroughly cooled, they should be stored with the same care as yeast breads—securely wrapped in plastic wrap or foil.

Muffins, Biscuits, Popovers, and Cream Puffs

Muffins, biscuits, popovers—their very names evoke thoughts of warm miniature breads that are enjoyed by themselves as satisfying snacks, or dappled with melting butter or jam for breakfast, or served as an elegant touch at dinner. Hot muffins or biscuits are popular quick breads, easily made from drop batters. Both rely on baking powder or baking soda for leavening and require minimal mixing. Too much mixing will cut down on the volume. Muffins, often sweetened and dessertlike, should have a smooth, moist crumb, while biscuits tend to be crustier on the surface and dryer inside.

Popovers are crusty hot breads that owe their dramatic increase in volume to the large amount of liquid in their batter and the leavening action of steam. Baked at high temperatures, popover batter will yield a large muffin with a hollow interior and crisp sides.

Cream puffs, like popovers, are a light, airy product steam-leavened in a hot oven, but there are some slight differences in the amount of fat and the number of eggs used in the batter.

Converting Old Recipes to Natural Sweeteners and Whole Grains

Most bread recipes can be converted easily for using natural sweeteners and whole grains by making several slight adjustments. Honey or molasses can usually be substituted for sugar as a sweetener. Honey and molasses have twice the sweetening power of sugar, so when you use them instead of sugar in a recipe, use half as much as the amount of sugar called for. Molasses is a good substitute for brown sugar, as the flavors are similar.

You may also substitute whole wheat flour in any recipe that calls for white flour. Though whole flour tends to absorb more liquid than white, the use of a liquid sweetener instead of a dry one will compensate for this tendency, so the amount of flour need not be changed.

If you are converting the sweetener in a recipe from dry to liquid but not changing from white flour to whole wheat, you may compensate by reducing to about half any liquid called for. However, this adjustment is best made by judging the consistency of the batter.

Pancakes, Waffles, and Crepes

Pancakes and waffles are a breakfast tradition most Americans have enjoyed many times. When made with whole grain flours, they become even more wholesome and delicious. Laced with honey or maple syrup or topped with fresh fruit, nuts, and yogurt, they can be either light or very substantial meals.

Crepes are very thin pancakes that serve as a modest foundation for myriad sauces, toppings, or fillings. They are often stuffed with cooked vegetables, fresh fruit, or chunks of meat or fish,

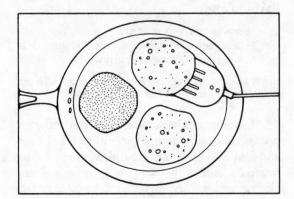

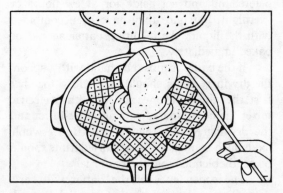

and then topped with a sauce. They can serve as the main course or, with sweet fillings, become appetizing desserts.

Pancakes, waffles, and crepes all are made easily from a sufficiently fluid batter spooned onto a hot, oiled griddle. Pancakes usually are lightened with baking powder or soda or beaten egg white, though they may use yeast.

Before the batter for pancakes, waffles, or crepes is poured, the griddle or waffle iron should be hot enough to cause drops of cold water to dance when dropped on the surface.

Because they are much thinner and made from a lighter batter, crepes are cooked a little differently than pancakes. To cook crepes, heat a heavy skillet or a crepe pan to medium-high heat, and add a bit of butter or oil to the pan. Take the pan from the heat when it is very hot, pour in just enough batter to cover it lightly, and swirl to distribute the batter evenly. For a 6-inch pan use about one-third cup of batter. Pour the excess batter, if any, back into the bowl.

Cook the crepe over medium heat for about one minute, then loosen the edges gently with a spatula. It should be golden brown on the bottom and dry on top. Turn the crepe over and cook it until the other side is also brown. After the first crepe or two, you will need very little oil for the pan. You may stack the crepes as they are cooked, one on top of the other on an ovenproof platter, and keep them warm in a low oven (150 to 200°F) until they are needed.

Pancakes are turned over when the bubbles formed during the cooking of the first side have popped, and the bottom is a pleasing brown. The second side is then browned.

Waffles should be cooked without opening the iron until the iron stops steaming.

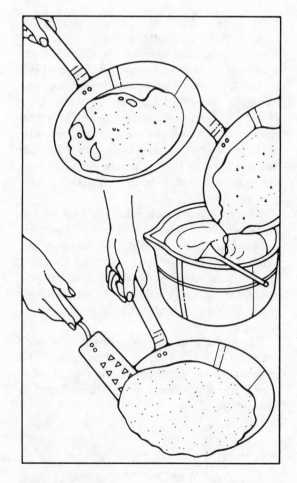

Flatbreads

Long before the world ever savored yeast-risen breads, simple flour-and-water flatbreads were the basic daily nourishment for the people of many cultures. Taste and texture could be varied by the use of many nonwheat flours—barley, millet, oat, rye—because there was no yeast involved. Flatbreads still dominate the fare in many parts of the world; sometimes they are enriched with eggs, butter, or oil.

In Mexico tortillas still are made daily from a mixture of water and cornmeal that has been cooked with lime. The mixture is flattened and cooked on a hot griddle until slightly brown, then served with beans, rice, and/or meat. The Indian chapati, served warm as scoops for other foods, are puffed up on a hot griddle. *Injera,* Ethiopian flatbreads made from a thin millet-and-water batter, are dark, subtle-tasting breads cooked on a ceramic griddle.

In this country jonnycakes are a traditional flatbread whose origin is traced to American Indian cookery. They are made from thin cornmeal batter cooked quickly on a hot surface. Crackers are a popular savory type of flatbread that also can be cooked fairly quickly from a simple dough incorporating any combination of grain, seed, or nut flour.

Most flatbreads are descendants of a more primitive type of bread, all utilizing almost the same balance of ingredients. The type of grain used is primarily what differentiates one flatbread from another.

Make Your Own Melba Toast

To make melba toast, simply slice bread thinly—about one-quarter inch thick—then toast it in a toaster oven or on both sides under an oven broiler until it is evenly browned, two to three minutes on each side. Choose a fine-grained bread, and use a very sharp knife to make thin slices without tearing. Slightly stale bread works better than fresh bread. Allow toast to cool completely before it is stored. Wrap melba toast in plastic wrap or foil, and store it in a bread box or another dry place.

Yeast Breads

Amaranth Sweet Rolls

Do try amaranth in your baking. The flavor is distinctive and rewarding.

Dough
½ cup butter
⅓ cup honey
¾ cup milk, scalded
1 tablespoon dry yeast
½ cup warm water
2 eggs, beaten
  juice and grated rind of ½ lemon
2 cups amaranth flour
3 to 3½ cups whole wheat flour

Filling
¼ cup butter, melted
3 tablespoons honey
2 tablespoons molasses
1½ teaspoons ground cinnamon
1 cup chopped walnuts
1 cup popped amaranth

To make the dough: In a large bowl combine butter, honey, and hot milk. Let cool to lukewarm.

Dissolve yeast in warm water. Let proof, then add to milk mixture. Add eggs, then add lemon juice and rind.

Combine flours and add to liquid, 1 cup at a time, using only enough flour to make a manageable dough. Turn out onto a floured surface and knead until smooth and elastic, 8 to 10 minutes. Place in an oiled bowl, and turn once to coat top of dough. Cover and let rise in a warm place until doubled in bulk, about 1 hour.

To make the filling: Mix butter, honey, molasses, cinnamon, nuts, and amaranth together.

Roll out dough on floured surface to form an 18 × 12-inch rectangle. Spread ½ of the filling evenly over dough. Roll as for a jellyroll, then cut into 1-inch slices.

Butter 2 12-cup muffin tins and cover bottom of each with remaining filling. Place rolls cut-side down in prepared tins. Cover with a cloth and let rise again until light, about 1 hour.

Preheat oven to 375°F.

Bake for about 25 minutes.

Makes 2 dozen rolls

Apple-Maple-Oatmeal Batter Bread

1¼ cups milk
1¼ cups quick-cooking rolled oats
¼ cup sweet butter
1 tablespoon dry yeast
¼ cup warm water
¼ cup maple syrup
1 egg
¼ cup wheat germ
½ teaspoon ground cinnamon
2½ cups whole wheat flour
½ cup dried currants or raisins
½ cup diced dried apple
sunflower seeds

Bring milk to a boil in a medium-size saucepan. Remove from heat. Stir in 1 cup rolled oats and butter. Cool to lukewarm.

In a large bowl dissolve yeast in warm water. Stir in 1 teaspoon maple syrup. Let proof. Then add oat mixture, remaining maple syrup, egg, wheat germ, cinnamon, and 1 cup flour. Beat with electric mixer at medium speed for 3 minutes. Stir in currants or raisins and apples. Beat in remaining flour gradually with a wooden spoon to make a smooth and elastic dough. Scrape down sides of bowl. Smooth top, cover, and let rise in a warm place until doubled in bulk, about 45 minutes.

Butter a 1½-quart soufflé or baking dish, and sprinkle with remaining rolled oats.

Stir down batter. Turn into prepared dish, smooth top, and sprinkle with sunflower seeds. Let rise again until doubled in bulk, 30 to 45 minutes.

Preheat oven to 350°F.

Bake for 40 minutes, or until bread is golden brown and sounds hollow when tapped. Cool for a few minutes on a wire rack. Remove from baking dish. Serve warm.

Makes 1 loaf

NOTE: While most batter breads do not call for a double rise, it does give this bread a better texture.

Apricot Braid

1 cup milk, scalded
¼ cup butter or vegetable oil
3 tablespoons honey
¼ cup water
1 tablespoon dry yeast
1 egg
1 teaspoon grated lemon rind
½ cup chopped raisins
¼ cup chopped nuts
½ cup slivered dried apricots
4 cups whole wheat flour

In a large bowl combine milk, butter or oil, honey, and water. Allow to cool to lukewarm. Add yeast and mix well. Set aside to proof. Then blend in egg, lemon rind, raisins, nuts, and apricots. Add flour and mix until dough is well blended and soft.

Lightly oil a baking sheet. Divide dough into 5 equal parts, and shape each into an 18-inch strip. Place 3 strips on prepared baking sheet and form into braid. Seal ends together. Twist 2 remaining strips together, and place on top of braid. Seal ends. Cover with a damp cloth, and let rise in a warm place until doubled in bulk, about 1 hour.

Preheat oven to 350°F.

Bake for 45 minutes.

Makes 1 braid

Bagels

    1 medium-size potato, thickly sliced
2 to 2½ cups water
    1 tablespoon dry yeast
    3 teaspoons honey
4 to 4½ cups whole wheat flour, sifted
    2 eggs
    3 tablespoons vegetable oil

    Glaze
    1 reserved egg yolk
    1 teaspoon cold water
      poppy or sesame seeds (optional)

Place potatoes in a medium-size saucepan, and cover with 2 to 2½ cups water. Bring to a boil and cook for about 15 minutes, or until tender. Remove potatoes and set aside for another use. Measure out 1 cup potato water, and let cool to about 90°F. Then place ½ cup potato water in a small bowl. Stir in yeast and 1 teaspoon honey, and set aside to proof.

Place 4 cups flour in a large bowl. Stir yeast mixture into flour, then add 1 egg, egg white (reserve yolk for glaze), remaining ½ cup potato water, remaining honey, and oil. Blend to make a firm dough, adding more flour if necessary.

Turn out onto a floured surface and knead until dough springs back when touched, 8 to 10 minutes. Place dough in an oiled bowl, turn once to coat top, and cover with a towel. Let rise in a warm place until dough has doubled in bulk, about 1½ hours. Dough is ready when you push down with 2 fingers and indentations remain. If dough springs back, let rise a bit longer.

Punch down dough, and knead for 2 to 3 minutes. Pull off or cut dough into 14 or 15 pieces. Roll each piece between floured hands until about 7 inches in length and ¾ inch thick. Coil each length into a ring, moistening the ends so that they stick when turned onto each other. Oil a board or pan. Place rings on it and let stand for about 10 minutes.

Preheat oven to 425°F. Lightly oil a baking sheet.

Bring 3 quarts water to a boil in a large pot. Using a slotted spoon, slide each bagel into boiling water, being careful not to crowd them. When bagels begin to float, boil for 2 minutes on each side. Remove with slotted spoon, and place on prepared baking sheet. (They will be very slippery.)

To make the glaze: Mix reserved egg yolk with 1 teaspoon water. Brush each bagel with mixture and sprinkle with poppy or sesame seeds (if used).

Bake for 20 to 25 minutes, or until golden brown. Place on wire racks to cool.

Makes 14 to 15 bagels

Baked Doughnuts

    1 large potato
    ½ cup milk, scalded
    ⅓ cup butter
    ½ cup honey, warmed
    2 teaspoons dry yeast
    1 egg, beaten
    2½ cups whole wheat flour
      softened butter
      Coconut Sugar (page 698)

Cook potato in enough water to cover until tender. Drain, reserving 2 tablespoons cooking water. Mash potato.

Combine milk, butter, and honey in a large bowl. Stir well and cool to lukewarm.

Dissolve yeast in warm reserved potato water. Let proof, then add to milk mixture. Add ½ cup mashed potatoes and egg, then work in flour. Place in an oiled bowl, turn once to oil top, cover, and let rise in a warm place until light, about 1 hour.

Turn out onto a floured surface, and knead for 5 to 8 minutes. Roll to ½-inch thickness and cut into circles, using a 3-inch doughnut cutter.

Lightly oil a baking sheet. Place doughnuts on baking sheet and let rise again for about 45 minutes.

Preheat oven to 425°F.

Bake for about 12 minutes, or until lightly browned. Remove from oven, brush immediately with butter, and dust with coconut sugar.

Makes 1½ dozen doughnuts

Bran Bread

    1 tablespoon dry yeast
    4 tablespoons honey

2¼ cups warm water
5½ cups whole wheat flour
⅓ cup butter, melted
2 cups bran
melted butter

In a large bowl dissolve yeast and 2 tablespoons honey in 2 cups warm water. Add 3 cups flour and blend well. Set aside for 20 minutes to proof.

Combine remaining water and honey and butter. Mix and let cool to lukewarm. Stir into yeast mixture.

Add ¾ cup bran and 2 more cups flour. Dough will be very soft and sticky. Pour all but ¼ cup remaining bran onto a floured surface. Remove ⅓ of the dough from bowl and knead into bran. Shape dough into a ball, place in a small oiled bowl, and turn once to oil top.

Begin to knead remaining flour into remaining dough. Add flour just until dough loses its stickiness. Knead about 10 minutes, then place dough in a second oiled bowl. Turn once to oil top. Cover both bowls and let dough rise in a warm place until doubled in bulk, 40 to 50 minutes.

Butter 2 8½ × 4½-inch loaf pans.

For each ball of dough, punch down, turn out onto a floured surface, and knead again. Divide larger dough ball in half, and shape each half into an 8-inch-long loaf. Set aside. Divide the smaller dough ball in half. Roll out each half into a 10-inch square on top of remaining ¼ cup bran. Wrap dough-and-bran squares around 8-inch loaves. Pinch seams together. Place loaves seam-side down in prepared loaf pans.

Cover and let rise again until doubled in bulk, 20 to 30 minutes. Be careful not to let bread rise too high.

Preheat oven to 350°F.

Bake for 30 minutes. Brush tops of loaves with melted butter, and return to oven for 5 to 10 minutes more, or until loaves sound hollow when tapped. Remove from pans and cool on wire racks.

Makes 2 loaves

Cheese-Herb Twist

1 cup cracked wheat
1½ cups boiling water

2 tablespoons dry yeast
2 cups warm water
2 tablespoons honey
2 tablespoons vegetable oil
½ cup nonfat dry milk
½ cup wheat germ
5½ to 6 cups whole wheat flour
¼ cup chopped fresh parsley
1 teaspoon crumbled dried marjoram
½ teaspoon crumbled dried oregano
½ teaspoon crumbled dried thyme
½ to 1 teaspoon pepper
2 cups coarsely grated Gruyère or Swiss cheese

Place cracked wheat in a small bowl. Pour boiling water over wheat, and let stand until lukewarm.

In a large bowl dissolve yeast in warm water. Stir in honey and let proof. Then stir in cooled cracked wheat, oil, dry milk, wheat germ, and 1 cup flour. Add parsley, marjoram, oregano, thyme, and pepper. Gradually stir in enough remaining flour to make a soft dough.

Turn out onto a floured surface, and knead until smooth and elastic, 8 to 10 minutes, using only as much flour as needed to keep dough from sticking. Place dough in an oiled bowl, and turn dough over to oil top. Cover with wax paper and a clean towel, and let rise in a warm place until doubled in bulk, about 1 hour.

On a floured surface punch down dough, and knead in cheese, reserving about ¼ cup cheese for tops of loaves. Invert bowl over dough, and let rest for 10 minutes.

Divide dough into 4 equal pieces. Roll each piece with hands to form a thick rope about 12 inches long. Twist 2 ropes together, pinch ends, and place each twist in an 8½ × 4½-inch clay loaf pan. If you do not have a clay loaf pan, place twists on a lightly oiled baking sheet. Cover and let rise again until doubled in bulk, about 45 minutes. Sprinkle with reserved cheese.

Preheat oven to 375°F.

Bake for 35 to 40 minutes, or until loaves are golden brown and sound hollow when tapped. Remove from pans to a wire rack and cool completely.

Makes 2 loaves

Cracklin' Corn and Wheat Bread

Cracklings
1 to 1½ pounds uncured pork belly fat or back fat, finely chopped
½ to ¾ teaspoon pepper

Bread
2 tablespoons dry yeast
2¼ cups warm water
¼ cup molasses
¼ cup vegetable oil
1 egg
½ cup nonfat dry milk
1½ cups cornmeal
¾ cup wheat or corn germ*
½ cup soy flour
5 to 6 cups whole wheat flour

To make the cracklings: Place fat in a large heavy saucepan and slowly cook over low to medium heat, stirring occasionally, for 1 to 1½ hours, until fat is rendered and cracklings are golden and crisp. Drain off lard and reserve for another use. Drain cracklings on paper towels. Sprinkle pepper over cracklings and toss to mix.

To make the bread: In a large bowl dissolve yeast in warm water. Add molasses and let proof. Stir in oil, egg, dry milk, cornmeal, wheat or corn germ, and soy flour until smooth. Gradually beat in 2 cups whole wheat flour. Cover bowl and let dough rise in a warm place until almost doubled in bulk, about 30 minutes.

Stir in enough remaining flour to make a stiff dough. Turn out onto a floured surface. Knead until smooth and elastic, 8 to 10 minutes. Place in an oiled bowl, and turn once to oil top. Cover with wax paper and a towel, and let rise again until doubled in bulk, about 1 hour.

Butter 2 9 × 5-inch loaf pans.

Punch down dough. On floured surface knead in cracklings. Divide dough in half and shape each half into a loaf. Place in prepared loaf pans. Cover and let rise again until doubled in bulk.

Preheat oven to 375°F.

Bake for 35 to 40 minutes, or until loaves are golden and sound hollow when tapped. Remove from pans and cool completely on wire racks.

Makes 2 loaves

*Corn germ is available in natural foods stores.

Fruit Bread

This bread requires advance planning—not extra work. The fruit must be left to soak in the prepared liquid for at least 12 hours, and the finished bread is best after "ripening" overnight.

1½ cups diced dried pears
½ cup diced dried figs
1½ cups diced mixed dried fruits (prunes, apples, peaches, or apricots)
½ cup raisins
¾ cup apple cider
¼ cup honey
2 teaspoons grated lemon rind
2 tablespoons lemon juice
3½ to 4 cups whole wheat flour
1 tablespoon dry yeast
1 cup milk
1 egg
1 tablespoon ground cinnamon
1 teaspoon aniseed, ground
½ cup coarsely chopped walnuts
½ cup coarsely chopped almonds
½ cup sunflower seeds
1 egg, beaten

At least 12 hours before making dough, place pears, figs, mixed fruits, and raisins in a medium-size bowl. Heat cider and honey in a small saucepan until bubbles appear around edge. Pour over fruits. Add lemon rind and juice. Toss to mix and coat fruits. Cover bowl with plastic wrap and leave to steep, stirring once or twice. Fruits will absorb all or most of liquid.

In a large bowl mix 1 cup flour with yeast. Heat milk to 120 to 130°F, and gradually add to dry ingredients. Beat for 2 minutes with electric mixer at medium speed. Add egg, ½ cup flour, cinnamon, and aniseed. Beat for 2 minutes. Stir in enough remaining flour to make a soft dough.

Turn out onto a floured surface, and knead until smooth and elastic, 8 to 10 minutes, using only enough flour to keep dough from sticking. Place in oiled bowl, and turn to oil top. Cover with wax paper and a towel. Let rise in a warm place until doubled in bulk, about 1 hour.

Lightly oil a baking sheet.

Punch down dough. Turn out onto floured surface, and gradually knead in fruit mixture, nuts, and seeds, using only as much flour as needed to keep dough from sticking. Divide in half and shape each half into a loaf about 12 inches long. Place on prepared baking sheet. Cover with a towel, and let rise again until doubled in bulk, 1 to 1½ hours.

Preheat oven to 350°F.

Brush loaves with egg, and bake for 35 to 40 minutes, or until golden brown. Cool completely on wire racks. Wrap in plastic wrap and leave in a cool place to "ripen" overnight or longer. Slice thin and serve with sweet butter and honey.

Makes 2 loaves

Golden Saffron Braid

½ teaspoon saffron threads, crushed
2 tablespoons boiling water
3½ to 4 cups whole wheat flour
1 tablespoon dry yeast
1 cup milk
½ cup butter
¼ cup honey
3 eggs
¾ cup brown rice flour
⅓ cup ground millet
1 teaspoon ground coriander
1 cup raisins or dried currants
poppy seeds or sesame seeds

In a small bowl soak saffron in boiling water for 15 minutes.

In a large bowl combine 1¼ cups whole wheat flour with yeast.

In a small saucepan heat milk, butter, and honey to 120 to 130°F. Gradually add to dry ingredients, and beat for 2 minutes with electric mixer at medium speed. Add saffron-water mixture, 2 eggs, rice flour, millet, coriander, and ½ cup whole wheat flour. Beat for 2 minutes. Stir in enough remaining flour to make a soft dough.

Turn out onto a floured surface, and knead until smooth and elastic, 8 to 10 minutes. Place in an oiled bowl, and turn once to oil top. Cover with wax paper and a clean towel. Let rise in a warm place until doubled in bulk, about 1 hour.

Lightly oil a large baking sheet.

Punch down dough and turn out onto floured surface. Knead in raisins or currants until evenly distributed throughout dough. Divide into 4 pieces. Set 1 piece aside. Roll each of 3 pieces into an 18-inch rope. Braid ropes together. Place on prepared baking sheet. Divide last piece of dough in half, and roll each half into a 24-inch-long rope. Twist ropes together and place lengthwise on top of braid. Pinch ends together to seal. Cover with towel and let rise again until doubled in bulk, 30 to 45 minutes.

Preheat oven to 350°F.

In a cup lightly beat remaining egg. Brush loaf with egg, sprinkle with poppy or sesame seeds, and bake for 40 to 45 minutes, or until loaves are golden brown and sound hollow when tapped. Remove to a wire rack. Cool completely.

Makes 1 loaf

NOTE: To make 2 smaller loaves, divide dough in half and shape each half as directed above, making ropes about 12 and 16 inches long. Bake for about 35 minutes.

Golden Sweet Potato Buns

        2 tablespoons dry yeast
        ⅔ cup warm water
        ½ cup maple syrup
6 to 7 cups whole wheat flour
        ½ cup cornmeal
        ½ cup soy grits
        ½ cup wheat germ
        1 teaspoon ground cinnamon
        ½ teaspoon ground ginger
        1 cup orange juice
        2 eggs
        3 tablespoons safflower oil
1 to 1½ cups mashed cooked sweet potatoes
        ½ cup soft tofu, drained
        2 tablespoons grated orange rind
           finely chopped pecans

In a small bowl dissolve yeast in warm water. Stir in 1 teaspoon maple syrup and let proof.

In a large bowl combine 1 cup flour, cornmeal, soy grits, wheat germ, cinnamon, and ginger.

Heat orange juice and remaining maple syrup to 120 to 130°F in a small saucepan. Gradually stir into dry ingredients and beat with a wooden spoon until smooth. Stir in yeast, 1 egg, oil, and 1 cup flour. Blend in sweet potatoes, tofu, and orange rind. Gradually beat in enough remaining flour to make a soft dough.

Turn out onto a floured surface, and knead until smooth and elastic, 10 to 12 minutes. Dough will be heavy and slightly tacky. Place in an oiled bowl, and turn dough to oil top. Cover with a clean towel, and let rise in a warm place until doubled in bulk, 1 to 1½ hours.

Generously butter 2 9-inch-square baking pans.

Punch down dough. Turn out onto floured surface and knead a few times. Divide dough in half. Then shape each half into 16 uniform smooth balls. Place in prepared baking pans. Cover and let rise again until doubled in bulk, about 1 hour.

Preheat oven to 400°F.

In a cup beat remaining egg lightly with a fork and brush tops. Sprinkle with pecans. Bake for 20 to 25 minutes, or until buns are golden brown and sound hollow when tapped. Remove from pans to wire racks. Serve warm.

Makes 32 buns

NOTE: These buns reheat nicely. Place in preheated 350°F oven for 5 to 8 minutes.

Green Cabbage-Stuffed Bread

   Dough
1½ teaspoons dry yeast
    2 tablespoons warm water
    1 tablespoon plus ½ teaspoon honey
    ½ cup milk
    ¼ cup butter
    1 egg
    ½ teaspoon caraway seeds
    ½ cup rye flour
1¾ cups whole wheat flour

   Filling
    1 medium-size onion, finely chopped
    2 tablespoons butter
3½ cups finely chopped Chinese cabbage,
       including ribs
    1 tablespoon minced fresh dill
    ¼ teaspoon pepper
    ½ cup creamed cottage cheese
    1 egg, beaten
       melted butter (optional)

To make the dough: Dissolve yeast in warm water. Add ½ teaspoon honey, stir, and set aside to proof.

Warm milk and melt butter in it. Set aside to cool.

In a large bowl beat egg with 1 tablespoon honey. Stir in milk and yeast mixtures. Add seeds and rye flour, and mix well into liquid. Then gradually mix in whole wheat flour, kneading briefly. Although dough might still be a little sticky, don't add any more flour.

Place dough in an oiled bowl, and turn so both sides are oiled. Cover and let rise in a warm place until doubled in bulk, about 45 minutes.

To make the filling: In a large skillet sauté onions in butter for about 3 minutes. Add cabbage and continue to sauté until wilted and soft but not browned. Add dill and pepper. Remove from heat and stir in cottage cheese and egg. Set aside.

Punch down dough, and knead well on a floured surface for 5 to 10 minutes. Return to bowl and allow to rise again until doubled in bulk. Punch down, knead briefly on floured surface, and divide into 2 equal parts.

Butter a 10-inch pie plate. Press or roll out part of dough so it fits bottom of pie plate and just starts to come up sides. Spread filling over bottom, leaving a ½-inch space along edge. Roll or press out remaining dough, and fit it over top of filling. Press the 2 layers of dough together around edge. Prick top with a fork to allow steam to escape. Let rise again until doubled in bulk.

Preheat oven to 350°F.

Bake for 20 minutes. Brush with butter (if used). Serve warm or cold.

8 servings

Herb Casserole Bread

    1 tablespoon dry yeast
    ¼ cup warm water
    3 teaspoons honey
    ¼ cup milk
    2 tablespoons butter
    1 cup creamed cottage cheese
    1 egg
    ½ cup rolled oats
    2 tablespoons soy flour
    2¼ cups whole wheat flour
    ¼ teaspoon baking soda
    ½ cup sliced scallions, with tops
    ¼ cup chopped fresh mint
    ½ teaspoon dried oregano
    ½ teaspoon grated lemon rind
      melted butter

In a large bowl dissolve yeast in warm water. Stir in 1 teaspoon honey. Set aside to proof.

Combine remaining honey, milk, and butter in a small saucepan, and heat until bubbles appear around edge. Remove from heat. Stir in cottage cheese and egg. Add to yeast. Then stir in ¼ cup oats, soy flour, 1 cup whole wheat flour, and baking soda. Beat with electric mixer at medium speed for 2 minutes. Stir in remaining flour to make a stiff dough. Cover bowl with wax paper and a clean towel, and let dough rise in a warm place until doubled in bulk, about 1 hour.

Generously butter a 1½-quart ovenproof casserole. Sprinkle with remaining rolled oats.

Stir down dough. Add scallions, mint, oregano, and lemon rind and stir in. Turn into prepared casserole. Cover and let rise again until doubled in bulk, about 45 minutes.

Preheat oven to 350°F.

Bake for 35 to 40 minutes, or until loaf sounds hollow when tapped. Brush top with melted butter for soft crust. Turn out of casserole, and cool on a wire rack. Serve warm.

Makes 1 loaf

Honey and Nut-Filled Buns

Dough
3 to 3¼ cups whole wheat flour
    ¼ teaspoon ground mace or nutmeg
    1 tablespoon dry yeast
    ½ cup water
    ½ cup milk
    ¼ cup plus 2 tablespoons butter
    ¼ cup honey
    2 eggs, at room temperature

Filling
    ¼ cup plus 1 tablespoon butter, softened
    ⅓ cup honey
    1 tablespoon plus 1 teaspoon grated orange rind
    1 teaspoon ground cinnamon
    1 cup chopped pecans or walnuts
    ½ cup raisins

To make the dough: In a large bowl combine 1 cup flour, mace or nutmeg, and yeast.

In a small saucepan heat water, milk, butter, and honey over low heat until very warm (120 to 125°F). Gradually add to dry ingredients, and beat for 2 minutes with electric mixer at medium speed, scraping bowl often. In a small bowl beat eggs together. Reserve about 2 tablespoons for brushing buns; add remainder to dough mixture. Add ¾ cup flour and continue beating for 3 minutes, scraping bowl often. Stir in enough remaining flour to make a fairly stiff dough.

Turn out onto a floured surface, and knead until smooth and elastic, 8 to 10 minutes, using only enough flour to keep dough from sticking. Place in a large oiled bowl, turn to oil top, cover, and let rise in a warm place until doubled in bulk, 1 to 1½ hours.

To make the filling: Place butter in a small bowl. Gradually beat in honey. Blend in orange rind and cinnamon. Then fold in nuts and raisins.

Preheat oven to 375°F. Lightly oil a baking sheet.

Punch down dough. Divide into 16 equal pieces. Shape each into a 4- to 5-inch round. Place about 1 rounded teaspoon filling on center of each, fold dough up and around filling, and pinch together tightly to enclose filling. Place buns pinched-side down on prepared baking sheet. Cover with clean towel, and let rise again until doubled in bulk, about 45 minutes. Brush with reserved egg.

Bake for 20 to 25 minutes, or until golden. Cool on a wire rack.

Makes 16 buns

Honey-Wheat Loaf

    1 tablespoon dry yeast
 2½ cups warm water
  ¼ cup plus 2 tablespoons honey
    3 tablespoons vegetable oil
    6 cups whole wheat flour
    1 teaspoon ground cinnamon
  ½ cup raisins
  ¼ cup sunflower seeds

In a large bowl dissolve yeast in warm water. Add ¼ cup honey and set aside to proof. Add oil.

In a medium-size bowl blend flour, cinnamon, raisins, and sunflower seeds. Mix them with liquid mixture. Knead until smooth, cover, and let rise in a warm place until doubled in bulk. Butter 2 9 × 5-inch loaf pans.

Punch down dough and form into 2 loaves. Place in prepared loaf pans, and let rise again until doubled in bulk.

Preheat oven to 350°F.

Bake for about 30 minutes. Brush with remaining honey and return to oven for 5 to 10 minutes to set glaze.

Makes 2 loaves

Hot Cross Buns with Cream Cheese Glaze

    2 tablespoons dry yeast
  ⅓ cup warm water
  ¼ cup honey
  ¾ cup half-and-half or light cream
  ¼ cup plus 2 tablespoons butter
    1 tablespoon molasses
    3 eggs
    1 cup quick-cooking rolled oats
  ¼ cup wheat germ
3 to 3½ cups whole wheat flour
  ½ teaspoon ground cinnamon
  ½ teaspoon ground cardamom
  ¾ cup dried currants or chopped raisins
      Cream Cheese Glaze (see opposite)

In a large bowl dissolve yeast in warm water. Stir in 1 teaspoon honey and let proof.

In a small saucepan heat half-and-half or cream and butter to 105 to 115°F. Add to yeast. Stir in remaining honey, molasses, 2 eggs, oats, wheat germ, 1 cup flour, cinnamon, and cardamom. Beat 2 minutes and then stir in currants or raisins and enough remaining flour to make a soft dough.

Turn out onto a floured surface, and knead until smooth and elastic, 6 to 8 minutes, adding only enough flour to keep dough from sticking. Place in oiled bowl, and turn dough to oil top. Cover with wax paper and a clean towel, and let rise in a warm place until doubled in bulk, 45 to 60 minutes.

Generously butter 2 8-inch-square baking pans.

Punch down dough. Divide into 18 equal-size pieces, and shape each into a smooth ball. Place 9 pieces in each prepared baking pan. Let rise again until doubled in bulk, 30 to 45 minutes. Cut a cross into top of each bun with a sharp razor blade. In a cup lightly beat remaining egg and brush top of each bun.

Preheat oven to 375°F.

Bake for 25 to 30 minutes, or until golden brown. Remove from pans and place on wire racks. While still warm, draw a cross on top of each with the glaze. Best served warm.

Makes 1½ dozen buns

Cream Cheese Glaze

    3 ounces cream cheese, softened
    1 tablespoon butter, softened
    2 tablespoons honey
  ¼ teaspoon grated lemon rind

In a small bowl beat cream cheese and butter until smooth. Then beat in honey and lemon rind. Refrigerate until ready to use.

Yields enough for 1½ dozen buns

Granola Bread

    2 tablespoons dry yeast
    2 cups warm water
    1 cup milk, warmed
  ½ cup vegetable oil
  ¼ cup honey
    8 cups whole wheat flour
  ½ cup granola
  ½ cup sunflower seeds
  ½ cup raisins
    2 tablespoons grated orange rind
    1 egg, beaten with 1 tablespoon milk

In a large bowl combine yeast, warm water, milk, oil, honey, and 4 cups flour. Stir in granola, sunflower seeds, raisins, orange rind, and 4 cups flour. Knead until smooth, 8 to 10 minutes. Place in an oiled bowl, turn to oil top, cover, and let rise in a warm place until doubled in bulk, 45 to 60 minutes.

Turn out onto a floured surface, punch down, return to bowl, cover, and let rise again until doubled in bulk, about 1 hour.

Butter 3 8½ × 4½-inch loaf pans.

After second rise turn out dough onto floured surface, punch down, and knead for just a couple of minutes. Divide into 3 equal loaves and place in prepared loaf pans. Cover and let rise again until doubled in bulk, 45 to 60 minutes.

Preheat oven to 350°F.

Slash tops with a sharp floured knife. Brush egg mixture over loaves, and bake for 45 to 50 minutes, or until loaves sound hollow when tapped. Turn out onto wire racks.

Makes 3 loaves

Millet-Wheat Bread

    2 tablespoons dry yeast
    ¼ cup warm water
    ⅔ cup honey
    2 cups milk, scalded
    2 tablespoons vegetable oil
    3 cups ground millet
    ½ cup soy flour
4 to 5 cups whole wheat flour
      cornmeal (optional)

In a small bowl dissolve yeast in warm water. Mix in 1 teaspoon honey. Set aside to proof.

Combine milk, oil, and remaining honey. Pour this mixture over millet in a large bowl and allow to cool, stirring occasionally.

When mixture has cooled, add yeast, soy flour, and 3 cups whole wheat flour. Blend well. Keep adding more flour until dough is thick and fairly dry.

Turn out onto a floured surface, and knead until dough seems moist and stretches without tearing, about 10 minutes. Shape dough into a ball, place in an oiled bowl, and turn over once to oil top. Cover bowl with a clean towel, and let rise in a warm place until doubled in bulk, about 1½ hours.

Generously butter 2 9 × 5-inch loaf pans.

Punch down dough, place on floured surface, and shape into 2 loaves. Score top of each loaf with a sharp knife, and place in prepared loaf pans. (Or shape into round or oblong loaves and place on a baking sheet sprinkled generously with cornmeal.) Cover loaves and let rise again for 45 minutes.

Preheat oven to 375°F.

Bake for about 50 minutes.

Makes 2 loaves

Multigrain–Sprouted Wheat Bread

    2 tablespoons dry yeast
   2½ cups warm water
    4 tablespoons molasses
    1 egg
    ¼ cup safflower oil
    2 tablespoons cider vinegar
4 to 5 cups whole wheat flour
    ¾ cup rye flour
    ½ cup amaranth flour
    ½ cup brown rice flour
    ½ cup soy flour
    ½ cup barley flour
    ¼ cup ground millet
    ½ cup rolled oats
    2 cups wheat sprouts, finely chopped

In a large bowl dissolve yeast in 1 cup warm water. Stir in 1 tablespoon molasses. Let stand to proof.

Stir in remaining water and molasses, egg, oil, vinegar, 1 cup whole wheat flour, the rye flour, amaranth flour, rice flour, soy flour, barley flour, millet, and oats. Beat until smooth. Gradually beat in enough remaining whole wheat flour to make a stiff dough that can be kneaded.

Turn out onto a floured surface and knead until smooth and elastic, about 10 minutes, adding enough flour to keep dough from sticking. Place in an oiled bowl, and turn to oil top of dough. Cover with wax paper and a clean towel, and let rise in a warm place until doubled in bulk, 1 to 1½ hours.

Butter 2 9 × 5-inch loaf pans.

Turn out dough onto floured surface, and knead in wheat sprouts. Divide dough in half and shape into 2 loaves. Place in prepared loaf pans. Cover and let rise again for 45 to 60 minutes. (They do not quite double.)

Preheat oven to 350°F.

Bake for 50 minutes, or until loaves sound hollow when tapped. Cool completely on a wire rack.

Makes 2 loaves

No-Knead Triticale Bread

1 tablespoon dry yeast
2⅔ cups warm water
2 teaspoons honey
2 cups triticale flour
3 cups whole wheat flour
3 tablespoons molasses
⅓ cup wheat germ
1 tablespoon unhulled sesame seeds

In a small bowl dissolve yeast in ⅔ cup warm water and then add honey. Leave to proof.

Warm flours by placing them in a 250°F oven for 20 minutes.

Combine molasses with ⅔ cup warm water and add to yeast mixture. Place warmed flours in a large bowl. Stir in yeast mixture, then add wheat germ and 1⅓ cups warm water. Dough will be sticky.

Butter a 9 × 5-inch loaf pan, taking care to butter corners well. Turn dough into pan. No kneading is necessary. Smooth dough with a spatula which has been held under cold water to prevent stickiness. Sprinkle sesame seeds over top of loaf. Let rise to top of pan in a warm place.

Preheat oven to 400°F.

Bake for 30 to 40 minutes, or until crust is brown and sides of loaf are firm and crusty. Cool pan on a wire rack for 10 minutes before removing loaf. Cool completely before slicing.

Makes 1 loaf

No-Knead Whole Wheat Bread

7½ cups whole wheat flour
2 tablespoons dry yeast
4 cups warm water
1 tablespoon honey
¼ cup molasses

Place flour in a large bowl and place in a warm oven for about 20 minutes to warm flour and bowl. If it is a gas oven, the pilot light will give sufficient heat; if electric, set at lowest temperature.

In a small bowl dissolve yeast in 1 cup warm water and then add honey. Let proof.

Mix molasses with 1 cup warm water. Combine yeast mixture with molasses mixture and add to flour. Add enough warm water to make a sticky dough, about 2 cups.

Butter 2 large loaf pans, at least 9 × 5 inches, or 3 small loaf pans, and place entire mixture directly into pans. No kneading is necessary. Let rise in a warm place for 1 hour.

Preheat oven to 400°F.

Bake for 30 to 40 minutes, or until crust is brown. Remove pans from oven and let cool on wire racks for 10 minutes. Remove loaves from pans and let cool completely on wire racks before slicing.

Makes 2 large or 3 small loaves

Old-Country Soft Pretzel Sticks

1 tablespoon dry yeast
1¼ cups warm water
1 tablespoon honey
4½ cups rye flour
1 egg, beaten with ½ teaspoon water
1 medium-size onion, chopped and sautéed
   (caraway, sesame, or poppy seeds may
   be substituted)

In a large bowl dissolve yeast in warm water. Add honey and let proof. Then stir in 4 cups flour.

Lightly oil a baking sheet.

Turn out dough onto a floured surface and knead in ½ cup flour until smooth. Divide dough into 48 pieces, and roll each into a rope about ½ inch in diameter and 5 inches long. Place on prepared baking sheet. Brush with egg and sprinkle with onions. Let rise in a warm place for 20 to 30 minutes.

Preheat oven to 425°F.

Bake for 15 to 20 minutes. Cool on wire racks.

Makes 4 dozen sticks

Pizza

  1½ cups warm water
    1 tablespoon honey
    2 tablespoons dry yeast
    3 tablespoons vegetable oil
 5 to 6 cups whole wheat flour
2½ to 3 cups tomato sauce
    4 cups shredded mozzarella cheese
    ¾ cup grated Parmesan cheese
      dried oregano, to taste

In a large bowl combine warm water, honey, and yeast and let proof. Then add oil and enough flour to make a firm dough. Turn dough onto a floured surface and knead until smooth and elastic, adding flour as needed. Place dough in an oiled bowl, and turn over once to oil top. Cover bowl with a damp towel, and let rise in a warm place until doubled in bulk, about 1 hour.

Punch down dough, knead briefly, cover, and let rise again until doubled in bulk.

Divide into 2 balls. Form each ball into a circle. Roll out each circle to fit a 16-inch-round pizza pan. (Or divide dough into 4 pieces and roll out each one to fit an 8-inch-round pan.) Place rolled dough on pans. Form a small raised ridge with dough around edge of each pan, to hold sauce. Allow dough to rise on pans another 30 minutes.

Preheat oven to 450°F.

Spoon sauce evenly over each pizza. Distribute mozzarella and Parmesan equally over each. Sprinkle oregano over tops.

Bake for 15 to 20 minutes, or until outer crust is crisp and cheese has melted.

Makes 2 large or 4 small pizzas

Variations:

Spread any 1 or a combination of the following toppings, to taste, over pizza before baking:
    diced green or sweet red peppers
    diced onions
    lightly sautéed sliced mushrooms
    crumbled cooked sausage

Poppy Seed Roll

     2 tablespoons dry yeast
5½ to 6 cups whole wheat flour
   1½ cups milk
    ½ cup honey
    ⅓ cup butter
    3 eggs
    1 cup boiling water
    ¾ cup poppy seeds
    ½ cup chopped nuts
    1 teaspoon grated lemon rind
    1 egg white

In a large bowl combine yeast with 2 cups of flour.

In a medium-size saucepan heat milk, ½ of the honey, and butter until lukewarm. Add mixture to dry ingredients. Add eggs. Stir in enough flour to make a stiff dough.

Turn out onto a floured surface, and knead for about 10 minutes. Shape into a ball, place in an oiled bowl, and turn once to oil top. Cover lightly and let rise in a warm place until doubled in bulk.

Pour boiling water over poppy seeds, and let stand for 30 minutes. Then drain thoroughly. Place poppy seeds in a blender, and blend until ground. Combine with nuts, remainder of honey, and lemon rind in a small bowl. Beat egg white until stiff, and fold into poppy seed mixture.

Turn out dough onto floured surface and punch down. Divide into 2 parts. Let rest for 10 minutes.

Butter 2 9 × 5-inch loaf pans.

Roll 1 part of dough into an 8 × 24-inch rectangle. Spread with ½ of the poppy seed mixture. Roll up jelly-roll style, starting with 8-inch side. Place seam-side down in prepared loaf pan. Repeat with rest of dough. Cover with a towel. Let rise again until doubled in bulk.

Preheat oven to 350°F.

Bake for 35 to 40 minutes.

Makes 2 loaves

Raisin-Rye Rolls from Potato Starter

The potato starter used to make these rolls needs a minimum of 24 hours (two to three days is better) to develop flavor before it can be mixed with the other ingredients to make the dough.

  1 tablespoon dry yeast
1¼ cups warm water
  ⅓ cup molasses
  1 cup Potato Starter (see opposite)
  3 tablespoons vegetable oil
  1 tablespoon caraway seeds
  1 tablespoon grated orange rind
  ½ cup bran
  ¼ cup sifted powdered carob
2½ cups rye flour
2 to 2½ cups whole wheat flour
  1 cup raisins
    cornmeal
  1 egg white, lightly beaten
    sesame seeds (optional)

In a large bowl dissolve yeast in warm water. Stir in 1 tablespoon molasses and let proof.

Stir in remaining molasses, potato starter, oil, caraway seeds, orange rind, bran, and carob. Gradually stir in rye flour and enough whole wheat flour to make a soft dough.

Turn out onto a floured surface, and knead until smooth and elastic, 8 to 10 minutes, using only enough remaining flour to keep dough from sticking. Dough will be slightly tacky. Place dough in a large oiled bowl, and turn once to oil top. Cover with a clean towel, and let rise in a warm place until doubled in bulk, about 45 minutes.

Punch down dough on floured surface and knead a few times. Knead in raisins. Invert bowl over dough and allow to rest for 10 minutes.

Lightly oil a baking sheet. Sprinkle with cornmeal.

Divide dough into 18 equal pieces, and shape into smooth balls. Place balls 2½ to 3 inches apart on prepared baking sheet. Let rise again until doubled in bulk, 30 to 45 minutes.

Preheat oven to 375°F.

Brush rolls with egg white, and sprinkle with sesame seeds (if used). Bake for 20 minutes, or until rolls sound hollow when tapped. Cool on a wire rack.

Makes 1½ dozen rolls

Potato Starter

1 large potato
1 tablespoon dry yeast
2 cups whole wheat flour or rye flour, or 1 cup each

Cut potato into quarters, and boil in enough water to cover until tender. Drain, reserving water. Add more water to equal 2 cups, if necessary. Cool to lukewarm. Mash potatoes with a fork.

In a large bowl dissolve yeast in reserved water. Stir in potato and flour to make a smooth dough. Cover tightly and let stand at room temperature (75°F) for at least 24 hours, preferably for 2 to 3 days for a fully developed flavor. Stir down once a day.

Yields 3 cups

NOTE: Starter should be stored in the refrigerator, then taken out and brought to room temperature before being used. After each use, replenish starter by adding equal amounts of flour and warm water.

Pumpernickel Bread

  1 cup milk
  ¾ cup water
  ¼ cup butter
  3 tablespoons sifted powdered carob
  ¼ cup unsulfured molasses
  1 tablespoon dry yeast
  2 eggs
  2 tablespoons caraway seeds
3½ cups whole wheat flour
  2 cups rye flour

Heat milk, water, butter, and carob in a medium-size saucepan until butter is melted. Cool to lukewarm in a large bowl. Stir in molasses. Stir yeast into milk mixture and allow to proof.

With an electric mixer or by hand, beat in 1 whole egg, 1 egg yolk, ½ of the caraway seeds, and 2 cups whole wheat flour. Gradually add rye flour. Stir in some remaining whole wheat flour until mixture becomes too thick to stir.

Turn out onto a floured surface, and knead in remaining whole wheat flour until dough is firm and elastic, 8 to 10 minutes. Place dough in an oiled bowl. Turn once to oil top and cover with plastic wrap. Let rise in a warm place until doubled in bulk, about 35 minutes.

Punch down dough and shape into 2 loaves. Place on a lightly oiled baking sheet. In a cup beat egg white lightly with a fork. Brush tops with egg white, and sprinkle with remaining caraway seeds. Let rise again until doubled in bulk, about 35 minutes.

Preheat oven to 375°F.

Bake for 30 minutes, or until loaves sound hollow when tapped.

Makes 2 loaves

Rye Bread

    3½ cups rye flour
     4 cups whole wheat flour
    1½ teaspoons baking soda
     2 tablespoons baking powder
     ½ cup caraway seeds
     4 cups buttermilk, at room temperature

In a large bowl mix dry ingredients. Then add buttermilk to make a sticky dough. Mix with a wooden spoon or with floured hands. If dough seems too sticky, add more flour.

Lightly oil and flour a baking sheet.

Form dough into 3 loaves of any of the basic shapes—long, oblong, oval, or round. Shape the loaves smoothly with your hands, and place on prepared baking sheet, leaving room between them for expansion. With a floured knife, cut a design in tops. Do it deeply—a cross, star, anything that will allow bread to expand evenly instead of bursting open at seams.

Dust tops with flour, then blow off excess.

Preheat oven to 425°F.

Bake for about 50 minutes, or until tops have browned nicely and bottoms sound hollow when tapped. Cool on wire racks.

Makes 3 loaves

Sage Pizza Bread

    2½ to 3 cups whole wheat flour
     2 tablespoons crumbled dried sage
     1 tablespoon dry yeast
    1¼ cups water, heated to 120 to 130°F
     3 tablespoons olive oil
       freshly ground pepper, to taste

Place 1 cup flour, sage, and yeast in a large bowl. Gradually add heated water, and beat well with a wooden spoon for 2 minutes. Beat in 1 tablespoon olive oil and enough remaining flour to make a soft dough.

Turn out onto a floured surface, and knead until smooth and elastic, about 10 minutes, using only as much remaining flour as needed to keep dough from sticking. Place in an oiled bowl. Turn once to oil top. Cover with a clean towel, and let rise in a warm place until doubled in bulk, about 1 hour.

Lightly oil a baking sheet.

Punch down dough, knead a few times on floured surface, and roll out to ½-inch thickness. Place on prepared baking sheet. Using fingertips, make a series of indentations in dough, drizzle with remaining oil, and sprinkle with pepper. Let rise again until doubled in bulk, about 20 minutes.

Preheat oven to 400°F.

Bake for 25 to 30 minutes, or until golden. Cool on a wire rack. Cut into wedges or tear off pieces for serving. Serve hot.

Makes 1 loaf

Variation:
Rosemary-Garlic Pizza Bread: Add 2 teaspoons crumbled dried rosemary instead of sage to dough. Place thin slivers of garlic (about 2 cloves) in indentations before baking. Remove garlic before serving.

Sally Lunn

Some say this bread was named for an eighteenth-century English woman who created it. Others with a more romantic turn of mind say it was named "Soleil et Lune" by the French, who thought it had the universal appeal of both the sun and the moon.

      ½ cup plus 1 teaspoon honey
      ¼ cup warm water
      2 teaspoons dry yeast
    1¾ cup milk, scalded
      1 cup dried currants (optional)
      ½ cup butter
      2 teaspoons ground cinnamon
      1 cup chopped walnuts (optional)
      3 cups whole wheat flour, at room temperature
      4 eggs, at room temperature, separated

Combine 1 teaspoon honey and warm water in a small bowl. Dissolve yeast in mixture and set aside to proof. Mix together milk, currants (if used), and butter. Mix cinnamon and walnuts (if used) with flour.

Using an electric mixer, beat egg yolks briefly in a large bowl. Add ½ cup honey and beat until fluffy. Beat in yeast and milk mixtures. Gradually add flour mixture, and beat hard for 3 minutes.

Beat egg whites until stiff. Fold ¼ of them thoroughly into batter. Then gently fold in remaining egg whites.

Generously butter 2 9 × 5-inch pans or 1 9-inch tube pan.

Gently turn batter into prepared pans. Set pans into a larger pan of warm water and let rise in a warm place for about 1 hour. Carefully lift pans out of water and into cold oven.

Preheat oven to 400°F.

Bake for 15 minutes. Reduce heat to 325°F and continue to bake for 25 to 30 minutes, or until a wooden pick inserted into center comes out clean. Remove pans from oven, and cool for 5 minutes on a wire rack. Gently loosen bread from sides of pans, and carefully turn out bread. Cool completely on a wire rack.

Makes 2 rectangular loaves or 1 round loaf

Soft Breadsticks

         1 tablespoon dry yeast
         ½ cup warm water
         1 teaspoon honey
         ½ cup vegetable oil or butter, melted
      1½ tablespoons honey
         ½ cup boiling water
         2 eggs
  3½ to 4 cups whole wheat pastry flour
           sesame, poppy, or caraway seeds

In a small bowl dissolve yeast in warm water. Add 1 teaspoon honey. Set aside to proof.

In a large bowl mix together oil or butter, 1½ tablespoons honey, and boiling water. Cool to lukewarm.

Lightly beat 1 egg and add to cooled liquid. Then add dissolved yeast. Gradually stir in 3½ cups flour, mixing well, but do not knead. If dough is too soft and sticky, add a bit more flour. Place in refrigerator to chill until firm.

Lightly oil a baking sheet.

Divide dough into 12 equal parts. On a floured surface and in hands, roll into sticks about 12 inches in length. Place 1½ inches apart on prepared baking sheet. In a cup beat remaining egg lightly with a fork, and brush tops of breadsticks. Then sprinkle with seeds. Let rise in a warm place for about 30 minutes.

Preheat oven to 425°F.

Bake for 15 minutes. Cool on a wire rack or serve warm.

Makes 1 dozen sticks

NOTE: For shorter sticks divide dough into 24 equal parts.

Sourdough English Muffins

When you make these muffins, be sure to plan on the milk-flour-starter mixture setting overnight, before continuing with the recipe.

   3 cups milk, scalded
   1 cup Traditional Sourdough Starter (page 350)
   8 cups whole wheat flour
   1 tablespoon dry yeast
   ½ cup warm water
   1 tablespoon honey
   ¼ cup plus 2 tablespoons vegetable oil
   ¼ cup cornmeal

Pour milk into a large bowl. When it has cooled to lukewarm, add sourdough starter, and gradually stir in 4 cups flour until thoroughly mixed. Cover loosely and leave in a warm place overnight (a turned-off oven is a good spot).

Next morning, in a large bowl dissolve yeast in warm water. Add honey, ¼ cup oil, and remaining flour. Set aside to proof.

Stir down sourdough mixture and add to yeast mixture.

Turn out dough onto floured surface, and knead for 10 to 12 minutes. Sprinkle floured surface with cornmeal, and roll out dough to thickness of English muffins—about ⅜ inch. Cut with large round cutter, and place muffins on baking sheet. Let rise in a warm place until doubled in bulk.

Heat a large iron skillet over medium-low heat, add remaining oil, and cook muffins for about 5 minutes on each side. Be very careful not to burn them. Serve muffins hot, or cool and store them, splitting and toasting them before serving.

Makes 2 dozen muffins

Sourdough Pumpernickel Bread

The sourdough starter for this bread will have to set overnight with the liquid and flour before you continue with the recipe.

   ½ cup cornmeal
   1 cup cracked wheat
   2 cups cracked rye*
  3½ cups boiling water
   1 cup Handy Sourdough Starter (page 350)
  1½ cups warm water
   ½ cup molasses
   2 teaspoons dry yeast
  2¾ cups rye flour
   3 cups whole wheat flour

In a large bowl combine cornmeal, wheat, and rye. Pour boiling water over all, stirring briskly to avoid lumping. Cool to lukewarm and then add sourdough starter, stirring until dough is smooth. This is the sponge. Leave overnight in a warm place (a turned-off oven is a good spot).

Next morning, remove 1 cup sponge, combine with 1 cup warm water, and refrigerate for future use.

In a small bowl combine ½ cup warm water and 1 tablespoon molasses. Dissolve yeast in this mixture. Set aside to proof.

Add yeast mixture and remaining molasses to remaining sponge. Then add flours, reserving some for kneading.

On a floured surface knead dough until no longer sticky. Place in a large oiled bowl, and turn to oil top. Cover with a cloth and let rise in a warm place for 2½ hours.

Butter 1 large ovenproof casserole or 2 small ones.

Punch down dough, and form into 1 large loaf or 2 smaller loaves. Place each in a prepared casserole. Cover with cloth, and let rise again for 1 hour.

Preheat oven to 200°F.

Cover casseroles tightly with foil and/or lid, and bake bread for 3 to 4 hours with a pan of water on lowest shelf of oven. Bread is done when a wooden pick inserted into center comes out clean. Remove from casseroles and cool before slicing.

Makes 1 large loaf or 2 small loaves

*If cracked rye is not available for purchase, you can make your own by coarsely grinding rye berries in a blender.

Sourdough Rye Bread

Plan to let the starter-liquid-flour mixture set overnight before going on with the rest of this recipe.

1 cup Handy Sourdough Starter (page 350)
1½ cups water
4 cups rye flour
1 tablespoon molasses
½ cup warm water
1 tablespoon dry yeast
2 tablespoons vegetable oil
4 cups brown rice flour
⅓ cup oat flour

Combine sourdough starter, water, and 2 cups rye flour in a large bowl. Cover and set in a warm place overnight (a turned-off oven is a good place).

Next morning, in a small bowl dissolve molasses in warm water, then stir in yeast. Set aside to proof.

Stir down sourdough mixture, add oil, yeast mixture, and rice flour. Mix in as much remaining rye flour by hand as possible, then turn out dough onto a surface which has been well floured with rye flour. Knead dough briefly to incorporate all the flour, and finish with oat flour to reduce stickiness of dough. Place in an oiled bowl, and turn dough to oil top. Cover and let rise in a warm place until doubled in bulk, about 1 hour.

Form dough into 2 round loaves, place on an oiled baking sheet, and let rise until almost doubled in bulk, 45 to 60 minutes.

Preheat oven to 375°F.

Bake for 35 minutes, or until loaves sound hollow when tapped. Cool on wire racks.

Makes 2 loaves

Sticky Cinnamon Buns

2 tablespoons dry yeast
⅓ cup light honey
¼ cup warm water
1 cup buttermilk
4½ to 5 cups whole wheat flour
2 eggs
¼ cup butter, softened

Filling
1 cup light honey
½ cup maple syrup
⅔ cup raisins
3 cups finely chopped nuts
2 teaspoons ground cinnamon
2 tablespoons butter, melted

In a small bowl dissolve yeast and 1 teaspoon honey in warm water. Set aside to proof.

In a large bowl combine buttermilk and remaining honey. Beat 1½ cups flour into buttermilk mixture. Add yeast mixture and continue beating to blend well. Add eggs, butter, and more flour, a little at a time, blending until dough begins to come away from sides of bowl. Dough will be soft.

Turn out onto a floured surface, and knead until smooth and elastic, 8 to 10 minutes. Shape into ball, place in an oiled bowl, and turn once to oil top. Cover and let rise in a warm place until doubled in bulk, about 1 hour.

Butter 3 8-inch-round pans.

To make the filling: Mix together all ingredients except butter. Divide filling in half and reserve half. Divide other half into 3 parts, and spread evenly over bottom of prepared pans.

Punch down dough, turn out onto floured surface, and divide into 2 parts. Keep 1 part covered with a cloth and roll out other into a 10-inch square. Brush with melted butter and spread with reserved filling. Roll up like a jellyroll, pinching edges of dough into roll. Roll dough a few times to secure edges, and then cut into 1-inch slices. Repeat procedure with remaining dough. Arrange slices around bottom of pans with each slice nearly touching the next. Cover and let rise again until doubled in bulk, about 45 minutes.

Preheat oven to 400°F.

Bake for 20 minutes. Carefully turn out onto wire racks to cool.

Makes 2 dozen rolls

Three-Grain Country Loaf

2 tablespoons dry yeast
2¼ cups warm water
2 tablespoons honey
¼ cup molasses

¼ cup butter, softened
1 cup cornmeal, rye flour, or finely ground barley
½ cup nonfat dry milk
6 cups whole wheat flour
2 cups cooked brown rice, cooled
⅓ cup sunflower seeds
1 egg, beaten

In a large bowl dissolve yeast in 1 cup warm water. Stir in honey and set aside to proof.

Stir in remaining water, molasses, butter, cornmeal or rye flour or barley, dry milk, 1 cup whole wheat flour, and rice. Gradually beat in enough remaining flour to make a soft dough.

Turn out onto a floured surface, and knead until smooth and elastic, 8 to 10 minutes, using only as much flour as needed to keep dough from sticking. Place in an oiled bowl, and turn to oil top. Cover with wax paper and a clean towel, and let rise in a warm place until doubled in bulk, about 1 hour.

Punch down dough, turn out onto floured surface, and knead in sunflower seeds. Invert bowl over dough, and allow to rest for 10 minutes.

Lightly oil 2 baking sheets.

Divide dough in half, shape each into a round loaf, and place on prepared baking sheets. Cover with towel, and let rise again until doubled in bulk, about 45 minutes.

Make crisscross slits 1½ inches apart on tops of loaves with a very sharp knife or razor blade. Brush with egg, and sprinkle with additional flour or sunflower seeds.

Preheat oven to 375°F.

Bake for 35 to 40 minutes, or until loaves are golden brown and sound hollow when tapped on bottom. Remove to a wire rack. Cool completely.

Makes 2 loaves

Walnut-Onion-Bran Bread

1 tablespoon yeast
1¼ cups warm water
4½ to 5 cups whole wheat flour
1 cup warm milk
4 tablespoons dark molasses
1 medium-size onion, minced
⅓ cup butter
2 teaspoons caraway seeds
2 cups bran
1 cup rye flour
¾ cup chopped walnuts
melted butter

In a small bowl dissolve yeast in ¼ cup warm water and set aside to proof. In a large bowl mix together remaining water, 3 cups of whole wheat flour, milk, and 2 tablespoons molasses. After yeast foams, add it to flour mixture. Beat until batter is completely smooth. Cover bowl and let stand in a warm place for about 20 minutes. (Batter should be bubbly and light.)

In a small skillet cook onions in butter over low heat until soft. Then add onions, caraway seeds, and 2 tablespoons molasses to yeast mixture. Beat ¾ cup bran and 1 cup whole wheat flour into batter.

Spread 1 cup bran on a floured surface. With a rubber spatula, scrape ⅓ of the batter onto bran. Knead bran into batter to form a rather stiff dough. Place dough in a small oiled bowl, and turn once to oil top.

Knead rye flour into remaining dough on floured surface. Knead in just enough whole wheat flour to make dough manageable. Dough will remain slightly sticky. Continue until dough feels smooth and lively. Work in walnuts. Form dough into a ball, place in a large oiled bowl, and turn once to oil top.

Cover both bowls, and let dough rise in a warm place until doubled in bulk, 40 to 50 minutes.

Butter 2 8½ × 4½-inch loaf pans.

Punch down both balls of dough, turn out onto floured surface, and knead each again briefly. Divide larger dough ball in half, shape each half into 8-inch-long loaf, and set aside.

Sprinkle floured surface with remaining bran. Divide smaller dough ball in half. Roll out each half on bran to form 2 10-inch squares. Wrap squares around 8-inch loaves. Pinch seams together. Place loaves seam-side down in prepared loaf pans. Cover and let rise again until doubled in bulk, about 30 minutes.

Preheat oven to 350°F.

Bake for 30 minutes. Brush tops of loaves with melted butter, and return to oven for 5 to 10 minutes more, or until loaves sound hollow when tapped. Remove from pans and cool on wire racks.

Makes 2 loaves

Whole Wheat Anadama Bread

*This is the bread an anonymous "Anna"
is said to have baked with such monotonous
regularity that her husband was driven to violence.
One night when it was served, he picked up a
sack of cornmeal and hurled it at her, shouting,
"Anna damn ya!" But she kept baking it and her
husband's unintentional christening has persisted
through the centuries.*

    1 tablespoon dry yeast
4½ to 5 cups whole wheat flour
    2½ cups water
    ½ cup molasses
    ¼ cup butter
    ½ cup cornmeal
    ⅓ cup nonfat dry milk

In a large bowl combine yeast and 2 cups flour.

In a medium-size saucepan combine water, molasses, and butter, and bring to a boil. Slowly stir in cornmeal. Cook 2 minutes, stirring constantly. Add nonfat dry milk. Cool mixture about 30 minutes.

Using an electric mixer at low speed, gradually beat cornmeal mixture into dry ingredients until just blended. Increase speed to medium, and beat 2 minutes. Beat in more flour, enough to make a thick batter. Continue beating 2 minutes, occasionally scraping bowl. With a spoon stir in enough additional flour to make a soft dough.

Turn dough onto a floured surface, and knead until smooth and elastic. Shape dough into a ball, place in a large oiled bowl, and turn over to oil top. Cover with a towel and let rise in a warm place for about 1 hour.

Punch down dough and turn out onto a floured surface. Cover with towel and let rest for 15 minutes.

Butter 2 8½ × 4½-inch loaf pans.

Roll half the dough into a 12 × 8-inch rectangle. Starting at 8-inch end, tightly roll dough, jelly-roll fashion. Place seam-side down in prepared loaf pan. Repeat with remaining dough. Cover with towel and let rise again for about 40 minutes.

Preheat oven to 375°F.

Bake loaves for 40 minutes. Cool on wire racks.

Makes 2 loaves

Whole Wheat Crescent Rolls

    2 tablespoons dry yeast
    1 cup warm water
    3 tablespoons plus 1 teaspoon honey
    1 cup vegetable oil
    1 cup boiling water
    3 eggs
    6 cups whole wheat flour
    ½ teaspoon water
    ¼ cup sesame seeds, roasted

In a small bowl dissolve yeast in warm water. Add 1 teaspoon honey. Let proof.

In a large bowl mix oil, 3 tablespoons honey, and boiling water. Cool to lukewarm.

Lightly beat 2 eggs and add to cooled liquid. Then add yeast mixture. Gradually stir in flour, mixing well, but do not knead. Place in refrigerator to chill until firm.

Lightly oil a baking sheet.

Turn out dough onto a floured surface. Divide into 3 parts and roll each into a large circle, as thinly as possible. In a cup beat remaining egg with ½ teaspoon water and brush evenly over rolled-out dough. (Reserve a little for dipping tops of rolls.) Sprinkle ½ of the sesame seeds over surface. Cut each circle into wedges about 2 inches wide at outside edge. Roll each wedge toward center, and dip top in reserved egg mixture and then in sesame seeds. Place on prepared baking sheet, leaving enough room for each crescent to rise. Let rise in a warm place for 1½ hours.

Preheat oven to 425°F.

Bake for 25 minutes, or until golden brown. Serve warm.

Makes about 4 dozen rolls

Whole Wheat-Walnut Bread

    1 tablespoon dry yeast
    ¼ cup warm water
    2 tablespoons plus 1 teaspoon honey
    1 cup buttermilk
    1 tablespoon vegetable oil
    ¼ teaspoon baking soda
    ¼ cup wheat germ
    2 tablespoons sifted powdered carob
    3 cups whole wheat flour
    1 cup coarsely chopped walnuts

In a large mixing bowl dissolve yeast in warm water. Stir in 1 teaspoon honey. Let proof.

Heat buttermilk with remaining honey in a small saucepan over low heat until just lukewarm. Add to yeast mixture. Stir in oil, baking soda, wheat germ, carob, and 1 cup flour until smooth. Beat with a wooden spoon for 2 minutes. Stir in enough remaining flour to make a stiff dough.

Turn out onto a floured surface, and knead until smooth and elastic, about 10 minutes, using only as much flour as needed to keep dough from sticking. Place dough in an oiled bowl, and turn to oil top. Cover with wax paper and a clean towel, and let rise in a warm place until doubled in bulk, 1 to 1½ hours.

Butter an 8½ × 4½-inch or 9 × 5-inch loaf pan.

Punch down dough, turn out onto floured surface, and knead a few times. Roll into a 15 × 9-inch rectangle. Sprinkle nuts evenly over dough. Roll up, jelly-roll fashion, from 1 short end. Pinch ends together to seal, and place seam-side down in prepared loaf pan. Let rise again until doubled in bulk, about 1 hour.

Preheat oven to 350°F.

Bake for 40 minutes, or until loaf is golden and sounds hollow when tapped. Remove from pan to a wire rack. Cool completely.

Makes 1 loaf

International Breads

Bavarian Onion Flatbread

- 2 teaspoons dry yeast
- ½ teaspoon honey
- ½ cup warm water
- 2 cups plus 1 tablespoon whole wheat flour, sifted
- 5 tablespoons vegetable oil
- 5 large onions, chopped
- 3 tablespoons vegetable oil
- ½ cup water
- 1 cup cottage cheese
- ½ cup yogurt

In a small bowl dissolve yeast and honey in warm water. Set aside to proof.

Place 2 cups flour in a large bowl. Pour yeast mixture and 5 tablespoons oil into flour, and knead to form a soft elastic dough, about 10 minutes. Cover with a damp cloth, and let rise in a warm place for 1 hour.

Sauté onions in 3 tablespoons oil in a large covered skillet over low heat until just soft but not brown. Add 1 tablespoon flour, stirring, and then add ½ cup water. Cook until thick. In a blender combine

cottage cheese and yogurt, and process until smooth. Combine cottage cheese mixture and onion mixture.

Preheat oven to 400°F. Lightly oil and flour a baking sheet.

Punch down dough and place on prepared baking sheet. Roll dough evenly over sheet to whatever thickness you prefer (usually ½ to ¼ inch). Spread cheese mixture evenly over dough, and bake for 30 minutes. Cut into 4-inch squares and serve warm or cold.

Makes about 8 squares

Kartoffel (Potato) Fruit Bread

- 1 medium-size potato
- ¼ cup plus 1 teaspoon honey
- 4 cups plus 1½ teaspoons whole wheat flour
- 1 tablespoon dry yeast
- 2 eggs
- ¼ cup butter, melted
- ½ cup warm milk
- ½ cup raisins
- ¼ cup chopped walnuts
- 1 tablespoon water
  honey (optional)
  chopped walnuts (optional)

Cook potato in enough water to cover. Drain, reserving ½ cup cooking water. Mash potato. Combine ¼ cup mashed potatoes, reserved potato water, 1 teaspoon honey, and 1½ teaspoons flour. When mixture is lukewarm, stir in yeast, and set aside to proof.

In a large bowl beat 1 egg slightly and combine with ¼ cup honey, butter, ¼ cup mashed potatoes, and warm milk. Mix well. Add yeast mixture and then add 2 cups flour. Stir well, cover, and set in a warm place to rise until doubled in bulk, about 1 hour.

Stir down dough. Add 2 cups flour, raisins, and nuts. Let rise again for 30 minutes.

Generously butter a 9 × 5-inch loaf pan.

Stir down dough and place in prepared loaf pan. Let rise again to top of pan, 20 to 30 minutes.

Preheat oven to 375°F.

Beat remaining egg with 1 tablespoon water, and brush surface of loaf. Bake for 30 to 35 minutes, or until loaf is brown on top and sounds hollow when tapped with fingers. Remove loaf from pan, and cool on a wire rack. If desired, brush surface with honey and sprinkle with chopped nuts.

Makes 1 loaf

Brioche à Tête

A lightly sweet French pastry made from an egg-rich dough.

       1 tablespoon dry yeast
     ⅓ cup warm water
       3 tablespoons honey
       7 eggs, at room temperature
   4¼ cups whole wheat flour
       1 cup butter
     ½ cup finely chopped hazelnuts or almonds
          (optional)

In the large bowl of an electric mixer, dissolve yeast in warm water. Stir in 1 teaspoon honey and let proof.

Add remaining honey, 6 eggs, and 2 cups flour. Beat at medium speed for 2 minutes, scraping bowl often. Add 1 cup flour and beat 1 minute. Add butter, about 2 tablespoons at a time, and beat until each piece is incorporated into batter. Gradually beat in remaining flour at low speed until smooth, about 2 minutes. Stir in nuts (if used). Cover bowl with wax paper and a damp towel, and let rise in a warm place until doubled in bulk, 1 to 1½ hours.

Punch down dough, cover again, and refrigerate several hours or overnight.

Punch down dough. Turn out onto a floured surface, and divide in half. Return 1 piece to refrigerator.

Butter enough fluted miniature brioche tins for 18 small brioche. You can also use muffin tins.

Knead remaining dough a few times, then roll it into a rope 12 inches long. Cut into 12 equal pieces. Shape 9 pieces into balls, and place in prepared tins. Divide each remaining piece into thirds. Shape into 9 small balls. Press 2 fingers into center of each large ball, almost to the bottom, and place 1 small ball in each depression. Cover with towel and let rise again until doubled in bulk, about 1 hour. Repeat procedure for remaining half of dough.

Preheat oven to 400°F.

In a cup beat remaining egg lightly with a fork, and brush tops of brioche. Bake for 20 to 25 minutes, or until golden brown. Serve warm or cold.

Makes 1½ dozen brioche

NOTE: To make 2 large brioche: Pull off ¼ of the dough and set aside for "topknot." Divide remaining dough in half and shape each half into a smooth round ball. Place in 2 buttered 7- or 8-inch fluted brioche pans. Divide remaining dough into 2 pieces and form each into a large teardrop. Cut a small slash in top of each larger piece and insert pointed end of smaller pieces into indentation. Push edges together to secure. Cover with a towel, and let rise until doubled in bulk. Bake at 400°F for 40 minutes, or until loaves are golden brown and sound hollow when tapped.

Dresden Stollen

A traditional German Christmas loaf, this rich, fruited sweet bread is ideal as a company snack with tea or coffee.

     ¾ cup raisins
     ⅓ cup chopped dried pineapple
       2 tablespoons grated orange rind
     ¼ cup orange juice
       1 tablespoon dry yeast
     ¼ cup honey
     ¼ cup warm water
       1 cup milk
     ⅔ cup butter
       2 tablespoons grated lemon rind
     ½ teaspoon almond extract (optional)
     ¾ cup chopped almonds
       2 eggs, beaten
5 to 6 cups whole wheat flour
          melted butter

Place raisins, pineapple, and orange rind in a bowl. Add orange juice and let fruits soak for 1 hour. Drain.

In a small bowl dissolve yeast and 1 teaspoon honey in warm water and let proof.

In a small saucepan heat milk, butter, and remaining honey. Pour into a large bowl, and let cool to lukewarm. Add lemon rind, almond extract (if used), fruit mixture, and almonds. Beat in eggs and yeast mixture. Add enough flour to make a soft dough.

Turn out onto a floured surface, and knead until smooth, 8 to 10 minutes. Place in an oiled bowl, and turn once to oil top. Cover and let rise in a warm place until doubled in bulk, 45 to 60 minutes.

Lightly oil a baking sheet.

Turn out dough onto a floured surface, and divide into 2 parts. Roll each piece into a flat oval about ¾ inch thick. Brush with melted butter. Roll up and place on prepared baking sheet. Brush tops with melted butter, cover lightly with wax paper, and let rise again until doubled in bulk.

Preheat oven to 350°F.

Bake for 40 minutes.

Makes 2 loaves

Kugelhopf
(Austrian Sweet Yeast Bread)

This festive holiday bread is excellent for breakfast. It is traditionally baked in a special fluted pan that adds to the appeal of the finished product.

- 1 tablespoon dry yeast
- 1 cup warm milk
- 4 cups whole wheat flour
- 16 whole blanched almonds
- 1 cup butter, softened
- ½ cup honey
- 4 eggs
- 2 teaspoons grated lemon rind
- ½ teaspoon ground cardamom
- ¾ cup finely chopped almonds
- ¾ cup golden raisins

In a medium-size bowl dissolve yeast in warm milk, stir in 1 cup flour until smooth. Let rise in a warm place until bubbly and doubled in bulk, 1 to 1½ hours.

Generously butter a 10-cup Kugelhopf pan, Bundt pan, or 10-inch tube pan. Arrange whole almonds in attractive pattern on bottom.

Beat butter and honey in a large bowl. Add eggs, one at a time, beating well after each addition.

Stir down yeast mixture. Add to butter-egg mixture and stir in. Add lemon rind, cardamom, 2 cups flour, chopped almonds, and raisins. Stir with a wooden spoon until well blended. Knead in remaining flour, and place in prepared pan. Cover with wax paper and a clean towel, and let rise until doubled in bulk, 1 to 1½ hours.

Preheat oven to 400°F.

Bake for 10 minutes, reduce oven temperature to 350°F, and continue baking 40 minutes longer, or until nicely browned and a wooden pick comes out clean. (If loaf browns too quickly, cover loosely with a square of foil.) Leave in pan for 3 minutes, then invert onto a wire rack. Cool completely.

Makes 1 loaf

Scottish Scones or Bannock

This Scottish bread is baked either as biscuits (scones) or as a single rounded bread (bannock) to be cut into wedges.

- 2 tablespoons dry yeast
- 6 tablespoons warm water
- 6 teaspoons honey
- 2 cups rolled oats, ground to a coarse flour in a blender
- 2 tablespoons warm milk or light cream
- 2 eggs, beaten
- 2 tablespoons butter, melted

In a small bowl dissolve yeast in warm water. Add 2 teaspoons honey. Let proof.

In a large bowl add yeast mixture to oats along with milk or cream and remaining honey. Mix well, cover, and set aside to rise in a warm place for 1 hour.

Combine eggs and butter, and stir into batter. Cover again and set aside for 1 more hour.

Preheat oven to 400°F. Oil a 10-inch iron skillet.

For scones drop batter by tablespoons into skillet, and bake for 10 minutes. For bannock pour batter all at once into skillet, and bake as for scones. Cut into wedges before serving. Serve hot with butter and honey.

Makes about 2 dozen scones or 1 bannock

Poteca
(Polish Nut-Filled Coffee Cake)

    4 cups whole wheat flour
    1 tablespoon dry yeast
    ¼ cup wheat germ
    ½ teaspoon ground cinnamon
    ¾ cup milk
    ¼ cup honey
    ¼ cup butter
    1 egg

       Filling
    ¼ cup butter
    ½ cup honey
    1 tablespoon grated orange rind
    ½ teaspoon ground cinnamon
    1 egg
    2 cups finely chopped walnuts

In a large bowl combine 1 cup flour, yeast, wheat germ, and cinnamon.

Heat milk, honey, and butter in a small saucepan until very warm (120 to 130°F). Gradually add to dry ingredients, and beat 2 minutes at medium speed of electric mixer, scraping bowl often. Add egg and ½ cup flour and beat 2 minutes. Stir in enough remaining flour to make a soft dough.

Turn out onto a floured surface, and knead until smooth, adding only enough flour to keep dough from sticking, 6 to 8 minutes. Place in an oiled bowl, and turn dough over to oil top. Cover and let rise in a warm place until doubled in bulk, about 1 hour.

To make the filling: Blend butter and honey in a medium-size bowl. Add orange rind, cinnamon, and egg. Beat well. Stir in nuts.

Lightly oil a baking sheet.

Punch down dough. Turn out onto a floured surface, and knead a few times. Roll out to a 26 × 11-inch rectangle. Spread with filling, and roll up, jelly-roll fashion, starting from 1 long side. Place seam-side down on prepared baking sheet, and shape into a coil or snail, leaving enough space to allow dough to rise. Cover with a clean towel, and let rise again until doubled in bulk, about 1 hour.

Preheat oven to 350°F.

Bake for 40 minutes. Remove to a wire rack. Serve slightly warm.

Makes 1 cake

Pita Bread

While they are baking, these breads puff up, forming a pocket into which you can stuff your favorite sandwich combinations.

    1 tablespoon dry yeast
    1¼ cups warm water
    1 tablespoon corn oil
3 to 3½ cups whole wheat flour

In a large bowl dissolve yeast in warm water. Add oil and 2 cups flour. Beat until dough is smooth. Add remaining flour as you knead dough in bowl. Place dough on a floured surface, and knead in some additional flour until dough is firm. Rub bowl with oil, return dough to bowl, and turn to oil dough on all sides. Cover and let dough rise in a warm place until doubled in bulk.

Punch down dough and divide into 12 equal pieces. Form dough into balls. Cover with wax paper or a towel to prevent them from drying out, and let them rest for at least 10 minutes.

Lightly oil a large baking sheet.

Roll out balls until they are ⅛ to ¼ inch thick and 4 to 4½ inches in diameter. (If rolled to a larger diameter, rounds may not puff all the way to the edges.) Place rounds on baking sheet.

Preheat oven to 500°F.

For rounds to bake properly, heat source must be directly beneath them. If you have an electric oven, this might mean removing the top heating element. These are usually removable for cleaning. Bake rounds on lowest rack. In a gas oven raise racks and place baking sheet directly on oven floor.

Place baking sheet on lowest rack or floor of oven, and bake for 5 minutes. Do not open the oven during this first baking. After 5 minutes, open oven, place baking sheet on a higher rack, and bake rounds for 3 to 5 more minutes or until pockets have puffed up and begin to brown.

Remove from oven and place pockets on wire racks to cool.

Makes 1 dozen pita bread pockets

NOTE: Reheat pita bread pockets by sprinkling lightly with water, wrapping them in foil, and placing in a 400°F oven for a couple of minutes.

Swedish Limpa Rye Bread

A sweet, and sweet smelling, bread with good keeping qualities—a nice change from wheat-based breads.

    2 tablespoons dry yeast
    ½ cup warm water
    ⅓ cup honey
    1 tablespoon grated orange rind
    1 teaspoon aniseeds
    1 teaspoon caraway seeds
    ⅓ cup molasses
    2 tablespoons vegetable oil
    1¼ cups hot water
    4 cups rye flour
    2½ cups whole wheat flour
    1 egg, beaten

In a small bowl dissolve yeast in warm water. Add 1 teaspoon honey and let proof.

In a large bowl combine remaining honey, orange rind, aniseeds, caraway seeds, molasses, and oil. Pour in hot water and stir well. Cool to lukewarm.

Blend in 1 cup rye flour, beating until smooth. Stir in yeast mixture, beating well. Add remaining rye flour, and mix until smooth. Beat in whole wheat flour with a spoon, turning dough out onto a floured surface to knead in rest of flour, if necessary. Let rest for 10 minutes.

Knead dough until smooth and no longer sticky. Place in an oiled bowl, turn once to oil top, cover with a damp cloth, and let rise in a warm place until doubled in bulk, about 1 hour.

Punch down dough. Cover and let rise again until nearly doubled in bulk, about 1 hour.

Butter 2 8½ × 4½-inch loaf pans, or lightly oil a baking sheet.

Shape dough into 2 loaves, and place either in prepared loaf pans or on baking sheet. Brush with egg and let rise about 1 hour.

Preheat oven to 350°F.

Bake for 45 to 50 minutes, or until a deep golden brown. Remove from pan and cool on a wire rack. Store in refrigerator.

Makes 2 loaves

Traditional Irish Oatmeal Bread

    3 tablespoons dry yeast
    1 cup warm water
    ¼ cup plus 1 tablespoon honey
    ¼ cup nonfat dry milk
    1 cup cold water
    ½ cup vegetable oil
    ¼ cup honey
    3 eggs
    2 cups rolled oats
    6½ cups whole wheat flour
    1 cup dried currants

In a small bowl dissolve yeast in warm water. Add 1 tablespoon honey. Let proof.

In a small saucepan combine dry milk and cold water with a wire whisk, and heat almost to scalding point. Add oil and remaining honey. Cool to lukewarm.

In a large bowl beat 2 eggs and add milk and yeast mixtures. Mix in oats and 6 cups flour, 3 cups at a time.

Turn out onto a floured surface, and knead until smooth and elastic, about 10 minutes. Place in an oiled bowl, turn once to oil top, and cover with a damp cloth. Let rise in a warm place until doubled in bulk, about 1½ hours.

Lightly oil 3 baking sheets.

Punch down dough and knead with remaining flour, gradually working in currants. Shape into 3 round loaves. In a cup beat remaining egg lightly with a fork and brush tops of loaves. Place on prepared baking sheets and let rise again for 1 hour.

Preheat oven to 375°F.

Bake for 25 minutes, or until golden brown. Remove from baking sheets and cool before slicing.

Makes 3 loaves

Tibetan "Prayer Wheel" Barley Bread

  1 tablespoon dry yeast
  ½ cup warm water
  1 teaspoon honey
  4 tablespoons sesame oil or other vegetable oil
  2 cups barley flour
  ¾ cup unhulled sesame seeds
  4½ cups whole wheat flour
  3 cups hot water
  1 egg, beaten

In a small bowl dissolve yeast in warm water. Stir in honey and set aside to proof.

Place 2 tablespoons oil in a large heavy iron skillet. Add barley flour and ½ cup sesame seeds, and brown over medium-high heat, stirring constantly, until flour is an even tan color. Take care to prevent it from burning. Remove mixture from skillet, and place in a large bowl. Stir in 4 cups whole wheat flour.

Mix hot water with remaining oil, and stir into flour mixture until ingredients are completely combined. Allow mixture to cool to lukewarm.

Stir in yeast mixture. Using ½ cup whole wheat flour, knead dough on a floured surface until smooth to the touch, about 15 minutes. Place dough in a large oiled bowl, and turn to oil top. Cover with a damp cloth, and let rise in a warm place overnight.

In the morning lightly oil a baking sheet. Carefully place dough on baking sheet, keeping shape of risen dough. Do not punch down, knead again, or reshape in any way. Brush top of dough with egg. Sprinkle remaining sesame seeds over surface. With tip of a sharp knife, score a large cross on surface of loaf. Allow loaf to spread on baking sheet for 1 hour in a warm place. After an hour the loaf should resemble a large wheel.

Preheat oven to 450°F.

Bake for 1 hour. The high temperature produces a crusty exterior and tender interior. Cool loaf on a wire rack before slicing.

  Makes 1 loaf

Quick Breads

Buttermilk-Nut Bread

  2¼ cups whole wheat flour
  ¾ teaspoon baking soda

  1½ teaspoons baking powder
  1 cup chopped walnuts
  2 eggs
  ¼ cup honey
  2 tablespoons butter, melted
  ⅓ cup molasses
  1 cup buttermilk

Preheat oven to 350°F. Butter a 9 × 5-inch loaf pan.

Sift together flour, baking soda, and baking powder. Add walnuts and mix well.

In a large bowl beat together eggs, honey, butter, molasses, and buttermilk. Fold dry ingredients into wet ingredients, and pour into prepared pan.

Bake for 50 to 60 minutes.

  Makes 1 loaf

Date-Nut Bread

  1 cup yogurt
  ½ cup honey
  2 eggs
  2 tablespoons vegetable oil
  2 cups whole wheat flour
  1 scant teaspoon baking soda
  1 pound pitted dates, quartered
  1 cup chopped walnuts

Preheat oven to 350°F. Generously butter 2 7½-inch loaf pans.

In a large bowl mix together yogurt, honey, eggs, and oil.

Combine flour and baking soda, and then add them to liquid ingredients, stirring to blend. Stir in dates and nuts. Pour batter into prepared pans.

Bake for 40 minutes, or until a wooden pick inserted into center comes out clean.

  Makes 2 loaves

Cranberry-Nut Bread

  ¼ cup butter
  ½ cup honey
  2 eggs, beaten
  ½ cup orange juice
  1 teaspoon grated orange rind
  1½ cups whole wheat flour

2 teaspoons baking powder
¾ cup chopped fresh or frozen cranberries
½ cup chopped walnuts

Preheat oven to 350°F. Butter and flour a 9 × 5-inch loaf pan.

In a large bowl cream butter and honey. Add eggs, orange juice, and orange rind. Mix flour with baking powder. Add to butter mixture, ⅓ at a time, blending after each addition. Stir in cranberries and walnuts. Pour into prepared pan.

Bake for 50 to 60 minutes.

Makes 1 loaf

Steamed Brown Bread

⅔ cup butter
1 cup molasses
1 cup sour milk, buttermilk, or yogurt
1 cup chopped raisins or dried currants
½ cup chopped walnuts
2½ cups whole wheat flour
2 teaspoons wheat germ
1 teaspoon baking soda
¼ teaspoon ground nutmeg

Cream butter with molasses in a large bowl. Add sour milk or buttermik or yogurt, raisins or currants, and walnuts.

In a small bowl combine flour, wheat germ, baking soda, and nutmeg. Stir into molasses mixture.

Pour into 5 oiled 8- to 10-ounce soup cans, filling two-thirds full. Cover tightly with oiled brown paper or foil. Set in a large pot, and add boiling water until it comes halfway up cans. Cover pot with a tight-fitting lid.

Bring to a boil and steam for 1 hour. Unmold, slice, and serve warm with cream cheese.

Makes 5 loaves

Crunchy Apple-Nut Butter Bread

1¼ cups whole wheat flour
¾ cup rolled oats
¼ cup wheat germ
1½ teaspoons baking soda
1 teaspoon ground cinnamon
½ cup finely chopped dates or dried prunes
⅓ cup peanut or cashew butter
3 tablespoons butter
⅓ cup honey

2 eggs
¾ cup yogurt
1 cup finely chopped apples
¼ cup chopped nuts or sunflower seeds
wheat germ

Preheat oven to 350°F. Butter an 8½ × 4½-inch or 9 × 5-inch loaf pan. Line bottom with wax paper and then butter paper.

In a small bowl mix together flour, oats, wheat germ, baking soda, and cinnamon. Blend in dates or prunes, separating them with your fingertips. In a large bowl beat peanut or cashew butter, butter, and honey until smooth. Beat in eggs, one at a time. Stir in ½ of the flour mixture, then yogurt, and then apples. Stir in remaining flour and nuts or sunflower seeds. Spoon batter into prepared pan, smooth top, and sprinkle with additional wheat germ.

Bake for 60 to 70 minutes, or until a wooden pick inserted into center comes out clean. Remove from pan. Cool completely. Wrap in plastic wrap overnight.

Makes 1 loaf

Crusty Brown Bread

1½ cups whole wheat pastry flour
1½ teaspoons baking soda
1 teaspoon baking powder
1 cup chopped dates
½ cup raisins
½ cup sunflower seeds
1 cup wheat germ
¾ cup cornmeal
¾ cup rolled oats
1 egg, lightly beaten
1 cup buttermilk
2 tablespoons maple syrup
½ cup blackstrap molasses
2 tablespoons vegetable oil

Preheat oven to 350°F. Butter a 9 × 5-inch loaf pan.

In a large bowl sift together flour, baking soda, and baking powder. Add dates, raisins, sunflower seeds, wheat germ, cornmeal, and oats.

In a medium-size bowl combine egg, buttermilk, maple syrup, molasses, and oil. Add to dry ingredients and stir until flour is moistened. Pour batter into prepared pan.

Bake for 50 to 60 minutes. Allow bread to cool in pan for 10 minutes before removing.

Makes 1 loaf

Chili-Cheese Skillet Corn Bread

    4 jalapeño peppers
    1 medium-size onion, chopped (½ cup)
    ½ sweet red pepper, finely chopped
    5 tablespoons vegetable oil
    1 cup cornmeal
    ½ cup whole wheat flour
    3 tablespoons baking powder
    ½ teaspoon baking soda
    ½ teaspoon crumbled dried oregano
    1 cup corn
    ½ cup heavy cream
    2 eggs
    1 cup buttermilk
   1½ cups shredded sharp cheddar cheese

Roast, peel, and seed jalapeño peppers (see page 54), then chop them.

In a 10-inch cast-iron skillet sauté onions and sweet peppers in 2 tablespoons oil for 5 minutes. Remove to a small plate. Cool.

Preheat oven to 400°F.

Oil skillet lightly and keep hot.

In a large bowl combine cornmeal, flour, baking powder, baking soda, and oregano.

In a small saucepan heat corn for 2 to 3 minutes. Place ⅔ of the corn in a blender. Add cream and blend at medium speed for 5 seconds, or just until kernels are coarsely chopped. Blend in eggs, buttermilk, and remaining oil. Pour over dry ingredients in bowl, add remaining corn, and stir. Add onion mixture, 1 cup cheese, and jalapeño peppers and blend. Pour into hot skillet, and sprinkle remaining cheese over top.

Bake for 30 to 35 minutes, or until golden brown. Cool in skillet on a wire rack for 15 to 20 minutes. Cut into wedges and serve warm.

8 to 10 servings

Dutch Pumpernickel Quick Bread

    1 cup rye flour
    ½ cup cornmeal
    ½ cup whole wheat flour
    2 teaspoons baking powder
    ¼ teaspoon baking soda
   1½ teaspoons caraway seeds, crushed
    2 eggs, beaten
    ¼ cup molasses
    ¾ cup milk
    ¼ cup vegetable oil
    1 small onion, finely chopped
       sesame seeds

Preheat oven to 350°F. Butter a 9 × 5-inch or 8½ × 4½-inch loaf pan. Line bottom with wax paper and butter paper.

Combine rye flour, cornmeal, whole wheat flour, baking powder, baking soda, and caraway seeds in a large bowl. Mix well.

In a small bowl beat eggs, molasses, milk, and oil. Pour over dry ingredients, and stir to blend well. Stir in onions. Pour into prepared pan, and sprinkle with sesame seeds.

Bake for 50 to 60 minutes, or until a wooden pick inserted into center comes out clean. Remove from pan. Cool completely.

Makes 1 loaf

Irish Soda Bread

    4 cups buttermilk, at room temperature
    2 eggs
    ½ teaspoon baking soda
 7 to 8 cups whole wheat flour
    2 cups raisins
    3 tablespoons honey
    ½ cup caraway seeds
    2 tablespoons plus 2 teaspoons baking powder

Preheat oven to 375°F. Butter and flour 2 9 × 5-inch loaf pans or small round ceramic bowls.

In a medium-size bowl combine buttermilk, eggs, and baking soda. Stir vigorously with a wooden spoon.

In a large bowl combine 7 cups flour, raisins, honey, caraway seeds, and baking powder, stirring with wooden spoon after each ingredient is added. Pour buttermilk mixture into flour mixture and stir well. If you like, flour your hands and then complete mixing. Dough does not require kneading, however. If dough seems too damp, add more flour.

Divide batter into 2 equal parts and place in prepared pans or bowls.

Bake for 1¼ hours or until well browned and a wooden pick comes out clean. Let loaves cool in pans for 15 minutes, then turn out onto wire racks. Cool thoroughly before freezing.

Makes 2 loaves

Pumpkin Bread

4 eggs
1 cup honey
2 cups mashed cooked pumpkin
1 cup vegetable oil
2 teaspoons baking soda
½ cup yogurt or buttermilk
3¾ cups whole wheat flour
1 teaspoon ground nutmeg
1 teaspoon ground cloves
1 teaspoon ground cinnamon

Preheat oven to 325°F. Butter 2 9 × 5-inch loaf pans.

In a large bowl beat eggs and honey together. Add pumpkin and oil.

Dissolve baking soda in yogurt or buttermilk.

Sift flour with spices, and add to pumpkin mixture alternately with soda mixture, blending after each addition. Pour into prepared pans.

Bake for 1½ hours. Remove from pans. Cool on a wire rack.

Makes 2 loaves

Zucchini-Raisin Quick Bread or Muffins

2 eggs, beaten
½ cup vegetable oil
½ cup honey
1 teaspoon vanilla extract
1 cup whole wheat flour
2 tablespoons wheat germ
2 tablespoons bran
1 teaspoon ground cinnamon
½ teaspoon baking powder
½ teaspoon baking soda
1 cup shredded zucchini
½ cup raisins

Preheat oven to 350°F. Butter an 8½ × 4½-inch loaf pan or a 12-cup muffin tin.

In a small bowl combine eggs, oil, honey, and vanilla.

In a large bowl combine flour, wheat germ, bran, cinnamon, baking powder, and baking soda. Add liquid ingredients and stir just until mixed. Blend in zucchini and raisins.

To make a bread, pour batter into prepared pan and bake for 45 minutes.

To make muffins, pour batter into prepared muffin tin and bake for 25 minutes.

Remove from pan or muffin tin and cool on a wire rack.

Makes 1 loaf or 1 dozen muffins

Variations:

Applesauce-Raisin Muffins: Substitute 1 cup unsweetened applesauce for zucchini, and add ¼ cup more flour, ¼ teaspoon ground cloves, and ½ teaspoon ground nutmeg.

Banana-Raisin Muffins: Substitute 1 cup mashed bananas (2 medium) for zucchini.

Blueberry Muffins: Substitute 1½ cups fresh blueberries for zucchini, and omit raisins and cinnamon. (If using frozen blueberries, add ¼ cup more flour.)

Carrot-Raisin Muffins: Substitute 1 cup grated carrots for zucchini.

Cranberry-Nut Muffins: Substitute 1½ cups chopped fresh cranberries for zucchini, substitute ½ cup chopped nuts for raisins, omit cinnamon, and add ¼ cup more flour.

Nut and Raisin Muffins: Substitute 1 cup chopped nuts for zucchini and omit cinnamon.

Pumpkin-Raisin Muffins: Substitute 1 cup pureed pumpkin or squash for zucchini, and add ¼ cup more flour, ¼ teaspoon ground cloves, and ½ teaspoon ground nutmeg.

Muffins, Biscuits, and Popovers

Apple-Honey-Oatmeal Muffins

1 cup whole wheat flour
1 cup rolled oats
2 teaspoons baking powder
½ teaspoon baking soda
½ teaspoon ground cinnamon
⅛ teaspoon freshly ground nutmeg
1 egg, beaten with ½ cup milk
1 cup unsweetened applesauce
¼ cup honey
2 tablespoons butter, melted

Preheat oven to 375°F. Generously butter a 12-cup muffin tin.

Combine flour, oats, baking powder, baking soda, cinnamon, and nutmeg in a medium-size bowl and mix well.

In a small bowl blend egg and milk with apple-sauce, honey, and butter. Pour over dry ingredients and mix with a fork just until moistened. Fill prepared muffin tin two-thirds full.

Bake for 25 minutes, or until a wooden pick inserted into center comes out clean. Loosen with a small spatula. Remove to a wire rack. Serve warm.

Makes 1 dozen muffins

Banana-Nut Muffins

1 egg
¾ cup mashed very ripe bananas (2 medium-size)
⅓ cup corn oil
¼ cup unsulfured molasses
¼ cup yogurt
1 cup whole wheat pastry flour
1 cup wheat germ
½ cup finely chopped walnuts
½ teaspoon baking soda
½ teaspoon baking powder
½ teaspoon ground cinnamon

Preheat oven to 375°F. Lightly butter a 12-cup muffin tin.

Beat egg in a large bowl. Then add bananas, oil, molasses, and yogurt.

In a small bowl thoroughly mix together flour, wheat germ, walnuts, baking soda, baking powder, and cinnamon. Add to liquid ingredients and stir until combined. Pour batter into prepared muffin tin.

Bake for about 20 minutes. Cool on a wire rack.

Makes 1 dozen muffins

Bran Muffins

1 cup bran
1 cup whole wheat pastry flour
1 teaspoon ground cinnamon
2 tablespoons vegetable oil
1 cup milk
4 eggs, separated
3 tablespoons honey or molasses
½ cup raisins, sunflower seeds, or nuts

Preheat oven to 375°F. Butter muffin tins.

In a medium-size bowl combine bran, flour, and cinnamon.

In a small bowl combine oil, milk, egg yolks, and honey or molasses. Add to dry ingredients. Add raisins, seeds, or nuts, or a combination of them.

Beat egg whites until stiff, and fold them into batter. Pour into prepared tins.

Bake for 25 minutes. Cool on a wire rack.

Makes 1 to 1½ dozen muffins

Buckwheat-Corn Muffins

⅓ cup boiling water
2 tablespoons bulgur
1 cup buckwheat flour
½ cup cornmeal
2 teaspoons baking powder
2 eggs, beaten
½ cup yogurt
¼ cup safflower oil
¼ cup honey
1 teaspoon grated orange rind
½ cup fresh blueberries (optional)

Pour boiling water over bulgur in a small bowl, and let stand for 30 minutes, or until water is absorbed and bulgur is fluffy. Drain on paper toweling. (You should have about ½ cup.)

Preheat oven to 375°F. Generously butter a 12-cup muffin tin.

Combine flour, cornmeal, and baking powder in a medium-size bowl.

In a small bowl stir together eggs, yogurt, oil, honey, orange rind, and soaked bulgur. Pour over dry ingredients, mixing with a fork just until moistened. Stir in blueberries (if used). Fill prepared muffin tin two-thirds full.

Bake for 20 minutes, or until a wooden pick inserted into center comes out clean. Loosen with a small spatula. Remove to a wire rack. Serve warm.

Makes 1 dozen muffins

Corn Muffins

    ¾ cup milk
    ¼ cup sour cream
    ⅓ cup maple syrup or honey
    2 eggs
    1 cup whole wheat pastry flour
    ¾ cup cornmeal
    ½ teaspoon baking soda

Preheat oven to 450°F. Butter a 12-cup muffin tin.

In a medium-size bowl combine milk, sour cream, maple syrup or honey, and eggs. Blend well.

Mix together flour, cornmeal, and baking soda, and add to liquid ingredients. Spoon batter into prepared muffin tin, filling about two-thirds full.

Bake for about 15 minutes. Cool on a wire rack.

Makes 1 dozen muffins

High-Energy Muffins

    1½ cups whole wheat flour
    ½   cup soy flour
    2   teaspoons baking powder
    ¼   cup nonfat dry milk
    3   tablespoons wheat germ
    ¼   cup chopped roasted peanuts
    ½   cup finely chopped dates
    2   eggs, beaten
    ¼   cup safflower oil
    ¾   cup milk
    ½   cup grated or finely shredded carrots
    2   tablespoons molasses

Preheat oven to 375°F. Butter a 12-cup muffin tin.

Combine whole wheat flour, soy flour, baking powder, nonfat dry milk, 2 tablespoons wheat germ, and peanuts in a medium-size mixing bowl. Mix well. Add dates and mix with your fingers to separate pieces.

In a small bowl stir together eggs, oil, milk, carrots, and molasses. Pour over dry ingredients, and mix with a fork just until moistened. Fill prepared

muffin tin two-thirds full. Sprinkle with remaining wheat germ.

Bake for 20 minutes, or until a wooden pick inserted into center comes out clean. Loosen with a small spatula. Remove to a wire rack. Serve warm.

Makes 1 dozen muffins

Molasses Muffins

    2 cups whole wheat flour
    2 teaspoons baking powder
    1 egg, beaten
    ½ cup milk
    ¼ cup vegetable oil
    ½ cup molasses
    ½ cup raisins

Preheat oven to 400°F. Butter a 12-cup muffin tin.

In a medium-size bowl combine flour and baking powder.

In a small bowl combine egg, milk, oil, molasses, and raisins and blend. Add to dry ingredients, and mix just until moistened. Fill prepared muffin tin two-thirds full.

Bake for 15 to 20 minutes. Cool on a wire rack.

Makes 1 dozen muffins

Whole Wheat Muffins

    2¼ cups whole wheat flour
    2   teaspoons baking powder
    1   cup milk
    1   egg
    ¼   cup honey
    3   tablespoons vegetable oil

Preheat oven to 350°F. Butter a 12-cup muffin tin.

Combine flour and baking powder in a medium-size bowl.

In a small bowl combine milk, egg, honey, and oil. Beat well. Add liquid ingredients to dry ingredients, and stir just until moistened. Fill prepared muffin tin half full.

Bake for 15 to 20 minutes, or until a wooden pick inserted into center comes out clean. Remove to a wire rack.

Makes 1 dozen muffins

Buttermilk Biscuits

   2 cups whole wheat flour
2¼ teaspoons baking powder
  ¼ teaspoon baking soda
  ¼ cup plus 2 tablespoons butter
  ¾ cup buttermilk
  1 tablespoon milk

Preheat oven to 450°F. Lightly oil a baking sheet.

In a medium-size bowl sift together flour, baking powder, and baking soda. Cut in butter with a pastry blender. Then add buttermilk and mix lightly. Turn out onto a floured surface, and knead gently for a few seconds. Roll out to ½-inch thickness, and cut into 2-inch circles. Place on prepared baking sheet, and brush biscuits lightly with milk.

Bake for 12 to 15 minutes, or until brown.

Makes 20 biscuits

Sesame Biscuits

  ½ cup butter
  ¼ cup honey
  ¼ cup light cream
  3 eggs
  3 cups whole wheat pastry flour
  2 teaspoons baking powder
    grated rind of 1 orange
  ¼ cup orange juice
1½ cups sesame seeds, toasted
  1 tablespoon milk

Preheat oven to 375°F. Lightly oil a baking sheet.

In a large bowl cream butter and honey together. Add cream and eggs, and beat thoroughly. Gradually add dry ingredients and orange rind and juice.

Turn out onto a floured surface. Add enough flour to make a smooth dough. Form into long rolls about 1 inch in diameter. Sprinkle area generously with sesame seeds. Roll each length through seeds, pressing them into dough. Reroll several times, if necessary. When finished, rolls should be ½ inch in diameter. Diagonally slice into 4-inch lengths. Brush with milk. Place on prepared baking sheets.

Bake for 10 to 15 minutes, or until golden brown.

Makes about 5 dozen biscuits

Barley-Buttermilk Biscuits

  1 tablespoon dry yeast
  ¼ cup warm water
  1 tablespoon honey
1¼ cups barley flour
  2 tablespoons butter
  ¼ cup buttermilk
  1 egg

In a small bowl dissolve yeast in warm water. Add honey and let proof.

Place flour in a medium-size bowl. With 2 knives or a pastry blender, cut butter into flour.

Combine buttermilk and egg and beat slightly. Then stir into flour mixture. Add yeast mixture, mix thoroughly, and let mixture stand for 20 minutes.

Preheat oven to 400°F. Lightly oil a baking sheet.

Drop dough by tablespoons onto prepared baking sheet. Pat into 2-inch rounds.

Bake for 15 to 18 minutes, or until browned.

Makes 1 dozen biscuits

Whole Wheat Popovers

1⅓ cups milk
1½ tablespoons vegetable oil
1½ cups whole wheat pastry flour
  3 eggs

Preheat oven to 450°F. Generously butter a 12-cup muffin or popover tin.

In a medium-size bowl combine milk, oil, and flour. Beat until smooth. Then add eggs, one at a time, beating only until batter is smooth. Fill prepared tin three-quarters full.

Bake for 15 minutes, then reduce heat to 350°F, and bake about 20 minutes longer.

Makes 1 dozen popovers

Crackers and Flatbreads

Barley-Sesame-Onion Crackers

These large decorative crackers are rimmed with Japanese black sesame seeds. If you must avoid eating anything made with wheat, these are a most satisfying compromise.

1 cup barley flour

⅓ cup sesame seeds, ground to a meal in a
blender

1 teaspoon sesame oil

1 teaspoon soy sauce

2 tablespoons finely minced onions

¼ cup cold water

2 tablespoons Japanese black sesame seeds*

1 egg white, lightly beaten

Place flour and sesame seed meal in a large bowl.

In a cup mix oil, soy sauce, and onions together, and then add to flour mixture. Slowly add water, a bit at a time, working with hands until dough holds together. It will be dry. Divide into 4 balls and set aside.

Toast 1 tablespoon black sesame seeds in a small skillet until lightly browned, about 10 minutes. Set aside.

Preheat oven to 400°F. Lightly oil a baking sheet.

Roll each ball to ¼-inch thickness with a rolling pin. Using a rice or cereal bowl that measures 4½ inches in diameter as a guide, cut circles out of dough. Scraps are added and rerolled until 7 large crackers are cut. (A smaller bowl will, of course, yield more crackers.) Using a spatula, carefully place crackers on prepared baking sheet, and brush with egg white. Rim outside of each cracker with 1 tablespoon untoasted black sesame seeds and sprinkle inside with toasted ones. Press gently with rolling pin so they adhere.

Bake for 10 to 15 minutes, or until light brown and crisp.

Makes 7 crackers

*Japanese black sesame seeds (*Irigoma*) are available in oriental grocery stores.

Bran-Sesame Crackers

¾ cup rolled oats, ground to a coarse flour in a
blender

½ cup bran

1 cup whole wheat flour

¼ cup plus 2 tablespoons vegetable oil

1 tablespoon honey

½ cup water

2 tablespoons sesame seeds

Preheat oven to 350°F. Lightly oil a baking sheet.

Combine oats, bran, and flour in a medium-size bowl.

In a large bowl blend oil and honey together. Stir in flour mixture and water, and mix just until dough is smooth.

Press or roll dough to ⅛-inch thickness on prepared baking sheet. Sprinkle top with sesame seeds, and press them lightly into dough so they adhere. Cut dough into 2-inch squares with a sharp knife.

Bake for 12 to 15 minutes, or until lightly golden. Cool for 5 minutes, then remove from pan.

Makes about 4 dozen crackers

Oatmeal Crackers

1½ cups rolled oats, ground to a coarse flour in
a blender

1 cup whole wheat flour

¼ cup plus 1 tablespoon vegetable oil

1 tablespoon honey

½ cup water

Preheat oven to 350°F. Lightly oil a baking sheet.

Combine oats and flour in a medium-size bowl.

In a large bowl blend oil and honey together. Stir in flour mixture and water, and mix just until dough is smooth.

Press or roll dough to ⅛-inch thickness on prepared baking sheet. Cut dough into 2-inch squares with a sharp knife.

Bake for 12 to 15 minutes, or until lightly golden. Cool for 5 minutes, then remove from pan.

Makes about 4 dozen crackers

Sesame Crisp Crackers

1 cup oat flour

¾ cup soy flour

¼ cup unhulled sesame seeds

¼ cup vegetable oil

½ cup water

Preheat oven to 350°F. Lightly oil a baking sheet.

In a medium-size bowl combine flours and sesame seeds. Add oil and blend well. Add water and mix to pie-dough consistency. Roll out dough to ⅛-inch thickness on prepared baking sheet. Score with a knife into square or diamond shapes.

Bake about 15 minutes, or until crackers are golden brown. Cool on wire racks.

Makes 3 to 4 dozen crackers

Graham Crackers

3 tablespoons honey
2 tablespoons molasses
¼ cup peanut butter
¼ cup butter
½ cup buttermilk
1 teaspoon vanilla extract
2¼ cups whole wheat flour
½ teaspoon baking powder
½ teaspoon baking soda

In a medium-size bowl beat honey, molasses, peanut butter, and butter together until smooth.

Combine buttermilk and vanilla and set aside.

Combine dry ingredients. Stir them and buttermilk mixture into butter mixture, alternately, stirring well after each addition. Let dough rest for a few minutes.

Preheat oven to 400°F. Lightly oil a baking sheet.

Divide dough into 3 pieces. Roll out each piece on prepared baking sheet to a thickness of $\frac{1}{16}$ inch. Cut into 2½-inch squares, and prick with a fork.

Bake for 6 to 8 minutes, or until lightly browned. Cool on wire racks. Store in an airtight container.

Makes 4 dozen crackers

Whole-Millet Crackers

¼ cup plus 1 tablespoon vegetable oil
1 tablespoon honey
½ cup water
¼ cup whole millet
½ cup finely ground millet
1 cup whole wheat flour

Preheat oven to 350°F. Lightly butter a baking sheet. (Do not use oil, as crackers may be difficult to loosen.)

In a medium-size bowl combine oil, honey, and water. Stir in whole millet, ground millet, and flour. (It may be necessary to knead dough to work in last of flour.)

Roll out dough to ⅛-inch thickness on prepared baking sheet. Score crackers with a knife in square or diamond shapes.

Bake for 20 minutes, or until golden brown. Cool on wire racks.

Makes 4 dozen crackers

Chapati

These thin bread disks are basic to the diet of India, where they are eaten with breakfast tea and used as a scoop for foods at other meals and for sopping up juices and gravies.

1 cup whole wheat flour
1 cup corn flour
1 cup cold water

Mix flours together in a medium-size bowl. Add water gradually, adding just enough to keep dough from sticking to hands (about 1 cup). Divide into 8 portions, and roll out each portion on a floured surface until it is about 5 inches in diameter.

Cook over medium-high heat in a large, dry, cast-iron skillet for about 30 seconds on each side, or until lightly toasted and cooked through.

Makes 8 chapati

Corn Tortillas

This standard Mexican flatbread is used as is or to encase a variety of fillings, as crepes are used in other cultures.

2 cups masa harina*
1 cup plus 2 tablespoons water
2 tablespoons corn oil

In a medium-size bowl mix masa harina with water and oil until it forms a ball. Divide into 10 balls, and cover to prevent from drying. Place 1 ball between 2 sheets of plastic wrap. Roll out into a 6-inch circle, or press in a tortilla press.

Cook on a hot ungreased griddle or in a medium-size heavy skillet for 30 seconds. Turn and continue cooking for 1 minute. Turn again and continue cooking for 15 to 30 seconds. Tortillas should be soft and pliable.

Makes 10 tortillas

*Masa harina is available in Mexican or Spanish grocery stores.

Flour Tortillas

2 cups whole wheat flour
⅓ cup butter
⅓ cup milk

In a medium-size bowl blend flour and butter together with a fork or pastry blender until mixture resembles coarse crumbs. Add milk until dough can be formed into a ball.

Knead thoroughly, about 5 minutes, and form into small balls of dough 1½ inches in diameter. Roll out balls until they are very thin and about 5 inches in diameter.

Cook on a hot ungreased griddle until slightly browned on each side.

Makes about 10 tortillas

Herb Garlic Bread

 ¼ cup butter, softened
 ½ teaspoon dried oregano
 ½ teaspoon dried basil
 4 cloves garlic
 1 small loaf whole grain bread, thickly sliced

In a small bowl mix together butter, oregano, and basil. Mince garlic and add to butter mixture. Mix well and refrigerate overnight to blend flavors.

Preheat oven to 350°F.

Spread herb butter on both sides of sliced bread. Rearrange into a loaf, and wrap with foil.

Bake for 20 minutes. Serve immediately.

Makes 1 loaf

Pancakes and Waffles

Barley Pancakes

 1 tablespoon dry yeast
 ½ cup warm water
 2 tablespoons honey
 2 eggs
 1 cup yogurt
 1 cup barley flour
 2 tablespoons vegetable oil

In a medium-size bowl dissolve yeast in warm water. Stir in honey and set aside to proof.

Blend together eggs and yogurt in a small bowl. Add to yeast mixture. Then add flour and oil. Leave batter in a warm place for 20 minutes.

Ladle batter onto a hot oiled griddle, and cook until golden brown and puffy. Turn pancake and cook until other side is golden brown. Serve with honey or maple syrup.

Makes about 10 pancakes

Blueberry Pancakes

 1½ cups whole wheat pastry flour
 2 tablespoons baking powder
 ½ cup wheat germ
 1½ cups milk
 2 eggs, beaten
 2 tablespoons vegetable oil
 2 tablespoons honey
 1½ cups fresh blueberries

Mix flour, baking powder, and wheat germ together in a large bowl.

In a medium-size bowl combine milk, eggs, oil, and honey. Mix this gently with dry ingredients. Then fold in blueberries. Pour batter onto a hot oiled griddle, and cook on both sides until golden brown. Serve with honey or maple syrup.

Makes about 16 pancakes

Buckwheat Pancakes

 ½ cup whole wheat flour
 ½ cup buckwheat flour
 1 teaspoon baking powder
 1 cup milk
 ¼ cup water
 2 tablespoons honey
 1 egg
 2 tablespoons vegetable oil

Combine whole wheat and buckwheat flours in a large bowl. Add baking powder, mix, and set aside.

Beat together remaining ingredients in a small bowl, and add to flour mixture. Stir until all dry ingredients are just moistened. Do not overmix. Batter will be thin.

Pour batter onto a hot oiled griddle to form pancakes. Cook until top is bubbly. Turn and brown other side. Serve with maple syrup or honey.

Makes about 14 pancakes

Cornmeal Griddle Cakes

1 cup cornmeal
1 cup whole wheat pastry flour
1 teaspoon baking powder
½ teaspoon ground cinnamon
2 cups yogurt or buttermilk
3 eggs, separated
2 tablespoons butter, melted

In a large bowl combine cornmeal, flour, baking powder, and cinnamon. Using a wooden spoon, stir in yogurt or buttermilk then egg yolks and butter.

In a small bowl beat egg whites until stiff but not dry. Then gently fold them into batter with a rubber spatula.

Pour batter onto a hot oiled griddle and cook for about 3 minutes on each side or until golden brown.

Serve with yogurt, cottage cheese, applesauce, fresh berries, or maple syrup. If you enjoy extra crunch, top them with lightly toasted sesame seeds.

Makes about 16 pancakes

Cottage Cheese and Cornmeal Pancakes

¾ cup white cornmeal
1 tablespoon corn germ*
⅔ cup low-fat cottage cheese
¾ cup skim milk
1 egg

Mix cornmeal and corn germ together in a medium-size bowl.

Using a blender or food processor, mix cottage cheese, milk, and egg together until well blended. Add to dry ingredients and mix.

Pour batter onto a hot oiled griddle. When pancakes start to bubble, turn carefully and cook on reverse side until lightly browned. Serve with applesauce, honey, or maple syrup.

Makes about 10 pancakes

*Corn germ is available in natural foods stores.

Featherlight Pancakes with Apricot-Prune Whip

2 eggs
1½ cups yogurt
1 cup whole wheat flour
¼ cup soy flour
2 tablespoons bran
3 tablespoons butter, melted, or vegetable oil
1 teaspoon baking powder
½ teaspoon baking soda

Apricot-Prune Whip (see below)

Place all ingredients in a blender, and process only until smooth. Pour batter onto a hot oiled griddle. Cook until bubbly, then turn over and cook reverse side for about 2 minutes. Serve with Apricot-Prune Whip.

Makes about 10 pancakes

Variation:
■ Add sunflower seeds or chopped apples to batter.

Apricot-Prune Whip

6 dried prunes
6 dried apricots
5 tablespoons yogurt

Soak prunes and apricots in enough cool water to cover in refrigerator for 2 days. Drain. Remove prune pits and process prunes and apricots in a blender.

Combine fruit mixture with yogurt, and serve as topping for pancakes.

Yields about ⅓ cup

Fluffy Cottage Cheese Pancakes

5 eggs, separated
2 cups creamed cottage cheese
½ cup whole wheat flour
2 tablespoons wheat germ

In a medium-size bowl blend together egg yolks, cottage cheese, flour, and wheat germ.

Beat egg whites until stiff but not dry. Then fold them into batter. Ladle batter onto a hot oiled griddle, and cook until browned on both sides.

Makes 10 to 12 pancakes

Yogurt Pancakes

2 cups whole wheat flour
1 teaspoon baking soda
1 teaspoon baking powder
¼ teaspoon ground cinnamon
3 eggs, separated
2 tablespoons honey
2 cups yogurt

In a large bowl sift together flour, baking soda, baking powder, and cinnamon.

Beat egg yolks in a small bowl. Then add honey and yogurt and mix well. Stir lightly into dry ingredients. Beat egg whites until stiff but not dry, and fold into batter.

Pour batter onto a hot oiled griddle, and cook pancakes until brown on both sides.

Makes about 14 pancakes

All-Corn Waffles

    4 eggs, separated
    2 tablespoons vegetable oil
1½ cups milk
    2 cups finely ground corn

In a medium-size bowl blend egg yolks and oil. Add milk gradually. Then add ground corn.

Beat egg whites beyond frothy stage but not until stiff. Then mix them into batter, and beat until batter is very light and has increased in bulk by about one-third. (Batter will be thin.)

Heat waffle iron, brush lightly with oil, if necessary, and pour in enough batter to just fill. Close and cook until steaming stops and waffles are crisp. Serve with honey or honey-fruit syrup.

Makes 6 waffles

Buttermilk Waffles

    2 cups whole wheat flour
    2 teaspoons baking powder
½ teaspoon baking soda
    2 eggs, separated
    2 tablespoons honey
¼ cup butter, melted
    2 cups buttermilk

In a medium-size bowl sift together flour, baking powder, and baking soda.

Combine egg yolks, honey, butter, and buttermilk in a small bowl. Add to dry ingredients and mix well.

Beat egg whites until stiff but not dry, and then fold into batter.

Heat waffle iron, brush lightly with oil, if necessary, and pour in enough batter to just fill. Close and cook until steaming stops and waffles are crisp. Serve with maple syrup or honey.

Makes 4 to 6 waffles

Whole Wheat Waffles

    1 cup whole wheat flour
¼ cup wheat germ
    2 teaspoons baking soda
    2 tablespoons corn oil
1½ cups buttermilk
    1 egg, beaten

Combine dry ingredients in a medium-size bowl.

In a small bowl blend oil, buttermilk, and egg together. Add to dry ingredients, and mix until combined. Do not beat.

Heat waffle iron, brush lightly with oil, if necessary, and pour in enough batter to just fill. Close and cook until steaming stops and waffles are crisp. Serve with applesauce or fresh fruit topping.

Makes 4 waffles

Crepes

Whole Wheat Crepes

    4 eggs
    1 tablespoon honey
    2 tablespoons butter, melted
    1 cup milk
    1 cup water
1¾ cups whole wheat pastry flour

Combine all ingredients in a blender, and process until batter is smooth. Let rest for 2 hours to allow particles of flour to expand in liquid, resulting in a tender crepe. Just before cooking crepes, process batter again briefly to blend ingredients.

Heat a small heavy skillet or crepe pan to medium-high heat. Pan is ready when a drop of water "dances" on it. Oil pan well. Stir batter and then pour about ¼ cup into pan. Add more liquid to batter, if necessary, to make a thin crepe. Cook crepe for about 2 minutes, or until golden brown underneath and dry on top. Flip crepe over with fingers and brown other side for about 1 minute. Slide crepe onto heatproof plate, and keep warm in low oven until ready to fill and serve. Crepes may be stacked on top of each other.

Makes 16 crepes

Oat Crepes

  4 eggs
  1 tablespoon honey (optional)
  2 tablespoons vegetable oil or butter
  2 cups milk
  1½ cups oat flour

Combine all ingredients in a blender, and process until batter is smooth. Let rest for 2 hours to allow particles of flour to expand in liquid, resulting in a tender crepe. Just before cooking crepes, process batter again briefly to blend ingredients.

Heat a small heavy skillet or crepe pan to medium-high heat. Pan is ready when a drop of water "dances" on it. Oil pan well. Stir batter and then pour about ¼ cup into pan. Add more liquid to batter, if necessary, to make a thin crepe. Cook crepe for about 2 minutes, or until golden brown underneath and dry on top. Flip crepe over with fingers and brown other side for about 1 minute. Slide crepe onto heatproof plate, and keep warm in low oven until ready to fill and serve. Crepes may be stacked on top of each other.

Makes 16 crepes

Rice and Soy Crepes

  4 eggs
  2 tablespoons sesame oil
  2 cups water
  1 cup brown rice flour
  ½ cup soy flour

Combine all ingredients in a blender, and process until batter is smooth. Let rest for 2 hours to allow particles of flour to expand in liquid, resulting in a tender crepe. Just before cooking crepes, process batter again briefly to blend ingredients.

Heat a small heavy skillet or crepe pan to medium-high heat. Pan is ready when a drop of water "dances" on it. Oil pan well. Stir batter and then pour about ¼ cup into pan. Add more liquid to batter, if necessary, to make a thin crepe. Cook crepe for about 2 minutes, or until golden brown underneath and dry on top. Flip crepe over with fingers and brown other side for about 1 minute. Slide crepe onto heatproof plate, and keep warm in low oven until ready to fill and serve. Crepes may be stacked on top of each other.

Makes 1 dozen crepes

Orange-Buckwheat Crepes

  5 eggs
  1 tablespoon honey (optional)
  2 tablespoons vegetable oil or butter
  1 cup buttermilk
  1 cup water
  1¼ cups buckwheat flour
  ½ cup whole wheat pastry flour
  1 teaspoon grated orange rind

Combine all ingredients in a blender, and process until batter is smooth. Let rest for 2 hours to allow particles of flour to expand in liquid, resulting in a tender crepe. Just before cooking crepes, process batter again briefly to blend ingredients.

Heat a small heavy skillet or crepe pan to medium-high heat. Pan is ready when a drop of water "dances" on it. Oil pan well. Stir batter and then pour about ¼ cup into pan. Add more liquid to batter, if necessary, to make a thin crepe. Cook crepe for about 2 minutes, or until golden brown underneath and dry on top. Flip crepe over with fingers and brown other side for about 1 minute. Slide crepe onto heatproof plate, and keep warm in low oven until ready to fill and serve. Crepes may be stacked on top of each other.

Makes 16 crepes

Crepe Fillings

The above basic crepe recipes may be served with any filling of your choice. To get you started, we have included two favorites here. For other crepe recipes, see Index.

Spinach Filling

    1 cup cottage cheese
    3 eggs, beaten
    ¼ cup grated cheddar cheese
    1 pound fresh or frozen chopped spinach
    2 tablespoons butter, melted
    ¼ cup grated Romano cheese

Preheat oven to 350°F. Butter a shallow medium-size baking dish.

In a medium-size bowl mix together cottage cheese, eggs, and cheddar cheese. Cook spinach and drain well by placing it in a strainer and pushing it with back of a spoon. Mix spinach into cheese mixture.

Place about 1 cup mixture onto each crepe, roll up, and arrange in prepared dish. Brush with butter, sprinkle with Romano cheese, and bake until heated through, about 20 minutes.

Yields about 10 cups

Mozzarella-Mushroom Filling

    3 tablespoons butter
    1 pound mushrooms, sliced
    1 large onion, chopped
    1 cup ricotta cheese
    4 ounces mozzarella cheese, grated
    3 cups tomato sauce

In a large skillet melt butter. Add mushrooms and onions, and sauté until most of liquid has evaporated. Mix in ricotta and mozzarella. Place about 1 cup mixture onto each crepe and roll up.

Preheat oven to 350°F.

Spread a thin layer of sauce on bottom of a shallow ovenproof casserole. Place crepes over sauce in a single layer. Top with remaining sauce, and bake until hot and bubbly, about 25 minutes.

Yields about 8 cups

Nuts and Seeds

Nuts and seeds are nature's very own "fast food"—and healthful, too. Except for removing an outer shell, you need do very little to enjoy them. Each seed—and each nut—contains within itself all the ingredients necessary to nourish and sustain a new plant. In fact, they hold even more nutrients in greater concentrations than do the plants on which they grow. Protein, fiber, several B vitamins, vitamin E, and various minerals make up a good part of the nutritional profile of most nuts and seeds. Energy foods that serve as wholesome and satisfying snacks, nuts and seeds are worth their weight in calories—unlike many commercial snack foods. However, because of the high fat content of nuts and seeds (except for chestnuts, which are mostly starch), many people are careful to monitor their intake of these foods.

Though nature produces them ready to eat, nuts and seeds lend themselves without limit to creative uses in the kitchen. For centuries cooks in most countries have enhanced dishes by adding nuts and seeds. People of the Middle East still use ground almonds and pine nuts to thicken their sauces. They also add them to stuffings for lamb, chicken, and large vegetables, and they fill pastries and sweets with them. Walnut-stuffed dates inspired some of our earliest confections.

In Europe, chestnuts, once the only food available during famines, serve as a distinguished accompaniment to turkey and other game. Pine nuts find their way into Italy's pesto sauce, a mouth-watering blend that features garlic, basil, and olive oil. The French dress trout and green beans with crisp almond slivers, and they like to top green salads with chopped walnuts; ground almonds or hazelnuts are featured in the rich nut cakes of Eastern Europe.

In America, nuts find their way into everything from ice cream and confections to baked goods and stuffings. Think of pecan pie and nut breads. Around Thanksgiving and Christmas, when traditional cooking is especially popular and nuts are in season, they appear in all types of puddings, pies, and dressings. Eating nuts with fresh fruit or by themselves at the end of a meal is also a pleasurable custom that resurfaces around that time of year.

Sliced, halved, chopped, or ground, nuts are a welcome addition to almost any kind of recipe. Their unexpected burst of flavor and crunch enlivens such familiar dishes as turkey dressing or steamed green beans. Add walnuts or cashews to the mixture to perk up a soufflé. Sprinkle ground nuts over casseroles before baking, or mix sunflower seeds and various chopped nuts into cold cereals or cooked grains for added appeal. Moreover, when they are stirred into batters and bread doughs, stews, ground meats, salads, or sauces, nuts and seeds combine with the basic protein source in the recipe to round out and enhance the protein content of the dish.

Sunflower seeds and pumpkin seeds are the most popular seeds used as snacks or for cooking. Sunflower seeds are a powerhouse of nutrition containing a good supply of protein, vitamins, minerals, and a highly digestible polyunsaturated oil. They are great as a snack food or can be added easily to cereals, casseroles, grainburgers,

398

and baked goods, for a nutty flavor, crunchy texture, and a good dose of nutrition.

Oriental people have long eaten the nutritious seeds of pumpkin, squash, and larger melons. Roasted or raw, they make an excellent snack food, and they can be lively additions to dried fruit-and-nut mixes, fresh fruit salads, and bean or grain dishes.

Sesame seeds and poppy seeds, though not eaten alone as snacks, are commonly used in cooking. Sesame seeds appear in Chinese chicken dishes and are an indispensable ingredient in the popular Middle Eastern appetizer *Baba Ghannouj*. They are frequently baked into the tops of breads as a flavorful garnish.

Poppy seeds are used as a filling in sweet loaves or strudels or on top of baked breads and buns. They impart a very special flavor that is released better if the seeds are steamed or crushed before they are used in cooking. White poppy seeds are actually a sunny yellow and have many uses in Indian cooking—as a seasoning and thickening for curries or for sprinkling in unleavened breads or in chutneys.

Buying Nuts and Seeds

Nuts are in season in autumn and early winter, so that is the time to find the best-quality nuts. But you can usually buy several common types of nuts and some kinds of seeds in supermarkets throughout the year. Specialty shops and natural foods stores are likely to have a good supply of the more unusual kinds. Buy nuts and seeds in stores that seem to sell a lot of them. That means quick turnover and less chance that the stock has become stale or rancid. Nuts and seeds tend to spoil quickly because of the oils they contain.

Whole nuts can be purchased either shelled or unshelled with the exception of cashews and macadamia nuts, which are sold only shelled. Roughly speaking, one pound of unshelled nuts will yield about one-half pound of shelled nuts.

Shelled nuts are sold raw or roasted and sometimes blanched (skins removed).

Raw nuts, shelled and unshelled, are generally sold either in loose form or in cellophane bags. When possible, examine them for any visible defects before purchasing. When buying unshelled nuts, choose clean ones free from splits, cracks, stains, and holes. Guard against buying moldy nuts (they may be harmful) or nuts that feel very light (probably old and shriveled) in their shells.

Shelled nutmeats should be plump and fairly uniform in color and size, and they should look firm, not limp or rubbery. Dark or shriveled kernels suggest staleness and poor quality.

Sunflower seeds, pumpkin seeds, and sesame seeds can be purchased hulled or unhulled. If buying hulled pumpkin or sunflower seeds, read the label to determine whether they are raw or have been roasted or salted. Hulled sesame seeds are a pearly white; unhulled ones are a light tan.

Poppy seeds can be found in most natural foods stores, gourmet foods shops, and supermarkets. Look for bluish black seeds packaged in plastic bags or glass jars.

Storing Nuts and Seeds

Due to their high fat content, the chemical changes that lead to rancidity in nuts begin almost as soon as the outside hull is removed. Pine nuts are especially susceptible to spoilage because they contain unstable resinous oils. Most shelled nuts will keep at least four months in the refrigerator, a good place to store them. (Nutmeats, packed airtight, also freeze well for up to a year.) If not refrigerated, shelled nutmeats and seeds are best stored in tightly covered glass jars or bottles, preferably ones tinted green or brown to block the light, because light also attacks the fats in nuts. At room temperature shelled nuts and seeds packed this way will keep for about two months. Unshelled nuts will keep longer—about one year—in a cool, dry place and even longer under refrigeration.

Nut and Seed Mixes

Nut and seed mixes are ideal foods for picnics, camping trips, bicycling tours, hikes, and similar outings. They also make tasty, filling snacks for children or quick appetizers for buffets and dinner parties.

Try the recipes below, or combine your own favorite nuts and seeds.

NOTE: All nuts should be raw and unsalted.

Basic Nut and Seed Mix

    1 cup almonds
    1 cup cashews
    1 cup walnuts
    1 cup Brazil nuts
    1 cup sunflower seeds
    1 cup pumpkin seeds
    ½ cup sesame seeds
    2 cups raisins (optional)

Toss nuts and seeds together. Stir in raisins (if used). Store in an airtight container.

Yields 4 to 6 cups

Curried Mixed Nuts

    2 cups mixed nuts, toasted
    ½ cup sunflower seeds
    ¼ cup butter
    1 tablespoon curry powder
    ½ teaspoon ground cumin
      dash of cayenne pepper
    ½ to ¾ cup raisins
    1 cup unsweetened shredded coconut, toasted (optional)

Sauté nuts and seeds in butter in a large skillet over medium-high heat, stirring constantly, for 2 to 3 minutes. Stir in curry powder, cumin, and cayenne. Continue cooking and stirring for 1½ to 2 minutes. Stir in raisins and coconut (if used). Remove from heat and cool, stirring often, for 30 minutes. Transfer nut mixture to paper towels to drain. Store in airtight container.

Yields about 3 cups

Cracking Nuts

Peanuts (actually legumes that are enjoyed in the same ways as nuts) and most seeds are easily shelled by using your fingers alone, but when it comes to cracking hard-shelled nuts without smashing the nutmeats, more sophisticated measures may be required. Many types of nutcrackers are available to make this chore a little easier. To crack a hard-shelled nut: Keep turning the nut in the nutcracker's jaws, bearing down on it in different places to spread the stress on the shell and avoid crushing the kernel inside. If time permits, soak unshelled nuts in warm water for several hours or overnight to make them easier to crack without crushing the nutmeats.

Blanching Nuts

The process that exposes the creamy white nutmeat by removing the thick skin that clings to the kernel is called blanching. Although this skin contains nutrients, some cooks remove it simply for the sake of appearance; others to better savor the nut's own delicate flavor.

To blanch shelled almonds: Place them in boiling water and let them stand for three minutes. Then, drain them, and slide the skins off with your fingers. Spread the blanched nuts on paper towels to dry.

To blanch chestnuts: Place them, shelled, in boiling water and let them stand for two minutes. Remove a few at a time and let them cool; then peel them with a paring knife. If they don't peel easily, return them to the boiling water for a minute or two.

Hazelnuts are the most difficult to blanch. Roasting or broiling them can facilitate the job. To blanch hazelnuts by roasting: Spread them, shelled, in a single layer in a shallow baking pan. Bake them at 300°F for 10 to 15 minutes or until heated through, stirring occasionally to keep them from burning. Cool them slightly and slip the skins off with your fingers.

To blanch hazelnuts by broiling: Toast shelled nutmeats under the broiler until the skins begin to color and loosen, being very careful not to burn them. Then put them in a paper bag and rub them against one another to free the skins from the kernels.

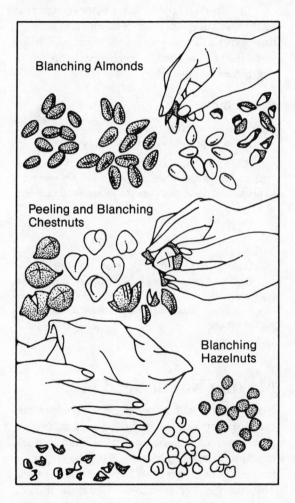

Blanching Almonds

Peeling and Blanching Chestnuts

Blanching Hazelnuts

Slivering or Slicing Nuts

Slivered nuts, an appetizing addition to salads or steamed vegetables, are also visually pleasing. Slice the nuts using a thin, sharp knife blade, while they are still warm and moist from blanching.

Chopping Nuts

Chopped nuts make an attractive garnish as well as a delectable ingredient for many dishes. They can be chopped as desired in a nut chopper. You can also chop them on a board or on a clean dish towel on a flat surface, using a knife that has a long, straight cutting edge. Some cooks prefer a wooden bowl with a rounded chopper for this. You may also use a blender or food processor, but the nuts may not be as coarsely chopped as with a manual tool.

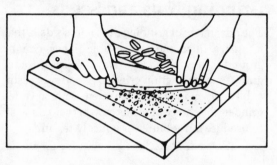

Roasting or Toasting Nuts and Seeds

Slight roasting or toasting of nuts and seeds heightens their rich flavor. They must not be overcooked, however, because their nutritional values can be impaired or destroyed and their flavors can become bitter.

Roasting and toasting can be done with the nuts dry. Nuts and seeds, rich in their own oils, need no extra fat for roasting or toasting. However, if you like the extra richness (and don't mind the calories), add one scant teaspoon of cooking oil to each cup of nutmeats, coating them evenly before cooking. To roast them: Spread the nuts or seeds in a shallow pan or on a baking sheet, and slide it into an oven preheated to 350°F. Heat, stirring them occasionally, until fragrant and lightly browned, five to ten minutes. Nuts and seeds continue to brown slightly after being removed from the heat, so be careful not to overcook them. Cool them on paper towels.

To roast chestnuts: Slash an X through the shells on the flat sides of the nuts. Place them, cut-side up, on baking sheets and roast them at 400°F until tender, about 20 minutes. Insert a fork to test them for tenderness.

To toast nuts and seeds: Spread them evenly in a heavy pan on top of the range. Heat them slowly over low heat, stirring frequently or shaking the pan from side to side as with popcorn, until lightly browned or fragrant, 10 to 15 minutes.

Grinding Nuts and Seeds

The advantage of grinding nuts and seeds is that it makes them more digestible. They can be ground in any number of ways—with a rotary grater, a meat or grain grinder, a food processor, a blender, a food mill, or even with a coffee grinder; the choice depends on whether you wish to produce a nut butter or a mealy texture.

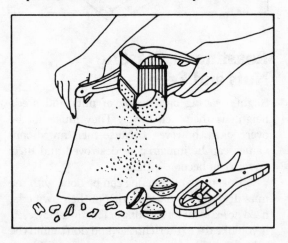

Making Nut or Seed Butter

When ground under pressure, peanuts, cashews, sunflower seeds, or sesame seeds make excellent butters. Grinding extracts the oil from the nut or seed meal to create the irresistible buttery texture. A meat grinder or food processor is effective in bringing out the oil. If nuts or seeds are ground without pressure (for example, in a blender), oil or water can be added to give a consistency that can be spread. Nut butters can be used as spreads, in drinks, or as bases for soups and sauces and can be made from roasted, as well as raw, nuts and seeds.

Store nut and seed butters in the refrigerator so they will keep their fresh flavors and will not turn rancid. They will spread and mix more easily if you allow them to reach room temperature just before you use them.

Peanut Butter

    1 cup roasted peanuts
    1 tablespoon plus 1 teaspoon vegetable oil

Place peanuts and oil in a blender. Process on medium to high speed, scraping down sides of container as necessary. Blend until smooth. Store tightly covered in a cool place.

    Yields 1 cup

Variations:
    Cashew Butter: Substitute roasted or raw cashews.
    Sesame Seed Butter (Tahini): Substitute roasted sesame seeds.
    Sunflower Seed Butter: Substitute roasted sunflower seeds.

Making Nut or Seed Meal

Nut or seed meal makes exceptionally nutritious bread or porridge, or it can be used in sauces, piecrusts, cakes, or torten. Almond meal, containing no starch and very little sugar, is frequently used as a flour in bread for diabetics. To make a nut or seed meal: Grind the nuts or seeds, one-quarter cup at a time, with either a small hand grinder or a blender at high speed. This will help keep the meal dry rather than release its oil. To use the meal in breads, replace two or three tablespoons of wheat flour with meal for every cup of wheat flour called for in the recipe. The texture of the bread will be changed only slightly.

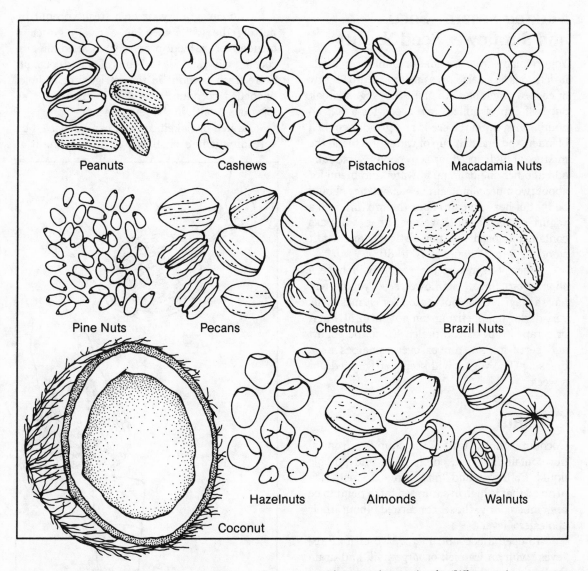

Peanuts   Cashews   Pistachios   Macadamia Nuts

Pine Nuts   Pecans   Chestnuts   Brazil Nuts

Hazelnuts   Almonds   Walnuts

Coconut

Making Nut or Seed Milk

Nuts and seeds brought to a liquid state are as nutritious and good tasting as whole nuts. Nut milk, which incidentally is as perishable as cow's milk, can be used as a quick energy drink or for sauces and soups. To make nut or seed milk: Lightly roast and grind any nuts or seeds. While grinding, gradually add water (whole or reconstituted dry milk can also be used) until a potable consistency is attained. (When using sesame seeds, strain the blended mixture.) One-quarter cup of nuts or seeds will yield one cup of milk. Sweeten it with honey or molasses, and add a few drops of vanilla extract if you desire.

You also can enhance the flavor of nut milk with any of these: one tablespoon of carob powder, honey, or molasses, or a few pitted dates, raisins, or banana slices. After adding them, reblend the mixture thoroughly.

Making Sesame Seed and Sunflower Seed Yogurt

Yogurt made from sesame or sunflower seeds is delicious as a salad dressing or as a dip for raw or cooked vegetables. To make this yogurt: Soak one-half cup of hulled, raw seeds for a full 24 hours. Then drain the seeds and grind them in a blender; add one-half cup of water and blend the mixture at high speed for 20 seconds. Gradually add another one-half cup of water and blend for about two more minutes. The consistency should be that of heavy cream. Pour the mixture into a yogurt maker, if you have one, or into a glass container (closed but not airtight), and let it stand for 8 to 24 hours at 70 to 80°F.

When it is ready, the yogurt will have a slightly tart flavor. Sunflower seed yogurt will have a grayish color, but the top sometimes turns very dark—unappetizing, but not harmful. Eat it or scrape it off, as you prefer. Spice the yogurt and serve it as a dip or over tomatoes as a dressing. The yogurt will keep, refrigerated, for a week.

Coconut

Coconut from the fruit of the palm is a tropical nut containing thick, edible meat and potable liquid. Both fruit and "milk" are extremely rich in an oil that is high in saturated fat, a point to be remembered by those concerned about their cholesterol level.

To open a coconut: Pierce two of its three "eyes" with an ice pick or large nail, and drain the liquid from the coconut. Refrigerate the liquid and use it for a refreshing drink. To remove the shell easily, bake the drained coconut at 350°F for 20 to 30 minutes or put it in the freezer for an hour. Then place the coconut on a firm surface and give the shell a quick, sharp blow with a hammer; it should break cleanly in two. Separate the meat from the shell with a sharp knife. The dark brown skin that clings tightly to the white meat can be peeled off, if desired.

You can grate your own fresh coconut by putting the white meat in a rotary grater, a blender, or a food processor. A medium-size coconut will yield 3½ to 4 cups of grated coconut. Store fresh coconut in the refrigerator. Whole, unshelled coconuts retain their quality for as long as a month in the refrigerator.

Grated or flaked coconut can be toasted by spreading it in a shallow pan and baking it at

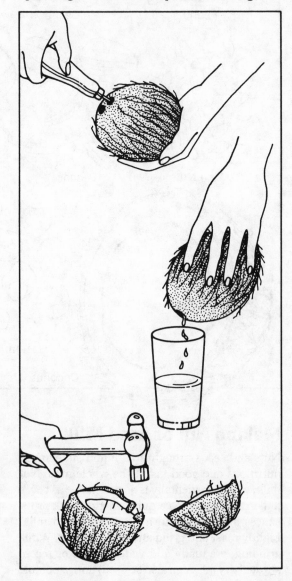

350°F, stirring frequently, until it is delicately brown, 10 to 20 minutes.

Though much of the grated or flaked coconut sold in stores is sweetened, you can usually find it unsweetened in natural foods stores.

Making Coconut Milk and Cream

To make coconut milk: Either chop or grate coconut meat freshly removed from the shell. In a blender process no more than one-half cup of coconut with about one-quarter cup of hot water at a time. Scrape down the sides of the blender, and add another one-half cup of water and blend again. Strain and measure. To make coconut cream: Simply replace the hot water with hot milk. You should end up with one cup of milk or cream. If not, add enough water to equal one cup and blend again.

Guide to Nuts and Seeds

Nut or Seed	Primary Sources	Appearance	Characteristics	Most Common Uses
Almond	Spain, Italy	oval-shaped, woody shell; smooth, white nutmeat; reddish brown skin	Sweet or bitter varieties. Bitter almonds yield extract only. Sweet almonds yield high-protein flour and oil.	eaten alone; in baked goods; as garnish for vegetables; as chief flavoring ingredient in marzipan
Brazil	South America	dark brown, very hard, rippled shell resembling orange segment; large, beige nutmeat; thick woody skin	Tastes best in winter. Rich and creamy flesh.	eaten alone; in baked goods, in stuffings, with rice dishes
Cashew	India	wrinkled, crescent-shaped, eggshell-colored nutmeat	Available shelled only. Sweet-tasting with a high fat content.	eaten alone; in baked goods, casseroles, in Middle Eastern, Indian, and Chinese dishes
Chestnut	United States	mound-shaped; mahogany-colored skin	Grows inside hard, outer husk. Contains much less oil than other nuts.	eaten roasted; cooked with moist, leafy vegetables; used in confections, stuffings; with game meat
Hazelnut (filbert)	northwestern United States	hard, reddish brown shell; long or squat, roundish oval nutmeat	When ground, contains enough oil and mealiness to replace flour and fat in cookie and cake making.	eaten alone; in baked goods, meat dishes; as garnish for fish
Hickory (butternut)	eastern United States	similar to walnuts and pecans	Sweet nutmeat is rich in oil. Similar to black walnut.	eaten alone; in baked goods; sometimes boiled or pickled
Macadamia	Australia, Hawaii	light beige; large, uneven, sphere-shaped nutmeat	Available shelled only. Sweet and buttery; often roasted in coconut oil.	eaten alone; in salads; as garnish for sweet dishes

[continued]

Guide to Nuts and Seeds—*Continued*

Nut or Seed	Primary Sources	Appearance	Characteristics	Most Common Uses
Peanut	southern and western United States	soft, papery shell; two bean-shaped nutmeats	Technically not a nut, but a member of legume family. Rich in cooking oil.	eaten alone; roasted; raw; as butter; in baked goods, casseroles, sauces, soups, stews
Pecan	southern United States	semihard shell; squat, irregular, curly halves (nutmeats)	Sweet, pulpy texture; can be used alternately with walnut.	eaten alone; in baked goods—especially pie; as meal to thicken sauces, soups, stews
Pine (pignolo)	Spain, Italy	white; long, thin, pellet-shaped nutmeat	Comes from pinecones and has sweet, pine taste. Very expensive.	used in Mediterranean dishes, pesto sauce; in stuffing for poultry, vegetables, vine leaves (dolmas)
Pistachio*	Middle East and California	hard off-white shell; naturally split at 1 end; pale green nutmeat; thin reddish skin	Mild flavor; noted especially for its color.	eaten alone; in halvah, ice cream, Middle Eastern pastries, stuffings
Walnut				
Eastern black	North America	resembles English walnuts, but not as plump and with a dark skin covering white nutmeat	Shell is very hard; difficult to crack. Stronger tasting than English walnut.	used in baked goods, candy, ice cream
English	western United States and France	hard shell; squat, irregular, curly halves (nutmeats)	Mild and sweet tasting; rich in cooking oil. Called green walnut when fresh; sometimes pickled.	eaten alone; in baked goods, desserts, sandwich spreads, stuffings, sweet loaves
Poppy seeds	central Europe	tiny, bluish black spheres (sometimes available white)	Pleasantly nutty when baked.	used in filling for sweet loaves, strudels; in or on raised breads
Pumpkin seeds	United States	long, flat, dark green seeds with white outer shells	Shelled, unshelled, raw, roasted, salted, unsalted; pressed into oil.	eaten alone; in baked goods; in dried fruit-nut mixes; in fresh fruit and vegetable salads
Sesame seeds†	Mexico	unhulled—small, tan ovals; hulled—white	Hulled, unhulled, raw; pressed into oil.	on raised breads; in *Baba Ghannouj,* Chinese chicken dishes; as tahini (sesame butter); as garnish on salads
Sunflower seeds	United States	grayish oval seeds in soft black and white seed coats	Shelled, unshelled, raw, roasted, salted, unsalted; pressed into oil.	eaten alone; in baked goods, bean or vegetable casseroles, patties, salads

*Pistachios are often sold covered with a red dye, but natural, undyed pistachio nuts may be obtained at natural foods stores and are well worth seeking out.
†Hulled sesame seeds are a little more digestible than unhulled, but unlike the larger seeds, sesame seeds need not be hulled before being eaten or used for cooking.

406

Sprouts

Growing sprouts in your kitchen is almost like growing vegetables in your yard, but without all the work. They are vegetables that can be grown and harvested at any time of the year and added to your diet in many novel ways. Most sprouts require no cooking, and those that do are ready after only a few minutes of stir-frying. You can add them to soups, breads, and main dishes, or eat them as is in salads or on sandwiches. Once you learn how simple it is to unlock the tremendous store of good nutrients that lie dormant in every seed (nuts, grains, and legumes are all seeds), you can enjoy fresh produce in every season.

Home-grown sprouts develop rapidly and are among the most economical foods available. Just one cup of mung beans will yield about four cups of sprouts. Three tablespoons of alfalfa seeds will expand into four cups of sprouts.

Sprouts actually are seeds that have begun to germinate. Soaking the seed activates the life forces packed away for its growth. Feeding itself on the starch containing its embryo, the seed can grow for several days without acquiring nutrients from soil, increasing its own protein and vitamin value in the process. Sprouting generates significant increases in vitamins A, B, C, and E, as well as in the amino acid content of the seed.

For people on weight-control diets, sprouts are a happy discovery. Because the growing sprout uses up the starch in the seed, sprouts are very low in carbohydrates. Sprouts also have a high water content. Consequently a cup of mung bean sprouts or alfalfa sprouts has only about 37 calories.

What to Sprout

Not all seeds and beans yield edible or palatable sprouts. Potato sprouts are considered poisonous. The sprouts of fava beans and lima beans require so much cooking to deactivate a potentially toxic substance that they become mushy and unpleasant by the time they are safe to eat. Many spice and herb seeds—coriander and pepper, for example—will sprout well, but the sprout is unpalatable. However, seeds, grains, and legumes that can be successfully sprouted still present an impressive choice (see Guide to Sprouting Seeds, page 411). Mung and alfalfa are the most popular, perhaps because they are the easiest to sprout. Wheat sprouts are nutty and sweet; radish sprouts have a crisp, tangy taste. Rye sprouts taste a lot like wild rice.

For improved flavor and nutrition, add a handful of sprouts to brown rice dishes, or add them to the dough or batter in bread recipes. You can keep jars of sprouts in the refrigerator for snacking and for salads. Drop some into soups just before serving, or garnish a cooked vegetable dish with a small handful of sprouts.

How to Sprout

Sprouting is very simple, even for beginners. All you need are seeds, a jar, a piece of cheesecloth, a rubber band, and clean water. You can also use a bowl, a pie plate, or a colander. Just about any container will work, but avoid those made of wood or metal, because wood absorbs moisture and may grow mold or mildew, and some metals may give sprouts a bad taste.

Most natural foods stores carry a good variety of seeds, grains, and legumes to sprout and they often stock sprouting equipment as well. You may also want to check on mail-order sources (see Appendix 4) if you intend to keep a variety of seeds sprouting. Buy seeds that are of the best quality, untreated with mold retardants, fungicides, or insecticides. As you measure the seeds, wash them thoroughly, removing any chaff or broken or cracked seeds.

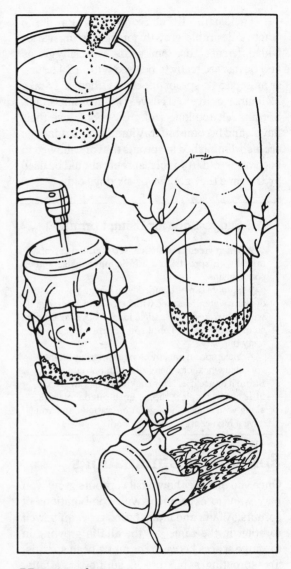

1. To begin the sprouting process, soak the seeds in a one-quart jar filled with warm water (70 to 80°F) at a ratio of one part seeds to four parts water. Seeds should be soaked for 8 to 12 hours, with small seeds taking a little less time and beans a little longer. Put the soaking seeds in a dark, warm place—under the sink, in the oven, or in a drawer.

After soaking the seeds, pour off the water and reserve it for cooking soups or for drinks; it has a mild flavor and some nutrients.

2. Rinse the soaked seeds in a strainer or colander or in the jar, straining the water through a piece of cheesecloth. Stretch the cheesecloth over the top of the jar, holding it in place with a rubber band, allowing air and water to pass through freely. Return the jar of seeds to the same dark, warm place as before, resting it on its side, slightly tilted so excess moisture will drain through the cheesecloth.

3. Sprouts should be rinsed at least twice a day, but they will thrive even better on more rinsings. The rinsing provides them with water and washes away any by-products of growth that encourage spoilage. To rinse the sprouts, simply fill the jar with water, swish it around briskly, then drain it thoroughly. Water permitted to stay in the jar can cause mold.

Harvesting

The sprouts can be harvested in three to five days. They may benefit from a few hours of direct sunlight before harvesting. It enables the sprouts to produce additional chlorophyll, thus increasing their nutritional value and coloring them a pleasant green.

The length of time required for sprouts to reach a desirable growth for harvesting varies with different seeds. Some seeds, especially grains and beans, are ready to be used within 24 hours, or as soon as a sprout appears. Others may take 72 hours — or five to six days. Timing is important. Sprouts left too long will grow roots, lose their flavor, and become bitter. Vitamins and minerals are also diminished in sprouts that are allowed to become too old. As a rule, sprouts should be used by the time they are five or six days old.

Suggestions for Using Sprouts

- When greens are scarce, serve grated carrots mixed with sprouts; add a little mayonnaise and some raisins.
- Sprouts can be blended with an equal amount of warm water, seasoned with herbs, and garnished with watercress for a delicious, body-warming soup full of vitality. Lentil sprouts are particularly tasty this way.
- Make sprout milk by blending one cup slightly sprouted wheat or other grain with one cup water. Strain it or use it as is for cooking or baking. Add a little honey, maple syrup, or unsulfured molasses, along with some wheat germ or granola, and you have a high-energy breakfast food.

Sprouting Combinations

Once you discover how easily sprouts grow, you may want to experiment with combinations of sprouts. Alfalfa and mung beans grow quite well together in the same jar, the alfalfa growing in the large spaces between the mung bean sprouts. Try sprouting a mixture of sunflower, alfalfa, lentil, fenugreek, and mung bean. It is also a good idea to have at least three jars of sprouts growing at once — a bean, a grain, and a small seed — because their protein patterns complement each other when they are used in the same meal.

Storage

Sprouts are best when used as soon as they are harvested. If you choose to store sprouts, place them loosely in a covered plastic or glass container, with a folded paper towel in the bottom of the container to absorb any remaining moisture. Do not use plastic bags, as tender shoots are easily crushed or broken in nonrigid containers and the sprouts will quickly spoil. Do not store them for more than two or three days, and store them in the coldest part of the refrigerator. Some sprouts continue to grow even under refrigeration.

Leftover Sprouts

If you find that you are growing sprouts faster than you can consume them and they are accumulating, freezing them is not the answer — the shoots become soggy and limp when thawed. However, an oversupply of sprouts can be dried quickly in a warm oven (about 250°F for 45 minutes) without losing many nutrients. Then you can whirl the dried sprouts into powder in a blender and store the powder in airtight jars. Use it as a nutritional supplement to regular flour in baking. Sprouted dried beans — chickpeas or soybeans — can be chopped or ground and used to replace nuts in recipes.

Wheat Flour from Sprouts

Sprouts made from wheat are very sweet, because the starches in the grain have been converted to simple sugars in the process of sprouting. When wheat sprouts are used in breads and pancakes, you will find little need for additional sweetener. Wheat sprouts can be dried or roasted, then finely ground and used to replace flour in baked products.

To make flour from wheat sprouts: Dry the sprouts in a very low oven for about eight hours. The pilot light may suffice if the oven is gas. When they are dry, run the sprouts through a seed mill or a blender. This product is known as diastatic malt, the elusive factor that characterizes many of the good-tasting breads baked in Europe. It can be blended with unsprouted wheat flour in the ratio of one part malt to four parts flour. The malt can also be used as a natural sweetener for cereal, bread, cookies, and other baked products.

Guide to Sprouting Seeds

Seed	Rinses (per day)	Harvest Sprout Length	Sprout Time (days)	Approximate Yield (seeds-sprouts)	Comments
Alfalfa	2	1-2 inches	3-5	3 tablespoons = 4 cups	Easy to sprout. Pleasant, light taste.
Almond	2-3	¼ inch	3-5	1 cup = 1½ cups	Similar to unsprouted nuts. Crunchy, nutty flavor.
Amaranth	3	¼ inch	2-3	3 tablespoons = 1 cup	Mild taste.
Anise	6	1 inch	2	3 tablespoons = 1 cup	Strong, anise flavor. Good if used sparingly.
Barley	2-3	Sprout is length of seed.	3-4	½ cup = 1 cup	Chewy texture, pleasant taste, not sweet. Toasting enhances flavor.
Bean (all kinds except those listed individually in table)	3-4	1 inch	3-5	1 cup = 4 cups	For tender sprouts, limit germination time to 3 days.
Buckwheat	1	¼-½ inch	2-3	1 cup = 3 cups	Easy to sprout. Buy raw, hulled groats for sprouting.
Chia	1	¼-1 inch	1-4	2 tablespoons = 3-4 cups	Hard to sprout. Tend to become gelatinous where wet. Sprinkle rather than rinse. Strong flavor.
Chick-pea	4	½ inch	3	1 cup = 3 cups	Best lightly cooked.
Clover (red)	2	1-2 inches	3-5	1½ tablespoons = 4 cups	Similar to alfalfa sprouts.
Corn	2-3	½ inch	2-3	1 cup = 2 cups	Sweet corn taste, with chewy texture. Difficult to find untreated kernels for sprouting.
Cress	2	1-1½ inches	3-5	1 tablespoon = 1½ cups	Gelatinous seed. Strong, peppery taste.
Fenugreek	1-2	1-3 inches	3-5	¼ cup = 1 cup	Spicy taste, good in curry dishes. Bitter if sprouted too long.
Flax	2-3	1-2 inches	4	2 tablespoons = 1½-2 cups	Tend to become gelatinous when wet. Sprinkle rather than rinse. Mild flavor.
Lentil	2-4	¼-1 inch	3	1 cup = 6 cups	Chewy bean texture. Can be eaten raw or steamed lightly.

[*continued*]

Guide to Sprouting Seeds—*Continued*

Seed	Rinses (per day)	Harvest Sprout Length	Sprout Time (days)	Approximate Yield (seeds-sprouts)	Comments
Millet	2-3	¼ inch	3-4	1 cup = 2 cups	Similar to barley sprouts.
Mung bean	3-4	1½-2 inches	3-5	1 cup = 4-5 cups	Easy to sprout. Popular in oriental dishes. Sprouts begin to lose crispness after 4 days of storage.
Mustard	2	1-1½ inches	3-4	2 tablespoons = 3 cups	Spicy, tangy taste, reminiscent of fresh English mustard.
Oat	1	Sprout is length of seed.	3-4	1 cup = 2 cups	Only unhulled oats will sprout. Water sparingly; too much water makes sprouts sour.
Pea	2-3	Sprout is length of seed.	3	1½ cup = 2 cups	Taste like fresh peas. Best when steamed lightly.
Pumpkin	2-3	¼ inch	3	1 cup = 2 cups	Hulled seeds make best sprouts. Light toasting improves flavor.
Radish	2	⅛-2 inches	2-6	1 tablespoon = 1 cup	Taste like the vegetable.
Rice	2-3	Sprout is length of seed.	3-4	1 cup = 2½ cups	Similar to other sprouted grains. Only whole grain brown rice will sprout.
Rye	2-3	Sprout is length of seed.	3-4	1 cup = 3½ cups	Easy to sprout. Very sweet taste, with crunchy texture.
Sesame	4	Sprout is length of seed.	3	1 cup = 1½ cups	Only unhulled seeds will sprout. Delicious flavor when young; sprouts over 1/16 inch turn bitter.
Soybean	4-6	1-2 inches	4-6	1 cup = 4-5 cups	Need frequent, thorough rinses. Should be cooked before eating for optimum protein availability.
Sunflower	2	Sprout is no longer than seed.	1-3	½ cup = 1½ cups	Good snacks, especially if lightly roasted. Become bitter if grown too long.
Triticale	2-3	Sprout is length of seed.	2-3	1 cup = 2 cups	Similar to wheat sprouts.
Wheat	2-3	Sprout is length of seed.	2-4	1 cup = 3½-4 cups	Easy to sprout. Very sweet taste.

Alfalfa Sprout Gazpacho

1 cup alfalfa sprouts
4 cups tomato juice
½ cucumber, chopped
1 stalk celery, chopped
1 scallion, chopped
1 slice green pepper, 1 inch thick, chopped
2 medium-size tomatoes, peeled and chopped

Combine all ingredients in a blender and process until completely liquefied. Chill for 1 hour. Serve as a beverage or a soup.

4 to 6 servings

Beef and Sprout Patties

1 pound lean ground beef
1 cup chopped mung bean sprouts
1 clove garlic, minced
¼ medium-size onion, minced
¼ cup tomato juice
2 tablespoons soy sauce
1 tablespoon dried basil

In a large bowl combine all ingredients, mixing by hand until you have a soft, moist, well-blended mixture. Form into patties and broil in a broiler or sauté in a large skillet on both sides until they are cooked through.

4 servings

Chick-pea Sprout Snack

A nutritious, no-sugar snack children enjoy; adults find it unusual and appealing, too. This is a sure-fire way to introduce sprouts.

2 cups chick-pea sprouts
1½ cups peanuts
¾ cup peanut butter
1 cup milk
1½ cups sesame seeds
1½ cups sunflower seeds
1½ cups whole wheat flour

In a medium-size bowl chop sprouts and peanuts together, or put through a meat grinder using blade with large holes. Cut in peanut butter and then add milk. Mix thoroughly.

In a large bowl, combine seeds and flour. Mix together the sprout and seed mixtures to form a stiff dough.

Preheat oven to 275°F.

Divide dough in half and spread each half on a greased baking sheet. Cover with wax paper and roll out to ¼-inch thickness. Cut into 1½-inch squares and bake for 1 hour, or until browned. Remove from pan and cool on rack. Store in an airtight container.

Makes 80

Coconut and Sprouts Custard Pie

2 cups milk
4 eggs
¼ cup honey
½ cup wheat sprout flour (see page 410) or ¼ cup whole wheat flour and ¼ cup soy flour
2 teaspoons baking powder
¼ cup butter
1½ teaspoons vanilla extract
1 cup wheat sprouts
1 cup unsweetened shredded coconut

Preheat oven to 325°F.

Place all ingredients in a blender except wheat sprouts and coconut. Blend on low for 3 minutes.

Butter a 10-inch pie plate. Spread wheat sprouts over the bottom. Pour in custard mixture and let stand for 5 minutes. Sprinkle coconut on top.

Bake for 30 minutes. Allow to cool and then refrigerate.

6 to 8 servings

Spicy-Hot Soy Sprouts

A nice alternative to green salads.

2 tablespoons sesame or vegetable oil
1 pound soy sprouts
2 or 3 scallions, chopped
2 or 3 cloves garlic, minced
½ teaspoon cayenne pepper
sesame seeds, toasted

Heat oil in a large skillet. Cook sprouts in oil, covered, for a few minutes over medium heat, shaking the pan occasionally. Add scallions, garlic, and cayenne. Cook until barely tender. Garnish with sesame seeds.

4 servings

Sprouted Wheat Bread

    2 cups wheat sprouts
    ½ cup vegetable oil
    1¼ cups milk
    2 cups whole wheat flour
    2 cups wheat germ

Put wheat sprouts through a meat grinder, using the fine blade, or process in a blender. In a large bowl combine all ingredients and let stand at room temperature for 20 minutes.

Preheat oven to 325°F.

Form sprout mixture into 2 oval loaves and place on an oiled baking sheet. Bake for 1 hour. Cool on a wire rack.

Makes 2 small loaves

Sprouted Wheat Sticks

    3 to 4 cups wheat sprouts
    2 tablespoons crushed caraway seeds
    1 egg, beaten
       cornmeal, for dredging

Put wheat sprouts through a meat grinder, using the fine blade, or process in a blender. Mix with seeds and egg in a medium-size bowl.

Preheat oven to 400°F.

Form sprout mixture into cigar shapes, roll in cornmeal, and place on an oiled baking sheet. Let dry for 5 minutes.

Bake for 10 minutes. Then reduce heat to 325°F and continue baking until done, about 5 more minutes.

Makes 1 dozen

Sprout Omelet with Tomatoes

    6 eggs
    2 scallions, chopped
    1 to 2 tablespoons fresh dill or parsley
    ¼ cup milk
    1 medium-size tomato, chopped
    ½ cup sunflower sprouts, or more if desired
       alfalfa sprouts

In a large bowl beat eggs, scallions, dill or parsley, and milk together with a wire whisk.

Heat mixture in a large buttered pan until it begins to set. Add tomatoes and sunflower seed sprouts; cover. When set, fold omelet over and top with alfalfa sprouts.

3 to 4 servings

Sprout Slaw

    ½ cup shredded red and/or green cabbage
    1 medium-size carrot, grated
    1 stalk celery, thinly sliced
    ½ medium-size green pepper, chopped
    2 scallions, chopped
    1 small parsnip, grated
    ¼ cup sunflower sprouts
    ½ cup alfalfa sprouts
    ½ cup bean sprouts (adzuki, mung, and lentil
       are a colorful combination)

Combine ingredients in a large bowl. Toss with Almost a Miracle Dressing (page 181) or Sour Cream Salad Dressing (page 184).

6 servings

Sprouts, Vegetables, and Cheese

    ½ cup chick-pea sprouts
    1 cup tightly packed alfalfa sprouts
    ½ cup chopped spinach
    ½ cup chopped lettuce
    ½ cup sliced scallions
    1 cup chopped green peppers
    ½ cup fresh peas
    ¾ cup diced zucchini
    ½ cup chopped cucumbers
    ⅔ cup cubed sharp cheddar cheese

Combine ingredients in a large bowl. Just before serving, toss with Herb Dressing (page 182) or Vinaigrette (page 184).

6 servings

Sprouts with Italian Herbs

    4 medium-size tomatoes, coarsely chopped
    6 medium-size okra, thinly sliced
    2 scallions, chopped

½ green pepper, sliced
½ teaspoon dried basil
¼ teaspoon dried oregano
1 clove garlic, minced
¼ cup grated Parmesan cheese
3 tablespoons lemon juice
    sprouts (alfalfa, mung bean, or soy)

Place vegetables in a large bowl. In a small bowl mix herbs, garlic, and cheese. Add lemon juice and toss with vegetables.

Serve over a large bowl of sprouts.

4 to 6 servings

Stir-Fried Bean Sprouts

This is a fine accompaniment to poultry and fish dishes, or it can serve admirably as a nonmeat main course.

½ large head broccoli
¼ cup vegetable oil
4 scallions, thinly sliced
4 cups coarsely chopped Chinese cabbage
2 cups sliced peeled turnips
2 tablespoons minced peeled ginger root
2 cups mung bean sprouts
¼ cup soy sauce
¼ cup water

Separate broccoli head into stalks. Trim stalks and cut stem off below the floret. Reserve the florets. Slice stalks ¼ inch thick.

Heat oil to medium-hot in a large skillet or wok. Stir-fry scallions for 1 to 2 minutes, then add cabbage, broccoli stalks, turnips, and ginger. Stir-fry for about 5 minutes. Finally, add broccoli florets, sprouts, soy sauce, and water. Stir-fry for a few more minutes, until vegetables are tender but still firm. Pan may be covered briefly toward the end of the cooking period to hasten tenderizing. Serve immediately.

6 servings

Vegetable-Sprout Medley with Cottage Cheese

1 cucumber, sliced
1 small zucchini, sliced
2 medium-size tomatoes, sliced
½ cup mung bean sprouts
¼ cup sunflower sprouts or seeds
¼ teaspoon dried oregano
¼ teaspoon dried basil
¼ teaspoon dried thyme
2 tablespoons vegetable oil
2 tablespoons vinegar or lemon juice
1 cup cottage cheese

In a large bowl combine cucumbers, zucchini, tomatoes, mung bean sprouts, sunflower sprouts or seeds, and herbs. Add oil and vinegar or lemon juice and mix well.

Make a well in center of salad and put cottage cheese in well.

6 servings

Wheat Sprout Candy

A healthful sweet that children enjoy.

1 cup wheat sprouts
1 cup walnuts
1 cup unsweetened shredded coconut
1 cup raisins
    sesame seeds

Put all ingredients except sesame seeds through a meat grinder, using the fine blade. Mix well in a medium-size bowl and shape into balls the size of marbles. Roll in sesame seeds and refrigerate before serving.

Makes 30

Eggs

Eggs are surely the most useful and adaptable of all foods. They are the core of such impressive convenience dishes as Eggs Provençale and provide the airy substance for such elegant presentations as Springtime Soufflé. With bread crumbs they become a coating for baked fish. Eggs keep oil and vinegar from separating in mayonnaise and crystals from forming in candies. They bind hearty meat loaves together and can be spun out into feathery meringues. Of course, they are indispensable for thickening rich, smooth custards. Team them with milk and flavoring and you have a tasty, healthful meal-in-a-glass.

Along with the versatility cooks love, a shape that artists adore, and an economy penny-pinchers crave, eggs are also low in calories and loaded with nutrients. They are relatively rich in cholesterol, however, a fact that is significant to those concerned about increased cholesterol levels in the blood.

Buying Fresh Eggs

Most supermarkets carry eggs in two or more sizes, grades, and, sometimes, colors. Which you buy depends on how you plan to use the eggs.

Egg sizes, established by the United States Department of Agriculture (USDA) in the 1930s, are based not on the measurement of the eggs,

Market Sizes for Eggs

Egg Size	Approximate Weight of 1 Dozen (ounces)
Jumbo	30
Extra large	27
Large	24
Medium	21
Small	18
Peewee	15

but on the weight of a dozen (see Market Sizes for Eggs table, above). To get the most egg for your money, buy the larger size when the price difference between two sizes is less than 10 percent.

Although most recipes call for either medium-size or large eggs—the sizes most readily available in markets—don't let that keep you from buying other sizes (see Egg Size Equivalents table, page 417). The recipes in this book were developed and tested with large eggs.

Do not pay extra for eggs with a particular shell color. The quality and nutritive value of brown eggs and of white ones are virtually identical.

When you shop for eggs, check the grade stamped on the carton. Grading gives you a general idea about the quality of the egg in the

416

box. Depth of the yolk, thickness of the white, size of the air sack, and position of the yolk determine whether the egg is graded AA, A, B, or C. Eggs AA and A, with high, firm yolks, thick whites, and obvious ropelike strands (chalazae) anchoring the yolk, are the ones found most frequently in markets. Grades B and C, which have flat, watery whites, usually go to commercial bakeries and food producers. Since Grade A eggs can drop to Grade B eggs if they are stored improperly or kept too long, always buy fresh eggs that have been kept under refrigeration.

Once home, you can check the freshness of the eggs you bought by floating them in water. If the eggs sink, they are fresh. If they float upright with the large end on top, they are not the freshest. If they rise to the surface, return them to the store or throw them out.

Although eggs are inspected by the producers for cracks or other defects, you may occasionally come across one that is cracked. Check the eggs in the carton before you buy them, to be sure none is cracked, since bacteria that cause food poisoning can enter the egg through any opening in the shell. If you do find that you are somehow stuck with cracked eggs, hard-cook them or use them in a cake. It is not safe to use cracked, raw eggs in something like eggnog or in a lightly cooked dish such as scrambled eggs.

Storing Eggs

Whole Eggs

Store eggs with the large end of the shell up (to keep the yolks centered in their shells) in a covered container in the refrigerator. Since the shells are porous, eggs tend to absorb odors, so keep eggs away from strong-smelling foods such as onions and garlic. For best quality, use fresh eggs within a week. You can keep shelled eggs in the freezer for four months. Add one teaspoon honey to one cup eggs before freezing in a tightly covered container.

Yolks

Cover with cold water and store in the refrigerator in a tightly covered container. Use within two days. Pour off water before using. To store yolks in the freezer, add one teaspoon honey to one cup yolks before freezing in a tightly covered container. Use within four months.

Whites

Refrigerate extra whites in a tightly covered container. Ideally, the whites should be used within two days. To freeze, put them in a sealed container for future use. Whites will keep this way for six months.

Egg Size Equivalents

	Equivalents			
Number of Large Eggs	Extra Large Eggs	Medium Eggs	Small Eggs	Approximate Volume
1	1	1	1	3 tablespoons
2	2	2	3	¼ cup plus 2 tablespoons
3	3	4	4	½ cup plus 2 tablespoons
4	3	5	6	¾ cup plus 1 tablespoon
5	4	6	7	1 cup
6	5	7	8	1 cup plus 3 tablespoons
8	6	10	11	1½ cups plus 2 tablespoons
10	8	12	14	2 cups
12	10	14	17	2¼ cups plus 2 tablespoons

Dried Eggs

Dried egg yolks, egg whites, and whole egg solids are used primarily by commercial bakers and institutions, though some family cooks like to keep dried eggs on hand for an emergency. If you do buy them (many grocery stores stock dried eggs), check the label, which will tell you if they have been pasteurized, inspected, and dried under sanitary conditions.

This guide will help you determine the quantity to buy:

> 8 ounces dried whole eggs = 16 large or 18 medium-size whole eggs
> 8 ounces dried yolks = 17 yolks
> 8 ounces dried whites = 50 whites

Store dried eggs in a tightly covered container so that they do not absorb odors or take on moisture, which makes them lumpy and hard to mix. If kept in the refrigerator, they should stay sweet for about a year.

Reconstituting dried eggs is simple. For scrambled eggs or custards, sift the solids and measure just the amount you need. Measure the correct amount of water; add it to the eggs and stir thoroughly to moisten the solids. Use the eggs immediately. If you want to use dried eggs in baking, you will find it is easier to mix the egg solids with the other dry ingredients and simply increase the liquid called for in the recipe by the amount needed to reconstitute the eggs. These are the specific proportions for reconstituting:

> 1 large whole egg = 2½ tablespoons dried eggs plus 2½ tablespoons water
> 1 yolk = 2 tablespoons dried yolk plus 2 teaspoons water
> 1 white = 2 teaspoons dried whites plus 2 tablespoons water

Basic Cooking

No matter how much you are tempted to do so, never hurry the cooking of an egg. Always cook it at low to moderate heat; high temperatures set the protein in the white and the yolk much too rapidly. As the protein sets, it shrinks, and the egg—scrambled, baked, hard-cooked, poached, or fried—becomes tough and rubbery. If the egg is part of a sauce when the shrinking takes place, it won't hold any liquid, and the mixture will curdle, showing small, tough lumps of egg. If the egg is in a soufflé, angel food cake, or meringue, it will not expand; the finished dish will lack volume and lightness.

You can avoid overheating eggs in sauces, puddings, and soft custards by using a double boiler, and by tempering the eggs (see Tempering Eggs, page 427). For sauces and puddings, cook the starch first—it needs extra time to thicken and lose its raw taste—then add the eggs.

Just slightly undercooked eggs are tender and moist. To serve yours that way, remove them from the heat a second or two before they actually finish cooking. The residual heat the eggs hold will finish them just right by the time you get them to the table.

Separating Egg Whites from Egg Yolks

Some recipes require only the white or the yolk of an egg; some call for adding the white and the yolk at different times. The technique for separating eggs is easily mastered.

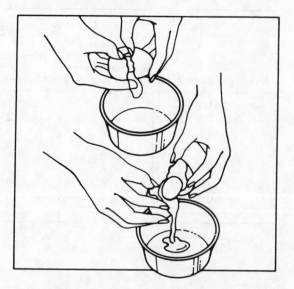

Use a knife blade to crack the shell of a cold egg in the middle, or tap the middle of the egg against the edge of a bowl. While holding the egg over a cup or small bowl, gently pull the shell into two pieces with your thumbs. Very carefully pass the yolk from one half of the shell to the other, letting the white drop into the cup or bowl. If a fragment of shell falls into the white, pick it out with a piece of the shell, paper toweling, or a teaspoon. If the yolk breaks and runs into the white, set the egg aside, since even a tiny speck of yolk will ruin the white for beating. Use the egg to make scrambled eggs or a plain omelet. Pour the perfectly separated whites into a large bowl. Repeat until you have the number of whites or yolks needed for the recipe.

Measuring Eggs

Number to Make 1 Cup

Egg Size	Whole Eggs	Whites	Yolks
Small	7	10	18
Medium	6	8	16
Large	5	7	14
Extra large	4	6	12

NOTE: If you should need half an egg when halving a recipe, break a large egg, beat it slightly, and use half of it (about 1½ tablespoons).

Beating Egg Whites and Yolks

Under the right conditions egg whites, properly beaten, can inflate to six times their original volume. To get the kind of expansion necessary for creating light, airy dishes, several things are critical: temperature, humidity, bowl, beaters, and ingredients.

Egg whites beat best on a day when the humidity is low and when they have been held at room temperature for 45 minutes. Add a pinch of cream of tartar or several drops of lemon juice to the whites if you are using honey to sweeten a meringue. (Though many cookbooks recommend using salt or refined sugar, results are excellent without them.) Place the whites in a bowl made of glass, stainless steel, ceramic, or copper. Some cooks prefer a copper one because the slight acidity of copper seems to make a fuller, longer-lasting foam. Never use an aluminum bowl (it turns the whites gray) or a plastic one (it may prevent foaming). Select a bowl that has a rounded bottom so that the beaters pick up all the white. The bowl and beaters must be absolutely clean. Even the slightest specks of fat (including egg yolk, which contains fat) seriously hinder the beating process.

You can use either a wire whisk, a hand-held rotary beater, or an electric mixer for beating egg whites. Gourmet cooks prefer balloon wire whisks, which do not cut the foam the way a rotary beater does. If you are in a hurry, you may decide to use the electric mixer. Start the mixer at low speed until the whites are foamy; then increase to medium speed. Be wary of overbeating when using an electric mixer.

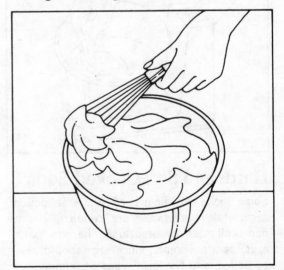

Beat the whites until they are glossy and moist, not dry. If they become dry, they have been overbeaten; they will lack volume and elasticity. Fortunately, you can rescue overbeaten whites by adding one to two tablespoons of cold water and beating again, briskly and briefly. Underbeaten whites create as many problems for the cook as do their overbeaten counterparts.

They leak water and added ingredients, and they do not hold their shape. Well-beaten whites should stand in either soft or stiff peaks. Follow the recipe for directions concerning the degree of stiffness desired.

Beaten egg yolks are not nearly as fragile as whites are. They can be beaten successfully in any bowl, at any time, with any type of beater. Yolks might be lightly beaten just to blend several together. With more beating they become thick and lemon colored. With still more beating yolks become thick enough to form a thin, flat ribbon that doubles back on itself when dropped from the beater.

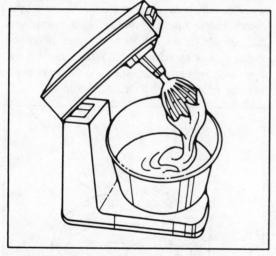

Hard- and Soft-Cooked Eggs

Some cooks call them hard- and soft-"boiled" eggs, while to others they are "coddled," but the names all mean the same thing. The term "boiled eggs" is a misnomer, since eggs should never be boiled, and "coddled" eggs are simply eggs that were started in boiling water instead of cold water. Whatever you call them, they are useful in dozens of ways. Sliced hard-cooked eggs make attractive garnishes; chopped ones make tasty salads; stuffed ones, quick hors d'oeuvres; and whole ones, great lunch-bag fillers. In a pinch you can even substitute a soft-cooked egg for a poached one.

Prepare hard- and soft-cooked eggs in one of these two ways:

Method One: Place cold eggs in a saucepan or a pot and cover them with cold water. Since both the eggs and the water are cold, there is no need to worry about the shells cracking. Bring the water just to a boil, then reduce the heat to simmer. For soft-cooked eggs simmer for 3 to 5 minutes, depending on how firm you want the whites; for hard-cooked eggs simmer for 10 to 15 minutes. Serve soft-cooked eggs while they are hot; hard-cooked ones should be plunged into cold water immediately to stop the cooking. If a hard-cooked egg is not cooled rapidly (or if it is cooked in boiling water), the white sticks to the shell, and the iron in the yolk combines with the sulfur in the white to form an unattractive green ring on the outer edge of the yolk. A dry, mealy yolk shows that the hard-cooked egg was cooked just right. If the yolk is waxy, the egg was under-cooked. A soft-cooked egg properly done will have a moist, tender white and a runny yolk.

Method Two (coddled eggs): Reduce the chances of cracking the shells by piercing the large ends of the shells with a pin or an egg piercer to release trapped air and by letting the eggs warm to room temperature (it takes about 45 minutes). Bring a pot of water to a boil and, with a tablespoon or wire basket, carefully lower the eggs into the water. Cover the pan and remove it from the heat. For soft-cooked eggs let them stand for 4 to 5 minutes, and for hard-cooked ones 10 to 15 minutes. Cool hard-cooked eggs instantly by dipping them into cold water.

Peel a hard-cooked egg by first tapping it on a hard surface to crack the shell. Then roll it between your hands until you loosen the shell. Starting at the large end, remove the shell and the thin membrane under it. If the shell is stubborn—an egg three or four days old is usually easier to peel than a fresher one—try holding it under cold running water as you peel.

Crack the shell of a soft-cooked egg by tapping it around the middle with a knife handle. Carefully remove the shell from the small end.

Next, use a spoon to scoop the egg from the large end.

Store hard-cooked eggs in the refrigerator for use within a few days. If you forget which eggs are cooked and which are raw, spin them on the counter. Raw ones roll neatly; cooked ones wobble. (Some cooks simply pencil HC on hard-cooked ones before refrigerating.)

Poached Eggs

Poached eggs have much to recommend them— delicate flavor, no added fat, silken texture, few calories, quick preparation. They are a little tricky for beginners, so it is a good idea to make them once or twice for yourself before preparing them for a crowd.

Always use the freshest eggs available. They will poach into compact, tidy spheres with the whites piled high around the yolks; older ones will not. To help shape those spheres perfectly and prevent streamers of white from forming, some cooks use poaching rings (which mold the eggs into neat rounds) or an egg poacher (which actually steams instead of poaching the eggs). But neither is really necessary if you follow this simple method.

Fill a shallow pan with just enough boiling water (or milk or broth) to cover the egg or the eggs. Break one egg, still cold from the refrigerator, into a saucer or small sauce dish; then place the edge of the dish at the side of a little whirlpool created by swirling the water with a wooden spoon, and gently slip the egg into it. Adding salt, vinegar, or lemon juice to hasten the setting of the whites, as many cookbooks suggest, is not necessary. In fact, acids and salt make the surface of the egg shrivel and pucker. Let the water return to a gentle simmer (boiling water leaves poached eggs with tough whites and a misshapen appearance). Either cover the pan and let the eggs stand until they are done, three to five minutes, or gently spoon the hot water over the eggs occasionally for two to three minutes.

When the eggs are done, use a slotted spoon to remove them from the water. They should have opaque, tender, jellylike whites and runny yolks covered by thin veils of white. Drain them and serve at once on toast points.

If you must delay serving, cool the eggs instantly in cold water. You can store poached eggs for up to 24 hours in refrigerated ice water. When ready to serve, immerse them in hot water for one minute.

For variety try poaching eggs in milk or Poultry Stock (page 110) instead of water. The eggs may be served on a bed of baked potatoes, cottage cheese, fresh pineapple rings, or pureed collards, pumpkin, or spinach. For added flavor top with Mornay Sauce (page 142), grated cheese, Sauce Béarnaise (page 144), toasted almonds, or tomato sauce, or garnish with snipped chives, dill, tarragon, or thyme.

Baked and Shirred Eggs

Baking is one of the easiest ways to prepare tender, tasty eggs. Even an inexperienced cook will have no trouble achieving first-class results by following these simple directions. Break eggs into lightly buttered individual ramekins, custard cups, or muffin tins. Cover each container with parchment paper and place the containers in a pan of hot water. Both of those steps help distribute heat evenly during cooking and ensure moist, tender eggs. To lock in moisture without covering the containers, top each egg with a dab of butter or a dollop of cheese sauce or cream. Bake the eggs at a moderate temperature (325°F) until the whites are a milky color and the yolks are soft but not runny, 5 to 15 minutes. Remove the still-soft eggs from the oven right away, since the containers will hold enough heat to continue the cooking for several seconds.

Shirred eggs are a cross between baked eggs and fried eggs, and they are also very easy to make. First, cook the eggs on top of the stove in a lightly buttered ovenproof dish until the whites just start to set; then, transfer the dish to the oven and bake for about five minutes.

If you use individual custard cups or ramekins for baking, you will have ready-made serving dishes; or you can use edible baking cups—hollowed baked potato shells, baked sweet potato shells, or tomato cups. Garnish the eggs with snipped chives, dill, tarragon, or another fresh herb, or top with broken nuts, grated cheese, Sauce Béarnaise (page 144), sautéed mushroom caps, tomato sauce, or yogurt. You may also want to try spooning the shirred eggs onto a bed of pureed peas or squash, sliced boiled herbed potatoes, sliced sautéed mushrooms or tomatoes, or cooked spinach.

Fried Eggs

The perfect fried egg—tender white, pliant yolk, greaseless—is within the grasp of every cook. The secret is a simple one: Replace most of the frying fat with water. Here is the method.

Lightly grease a heavy skillet with one-quarter to one-half teaspoon oil or butter—just enough to prevent the eggs from sticking. Warm over low heat until a few drops of water sprinkled in the pan bounce. Carefully break the eggs, one at a time, into a saucer or custard cup; then slide the egg into the skillet. As each egg is added to the pan, be certain to allow enough room between the eggs to keep them separate. (Otherwise, you will have to cut the whites apart when you turn the eggs or serve them.) Add one tablespoon of water to the pan for each egg. Cover with a tight-fitting lid and steam-fry the eggs until the whites are set and slightly thick and the yolks are covered by a thin veil of white, two to three minutes. While the eggs are cooking, you can baste them once or twice with the water if you like your eggs sunny-side up. If you prefer them "over easy," use a spatula to lift them carefully, so that the yolk will not be broken, and turn them over for the last few seconds of cooking.

For interesting variations try serving fried eggs on a bed of brown rice or bulgur, or on Buttermilk Biscuits (page 390) or Sourdough English Muffins (page 375). You can also season them with chives, grated cheese, lemon or lime juice, minced green pepper, wheat germ, or white pepper.

Scrambled Eggs

Mention scrambled eggs and most people think of breakfast, *only* breakfast. But add minced cheese, vegetables, or cooked meat to those light yellow, softly textured eggs, and you have a welcome main dish for a light lunch or supper.

Although most recipes call for adding water, cream, or milk, the only ingredient that is really necessary for scrambled eggs is eggs! If you like, you can add a tablespoon of liquid for each egg you are cooking (1½ to 2 eggs per person) but don't use more. Too much added liquid will turn tender, fluffy scrambled eggs into watery, lumpy ones.

The size of the pan and how evenly it distributes heat also influence volume and texture. If the pan is too large, the scrambled egg mixture spreads out too thin and cooks too quickly; in a pan that is too small, the mixture is too thick (more than an inch deep), and, inevitably, the bottom cooks too quickly. The 8-inch pan is ideal for cooking four scrambled eggs. But if you want extra-creamy, soft scrambled eggs, a double boiler is the perfect utensil. It solves the heat problem nicely, since the simmering water maintains an even temperature.

You can mix eggs in three different ways to get scrambled eggs just the way you like them. With a fork or wire whisk, blend them thoroughly if you like eggs that are solid, delicate yellow; blend only lightly if you prefer flecks of white and yellow; or beat whites separately if you want maximum lightness and volume. (Adding an extra white also helps.)

After blending the eggs and any optional liquid or seasonings, pour the mixture into a lightly buttered pan over low heat. As the eggs begin to set, stir only enough to keep them from sticking to the pan and to let the uncooked portion flow to the bottom. Too constant stirring makes dry, crumbly scrambled eggs. When they are puffy and hold their shape but are still moist and slightly undercooked, in two to three minutes, take them off the heat. The eggs will continue to cook for a few seconds after they are removed from the heat, so they will be done by the time you serve them. Add any desired vegetables, cheese, meat, or yogurt—usually one-third to one-half cup is a good amount for six to eight eggs—a minute before you take the eggs off the stove

Scrambled eggs chill rapidly, so pile them quickly, but gently, onto heated plates. Garnish with a sprig or two of parsley for an attractive color combination.

Plain Omelets

The classic plain omelet, very delicately browned on the outside and creamy yellow on the inside, is versatile enough to be served at any meal. With a little knowledge and some practice, you can have one ready to eat in just minutes.

A plain omelet has three basic ingredients—eggs, a liquid, and butter. Two or three eggs will make a small omelet that serves one person. Eggs allowed to warm to room temperature before cooking make an omelet with the best volume. Most recipes call for one tablespoon of water or milk for each egg used (fruit or vegetable juice can be substituted). Water makes a tender omelet; milk makes one that is firmer.

A simple way to enhance the flavor of the eggs in a plain omelet is to add a small amount —about one-quarter teaspoon—of an herb or spice. Chives, oregano, basil, tarragon, dillweed, parsley, marjoram, white pepper, and thyme, alone or in combination, complement eggs. Before cooking, blend herbs or spices with the eggs and the liquid. If you choose to add salt to your eggs

as they cook, you should know that it will toughen them.

The quality and type of pan you use has a lot to do with the success of your omelet. The pan should be heavy enough for even cooking, but light enough to manipulate easily. Omelet pans range from 6 to 10 inches in diameter and have 2-inch sloping sides. A 6- or 7-inch pan, which nicely cooks a two-egg omelet, is best for home use. Larger omelets, slightly more difficult to handle, require close monitoring or they will cook unevenly. Small ones cook so rapidly you can make another in a jiffy. Season the pan before using by pouring one inch of oil into it, then warming it over low heat for 20 minutes. Drain off the excess oil and wipe the pan dry. Then fill the pan with eggs—no more than one-quarter inch deep. After making an omelet, do not wash the pan; simply wipe it with a paper towel. If you do decide to wash it, reseason before cooking again.

Because the actual mixing and cooking of an omelet is quick, it is wise to assemble the ingredients before you break the eggs. You may also want to heat fillings (except cheese) before adding them. Use a light touch with a wire whisk or fork to beat the eggs and the liquid only until there are no visible lumps of white or yellow, 20 to 30 seconds. Overbeating makes a tough omelet. Add a pat of butter to the pan, and pour the mixture (no more than one-quarter inch deep) into the moderately hot pan when the butter stops foaming but before it starts to brown. (Omelets are an exception to the rule that says eggs should be cooked at a low temperature.) As the eggs cook, use a fork or a spatula to draw the edges of the eggs toward the center of the pan. At the same time, tilt the pan to let the uncooked portion flow underneath. Continue until the top of the omelet is moist but no longer runny, about 15 to 30 seconds. If you are adding a filling— one-third to one-half cup is plenty—spread it on half of the omelet. Remove the finished omelet from the heat and fold it in half as you slide it onto a warm plate.

Fluffy Omelets

To shape the framework for tender fluffy omelets, beat egg whites and yolks separately. Beat the yolks to a thick, yellow foam and the whites to airy peaks. After beating, immediately fold the yolks into the whites (see Folding Beaten Egg Whites, opposite). Now you must work swiftly. Delaying a minute or two before cooking gives the liquid time to seep from the mixture and collect on the bottom of the pan. Pour the mixture immediately into a hot ovenproof skillet in which butter is bubbly but not brown.

The two steps in cooking a fluffy omelet are simple. First you partially cook the omelet as you would a plain omelet. Then you bake it uncovered in a 350°F oven.

Switch the omelet to the oven when the bottom is set but the top is still moist, three to five minutes. After the omelet is in the oven for a few minutes and looks puffy, touch the surface lightly to see if it is done. If done, it will spring back; it will also look slightly dry on the surface.

As soon as you remove the omelet from the oven, fold it in half, slip it onto a warm plate, and serve at once.

Frittatas

In making a frittata, the famous Italian omelet, you mix the filling with the eggs and cook everything at once. For the filling use about one cup cooked, chopped vegetables, meat, poultry, or flaked fish to three eggs for three servings. Cook the frittata the way you would a plain omelet, but when the bottom is set, lightly brown the top by flipping the omelet over or by placing it under a hot broiler for one to two minutes. Serve the frittata unfolded on a warm plate.

Soufflés

Light, high, feathery, yet creamy—a soufflé is actually a version of the fluffy omelet made with a sauce that contains the egg yolks. It is baked in a deep dish that permits it to rise as its top bakes into a crusty dome. Like omelets, soufflés make elegant main courses or grand desserts.

Soufflés puff to impressive heights when air bubbles trapped in beaten egg whites expand during baking. The degree of expansion depends on the way you handle the egg whites and sauce and how you bake the soufflé. For maximum volume and lightness, use an extra egg white for every two whole eggs. Beat the whites until they form a thick, glossy foam with peaks that have slightly rounded tips. Be careful not to overbeat or your delicate foam is likely to disintegrate into small, dry curds. Immediately after beating, gently fold the sauce, thinned with a small portion of the beaten whites, into the whites. Do this quickly or the whites will deflate.

Folding Beaten Egg Whites

When the success of a recipe depends on keeping beaten egg whites light and airy, beaten egg yolks —and sauces or other ingredients—are folded into the whites. To fold: Carefully spoon yolks over the whites. With a spatula, gently spread the yolks; then lift the whites from the bottom and gently turn them over the yolks. Repeat until there are no streaks of white or yellow.

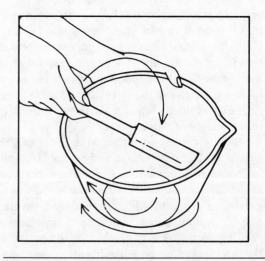

If you are making one of the elegant soufflé recipes that call for vegetables, fruits, meat, poultry, fish, or cheese, blend those foods with the sauce; then fold the mixture into the beaten whites. Cooked foods give better results than raw ones, because the moisture raw foods hold unbalances the liquid-to-eggs ratio. Also, use pureed or minced ingredients for a soufflé, since large pieces interfere with rising.

As soon as the sauce base is thoroughly folded into the beaten whites, gently pour the soufflé mixture into a prepared baking dish. For the classic high soufflé, use a standard porcelain soufflé dish that holds six cups or less. Huge soufflés (over six cups) tend to be overly dry and to collapse easily. If you need more, it is better to make two smaller ones. When the traditional appearance is of no concern, any deep, straight-sided baking dish will serve. Stay away from dishes with sloping sides unless you are prepared to deal with a soufflé that slumps.

Prepare the soufflé dish by buttering the bottom only, or by buttering the entire inside and then lightly sprinkling flour over it. (If you are making a cheese soufflé, sprinkle with grated Parmesan cheese as a tasty substitute for this flour.) The soufflé clings to the flour granules as it rises in the dish. After baking is done, the same granules keep the crust from sticking to the dish.

Will your soufflé wear a two-inch cap or a high hat? For a small cap, fill the dish almost to the top, level the mixture with a spatula, and make a groove around the edge with your thumb. For the impressive high hat, choose a soufflé dish that is one to two cups smaller than what the recipe calls for and tie a two- to three-inch collar around the top (see Procedure for Making a Soufflé Collar, page 636).

After filling the dish, rush the soufflé to a preheated oven. Center the soufflé on a rack six inches from the bottom of the oven and bake for 40 to 50 minutes. Do not open the oven to check on the soufflé's progress. A cool draft can cause instant collapse!

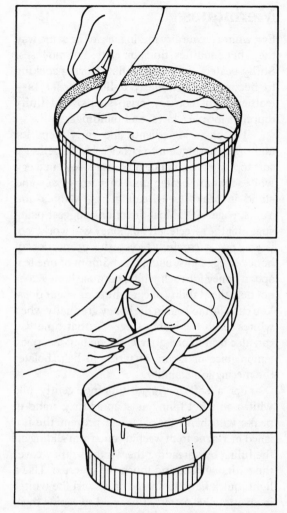

Most Americans like dry soufflés, considered done when a knife inserted in the center comes out clean. The European preference is for slightly underbaked, unstable soufflés, with the sauce still runny in the center.

When the soufflé is done as you like it, remove the parchment collar. Hurry your steaming soufflé to the table while it is still high, and divide it so that each serving has some of the crust. In an emergency you can hold a soufflé in the oven for up to 10 minutes after baking is done, but be sure to turn off the heat, and do not open the oven door.

Meringues

Egg whites create airy meringues in the same way they shape soufflés, fluffy omelets, and mousses. Stiffly beaten, the whites inflate during cooking to become exceptionally delicate desserts— featherweight cookies, crisp shells, and fluffy toppings for pies, tarts, and puddings.

The basic ingredients and early steps for making a meringue into either a hard shell or a soft topping are similar. Both use sweetened egg whites that are beaten until they are glossy and stand in peaks (see Beating Egg Whites and Yolks, page 419). Most directions suggest using sugar for the sweetener, but honey will work, too, if you use it carefully. Keep the proportion of honey to eggs low, using a maximum of one teaspoon honey for each white, because honey does not help the stability of egg whites as sugar does. You can start to beat in the honey gradually when whites reach the foamy stage. At that time you can also beat in one-quarter to one-half teaspoon lemon juice or cream of tartar to help bolster the meringue's stability.

For a soft meringue topping, gently pile whites on a hot filling as soon as they stand in peaks with bent tips. You can prevent the finished meringue from weeping and from sliding off the filling by spreading the whites so they cover the entire surface and touch the piecrust. Use a light, quick hand to spread and swirl the whites in an attractive pattern. But avoid sweeping them into sharp peaks, which may burn before the rest of the meringue browns. If you dip the spatula into cool water occasionally, the whites will not stick to the spatula as you spread them.

Bake a soft meringue in a preheated moderate oven (375°F) until the background is a pleasing light brown and the peaks are slightly darker. When your meringue cools, you will know if it was underbaked (it weeps), or overbaked (the surface is tough and hard to cut).

Serve soft meringues within an hour or two after baking. As more time lapses, the meringue becomes sticky and clings to the serving knife. To prevent tearing a tender, soft meringue, cut it with a buttered knife.

The appearance of a hard meringue depends on how tenderly you treat the whites. After beating them until they stand in stiff, pointed peaks, shape the whites on baking sheets lined with parchment paper to diffuse heat and prevent sticking. A spoon and a spatula or a pastry bag can be used to form three-inch shells or bite-size cookies. To keep the whites from deflating, work quickly and handle them as little as possible. While you are shaping the meringues, preheat the oven to a low temperature—225°F for soft, crunchy meringues or 275°F for chewy ones. The low temperature will dry the meringues without browning them. After 1½ hours of baking, turn off the oven and let the meringues cool slowly as they continue to dry for another hour or two. Remove them from the oven and let them finish cooling away from drafts.

Good meringues are easy to cut. They are never brittle, tough, or gummy. If yours are gummy, try using less honey, beating longer, or baking longer; if they are tough, bake them for a shorter time.

When the meringues are dry and cool, you can fill them with a colorful raspberry or blueberry sauce and serve right away. Store unused, unfilled meringues in tightly covered containers; otherwise, they will absorb moisture and disintegrate rapidly. Never freeze meringues, because they will turn into a gummy mess.

Custards (Soft and Baked)

Many of the most delightful dishes—pumpkin pies, coconut custard pies, quiches, Bavarian creams, éclairs, fruit sauces—are based on creamy, satiny custards. Either soft or baked, true custards gain their tender firmness from eggs that are slowly cooked with milk, a sweetener, and a flavoring. No starchy thickener is ever used.

You can use homogenized, nonfat dried, or evaporated milk to make successful, tasty custards, although those made with homogenized milk take longer to cook. If you scald the milk (not necessary when using pasteurized milk), the cooking time decreases. When using scalded milk, take care not to curdle your custard. Always cool the milk and temper the eggs.

Tempering Eggs

Tempering, often referred to as a liaison, prevents curdling when raw eggs are combined with hot liquids or sauces. Temper eggs by adding two to three tablespoons of the hot liquid, partially cooled, to beaten eggs. Mix. Then, add the egg mixture to the remaining liquid. Blend thoroughly.

Soft custards (stirred custards): These sauces have the consistency of thick, heavy cream and can curdle without warning if you cook them over high heat or too long. Although you can rescue a curdled custard by beating it vigorously and then straining, the taste of most "saved" custards is slightly inferior. To prevent curdling, use a double boiler over simmering water and stir constantly to distribute the heat evenly. Cook until the sauce forms a thick coating on a spoon. Add fruits after cooking is complete, since acids also curdle a cooking custard. When it is done, quickly cool the custard over cold water and continue stirring to release trapped steam—the cause of a watery custard.

Baked custards: Such custards are firm, yet tender—a wedge cut from a custard pie holds its shape—because they're cooked without stirring. Unlike soft custards they rarely curdle, but they often become weepy from too much heat. To avoid overcooking the outside before the center is set, place filled custard cups on a rack or a folded towel in a pan with an inch of hot water. When you think the custard is done, insert a knife halfway between the edge and the center of the custard. If the blade comes out clean, remove the custard from the oven and put it on a wire rack to cool. (There is so much heat in a custard that it will continue cooking; by the time it cools, the center will set.) If the center is firm when tested, cool the custard swiftly by setting the pan in an inch of cold water.

To unmold a baked custard, first let it cool for 10 to 15 minutes. Then run a knife around the inside edge of the mold. Hold an inverted dish over the mold, then turn both over, and lift away the mold.

Custard pies tend to suffer from soggy crusts, but you can keep yours crisp by cooling it as soon as it comes out of the oven. Place the pie on a wire rack or inverted colander to allow the air to circulate freely. You may also bake the shell and the filling separately. Later, when both are cool, simply ease the custard into the baked crust.

Store custards in the refrigerator. They are susceptible to spoilage in a warm room.

Timbales

Timbales comprise a variety of creamy entrées made from eggs—baked eggs covered with a sauce, creamy custards made with meats or vegetables, soufflés, and mousses. Timbales are steamed in individual ramekins or in large molds placed in a pan of hot but not boiling water in a 350°F oven, then unmolded, garnished with a tasty sauce, and served hot. A timbale can also be a filled pastry shell or a pastry fried with a timbale iron and filled with a sauce.

Hard-Cooked Eggs

Curried Eggs and Avocados

    3 tablespoons butter
    ¼ cup minced onions
    3 tablespoons whole wheat flour
    2 teaspoons curry powder, or to taste
    2 cups milk
  12 hard-cooked eggs, quartered
    2 avocados, cut into thick slices
      chopped fresh parsley

In a medium-size skillet or saucepan melt butter until bubbling but not brown. Add onions and sauté for about 5 minutes, or until tender and translucent but not brown.

    Add flour and curry powder and cook to a smooth paste, stirring constantly so mixture will blend but not brown. Add milk gradually and continue to stir until sauce is smooth and medium thick, about 8 minutes. Add eggs and avocados. Stir gently just until heated through.

    Serve over rice, bulgur, or whole wheat toast. Garnish with parsley.

    6 servings

Deviled Eggs

    8 hard-cooked eggs, cut in half lengthwise
    1 tablespoon prepared mustard
    3 tablespoons mayonnaise
      white pepper, to taste
      minced fresh parsley
      paprika

In a food processor or blender combine egg yolks, mustard, mayonnaise, and pepper. Process until smooth and creamy.

    Fill egg whites with mixture.

    Garnish 8 egg halves with parsley and remainder with paprika.

    4 servings

Egg and Sour Cream Casserole

This dish is primarily intended to be served hot, but it is also delicious cold.

    6 hard-cooked eggs, cut in half lengthwise
    2 tablespoons butter, softened
    1 tablespoon grated onions
    1 tablespoon chopped fresh parsley
    1 teaspoon prepared mustard
      dash of pepper
    ¾ cup sour cream
    ¼ cup whole grain bread crumbs
    1 tablespoon butter

Preheat oven to 350°F. Butter a shallow 8-inch-round ovenproof casserole.

    Remove egg yolks and mash them. Add softened butter, onions, parsley, mustard, and pepper. Mix well.

    Fill egg whites with yolk mixture and place cut-side down in prepared casserole. Spread sour cream over eggs, sprinkle with crumbs, dot with 1 tablespoon butter, and bake for 25 minutes.

    4 servings

Red Beet-Pickled Eggs

    1 teaspoon dry mustard
    1 teaspoon ground allspice
    1 teaspoon ground ginger
    2 tablespoons honey
    1 cup cider vinegar
    2 cups sliced cooked red beets
    4 hard-cooked eggs
      lettuce leaves

Mix together mustard, allspice, ginger, honey, and vinegar. Heat to boiling. Pour over beets and set aside to cool. When cool, add eggs and refrigerate overnight. Shake container occasionally so eggs will color evenly.

    To serve, cut eggs in half lengthwise and place on lettuce leaves with beet slices.

    4 servings

Eggs San Sebastián

Eggs in aspic always suggest a festive event, particularly when eggs are paired with flavorful and decorative vegetables, as in this recipe.

1 envelope unflavored gelatin
¼ cup cold water
2 cups boiling rich Poultry Stock (page 110)
2 tablespoons lemon juice
4 hard-cooked eggs, cut in half lengthwise
1½ cups diced cooked carrots
1½ cups diced cooked turnips
½ cup chopped fresh parsley
    lettuce leaves

Soak gelatin in cold water. Then dissolve it in boiling stock. Add lemon juice and chill.

When mixture begins to set, rinse a 6-cup ring mold in cold water and fill with a ¼-inch layer of aspic. Chill. When gelatin is set, arrange egg halves cut-side down on aspic. Cover with a ½-inch layer of aspic. Chill again.

Add carrots, turnips, and parsley to remaining jelly and spoon onto mixture in mold. Chill until completely set.

When ready to serve, unmold onto crisp lettuce leaves.

4 to 6 servings

Egg Balls

As a soup garnish, these add flavor and texture.

2 hard-cooked eggs
1 raw egg yolk
1 tablespoon whole grain bread crumbs

Rub hard-cooked eggs through a sieve. Add raw egg yolk. Mix into a paste, then shape into small balls and roll in bread crumbs.

Drop balls into very hot, but not boiling, soup and simmer, covered, for about 7 minutes.

Makes about 8

NOTE: For crisp-coated egg balls, sauté them in butter and drop into soup just before serving—before they lose their crispiness.

Pesto Deviled Eggs

The pungent flavor of basil brings an attractive zip to this buffet standby.

1 small clove garlic, minced
½ cup chopped fresh parsley
¼ cup grated Parmesan cheese
3 tablespoons coarsely chopped fresh basil or
    2 teaspoons dried basil
⅓ cup chopped walnuts
⅓ cup olive oil
8 hard-cooked eggs, cut in half lengthwise
    lettuce leaves

In a blender combine garlic, parsley, cheese, basil, nuts, and oil. Process until mixture becomes fine.

Cover each egg half with pesto and arrange on lettuce leaves.

4 servings

Soft-Cooked Eggs

Eggs Crécy

These eggs are served on a bed of carrot puree.

1 pound carrots
½ teaspoon dried basil
2 tablespoons grated cheddar cheese
4 soft-cooked eggs
2 tablespoons chopped fresh parsley
1 tablespoon chopped scallions

Cook carrots in enough water to cover. Drain, reserving liquid.

Place carrots in a blender and add enough reserved liquid to permit blending. Add basil and cheese. Process until smooth and thick. Transfer puree to a saucepan and warm.

Spoon puree onto a hot platter, place eggs evenly on surface, and garnish with parsley and scallions.

4 servings

Eggs Renaissance

8 soft-cooked eggs
8 globe artichoke bottoms, boiled and trimmed
1 cup tomato sauce, heated
¼ cup chopped fresh parsley

Place 1 egg in each artichoke bottom, cover with tomato sauce, top with parsley, and serve immediately.

4 servings

Eggs Stanley

Tasty tartlets of soft-cooked eggs resting on a bed of curried onions provide a memorable treat for guests who delight in unusual and sophisticated combinations.

pastry for 1 Basic Rolled Piecrust (page 718)
2 cups sliced onions
2 tablespoons butter
½ cup Poultry Stock (page 110)
1⅛ teaspoon curry powder
4 soft-cooked eggs
½ cup Béchamel Sauce (page 141)

Preheat oven to 450°F.

Divide pastry dough into 4 parts. Roll each section to a 6-inch circle. Position circles over cups of an overturned muffin tin and prick holes in dough with a fork. Bake for 8 to 10 minutes. Remove from oven and set aside to cool.

In a medium-size skillet sauté onions in butter for about 5 minutes. Add stock and 1 teaspoon curry powder and simmer for 5 minutes. Pour into a blender and process until smooth.

Spoon puree into shells and top each with 1 egg. Heat sauce with remaining ⅛ teaspoon curry powder and spoon over eggs.

4 servings

Poached Eggs

Eggs, Chantilly Style

Yogurt replaces the traditional heavy whipping cream as the sauce with peas and curry in this colorful dish of poached eggs over crepes. Ideal for breakfast, brunch, or luncheon.

8 poached eggs
4 Whole Wheat Crepes (page 395)

1½ cups cooked fresh peas
1 cup yogurt
¼ teaspoon curry powder

Arrange 2 poached eggs on top of each crepe. Mix peas with yogurt and curry powder and heat without boiling. Cover eggs with peas-yogurt mixture and serve immediately.

4 servings

Eggs Chanticleer

This is a captivating variation on Eggs Benedict, particularly for those who would like to avoid the saltiness and added calories of ham.

4 Sourdough English Muffins (page 375)
8 thin slices cooked chicken
8 poached eggs
1½ cups Hollandaise Sauce (page 143)

Split and toast muffins. Place a slice of chicken on each muffin half. Top with a poached egg and cover with sauce. Serve very hot.

4 servings

Eggs Parmentier

Scooped-out baked potato shells serve as the containers for eggs covered with grated cheese and placed under the broiler.

2 medium-size potatoes, baked
2 tablespoons butter, melted
½ cup grated cheddar cheese
4 poached eggs
2 to 3 tablespoons milk or rich Poultry Stock (page 110)

Cut potatoes in half crosswise and scoop out part of the center of each half, making a well large enough to hold an egg. Pour a little melted butter into each well and then sprinkle with half the cheese. Place 1 egg in each prepared well.

Mash potato pulp removed from each half, thinning with milk or stock until it can be piped or spooned around edge of potatoes.

Sprinkle remaining cheese over all and place in a hot oven or under the broiler until cheese is melted and brown. Serve immediately.

4 servings

Baked Eggs

Baked Chilies Rellenos

These green chilies stuffed with cheese and covered with a milk and egg mixture puff up firm and brown in the oven.

    1 can (7 ounces) green chilies
    2 cups grated sharp cheddar cheese
    2 eggs
    1 cup milk
    1 cup tomato sauce (optional)

Preheat oven to 350°F. Butter a 9 × 5-inch loaf pan.

Slit chilies lengthwise and open flat. Remove seeds, rinse chilies under hot water, and place in prepared pan. Measure 1½ cups cheese and divide evenly over chilies.

Beat eggs, then add milk. Pour egg mixture over chilies and sprinkle with remaining cheese. Bake for 35 to 40 minutes, or until puffed, firm, and brown.

Heat tomato sauce (if used) and pour over chilies.

    4 servings

Egg Baked in a Nest

    1 egg, separated
      grated sharp cheddar cheese
      dash of paprika
    1 slice whole grain toast, buttered

Preheat oven to 350°F. Butter 1 individual ramekin or baking dish.

Beat egg white until stiff but not dry. Place in prepared ramekin and very carefully press a dent in the top of the mound of egg white. Carefully slip egg yolk into dent and sprinkle with cheese and paprika. Bake until egg is set and cheese is melted.

Serve on toast.

    1 serving

Eggs Columbus

Eggs baked in whole sweet peppers make an engaging presentation for a Sunday brunch, and the garlic-flavored tomato sauce is an unusual note in an egg dish.

    4 green or sweet red peppers
    ½ teaspoon minced garlic

    1 cup tomato sauce
    4 eggs
    4 slices whole grain toast

Preheat oven to 350°F. Butter a small ovenproof casserole.

Plunge peppers into boiling water and simmer for 5 to 7 minutes. Drain and dry well. Cut off entire stem section and remove seeds and ribs.

Stand peppers upright in prepared pan. Add garlic to tomato sauce and spoon 2 tablespoons of mixture into each pepper. Break an egg into each, and bake for 12 to 15 minutes, or until eggs are set.

Put 1 pepper carefully on each slice of toast. Top eggs with remaining tomato sauce and serve immediately.

    4 servings

Eggs Lyonnaise

    2 cups chopped onions
    2 tablespoons butter
    ½ cup milk
    4 eggs
    ½ cup grated Swiss cheese

Preheat oven to 350°F. Butter an 8-inch-square baking dish.

In a medium-size skillet sauté onions in butter over medium heat until translucent. Add milk and cook, stirring constantly, to make a thin onion sauce. Spoon into prepared baking dish and break eggs over top, spacing evenly. Cover with cheese and bake for 12 to 15 minutes, or until nicely browned.

    4 servings

Swiss Eggs

    3 tablespoons butter
    6 eggs
    6 thin slices Swiss cheese
    ½ cup light cream or milk
      dash of ground nutmeg

Preheat oven to 350°F.

Melt butter in an ovenproof casserole, break eggs into it, and cover each one with a slice of cheese. Combine cream or milk with nutmeg and pour over cheese.

Bake until eggs are set and cheese is melted, about 12 minutes.

    4 servings

Eggs Provençale

> 1 tablespoon olive oil
> 4 medium-size tomatoes, chopped
> 1 clove garlic, minced
> 1 teaspoon chopped fresh parsley
> 6 eggs
> 2 tablespoons grated Parmesan cheese

Preheat oven to 350°F. Butter a medium-size oven-proof casserole.

Heat oil in a medium-size skillet. Add tomatoes, garlic, and parsley and cook slowly for 20 minutes.

Transfer tomato mixture to prepared casserole. Break one egg at a time into a small saucer. Slip each egg carefully from saucer onto tomato mixture, spacing evenly and allowing egg to rest on top of mixture.

Cover eggs, but not tomato mixture, with cheese and bake for 8 minutes, or until eggs are set and cheese is melted.

6 servings

Fried Eggs

Huevos Rancheros

This classic Mexican egg dish is a grand brunch feature that also works well as a low-cost main course for lunch or dinner.

> 3 tablespoons vegetable oil
> 4 Corn Tortillas (page 392)
> ½ cup chopped onions
> 2 cloves garlic, minced
> 1½ cups tomato sauce
> 1 can (4 ounces) green chilies, minced
> ½ teaspoon ground cumin
> 4 eggs
> ¾ cup shredded sharp cheddar cheese
>   Guacamole (page 80)

Heat oil in a medium-size skillet. Fry tortillas, one at a time, on both sides just until heated. Drain on paper towels and keep warm.

In the same skillet sauté onions and garlic. Add tomato sauce, chilies, and cumin. Heat to boiling, then reduce heat and simmer for 15 minutes.

Meanwhile, in a small skillet fry one egg at a time, sunny-side up. Place one egg on each tortilla, then on ovenproof serving plates. Top each egg with sauce, sprinkle with cheese, and place under broiler until cheese melts. Top with a dollop of Guacamole and serve.

4 servings

Scrambled Eggs

Basic Scrambled Eggs

> 1 tablespoon butter
> 3 eggs
> 3 tablespoons water, milk, or light cream
>   (optional)

Melt butter in a medium-size skillet over low heat.

Beat eggs lightly with water, milk, or cream (if used). Pour into skillet. Stir the mixture with a wooden spoon occasionally. Continue until entire mixture is softly set and moist. Remove from heat and serve immediately.

2 servings

Variations:

Cheese and Egg Scramble: Stir ¼ cup cottage cheese or diced cheddar cheese into beaten eggs.

Eggs with Fresh Herbs: Add 1 tablespoon minced fresh herbs (parsley, basil, tarragon, or thyme) to beaten eggs.

Scrambled Eggs with Seafood: Stir ¼ cup tuna or cooked shrimp into egg mixture a minute before eggs are done.

Vegetable-Egg Medley: Stir ¼ cup cooked vegetables (chopped onions, diced tomatoes, sliced mushrooms, sliced carrots, or peas) into egg mixture a minute before eggs are done.

Creamy Scrambled Eggs with Sweet Pepper

> 8 eggs
> ½ cup milk
> 1/3 cup chopped green peppers
> 1/3 cup chopped sweet red peppers
> ½ teaspoon soy sauce
> 1 tablespoon butter

In a medium-size bowl whisk eggs until foamy. Add milk, peppers, and soy sauce.

In a large skillet melt butter over medium heat. Add egg mixture and cook for 4 to 5 minutes, stirring occasionally.

4 servings

Eggs and Broccoli Scramble

1 tablespoon vegetable oil
¼ pound diced chicken livers
2 tablespoons chopped onions
2 cups chopped cooked broccoli
1 tablespoon sesame seeds
2 tablespoons chopped almonds
4 eggs, beaten

In a large heavy skillet heat oil. Add chicken livers and onions and sauté for 8 minutes. Add broccoli, sesame seeds, and almonds. Cook for 3 more minutes.

Add eggs and cook, stirring gently, until eggs are almost dry. Serve immediately.

4 servings

Mexican Scramble

A satisfying one-dish meal for the cook who is on a budget and in a hurry.

2 tablespoons butter
1 green pepper, diced
1 medium-size onion, diced
1/3 cup diced green chilies
4 medium-size tomatoes, diced
1 cup corn
8 eggs, beaten
8 slices Monterey Jack cheese

Heat butter in a large skillet. Add peppers, onions, chilies, tomatoes, and corn. Cook until vegetables are tender.

Add eggs and cook over medium heat, stirring occasionally, until eggs are set but not dry. Top with slices of cheese, cover, and let cook for 1 to 2 more minutes, or until cheese is melted.

4 servings

Omelet-Julienne Egg Salad

3 eggs
2 tablespoons milk
1 tablespoon chopped fresh parsley
1 tablespoon butter
¼ cup mayonnaise
½ cup yogurt
1 teaspoon French-style mustard
¼ teaspoon curry powder
6 cups salad greens, torn into bite-size pieces

Beat together eggs, milk, and parsley.

In a 10-inch skillet melt butter over medium heat. Pour in egg mixture and cook, without stirring, until eggs are set.

Remove from skillet and cut into ½-inch julienne strips and chill.

Combine mayonnaise, yogurt, mustard, and curry powder and chill.

Place greens in a salad bowl and toss with chilled dressing. Top with egg pieces and serve.

4 servings

French Toast

French Toast with Sesame Seeds

1 egg
¼ cup milk
1 tablespoon molasses
     butter or vegetable oil
2 tablespoons sesame seeds
2 tablespoons wheat germ
3 slices whole grain bread

In a shallow bowl beat together egg, milk, and molasses. In a large skillet heat butter or oil.

Combine sesame seeds and wheat germ on a plate. Dip bread slices in egg mixture, turning to coat both sides. Then dip in sesame seeds and wheat germ mixture, again coating both sides.

Place bread slices in skillet and cook on each side until golden brown. Serve with maple syrup and sour cream, yogurt, or applesauce.

Makes 3 slices

French Toast Parmesan

    3 eggs
    ½ cup milk
    ¼ cup grated Parmesan cheese
        butter or vegetable oil
    8 slices whole grain bread

In a shallow bowl beat together eggs, milk, and cheese. In a large skillet melt butter or oil over medium heat until bubbly.

Dip bread slices in egg mixture, turning to coat boat sides. Place bread slices in skillet and cook on each side until golden brown. Serve with sour cream or yogurt.

    Makes 8 slices

French Toast with Sliced Bananas

A quick and easy meal. Great for a festive breakfast or a light and satisfying supper.

    1 egg, beaten
    ½ cup milk
    ¼ teaspoon ground cinnamon
    ½ teaspoon vanilla extract
    2 tablespoons butter or vegetable oil
    8 slices whole grain bread
    ¼ cup sesame seeds
    2 ripe bananas

In a shallow bowl beat together egg, milk, cinnamon, and vanilla. In a large skillet heat butter or oil.

Dip bread slices one at a time into egg mixture, turning to coat both sides. Place in skillet immediately and sprinkle with sesame seeds. Continue with as many slices as the skillet will hold, turning once to brown the other side.

Slice the bananas over 4 pieces of toast. Cover each piece with another, making a sandwich. Serve hot with maple syrup and yogurt or applesauce.

    4 servings

Fruited French Toast

    1 can (15½ ounces) unsweetened pineapple
        slices
    3 eggs
        butter or vegetable oil
    8 slices whole grain bread

Drain pineapple and reserve juice.

In a shallow bowl beat eggs and then add ½ cup pineapple juice. In a large skillet melt butter or oil over medium heat until bubbly.

Dip bread slices into egg mixture, turning to coat both sides. Place bread slices in skillet and cook on each side until golden brown. Keep warm.

Heat pineapple slices in skillet and place 1 slice on top of each piece of toast. Serve with yogurt or sour cream.

    Makes 8 slices

Omelets

Basic Plain Omelet

    ½ tablespoon butter
    4 eggs
    3 tablespoons milk
        dash of white pepper

Heat butter in an omelet pan.

Beat eggs until fluffy; add milk and pepper. Pour egg mixture into pan. Cook quickly over medium heat. When underside is set, lift omelet slightly with a fork or a spatula to let uncooked portion flow underneath.

As soon as mixture is set, fold omelet in half and serve immediately. For a filled omelet spread any of the following fillings on ½ of the omelet before folding.

    2 servings

Variations:

    Avocado-Sprout Omelet: Spread ½ cup alfalfa or mung bean sprouts and ½ avocado, sliced, on ½ of the omelet before folding.

    Brunch Omelet with Poultry: Spread ¾ cup diced cooked chicken or turkey on ½ of the omelet before folding.

    Cheese Omelet: Spread ½ cup cottage cheese or grated Swiss, Muenster, or cheddar cheese on ½ of the omelet before folding.

    Chicken Liver Omelet: Spread ½ cup chopped cooked chicken livers on ½ of the omelet before folding.

    Fruit-filled Omelet: Spread ½ cup applesauce, pureed apricots, or pureed peaches on ½ of the omelet before folding.

Seafood Omelet: Spread ¾ cup flaked cooked flounder, salmon, tuna, or other firm-fleshed fish on ½ of the omelet before folding.

Vegetarian Omelet: Spread ½ cup sautéed mushrooms, chopped cooked broccoli, cooked asparagus, cooked sliced green beans, or cooked fresh peas (or any ½-cup combination of the preceding) on ½ of the omelet before folding.

Basic Fluffy Omelet

3 egg yolks
1 tablespoon water, milk, or light cream
1 teaspoon butter
4 egg whites

Preheat oven to 375°F.

Combine egg yolks and water, milk, or cream. Beat with a fork or small wire whisk until lightly blended. Set aside.

Place butter in an ovenproof omelet pan and melt over medium-high heat. With a wire whisk, beat egg whites until they are glossy and form soft peaks. Fold egg yolk mixture lightly into whites.

When butter is bubbly, gently pour egg mixture into pan. Cook until bottom is set but top is still moist, about 5 minutes. Transfer to oven. Bake until omelet is puffy and firm to the touch, about 11 minutes. Remove from oven and fold in half. Slide onto a warm plate and serve immediately.

2 servings

Cauliflower Omelet Mornay

1 cup cauliflower florets
2 tablespoons butter
¼ cup whole grain bread crumbs
2 tablespoons sesame seeds
4 eggs
¼ cup water
½ teaspoon soy sauce
1 teaspoon chopped fresh chervil or parsley
Mornay Sauce (page 142)

Steam cauliflower for about 7 minutes, or until slightly tender. Drain. Melt butter in a large skillet, add cauliflower, and sauté for 5 minutes. Add bread crumbs and sesame seeds and sauté for 3 minutes longer.

Beat eggs with water, soy sauce, and chervil or parsley. Pour over cauliflower mixture and cook, turning once to cook second side. Serve topped with sauce.

4 servings

Garden Omelet

1 tablespoon vegetable oil
¼ cup chopped scallions
½ cup shredded lettuce
1 cup cooked fresh peas
6 eggs
¼ cup cold water
½ teaspoon dried mint
2 teaspoons butter

In a small skillet heat oil and then sauté scallions. Add lettuce and peas and set aside.

Beat eggs until light and fluffy. Add water and mint, and mix well. Heat butter in an omelet pan until bubbly. Add eggs and cook until omelet is set. Spread filling over half the omelet. Fold other half over filling, and serve immediately.

4 to 6 servings

Potato-Cheese Omelet

3 tablespoons butter
¼ cup chopped onions
1 cup sliced cooked potatoes
6 eggs
¼ cup milk
1/3 cup diced green peppers
½ cup shredded cheddar cheese
¼ teaspoon dried thyme
dash of paprika
fresh parsley

Heat butter in a 10-inch cast-iron skillet. Add onions and potatoes. Cook and stir until potatoes are golden brown.

Beat eggs and then add milk. Stir in peppers, cheese, and thyme. Pour over potatoes and onion. Cook over low heat until omelet is set. Fold omelet and turn onto serving plate. Garnish with paprika and parsley.

4 servings

Frittatas

Basic Frittata

1½ tablespoons olive oil or butter
1 clove garlic, minced
6 eggs
2 cups grated cheddar cheese, sautéed chopped
    mushrooms, or diced cooked potatoes
    minced fresh basil, parsley, tarragon, or
    thyme (optional)

Heat oil or butter in a large skillet. Add garlic and sauté for 2 minutes.

Beat eggs lightly, add filling and herbs (if used), and pour all into skillet. Cook slowly until bottom is set. Turn over and cook other side, or place under the broiler for several minutes until top is lightly browned.

Cut into wedges and serve immediately.

3 servings

Creole Frittata

1½ tablespoons butter
1 tablespoon chopped onions
1 tablespoon diced pimientos
1 clove garlic, minced
½ cup chopped okra
1 tablespoon chopped fresh parsley
2 tablespoons chopped tomatoes
6 eggs, beaten
1 tablespoon vegetable oil

Melt butter in a large skillet. Add onions, pimientos, garlic, and okra and sauté for about 10 minutes, or until okra is tender. Add parsley and tomatoes and sauté for 1 minute longer. Place vegetable mixture in a large bowl and stir in eggs.

Wipe out pan, then add oil, and heat. Pour in vegetable-egg mixture and cook slowly until bottom is set. Turn and cook other side. Cut into wedges and serve immediately.

4 servings

Eggs Foo Yong
(Chinese Frittata)

6 eggs
¼ cup milk or water (optional)
¼ cup chopped onions
1½ cups mung bean sprouts
½ cup sliced mushrooms
2 teaspoons soy sauce
1 to 2 tablespoons vegetable oil

Beat eggs and milk or water (if used). Add onions, sprouts, mushrooms, and soy sauce and stir.

Heat about 1 teaspoon oil in a 6-inch skillet. Pour in ⅓ cup egg mixture and cook for about 3 minutes on each side, or until egg is set. Continue to cook mixture until used up, adding oil as needed. Serve hot with cooked brown rice.

4 to 6 servings

Oven-Baked Beef-Mushroom Frittata

½ pound lean ground beef
1 teaspoon butter
4 mushrooms, sliced
¼ cup sliced onions
1 pound spinach, chopped
6 eggs, beaten
½ cup milk
1 cup shredded mozzarella cheese (4 ounces)
¼ teaspoon dried oregano or basil

Preheat oven to 350°F. Generously butter a 13 × 9-inch baking dish.

Crumble beef into a large skillet and sauté over medium heat, stirring occasionally, until slightly browned. Transfer to a medium-size bowl.

Wipe out skillet. Add butter and melt over medium heat. Add mushrooms and onions and sauté until onions are soft but not brown. Add spinach and continue to cook until spinach is wilted. Turn into bowl containing beef.

Combine eggs, milk, cheese, oregano or basil, and then add to beef-spinach mixture. Turn into prepared dish and bake until a knife inserted in center comes out clean, about 35 minutes.

4 to 6 servings

Spinach Frittata

    3 tablespoons olive oil
    ¼ cup chopped onions
    1 clove garlic, minced
    1 pound spinach, chopped
    ¼ cup wheat germ
    ½ teaspoon dried basil
    ¼ teaspoon dried oregano
    1 cup grated Parmesan cheese
    6 eggs, beaten

In a large skillet heat 1 tablespoon oil over medium heat. Add onions and garlic and sauté for 5 minutes. Add spinach and stir until wilted. Remove from pan and keep warm.

Combine wheat germ, basil, oregano, cheese, and eggs.

In same skillet heat remaining oil over medium heat. Add spinach mixture to egg mixture and pour into skillet. Reduce heat and cook until top of frittata is set.

Turn out onto a warm plate, cut into wedges, and top with warmed Duxelles Velouté (page 142) or Mornay Sauce (page 142).

4 to 6 servings

Zippy Zucchini Frittata

    1½ tablespoons olive oil
    3 to 4 medium-size zucchini, cut into ¼-inch slices
    3 tablespoons chopped sweet red peppers, or 1
        teaspoon chopped hot peppers
    4 scallions, sliced
    1 clove garlic, minced
    1 tablespoon chopped fresh sage or 1 teaspoon
        ground sage

    2 tablespoons butter
    4 eggs, beaten
    1½ cups shredded provolone cheese

In a 10-inch cast-iron skillet heat oil and add zucchini, peppers, scallions, garlic, and sage. Sauté, stirring occasionally, until zucchini is slightly browned.

Add butter. When foamy, pour in eggs, reduce heat to medium, and cook until bottom is set. Slip pan under broiler and cook until top is puffed and golden.

Sprinkle with cheese and broil again to melt cheese, or cover pan, turn off heat, and let cheese melt. Cut into wedges and serve.

4 servings

Zucchini Parmesan Frittata

    1 cup diced zucchini
    2 tablespoons whole grain bread crumbs
    3 tablespoons milk
    ¼ cup grated Parmesan cheese
    ¼ teaspoon grated lemon rind
    1 tablespoon chopped fresh parsley
    1 teaspoon chopped fresh chives
    ½ teaspoon soy sauce
    4 eggs
    1 tablespoon butter

Steam zucchini for 3 to 4 minutes, or until slightly tender. Set aside.

In a large bowl soak bread crumbs in milk for 5 minutes. Add zucchini, cheese, lemon rind, parsley, chives, and soy sauce.

In another bowl beat eggs until just blended and then add to zucchini mixture.

Melt butter in a 10-inch cast-iron skillet over medium heat. Pour in egg-zucchini mixture and cook for 3 to 5 minutes, or until dry and brown on top. Slice into wedges and serve immediately.

4 servings

Soufflés

Basic Soufflé

3 tablespoons butter
3 tablespoons whole wheat flour
1 cup milk, or ½ cup Poultry Stock (page 110)
    plus ½ cup milk
4 eggs, separated, at room temperature

Preheat oven to 350°F. Butter bottom and sides of a 1- or 1½-quart soufflé dish and dust with flour.

Melt butter in a small saucepan. Add flour and mix quickly and thoroughly. Continue stirring and gradually add milk or stock and milk, cooking over low heat. Stir constantly until sauce is thick and smooth, about 20 minutes. Remove from heat.

Beat egg whites until stiff but not dry. Set aside.

Beat egg yolks until light. Add 3 tablespoons white sauce to yolks; then stir egg yolk mixture into rest of white sauce.

Gently and thoroughly fold egg whites into white sauce mixture. Pour soufflé mixture into prepared soufflé dish and bake until firm, puffed, and brown, about 35 minutes. Serve immediately.

4 to 6 servings

Variations:

Fall-Garden Soufflé: Add 1⅓ cups pureed cooked broccoli, carrots, cauliflower, pumpkin, sweet potatoes, or butternut squash to sauce before folding in beaten egg whites.

Soufflé aux Fines Herbes: Add 1 tablespoon chopped fresh herbs (parsley, basil, tarragon, thyme, and chives) to sauce before folding in beaten egg whites.

Soufflé Lyonnaise: Add 1 tablespoon finely chopped onions to sauce before folding in beaten egg whites.

Cheese and Scallion Soufflé

6 tablespoons grated Parmesan cheese
5 eggs, separated
1 cup ricotta or cottage cheese
¼ cup plus 2 tablespoons whole wheat flour
⅔ cup finely chopped scallions
    dash of cayenne pepper
1 tablespoon French-style mustard

Preheat oven to 350°F. Butter bottom and sides of a 1½-quart soufflé dish and sprinkle with 3 tablespoons Parmesan cheese.

Beat egg yolks until thick. Add ricotta or cottage cheese, flour, scallions, cayenne, and mustard. Beat egg whites until stiff and fold into egg yolk mixture. Pour into prepared soufflé dish, sprinkle with remaining 3 tablespoons Parmesan cheese, and bake for 45 minutes, or until set. Serve immediately.

4 servings

Cheese-Mustard Soufflé

3½ tablespoons butter
¼ cup whole wheat flour
1½ cups hot milk
6 eggs, separated
1½ teaspoons French-style mustard
    dash of cayenne pepper
    dash of ground nutmeg
1½ cups grated cheddar or Swiss cheese

Preheat oven to 325°F. Butter bottom and sides of a 2-quart soufflé dish and dust with flour.

Melt butter in a medium-size saucepan over medium heat. Add flour and blend until smooth. Then add hot milk and stir briskly until smooth. Bring almost to a boil, remove from heat, and cool slightly.

In a mixing bowl beat egg yolks vigorously. Add mustard, cayenne, and nutmeg, and then stir into sauce. Beat egg whites and fold into mixture alternately with cheese. When mixture is smooth and light, pour into prepared soufflé dish and bake for 50 to 55 minutes, or until set. Serve immediately.

4 to 6 servings

Corn Soufflé

1 tablespoon butter
2 tablespoons whole wheat flour
1 cup milk
2 cups corn
½ teaspoon ground celery seeds
2 egg yolks, beaten
2 egg whites

Preheat oven to 325°F. Butter bottom and sides of an 8-inch soufflé dish and dust with flour.

Melt butter in a small saucepan, add flour, and mix until smooth. Pour in milk gradually. Bring almost to a boil, stirring constantly. Remove from heat. Stir in corn, celery seeds, and egg yolks. Beat egg whites until stiff, then fold into sauce mixture. Pour into prepared soufflé dish and bake for 30 minutes. Serve immediately.

4 servings

Crown Soufflé

¼ cup butter
¼ cup whole wheat flour
¾ cup milk
¼ cup lemon juice
⅛ teaspoon pepper
   dash of ground nutmeg
3 egg yolks
6 egg whites
1 cup grated Port du Salut cheese (4 ounces)

Preheat oven to 350°F. Butter bottom and sides of a 2-quart soufflé dish and dust with flour.

Melt butter in a small saucepan, add flour, and mix until smooth. Gradually stir in milk, lemon juice, pepper, and nutmeg. Cook over low heat, stirring constantly, until sauce thickens, about 15 minutes. Cool slightly and beat in egg yolks. Beat egg whites until stiff. Fold in ¼ of egg whites. Add cheese and remaining egg whites and fold gently into sauce mixture. Pour into prepared soufflé dish. Set dish in a pan containing hot water 1 inch deep. Run tip of a spoon in a circle on outer top edge of soufflé. This will make top rise to a crown effect.

Bake for 1¼ hours, or until puffed and golden brown. Serve immediately.

6 servings

Roquefort or Blue Cheese Soufflé

6 eggs
½ cup milk or light cream
1 teaspoon soy sauce
   dash of cayenne pepper
½ pound Roquefort or blue cheese
11 ounces cream cheese

Preheat oven to 375°F. Butter bottom and sides of a 1½-quart soufflé dish and dust with flour.

In a blender combine eggs, milk or cream, soy sauce, and cayenne. Process until smooth. With blender running, add small pieces of the Roquefort or blue cheese, and then gradually add chunks of cream cheese. After all the cheese has been incorporated, blend at high speed for another 5 seconds.

Pour mixture into prepared soufflé dish and bake for 40 to 45 minutes. Serve immediately.

4 servings

Springtime Soufflé

⅓ cup whole grain bread crumbs
4 tablespoons butter
2 tablespoons chopped shallots
1 pound fresh spinach, chopped
3 ounces cream cheese
   dash of ground nutmeg
2 tablespoons whole wheat flour
1 cup milk
4 eggs, separated
½ cup grated Swiss cheese (4 ounces)
¼ cup plus 2 tablespoons grated Parmesan cheese
6 hard-cooked eggs, cut in half lengthwise

Preheat oven to 375°F. Butter bottom and sides of a 2-quart soufflé dish and dust with bread crumbs.

Melt 2 tablespoons butter in a saucepan. Add shallots and sauté for 2 minutes. Add spinach and cook just until wilted and heated through. Melt in cream cheese and add nutmeg. Set aside.

In a clean saucepan melt 2 tablespoons butter. Add flour and cook until foamy. Whisk in milk and cook slowly, stirring constantly, until thickened. Remove from heat. Beat egg yolks lightly and slowly blend into sauce. Return to moderate heat and cook slowly until thickened, about 15 minutes. Do not let mixture get too hot or it will curdle. Remove from heat again, stir vigorously until slightly cooled, and then add Swiss cheese and ¼ cup Parmesan cheese. Set aside to cool to just above room temperature.

Pack spinach mixture into prepared dish. Arrange hard-cooked eggs around outside with yolk pressed against sides of dish. Beat egg whites until stiff but not dry and fold into cheese sauce. Pour over eggs and spinach in dish. Sprinkle with remaining Parmesan and bake for 30 to 45 minutes. Serve immediately.

4 to 6 servings

Vegetable Soufflé

½ pound mushrooms, sliced
2 tablespoons butter
4 medium-size carrots, diced
1 cup fresh peas
⅓ cup butter, softened
5 eggs, separated
½ cup sour cream
¼ cup whole wheat flour
¼ teaspoon pepper
¼ teaspoon ground nutmeg
½ cup grated Parmesan cheese

Preheat oven to 350°F. Butter bottom and sides of a 7 × 11-inch baking dish and dust with flour.

Sauté mushrooms in 2 tablespoons butter for about 5 minutes. Set aside.

Steam carrots and peas until carrots are just tender. Drain and add to mushrooms.

Beat softened butter until creamy, then beat in egg yolks, sour cream, flour, pepper, nutmeg, and 2 tablespoons cheese.

In a large bowl beat egg whites until stiff. Fold into egg yolk mixture.

Spread ½ of the egg mixture in prepared baking dish and cover with ½ of the vegetable filling and 2 tablespoons of the cheese. Spread with remaining egg mixture. Spoon remaining filling in a strip down the center lengthwise. Sprinkle remaining cheese on top.

Bake for 30 to 35 minutes, or until golden brown. Serve immediately.

4 to 6 servings

Meringues

Soft Meringue Topping

3 egg whites
½ teaspoon cream of tartar
1 teaspoon honey, warmed
1 teaspoon lemon juice or vanilla extract

Beat egg whites until foamy. Add cream of tartar and beat until texture is smooth. Add honey, a drop at a time, beating constantly. Add lemon juice or vanilla and continue beating for 5 to 10 minutes, or until whites are very smooth and shiny and stand in soft peaks.

Makes topping for one 9-inch pie or six 3-inch meringues

Variations:
■ For soft meringue pie topping: Spread meringue over entire surface of a warm pie filling so that it forms a seal with the crust. Bake at 375°F until lightly browned, about 12 to 15 minutes. Cool. Serve within 2 hours.
■ For individual toppings for custards, puddings, or gelatins: Fill cups of a muffin tin half full with hot water. Gently heap meringue on top of water and bake at 325°F for 10 to 12 minutes. Carefully lift meringues from water with a spatula and place on top of desserts.
■ For meringue shells: On a baking sheet lined with parchment paper, form meringue into 3-inch circles. Use back of a spoon to make a well in center of each. Place sheet in preheated 250°F oven for about 45 minutes. Turn off oven and allow meringues to cool for an hour. Remove from oven and finish cooling.

Custards

Basic Baked Custard or Cup Custard

3 eggs
¼ cup honey, warmed
2 cups milk
1 teaspoon vanilla extract
dash of ground nutmeg (optional)

Preheat oven to 300°F.

In a medium-size bowl beat eggs lightly. Then stir in honey and gradually add milk and vanilla.

Butter a large mold or 6 small individual custard cups.

Pour mixture into mold or cups, top with nutmeg (if used), and set on a wire rack in a larger pan. Pour boiling water around mold or cups and place in oven. Bake for 40 to 60 minutes for large mold, 25 minutes for individual cups, or until a knife inserted halfway between edge and center of custard comes out clean. Remove custard from water bath, allow to cool, and unmold. Serve immediately or chill first.

4 to 6 servings

High-Protein Custard

The dry milk increases nutrition in this dish without adding fats. A good get-well idea for a child who is on the mend.

3 cups milk
¾ cup nonfat dry milk
3 eggs
3 tablespoons honey, warmed
½ teaspoon vanilla extract
 dash of ground nutmeg

Preheat oven to 350°F.

In a saucepan combine milk and dry milk. Place over medium heat and bring to a boil, stirring constantly to dissolve dry milk.

In a small bowl beat eggs lightly. Add honey and vanilla and then stir into heated milk very slowly. Pour into custard cups, sprinkle with nutmeg, and place in a shallow pan of hot water. Bake for 40 minutes.

4 to 6 servings

Variation:

Coconut Custard: Omit nutmeg and add ⅓ cup unsweetened shredded coconut to hot mixture before pouring into cups.

Double-Boiler Custard

1½ cups milk
2 tablespoons butter
6 eggs
1 teaspoon soy sauce
 dash of cayenne pepper
2 tablespoons chopped parsley

Heat milk and butter in top of a double boiler.

Meanwhile, in a medium-size bowl beat eggs until very light. Add soy sauce and cayenne.

Pour hot milk slowly into egg mixture and beat thoroughly. Return hot mixture to double boiler, cover, and cook over simmering water for 30 minutes.

Serve hot with Duxelles Velouté (page 142), Mornay Sauce (page 142), or Velouté Sauce (page 142). Garnish with chopped parsley.

4 to 6 servings

Soft Custard

3 or 4 egg yolks or 2 whole eggs
¼ cup honey, warmed
2 cups milk
1 teaspoon vanilla extract
1 teaspoon grated lemon rind

Beat eggs lightly, add honey, and place in top of a double boiler.

Scald milk and cool slightly.

Temper eggs (see page 427 for tempering directions) and gradually add milk. Place over hot (not boiling) water and stir constantly until thick and smooth, about 7 minutes. Remove from heat and cool.

Add vanilla and lemon rind, then chill thoroughly.

Yields 2½ cups

Spinach Custard

1 pound spinach, coarsely chopped
3 tablespoons chopped onions
1 cup yogurt
 dash of nutmeg
 dash of cayenne pepper
3 eggs, beaten
2 tablespoons butter

Preheat oven to 350°F.
Butter an 8-inch-round baking dish.
Combine spinach with onions, yogurt, nutmeg, and cayenne. Fold eggs into spinach mixture. Spoon into prepared baking dish, dot with butter, and bake for 40 to 45 minutes.

4 servings

Quiches

Cheese-Mushroom Quiche

    pastry for 1 Basic Rolled Piecrust (page 718)
3 eggs
1 teaspoon chopped chives
2 cups milk or light cream, scalded
1 egg white, lightly beaten
½ cup grated Parmesan cheese
½ cup sautéed sliced mushrooms

Preheat oven to 375°F.

Roll out pastry and line a 9-inch pie plate.

Beat eggs with chives and then add to milk or cream. Brush egg white over piecrust. Sprinkle Parmesan cheese over bottom of piecrust and then add a layer of mushrooms.

Gently pour egg mixture over cheese and mushrooms. Bake for 35 to 40 minutes, or until top is golden brown.

    6 servings

Variations:

Chicken-Swiss Cheese Quiche: Substitute ¼ pound slivered cooked chicken and ½ cup diced Swiss cheese for Parmesan and mushrooms.

Green Vegetable Quiche: Substitute 1 cup lightly steamed chopped spinach, kale, or Swiss chard and 1 teaspoon grated onions for mushrooms.

Onion-Cheddar Quiche: Substitute 1 cup sautéed sliced onions and 1 cup grated cheddar cheese for Parmesan and mushrooms.

Onion Quiche

    Crust
1 cup whole wheat flour
1 cup cornmeal
¾ cup butter
2 or 3 drops lemon juice
1 to 3 tablespoons ice water

    Filling
½ cup chopped scallions
1 tablespoon butter
6 to 8 ounces Gruyère cheese, cubed

3 eggs, beaten
1½ cups light cream
¼ teaspoon ground nutmeg

To make the crust: Combine flour and cornmeal. Cut butter into flour mixture with a pastry blender or 2 knives until mixture resembles coarse crumbs. Add lemon juice and water and mix until dough can be formed into a ball. Chill before rolling.

Preheat oven to 450°F.

Roll out piecrust between 2 pieces of lightly floured wax paper and fit crust into a 9-inch pie plate. Prick with a fork and bake for 5 minutes.

To make the filling: Sauté scallions in butter in a small skillet. Then sprinkle scallions and cheese over bottom of crust.

Mix together eggs, cream, and nutmeg, pour over scallions and cheese, and bake for 15 minutes. Reduce oven temperature to 350°F and bake for 10 to 15 minutes longer.

    6 servings

Swiss Flan

    Pastry
2 cups whole wheat pastry flour
½ cup butter, cut into small cubes
2 egg yolks
1 tablespoon honey
1 teaspoon finely grated lemon rind
2 teaspoons ice water

    Filling
2 cups grated Emmenthal or Swiss cheese
4 eggs
2 tablespoons butter
    dash of ground nutmeg
2 cups milk or light cream

To make the pastry: Sift flour into a medium-size bowl. Make a well in the center. Place butter, egg yolks, honey, and lemon rind in well. With a wooden spoon mix ingredients together. Add water and work into mixture until dough is smooth. Form into a ball, dust with flour, cover with a cloth, and allow to stand for 40 minutes.

Preheat oven to 350°F. Butter and flour a 9-inch flan ring or pie plate. Roll dough very thin and press into ring.

To make the filling: Spread cheese evenly over dough.

In a bowl beat eggs until light. Add butter, nutmeg, and milk or cream. Pour over cheese in piecrust and bake for 20 to 25 minutes, or until custard is set and lightly browned.

6 servings

Tuna-Yogurt Quiche

1 cup yogurt
3 eggs
¾ pound sliced mushrooms, sautéed and drained
1 baked Basic Rolled Piecrust (page 718)
1 can (6½ ounces) water-packed tuna, flaked
1 tablespoon lemon juice
2 tablespoons grated Parmesan cheese

Preheat oven to 375°F.
Combine yogurt and eggs and beat well.
Place mushrooms in bottom of piecrust. Top with tuna and sprinkle with lemon juice.

Pour yogurt mixture over ingredients in shell, sprinkle with cheese, and bake for 25 to 30 minutes, or until puffed and set. Cool slightly before serving.

6 servings

Timbales

Basic Egg Timbale

1½ cups light cream, warmed
4 eggs, beaten
½ teaspoon paprika (optional)
1 tablespoon minced fresh parsley

Preheat oven to 325°F. Lightly butter a 1½-quart mold or 4 individual molds.

Combine all ingredients and mix well. Fill molds ⅔ full of mixture and place on a rack in a large pan of water. The water should be at least 1 inch in depth.

Cover all with a loose-fitting lid or a piece of parchment paper. Bake the timbales for 20 to 45 minutes, or until a knife inserted in center comes out clean.

4 servings

Variations:

Green Confetti Timbale: Add 2 cups chopped stir-fried celery or green peppers to egg mixture, mix well, and bake as above.

Light Vegetarian Timbale: Add 2 cups chopped steamed asparagus, broccoli, cauliflower, or spinach to egg mixture, mix well, and bake as above.

Luncheon Timbale with Meat or Poultry: Add 2 cups chopped cooked meat or poultry to egg mixture, mix well, and bake as above.

Mushroom–Onion Timbale: Add 2 cups sliced stir-fried mushrooms or onions to egg mixture, mix well, and bake as above.

Timbale à la Neptune: Add 2 cups flaked cooked firm-fleshed fish to egg mixture, mix well, and bake as above.

Cheese Timbale with Green Peas

4 eggs
1 cup Beef Stock (page 110)
⅓ cup shredded sharp cheddar cheese
2 ounces garlic Monterey Jack cheese, cut into ¼-inch cubes
1 cup cooked fresh peas
dash of ground nutmeg
1 cup tomato sauce

Preheat oven to 350°F. Butter 6 custard cups or timbale molds.

With a wire whisk, beat eggs and then add broth and cheddar cheese. Stir in cheese cubes, peas, and nutmeg. Spoon into custard cups or molds, set cups in a pan of hot water, place pan in oven, and bake for 25 to 30 minutes.

While timbales are baking, heat tomato sauce. Unmold baked timbales onto a hot serving platter, cover with tomato sauce, and serve immediately.

6 servings

Dairy Foods

Among foods, milk has a unique distinction. In itself it can provide the entire diet for young mammals. Naturally, the composition of each animal's milk is especially suited to the best nourishment of its species, but all the milks are interchangeable as a satisfying food or beverage. Cow's milk and its products—creams, yogurts, cheeses—are the most popular dairy foods in the United States, with goat's milk foods ranking second.

Milk lends its distinctive flavor and pleasing, smooth texture to a range wide enough to include hot carob drinks that warm body and soul on chilly mornings and ice cream desserts that take the heat out of a hot summer's night. The tastes of milk products run the gamut from tangy fermented yogurts and kefirs to rich, sweet cream fillings for pastries.

Milk

An excellent buy in terms of nutrition, milk is just about the most concentrated food source of calcium known. It is also an excellent source of vitamin A, riboflavin, thiamine, and protein. Many people allergic to the lactose in milk can still take advantage of milk's nutrients by using one of the cultured milks in which the lactose is tamed into lactic acid.

Cooking with Milk

Milk is exceptionally sensitive to heat. When warmed, it coats the bottom of the pan with a type of gel that can easily scorch and leave milk with a light brownish color and unpleasant, burnt taste. You can avoid scorching milk by heating it over a very low setting for a short time. Better yet, heat milk in a double boiler or in a heavy-bottom saucepan.

Even the most carefully warmed milk usually evaporates a little to form a "skin" on the top. Frequent stirring or whisking helps prevent its appearance on delicate white sauces, thick cream soups, and creamy puddings. (Constant stirring keeps those mixtures from lumping, too.) Cover puddings and cream pies with wax paper as they cool to eliminate this skin that spoils the appearance and texture of silky, rich, chilled desserts.

Curdling often occurs in casseroles and soups made with milk. To avoid this, use a low temperature and wait to blend tomatoes, lemon juice, or other acid foods with hot or cold milk until just before serving. Slowly add the acid foods to the milk, rather than the reverse order. You will find that evaporated milk, which is thick and rich, is more stable than homogenized milk when heated and mixed with vegetables and fruits. Salted, cured foods such as ham added to scalloped potatoes often cause curdling. Though cured foods are best avoided, add shortly before cooking is done, if used.

Scalding Milk

When using pasteurized milk, scalding to destroy bacteria is unnecessary. Some recipes, however, call for scalding to improve texture or hasten fermentation.

To scald milk, first rinse a saucepan with

cold water to lessen sticking; then, heat the milk over very low direct heat, or in the top of a double boiler, until tiny bubbles form around the edge of the pan and the milk reaches 180°F. Do not let the milk boil up. Cool the milk slightly before adding it to other ingredients.

Reconstituting Dry Whole or Nonfat Milk

Dry milk works well, either reconstituted or used in powdered form, to enrich white sauces, breakfast cereals, and cakes, breads, biscuits, and muffins. Follow the package directions or use three to four tablespoons of powder to one cup of water to reconstitute. Mix together at least two hours before using and refrigerate for full flavor. If you are substituting reconstituted nonfat milk for fresh whole milk and want to retain richness in sauces and puddings, add two teaspoons of butter for each cup of reconstituted milk used. In breads and other baked goods, reconstituted milk works fine without the added butter.

For enriching sauces, use no more than three tablespoons of milk solids to each cup of liquid. To avoid lumping, mix the milk solids with the flour; gradually pour in the warm liquid. To cereals, add three tablespoons of solids to each one-half cup of dry, whole grains. Then cook the cereal with the usual amount of fluid milk or water.

You can boost the quality of protein in baked goods by adding nonfat dry milk solids along with the flour. For each cup of flour used, substitute up to one-quarter cup of flour with dry milk. Bran muffins, whole wheat breads, and carrot cakes made with added dry milk have nicely browned crusts.

Pasteurizing Milk

Pasteurization is a safeguard against harmful milk-borne bacteria and diseases. If you have access to raw milk and want to pasteurize it yourself, here is a recommended method.

Place sterile, heatproof glass jars in a large kettle. Fill the jars with fresh milk to two inches from the top. Then pour water into the kettle until it reaches the fill-line of the milk. Heat the kettle until the milk reaches 145°F and hold that temperature for 30 minutes. Remove the jars and place them in chilly water to cool the milk rapidly to 40°F; then refrigerate.

Storing Milk

Store milk in the refrigerator. Do not freeze milk unless necessary—it may separate and develop an off-flavor. Store milk in opaque containers to protect it from bright light, which causes a loss of riboflavin, ascorbic acid, and vitamin B_6. Keeping the containers tightly closed will prevent absorption of flavors from other foods in the refrigerator.

Always return milk to the refrigerator immediately after pouring. Exposure to temperatures above 40°F for even a few minutes quickly reduces milk's shelf life. Never return a small portion of unused milk to the original container. Store it separately. (For more information see Storing Dairy Products table, page 449.)

Whipping Cream

Properly whipped, heavy cream forms glistening, soft mounds as it doubles in volume. A dollop of whipped cream mellows the tartness of fresh fruit. Folded gently with gelatin, it makes airy, rich Bavarian creams and lush mousses. For maximum fluffiness and velvety smoothness, cream should be a day old and chilled for at least two hours before whipping.

Use a bowl of appropriate size; one that is neither too large nor too small. One that will, at most, be half full with cream is just right—a glass, quart-size measuring cup works well too. The cream needs room to expand, but too much space results in prolonged whipping and poor volume. Whip large quantities (more than one-half quart) in two or more batches.

Chill the bowl and beaters for two hours before whipping as an aid to achieving good volume. Another trick: Just before whipping, rinse the bowl with cold water and dry it. On hot summer days place the bowl over ice to keep the cream cool. When the temperature rises above 45°F, the butterfat in cream tends to become oily, and it readily separates into butter and buttermilk.

Though whipping must be vigorous and rapid, a blender is not well-suited to the job, since it does not incorporate much air into the cream. A hand rotary beater or an electric mixer performs best. If you use the electric mixer, watch the process carefully—it is easy to overdo and create butter instead of the intended fluff. Stop beating the instant the cream forms soft peaks.

A good foam glistens and appears uniformly smooth. One that looks granular and watery is overwhipped and is about to become butter.

If your cream threatens to turn into butter, beat in two or more additional tablespoons of cream. Continue to whip. The resulting foam will be smooth but stiff.

For a tasty change, flavorings can be added to whipped cream. Small amounts of honey, vanilla, lemon juice and rind, orange juice and rind, and purees of other fresh fruits are exceptionally delightful. Add flavorings near the end of the whipping; otherwise, they will raise the temperature of the cream and interfere with whipping.

Making Butter

For those special occasions when you want butter with a creamery-fresh, delicate taste, try your hand at making butter. Though cream from either cow's milk or goat's milk is delicate and sweet, goat's milk, with its low yield and heavenly taste, is the most luxurious. If cream straight from the farm is not handy, the standard whipping cream found in any supermarket will still make excellent unsalted (sweet) butter.

Gourmet cooks favor the natural, sweet taste of butter without salt. In the past salt was used as a preservative, but with today's careful handling and refrigeration it is no longer necessary. Besides, foods cooked with salted butter are more likely to stick to baking pans and skillets.

Before starting, allow the cream to warm to churning temperature—58 to 62°F. If it is too cold, much of the butterfat will end up in the buttermilk; if it is too hot, the butter will be soft and greasy.

To churn the cream, fill a regular butter churn half full, or a five-cup blender jar three-quarters full. Run the churn, the blender, or a powerful mixer full tilt until the globules of fat have separated out to form the butter.

With a wooden spoon or a rubber spatula, pat the butter into a ball and lift it out of the buttermilk. Press the ball of butter to squeeze out any remaining buttermilk. You can also wash it under cool running water or churn it again in cold water. Press out the water and wrap the butter tightly for storing in the refrigerator or freezer.

Cultured Milks

For centuries European and Asian peoples have enjoyed the zing of cultured milks. Yogurt, kefir, piima, and buttermilk are among those most favored.

The live cultures in these fermented milks are purported to have special healthful properties, such as establishing a balance of beneficial bacteria in the intestines. Because fermentation results in a small, tender curd, and because lactose is transformed into lactic acid, many people who are allergic to fresh milk are able to digest cultured milks easily.

Drinks made with cultured milks and fresh peach, pineapple, or orange flavorings are filling and sweet with just a hint of tang. Cultured milks give sauces and soups a luscious smoothness. And, when used in breads, cakes, and biscuits, the acid in cultured milks interacts with the protein in flour to all but guarantee a tender crumb.

Yogurt

Yogurt, a tangy, custardlike fermented milk, has long been a popular dietary staple in the Middle East and Russia. Though middle America was introduced to yogurt in the 1930s, it was not until the 1960s that yogurt gained real acceptance.

It takes only two ingredients to make yogurt: milk and a starter.

Just about any milk—goat's, mare's, water buffalo's, cow's, reindeer's, soybean—will produce a tasty yogurt, though the texture and flavor will vary with each. Whole cow's milk (the one most commonly used in the United States) makes a smooth, custardlike, tart yogurt; skim milk makes a fairly thin one; and a combination of half milk and half light cream (or three cups milk with one cup heavy cream) yields a rich, thick, sweet product. Adding one-third cup of dry milk solids to one quart of skim milk will produce a firmer, more nutritive yogurt.

The starter can be a packet of freeze-dried culture (bacteria) that is available in natural foods stores, or yogurt from a previous homemade (or commercial) batch. Though the freeze-dried culture is the most reliable, the reserved tablespoon or two of yogurt will give excellent results most of the time. The special bacteria that turn milk into yogurt are *Lactobacillus bulgaricus* and *Streptococcus thermophilus*.

If you use a commercial yogurt as a starter, be absolutely certain it contains a live culture. Today, many commercial yogurts have been pasteurized to increase their shelf life, but, unfortunately, the heat treatment inactivates the bacteria. Freshness of the yogurt is also important: Old cultures tend to be weak. Select a yogurt without added gelatins, flavors, or sweeteners. The extras interfere with the growth of the bacteria.

The equipment needed for making yogurt is relatively simple. Use an enameled, stainless steel, or glass vessel for heating the milk, since none of those materials taint the taste. A glass bowl or jar works best for the incubation period.

To make yogurt, slowly heat a quart of milk until it just reaches the boiling point. Do not let it actually boil and foam. (Pasteurize the milk if it is raw. Bacteria in raw milk will interfere with the yogurt culture.) Cool the milk to between 105 and 110°F. At that temperature a drop of milk on your wrist should feel lukewarm and you

should be able to keep your little finger in the milk for a slow count of ten.

Stir into the milk one packet of freeze-dried culture or two tablespoons of yogurt from a previous batch. Incubate the mixture—do not jiggle it during incubation—in a covered container at 105 to 110°F for five to ten hours. (See Heat Sources for Incubating Yogurt, below.) The longer the incubation, the tarter the yogurt.

Heat Sources for Incubating Yogurt

Insulated picnic cooler: Place filled jars in the cooler and surround them with warm water (105 to 110°F). If possible, the water should be up to the midpoint of the jars. However, too much water will make the cooler unwieldy. Check the temperature every hour and add or subtract water as needed.

Oven: An electric oven set on very low heat will do the job. So will a gas oven with only a pilot light. In both cases use a thermometer, and set the jars in a pot of water to be sure the temperature remains constant.

Heat tray: A thermostatically controlled tray used for keeping food warm works well. A thermometer and a jar of water will help you find the right temperature setting.

Thermos: This is a good method if you are making only one quart of yogurt. Pour the inoculated milk into a prewarmed, widemouthed thermos, cap it, and let it sit undisturbed.

Electric yogurt maker: Pour the heated, inoculated milk into the jars that come with the unit and follow the manufacturer's operating directions.

Chill the thickened yogurt in a covered container at 40°F for at least 12 hours before serving. Yogurt will stay fresh for four to five days, though it will taste tarter on the fifth day than on the first. If a watery, yellowish liquid (whey) accumulates on the top, drain it off if you like a thick consistency, or stir it in if you prefer a thin one.

Flavorings should be added to yogurt right before serving. If you want to retain a thick yogurt consistency, gently fold instead of stirring. Pureed fruits, homemade preserves, honey, vanilla, and cinnamon combine deliciously with yogurt for light desserts and snacks.

Cooking with yogurt can be somewhat tricky. Always heat it over low heat. And to reduce the chances of its separating or curdling, do not add it to hot foods until shortly before they are finished cooking. If lengthy cooking should be required, one tablespoon of flour, cornstarch, or arrowroot blended with one quart of yogurt or one slightly beaten egg white works well as a stabilizer. Bring the mixture to a boil slowly, stirring continuously in one direction. Reduce the heat and simmer gently, uncovered, for ten minutes. Cool and refrigerate until needed.

Why the Yogurt Did Not Set

If your yogurt did not set, look for the cause:

- Was the incubation temperature between 105 and 110°F?
- Was the incubation period long enough?
- Did someone agitate the container during incubation or before the yogurt cooled?
- Was the milk too cool?
- Was the milk unpasteurized?
- Was either the starter or the milk old?
- Was the starter yogurt pasteurized?
- Did high heat inactivate the culture?
- Were there antibiotics in the milk?
- Was the equipment less than perfectly clean?

In recipes yogurt makes a fine substitute for milk, cream, buttermilk, or sour cream. As a replacement for sour cream, it has a thinner texture and less intense but sharper flavor. When used in place of milk in biscuits and breads, it yields a more tender crumb. (In baking be sure to add one-half teaspoon of baking soda for each cup of yogurt used.) You can also fold yogurt into whipped cream, and you can use yogurt to replace either all or half of the mayonnaise called for in a recipe.

Kefir

Popular in the Middle East, Eastern Europe, and Russia, kefir is one of the oldest-known fermented milks, yet it is a rarity in the United States. In many ways kefir resembles yogurt, but its flavor is somewhat milder and sweeter. Because the curd of kefir is fairly loose, many of the people who are allergic to sweet whole milk can digest it easily.

To make kefir, heat milk; then let it cool to room temperature. Add the culture and put the mixture in containers to incubate at room temperature for 12 to 24 hours. (For information on where to obtain culture, see Appendix 4.) Successive batches of kefir can be made with small amounts of kefir set aside from each previous batch.

Serve kefir chilled. Blended until frothy with fresh fruit, it makes a delectable drink.

Piima

In the Scandinavian countries piima is a favored cultured milk. It is milder tasting than either yogurt or kefir and is extremely easy to prepare. As for yogurt and kefir, once you have made piima from a freeze-dried culture, you can go on indefinitely, making new batches with a few spoonfuls from a previous batch.

To make piima, simply stir the culture into milk at room temperature (about 70°F). (For information on where to obtain culture, see Appendix 4.) Use only pasteurized milk—piima bacteria grow best when they have no competition. Let the mixture incubate for 8 to 24 hours. The piima will ferment more slowly in a cool room (one below 70°F).

Since piima is milder than kefir, it can be used as a direct substitute in any recipe that calls for milk. Blend it with egg and gelatin for a delicious, quick custard. Or serve it instead of sour cream on baked potatoes. It mixes well with mayonnaise and enhances salad dressings and dessert toppings. Mix it with fruit juice or concentrate for a refreshing drink.

Buttermilk

Real buttermilk, thick and mildly acidic with flecks of butter, was originally the liquid residue from butter making. Today it is a cultured (soured) milk made from pasteurized skim milk. Lactic acid bacteria are added to the milk and the mixture is left to clabber at room temperature.

You can make a quart of cultured buttermilk at home by simply adding a packet of freeze-dried culture (available in some natural foods stores) or one-half cup of buttermilk to fresh skim milk. Let the mixture ferment at room temperature. Store it in the refrigerator as you would fresh milk.

In recipes buttermilk and sour milk are readily interchangeable. However, if you replace fresh milk with buttermilk in baking, you must remember to adjust the recipe to accommodate the acidity of the buttermilk. Use one-half teaspoon of baking soda for each cup of buttermilk. Biscuits, waffles, muffins, and breads made with buttermilk have an exceptionally tender crumb and pleasing brown crust. Cold buttermilk soup is a great way to spark summer appetites. You can substitute buttermilk in any recipe that calls for yogurt and stock.

Storing Dairy Products

Dairy Product	Storage Conditions	Length of Storage
Fresh milk, cream, and butter		
Skim milk	covered and refrigerated	3-5 days
Whole milk	covered and refrigerated	3-5 days
	frozen	1-6 months
Cream		
Light and heavy	covered and refrigerated	3-5 days
Whipped	covered and refrigerated	2-3 days
	frozen	1 month
Butter	tightly wrapped and refrigerated	1 week (unsalted), 10 days (salted)
	tightly wrapped and frozen	6 months
Cultured milks		
Buttermilk	covered and refrigerated	3-5 days
Kefir	covered and refrigerated	3-5 days

Storing Dairy Products—Continued

Dairy Product	Storage Conditions	Length of Storage
Piima	covered and refrigerated	3-5 days
Yogurt	covered and refrigerated	3-5 days
Dry milks		
Dry milk solids		
Whole	refrigerated	2-4 weeks
Nonfat	room temperature	3-6 months
Reconstituted nonfat dry milk	covered and refrigerated	3-5 days
Canned milks		
Evaporated milk		
Unopened can	room temperature (Invert can every 2 weeks.)	6 months
Opened can	covered and refrigerated	3-5 days
Sweetened condensed milk		
Unopened can	room temperature (Invert can every 2 weeks.)	3-6 months
Opened can	covered and refrigerated	3-5 days
Cheeses		
Cheddar, Swiss, and other hard varieties	tightly wrapped and refrigerated	2-4 weeks (unless mold develops)
	tightly wrapped and frozen	6 months
Commercial cheese spreads and cheese foods	tightly covered and refrigerated	4-6 months (unless mold develops)
Cottage, fresh ricotta	covered and refrigerated	3-5 days
Cream, Neufchatel, and other soft varieties	covered or tightly wrapped and refrigerated	2 weeks

Making Crème Fraîche (Cultured Heavy Cream)

A delicious alternative to sour cream and yogurt, crème fraîche is a thick, subtly tart fermented cream. Use two tablespoons of cultured buttermilk to transform one cup of heavy cream into crème fraîche. Combine the buttermilk and cream in a clean, warm jar with a screw-top. Cover the jar tightly and set it in a warm place for 12 to 24 hours. When the mixture has set or is almost firm, transfer it to the refrigerator to complete thickening. Crème fraîche will keep nicely in the refrigerator for up to ten days.

Cheeses

Hundreds of types of cheeses with individual flavors and textures are made all over the world, and they adapt readily to countless uses. Colby or cheddar cheese can be combined with macaroni to make a simple main dish that is a universal favorite with both children and adults. Roquefort and blue cheeses lend tang to dressings destined for tossed salads. Parmesan or Romano cheese, grated and sprinkled over a plate of pasta or blended into a plain white sauce, adds a zest that is incomparable. Fresh ricotta, cottage, and cream cheeses give smoothness and body to rich cheesecakes and pies. Other soft and aged cheeses can be used as a base or as a flavoring for dips, spreads, breads, and pastries. In addition, many cheeses are perfect eaten out of hand just as they are, with no embellishment.

Natural Cheeses

Natural cheeses come in more than 400 varieties. Their textures range from the very hard, granular cheeses to the creamy, soft ones—from Romano to cheddar to Brie; their flavors—from mild cream cheese to nippy Swiss to Limburger.

Though no two types of cheese are alike, all cheese makers start the cheese-making process in the same way. First, they add a culture (bacteria) or rennet (an enzyme from the lining of a calf's stomach) to coagulate (curdle) the protein in milk.

Then, they cut or break up the resulting solid (curd) and drain off the liquid (whey). After a brief draining, soft, fresh cheeses such as cottage cheese are ready for eating. Firmer cheeses require additional steps such as pressing and ripening (curing). The unique flavor and texture of each cheese depend on many factors including: the amount of whey drained and pressed from the curd, the seasonings used, the type of bacteria added during curing, and the ripening conditions —temperature, humidity, and length of time.

Natural cheeses—rich in protein, vitamins, calcium, and other minerals—find a welcome place in our diets. Yet, many of them contain relatively large amounts of fat from the whole milk and cream used to make them, a serious concern for some (see Fat Content in Cheeses table, below). Likewise, people who are limiting

Fat Content in Cheeses

Cheese	Fat Content (grams in 1 ounce)
Blue	8.15
Brick	8.41
Brie	7.85
Camembert	6.88
Cheddar	9.40
Colby	9.10
Cottage, creamed	1.27
Cottage, dry-curd	0.12
Cottage, low-fat, 2 percent	0.53
Cream	9.89
Edam	7.88
Gouda	7.78
Gruyère	9.17
Limburger	7.72
Monterey Jack	8.58
Mozzarella	6.12
Mozzarella, part-skim	4.51
Muenster	8.52
Neufchatel	6.64
Parmesan	8.51
Port du Salut	8.00
Provolone	7.55
Romano	7.64
Roquefort	8.69
Swiss	7.78

their intake of sodium should avoid certain cheeses. The natural sodium content of milk and its products is substantial; further, liberal quantities of salt are often added during curing to flavor, to inhibit unwanted mold growth, and to draw out excess moisture. (See Appendix 3 for more information on the sodium content of dairy products.)

Buying Cheeses

Specialty shops and well-stocked supermarkets carry a large assortment of imported and domestic cheeses. For top-notch cheeses shop in a market where the turnover is high, select only wrapped cheeses kept in chilled cases, and read the label carefully to check contents. Some cheeses, however, will also contain ingredients that are not always listed on the label:

- Bleaching agents: Benzoyl peroxide is sometimes used to bleach the milk in blue cheese, provolone, Parmesan, and Romano.
- Water-binding agents: A gum or gelatin is often used in cream cheeses and spreads to help bind moisture to the curd.
- Preservatives: Sorbic acid, potassium sorbate, or sodium sorbate is often added to slices of cheese to inhibit mold growth.

Determine freshness, too, by sampling cheese whenever possible. In specialty stores where cheeses are cut from large wheels and blocks, customers are usually permitted to sample the cheese. Take advantage of the opportunity to be sure the cheese you are considering is of peak quality.

Storing Cheeses

Since hard cheeses are fairly low in moisture, they store well for several months. Soft, fresh cheeses, on the other hand, have a high moisture content and keep for only three to five days.

Before you store a cheese in the refrigerator, the general rule is to wrap it snugly in foil or plastic wrap to keep it from drying out or from picking up unwanted moisture. Blue cheeses should be loosely wrapped or placed in a covered container because they keep best when surrounded by a small amount of air. Always store a strong cheese like Limburger in a tightly closed container; otherwise, the contents of your refrigerator will pick up Limburger's distinctive aroma.

For extended keeping you can seal the cut surfaces of cheese with hot paraffin. An alternative is freezing, but the texture of any cheese that has been frozen tends to be crumbly and either mealy or pebbly. The cheeses most successfully frozen are brick, cheddar, Edam, Gouda, mozzarella, Muenster, Port du Salut, provolone, and Swiss. Freeze the cheese in one-inch-thick pieces for no longer than six months, and use frozen cheese quickly after thawing.

If cheese becomes hard and dry during storage, all is not lost. Simply grate the cheese. It makes a fine topping for spaghetti, vegetables, soups, biscuits, or casseroles.

If mold grows on cheese you are keeping, however, it may be a matter for concern, since some molds contain dangerous aflatoxins. To be on the safe side, discard cheeses that grow moldy spots.

(For more information on storing cheeses, see Storing Dairy Products table, page 449.)

Serving Cheeses

Unadorned, perhaps with a simple cracker or with a wedge of apple, cheese lends itself to almost any occasion. It is ideal for children's snacks since it is high in several nutrients. For a host or hostess in a hurry, cheese is a quick, always welcome appetizer. As a dessert, cheese with fruit and nuts is a satisfying conclusion to the most elaborate dinner.

Serve hard (ripened) cheeses at room temperature to enjoy their full flavors and creamy textures. Allow 20 to 60 minutes for a cheese to warm up, and only warm the amount of cheese needed. Continual rewarming ages cheese. While the cheese is warming, keep it covered to prevent the surfaces from drying out. Fresh (unripened) cheeses are tastiest when cold. Present them directly from the refrigerator.

Whenever you serve cheese, use plain breads and crackers—no seasoned or salted ones. The flavorings tend either to fight with the flavor of the cheese or to mask it. And do not cut the cheese ahead of time. Precutting, which exposes many surfaces to the air, causes the cheese to dry out.

For a cheese tasting or a buffet, serve six to nine ounces of cheese per person. If you limit the selection to three or four cheeses, you will find that it is easy to savor each one. Depending upon the sophistication of the group in terms of cheese, you might present a wide variety of cheeses or variations on a single type—all sharp, all mild, all aromatic.

Cooking with Cheeses

Cooked cheeses add body and flavor to all types of dishes, but there are certain rules for ensuring smooth, creamy results.

Always cook cheese over warm, not high, heat and keep the cooking time minimal. At high temperatures, or during prolonged cooking, the protein in cheese separates from the fat and the cheese becomes a stringy, rubbery mass floating in an oily liquid.

When using cheese in sauces and fondues, shred, grate, crumble, or dice it. Cheese in small pieces blends readily and melts faster. Add cheese to a liquid or a sauce that is already hot and, if possible, cook the mixture over boiling water in a double boiler. Remove it from the heat as soon as the cheese and the liquid (or the sauce) are smoothly blended.

To broil cheese, place it four to five inches below the heat. It will melt in one to three minutes, so keep a close watch. Broiled cheese is delight-ful on an open-faced sandwich of meat, tomatoes, poultry, or fish.

In baked cheese dishes keep the oven temperature low to moderate—about 325 to 350°F is fine. Set cheese custards in water to prevent them from burning. And to help keep cheese toppings from toughening or hardening during baking, cover them with fine bread crumbs, or wait to add the cheese just a minute or two before removing the food from the oven.

Grating and Shredding Cheeses

Grated and shredded cheeses make nice garnishes on casseroles and blend readily into sauces. Shred, grate, or crumble four ounces (one-quarter pound) of cheese for every cup of cheese called for in a recipe. The very hard cheeses are excellent for fine grating and the softer ones work best when shredded. Trying to grate a soft cheese too finely will only result in a clogged grater. For easiest grating and shredding, use cheeses that are very cold.

Making Cheeses at Home

Tasty, salt-free soft cheeses are easy to make at home. Hard cheeses, on the other hand, require quite a bit of equipment and time. They also call for salt, as a rule.

It takes approximately ten pounds (or about five quarts) of milk to make one pound of cheese. You also need these seven items:

- an earthenware crock, glass casserole dish, or stainless steel or enameled pot
- a dairy thermometer
- a long-handled spoon (preferably made from glass, wood, stainless steel, or enamel)
- a spatula or wide knife
- a large pan or shallow pot that is larger than your crock
- a cheesecloth
- a colander

All equipment must be scrupulously clean. Unwanted bacteria will interfere with the curdling process and produce off-flavors and strange textures. Wash the equipment with soapy water and rinse it thoroughly with very hot water.

For more detailed instructions for making your own soft cheese, see the table on page 454.

Cottage Cheese

This is the cheese for beginners to try. The time element is a consideration, but it is not "work" time, and it does not require the cook's presence as the mixture sets. Only a minimum of skill is required. After the first batch, most cooks will feel confident about the procedure.

Small-Curd Cottage Cheese

This cheese can be made in 16 to 36 hours.

1 gallon skim or whole milk
¼ cup yogurt or ½ cup cultured buttermilk

Pour milk into a very clean, large, stainless steel or enameled pot. Set pot on a rack inside a larger pot. Fill outside pot with hot water. Warm on stove over low heat until milk reaches 85°F.

Stir yogurt or buttermilk into milk with a wire whisk. Cover with a towel. Incubate milk, without disturbing it, at a temperature of 72 to 85°F until milk becomes firm and yogurtlike. When curd pulls away from side of pot, it is ready to "set" by being heated. You will see a clear liquid around edges of pot. This will take between 12 and 36 hours. Temperature may fluctuate during this time but milk may not be jiggled.

It is now time to separate the whey, a clear liquid, from curds, which are white and made of coagulated proteins. With a long thin stainless steel knife, cut curd into ¼-inch squares. Next, hold knife at a 45-degree angle and slice diagonally through lines which are already made. These cuts will allow whey to seep out of curds and will facilitate even heating.

Place fresh hot water in outside pot and place pot containing curds in it. Over low heat raise temperature of curds to 90°F (check temperature near outside of pot). At no time allow water in outside pot to get hotter than 170°F. Slowly stir curds from outside edges into center and bring curd from bottom to top, using a rubber spatula or a large metal spoon. Curds are still soft at this point and easily broken. Continue to raise temperature of curds to 120°F, stirring gently every 10 minutes. Time needed to raise temperature to 120°F from room temperature should be regulated to take about 45 minutes.

Hold curds at 120°F until they feel firm, 10 to 20 minutes more. When curds show resistance to being squeezed and feel slightly springy but still a long way from being rubbery, they are ready to drain. Whey will be very clear with a golden tinge. Rinse a cheesecloth and line a colander with it. Gently ladle curds into colander. Pour whey through curds. Rinse gently with cool water. If water drains too slowly, shift curds about in cheesecloth. Rinse again to finish cooling curds. Tie ends of cheesecloth together and hang to drain for another 30 minutes. Refrigerate.

Yields 4 cups

Variation:

Large-Curd Cottage Cheese: Dissolve ¼ rennet tablet in 2 tablespoons water, and add to milk when stirring in yogurt or buttermilk. Follow directions above until mixture has curdled. Cut curd into ½-inch cubes in same manner as for small curd. Heat and stir as above, but remove from heat and drain as soon as curd begins to firm, or it will have a texture similar to mozzarella cheese. Test, drain, wash, and drain again as with small curd.

What Happened to the Cottage Cheese?

It is rubbery because:
- too high a temperature or too long a heating time was used.
- not enough rennet was added (for large curd).
- not enough acid was in the curd before heating.

The curd is soft and pasty because:
- too much acid was in the milk before heating.
- too much rennet was added (for large curd).
- too low a temperature or too short a heating time was used.
- the milk was pasteurized at too high a temperature and/or for too long a time.

Basic Steps for Making Soft Cheeses

Steps	Cottage Cheese	Farmer Cheese	Soft White Cheese	Mozzarella	
Start with basic ingredients.	skim or whole milk	skim or whole milk	skim or whole milk	skim or whole milk	
Add culture.	¼ cup yogurt or ½ cup buttermilk per gallon	same as for cottage cheese	½ cup buttermilk per gallon	½ cup buttermilk per gallon	
Warm.	Warm to room temperature.	same as for cottage cheese	Warm to 92-94°F.	Warm to 90°F.	
Add rennet (¼ tablet per gallon).	Add rennet for milky, large-curd cheese.	same as for cottage cheese	Add rennet.	Add only ½ rennet solution.	
Curd forms.	Cut curd after 12-36 hours at 72-85°F.	same as for cottage cheese	Cut curd after 30 minutes.	Cut curd after 20-30 minutes.	
Heat.	Stir 30-45 minutes at 95-120°F.	same as for cottage cheese	Stir 30 minutes at 92-94°F.	Stir 15 minutes at 90°F.	
Drain.	Drain in cheesecloth-lined colander; then hang; rinse.	same as for cottage cheese (becomes pot cheese at this step)	Pour off whey.	Pour off and reserve whey.	
Press.	. . .	Wrap in several layers of cheese-cloth, press with 1- or 2-pound weight.	Pack into weighted press 2-4 hours.	Pack curds, cut into 3 × 3-inch blocks.	
Cool.	. . .	. . .	. . .	Bathe in cool water 15 minutes.	
Refrigerate.	. . .	. . .	. . .	Tie in cheesecloth; refrigerate in whey 1-3 days.	
Reheat.	. . .	. . .	. . .	Bring curd to room temperature; heat whey to 180°F.	
Knead.	. . .	. . .	. . .	Knead curds in whey until smooth and plastic.	
Shape.	. . .	. . .	. . .	Form small balls; cool quickly in cold water.	

*Yogurt cheese is a fresh cheese made by allowing whey to drain from yogurt solids.
†Traditional ricotta is made from whey. It was originally produced in Italy and is still commonly found in many European countries.
‡New World ricotta is made from a combination of milk and whey. This type is generally more popular in the United States.

Cream Cheese	Neufchatel	Yogurt Cheese*	Mysost	Traditional Ricotta†	New World Ricotta‡
whole milk and cream	whole milk and cream	yogurt	whey and ¼ cup cream per quart	whey (2½ gallons yield 1 pound)	skim or whole milk plus ¼ cup whey powder per quart
½ cup buttermilk per gallon (optional)	. . .	. . .	. . .	. . .	. . .
Warm to 60-65°F.	Warm to 86°F.	Warm to room temperature.	Simmer until thick cream forms.	Heat until cream rises; add 1 cup milk per gallon at 200°F.	Warm to room temperature.
Add rennet.	Add only ½ rennet solution.	. . .	. . .	Add 6 table-spoons vinegar per gallon.	Add 2 table-spoons butter-milk or lemon juice or vinegar per quart.
Custard forms after 12 hours; do not cut.	Custard forms after 18-24 hours; do not cut.	. . .	. . .	Remove from heat; dip out curds.	Leave undisturbed 24 hours.
. . .	. . .	. . .	Continue to cook to apple butter consistency.	. . .	Heat very slowly to 200°F.
Drain in cheese-cloth-lined colander; then hang overnight.	Pack into molds; drain 12-24 hours.	Hang in cheese-cloth 6-8 hours to drain.	. . .	Drain in cheese-cloth-lined colander.	Dip out curds; drain through cheesecloth.
. . .	. . .	. . .	. . .	. . .	. . .
. . .	. . .	. . .	. . .	. . .	. . .
. . .	. . .	. . .	. . .	. . .	. . .
. . .	. . .	. . .	. . .	. . .	. . .
. . .	. . .	. . .	. . .	Knead 10 minutes at room temperature.	. . .
. . .	. . .	. . .	. . .	Pack into molds to harden.	. . .

Natural Cheeses and Their Uses

Cheese Variety and Origin	Description	Uses
Asiago (Italy)	whole or part-skim cow's milk; hard, granular; tiny holes; light yellow; piquant, sharp in aged cheese	seasoning
Bel Paese (Italy)	whole cow's milk; soft to medium firm, creamy; mild, sweet flavor; creamy yellow interior; gray brown surface; sometimes covered with yellow wax	appetizers, desserts, salad dressings, salads, sandwiches, snacks; good with crackers
Blue (France)	whole cow's milk; semisoft, pasty, sometimes crumbly; chalky white, streaked with blue green mold; tangy	desserts, dips, salad dressings, salads, sandwich spreads; good with crackers
Brick (United States)	whole cow's milk; semisoft to medium firm, elastic; creamy yellow to orange interior; brick shaped; mild to moderately sharp	appetizers, desserts, sandwiches, snacks
Brie (France)	whole cow's milk; soft, smooth; creamy yellow interior; brown, edible exterior; mild to pungent	appetizers, desserts, sandwiches, snacks; good with crackers, fruit
Caciocavallo (Italy)	cow's milk or mixture of cow's, ewe's, or goat's milk; firm to hard; light interior; tan surface; flavor similar to provolone but not smoked	desserts, sandwiches, seasoning, snacks
Camembert (France)	whole cow's milk; soft—almost runny when fully ripe; thin edible crust; creamy yellow interior; mild to pungent	appetizers, desserts, sandwiches; good with crackers, fruit
Cheddar (England)	whole cow's milk; firm, smooth; white to medium yellow-orange; mild to sharp	appetizers, casseroles, desserts, salads, sandwiches, sauces, seasoning; good with crackers, fruit, pasta, vegetables
Colby (United States)	whole cow's milk; firm, somewhat open texture; light yellow to orange; mild to mellow	appetizers, casseroles, desserts, salads, sandwiches, seasoning; good with crackers, fruit, pasta, vegetables
Cottage (uncertain)	whole or skim cow's milk; white to creamy white; soft, moist, delicate curds; mild, slightly acidic	appetizers, dips, salads; good with fruit, in cheesecakes
Cream (United States)	cream from cow's milk; smooth, buttery; white; mild, delicate, slightly acidic	appetizers, desserts, dips, snacks; good in cheesecakes and icings
Edam (Netherlands)	part-skim cow's milk; firm, rubbery; creamy yellow with red wax coating; mellow, nutlike	appetizers, desserts, salads, sandwiches, snacks; good with crackers, fruit
Feta (Greece)	mixture of cow's, ewe's, or goat's milk; soft, creamy, smooth; white; tangy, pleasantly salty	appetizers, pastry, pies, salads; good with citrus fruit, crackers, crusty bread
Gjetost (Norway)	whey from goat's milk or mixture of whey from goat's and cow's milk; very firm, buttery; golden brown color; sweet, caramel flavor	desserts, snacks; good with dark breads, crackers, biscuits, or muffins
Gorgonzola (Italy)	cow's milk, goat's milk, or mixture of both; semisoft, pasty, sometimes crumbly; creamy white interior, streaked with blue green mold; light tan exterior; tangy, spicy, rich	appetizers, desserts, dips, salads, sandwich spreads
Gouda (Netherlands)	whole or part-skim cow's milk; semisoft to firm, smooth; creamy yellow; usually with red wax coating; mellow, nutlike, sometimes slightly acidic	appetizers, desserts, salads, sandwiches, sauces, snacks
Gruyère (Switzerland)	part-skim cow's milk; firm, smooth, tiny holed; light yellow; nutlike, salty; melts easily	appetizers, desserts, fondues, snacks; good with crackers

Natural Cheeses and Their Uses—*Continued*

Cheese Variety and Origin	Description	Uses
Havarti (Tilsit) (Denmark)	whole cow's milk; semisoft, smooth, creamy; white paraffin coating, deep yellow rind, or rindless; ivory to light yellow interior; mild to tangy	appetizers, desserts, salads, sandwiches, snacks; good with crackers, fruit, whole grain bread
Jarlsberg (Norway)	whole and skim cow's milk; semisoft; irregular holes (eyes); light yellow; forms tears when cut; taste similar to Swiss	appetizers, fondues, sandwiches, snacks
Liederkranz (United States)	whole cow's milk; soft, smooth; creamy yellow interior, russet surface; robust	appetizers, desserts, snacks
Limburger (Belgium)	whole or part-skim cow's milk; soft, smooth; creamy white to yellow; highly pungent	appetizers, desserts, snacks
Monterey Jack (United States)	whole cow's milk; semisoft, smooth; creamy white; mild	sandwiches, snacks; good with crackers
Mozzarella (Italy)	whole or part-skim cow's milk (originally from buffalo's milk); slightly firm, plastic; creamy white; delicate; melts easily	appetizers, main dishes (casseroles, lasagna, pizza), sandwiches, snacks
Muenster (Germany)	whole cow's milk; semisoft, smooth; white interior; yellowish tan surface; mellow	appetizers, desserts, sandwiches, snacks
Mysost (Norway)	whey from goat's milk or a mixture of whey from goat's and cow's milk; firm, buttery; light brown; sweet, caramel flavor	desserts, snacks; good with dark bread
Neufchatel (France)	whole cow's milk; soft, smooth, creamy; white; mild	desserts, dips, salads, sandwiches; good in cheesecakes and pies
Parmesan (Italy)	part-skim cow's milk; hard, granular; yellowish white; sharp, distinctive flavor	seasoning
Port du Salut (France)	whole or partly acid cow's milk; semisoft, smooth, buttery; creamy yellow interior; russet surface; mild to robust	appetizers, desserts, snacks; good with crackers, fruit
Provolone (Italy)	whole cow's milk; hard, compact; light, creamy interior; brown or golden yellow surface; mild to sharp, smoked, salty flavor	appetizers, main dishes, sandwiches, seasoning, snacks
Ricotta (Italy)	whey and whole or skim cow's milk, or whole or part-skim cow's milk; soft, loose curds, moist or dry; white; bland, sweet	appetizers, lasagna, ravioli, noodles, salads, snacks; good as seasoning when dried
Romano (Italy)	cow's milk (sheep's milk in Italy); very hard, granular; yellowish white interior; greenish black surface; sharp, piquant	seasoning
Roquefort (France)	sheep's milk; semisoft, pasty, crumbly; white, marbled with blue green mold; sharp, peppery	appetizers, desserts, dips, salad dressings, salads, sandwich spreads; good with crackers
Stilton (England)	whole or part-skim cow's milk or cream; semisoft, crumbly; white interior streaked with blue green mold; spicy	appetizers, desserts, salads, snacks; good with bland crackers
Sapsago (Switzerland)	skim cow's milk; very hard; light green (clover leaves added); sharp, pungent	seasoning; good as spread when grated and blended with soft butter
Swiss (Switzerland)	part-skim cow's milk; firm, elastic interior with large holes; light yellow; sweet, nutlike	fondues, salads, sandwiches, snacks

Meats

For most Americans, a savory meat dish sets the tone for the main meal, and all other dishes—a tasty vegetable or two, a tender pasta, a crisp salad—are planned around it. Meat has attained this status, at least in part, because of its satisfying richness and abundant stores of protein. Unfortunately, meat is the most expensive item in the food budget, and that fact—plus a general concern about excessive dietary fat intake—has led many Americans to cut back on their meat consumption. An imaginative cook who is also a good shopper can stay within the budget and still serve meat regularly by using recipes that can accommodate the less-tender cuts, buying the specials, and serving dishes in which just a little meat stretches far and still remains the focus of the meal.

Buying Meat

If you can buy meat where you have the opportunity to discuss your purchase with the butcher—specialty meat markets, farmers' markets, co-ops, some supermarkets—by all means do so. You can learn a great deal about the right cut to buy. The costliest is not always the best for a given purpose. Butchers generally welcome inquiries, and they give sound advice that will save you money and keep you coming back.

If you shop where the meat is prepackaged, carefully examine the packages and labels. See-through trays that permit you to inspect both sides of the meat are ideal. The label should provide the name of the type of meat (beef, veal, lamb, pork), the name of the primal or wholesale cut (chuck, round, shank, loin), the specific retail name of the cut (steak, rib roast, chop), and the price per pound. In the better markets, the label will also include the grade of meat, a date, and a suggested cooking method. Avoid meat (and the market, too!) in which the label has been placed in such a way that it covers bone or fat, thereby creating the illusion that the meat is a better buy than it really is.

Since butchers throughout the country tend to give fanciful names—such as "his and hers" steaks—to many of the more than 300 official cuts of meat, it is essential to become familiar with the major primal (wholesale) cuts (see the diagrams for meat cuts on pages 460 and 461). That way you always know what you are really buying, and you can judge whether the price is good and determine the best methods for cooking the meat. (See Tender and Less-Tender Cuts, page 470.)

As you examine each piece of meat, look for these qualities:

Beef: A uniform, bright, light to deep red color is characteristic of good beef. The lean is firm and slightly moist, with a fine texture and some marbling (distribution of fat particles throughout the lean). Red, porous bones also indicate good-quality beef. Since the color of beef fat varies with age, feed, and breed, fat color is not a reliable clue to the quality of the beef.

Lamb: The lean of good, young lamb is pink to light red in color, and it is firm and fine textured. Bones are slender, red, moist, and porous. On good lamb the external fat is firm. Color of the fat varies with age, breed, and feed. The lean of somewhat older lamb is light red, and the bones are drier and less red than that of younger lamb.

Pork: Good-quality fresh pork has a high proportion of lean to fat and bone. The lean is firm, fine textured, and grayish pink to light red in color. A deep pink color is typical of the lean of cured pork.

Sodium nitrate and sodium nitrite are commonly used in curing pork as well as beef. Since studies indicate these additives may be harmful to your health, it is best to avoid cured meats, or at least to seek out meats cured without nitrite or nitrate. Cured meats also contain plenty of sodium chloride (salt)—another reason many health-conscious consumers avoid eating them.

Veal: The lean of very young veal is pale pink to grayish pink; that of somewhat older veal is slightly red. All veal should have a smooth texture and practically no fat.

When selecting from the many cuts of meat available, always try to figure the cost per serving. A cut with a high price per pound and with little waste is often more economical than one that is less expensive but has lots of waste (see Yield of Cooked Meat table, page 461). Of course, the actual number of servings in a pound depends on individual appetites. Choose well-trimmed meat; waste is costly.

Inspection and Grading of Meat

Before and after slaughter, all meat must be federally inspected for wholesomeness. (Some states have their own equivalent inspection for meat sold within the state.) Those meats passing the inspection have a round, purple mark to indicate that the meat came from a healthy animal and that it was processed under sanitary conditions. The stamp is put only on carcasses and major cuts, so it will rarely appear on small retail cuts. If the stamp does appear on a piece of meat you purchase, the marking fluid need not be trimmed off before cooking, since it is harmless.

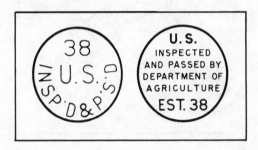

For a fee, the United States Department of Agriculture (USDA) offers grading of beef, lamb, mutton, and veal as a voluntary service to packers. The grade marking, a shield-shaped stamp, is a guide to quality—tenderness, juiciness, and flavor—in meat. U.S. Choice and U.S. Good are the grades of meats most commonly available to consumers. Other grades of meat are sold to restaurants and manufacturers.

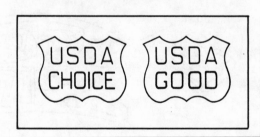

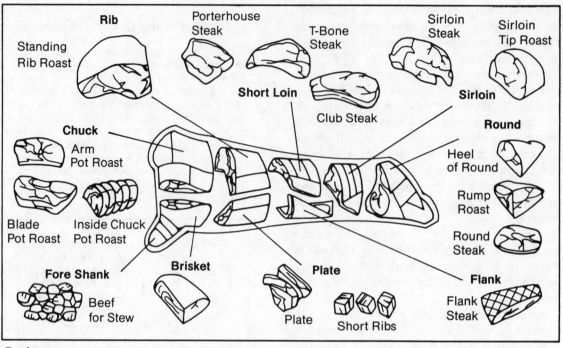

Beef

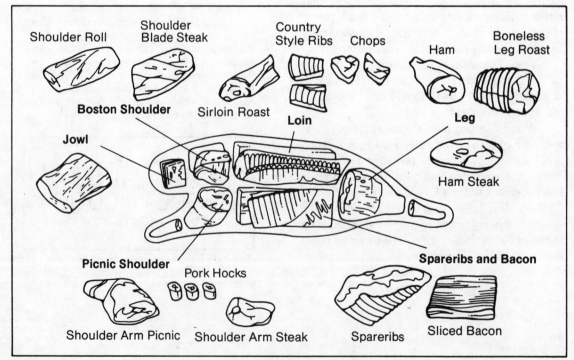

Pork

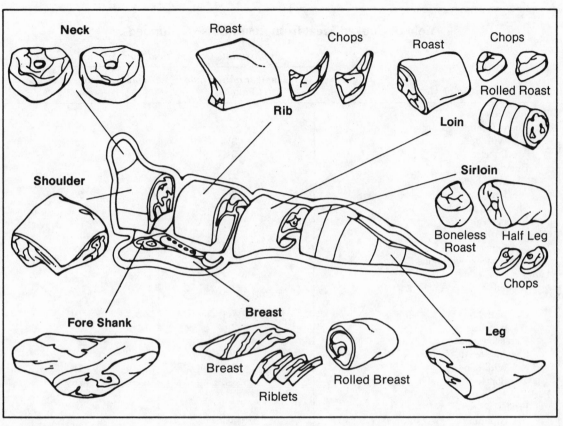

Lamb

Yield of Cooked Meat from Retail Cuts

| | Approximate Cooked Yield from 1 Pound of Meat | |
Cut of Meat	Number of Servings (3 ounces)	Volume, Chopped or Diced (cups)
Beef		
Brisket, boneless, fresh or corned	3	1½-2
Chuck roast		
With bone	2½	1½
Boneless	3-3½	2
Club steak, with bone	2	...
Flank steak, boneless	3½	...
Ground	4	...
Porterhouse steak, with bone	2¼	...
Rib roast		
With bone	2½	1½
Boneless	3	1½-2

[*continued*]

Yield of Cooked Meat from Retail Cuts—*Continued*

Cut of Meat	Approximate Cooked Yield from 1 Pound of Meat	
	Number of Servings (3 ounces)	Volume, Chopped or Diced (cups)
Beef *(continued)*		
Round steak		
With bone	3¼	...
Boneless	3¾	...
Rump roast		
With bone	2½	1½
Boneless	3½	2
Short ribs, with bone	1½	...
Sirloin steak		
With bone	2–2½	...
Boneless	2½–3	...
T-bone steak, with bone	2	...
Lamb		
Ground	3½	...
Leg		
With bone	2½–3	1½
Boneless	3½	2
Pieces for stew	3	2
Shoulder roast		
With bone	3	1½
Boneless	3–3½	2
Pork		
Fresh		
Ground	3¾–4	...
Ham		
With bone	2½–2¾	1½–1¾
Boneless	2¾–3	1¾–2
Heart	2¾–3	1¾
Liver	3½	...
Loin chop, with bone	2–2¼	...
Loin roast		
With bone	2–2¼	1¼
Boneless	2¾–3	1½–1¾
Picnic shoulder roast		
With bone	1¾–2	1–1¼
Boneless	2½	1½
Pieces for stew	3–3¼	...
Rib chop, with bone	1¾–2	...
Shoulder butt roast (Boston butt)		
With bone	2½–2¾	1½
Boneless	2¾–3	1¾

Yield of Cooked Meat from Retail Cuts—*Continued*

	Approximate Cooked Yield from 1 Pound of Meat	
Cut of Meat	Number of Servings (3 ounces)	Volume, Chopped or Diced (cups)
Spareribs	1¼-1½	...
Cured		
Ham		
Canned, boneless		
Served cold	4¾	2¾
Heated before serving	3½	2
Cook-before-eating		
With bone	2¼	1¼-1½
Boneless	2¾-3	1½-1¾
Fully cooked		
With bone	2¾-3	1½-1¾
Boneless	3¼	1¾-2
Picnic shoulder		
With bone	2-2¼	1¼
Boneless	2¾-3	1½-1¾
Shoulder butt		
With bone	2¾	1½
Boneless	3	1¾
Veal		
Breast		
With bone	2	1-1½
Boneless	3	1½-2
Cutlet		
With bone	3½	...
Boneless	4	...
Leg roast		
With bone	2½	1½
Boneless	3½	2
Loin chop, with bone	2¾	...
Loin roast		
With bone	2½	1½
Boneless	3½	2
Rib chop, with bone	2½	...
Rib roast		
With bone	2¼	1-1½
Boneless	3½	2
Shoulder roast		
With bone	2½	1½
Boneless	3½	2

Buying Ground Meat

Although ground beef (often called hamburger) is the most common and popular of the ground meats, lamb, veal, and pork are also available in ground form. When lamb and veal are ground and shaped into patties, they are labeled as lamb or beef patties. Ground pork combined with ground veal and ground beef is commonly sold as meat loaf mix.

Good ground beef contains 70 to 85 percent lean. Usually, ground round has the most lean; regular ground beef has the most fat; and ground chuck lies between these two.

As you buy ground meats, notice whether the meat is liberally specked with white. Fatty ground meats show a great deal of white throughout, causing the overall color to be light pink. By comparison, the white is less noticeable in lean ground meats, so they look fairly dark and red.

Buying Variety Meats and Oxtail

Variety meats (sometimes called organ meats) include the liver, heart, kidneys, tongue, and brains of beef, lamb, pork, and veal. Sweetbreads (thymus gland of beef or lamb) and tripe (stomach of beef or veal) also fall into this category. Oxtail, not actually a variety of meat, is simply the tail of beef.

In America the demand for variety meats is not great, so they are sometimes priced very economically. If the value is good, consider buying these cuts as a savings measure—they are all rich in protein and other nutrients as well as in flavor.

Liver: Fresh liver has no objectionable odor, but the livers of beef, pork, lamb, and calf do each have a distinctive scent. In beef liver check for a beefy smell, deep red-brown color, fairly firm feel, fine texture, and two unequal-size lobes. Whole beef liver, which weighs between 7 and 14 pounds, has a moist, smooth surface. Sliced liver looks somewhat porous. The most popular liver, calf's, is rosy red and quivery. Its texture and shape are similar to that of beef; it weighs 2½ to 5 pounds. High-quality pork liver has a bland, porky smell, deep red-brown color, fairly firm feel, fine texture, three equal-size lobes, and a moist, smooth surface. Pork liver is small— ¾ to 1¼ pounds. A distinctive yet mild flavor and smell accompany lamb liver. It has two unequal-size lobes, is a deep red color, and has a smooth, wet exterior. Pork and lamb livers are often about the same size. You can serve four with approximately 1 pound of liver.

Heart: This meat, whether from beef, lamb, pork, or veal, is firm and smooth textured. Beef heart has the most fat and weighs up to five pounds. Veal heart weighs about one pound; pork heart, eight ounces; lamb heart, five to six ounces. One pound of heart yields four servings.

Kidney: Beef and veal kidneys are made up of numerous, irregular lobes and deep clefts. Pork and lamb kidneys, which are smaller than either beef or veal, are smooth and resemble oversize kidney beans. Though a membrane covers all kidneys, it should be removed by the butcher. The best indication of freshness in kidneys is the smell. If it is disagreeable, the kidneys are past their prime. Fresh ones, in good condition, have a slight odor that is not objectionable. You can expect to get two to four servings from a beef kidney, one to two from a veal kidney, one to two from a pork kidney, and one-half to one from a lamb kidney.

Tongue: Tongue is firm, with a rough skin covering. Beef and veal tongues are available fresh, pickled, corned, or smoked. Pork and lamb tongues are often sold cooked and ready to serve.

Sweetbreads: Available from young beef, veal, and occasionally from lamb, this creamy white gland is covered with a thin, transparent membrane and has a soft, delicate consistency. Young beef and veal sweetbreads consist of two parts: the heart sweetbread and the throat, or neck, sweetbread. Together, they weigh ¾ to 1¼ pounds and are more desirable to eat as a pair than as parts. Lamb sweetbreads are very small. Buy only fresh, moist sweetbreads.

Brains: This soft, tender, and delicately flavored organ is pinkish in color and has a shiny, moist surface covered with a thin membrane. Brains from beef are the largest, weighing about three-quarters pound. Those from lamb weigh about one-quarter pound and are the smallest. Beef and veal brains are similar in flavor, texture, and tenderness. Since any aging quickly spoils brains, buy only the freshest. You will need one pound for four servings.

Tripe: Plain, or smooth, tripe is the tissue lining of the first stomach of beef or veal; honeycomb tripe comes from the second stomach. Tripe is available fresh, pickled, and canned. Although fresh tripe is actually partially cooked when sold, it must still be cooked for a couple more hours before it is edible. One pound will yield four servings.

Oxtail: Weighing under two pounds, fresh oxtail has a rosy appearance. Make certain the tail has been cut or cracked through the cartilage at the joints and that all exterior fat has been removed before you purchase it.

Buying Sausage

Buying sausage would be confusing, indeed, if the more than 200 varieties of sausage and luncheon meat made and sold today were available all at once in a single market. But most markets stock only one or two dozen varieties at a time.

Sausage varieties can be divided into two broad categories: (1) fresh and smoked sausage that must be cooked before eating, and (2) ready-to-serve, or fully cooked, sausage and luncheon meat.

Unlike sausage made at home, commercially made sausage is seldom merely fresh meat and seasonings stuffed into natural animal casings (pork, lamb, or beef intestines). Sausage found in the market usually includes several of the following federally approved ingredients: antioxidants, binders and extenders, salt, natural and artificial coloring, curing agents, emulsifying agents, flavoring agents, gases, sodium bicarbonate to neutralize excess acidity, calcium propionate to retard molding, and phosphates. Casings, too, may vary from the natural ones used in home production. Synthetic cellulose is a casing employed by some packers; others use paraffined cloth for certain types of sausage.

If you decide to buy sausage, rather than make your own, in spite of the above, be sure it is fresh. Quality deteriorates in all sausage during storage, even if it has been smoked and dried. Look at the links or patties. The fat (tasty sausage is about one-third fat) should be evenly distributed throughout, and the links should be unbroken and lightly packed. Broken or overstuffed sausage will split during cooking. Check the label to see whether the sausage is fully cooked or if it must be cooked before serving. The label will also list the ingredients. Examine the exposed surfaces. Do not buy if they seem slimy; such sausage is dangerous to eat.

Storing and Thawing Meat

All fresh and cooked meats are perishable. Store fresh meats, loosely covered with wax paper or foil, in the coldest part of your refrigerator. While some fresh meats will keep for five to seven days, most are best if used within one to three days. (See Storage of Meat table, page 466.) Cover cooked meats and meat dishes and keep them in the refrigerator for no more than four days. Always store gravy, stuffing, and meat in separate containers. For longer storage, freeze fresh and cooked meats as well as meat dishes, gravies, and stuffings (see Freezing Meats, page 755, and Freezing Prepared Foods, page 756).

Home Storage of Meat

Meat Product or Cut	Storage Period	
	Refrigerator	Freezer
Beef and veal		
Fresh		
Chop and cutlet	3-5 days	6-9 months
Ground	1-2 days	3-4 months
Pieces for stew	1-2 days	3-4 months
Roast		
Beef	3-5 days	6-12 months
Veal	3-5 days	6-9 months
Steak	3-5 days	6-12 months
Variety meats	1-2 days	3-4 months
Cured, smoked, ready-to-serve		
Corned beef	1 week	2 weeks*
Frankfurter	1 week	1 month*
Luncheon meat	3-5 days	not recommended
Sausage		
Dry and semidry	2-3 weeks	not recommended
Smoked	1 week	not recommended
Cooked		
Meat and meat dishes	3-4 days	2-3 months
Gravy and meat broth	1-2 days	2-3 months
Lamb		
Fresh		
Chop and steak	3-5 days	6-9 months
Ground	1-2 days	3-4 months
Roast	3-5 days	6-9 months
Pieces for stew	1-2 days	3-4 months
Variety meats	1-2 days	3-4 months
Cooked		
Meat and meat dishes	3-4 days	2-3 months
Gravy and meat broth	1-2 days	2-3 months
Pork		
Fresh		
Chop	3-5 days	3-4 months
Roast	3-5 days	4-8 months
Sausage	1-3 days	1-2 months
Variety meats	1-2 days	3-4 months
Cured or processed		
Bacon	1 week	1 month or less*
Frankfurter	1 week	2 weeks*
Ham		
Whole	1 week	1-2 months*
Half	3-5 days	1-2 months*
Slices	3 days	1-2 months*
Canned (unopened)	1 year	...

*Frozen cured meat loses quality rapidly and should be used as soon as possible.

Home Storage of Meat—*Continued*

| | Storage Period | |
Meat Product or Cut	Refrigerator	Freezer
Luncheon meat	3-5 days	not recommended
Sausage		
Dry and semidry	2-3 weeks	not recommended
Smoked	1 week	not recommended
Cooked		
Meat and meat dishes	3-4 days	2-3 months
Gravy and meat broth	1-2 days	2-3 months

To maintain safety and high quality, thaw fresh and cooked meats, still wrapped, in the refrigerator. For a quicker method you can immerse a package of raw meat in its watertight wrapper in cold water. Thaw until pliable. Meat that is cold enough to retain ice crystals may be safely refrozen, but quality will suffer.

Meat may also be cooked frozen. Allow at least 1½ times as long to cook frozen meat as thawed meat of similar weight and shape.

If, at any time, meat has an off-odor, slimy surface feel, or mold on it, throw the meat away. It is probably spoiled.

Preparing Meat

Generally speaking, meat requires very little preparation before cooking and will stay wholesome (and safe) if handled as little as possible and kept well chilled in the refrigerator until cooking time. When you are ready to use it, trim away excess fat and other waste, and wipe the meat with a clean, damp cloth.

Cutting and Grinding

The flavors and textures of stews, kabobs, patties, loaves, and casseroles benefit nicely from freshly cut or ground meats. Use a sharp knife and a clean cutting board to transform a large roast into well-trimmed, one-inch cubes. A meat grinder, food processor, or sharp knife works well for preparing finely chopped meat.

After handling raw meat, be certain to use hot, soapy water to wash your hands, the utensils, and the work surfaces thoroughly. Raw meat commonly contains bacteria that can make you ill if the bacteria spread and multiply.

Marinating

Marinating imparts flavor to meat and tenderizes it at the same time. Marinades contain oil, an acid ingredient—vinegar or juice—for tenderizing, and seasonings for flavor.

Use marinades on the less-tender cuts of meat that you plan to cook by dry heat. In moist cooking (braising, simmering, stewing), the liquid used tends to dilute the flavor of the marinade. Also, moist cooking in itself tenderizes meat and makes the use of a marinade unnecessary.

Since the tenderizing effect penetrates meat to only a shallow depth, steaks, kabobs, and other small or flat cuts are more successfully tenderized with a marinade than are large cuts such as a rump roast. Use moist heat for cooking large cuts.

Commercial meat tenderizers made from papain (an enzyme in papaya) will also tenderize meats. Like a marinade, papain works best on flat cuts because penetration is not deep. Use commercial tenderizers sparingly; they can easily give meats a mushy surface.

To marinate: Soak meat for 3 to 24 hours in enough seasoned liquid to cover. Meat soaked for 24 hours will have more marinade flavor and be more tender than meat soaked for 3 or 4 hours. However, avoid marinating very small cubes of meat or extremely thin cuts for more than 4 hours. During lengthier marinating of small cuts, juices are extracted from the meat. And without those flavorful juices, the cooked meat will have a dry texture. Though meat can be marinated at room temperature, refrigeration is safest. The same marinade doubles as a tasty liquid that can be used to baste the meat during cooking.

Basic Marinade for Meat

A typical marinade that nicely flavors and tenderizes beef, lamb, or pork starts with a simple vinaigrette dressing such as this. It may be varied according to taste and to the ingredients you have on hand in the kitchen. This recipe yields enough marinade for 1 to 1½ pounds of meat. Double or triple the recipe if needed in order to completely cover the cut.

½ cup safflower, olive, or corn oil
3 to 4 tablespoons vinegar* or lemon juice (several lemon slices may be substituted)
2 cloves garlic, minced
1 tablespoon chopped mixed fresh herbs or 2 teaspoons dried herbs (parsley, tarragon, chives)

Combine all ingredients and blend well. Pour over meat, cover, and set aside to marinate.

Yields about ¾ cup

*Cider vinegar, red or white wine vinegar, or herb vinegar are equally good and impart subtle differences in flavor.

If an herb vinegar is used, you may omit the herbs called for in the recipe.

Variations:

Barbecue-Style Marinade for Meat: Add 2 teaspoons minced onions, Worcestershire sauce, soy sauce, or mustard as well as 1 tablespoon chili sauce, catsup, honey, or molasses.

Hot Marinade for Meat: Add 1 teaspoon crushed red pepper.

Preparing Variety Meats

For optimum flavor, appearance, and tenderness, variety meats need some preparation before cooking. Also, variety meats are highly perishable, so keep them well chilled until you are ready to clean and cook them. They should be cooked according to your favorite recipe no longer than 24 hours after preliminary cleansing, soaking, and simmering—although for best results, cooking should immediately follow this process. All variety meats should be eaten within 24 hours after being cooked.

Acidulated water is used in the preparation of some variety meats to retain whiteness. (Recipes using fruits or some other foods may also call for this.) To make acidulated water, mix one tablespoon of lemon juice or white vinegar with one quart of water. Use as directed.

To prepare variety meats for cooking, follow these procedures:

Liver: Rinse in cold water and remove the outer membrane if the butcher has not already done so. (This prevents curling during cooking.) Cut away large blood vessels. Broil, panbroil, panfry, bake, or use in a tasty casserole recipe.

Heart: Wash in warm water and remove all fat. Split open lengthwise, leaving halves attached on one side if the heart is to be stuffed. Cut out vessels and large tubes. Slice or stuff, then braise or simmer.

Kidney: Rinse in cool water. Peel off the outer membrane (if not already done by the butcher) and fat; then split in half lengthwise. Remove inner lobes of fat and tubes. Soak beef and pork kidneys in cold acidulated water or buttermilk for one hour. Rinse well, then simmer for one minute in fresh water before use in a recipe.

Tongue: Unlike other variety meats, the preparation of tongue (removing skin, root, bones, gristle) occurs after, rather than before, cooking it. For directions, see Boiled Fresh Tongue recipe, page 513.

Sweetbreads: Soak in cold acidulated water for 2 to 24 hours, changing the water occasionally during soaking. Remove the outer membrane, blood vessels, and connective tissue. Rinse, place in a saucepan, and cover with cold water. Bring slowly to a boil, then simmer for two to five minutes. (Sweetbreads will change color and become firm after two minutes.) Drain and cover with cold water until cool enough to handle. Remove the outer tissue, separating sweetbreads into small sections. Then braise, sauté, or broil as your recipe suggests.

Brains: Rinse in cold water to remove blood; then soak in cold acidulated water for 30 to 50 minutes. Rinse again and cut away blood vessels and excess connective tissue. Simmer gently in fresh acidulated water for 15 to 20 minutes until firm and white. Brains are now ready for sautéing or broiling, or use in your favorite recipe.

Tripe: Although fresh tripe is cooked before it is offered for sale, further cooking is necessary to tenderize it. Pull or cut all fat from the tripe and discard. Wash well with cold water and simmer in water to cover for 1½ to 2 hours. For pickled tripe, soak in cold water for 2 hours before using. Tripe is now ready for frying, creaming, or cooking according to your recipe directions.

Making Fresh Sausage

Making your own seasoned sausage is fun and easy. And you know the ingredients are natural, fresh, and wholesome.

Basically, fresh, homemade sausage contains meat, fat, and seasonings. Vegetables, grains, and dry milk solids may be added to increase nutrients as well as to change texture and flavor. While pork is the meat most commonly used to make sausage, beef and poultry are also good. Fat is a necessary ingredient; it adds flavor, binds the meat and the seasonings, and lubricates the casings. As a rule, one part fat to two parts meat makes a moist, juicy sausage. Less fat can be added, but the results will be a drier, meatier sausage. Because of its sweet flavor, pork fat is the most common type used.

The only equipment needed for making sausage is a meat grinder, a sharp knife, and, if you are making links, a funnel or a stuffing attachment for the meat grinder. For links you will also need to make your own muslin casings or to purchase animal casings (see Sausage Casings, page 470).

To make fresh sausage: Grind meat and fat in a meat grinder or finely chop with a knife. Blend the meat mixture and seasonings together in a bowl. Next, shape patties and loaves by hand, or fill casings using a funnel and the long handle of a wooden spoon, or the stuffing nozzle on the meat grinder. Do not overfill since overly plump casings tend to burst during filling or cooking. Break air bubbles with a pin; then twist or tie sausage to desired lengths.

NOTE: Never taste raw sausage made with uncooked pork or poultry. The meat may contain trichinae or salmonellae.

Fresh sausage may be stored in the refrigerator up to 3 days. For longer storage, freeze it — but it is best not to keep longer than six weeks. The high fat content in sausage encourages rancidity.

Sausage Casings

Casings made from pork, lamb, or beef intestines as well as those made from cloth, chicken skin, or pig's stomach help sausages retain their shape during cooking. Pork or lamb casings are a good size for small sausages that will be fried, and beef casings work well for large, boiling sausages. For the occasional very large sausage, muslin or cheesecloth does a nice job. Chicken skin casings, while tricky to handle, marry perfectly with poultry sausage. Those made from pig's stomach require special preparation from a butcher.

Animal casings can be purchased fresh or packed in salt. They are available from butchers or meat wholesalers, and are generally sold by the hank (6 to 8 feet of edible intestine casing).

Most recipes call for approximately four feet of 1-inch-diameter pork or lamb casings for every three pounds of sausage; one foot of 1½-inch-diameter pork or lamb casings for each pound of sausage; or two feet of 3- to 4-inch-diameter beef casings for every five pounds of sausage. However, you may end up using twice the quantity cited in a recipe since casings from intestines tear easily.

To prepare animal casings for use: If originally packed in salt, first soak them in lukewarm water for about 30 minutes to remove the packing salt, changing the water two or three times during soaking. Rinse under running water; then open and run cold water through the inside several times. Remove the inner membrane. Fill casings and tie off lengths with string. Store unused casings, packed in table salt, in a sealed plastic bag in the refrigerator or freezer. They will keep this way indefinitely.

To make a cloth casing: Cut cheesecloth or muslin into a long, narrow rectangle (15 by 6 inches). Dip the cloth into cold water; then wring out excess water and spread the cloth on a flat surface. Spoon sausage meat lengthwise down the center of the rectangle and fold the cloth over the meat. Roll to form a long, regular shape. Use string to tie the ends shut.

To make a chicken skin casing: Remove the skin from the bird carefully. A skin with no tears is easiest to stuff. Use string and toothpicks to secure.

Guidelines for Cooking and Serving Meat

Purchasing a specific cut of beef, lamb, pork, or veal by no means predetermines the final flavor and texture of the cooked meat. It is only a starting point. The cooking method and temperature used as well as the degree to which the meat is cooked will all affect its taste, appearance, and tenderness.

Tender and Less-Tender Cuts

Select a method of cooking that suits the cut (see Methods of Cooking Meat, page 474). The tender cuts (leg of lamb, tenderloin steak, pork loin roast) do well with dry heat methods such as roasting or broiling. Less-tender cuts (chuck roast, breast of lamb, pork shoulder steak) benefit from the moisture of braising and simmering.

The table on page 471 lists the various commercial cuts according to general tenderness. The most tender meat, of course, comes from that part of the animal which is the least active.

Another method to keep in mind while shopping for meat is that the shape of the bone is usually a good guide to the tenderness of that piece (see illustration below).

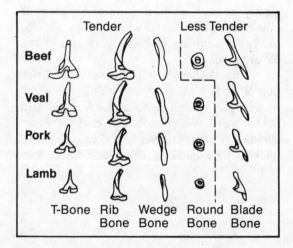

	Tender			Less Tender	
Beef					
Veal					
Pork					
Lamb					
	T-Bone	Rib Bone	Wedge Bone	Round Bone	Blade Bone

Tender and Less-Tender Cuts of Meat

Type of Meat	Tender Cut	Less-Tender Cut
Beef (mature cattle, 15-30 months old)	Rib — roast, steak Short loin — roast, steak Sirloin — steak	Brisket Chuck — roast, steak, pieces for stew Flank — steak Neck — pieces for stew Plate — short ribs, pieces for stew Round — roast, steak, pieces for stew Rump — roast Shank — pieces for stew
Lamb (young sheep, less than 1 year old)	Leg Loin — roast, chop Rib — roast, chop	Breast — roast, riblets Neck — slice Shank Shoulder — roast, chop, pieces for stew
Pork (hogs, less than 1 year old)	Bacon Ham, fresh or cured — whole, half, steak Loin — roast, chop, Canadian bacon, back ribs, tenderloin Spareribs	Boston shoulder, fresh or cured — roast, steak Feet Hock, fresh or cured Jowl Picnic shoulder, fresh or cured — roast, steak, pieces for stew
Veal (young cattle, less than 3 months old)	Loin — roast, steak, chop Rib — roast, steak, chop	Arm — roast, steak Breast — roast, riblets Leg — cutlet, steak, roast Neck — pieces for stew Rump — roast Shank Shoulder — roast, steak, pieces for stew

By looking at both bone shape and label information, you should be able to determine fairly accurately the best method of cooking your cut.

Temperature

As a rule, meats cooked at low to moderate temperatures (300 to 350°F) are the juiciest, most tender, and most flavorful. These meats have a pleasant aroma during cooking, and the color of the finished meat is fairly uniform throughout. Another advantage: The number of servings is maximized since there are fewer losses from shrinkage, dripping, and evaporation.

A few books still recommend searing meat to seal in juices (initially cooking meat at a high temperature, 400 to 500°F, then lowering the temperature for the remainder of the cooking period). In spite of this, it is generally accepted among food professionals that searing does not reduce dripping but actually encourages it. Meat exposed to a high temperature has a dark crust, excessive shrinkage, and often a tough, dry interior.

Always start cooking with meat at refrigerator temperature (32 to 40°F) or colder. While cooking is slightly faster and more even in meat at room temperature (60 to 80°F), allowing raw meat to warm to room temperature is an unsafe practice. During the time the meat takes to warm, bacteria — which thrive at temperatures between 50 and 140°F — will multiply rapidly. Large quantities of bacteria and their toxins can make you ill.

Cook meat without interruption until it is done. Never partially cook meat and then finish the cooking at another time. Partial cooking, which allows bacteria to build up, can make meat unsafe to eat.

Rare, Medium, or Well Done

When roasting or broiling beef or lamb, individual taste is the only important consideration guiding the degree to which the meat is cooked. Beef is tasty rare, medium, or well done. Rare beef has a brown exterior and deep red interior. Beef cooked to medium is light pink inside. Well-done beef is light brown throughout.

Americans tend to prefer lamb when it is either medium or well done. (It can also be served rare, as many Europeans enjoy it.) Medium-cooked lamb has a grayish tan interior with a tinge of pink. Well-done lamb is also grayish tan but it lacks the pink tinge.

To bring out the flavor and increase tenderness, veal and variety meats are generally cooked until they are well done. Veal roasted to this stage has a reddish brown exterior and gray interior. Well-done variety meats are brown, grayish, or creamy white, depending on the organ and species of meat.

To be sure that pork and sausage are safe to eat, they must be cooked until well done. Even with modern farming techniques and careful inspection, a small percentage of pork available on the market is infected with trichinae, microscopic organisms that can live in pork and be transmitted to you. If the organisms are not killed by thorough cooking, severe illness can result when the meat is eaten.

Cured pork (ham) labeled "cook before eating" must also be cooked until well done. Cured pork marked "fully cooked" may be heated to improve flavor. If you are uncertain whether a ham is fully cooked, cook it thoroughly, just as you would a cook-before-eating ham.

Although many meats are cooked to the well-done stage (in addition to pork, meats cooked by moist heat are always well done), it is essential to avoid overcooking. When overdone, meats become dry, stringy, and flavorless. Prevent overcooking by using a table of cooking times to estimate the length of cooking needed (see Roasting table, page 475, Broiling table, page 477, Braising table, page 479, or Simmering table, page 480) and by using a test to determine the stage of readiness of the meat.

Why Cooking Time of Meat Varies

The time it takes to cook meat will be longer or shorter depending on the following factors:

Temperature of the meat at the start of cooking: Frozen meat takes one-third to one-half longer cooking time than meat at refrigerator temperature.

Size of the roast: A small roast requires less time to cook than a large one, even though total cooking time is not directly proportional to size.

Thickness of the cut: A thick cut takes longer to cook than a thin one of the same weight.

Fat cover: A roast with an outside layer of fat takes longer to cook than one with little or no fat cover.

Amount of bone: Boneless and rolled roasts need more cooking time per pound than meats with the bone in.

Extent of aging: Aged meat cooks slightly faster than meat that has not been aged.

Testing Methods: There are four quick, easy ways to test how well cooked your meat is. One test is usually enough to determine doneness, but occasionally it is helpful to use two or more methods.

• *Internal temperature.* Checking the internal temperature with a meat thermometer is the most accurate means of knowing when the meat is done. Unfortunately, it is efficient only for testing large roasts cooked by dry heat. (See Using a Meat Thermometer, opposite.)

• *Fork-tenderness.* This method is best for testing braised, simmered, or stewed meats. Insert a slender, two-pronged fork into the meat near the end of the suggested cooking time. When the meat is cooked to tenderness, the fork will slide in easily.

• *Tenderness to touch.* An old-fashioned test still popular with some cooks is to prod the meat with your finger. If the meat feels soft, it is rare; if hard, it is well done. The feel of medium-done meat is in between.

• *Color of meat and juices.* Usually, this is the best way to test small cuts that are broiled, panbroiled, or panfried. With a sharp knife make a very small slit near the bone (if there is no bone, cut into the middle or thickest part). Check the color of the meat and its juice. Rare meat is dark red with red juice; medium-done meat is pink in the middle with light pink juice; and well-done meat is grayish brown throughout with clear to slightly yellow juice.

Pan Juice and Gravy

The drippings left in the pan after roasting, broiling, panbroiling, or panfrying meat can be used as the base for a flavorful gravy or deglazed and served as a natural juice topping for the meat.

To make pan juice: First, skim off any fat. Then, add a little water or stock, place the pan over medium heat, and use a wooden spoon to scrape the brown particles from the bottom and sides of the pan, mixing them into the liquid. Cook for a few minutes to reduce the juice if the flavor is too diluted, and serve.

To make pan gravy: See the directions on page 141, Gravy for Meat and Poultry.

Using a Meat Thermometer

A meat thermometer is the best guide to determining the degree to which a roast has been cooked—rare, medium, or well done. The cooking stages for different types of meat are noted on its head, but the number and completeness of these markings may vary among the different brands of thermometers. Because of this, it is best to look at a roasting table to locate the temperature needed for cooking your specific cut of meat to the desired stage.

To use the thermometer, insert it as near the center of the roast as possible, in the middle of the thickest part. The tip should not touch bone or fat.

Check the thermometer 20 to 30 minutes before the meat should be done. If the needle registers 5°F below the desired temperature, remove the roast from the oven and allow to rest. During this period, the internal temperature will rise to the correct degree.

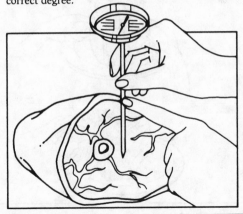

Carving Meat

Once your roast or steak has been cooked, carving it will be easy if you follow these basic steps:

1. Determine the direction of the grain in the meat and the position of the bone, if any.

2. Anchor the meat firmly with a curved, two-pronged fork. Because juices escape each

time the fork pierces the meat, place the fork so that you avoid moving it too often.

3. Use a sharp carving knife and, for most roasts, slice across the grain. Steaks which are very tender may be cut with the grain; brisket of beef and flank steaks should be sliced at a 45-degree angle to get large serving pieces. Use a gentle sawing motion as you slice, and do not change the angle of the knife once you have started cutting.

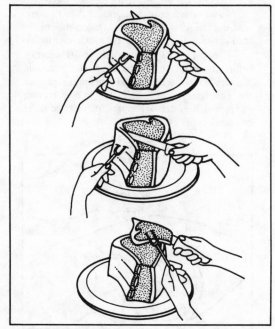

Carving Beef

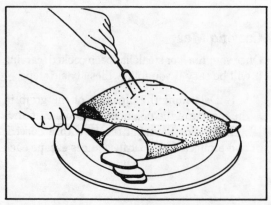

Carving Lamb

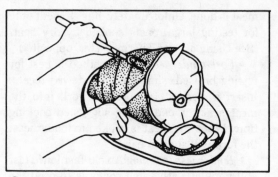

Carving Ham

Reheating Meat

Leftovers from roasts lend themselves best to new dishes such as casseroles and soups. However, they can be very tasty by themselves when reheated using any of these suggestions:

• Thinly slice the meat, place it on a heated plate, and smother with hot gravy or a tasty sauce. Serve the dish immediately.

• Put the roast on a rack in a shallow baking pan. Place it, uncovered, on the top shelf of a 300°F oven; set a pan of hot water on the lower shelf. Heat for about 30 minutes.

• Place thin slices of meat in a shallow, ungreased baking pan and top with a gravy or sauce. Cover the pan with foil and heat for 20 minutes in a 350°F oven.

• Combine thin slices of meat with gravy or sauce in a skillet. Cover tightly and warm over low heat for 5 to 10 mintues.

Methods of Cooking Meat

New cooks who are intimidated by the challenge of finishing meat just right can feel confident about results if they use the basic methods that follow. The aim of retaining moisture and flavor often depends on the choice of cooking method, so consider carefully the suggestions for the various kinds and cuts of meat before you begin.

Roasting

Roasting, which cooks meat by warm, dry air, is ideal for cooking large (over four pounds), tender roasts such as beef ribs, pork loin, and leg of lamb.

To roast: Place chilled meat, fat-side up, on a wire rack set in a large shallow pan. By putting the fat side on top, the melting fat bastes the meat during roasting. The shallow pan and the rack allow air to circulate around the entire piece of meat. The rack also keeps the meat away from any moist drippings. Rib roasts can be roasted without a rack since the bones act as a natural one.

A crown (rib) roast can be roasted without a rack if it is to be filled with a cooked vegetable. Just cook the roast upside down and the bones will act as a natural rack. If the roast is to be filled with a stuffing, place the meat on a rack with bone tips facing up, and cover the tips with foil before roasting. Remove the roast one hour before it is done and fill with a favorite bread stuffing, then continue roasting until the meat is cooked. (Each bone tip may be decorated with a paper frill before serving, for a festive touch.)

When roasting any cut, leave meat uncovered—a cover will lock in steam and result in cooking the meat with moisture. For the same reason, do not add liquid to the pan.

For juicy, tender roasts, an oven temperature between 300 and 350°F is best. Unfortunately, many ovens have faulty thermostats. If you suspect your meat is browning too quickly, check the oven temperature with an oven thermometer; then reset the oven to compensate for the difference.

You can season meats either before or after roasting since the flavors imparted by herbs and spices remain near the surface of the meat. But, seasoning at the beginning creates a delightful aroma during cooking.

A roast may be cooked until it is rare, medium, or well done (see discussion on page 472), depending on personal preference and on the type of meat (pork must always be well done). The amount of time needed for roasting depends on several factors (see Why Cooking Time of Meat Varies, page 472). Therefore, although some cooks follow a prescribed formula of minutes per pound to cook a roast, more accurate and consistent results can be achieved by using the Roasting table, below, to find the approximate cooking time needed for your cut of meat. Also inserting a meat thermometer into the roast is the safest way to determine when the meat is cooked to your liking (see Using a Meat Thermometer, page 473). Since roasts are large and therefore more expensive cuts, a thermometer is a good investment if you do not already have one.

Cooking Times for Meat: Roasting

Cut of Meat	Weight (pounds)	Approximate Cooking Time at 325°F* (hours)	Internal Temperature of Meat When Done (°F)
Beef			
Rib roast, boneless, rolled			
Rare	5–7	2⅔–3¾	140
Medium	5–7	3¼–4½	160
Well done	5–7	4–5⅔	170
Rump roast, boneless rolled	4–6	2–2½	150–170
Sirloin tip roast	3½–4	2⅓	140–170
	6–8	3½–4	140–170

*Time is based on meat being at refrigerator temperature at start of roasting.

[continued]

Cooking Times for Meat: Roasting—*Continued*

Cut of Meat	Weight (pounds)	Approximate Cooking Time at 325°F* (hours)	Internal Temperature of Meat When Done (°F)
Beef *(continued)*			
Standing rib roast†			
Rare	4-6	2¼-2½	140
Medium	4-6	2½-3½	160
Well done	4-6	2¾-4	170
Rare	6-8	2½-3	140
Medium	6-8	3-3½	160
Well done	6-8	3½-4¼	170
Lamb			
Leg	5-8	3-4	170-180
Leg, boneless, rolled	3-5	2-3	170-180
Rib roast (rack)	4-5	3-3⅓	170-180
Shoulder roast	4-6	2⅓-3	170-180
Shoulder roast, boneless, rolled	3-5	2¼-3⅓	170-180
Shoulder roast, boneless, cushion-style	3-5	1¾-2½	170-180
Pork			
Fresh‡			
Ham	12-16	5½-6	170-180
Half	5-7	5-5½	170-180
Boneless, rolled	10-14	4⅔-5½	170-180
Loin, center-cut	3-5	2-4	170-180
Picnic shoulder roast	5-8	3-5	170-180
Picnic shoulder roast, boneless, rolled	3-5	2-3	170-180
Shoulder butt roast (Boston butt)	4-6	3-4	170-180
Shoulder butt roast (Boston butt), boneless, rolled	3-5	2¼-3¼	170-180
Spareribs	3-4	2	. . .
Cured, cook-before-eating‡			
Canadian bacon	2-4	1⅓-2½	160
Ham	5-7	2-2½	160
	10-14	3½-4¼	160
Picnic shoulder, boneless	5-8	3-4⅔	170
Shoulder butt, boneless	2-4	1½-2⅓	170
Cured, fully cooked			
Ham	5-7	2	140
	12-16	3½-4	140
Ham, canned, boneless	6-10	1½-2½	140
Veal			
Leg roast	5-8	3-3⅓	170
Loin roast	4-6	2⅓-3	170
Rib roast	3-5	2-3	170
Shoulder roast, boneless, rolled	3-5	2¼-3½	170

*Time is based on meat being at refrigerator temperature at start of roasting.
†Roasting time is for 8-inch ribs; for 10-inch ribs allow about 30 minutes less time.
‡Pork must be cooked until well done.

Plan to finish roasting 20 to 30 minutes before serving time so that the meat can rest. During that time, the meat will continue to cook somewhat. Meat that has been allowed to rest retains juice when carved and cuts more easily.

Roasted meats are delightful when served plain with a simple garnish, crisp green salad, and hearty whole grain biscuits. On other occasions, present them lightly sauced with their own, warmed pan juice or a hot, savory gravy.

Broiling

Broiling cooks meat by dry, direct heat. This method is nicely suited to cuts that are at least three-quarters inch thick—beefsteaks, lamb chops, ham slices, and ground beef or lamb patties.

Thinner cuts, along with pork chops, which must be well done, and veal chops, which are very lean, become too dry under the intense heat.

To broil: Score fat every two inches around the edge of the meat to prevent curling. Place meat on a cold broiler grid. If the meat is very lean, oil the grid lightly to prevent sticking.

Use a preheated broiler and cook the meat two to five inches from the heat, depending on thickness. To avoid excessive browning on the outside, place thick pieces and frozen pieces, both of which take longer to cook, farther from the heat (or adjust the thermostat, if possible).

When the meat is half done and lightly browned on the top, turn it over. (See Broiling table, below, for cooking times.) To preserve tasty juices, use tongs for turning instead of a fork.

Cooking Times for Meat: Broiling

Cut of Meat	Thickness (inches)	Approximate Cooking Time* (minutes)		
		Rare	Medium	Well Done
Beef				
Ground (patty)	¾	. . .	12	14
Steak—club, porterhouse, rib, sirloin,				
T-bone, tenderloin	1	15-20	20-25	25-30
	1½	25-30	30-35	35-40
	2	35-40	40-45	45-55
Lamb				
Chop—loin, rib, shoulder	1	. . .	12	14
	1½	. . .	18	22
Ground (patty)	1	. . .	15-18	20
Steak—leg	1	. . .	12-14	16-18
Pork, cured				
Bacon (slice)	. . .	. . .	. . .	4-5
Canadian bacon (slice)	¼	. . .	. . .	6-8
	½	. . .	. . .	8-10
Ham (slice), cook-before-eating	¾	. . .	. . .	13-14
	1	. . .	. . .	18-20
Ham (slice), fully cooked	1	. . .	. . .	10
Veal†				
Ground (patty)	¾	. . .	. . .	15

*Time is based on meat being at refrigerator temperature at start of broiling.
†Except for veal patties, broiling is not recommended for cuts of veal.

Seasonings or sauces nicely accent broiled meats. Baste with the sauce (or marinade, if one was used) during the last few minutes of cooking. Add seasonings after the meat has browned on top and been turned over.

Charcoal broiling (grilling) over hot coals may cause harmful changes in the meat. Broiling *under* the heat source is therefore the preferred method.

Panbroiling

Panbroiling, which cooks meat over moderately hot, dry heat, is excellent for cooking tender beefsteaks, ham steaks, and lamb chops as well as ground meat patties. Cuts less than three-quarters inch thick are best suited to panbroiling.

To panbroil: Score the edge of the meat every two inches to prevent curling and, if the meat is very lean, rub the skillet lightly with vegetable oil. Preheat the skillet to a moderate temperature and then add the meat. For an even brown color, turn the meat frequently with tongs. Remove drippings as they accumulate; otherwise, moist heat will actually cook the meat. Continually regulate the heat under the skillet since an overly hot pan will burn the fat, producing an unpleasant aroma and flavor.

Seasonings lend variety to the flavors of panbroiled meats. Season with herbs and spices after cooking, or serve meat with a complementary chutney or other condiment.

Panfrying

Panfrying, sometimes called sautéing, is a tasty, quick way of cooking tender steaks, chops, and patties that are less than an inch thick. Because panfried meat is cooked, uncovered, in a small amount of fat, it has a nicely browned, crisp crust.

To panfry: Score the edges of the meat to prevent curling during cooking. For an extra-crisp exterior, coat the meat with whole grain flour, cornmeal, or fine, dry bread crumbs (mixed with crushed dried herbs for added flavor). Or, a thicker breading may be used (see page 528 for preparation directions). Chill breaded meat for several minutes to set the coating.

Meanwhile, melt one or two tablespoons of butter in a skillet (or use half butter and half vegetable oil). Add the meat when the pan is moderately hot. Turn occasionally with tongs to brown the meat evenly on both sides. When the meat is done, remove it with a slotted spoon or tongs and drain on paper towels.

Serve panfried meat plain or with a piquant sauce. Raw vegetable garnishes give pleasant texture and color contrasts to these meats.

Braising

Braising cooks meat very slowly with moist heat. It is ideal for cooking the less-tender beef, lamb, and pork roasts as well as chops and steaks.

To braise: Heat a small amount of vegetable oil in a heavy saucepan and brown the meat slowly and evenly on all sides. Use only enough oil to keep the meat from sticking to the pan and, for a rich brown color, flour the meat first. When the meat is brown, add up to one-half cup of liquid (some large cuts are so juicy they need no extra liquid). Then, cover the pan with a tight-fitting lid and simmer slowly on the stove top or in a 325 to 350°F oven (for cooking times, see Braising table, page 479). If the liquid cooks away, add more as needed. But avoid using too much—it dilutes the rich flavor of braised meat. Do not let the liquid boil since high heat causes meat to become tough and stringy.

Using broth or vegetable juices instead of water as the cooking medium enhances the taste

Cooking Times for Meat: Braising

Cut of meat	Weight (pounds)	Thickness (inches)	Approximate Cooking Time* (hours)
Beef			
Pieces for stew	. . .	1½ × 1½	1½-2½
Pot roast—chuck, round	3-5	. . .	3-4
Short ribs	. . .	2 × 4	1½-2½
Steak—chuck, round	. . .	¾-1	1-1½
Steak—flank	. . .	½	1½-2
Lamb			
Breast, boneless, rolled	1½-2	. . .	1½-2
Breast, stuffed	2-3	. . .	1½-2
Chop—shoulder	. . .	¾-1	¾-1
Neck (slice)	. . .	¾	1
Pieces for stew	. . .	1½ × 1½	1½-2
Riblets	. . .	. . .	1½-2
Shank	¾-1	. . .	1½-2
Pork			
Chop—rib, loin	. . .	¾-1½	¾-1
Pieces for stew	. . .	1 × 1	¾-1
Spareribs	2-3	. . .	1½
Steak—shoulder	. . .	¾	¾-1
Veal			
Chop	. . .	½-¾	¾-1
Pieces for stew—shoulder	. . .	1 × 1	1½-2
Shoulder roast, boneless, rolled	3-5	. . .	2-2½
Steak and cutlet	. . .	½-¾	¾-1

*Cooking time is for meat braised at simmering temperature. Time needed for braising in a pressure cooker is considerably shorter; follow pressure cooker manufacturer's directions. Time is based on meat being at refrigerator temperature at start of braising.

and richness of braised meats. And, adding finely chopped vegetables during the last few minutes of cooking mellows and merges the flavors of both the braised meat and the vegetables. Puree the vegetables together with the cooking liquid and use this as a sauce for the meat.

Simmering

Simmering, sometimes called poaching, cooks meat with moisture and is ideal for cooking large cuts of less-tender meats—brisket of beef; veal shanks; boneless pork shoulder butt; boneless, rolled breast of lamb.

To simmer: Brown the meat in a small amount of fat in a large, heavy saucepan. (Browning most cuts is optional, but never brown cured meat.) Pour in enough water or broth to cover the meat, then add your favorite seasonings—and, perhaps, a bay leaf, a few whole peppercorns, a celery stalk, a carrot, and a small, whole onion. Cover with a tight-fitting lid and cook slowly over low heat or in a 325°F oven (see Simmering table, page 480, to determine cooking time). Do not boil; high heat produces stringy meat that is difficult to cut and chew.

Cold, simmered meat has more flavor and juice if it has been chilled quickly in the stock in which it was cooked than if the stock were drained from the meat before chilling. These meats work well as the main ingredient in salads and sandwiches.

Stewing

As a moist heat method of cooking, stewing is ideal for tenderizing cuts of beef, lamb, pork, and veal that have been cut into either one-inch cubes or thin strips.

To stew: Trim excess fat from meat cubes and dredge the cubes in whole grain flour. In a heavy saucepan brown the cubes in one or two tablespoons of vegetable oil. (Veal, however, is usually not floured and browned.) Drain off any excess fat and cover the meat with liquid—water, broth, vegetable juice. Add seasonings, garlic, and onions; then cover the pot with a tight-fitting lid. Cook the meat slowly—do not allow it to boil (for cooking times, see Simmering table, below). If necessary, add more liquid.

Vegetables and grains such as rice or barley make tasty additions to any stew. Add these ingredients at appropriate times during cooking and increase the cooking liquid as needed.

Cooking Times for Meat: Simmering

Cut of meat	Weight (pounds)	Approximate Cooking Time* (hours)
Beef		
Fresh		
Brisket	8	4-5
Pieces for stew (1½-inch cubes)	...	2½-3
Plate	8	4-5
Shank	4	3-4
Corned		
Brisket (whole)	8	4-5
Brisket (piece)	3	3-3¾
Lamb		
Pieces for stew (1½-inch cubes)	...	1½-2
Pork		
Fresh		
Hock	¾-1	2½-3
Cured		
Ham, country-style (whole)	12-16	4-5
Ham—shank or butt	5-8	2-3
Picnic shoulder	5-8	3-4
Shoulder butt, boneless	2-3	1½-2
Veal		
Pieces for stew (1½-inch cubes)	...	2-3
Shank	¾-1	2-3

*Time is based on meat being at refrigerator temperature at start of simmering.

Using a Slow Cooker or Pressure Cooker

Slow cookers and pressure cookers both cook meat by moist heat and are ideal for the busy person who has little time to spend in the kitchen. Because slow cookers are regulated by a thermostat, they can be left untended to cook meat gently for several hours. Temperatures are kept low, so the cooked meat is tender, flavorful, and juicy. Pressure cookers, on the other hand, cook meat in just minutes, using 10 to 15 pounds of pressure. Here, the temperatures are fairly high, so pressure-cooked meat tends to be slightly stringy and light on flavor and juice. To use either appliance to best advantage, follow the manufacturer's instructions.

Cooking Variety Meats

Depending on tenderness, variety meats can benefit from cooking with either dry or moist heat. All lamb variety meats, as well as pork brains, beef brains, beef sweetbreads, calf's liver, and veal kidney, are tender and well suited to panfrying and broiling. On the other hand, pork liver, kidney, and heart, along with beef heart, tongue, tripe, liver, kidney, and oxtail, are less tender and do best with braising and simmering, although sometimes dry heat methods are used in a recipe. (See Preparing Variety Meats, page 468, for preliminary cooking procedures.) Variety meats work well in casseroles and with chutneys, piquant sauces, and other condiments.

Cooking Sausage

Fully cooked sausage: Fully cooked sausage is tasty when broiled, panfried, or simmered. Since it needs only to be heated, cooking time will be short.

To broil: Brush either links or patties with vegetable oil and place them on a lightly oiled broiler pan. Broil three inches from the heat for four to five minutes, turning often with tongs. Heat until evenly browned. Links are also tasty when split lengthwise, brushed with melted butter, and broiled for two minutes on each side.

To panfry: Heat one to two tablespoons of butter or vegetable oil in a heavy skillet and fry links or patties for three to five minutes. Turn them frequently to brown evenly. Links can also be split lengthwise and browned on each side for about two minutes.

To simmer: Bring water to a simmer; then drop in links. Cover pan and simmer gently for five to eight minutes. Do not boil.

Fresh sausage: Fresh sausage containing pork must be cooked until well done. For moist, nicely browned sausage, cook in liquid first; then broil or panfry. Baking sausage slowly also preserves juiciness and enhances color.

To simmer: Place links or patties in a cold skillet with two to four tablespoons of water. Cover the pan with a tight-fitting lid and simmer the sausage until thoroughly cooked (10 to 30 minutes, depending on size). Drain and serve immediately, or brown first, by broiling or panfrying. If the sausage has a cheesecloth or muslin casing, remove it before browning. Otherwise, puncture cased sausage with a fork in several places to keep skins from bursting while browning.

To broil: Brush simmered sausage with melted butter or vegetable oil and place on a lightly oiled broiler pan. Broil until evenly browned (five to eight minutes), turning often with tongs.

To panfry: Brown simmered sausage in one to two tablespoons of melted butter or vegetable oil in a heavy skillet. For convenience, use the same pan in which the sausage was simmered. Turn sausage often for an even color. (For extra crispness, dry the sausage and dredge in flour before panfrying.)

To bake: Spread links or patties in a single layer in a shallow roasting pan. (Prick cased sausage with a fork in several places.) Cover with foil and bake at 350°F for 10 to 15 minutes, depending on size. Uncover and continue to bake 10 to 15 minutes longer, until lightly browned and thoroughly cooked. During baking, turn sausage often with tongs and remove the drippings as they accumulate.

Cooking Game

When purchased from the butcher, game—venison, rabbit, squirrel—generally needs no special preparation since it has already been cleaned. Wild game, on the other hand, needs careful cleaning that is best described in a good hunting manual.

Game can be roasted, braised, or stewed in the manner described for beef, lamb, pork, and veal. Choose the method of cooking appropriate to the age of the animal and the tenderness of the meat. Roast the tender ones, and braise or stew the less tender.

Beef

Basic Beef Pot Roast

3 to 4 pounds chuck roast, blade roast, boneless
      neck, rump roast, or lean brisket
  1 clove garlic, halved
  ½ cup whole wheat flour
  2 tablespoons vegetable oil
    pepper, to taste
  1 teaspoon dried thyme
  1 teaspoon dried marjoram
  ½ teaspoon dried basil
  ½ teaspoon Worcestershire sauce
1½ cups water, Beef Stock (page 110), or tomato
    juice

  1 bay leaf
  1 small onion, stuck with 2 cloves
  ¼ cup chopped green peppers
  4 carrots, cut into 1½-inch pieces
  2 medium-size potatoes or sweet potatoes,
    quartered
  ½ cup cold water

Trim fat from meat. Rub meat on all sides with garlic, then dredge in ¼ cup flour.

Heat oil in a Dutch oven or roasting pan and brown meat slowly on all sides. Pour off excess fat.

Sprinkle meat with pepper, thyme, marjoram, basil, and Worcestershire sauce. Add water, stock, or tomato juice, then bay leaf, onion, and green peppers. Cover pan and simmer on top of stove for 1½ hours; or, bake, covered, at 325°F for 1½ hours. Add carrots and potatoes (and extra liquid, if needed). Cover and cook or bake for another 45 minutes, or until vegetables are tender.

Transfer meat and vegetables to a platter and keep warm. Remove onion and bay leaf and discard. Pour meat juice into a large measuring glass or bowl, and skim off fat from surface. Measure out 1½ cups, adding water if necessary to make the full amount, and return this to Dutch oven or roasting pan.

Blend water together with remaining ¼ cup flour in a measuring cup or bowl and stir until smooth. Add flour mixture to meat juice. Stir over medium heat until thickened and bubbly, then cook 1 to 2 minutes longer. Serve gravy with meat and vegetables.

8 servings

Boiled Beef with Dill Sauce

3 to 3½ pounds lean brisket
    1 medium-size onion, quartered
    1 carrot, quartered
    1 teaspoon celery seeds
    2 peppercorns
    Dill Sauce (see page 483)

Place meat, onions, carrots, celery seeds, and peppercorns in a Dutch oven. Add enough boiling water to cover. Bring water to a boil again, then reduce heat, cover, and simmer for 2½ hours, or until tender.

Drain meat (reserving liquid for use in a soup), then thinly slice across the grain. Serve with dill sauce.

6 servings

Dill Sauce

3½ cups Beef Stock (page 110)
3 tablespoons cornstarch
1 tablespoon butter
3 tablespoons lemon juice
¼ teaspoon garlic powder
¼ cup chopped fresh dill
1 cup sour cream
1 tablespoon horseradish, drained (optional)

Bring 3 cups stock to a boil in a 1-quart saucepan. Mix cornstarch with remaining ½ cup stock and add to saucepan gradually, stirring with a wire whisk. Continue to boil, stirring constantly, until mixture thickens. Add butter, lemon juice, garlic powder, and dill. Reduce heat and cook 5 minutes longer. Thin sour cream with some of the hot liquid and stir into saucepan along with horseradish (if used). Heat through but do not boil.

Yields about 3½ cups

Cider Chuck Roast with Vegetables

The combination of cider and spices in this recipe will present you and your guests with a flavorful chuck roast like no other. Be sure to allow for overnight marinating of the meat.

3 pounds boneless chuck roast, trimmed of fat
2 cups apple cider, or more as needed
1 tablespoon each peppercorns, whole cloves, and celery seeds
1 tablespoon whole allspice or ½ teaspoon ground allspice
1 tablespoon mustard seeds or ½ teaspoon dry mustard
3 bay leaves
1 tablespoon vegetable oil
1 large onion, chopped
4 large potatoes or sweet potatoes, cut into thirds
½ pound fresh green beans, cut into 2-inch lengths

Place meat in a glass or ceramic bowl and add enough cider to completely cover it. Add spices and bay leaves. Marinate overnight in refrigerator, turning meat over once.

Lift meat out of marinade and scrape all seeds off with the back of a table knife. Strain marinade and set aside.

Heat oil in a Dutch oven. Wipe meat dry with paper towels, then brown on all sides in hot oil, adding onions about halfway through browning. Pour enough marinade into pot to make a depth of 1 inch. Cover and simmer for 3 hours, or until meat is tender. Check liquid level from time to time, adding more marinade if needed.

Reduce remaining marinade to ½ cup by boiling it, uncovered, in a small saucepan. Add reduced marinade, potatoes, and green beans to meat. Cover and continue to simmer for 15 to 20 minutes, or until vegetables are tender. Skim fat from pan juice, then serve with meat and vegetables.

6 servings

Fruited Pot Roast

3 tablespoons vegetable oil
4 to 5 pounds rump or chuck roast, trimmed of fat
3 medium-size onions, coarsely chopped
¼ teaspoon ground cloves
2 cups apple juice or cider
10 ounces pitted dried prunes (1½ cups)
½ pound dried apricots (1½ cups)
2 to 4 tablespoons cornstarch, dissolved in ¼ cup cold water (optional)

Heat oil in a Dutch oven or roasting pan and brown meat on all sides. Add onions, cloves, and apple juice or cider. Cover tightly, then reduce heat and simmer for 2 hours, or until nearly tender. Or, cover and bake at 350°F for 2½ hours.

Add prunes and apricots and continue to cook or bake 30 minutes longer.

If desired, thicken liquid in pot by removing meat and adding cornstarch mixture. Cook until thickened, stirring constantly. Serve over meat and fruit.

10 servings

Sauerbraten

This is an entrée fit for a special dinner, and well worth the planning. Allow 48 hours for marinating the meat and another 3 hours of simmering to make it fork-tender.

3 to 3½ pounds boneless round or rump roast
    ½ teaspoon freshly ground pepper
    2 medium-size onions, sliced
    1 large carrot, shredded or sliced
    1 stalk celery, chopped
    6 whole cloves
    2 bay leaves
    4 whole allspice
    ½ teaspoon peppercorns
  1¾ cups red wine vinegar
  1½ cups water
    2 tablespoons vegetable oil

    Gravy
    2 cups reserved marinade
    2 tablespoons vegetable oil
  2½ tablespoons potato or rye flour
    ½ cup cold water
    ½ cup yogurt (optional)

    chopped fresh parsley

Trim fat from meat, then rub with pepper and place in a large glass bowl or deep earthenware crock. Add onions, carrots, celery, cloves, bay leaves, allspice, and peppercorns.

Combine vinegar and water in a saucepan and bring to a boil. Cool slightly, then pour over meat, vegetables, and spices. Cool completely. Cover and marinate in refrigerator for 48 hours or more, turning several times a day.

When ready to cook, lift out meat (reserving marinade) and wipe dry with paper towels. Heat oil in a Dutch oven and brown meat on all sides. Pour reserved marinade into pot so that it reaches not more than halfway up sides of meat. Cover tightly and simmer slowly for about 3 hours, or until fork-tender.

Transfer meat to a warm platter (again reserving marinade) and keep hot while preparing gravy.

To make the gravy: Strain hot marinade, measure 2 cups, and set aside. Heat oil in a 1-quart saucepan over medium heat. Add flour and stir until mixture bubbles. Gradually blend in water and marinade,

stirring constantly. Cook until mixture thickens. Add yogurt (if used).

Slice sauerbraten and ladle some hot gravy over meat. Garnish with parsley. Pour remaining gravy into sauceboat. Sauerbraten is traditionally served with Spaetzle (page 345) or *Lefse* (page 236).

6 servings

Marinated Chuck Roast with Mustard Sauce

The marinade tenderizes and flavors; then the sauce makes a company dish out of a budget cut of beef.

    3 pounds boneless chuck roast, 2 inches thick, or 3½ pounds chuck roast with bones
    1 cup white or cider vinegar
    1 large onion, finely chopped
    1 carrot, finely chopped
    1 stalk celery, finely chopped
    2 cloves garlic, minced
    1 tablespoon dried tarragon
    1 teaspoon dried thyme
    ¼ teaspoon pepper
    1 bay leaf
    1 tablespoon vegetable oil
    1 cup water

    Sauce
    reserved pan juice
    1 cup heavy cream
    1 tablespoon cornstarch, dissolved in ¼ cup cold water
    1 tablespoon French-style mustard
    1 teaspoon grated horseradish

Trim fat from meat.

In a large ceramic or glass bowl combine vinegar, onions, carrots, celery, garlic, tarragon, thyme, pepper, and bay leaf. With a sharp fork prick meat on both sides. Place meat in marinade, cover, and refrigerate for 6 hours or more, turning meat about 4 times during that period. When ready to cook, drain and discard liquid, reserving chopped vegetable mixture. Wipe meat dry with paper towels.

Preheat oven to 350°F.

Heat oil in a large ovenproof skillet or Dutch oven and brown meat on all sides. Add reserved vegetable mixture and water. Cover and bake for 2 hours, or until meat is tender.

Remove and slice meat, cover, and keep warm. Reserve pan juice.

To make the sauce: Strain pan juice; discard solids. Skim fat off, then measure juice and return it to pan. If there is more than ½ cup juice, reduce it to that amount by boiling rapidly, uncovered. Add cream and cornstarch mixture to the ½ cup pan juice and cook over medium heat, stirring constantly, until thickened and bubbly. Whisk in mustard and horseradish. To serve, pour some sauce over meat. Pass the rest in a gravy boat at the table.

6 servings

Chili Beef Hash in Baked Potato Shells

For a special brunch this combination is hard to beat. It is also a natural for hungry teenagers who thrive on hearty fare–and a good way to use that leftover roast.

    4 large baking potatoes
      vegetable oil
 1¾ cups diced cooked beef (about ½ pound)
    1 small onion, halved
    2 tablespoons butter
  ½ teaspoon Worcestershire sauce (optional)
    1 egg, beaten
  ½ cup coarsely grated cheese

    Topping
  ¼ cup olive oil
    1 medium-size onion, chopped
    3 large tomatoes, peeled and chopped
  ¼ teaspoon garlic powder
½ to 1 teaspoon chili powder, to taste
    1 cup cooked kidney beans, drained

Preheat oven to 400°F.

Rub potatoes with a small amount of oil, prick them with a fork, and bake for 1 hour. When potatoes are done, split them lengthwise and gently scoop out pulp without damaging skins. Place potato shells in a shallow baking dish. Cut pulp into pieces and set aside.

Coarsely chop beef and onion in a food processor. Melt butter in a large skillet. Add chopped beef and onions to skillet and sauté until onions are golden.

Add potato pulp and sauté until lightly browned. Stir in Worcestershire sauce (if used). Remove from heat and allow mixture to cool slightly, then stir in egg.

Divide hash evenly among potato shells and top each with a tablespoon of cheese. Bake at 350°F for 10 to 15 minutes, or until cheese melts. Meanwhile, prepare the topping.

To make the topping: Heat oil in a medium-size skillet. Add onions and sauté until golden. Add tomatoes, garlic powder, chili powder, and kidney beans. Cook until just heated through. To serve, spoon hot topping over hash-filled potato shells.

4 servings

Braised Short Ribs

    2 pounds lean short ribs
    2 cloves garlic, crushed
¼ to ⅓ cup whole wheat flour
    2 tablespoons vegetable oil
    1 large onion, chopped
  ½ pound mushrooms, sliced
  ½ cup Beef Stock (page 110) or water
    1 cup chopped tomatoes
    1 bay leaf
      pepper, to taste
    2 carrots, chopped
    2 stalks celery, chopped
    1 green pepper, cut into chunks
    2 tablespoons chopped fresh parsley
    2 potatoes, cut into chunks
    1 tablespoon sour cream (optional)

Cut ribs into serving pieces. Rub pieces with garlic and dredge in flour.

Preheat oven to 325°F.

Heat oil in a Dutch oven and brown floured ribs on all sides. Add onions, mushrooms, stock, tomatoes, bay leaf, and pepper. Cover and bake for 1½ to 2 hours, or until meat is nearly tender. (Or, cook over moderate heat on top of the stove.) Add carrots, celery, green peppers, parsley, and potatoes and continue baking or cooking until vegetables are tender. Remove from heat and skim off fat. Discard bay leaf. If used, add sour cream to pan liquid and stir until combined.

4 to 6 servings

Tzimmes

*Short ribs, squash, and dried fruits combine
to form this Jewish dish traditionally served
at harvesttime.*

     6 lean short ribs
     1 cup chopped onions
    1½ cups Beef Stock (page 110)
     1 teaspoon paprika
     ½ teaspoon ground ginger
     ½ teaspoon ground allspice
     6 small sweet potatoes, halved
     3 large carrots, halved
     1 small butternut squash, peeled, seeded, and
          cut into 6 chunks
     ¼ pound each pitted dried prunes and dried
          apricots or ½ pound mixed dried fruits
     ½ cup orange juice
     1 teaspoon grated orange rind

Heat a Dutch oven over medium heat. Add ribs
and quickly brown them on all sides in their own fat.
Add onions and continue to fry until they are golden
brown. Add stock, paprika, ginger, and allspice. Cover
and simmer stew for 1 hour.

Preheat oven to 350°F.

Add remaining ingredients to pot, placing ribs on
top of vegetables. Place covered pot in oven and bake
for 45 minutes. Uncover and continue to bake for
about 30 minutes, or until most of liquid is absorbed,
vegetables are tender, and top is brown.

6 servings

Budget Beef Stroganoff

*Using round steak instead of the traditional
filet mignon makes this dish an inexpensive treat;
using yogurt instead of sour cream makes it a
good choice for dieters.*

    1½ pounds round steak, 1 inch thick
     3 tablespoons vegetable oil
     1 cup chopped or thinly sliced onions
     1 clove garlic, minced
     ½ pound mushrooms, sliced ¼ inch thick
     2 tablespoons potato or rye flour
     ½ teaspoon pepper

    1½ cups Beef Stock (page 110)
     2 tablespoons tomato puree
     1 teaspoon chopped fresh dill (optional)
     2 teaspoons potato starch
     1 cup yogurt
       minced fresh dill or parsley

Trim fat from beef. Cut across grain to make strips
1 inch wide, ¼ inch thick, and about 2 inches long.

Heat 2 tablespoons oil in a large heavy-bottom
skillet. Add just enough beef strips to cover bottom of
skillet. Brown quickly on both sides, removing each
piece as it is done. Continue until all beef is browned.
Set aside.

Add remaining oil to the same skillet and sauté
onions, garlic, and mushrooms until barely tender,
about 5 minutes. Remove from heat. Add browned
beef strips. Sprinkle flour over mixture, tossing lightly.
Season with pepper. Place skillet over medium heat
and add stock slowly, stirring until smooth. Add
tomato puree. Bring mixture to a boil, then reduce heat
and simmer for about 45 minutes, or until steak is
fork-tender. Stir in chopped dill (if used).

In a small bowl blend potato starch with yogurt
and stir slowly into meat mixture. Simmer (do not
boil) for about 2 minutes. Transfer to a warmed
serving dish and garnish with minced dill or parsley.
Stroganoff goes well served over brown rice, whole
wheat noodles, or buckwheat groats.

6 servings

Stir-Fried Beef and Asparagus Mimosa

     2 tablespoons butter
     2 cloves garlic
     ½ cup coarse, fresh, whole grain bread crumbs
     1 hard-cooked egg, finely chopped
     ¼ cup chopped fresh parsley
     1 pound asparagus, cut into 1-inch pieces
     1 pound round steak, ½ inch thick
     2 tablespoons vegetable oil
       pepper, to taste

Melt butter in a small skillet. Slice 1 clove garlic
and sauté in butter until soft but not brown. Let stand
for 20 minutes, then remove garlic slices and discard.

Add bread crumbs and sauté until crisp. Gently toss together sautéed crumbs, chopped egg, and parsley. Reserve mixture.

Drop asparagus into a pot of boiling water and boil for 4 minutes, or until crisp-tender. Drain and reserve.

Trim fat from beef and cut into 1-inch squares. Heat oil in a 12-inch skillet. Slice remaining clove garlic and sauté in oil until soft but not brown. Remove garlic slices and discard. Over highest heat, stir-fry beef until browned, keeping pieces in 1 layer as much as possible. Add asparagus to skillet and heat through. Season with pepper. Serve beef and asparagus topped with egg-crumb mixture.

4 servings

Sukiyaki

This traditional Japanese dish is quick to cook once the ingredients have been assembled. If an electric skillet is used, the dish may be prepared right at the table. Note that the beef slices best if partially frozen.

  1½ pounds flank steak, beef tenderloin, or sirloin steak
  1 cup sliced scallions (diagonal slices ½ inch wide)
  1 cup sliced celery (diagonal slices 1 inch wide)
  1 cup thinly sliced mushrooms
  5 cups torn fresh spinach or shredded Chinese cabbage
  1 can (5 ounces) water chestnuts, drained and thinly sliced (⅔ cup)
  1 can (5 ounces) bamboo shoots, drained
  1½ cups bean sprouts
  ¼ cup soy sauce
  1 tablespoon honey
  ½ cup Beef Stock (page 110)
  3 tablespoons vegetable oil

Trim fat from meat and thinly slice it on the diagonal. (Partially freeze beef before slicing for best results.)

Before beginning to cook, arrange sliced meat and vegetables on a large platter or tray, ready for use.

Combine soy sauce, honey, and stock in a small bowl.

In a large cast-iron or electric skillet heat oil until hot but not smoking. Add beef strips and stir-fry for 1 to 2 minutes, or just until browned. Pour soy sauce mixture over beef and cook until mixture bubbles. Push meat to one side of skillet.

Add scallions and cook and stir over medium-high heat for 1 to 2 minutes. Push to one side. Repeat process with celery, and then with mushrooms.

Add spinach or Chinese cabbage. Cook and stir until just heated through. Repeat with water chestnuts, then bamboo shoots, and finally bean sprouts. Serve immediately with brown rice or Chinese noodles.

6 servings

Stuffed Flank Steak Baked in Buttermilk

  2½ cups soft whole grain bread crumbs
  ¼ cup butter, melted
  1 tablespoon chopped onions
    dash of pepper
  ½ teaspoon dried basil
  ½ teaspoon ground sage
  1 teaspoon vegetable oil
  1¼ pounds flank steak, 1½ inches thick
  3 cups buttermilk
  2 tablespoons whole wheat flour, mixed with 3 tablespoons cold water

Preheat oven to 350°F.

Combine bread crumbs, butter, onions, pepper, basil, and sage. Mix well.

Cut a large pocket into steak, stuff with crumb mixture, and fasten closed with small skewers.

Heat oil in a large skillet and brown steak on all sides. Transfer steak to a roasting pan, pour buttermilk over it, and cover with foil. Bake for about 1½ hours, or until tender.

Place steak on a serving platter and keep warm. With a wire whisk beat pan juice until well blended. Strain and return to pan.

Stir flour mixture into pan juice, place over medium heat, and cook until thickened, stirring constantly. Pour sauce over meat and serve immediately.

6 servings

Beef and Barley Bake

    2 tablespoons butter
    1 pound stewing beef, trimmed of fat and cut
        into ½-inch cubes
    1 medium-size onion, chopped
    5 cups Beef Stock (page 110)
    ½ teaspoon dried marjoram
    ¼ teaspoon dried rosemary
    1 cup barley

Melt butter in a large skillet. Add beef and brown on all sides. Add onions and sauté until golden. Transfer beef and onions to a 3-quart ovenproof casserole.

Preheat oven to 350°F.

In the same skillet combine stock, marjoram, rosemary, and barley. Bring to a boil and then pour mixture over beef. Cover and bake for 1 hour, or until beef is tender.

    4 servings

Beef and Pumpkin Stew

A fresh outlet for the next crop of pumpkins, this stew answers the prayers of many gardeners and provides a tempting variation on a low-cost standby.

    1 tablespoon vegetable oil
    1½ pounds stewing beef, trimmed of fat and cut
        into 1-inch cubes
    1 large onion, chopped
    1 stalk celery, with leaves, chopped
    1 green pepper, diced
    1½ cups boiling water
    2 pounds peeled pumpkin, cut into 3-inch
        chunks
    2 tablespoons lemon juice
    ¼ teaspoon each ground nutmeg, mace, allspice,
        cardamom, and pepper
    1 tablespoon cornstarch, dissolved in ¼ cup
        cold water
    2 tablespoons chopped fresh parsley
    ¼ cup pumpkin seeds, toasted (optional)
    1 cup whole wheat elbow macaroni, cooked
        (optional)

Heat oil in a 12-inch skillet or Dutch oven and brown meat on all sides. Add onions, celery, and green peppers. Continue frying until onions are golden. Add water and cover skillet, then reduce heat and simmer stew for 45 minutes.

Add pumpkin, lemon juice, and spices. Cover and continue to simmer for 30 minutes, or until meat and pumpkin are tender.

Add cornstarch mixture and parsley. Cook, stirring constantly, until gravy bubbles and thickens. Simmer 3 minutes longer. If used, add pumpkin seeds and cooked macaroni. Serve hot.

    4 servings

Beef, Bean, and Noodle Casserole

    3 tablespoons whole wheat flour
    1 teaspoon paprika
    2 pounds stewing beef, trimmed of fat
        and cut into 1-inch cubes
    ¼ cup vegetable oil
    1 medium-size onion, sliced
    2 carrots, cut into 1-inch pieces
    1½ cups Beef Stock (page 110)
    ¼ teaspoon ground thyme
    ¼ teaspoon pepper
    2 cups cut fresh green beans
    8 ounces uncooked whole wheat noodles

Preheat oven to 350°F.

Place flour and paprika in a large plastic bag. Add beef cubes and shake until pieces are well coated.

In a large skillet heat oil. Add beef and brown on all sides. When beef is almost finished browning, add onions and continue to stir and fry until onions are golden. Then add carrots, stock, thyme, and pepper and bring to a boil over high heat. Pour mixture into a 3-quart ovenproof casserole, cover, and bake for 1 hour. Add green beans, cover, and bake 15 minutes longer.

Meanwhile, cook noodles until tender. Drain and stir into casserole just before serving.

    4 servings

Beef Stew

    3 pounds stewing beef from chuck, round, lean
        brisket, or shin
    vegetable oil
    2 medium-size onions, coarsely chopped
    4 medium-size carrots, cut into chunks
    4 medium-size potatoes, cut into chunks
        (optional)
    3 to 4 tablespoons potato or rye flour, dissolved in
        ½ cup cold water
    chopped fresh parsley

Cut meat into 1½-inch cubes, trimming off any fat. Heat a small amount of oil in a large skillet and brown meat on all sides, adding more oil as needed. Lift meat out and place in a 5-quart heavy-bottom pot.

Brown onions in the same skillet. (Onions absorb browned-meat juice, adding to flavor of stew.) Add onions and pan juice to pot.

Add just enough cool water to pot to cover meat, then cover pot with a lid and bring slowly to a boil. Reduce heat and simmer for 1 to 2 hours, or until meat is almost tender.

Add carrots, and potatoes (if used), and continue to simmer 30 minutes longer, or until vegetables and meat are tender.

Before serving, thicken stew. Slowly add a little hot liquid from pot to flour mixture, stirring constantly, until it is a smooth sauce. Pour sauce into stew, stirring gently. Simmer for about 5 minutes. Garnish with parsley.

6 to 8 servings

Beef Stewed in Cranberry Chutney

This dish is fine to cook ahead, and is a welcome feature for a buffet. Just multiply the recipe for a crowd.

  2 tablespoons vegetable oil
1½ pounds stewing beef, trimmed of fat and cut into 1-inch cubes
  1 large onion, chopped
  1 stalk celery, with leaves, chopped
  1 clove garlic, minced
1¼ cups boiling water
  2 cups fresh cranberries
  ½ cup raisins
  ¼ cup walnuts (optional)
  1 tablespoon cider vinegar
  1 tablespoon honey
  ¼ teaspoon each ground cinnamon, ground ginger, and ground cloves
  ⅛ teaspoon cayenne pepper, or more to taste

Heat oil in a large skillet. Add beef and brown on all sides. Add onions and celery and sauté until golden brown. Add garlic and sauté mixture 1 minute longer, stirring constantly. (Do not let garlic change color.)

Stir water into mixture, then add remaining ingredients. Cover and simmer for 1¼ hours, or until beef is tender and liquid is reduced to ⅓ to ½ cup. If pan juice gets too low during cooking, add a little hot water. Or, if pan juice does not reduce sufficiently, uncover skillet during last 30 minutes of cooking and stir often. Taste to correct seasonings. Stew goes well with brown rice.

4 servings

Jachtschotel
(Dutch Hunter's Stew)

Apples and spices define the pleasurable character of this traditional European dish.

  2 tablespoons butter
1½ pounds stewing beef, trimmed of fat and cut into 1-inch cubes
  1 large onion, chopped
  2 cups Beef Stock (page 110)
  2 tablespoons chopped fresh parsley
  1 bay leaf
  4 large potatoes
  2 teaspoons cornstarch, dissolved in ¼ cup cold water
  ¼ teaspoon each ground cloves, allspice, nutmeg, and pepper
  2 large or 3 small apples, peeled, cored, and sliced
  ½ cup soft whole grain bread crumbs (about 1 slice bread)

Melt butter in a Dutch oven. Add meat and brown on all sides. Then add onions and sauté until golden brown. Stir in stock, parsley, and bay leaf. Cover and simmer stew for 1 hour.

Add whole potatoes, cover, and continue to cook stew until potatoes are just tender, 15 to 20 minutes.

Remove meat with a slotted spoon. Remove potatoes and cut into cubes. Set aside.

Cook pan juice over high heat until reduced to 1 cup. Remove bay leaf, then pour cornstarch mixture all at once into simmering liquid, stirring constantly until thickened. Add cloves, allspice, nutmeg, and pepper. Pour gravy into a bowl.

Preheat oven to 350°F.

Layer ½ of the potatoes in the same Dutch oven. Top with ½ of the apples, then all of the meat. Finish with remaining apples and remaining potatoes. Pour gravy over all and sprinkle with bread crumbs. Bake for 30 minutes, or until apples are tender.

4 servings

Biscuit and Beef Stew

The addition of fruit takes this beef stew out of the ordinary, and serving it over oat flour biscuits makes it even more special.

 2 tablespoons butter
 1 pound stewing beef, trimmed of fat and cut into ½-inch cubes
 1 medium-size onion, chopped
 4 cups Beef Stock (page 110)
 ½ cup chopped dried apricots
 ½ cup chopped dried prunes
 1 clove garlic, halved
 1 teaspoon ground ginger
 ¼ cup cornstarch, dissolved in ½ cup cold water
   Oat Flour Biscuits (see below)

In a Dutch oven melt butter. Add beef cubes and brown on all sides. Add onions and sauté until translucent. Stir in stock, apricots, prunes, garlic, and ginger. Simmer for about 2 hours, or until meat is tender.

Discard garlic. Remove meat with a slotted spoon. Add cornstarch mixture to pot and stir constantly over medium heat until gravy thickens. Return meat to gravy and keep stew warm while biscuits are prepared. To serve, split hot biscuits open and top with stew.

 4 servings

Oat Flour Biscuits

 2 cups oat flour
 1 tablespoon baking powder
 1⅓ cups light cream
 1 tablespoon plus 2 teaspoons yogurt

Preheat oven to 425°F.

Sift flour and baking powder together in a small bowl. Lightly mix in cream and yogurt. Drop dough by spoonfuls onto an oiled baking sheet and bake for 15 minutes.

 Makes 1 dozen biscuits

Beef Stew with Herb Dumplings

 2 tablespoons whole wheat flour
 ½ teaspoon paprika
 ¼ teaspoon pepper

 1¼ pounds stewing beef, trimmed of fat and cut into 1-inch cubes
 2 tablespoons vegetable oil
 2 large onions, chopped
 4 cups Beef Stock (page 110) or Poultry Stock (page 110)
 ½ teaspoon dried thyme
 1 bay leaf
 4 large potatoes, cut into 1-inch cubes
 4 carrots, sliced
 2 tablespoons chopped fresh parsley
   Herb Dumplings (see below)

Combine flour, paprika, and pepper in a plastic bag. Add beef cubes and shake to coat meat evenly. Heat oil in a Dutch oven. Add meat and brown on all sides over medium-high heat. Then add onions and sauté until golden brown. Add stock, thyme, and bay leaf. Bring to a boil, cover, and reduce heat. Simmer for 1¼ hours, or until meat is tender. Remove bay leaf and add potatoes, carrots, and parsley. Simmer stew 10 minutes longer, then add dumpling batter.

 4 servings

Herb Dumplings

 1⅓ cups whole wheat flour
 1 tablespoon plus ½ teaspoon baking powder
 1 tablespoon chopped fresh chives
 1 tablespoon chopped fresh parsley
 ¾ cup milk

Combine flour and baking powder in a small bowl and mix thoroughly. Stir in chives and parsley. When ready to cook, add milk to flour mixture all at once and stir just enough to blend. Drop batter by the tablespoon into pot of simmering stew. (Batter makes about 8 dumplings.) Cover pot tightly, raise heat slightly to a low boil, and cook without uncovering for 12 minutes. When fully cooked, dumplings should be puffed and dry inside.

 4 servings

Chili con Carne

 2 tablespoons corn oil
 2 pounds ground chuck or round
 1 medium-size onion, chopped

1 cup chopped celery
½ cup chopped green peppers
1 clove garlic, minced
2 cups chopped tomatoes
1 cup tomato puree
2 teaspoons ground cumin
2 teaspoons chili powder
2 cups cooked kidney beans, drained

Heat oil in a heavy skillet. Add beef, onions, celery, green peppers, and garlic and sauté until beef has browned.

Stir in tomatoes and tomato puree. Then add seasonings, cover, and simmer for 45 to 60 minutes. Add kidney beans and continue to simmer 30 minutes longer.

6 to 8 servings

Dilly Meatballs and Vegetables

1 pound lean ground beef
1 cup soft whole grain bread crumbs
1 egg, beaten
1 small onion, minced
1 clove garlic, minced
2 tablespoons vegetable oil
1¼ cups water
4 medium-size potatoes, sliced
2 small zucchini, sliced
1 tablespoon cornstarch, dissolved in ¼ cup cold water
1 cup sour cream
3 tablespoons minced fresh dill or 1 tablespoon dillweed

Combine beef, bread crumbs, egg, onions, and garlic in a medium-size bowl. Blend well. Form into 24 small balls.

Heat oil in a large skillet and brown meatballs on all sides. Remove them with a slotted spoon and place in a 2-quart ovenproof casserole.

Bring water to a boil in a large saucepan. Add potatoes and zucchini, cover, and boil gently for 5 minutes. Drain, reserving 1 cup water. Add potatoes and zucchini to casserole.

Pour reserved water into skillet in which meat was browned. Add cornstarch mixture and cook, stirring constantly, until mixture thickens. Reduce heat to low. Blend in sour cream and dill or dillweed.

Preheat oven to 350°F.

Pour sauce over meat and vegetables, mix gently, and bake for 30 minutes.

4 servings

Cabbage Rolls

8 to 10 large cabbage leaves

Stuffing
1 pound lean ground beef
1½ cups cooked brown rice
1 egg, beaten
¼ cup chopped onions
2 tablespoons milk
⅛ teaspoon pepper
⅛ teaspoon garlic powder

Sauce
1 cup tomato juice, or more as needed
1 tablespoon honey
1 tablespoon lemon juice

Place cabbage leaves in a large pot of boiling water. Cover, remove from heat, and let stand for 5 minutes. Drain well. Cut thick rib off back of each leaf and discard.

To make the stuffing: Combine beef, rice, egg, onions, milk, pepper, and garlic powder in a medium-size bowl. Mix well.

Place a large spoonful of stuffing on top of each cabbage leaf. Roll leaf over stuffing, snugly tucking in ends. Place cabbage rolls, seam-side down, in a large baking dish.

Preheat oven to 350°F.

To make the sauce: Combine tomato juice, honey, and lemon juice in a small saucepan. Stir over low heat until honey has melted. Pour sauce over cabbage rolls and bake for 45 to 60 minutes, or until cabbage is tender. Add more tomato juice if necessary to keep rolls moist during baking.

4 servings

Hearty Yogurt-Beef Patties

1¼ pounds lean ground beef
2 eggs, beaten
3 tablespoons yogurt or sour cream
2 tablespoons minced onions
2 tablespoons wheat germ
1 teaspoon paprika
¼ teaspoon dried thyme
¼ teaspoon ground sage
¼ teaspoon pepper
2 cups whole wheat cereal flakes
3 tablespoons vegetable oil
   yogurt or sour cream, for topping

Combine beef, eggs, yogurt or sour cream, onions, wheat germ, and seasonings and blend well. Form into 12 patties.

Crush cereal between 2 pieces of wax paper using a rolling pin. (A food processor may also be used, but do not reduce the cereal to powder.) Dip patties on both sides in crushed cereal and chill in refrigerator to firm them.

Heat 2 tablespoons oil in a 12-inch skillet and fry patties slowly over medium-low heat, a few at a time, until just cooked through, turning once. Add remaining oil as needed. Serve with additional yogurt or sour cream as a topping.

6 servings

Italian Meatballs and Noodles

1 pound lean ground beef
⅛ teaspoon pepper
1 tablespoon dried parsley
¼ cup grated Parmesan cheese
½ cup whole grain bread crumbs
2 cups Beef Stock (page 110)
1 egg, beaten
2 tablespoons wheat germ (optional)
¼ cup olive oil, or more as needed
1 clove garlic, minced
½ pound mushrooms, sliced
2 cups chopped canned tomatoes
1 teaspoon dried oregano
½ teaspoon dried basil
2 cups uncooked whole wheat noodles
2 tablespoons cornstarch, dissolved in ¼ cup cold water

In a large bowl mix together beef, pepper, parsley, cheese, bread crumbs slightly moistened with a little of the stock, egg, and wheat germ (if used). Form into balls about 1 inch in diameter.

Heat oil in a Dutch oven and sauté garlic. Add meatballs and brown on all sides, adding more oil if needed. Remove meatballs and reserve. Sauté mushrooms in the same pot, adding more oil if needed. Add tomatoes, remaining stock, oregano, and basil. Return meatballs to pot, cover, and simmer for 20 minutes.

While meatballs are simmering, cook noodles until tender. Drain.

When meatballs are done, add cornstarch mixture to pot and cook until liquid thickens, stirring constantly. Gently mix in drained noodles and serve.

6 servings

Mosaic Loaf

3 large carrots
1 tablespoon vegetable oil
1 medium-size onion, finely chopped
1 green pepper, diced
1 clove garlic, minced
1½ pounds lean ground beef
1 egg, beaten
¼ cup grated Parmesan or Romano cheese
2 tablespoons minced fresh parsley
1 tablespoon chili powder
2 cups cooked brown rice

Preheat oven to 350°F.

Slice carrots on the diagonal, ½ inch thick, and cook in a small amount of boiling water for 8 minutes. Drain and set aside.

In a small skillet heat oil and sauté onions, green peppers, and garlic until soft but not brown.

In a large bowl blend together beef, egg, cheese, parsley, chili powder, and rice. Gently stir in carrots and sautéed vegetables. Pack mixture into a 9 × 5-inch loaf pan and bake for 1 hour.

Drain off all fat. Place a platter upside down over loaf pan and invert to unmold. Let loaf stand for 10 minutes before slicing.

8 servings

Layered Beef Casserole

    2 tablespoons vegetable oil
    1 pound lean ground beef
    1 small onion, chopped
      pepper, to taste
    1 pound fresh green beans, cut into 1-inch
      lengths
    4 medium-size potatoes, sliced
    1 egg, beaten
    ¼ cup milk
    1 tablespoon butter
    ¼ teaspoon white pepper
    1 cup coarsely grated cheddar cheese (optional)
    2 tablespoons wheat germ

Heat oil in a large skillet. Add beef and stir over medium heat until browned. Add onions and sauté until golden. Remove mixture with a slotted spoon and place in a 1½-quart ovenproof casserole. Sprinkle with pepper.

Cook green beans in a small amount of boiling water for 5 minutes. Drain and spread over meat mixture.

Boil potatoes in a small amount of water until tender. Drain and mash them together with egg, milk, butter, and white pepper.

Preheat oven to 350°F.

Spoon potato mixture over beans, sprinkle with cheese (if used) and wheat germ, and bake for 30 minutes, or until top is golden brown.

    4 servings

Shepherd's Pie

    1 tablespoon vegetable oil
    1 medium-size onion, chopped
    1 pound lean ground beef
    1 teaspoon dried basil
    ½ pound fresh green beans, steamed until
      tender
    1 cup chopped canned tomatoes
    2 medium-size potatoes, cooked until tender
    1 egg, beaten
    ½ cup water

Heat oil in a large skillet and sauté onions until golden. Add beef and basil and cook until browned.

Stir in green beans and tomatoes, then turn mixture into a 1½-quart ovenproof casserole.

Preheat oven to 350°F.

Mash potatoes together with egg and water, spoon evenly over meat mixture, and bake for 15 minutes.

    4 servings

Stuffed Escarole Leaves

    Sauce
    2 stalks celery, with leaves
    ¼ cup olive oil or other vegetable oil
    2 cloves garlic, minced
    1 medium-size onion, chopped
    4 cups chopped peeled tomatoes
    1 carrot, grated
    ½ cup Poultry Stock (page 110)
    ½ cup golden raisins
    2 tablespoons cider vinegar
    ½ teaspoon pepper

    Stuffing
    1 pound lean ground beef
    2 cups cooked brown rice
      reserved minced celery leaves
    1 medium-size onion, chopped
    ¼ teaspoon pepper
    1 tablespoon minced fresh parsley

    2 heads escarole (large outer leaves only)

To make the sauce: Mince leaves from celery and reserve for stuffing. Finely chop celery stalks. Heat oil in a large skillet and sauté garlic, chopped celery stalks, and onions until soft but not brown. Add tomatoes, carrots, stock, raisins, vinegar, and pepper. Simmer mixture, uncovered, for 30 minutes, stirring occasionally.

Preheat oven to 350°F.

To make the stuffing: Mix together beef, rice, reserved celery leaves, onions, pepper, and parsley.

Cut out tough core of escarole leaves with a V-shaped notch. Place a rounded tablespoon of stuffing at large end of leaf. Fold sides over stuffing and roll up leaf. Repeat until all stuffing has been used. Place rolls, seam-side down, in an oiled 12 × 15-inch ovenproof casserole, in 1 or 2 layers as needed. Pour sauce over rolls. Cover casserole with foil, cut 2 slits in foil, and bake for 1 hour.

    6 servings

Stuffed Peppers

Stuffing
vegetable oil
1   pound lean ground beef
1   cup cooked brown rice
¼   cup wheat germ
2   tablespoons grated Parmesan cheese
1   teaspoon dried oregano
⅛   teaspoon garlic powder
1   cup chopped canned tomatoes, or more as needed

3   tablespoons olive oil
8   large green peppers

To make the stuffing: Heat a small amount of oil in a large skillet and brown beef. Add rice, wheat germ, cheese, oregano, garlic powder, and tomatoes. Mix well. If mixture seems too dry, add more tomatoes. Set stuffing aside.

Preheat oven to 350°F. Oil a large roasting pan with ½ of the olive oil.

Cut green peppers in half lengthwise and remove membranes and seeds. Drop halves into a large pot of boiling water and simmer for 5 minutes. Drain.

Arrange peppers, cut-side up, in a roasting pan and fill with stuffing. Drizzle remaining olive oil over tops and bake for 45 minutes, or until peppers are tender.

8 servings

Walnut and Herb-Stuffed Meat Loaf

Meat loaf takes on a new meaning in this recipe—a sort of meat-loaf roll. If you wait until you have some beef gravy from a previous meal, you will have a head start on this dish.

Stuffing
1   cup finely chopped walnuts
1   cup soft whole grain bread crumbs (about 2 slices bread)
2   tablespoons minced fresh parsley

¼   teaspoon each pepper, ground sage, dried thyme, and dried marjoram
1   large shallot, minced (about 1 tablespoon)
3 to 4   tablespoons thin beef gravy

Meat Loaf
2   pounds lean ground beef and pork (all ground beef may be substituted)
1   large shallot, minced (about 1 tablespoon)
2   eggs
2   tablespoons soy sauce
¾   cup thin beef gravy

To make the stuffing: Mix together walnuts, bread crumbs, parsley, pepper, sage, thyme, marjoram, and shallots. Moisten with just enough gravy so that stuffing holds its shape when pressed between fingers.

Preheat oven to 350°F.

To make the meat loaf: Blend together ground meat, shallots, eggs, soy sauce, and ¼ cup gravy (reserve remainder for topping).

On a large piece of wax paper, pat meat mixture into a 12 × 15-inch rectangle. Pat stuffing into a layer on top, to within 1 inch of all edges of meat. Lift 2 (lengthwise) corners of wax paper and roll meat over stuffing. Pinch seam and ends closed and pat together any breaks in meat cover. Lift wax paper to transfer roll to a roasting pan, placing it seam-side down. Pour remaining gravy over all and bake for 40 to 45 minutes. Allow to rest for 10 minutes before slicing.

6 to 8 servings

Lamb

Leg of Lamb with Nut-Herb Stuffing

Stuffing
½   pound spinach
1   tablespoon olive oil
½   cup chopped scallions
2   large cloves garlic, chopped
¼   cup chopped fresh parsley

3 tablespoons chopped fresh mint or 1 teaspoon
    dried mint
2 teaspoons finely chopped lemon rind
¾ cup finely chopped walnuts
¼ cup pine nuts
½ cup soft whole grain bread crumbs
1 egg, beaten

7½ to 9 pounds leg of lamb, boned and butterflied*
    freshly ground pepper, to taste
    juice of ½ lemon
1 tablespoon olive oil
2 teaspoons minced fresh rosemary

To make the stuffing: Steam spinach for 3 to 4 minutes. Drain and squeeze out water. Then chop. (There should be ½ cup). Heat oil in a small pan and sauté scallions and garlic for 2 to 3 minutes. Combine spinach, scallion mixture, parsley, mint, lemon rind, walnuts, pine nuts, bread crumbs, and egg. Blend well.

Place boned lamb on work surface, skin-side down. Make gashes in thick meaty parts to flatten if necessary. Grind pepper over lamb, then squeeze lemon half over it and rub juice in. Spoon nut-herb stuffing over lamb. Using your hands, work stuffing into folds or pockets of meat and spread evenly. Roll meat up, fasten with small skewers, and then sew edges together with a trussing needle and kitchen string. Tie lamb roll 2 or 3 times with string to make a compact oblong roast. Remove skewers. Rub outside of roast with oil and rosemary and place on a rack set in a roasting pan. Set aside to marinate at room temperature for 1 hour.

Preheat oven to 325°F.

Roast lamb, uncovered, for 12 to 15 minutes per pound for medium or 20 minutes per pound for well done. Baste often with pan juice during roasting. Allow roast to rest for 10 minutes on a heated platter before slicing. Serve with pan juice.

8 servings

*Your butcher can bone and butterfly the lamb upon request.

Lamb Hash with Curried Yogurt Sauce

Lamb and curry have been happily paired for generations. This time the combination is a bit different, but just as delectable as the traditional form. A good opportunity to use lamb or poultry gravy left from a previous meal.

3 cups cubed cooked lamb
2 large potatoes, cubed
1 medium-size onion, chopped
¼ cup lamb gravy, poultry gravy, or Poultry
    Stock (page 110)
¼ teaspoon pepper
    Curried Yogurt Sauce (see below)

Preheat oven to 350°F.

Coarsely grind lamb, potatoes, and onions in a food mill or food processor. Mix thoroughly with gravy or stock. Stir in pepper. Press hash into a well-oiled 9-inch baking dish. Bake for 40 minutes, or until crusty and well browned. Serve with sauce.

4 servings

Curried Yogurt Sauce

1 tablespoon vegetable oil
1 clove garlic, minced
½ cup peeled, seeded, and chopped tomatoes
2 teaspoons curry powder
1 tablespoon cornstarch, dissolved in 1 cup
    cold lamb stock or Poultry Stock (page 110)
1 cup yogurt
    cayenne pepper, to taste

Heat oil in a small skillet. Add garlic and sauté for 1 minute. (Do not allow to brown.) Add tomatoes and simmer, uncovered, for 5 minutes. Stir in curry powder and cornstarch mixture and bring to a boil. Cook, stirring constantly, until thickened. Then remove from heat and blend in yogurt and cayenne. Heat through but do not boil.

Yields about 2½ cups

Lamb Shanks with Lentils

½ cup oat flour
⅛ teaspoon pepper
½ teaspoon paprika
4 pounds lamb shanks, with bones cracked,
    trimmed of fat
3 tablespoons vegetable oil
1 clove garlic, minced
4 cups water
2 cups dried lentils
8 carrots, halved
1 cup chopped stewed tomatoes
2 cups shredded spinach (optional)
½ teaspoon dried basil
½ teaspoon dried oregano

Preheat oven to 350°F.

Mix flour, pepper, and paprika together in a shallow bowl. Dredge shanks in flour mixture. Heat oil in a large Dutch oven and sauté garlic. Add lamb shanks and brown on all sides. Add water, lentils, carrots, tomatoes, spinach (if used), basil, and oregano. Cover and bake for 2½ hours. If top of casserole seems greasy, skim before serving.

4 servings

Lamb and Chick-Peas

Chick-peas need overnight soaking and about two hours of simmering before they are ready for inclusion in this recipe, so plan ahead when you want to treat the family to this hearty dish.

2 cups dried chick-peas
4 cups water
1 tablespoon vegetable oil
1½ pounds lean meaty lamb riblets
1 small onion, chopped
1 stalk celery, with leaves, chopped
3 cloves garlic, minced
¼ cup chopped fresh parsley
1 teaspoon ground coriander
½ teaspoon dried oregano
¼ teaspoon pepper
1 medium-size potato, halved

Soak chick-peas (see page 261 for soaking directions). Drain and rinse. Place soaked chick-peas in a 4-quart pot, add the 4 cups water, cover, and simmer for 2 hours. Drain and reserve liquid. Leave chick-peas in pot.

Heat oil in a 12-inch skillet, and brown riblets on all sides, turning often. Add onions to skillet and cook with riblets until golden brown. Add celery and garlic and turn off heat as soon as they begin to sizzle.

Pour ½ cup reserved chick-pea cooking liquid into skillet to loosen brown bits, then transfer riblets, vegetables, and pan juice to pot containing chick-peas. Add parsley, coriander, oregano, and pepper. Cover and simmer mixture for 1½ hours. Add potato halves and cook 30 minutes longer. Remove potato halves, mash very well, and return them to pot. Stir to mix potatoes into liquid. If desired, meat can be deboned before serving.

6 servings

Lamb Shoulder Chops in Yogurt Sauce

1 large beet, peeled and cubed
2¾ cups water
4 cloves garlic
½ teaspoon pepper
1 teaspoon turmeric
1 teaspoon ground ginger
½ teaspoon ground nutmeg
4 large lean lamb shoulder chops, boned and
    cubed
½ cup butter
3 cups chopped onions
1 cup yogurt
1 teaspoon lemon juice
1 avocado
  acidulated water (page 468)
1 large tomato

Simmer beet cubes, uncovered, in ¾ cup water for about 20 minutes. Discard beets, reserving cooking liquid.

While beets are cooking, mince 2 cloves garlic. Combine with pepper, turmeric, ginger, nutmeg, and lamb in a large pot. Add remaining 2 cups water and bring to a boil. Reduce heat, cover, and simmer for 45 minutes.

In a large skillet clarify butter (see page 140 for directions), then cook until browned. Add onions and sauté until golden.

Drain lamb, reserving broth and discarding garlic. Add lamb to onions and butter and brown on all sides.

With a mortar and pestle work remaining 2 cloves garlic into a paste. Stir garlic paste into butter and onion mixture. Add reserved beet liquid, reserved lamb broth, yogurt, and lemon juice. Simmer for 20 minutes. (Yogurt will separate and appear to have soured.) Increase heat, bring to a boil, and cook sauce, stirring constantly, for 10 minutes, or until sauce reduces and looks glazed.

Peel avocado, cut it into wedges, and dip wedges in acidulated water. Cut tomato into wedges. Serve lamb garnished with avocados and tomatoes.

4 servings

Lamb Slivers with Peachy Yogurt

Marinating the lamb gives it an extra zing of flavor later complemented by a sauce of peaches and yogurt.

- ½ cup orange juice
- 1 tablespoon lemon juice
- 1 teaspoon soy sauce
- 4 large lean lamb shoulder chops, boned and cut into slivers
- 2 ripe peaches, peeled, pitted, and quartered
- 1 cup yogurt
- 2 tablespoons honey (optional)
- 2 tablespoons butter

Combine orange juice, lemon juice, and soy sauce. Pour over lamb slivers and marinate in refrigerator for at least 3 hours. Drain, reserving marinade.

In a food processor chop peaches together with yogurt, honey (if used), and 2 tablespoons reserved marinade.

Melt butter in a large skillet. Add lamb slivers and stir-fry just until lamb is cooked. Add peach-yogurt mixture and cook just until heated through. Delicious served with brown rice.

4 servings

Braised Lamb with Eggplant

- 3 to 5 tablespoons olive oil
- 4 large lean lamb shoulder chops
- 1 medium-size eggplant, peeled and cubed
- 2 sweet red peppers, cut into chunks
- 1 clove garlic, minced
- 1 teaspoon dried oregano
- ½ teaspoon dried thyme
- ⅛ teaspoon pepper
- ¼ cup water
- 2 tablespoons minced fresh parsley

Heat 1 tablespoon oil in a 12-inch skillet and brown chops on both sides. Remove chops and set aside. Add 2 tablespoons oil to skillet and stir-fry eggplant, red peppers, and garlic for about 5 minutes, or until eggplant begins to turn translucent. If necessary, add up to 2 more tablespoons oil during cooking if mixture is too dry and vegetables begin to brown. Remove and reserve vegetables.

Return chops to skillet. Add herbs and pepper. Pour in water, cover, and simmer chops for 25 minutes.

Return vegetables to skillet, add parsley, cover, and continue to simmer 20 minutes longer, or until chops are tender. Goes well with pita bread.

4 servings

Lamb Ragout

- ¼ cup vegetable oil
- 4 lean lamb shoulder chops (about 2 pounds)
- 1 large onion, chopped
- ⅛ teaspoon garlic powder
- ¼ teaspoon pepper
- ½ teaspoon celery seeds
- 2 tablespoons cornstarch, dissolved in 1 cup Poultry Stock (page 110)
- 4 medium-size potatoes, thinly sliced
- 4 carrots, thinly sliced
- parsley sprigs

In a large skillet heat oil and brown chops on both sides. Remove and set aside. Add onions to the same skillet and sauté until translucent. Stir in garlic powder, pepper, and celery seeds and sauté for 1 to 2 minutes. Add cornstarch mixture and cook, stirring constantly, until sauce bubbles and thickens. Remove from heat. Mix in potatoes and carrots.

Preheat oven to 350°F.

Layer ½ of the vegetables and sauce in a 4-quart ovenproof casserole. Add chops, then top with remaining vegetables and sauce. Bake, covered, for 1 hour. Garnish with parsley sprigs.

4 servings

Lamb Cassoulet

This traditional favorite of French peasants is a sturdy combination of white beans, lamb, and sausage, plus vegetables and a wonderful combination of herbs. Allow about four hours of preparation time.

2 cups dried white beans
4 cups cold water
5 carrots, cut into 2-inch pieces
6 small onions, whole or halved
2 cloves garlic, minced
½ cup chopped celery leaves
½ teaspoon pepper
1 large bay leaf
1 teaspoon dried thyme
1 teaspoon ground sage
4 cups Poultry Stock (page 110) or Beef Stock (page 110)
2 tablespoons butter or vegetable oil
1½ to 2 pounds lean lamb shoulder chops or stewing lamb, trimmed of fat and cut into cubes
  pepper, to taste
½ pound fresh sausage links
3 tablespoons chopped fresh parsley

In a 6- to 8-quart pot with cover, soak beans in the 4 cups water for at least 2 hours. Without draining beans, add carrots, onions, garlic, celery leaves, pepper, bay leaf, thyme, sage, and stock. Bring to a boil, then reduce heat, cover, and simmer for about 1 hour. Discard bay leaf.

Meanwhile, heat butter or oil in a large skillet. Brown lamb on all sides. Pepper lightly.

Preheat oven to 350°F.

Transfer lamb to an oiled 4-quart ovenproof casserole. Cover with bean mixture. Make deep diagonal cuts across tops of sausage links. Place sausages on top of beans. Cover tightly and bake for 50 minutes. Uncover and continue to bake about 10 minutes longer, or until sausages have browned. Garnish with parsley and serve from casserole.

4 to 6 servings

Lamb Curry with Condiments

This impressive dish will not tax the talents of even an inexperienced cook, yet it can be served with pride to family or guests, and the condiments add a festive touch.

2 tablespoons whole wheat flour
2 pounds stewing lamb, trimmed of fat and cut into chunks
2 tablespoons butter or vegetable oil
1 small onion, chopped
1 clove garlic, minced
1 can (16 ounces) tomatoes, chopped
1 tablespoon curry powder
1 cup yogurt
4 cups hot cooked brown rice
  Condiments for Curry (see below)

Preheat oven to 350°F.

Place flour in a large plastic bag. Add lamb and shake until well coated.

Heat butter or oil in a Dutch oven and brown lamb on all sides. Add onions and garlic and sauté for 3 minutes, then add tomatoes and curry powder. Cover and bake for 1 hour, or until meat is tender. Stir in yogurt. Serve over rice, accompanied by condiments.

4 servings

Condiments for Curry

2 bananas, sliced
¼ cup wheat germ
½ cup golden raisins
1 green pepper, chopped
½ cup sliced scallions
2 hard-cooked eggs, chopped

Coat banana slices with wheat germ and sauté lightly in a small amount of butter. Place sautéed bananas, raisins, green peppers, scallions, and eggs in individual small bowls and pass them at the table.

4 servings

Lamb Stew with Artichoke Hearts

¼ cup olive oil
2 pounds boneless lamb, trimmed of fat and cut into 1-inch cubes
1 cup finely chopped onions
½ cup white grape juice
3 cups water
1½ teaspoons lemon juice
1 teaspoon dried basil
¼ teaspoon garlic powder
1 can (6 ounces) tomato paste
3 medium-size potatoes, cubed
9 ounces frozen artichoke hearts, thawed

Heat oil in a Dutch oven and lightly brown lamb and onions.

Mix together grape juice, water, lemon juice, basil, and garlic powder. Pour over lamb. Stir in tomato paste, cover, and simmer for 1 hour.

Add potatoes and continue to simmer for another 30 minutes, or until lamb is tender. Add artichokes and simmer 30 minutes longer, or until vegetables are tender.

4 servings

Lamb Stew with Prunes

2 tablespoons butter
2 tablespoons vegetable oil
1 large onion, chopped
1 stalk celery, chopped
1½ pounds boneless lamb, trimmed of fat and cubed
½ teaspoon each ground cardamom, cumin, ginger, and coriander
¼ teaspoon pepper
1 cup water
¼ cup chopped fresh parsley
1 tablespoon honey
1 cup pitted dried prunes (dried figs may be substituted)
1 tablespoon cornstarch, dissolved in ¼ cup cold water

In a Dutch oven or large skillet heat butter and oil until butter melts. Add onions, celery, and lamb and sauté, while stirring, for about 10 minutes, or until meat changes color. Add spices and pepper and continue to cook for 5 minutes. Stir in water, parsley, and honey, then cover and bring to a boil. Reduce heat and simmer for 45 minutes.

Add prunes and cook 25 minutes longer.

Add cornstarch mixture and stir until sauce thickens. Cook an additional 3 minutes before serving.

4 servings

Moroccan-Style Lamb Stew

Almonds, raisins, and cinnamon bring an exotic, Near Eastern flavor to this very appealing dish.

2 pounds stewing lamb, with bone
1 tablespoon vegetable oil
2 large onions, chopped
1 clove garlic, minced
6 plum tomatoes or 4 medium-size tomatoes, peeled and sliced
½ cup golden raisins
½ teaspoon pepper
½ teaspoon dried thyme
¼ teaspoon ground cinnamon
¼ teaspoon ground allspice
½ cup Poultry Stock (page 110)
½ cup whole blanched almonds
4 cups hot cooked brown rice

Trim fat from lamb and cut meat into chunks.

Heat oil in a 12-inch skillet or Dutch oven and brown lamb and bone. Add onions and garlic and sauté for 3 minutes, then add remaining ingredients, except almonds and rice. Cover and simmer for 45 minutes.

Add almonds and simmer 15 minutes longer. Serve over rice.

4 servings

Stir-Fried Lamb and Cauliflower

1 tablespoon vegetable oil
3 dried hot chili peppers
3 slices peeled ginger root
1 clove garlic, sliced
1 small head cauliflower (1 to 1½ pounds)
1 pound boneless lamb, trimmed of fat and cut
    into ¼-inch-thick slices
3 tablespoons soy sauce
1 tablespoon cornstarch
½ cup cold Poultry Stock (page 110)

In a 12-inch skillet combine oil, peppers, ginger root, and garlic. Place skillet over lowest possible heat while preparing cauliflower and lamb. (Garlic should not brown.)

Bring a large pot half full of water to a boil. Meanwhile, trim cauliflower into florets. Cut small florets in half; cut large ones in quarters. Place florets in a pot of boiling water and boil gently for 5 minutes. Then drain and place in a bowl of cold water. Set aside.

Remove garlic from skillet and discard. Increase heat to high. When oil is hot, add lamb and stir-fry until browned. Remove and discard chili peppers and ginger.

Combine soy sauce, cornstarch, and stock in a small saucepan and stir until there are no lumps. Bring to a boil, stirring constantly. Pour sauce over lamb, add cauliflower, and heat through.

4 servings

Yogurt-Marinated Lamb with Melon Chunks

Begin marinating the lamb in the morning, then enjoy these kabobs for a quick yet special dinner that can be on the table in less than half an hour. The peanut sauce is an exotic highlight.

1½ cups yogurt
2 tablespoons honey
2 cloves garlic, halved
3 tablespoons lemon juice
1 small onion, quartered
2 pounds boneless lamb, trimmed of fat and cut
    into 1½-inch cubes
1 cantaloupe, cut into 1½-inch chunks

Sauce
1 cup yogurt
1 clove garlic, halved
½ cup peanuts

Place yogurt, honey, garlic, lemon juice, and onion in a food processor and blend well. In a large bowl combine lamb with yogurt mixture, cover, and refrigerate for 8 hours, stirring occasionally.

Remove lamb from marinade. Alternate lamb cubes and melon chunks on skewers. Broil for 8 minutes, then turn and broil 8 minutes longer, or until lamb is cooked to taste.

To make the sauce: Blend yogurt, garlic, and peanuts together in a food processor until pureed. Serve lamb and melon chunks with sauce for dipping.

4 servings

Eggplant Quiche

pastry for 1 Basic Rolled Piecrust (page 718)
¼ cup olive oil, or more as needed
1 clove garlic, minced
1 medium-size onion, finely chopped
1 medium-size green pepper, chopped
½ cup sliced mushrooms
1 small eggplant, peeled and diced
2 large tomatoes, peeled, seeded, and chopped
½ pound lean ground beef
½ pound lean ground lamb
2 eggs
1 cup half-and-half
1 cup grated mozzarella cheese

Preheat oven to 425°F.

Roll out pastry and line a 9-inch pie plate. Prick bottom of piecrust with a fork and add a handful of dried beans to weight down crust. Bake for 5 minutes. Set aside to cool.

Heat oil in a large skillet. Add garlic, onions, and green peppers and sauté until they start to soften. Add mushrooms and continue to cook, stirring frequently, until mushrooms have darkened. Add eggplant, and more oil if needed. Sauté for about 3 minutes, or until eggplant is lightly browned. Stir in tomatoes and cook until heated through. Drain mixture well and set aside in a large bowl to cool.

Discard oil in skillet and wipe it lightly with paper toweling. Then brown beef and lamb. Drain cooked meat well in a strainer, pushing it with the back of a spoon to eliminate grease. Set aside to cool. When cool, mix meat with vegetables.

Preheat oven to 350°F.

While meat is cooling, beat eggs together with half-and-half. Place ½ of the meat-vegetable mixture in cooled piecrust. Over this, layer ½ of the grated cheese, then remaining meat and vegetables, and finally remaining cheese. Pour egg mixture over all. Place on a baking sheet to catch any drippings and bake for about 45 minutes, or until knife inserted in center comes out clean. Allow to rest for 10 minutes before cutting and serving.

6 to 8 servings

Lamb Meatballs with Cucumber Sauce

1 pound lean ground lamb
2 eggs, beaten
¼ cup whole grain bread crumbs
¼ cup chopped fresh parsley
1 teaspoon paprika
½ teaspoon dry mustard
⅛ teaspoon pepper
1 tablespoon vegetable oil
1 medium-size onion, chopped
¼ cup water
1 cucumber
1 cup yogurt or sour cream

Combine lamb, eggs, bread crumbs, parsley, paprika, dry mustard, and pepper and blend well. Form into 12 to 14 small balls.

Heat oil in a 12-inch skillet and brown meatballs on one side over medium-low heat. Loosen and turn them, then cook on the second side for 1 minute. Add onions to skillet, cover, and cook for 20 minutes over low heat, checking and stirring from time to time to be sure they do not overbrown. When meatballs are cooked through, drain off fat. Add water to skillet, bring to a boil, and immediately turn off heat.

Cut ends off cucumber. Cut 4 thin unpeeled slices and reserve them for garnish. Peel, seed, and chop remainder. Mix chopped cucumbers with yogurt or sour cream, then stir into pan juice. Heat through but do not boil. Garnish each serving with a reserved cucumber slice.

4 servings

Lamb-Stuffed Acorn Squash

3 small acorn squashes (about ¾ pound each)

Stuffing
½ cup bulgur
1 cup boiling water
1 tablespoon vegetable oil
1½ pounds lean ground lamb
1 medium-size onion, chopped
1 green pepper, diced
¼ cup raisins
¼ cup pine nuts (optional)
½ teaspoon paprika
½ teaspoon ground thyme
¼ teaspoon each ground cinnamon, ground cumin, dried oregano, and pepper

Preheat oven to 375°F.

Cut squashes in half lengthwise, scoop out seeds, and lay them, cut-side down, in a roasting pan. Bake for 40 minutes, or until tender. Turn oven down to 350°F after squash halves are done.

While squash halves are baking, prepare stuffing.

To make the stuffing: Combine bulgur with water. Let mixture stand until all water is absorbed, 20 to 30 minutes. Meanwhile, heat oil in a large skillet and brown lamb, breaking up lumps with a fork. Drain off fat. Add onions and green peppers and continue to fry until vegetables are soft. Remove from heat and stir in raisins and nuts (if used). Mix spices into soaked bulgur until well blended, then stir into skillet.

Fill squash cavities with stuffing, mounding it so that stuffing covers squash. (It is easier to do this with hands than a spoon.) Stand stuffed squash halves in a roasting pan that will hold them upright, and bake for 30 minutes.

6 servings

Meatballs *Avgolemono*

1 pound lean ground lamb (ground beef may be substituted)
1 cup soft whole grain bread crumbs
1 egg, beaten
1 small onion, minced
¼ teaspoon garlic powder
2 teaspoons chopped fresh mint
1 tablespoon vegetable oil

Sauce
1½ cups Poultry Stock (page 110)
2 tablespoons cornstarch, dissolved in ¼ cup cold water
3 eggs
¼ cup lemon juice

Mix together lamb, bread crumbs, egg, onions, garlic powder, and mint. Form into 1-inch balls.

Heat oil in a large skillet and brown meatballs on all sides. Reduce heat and continue to cook until meatballs are done, about 10 minutes. Meanwhile, prepare sauce.

To make the sauce: Place stock in top of a double boiler over simmering water and heat well. Add cornstarch mixture and boil until thickened, stirring constantly.

Beat eggs in a small bowl with a wire whisk. Slowly beat in lemon juice, then add heated stock, a little at a time, beating constantly.

Transfer meatballs to a serving dish, pour sauce over them, and serve immediately.

4 servings

Pork

Braised Pork with Fennel

The subtle, licoricelike flavor of fennel adds an uncommon accent to the mildness of fresh pork meat.

2 tablespoons vegetable oil
4 to 5 pounds fresh ham, trimmed of excess fat
1 medium-size onion, chopped
1 green pepper, chopped
1 carrot, finely chopped
1 clove garlic, minced
1 bay leaf
1 cup Poultry Stock (page 110) or Beef Stock (page 110), or more as needed
1 bunch fennel (1 teaspoon fennel seeds and ½ bunch celery, cut into chunks, may be substituted)

Preheat oven to 300°F.

Heat oil in a Dutch oven and brown pork on all sides. Remove pork. Add onions, green peppers, carrots, and garlic and sauté until onions are golden. Return pork to pot and add bay leaf and stock. Cover and bake for 4 hours, or until pork is tender.

Cut lacy tops from fennel; mince and reserve them. Cut bulb portion into 1-inch pieces. Remove bay leaf from pot and add fennel pieces. Cover and continue to bake for 20 to 25 minutes, or until fennel is tender. If necessary, add more stock to pot.

When done, transfer pork and fennel to a platter. Strain pan juice and skim off fat. Pour strained juice over roast and sprinkle on reserved minced fennel tops.

8 to 10 servings

Oven-Barbecued Pork Shoulder

4 to 4½ pounds pork shoulder roast or any semi-boneless cut of pork
3 medium-size tomatoes, peeled, or 1 can (16 ounces) tomatoes
⅓ cup tomato paste, mixed with ⅓ cup water
⅓ cup cider vinegar
2 carrots, finely chopped
1 stalk celery, finely chopped
1 green pepper, finely chopped
2 cloves garlic, minced
2 tablespoons soy sauce
1 tablespoon Worcestershire sauce
1 teaspoon each dry mustard, dried oregano, and paprika
½ teaspoon pepper
½ teaspoon hot pepper sauce

Preheat oven to 375°F.

Place pork in a Dutch oven or set on a wire rack in a roasting pan. Roast, uncovered, for 1 hour.

Meanwhile, combine remaining ingredients in a large skillet and simmer mixture for 20 minutes. If it becomes too thick, add a little hot water.

After pork has cooked for 1 hour, spoon off accumulated fat from pot and discard. Pour sauce over and under pork. Reduce oven temperature to 325°F and continue to cook for 1¼ hours, basting several times.

8 servings

Braised Pork Chops with Apple Rings

    1 tablespoon butter
    4 lean pork chops or cutlets, ¾ inch thick
    2 medium-size onions, sliced into thick rounds
1 to 1¼ cups Poultry Stock (page 110)
    ½ teaspoon ground cinnamon
    ½ teaspoon dried thyme
    2 unpeeled apples, cored and sliced into
        4 rounds each

Heat butter in a 10-inch skillet. Add chops or cutlets and brown on both sides. Add onions and fry, turning occasionally, until rings begin to separate, about 5 minutes. Stir in 1 cup stock along with cinnamon and thyme. Cover and simmer for 45 minutes, or until meat is tender. Check during cooking to see that pan juice does not reduce below ¼ cup; add a little more stock if necessary.

When meat is tender, add apples, turning slices to coat them on both sides with pan juice. Cover and cook for 5 minutes, or until apples are tender but not mushy.

4 servings

Crepes Filled with Pork and Sour Cream

Leftover roast often provides the nucleus for a satisfying main dish, and here is an excellent idea for making the most of yesterday's riches.

    Whole Wheat Crepes (page 395)
3 to 3¼ cups diced cooked pork (cooked beef
        may be substituted)
    1 tablespoon butter

    1 small onion, minced
    ½ cup chopped mushrooms
    1 clove garlic, minced
    1 teaspoon paprika
    ⅛ teaspoon pepper
    1 cup sour cream

Prepare crepes and set aside. Finely grind meat in a food mill or food processor and set aside.

Preheat oven to 375°F.

Melt butter in a large skillet and brown onions, mushrooms, and garlic. Add ground meat, ½ teaspoon paprika, and pepper and sauté lightly. Add ½ cup sour cream and heat through, stirring constantly.

Divide filling between crepes, roll them up, and place in a shallow buttered baking pan. Butter a piece of foil slightly larger than pan. Place foil, butter-side down, over crepes and bake for about 10 minutes.

Mix remaining sour cream with remaining paprika and serve with crepes.

6 servings

Pork and Beans

    1¼ cups dried kidney beans
    1 medium-size onion, chopped
    1 green pepper, chopped
    2 lean pork chops, boned and halved
        pepper, to taste
    2 tablespoons molasses
    ½ teaspoon dry mustard
    ½ teaspoon chili powder

Place kidney beans in a medium-size saucepan. Cover with water to 1 inch above beans. Bring to a boil, then turn off heat, cover, and let stand for 1 hour. Drain, reserving soaking liquid.

Preheat oven to 350°F.

Spoon beans into a 2-quart ovenproof casserole and mix in remaining ingredients. Add reserved soaking liquid and enough boiling water to just cover beans. Bake, with cover ajar, for 2 to 2½ hours, or until beans are tender. Add more boiling water if beans seem too dry, but do not add so much as to make them soupy.

4 servings

Pork Chops with Orange Sauce

1 tablespoon butter
1 tablespoon vegetable oil
1 clove garlic, quartered
½ teaspoon ground sage
4 lean pork chops, 1 inch thick
 pepper, to taste
½ cup orange juice
1 teaspoon lemon juice

Sauce
2 navel oranges
2 tablespoons butter
½ cup seedless white grapes, halved
¼ cup orange juice
¼ cup white grape juice
1 tablespoon cornstarch

In a large skillet heat butter and oil. Add garlic and sage. Then add chops and brown on both sides, seasoning with pepper. Add orange juice and lemon juice. Reduce heat, cover, and simmer for 20 minutes. While chops are cooking, prepare sauce.

To make the sauce: Peel oranges and slice across segments. Cut each segment piece in half.

Melt butter in a large skillet. Add oranges and grapes and lightly sauté. (Do not overcook.) Combine orange juice, grape juice, and cornstarch in a jar with a tight-fitting lid and shake well. Mix into fruit and cook, stirring constantly, until thickened.

Remove chops from pan and place in sauce. Turn to coat both sides. Serve sauce poured over chops.

4 servings

Pork Chops with Pineapple

2 tablespoons vegetable oil
4 lean pork chops, ¾ inch thick
1 small green pepper, chopped
1 small onion, chopped
1 can (16 ounces) unsweetened pineapple
 chunks
1 tablespoon cornstarch
½ cup peanut butter

Preheat oven to 325°F.

Heat oil in a large skillet and brown chops on both sides. Remove from pan. In the same skillet sauté peppers and onions until soft.

Drain pineapple chunks, reserving juice in a 2-cup measure. Add enough water to equal 1½ cups liquid, then stir in cornstarch until dissolved. Pour cornstarch mixture into skillet, blend in peanut butter, and cook until sauce thickens, stirring constantly. Add pineapple chunks.

Pour a thin layer of sauce on bottom of a 2-quart ovenproof casserole. Add chops, then remaining sauce. Bake for 50 minutes, or until chops are cooked through. Serve with brown rice.

4 servings

Prune-Stuffed Pork Pockets

4 lean center-cut pork chops, 1 inch thick
1 tablespoon vegetable oil
1 tablespoon butter
12 to 16 pitted dried prunes
2 pears, peeled, cored, and quartered lengthwise
2 tablespoons cider vinegar

Preheat oven to 375°F.

With a thin sharp knife cut a slit about 2 inches long on outside edge (away from bone) of each chop. Enlarge each slit into a pocket about 2 inches deep by working knife almost through to bone and then sideways.

Heat oil in a 10-inch skillet and brown chops on both sides. Remove them from pan and allow to cool just enough so that they can be handled. Add butter to skillet and heat until melted.

Stuff each pocket with 3 to 4 prunes; use 2 wooden picks to hold each chop together. Lay chops in an oiled baking dish and surround them with pear quarters. Brush pears with butter-oil mixture from skillet, sprinkle chops with vinegar, and bake, uncovered, for about 40 minutes, or until cooked through. Remove wooden picks before serving.

4 servings

Sage Pork Chops with Lemon Sauce

½ cup whole grain bread crumbs
¼ cup wheat germ
1 teaspoon ground sage
1 teaspoon paprika
6 lean pork chops
  milk or water
1 tablespoon vegetable oil

Sauce
1 cup heavy cream
1 tablespoon cornstarch
¼ teaspoon white pepper
¼ teaspoon ground sage
½ cup cold rich Poultry Stock (page 110)
⅓ cup lemon juice

Preheat oven to 375°F.

In a plastic bag mix bread crumbs, wheat germ, sage, and paprika. Moisten chops with milk or water, drain, and shake them, two at a time, in bag with crumb mixture. Lay them in a single layer on an oiled baking sheet. Drizzle oil over all and bake until just cooked through; do not overcook. Half-inch chops should bake about 45 minutes; thicker ones will take longer.

To make the sauce: In a small saucepan heat cream. Stir cornstarch, white pepper, and sage into stock until there are no lumps. Pour cornstarch mixture into heated cream and stir constantly over medium heat until sauce is bubbly and thick. Gradually stir in lemon juice. Serve sauce over chops.

6 servings

Southern-Style Pork Chop Casserole

2 tablespoons vegetable oil
4 lean pork chops
½ cup chopped onions
4 medium-size sweet potatoes, sliced
2 cups sliced okra

2 cups Poultry Stock (page 110)
⅛ teaspoon pepper
2 tablespoons cornstarch

Preheat oven to 325°F. Oil a 3-quart ovenproof casserole.

Heat oil in a large skillet and brown chops on both sides. Add onions and brown them. Arrange sweet potatoes and okra in bottom of casserole. Top with chops and onions.

Pour 1½ cups stock into the same skillet, add pepper, and bring to a boil, scraping bottom and sides of skillet with a wooden spoon to loosen any brown bits.

Stir cornstarch into remaining ½ cup stock until dissolved. Add cornstarch mixture to skillet, stirring constantly, and cook until sauce bubbles and thickens. Pour sauce over chops and vegetables. Cover and bake for 1 hour, or until tender.

4 servings

Pork and Apple Stew

2 pounds boneless pork, trimmed of fat and cubed
¼ cup whole wheat flour
2 tablespoons vegetable oil
1 cup apple juice
2 cups Poultry Stock (page 110)
4 medium-size potatoes, quartered lengthwise
4 carrots, sliced lengthwise
½ teaspoon ground cinnamon
¼ teaspoon pepper
4 apples, peeled, cored, and quartered

Preheat oven to 325°F.

Shake pork cubes and flour together in a plastic bag until pork is well coated.

In a Dutch oven heat oil and brown pork cubes on all sides. Add remaining ingredients, except apples, and bring quickly to a boil. Cover and bake for 1¼ hours. Stir, add apples, and continue to bake 15 minutes more.

4 servings

Pork and Sweet Potato Casserole

1½ pounds boneless pork, trimmed of fat and
    cubed
2 tablespoons cornstarch
1 tablespoon vegetable oil
1 medium-size onion, chopped
1 cup Poultry Stock (page 110)
1 cup apple cider
1 bay leaf
2 apples, peeled, cored, and sliced
½ teaspoon ground cinnamon
4 large sweet potatoes, cooked until tender
2 tablespoons butter, melted

Place pork cubes in a bowl. Sprinkle them with
cornstarch and, using 2 forks, toss until all cubes are
lightly coated.

Heat oil in a large skillet and brown pork cubes on
all sides. Add onions and cook, stirring, until onions
are soft but not brown. Add stock, cider, and bay leaf.
Cover and simmer for 1 hour, or until pork is tender.
Stir occasionally during cooking.

Preheat oven to 350°F.

Discard bay leaf. Remove pork with a slotted
spoon (reserving pan juice) and place in a 10-inch
ovenproof casserole. Top with apples and sprinkle
with cinnamon. Add enough reserved pan juice to
reach apple layer. Mash sweet potatoes and layer them
on top of apples. Drizzle butter over potatoes and bake,
uncovered, for 30 minutes, or until apples are tender
and potatoes are browned.

    4 servings

Pork Casserole with Walnuts and Scallions

1½ cups walnut halves or pieces
2 tablespoons vegetable oil
3 stalks celery, thinly sliced
3 bunches scallions (white part only), cut into
    1-inch lengths
1½ pounds boneless pork, trimmed of fat and
    cubed
2 cups Poultry Stock (page 110), or more as
    needed
3 tablespoons soy sauce

1 tablespoon honey
1 teaspoon ground ginger
3 cups cut fresh green beans
1½ tablespoons cornstarch, dissolved in ½ cup
    cold water

Preheat oven to 350°F.

In a small saucepan cover walnuts with water,
bring to a boil, and continue to boil for 3 minutes.
Drain and rinse walnuts; set aside.

Heat 1 tablespoon oil in an ovenproof skillet or
Dutch oven and stir-fry celery for 3 minutes. Add
walnuts and scallions and continue to stir-fry for
2 minutes. Remove vegetables and nuts with a slotted
spoon and reserve them. Add remaining oil to pan,
heat, and brown pork cubes on all sides. Add stock,
soy sauce, honey, and ginger. Cover and bake for
1½ hours.

Stir green beans into pan and add more stock if
liquid level seems low. Bake 30 minutes longer. When
done, beans should be crisp-tender; do not overcook.

Place pan on range top over medium heat and stir
in cornstarch mixture until thickened. Add reserved
vegetables and nuts and heat through.

    4 to 6 servings

French Canadian Meat Pies
(Tourtières)

*The richly seasoned filling is what makes this
an international favorite.*

    Filling
1 tablespoon vegetable oil
1 pound lean ground pork
1 pound lean ground beef
1 cup chopped onions
1 clove garlic, minced
1 cup water
2 medium-size potatoes, cut in half lengthwise
½ teaspoon dillweed
¼ teaspoon each dried thyme, ground sage,
    celery seeds, ground cinnamon, ground
    allspice, pepper, and dry mustard

pastry for 4 Basic Rolled Piecrusts (page 718)

To make the filling: Heat oil in a 12-inch skillet. Brown pork and beef over medium-high heat, breaking up lumps with a fork. Drain off all fat. Add onions and garlic to meat and stir-fry for 3 minutes. Stir in remaining ingredients, except pastry. Cover skillet and simmer mixture for 20 minutes.

Uncover skillet, mash potatoes in pan, and blend throughout meat mixture. Chill thoroughly in refrigerator.

Prepare pastry in 2 batches. Then divide each batch in half so that you have 4 equal portions. Roll out 2 portions, one at a time, and line 2 9-inch pie plates. Trim away excess dough around edges with a knife. Chill in refrigerator for 20 minutes.

Preheat oven to 425°F.

Divide cold filling between piecrusts. Roll out remaining 2 portions of pastry and cover tops of pies, allowing a 1-inch overhang. Fold overhang over and underneath edges of bottom crusts. Seal edges with a flour-dipped fork. Cut 4 1-inch slits in top of each pie. Bake pies on top shelf of oven for 15 minutes. Reduce heat to 375°F and continue to bake 30 minutes longer, or until pies are golden brown. Allow to rest for 10 minutes before serving.

Makes two 9-inch pies

NOTE: Pies can be frozen, unbaked, and then wrapped in foil for storage. To bake: Remove foil, place still-frozen pies in preheated 375°F oven, and bake for 1 hour, or until golden brown.

Pork and Cabbage Dinner

1½ pounds lean ground pork
⅓ cup soft whole grain bread crumbs (1 small slice bread)
2 tablespoons chopped celery leaves
2 large shallots, minced (about 2 tablespoons)
1 teaspoon crushed fennel seeds
½ teaspoon freshly ground pepper
¼ teaspoon dried thyme
¼ teaspoon ground allspice
1 egg, beaten
1 tablespoon vegetable oil
1 large onion, chopped

6 medium-size tomatoes (2 pounds), peeled and diced
1 small head cabbage, shredded (4 to 5 cups)
½ teaspoon whole cloves

Mix pork with bread crumbs, celery leaves, shallots, fennel seeds, pepper, thyme, and allspice. Blend in egg. Form into 1 to 1½-inch balls.

Heat oil in a Dutch oven or large heavy-bottom pot and brown meatballs on all sides. Remove meatballs with a slotted spoon. Add onions to same pot and fry until golden brown. Stir in tomatoes and simmer, uncovered, for 10 to 15 minutes.

Add cabbage, cloves, and meatballs to pot. Cover and simmer for 15 to 20 minutes, or until cabbage is tender and meatballs are cooked through. Delicious served with brown rice.

4 servings

Pork Balls in Peanut-Tomato Sauce

1½ pounds lean ground pork
1 small onion, minced
1 cup soft whole grain bread crumbs (about 2 slices bread)
¼ cup peanut oil, or more as needed
1 medium-size onion, chopped
1 green pepper, chopped
3 large tomatoes, peeled and chopped
½ teaspoon cayenne pepper
2 cups water
1 cup peanut butter

Mix together pork, onions, and bread crumbs. Form into 1-inch balls.

Heat oil in a large skillet and brown meatballs well on all sides, adding more oil as needed. Reduce heat and continue to sauté until meatballs are cooked through. Transfer to a Dutch oven. Add onions, green peppers, tomatoes, cayenne, and water. Simmer for 20 minutes.

Remove 1 cup cooking liquid from pot, mix in peanut butter, and return mixture to Dutch oven, stirring gently to blend. Simmer 15 minutes longer, then serve immediately. Stew goes well with brown rice.

4 servings

Pork-Stuffed Mushrooms

Be sure to have very large mushrooms on hand for this recipe. If you like, this dish can be used as an appetizer with two or three mushrooms per serving.

24 large mushrooms
olive oil

Stuffing
3 tablespoons butter
1 medium-size onion, minced
1½ cups cooked ground pork, drained
1 cup whole grain bread crumbs
¾ to 1 cup heavy cream
2 tablespoons minced fresh parsley
¼ cup grated Parmesan cheese
½ teaspoon ground sage
white pepper, to taste
¼ cup butter

watercress

Preheat oven to 375°F. Butter a shallow baking pan.

Remove stems from mushrooms and chop them. Brush outsides of mushroom caps with olive oil.

To make the stuffing: In a small saucepan melt butter and sauté onions, then place in a large mixing bowl. Add pork, chopped mushroom stems, bread crumbs, and ¾ cup cream, mixing well. Stir in parsley, cheese, sage, and pepper. Add more cream if needed— stuffing should hold together but not be mushy.

Fill caps with stuffing and place in baking pan. Place a sliver of butter (about ½ teaspoon) on top of each cap and bake for 15 to 20 minutes. Garnish with watercress.

4 servings

Veal

Asparagus and Veal, Chinese Style

1 teaspoon honey
3 tablespoons soy sauce
½ teaspoon white wine vinegar
3 tablespoons plus 1 teaspoon vegetable oil, or more as needed
2 tablespoons white grape juice
3 teaspoons cornstarch
¼ teaspoon ground ginger
1½ pounds thin veal scallops, cut into 1-inch pieces
2 pounds asparagus, cut into 1-inch lengths

In a small cup dissolve honey in 2 tablespoons soy sauce. Add vinegar, 1 teaspoon oil, 1 tablespoon grape juice, and 2 teaspoons cornstarch. Mix well and set aside.

In a small bowl mix together 1 teaspoon cornstarch, ginger, 1 tablespoon soy sauce, and 1 tablespoon grape juice. Add veal and stir to coat well.

Heat 3 tablespoons oil in a large pan or wok and stir-fry asparagus for about 3 minutes. Remove and keep warm. Add more oil if needed and stir-fry veal just until it loses its pink color. Add asparagus along with sauce that has been set aside. Cook just until asparagus is heated through. Serve immediately.

4 servings

Veal Parmesan

8 thin veal scallops (about 1 pound)
1 egg, beaten
⅓ cup whole wheat flour
¼ cup olive oil
1½ cups thick tomato sauce or Marinara Sauce (page 328)
½ cup grated Parmesan cheese
8 ounces mozzarella cheese, sliced

Dip scallops into egg and then into flour.

Heat 2 tablespoons oil in a large skillet and brown scallops lightly on both sides, a few at a time. Add remaining oil as needed.

Pour tomato or marinara sauce over scallops in skillet and sprinkle with Parmesan cheese. Bring to a boil, then reduce heat, cover, and simmer for 15 minutes. Uncover and top with mozzarella cheese. Cover again and cook until cheese melts. If sauce is too thin, uncover and simmer for a few more minutes.

4 servings

Braised Veal and Vegetables

¼ cup olive oil or other vegetable oil
2 pounds stewing veal, cut into chunks
1 medium-size onion, sliced and separated into
  rings
1 carrot, thinly sliced
1 stalk celery, chopped
1 clove garlic, crushed
1 tablespoon chopped fresh parsley
1 can (16 ounces) tomatoes, drained and
  chopped
1 cup Beef Stock (page 110)
  pepper, to taste
  parsley sprigs

Preheat oven to 325°F.

Heat oil in a Dutch oven and brown veal on all sides. Add onion rings, carrots, celery, and garlic and sauté for 3 minutes. Add remaining ingredients, except parsley sprigs. Cover and bake for 1½ hours, or until meat is tender. Garnish with parsley sprigs. Goes well with whole wheat pasta.

4 servings

Veal Chops in Herb Sauce

3 tablespoons olive oil
4 green peppers, cut into strips
4 medium-size onions, sliced and separated into
  rings
4 veal shoulder chops (1½ to 2 pounds)
1 cup Poultry Stock (page 110)
⅛ teaspoon garlic powder
1 teaspoon dried basil
¼ cup chopped fresh parsley
1 tablespoon cornstarch, dissolved in ½ cup
  cold milk
  pepper, to taste
  lemon slices

Heat oil in a large skillet and sauté peppers and onion rings until soft. Remove them from pan with a slotted spoon and set aside. Add chops and brown on both sides. Remove and set aside.

Combine stock, garlic powder, basil, and parsley in the same skillet and bring to a boil. Stir in cornstarch mixture and pepper and simmer for 3 minutes, stirring constantly.

Preheat oven to 325°F.

Spread a little sauce in bottom of a 3-quart ovenproof casserole. Add 2 chops, ½ of the onions and peppers, and ½ of the remaining sauce. Repeat layers, ending with sauce. Bake for 1¼ hours, or until chops are tender. Garnish with lemon slices. Serve with brown rice or whole wheat pasta.

4 servings

Veal Scallops au Gratin

8 thin veal scallops
½ cup whole wheat flour
⅛ teaspoon pepper
½ cup plus 3 tablespoons butter
8 slices Swiss cheese
1 teaspoon dried basil
2 teaspoons chopped fresh parsley
½ cup grated Parmesan cheese
1 pound mushrooms, sliced

Preheat oven to 350°F.

Dredge veal in flour mixed with pepper.

In a large skillet melt ¼ cup butter. Add veal and sauté about 3 minutes on each side, or until lightly browned. Transfer to a large buttered shallow baking dish and top each scallop with a slice of cheese. Brown ¼ cup butter in the same skillet. Dribble browned butter over cheese slices, dividing evenly. Mix together basil, parsley, and Parmesan cheese and sprinkle over cheese. Bake for 10 minutes, or until cheese is slightly melted.

While veal is baking, heat 3 tablespoons butter in a large skillet and sauté mushrooms until all moisture has evaporated. Serve mushrooms on top of veal scallops.

4 servings

Veal and Chicken Paprikash

3 tablespoons whole wheat flour
1 tablespoon paprika
1 whole chicken breast, boned, skinned, and cut into bite-size pieces (about 1 pound boneless)
1 pound stewing veal, cubed
¼ cup vegetable oil, or more as needed
2 cups Poultry Stock (page 110)
1 tablespoon honey
2 tablespoons cornstarch
1 cup sour cream

Combine flour and paprika in a large plastic bag. Add chicken pieces and shake to coat, then repeat with veal.

Heat oil in a large skillet and brown chicken and veal on all sides, adding more oil as necessary. Remove meat with a slotted spoon and set aside.

In the same skillet heat 1½ cups stock. Add honey and stir to dissolve. Dissolve cornstarch in remaining ½ cup stock and add to skillet, stirring constantly. Cook until mixture bubbles and thickens.

Preheat oven to 350°F.

Combine meat and sauce in a 3-quart ovenproof casserole. Cover and bake for 1 to 1¼ hours. Stir in sour cream and bake an additional 5 minutes to heat through. Serve with whole wheat noodles.

4 servings

Variety Meats

Most variety meats require some preparation before they are ready to be cooked. Preliminary steps may take only a few moments, such as removing the membrane and veins from liver, or they may involve one to two hours of soaking or simmering. Preparing Variety Meats, page 468, describes these steps. Be sure to allow time for this when using the following recipes.

Beef Liver, Italian Style

The garlic and lemon juice, instead of a tomato sauce, suggest the northern Italian influence in this dish.

2 pounds beef liver
½ cup whole wheat flour
    pepper, to taste
3 tablespoons vegetable oil
2 cloves garlic, halved
2 tablespoons butter
2 tablespoons lemon juice
1 lemon, sliced
    parsley sprigs

Prepare liver for cooking (see page 468), then thinly slice it. Dredge slices in mixture of flour and pepper.

In a large skillet heat oil. Add garlic and sauté, stirring occasionally. Add liver and sauté quickly on both sides just until golden brown. Lift out liver, transfer to a heated serving platter, and keep warm. Discard garlic.

Melt butter in the same oil. Add lemon juice and stir with a wooden spoon, scraping up any brown bits in bottom of skillet. Pour pan juice over liver and garnish with lemon slices and parsley sprigs.

6 servings

Calf's Liver with Mustard Sauce

8 slices calf's liver
3 tablespoons butter
2 large onions, sliced and separated into rings
1 cup Poultry Stock (page 110)
1 tablespoon cider vinegar
½ teaspoon dried tarragon
½ cup sour cream
1 teaspoon French-style mustard
¼ teaspoon pepper

Prepare liver for cooking (see page 468).

Heat a large skillet and melt 2 tablespoons butter in it. Add liver slices and sauté quickly on both sides just until cooked through. (Do not overcook.) Lift out liver, transfer to a heated serving platter, and keep warm.

Add remaining butter to the same skillet, along with onion rings. Sauté, stirring, until soft. Then reduce heat, cover, and cook until tender, about 5 minutes.

Add stock, vinegar, and tarragon. Cook over high heat until stock is reduced to about ½ cup. Blend in sour cream, mustard, and pepper. Heat sauce through, but do not boil. Pour sauce over liver to serve.

4 servings

Fitness House Sautéed Liver

6 slices beef liver or calf's liver (about
    1½ pounds)
¾ cup rye flour
¼ cup vegetable oil

Prepare liver for cooking (see page 468), then dredge slices in flour, one at a time.

Heat oil in a large skillet over medium-high heat until hot but not smoking. Add liver slices and sauté quickly, turning each only once after the underside is golden brown. When both sides are golden brown and no more juice is coming out, transfer to a serving platter and serve immediately. May be accompanied by sautéed sliced onions.

6 servings

Liver in Sour Cream

1½ pounds liver
2 tablespoons butter
2 tablespoons whole wheat or rye flour
⅛ teaspoon pepper
1½ cups sour cream

Preheat oven to 300°F.

Prepare liver for cooking (see page 468), then cut into slices ¾ inch thick.

Melt butter in a large ovenproof skillet which has a tight-fitting lid. Add liver and sauté quickly on both sides just until golden brown, then lift out and set aside.

Stir flour and pepper into pan drippings. Blend over medium heat until smooth and lightly browned. Add sour cream and cook for 1 minute, stirring constantly.

Return liver to sauce in skillet, cover tightly, and bake for about 40 minutes, or until tender. Serve liver with sauce poured on top.

4 to 6 servings

Braised Stuffed Veal Hearts

2 veal hearts (1¼ to 1½ pounds)
4 tablespoons vegetable oil
3 scallions, chopped
½ cup cracker crumbs
2 tablespoons chopped fresh parsley
½ teaspoon dried thyme
½ teaspoon ground sage
    pepper, to taste
1 egg, beaten
1 tablespoon butter
2 cups mixed carrot sticks, celery sticks, and
    whole scallions
1 large tomato, peeled and chopped
½ cup Poultry Stock (page 110) or water
1 tablespoon cider vinegar

Prepare hearts for cooking (see page 468), leaving halves attached on one side.

Heat 3 tablespoons oil in a Dutch oven and sauté chopped scallions lightly. Empty contents of pot into a small bowl, add crumbs, 1 tablespoon parsley, thyme, sage, pepper, and egg and mix until well blended. Pack stuffing into each split heart, then press halves together so that all stuffing is in center, as if they were whole hearts. Tie in several places with kitchen twine to hold them together.

Add butter and remaining oil to pot and brown stuffed hearts lightly on all sides. Add carrots, celery, and whole scallions and stir-fry until they begin to brown. Stir in remaining parsley, tomatoes, stock or water, and vinegar. Cover and simmer for 2½ hours, or until tender. Remove twine, then slice and serve.

3 to 4 servings

Eggplant Shells Stuffed with Veal Kidney

    4 small veal kidneys
    2 medium-size eggplants
    4 tablespoons olive oil, or more as needed
    1 green pepper, chopped
    1 medium-size onion, chopped
    1 teaspoon minced garlic
    3 medium-size tomatoes or 1 can (16 ounces)
        tomatoes, chopped
    ½ teaspoon dried oregano
        freshly ground pepper, to taste
    1 cup soft whole grain bread crumbs (about
        2 slices bread)
    ½ cup grated Parmesan cheese

Prepare kidneys for cooking (see page 469).

Cut eggplants in half lengthwise. Scoop out flesh, leaving ½-inch-thick shells. Dice eggplant flesh.

Heat 1 tablespoon oil in a large skillet. Add kidneys and brown on both sides. (Do not overcook.) Lift kidneys out of skillet and set aside.

Heat remaining oil in the same skillet and sauté green peppers, onions, and garlic until soft but not brown. Add diced eggplant and continue to cook, stirring, until eggplant shrinks a bit and softens. If necessary, add a little more oil to keep pieces from sticking. Add tomatoes and oregano. Stir and cook, uncovered, until slightly thickened but not runny, about 10 minutes.

Preheat oven to 350°F.

Arrange kidneys in eggplant shells placed in a baking pan. Spoon vegetable mixture over them and sprinkle with pepper, crumbs, and cheese. Bake for 30 minutes, or until eggplant shells are easily pierced with a fork.

    4 servings

Kidneys en Brochette

    4 veal kidneys or 8 lamb kidneys
    ½ cup vegetable oil
    2 cloves garlic, minced
    1 teaspoon dried oregano
    2 tablespoons lemon juice
    16 cherry tomatoes
    2 large green peppers, cut into 1-inch pieces
    16 medium-size mushrooms
    2 bunches small scallions (white parts only)

Prepare kidneys for cooking (see page 469), then cut into 1-inch cubes.

Combine oil, garlic, oregano, and lemon juice in a deep bowl. Add kidney cubes and refrigerate, covered, for 1 to 2 hours, stirring occasionally.

Place marinated kidney cubes, tomatoes, peppers, mushrooms, and scallions alternately on skewers. Broil for about 15 minutes, or until vegetables are tender and kidneys are browned and juicy. Serve with brown rice.

    4 servings

Steak and Kidney Pie

No British pub could survive without having this on the menu. Its popularity persists through the centuries because the dish is so tasty and hearty.

    1 beef kidney (about 1 pound)
    2 tablespoons butter
    1 medium-size onion, chopped
    1 carrot, coarsely grated
    1 stalk celery, minced
1 to 1½ pounds chuck steak, trimmed of fat
        and cut into 1-inch cubes
    ¼ cup whole wheat flour
    1 teaspoon paprika
    ¼ teaspoon pepper
    2 tablespoons vegetable oil
    3 cups Beef Stock (page 110)
    1 medium-size potato, quartered

    Topping
    6 slices whole wheat bread
    3 tablespoons butter, melted
    2 tablespoons chopped fresh parsley

Prepare kidney for cooking (see page 469), then slice it thinly.

Melt butter in a large skillet and sauté kidney slices for 5 minutes. Remove with a slotted spoon and place in a 3-quart ovenproof casserole. Sauté onions, carrots, and celery in the same skillet for 3 minutes. Transfer to casserole.

Preheat oven to 350°F.

Shake beef cubes, flour, paprika, and pepper together in a large plastic bag until beef is well coated. Heat oil in the same skillet, add beef, and brown on all sides over medium-high heat. Transfer to casserole. Add stock to skillet and bring to a boil, scraping brown bits off bottom and sides of skillet. Add to casserole along with potato pieces. Cover and bake for 1½ hours, or until meat is tender. Remove potatoes, mash them with some cooking liquid, and return to casserole. Stir to mix.

To make the topping: Toast bread, brush with melted butter, and cut into triangles. Arrange triangles in overlapping rows on top of pie. Sprinkle with parsley and serve.

6 servings

Boiled Fresh Tongue

Sliced cold tongue makes excellent sandwiches. You may also want to cube it, for adding to salads and stews, or to serve it hot, complemented by a favorite sauce.

1 fresh beef tongue or 4 fresh veal tongues
1 medium-size onion, sliced
2 bay leaves
¼ teaspoon pepper

Place tongue in a large pot, cover with water, and add onions, bay leaves, and pepper. Simmer for 2 to 4 hours, or until tender.

Lift tongue out of broth and plunge briefly in cold water to loosen skin. While still warm, slit skin on underside lengthwise and peel off. With a sharp knife cut away root, bones, and gristle at thick end.

Tongue is now cooked and ready to serve hot, as is, or to use in a recipe. (Broth may be strained and used as a stock for soup.) If serving it cold, return tongue to cooking broth and allow to cool completely for added juiciness and flavor.

4 servings

Braised Sweetbreads with Scallions and Mushrooms

¾ to 1 pound sweetbreads
2 tablespoons butter
10 large mushrooms, sliced
6 scallions, thinly sliced
3 cloves garlic, minced
¼ teaspoon dried thyme
½ cup white grape juice

Prepare sweetbreads for cooking (see page 469).

Melt butter in a large skillet and sauté mushrooms and scallions. Stir in garlic and thyme, then add sweetbreads and grape juice. Cover and simmer for 25 to 30 minutes. Serve over cooked grains or buttered whole wheat toast points.

4 servings

Breaded Sweetbread Cutlets

Sweetbreads require several hours of preparation time for this recipe, most of the time being needed for soaking, then firming the cutlets before sautéing.

1 pound sweetbreads
½ cup rye or whole wheat flour
1 egg
2 tablespoons water
1 teaspoon plus 2 tablespoons vegetable oil
1¼ cups fine, soft, whole grain bread crumbs (2 to 3 slices bread)
2 tablespoons butter
pepper, to taste
lemon slices
parsley sprigs

Prepare sweetbreads for cooking (see page 469).

Slice sweetbreads into 8 cutlets. Cover with paper towels and place between 2 cutting boards, weighting them down with a heavy object. Let stand for several hours, to firm them. (This improves the texture.)

Dredge sweetbread cutlets on all sides in flour. Beat egg in a shallow bowl, then stir in water and 1 teaspoon oil. Place bread crumbs in another shallow bowl. Dip cutlets in egg mixture and then in bread crumbs. Coat thoroughly and pat to make crumbs adhere.

In a large skillet heat butter and remaining 2 tablespoons oil. Add sweetbreads and sauté until golden on both sides. Garnish with pepper, lemon slices, and parsley sprigs.

4 to 6 servings

Broiled Sweetbreads

¾ to 1 pound veal sweetbreads
    ¼ cup butter
    2 sweet red peppers, sliced into wide strips
 10 large mushrooms
    2 tablespoons soy sauce
    ½ cup grated Parmesan cheese

Prepare sweetbreads for cooking (see page 469).

Slowly brown sweetbreads in butter. (A pan that can go from stove top to oven will save a step.) Add red peppers and mushrooms and continue to sauté for a few minutes. Add soy sauce and toss.

Spoon mixture into a pan that can be placed under broiler. Top with cheese and place pan about 8 inches from heat source. Broil until cheese melts, about 5 minutes.

    4 servings

Variation:

Sweetbreads en Brochette: Prepare sweetbreads for cooking (see page 469), then cut into pieces. Arrange alternately on skewers with red peppers and mushrooms. Melt butter and stir in soy sauce. Brush mixture over skewered pieces, sprinkle with cheese, and broil about 5 minutes, or until cheese melts.

Veal Roast Stuffed with Sweetbreads

    ½ pound veal sweetbreads
 3 to 4 pounds boneless veal shoulder or leg roast
    ¼ teaspoon each dried marjoram, rosemary, and
        thyme
    2 cloves garlic, halved
    3 tablespoons olive oil
 1½ cups Poultry Stock (page 110)
        juice of 2 lemons
    ¼ cup butter, melted

Prepare sweetbreads for cooking (see page 469), then dice and set aside.

Untie cord that holds roast together. Make whatever cuts are necessary to cause roast to lie flat. Arrange diced sweetbreads over roast to within 1 inch of all edges. Mix and crush herbs and sprinkle them over sweetbreads. Reshape and tie roast securely with kitchen twine, using both lengthwise and crosswise ties 1 inch apart. Make 4 slits in roast and insert garlic halves into slits.

Preheat oven to 350°F.

Heat oil in a Dutch oven and brown roast on all sides. Combine stock with lemon juice and melted butter and pour ½ of the mixture over roast. Cover and bake for about 1½ hours.

Uncover roast and cook 1 to 1½ hours more, or until tender, basting from time to time with remaining stock mixture. Remove garlic with a knife point and allow roast to rest for 15 minutes before removing twine and slicing.

    8 to 10 servings

Brains and Eggs

    ½ pound veal brains
    2 tablespoons butter
    8 eggs
    ½ cup milk
    ¼ cup grated Parmesan cheese

Prepare brains for cooking (see page 469), then cut into bite-size pieces.

Melt butter in a large skillet. Beat eggs together with the milk and pour into skillet. When eggs begin to firm up, scramble them with a wooden spoon. Add brains and continue to stir until eggs reach desired dryness. Sprinkle with Parmesan and serve immediately.

    4 servings

Brains in Brown Garlic Butter

    1 pound veal brains
    ¼ cup plus 2 tablespoons butter
    2 cloves garlic, minced
    2 tablespoons lemon juice

Prepare brains for cooking (see page 469), then separate into 8 large pieces.

Melt ¼ cup butter in a large skillet. Add brains and brown them, then transfer to a heated platter.

Add garlic and remaining butter to skillet. Heat slowly until butter browns but does not burn. Stir in lemon juice, then pour browned butter over brains and serve.

4 servings

Sautéed Brains

2 pounds veal brains
  cornmeal
2 tablespoons vegetable oil
  lemon juice
  pepper, to taste
  chopped fresh parsley

Prepare brains for cooking (see page 469), then slice into serving pieces and dust with cornmeal.

Heat oil in a large heavy-bottom skillet. Add brains and sauté for 5 minutes on each side. Drizzle a few drops of lemon juice over each piece, sprinkle with pepper, and garnish with chopped parsley.

6 to 8 servings

Tripe with Herbs and Potatoes

2 pounds fresh tripe
¼ cup vegetable oil
1 small onion, chopped
2 cups cold Beef Stock (page 110)
1 tablespoon Worcestershire sauce
¼ teaspoon ground thyme
½ teaspoon dried basil
1 tablespoon minced fresh parsley
2 tablespoons cornstarch
4 medium-size potatoes, diced

Prepare, then fully cook, tripe (see page 469). Cool and cut into 1-inch pieces.

Heat oil in a large skillet and brown tripe. Add onions and sauté lightly. Then remove onions and tripe with a slotted spoon and place in a 3-quart ovenproof casserole.

In the same skillet combine 1½ cups stock, Worcestershire sauce, thyme, basil, and parsley and bring to a boil. Stir cornstarch into remaining ½ cup stock until dissolved. Pour cornstarch mixture into hot stock, stirring constantly, and cook until sauce bubbles and thickens.

Preheat oven to 350°F.

Combine sauce and potatoes with tripe and onions in casserole. Stir, cover, and bake for 45 minutes, or until potatoes are tender.

4 servings

Oxtails with Tomatoes and Bulgur

3 tablespoons vegetable oil
4 pounds meaty oxtails, trimmed of fat
2 large onions, chopped
2 stalks celery, with leaves, chopped
1 carrot, chopped
2 cloves garlic, minced
6 medium-size tomatoes, 2 pounds plum
    tomatoes, or 4 cans (16 ounces each) Italian-
    style tomatoes, chopped
8 sprigs flat-leaf parsley
1 teaspoon dried basil
½ teaspoon dried marjoram
¼ teaspoon pepper
½ teaspoon grated lemon rind
  juice of 1 lemon
1½ cups bulgur

Heat oil in a Dutch oven. Add oxtails and brown on all sides. Remove and reserve oxtails. Drain off all but 1 tablespoon oil from pan, then add onions, celery, carrots, and garlic and sauté until soft but not brown. Add reserved oxtails, tomatoes, stems from parsley (reserve leaves), basil, marjoram, pepper, and just enough water to cover. Cover and simmer (or bake at 350°F) for 3½ to 4 hours, or until meat is very tender.

Remove oxtails with a slotted spoon and set aside. Skim off and discard excess fat. Strain pan juice, then measure and add enough water to make 3 cups. Pour liquid into pan and add lemon rind and lemon juice. Bring to a boil, then gradually add bulgur, stirring constantly.

Preheat oven to 350°F.

Return meat to pot, cover, and bake for 30 minutes, or until bulgur is cooked and all liquid has been absorbed. Chop reserved parsley leaves and sprinkle over oxtails and bulgur before serving.

4 servings

Sausage

Farmer's Supper Sausage

After refrigerating overnight, these sausage patties make a filling supper dish when accompanied by a green salad and fresh fruit dessert.

1¾ pounds well-fatted boneless beef, cubed
¼ pound well-fatted boneless pork, cubed
1 tablespoon vegetable oil
1 large onion, finely chopped
1 green pepper, finely chopped
1 medium-size tart apple, peeled, cored, and finely chopped
3 medium-size potatoes, cooked until tender, cooled, and finely diced
¼ cup fine whole grain bread crumbs
¼ cup light cream
  generous pinch each of dried thyme, sage, and savory
¼ teaspoon pepper

Grind beef and pork together with a meat grinder.

Heat oil in a large skillet and gently sauté onions, green peppers, and apples until transparent and tender but not browned. Allow to cool.

Place ground meat, sautéed ingredients, potatoes, bread crumbs, cream, thyme, sage, savory, and pepper in a large bowl. Using hands moistened with water, gently blend ingredients. Mix thoroughly, being careful not to break potato dice.

Shape into patties 1 inch thick and 2½ to 3 inches across (or form into links if desired—see page 469). Cover loosely with wax paper and refrigerate overnight. Cook as desired (see page 481).

Makes 2½ to 3 pounds

NOTE: Because of the potatoes, this sausage does not freeze well. However, it may be prepared and frozen in bulk without the potatoes—which can then be added just before shaping into patties and cooking.

Mild Italian Sausage

Prepare this sausage the night before, then try it loose as a stuffing for green peppers for a quick, attractive meal, or add cut-up links to a favorite Italian dish with plenty of sautéed onions, peppers, and tomato sauce.

2 pounds well-fatted pork shoulder, cubed
4 whole chicken legs, boned, skinned, and cubed (about 1 pound boneless)
1 large clove garlic, diced
2 tablespoons rich Beef Stock (page 110)
1 teaspoon minced fresh oregano
2 teaspoons chopped fresh basil
1 teaspoon minced fresh marjoram
1 cup fine whole grain bread crumbs
3 to 4 feet pork or lamb casings

Grind pork, chicken, and garlic together in a meat grinder. Place in a large bowl and add stock, oregano, basil, marjoram, and bread crumbs. Blend thoroughly, using hands moistened with water.

Fill casings (see page 469) with mixture. (Or, use loose as a stuffing or shape into patties, if desired.) Cover with wax paper and refrigerate overnight. Cook as desired (see page 481).

Makes 3 pounds

Mexican Beef and Pork Sausage
(Chorizo)

Traditionally, chorizo is used loose in meat sauces or formed into links that are the size of a man's thumb. To fully blend flavors, the sausage is refrigerated for 48 hours before use.

1 pound well-fatted boneless beef, cubed
1 pound well-fatted boneless pork, cubed
2 cloves garlic, diced

1 teaspoon dried oregano
½ teaspoon ground cinnamon
2 tablespoons paprika
1 teaspoon ground cumin
¼ teaspoon crushed red pepper, or to taste
2 tablespoons vinegar
2 to 3 feet pork or lamb casings

Grind beef, pork, and garlic together with a meat grinder. Place in a large bowl and add oregano, cinnamon, paprika, cumin, red pepper, and vinegar. Mix thoroughly, using hands moistened with water.

Fill casings (see page 469) and tie off in 2-inch links. (Or, shape into patties or use loose in a meat sauce, if desired.) Cover with wax paper and refrigerate for 2 days. Then cook as desired (see page 481), or freeze.

Makes 2 pounds

Traditional English Liver Sausage

This sausage mixture is traditionally wrapped in squares of caul fat and formed into balls placed close together in a baking pan. Two other methods of shaping it are provided here instead, since a caul may not be easily obtainable. The sausage is baked, then refrigerated overnight before serving.

1½ pounds pork liver
½ pound good-quality pork fat
2 medium-size onions
1 clove garlic, chopped
1 teaspoon chopped fresh parsley
1½ teaspoons ground sage
½ teaspoon pepper
  generous pinch each of ground nutmeg, cloves, and cinnamon
1 cup fine whole grain bread crumbs, or more as needed
1 pig's stomach (optional)

Prepare liver for cooking (see page 468).

Grind liver, pork fat (reserve 2 or 3 strips), onions, and garlic together with a meat grinder. Place in a large bowl and stir in parsley, sage, pepper, nutmeg, cloves, and cinnamon. Add bread crumbs and blend well. Mixture will be rather runny but should plop when dropped from a spoon. Add a small amount of extra bread crumbs if necessary.

Preheat oven to 350°F.

Shape and bake sausage using one of the following methods:

1. Lightly oil a small ovenproof crock or pottery or ceramic casserole and pack sausage mixture into it. Top with reserved strips of pork fat and cover tightly. Set this in a deep baking pan and pour hot water into pan until it is ⅓ to ⅔ up the side of crock or casserole. Bake for about 1 hour, or until juice runs clear. (Check water level occasionally, adding more hot water as necessary.)

2. Tie off the three small orifices of a pig's stomach with string. Fill stomach with sausage mixture, then tie off the large opening. Pull all tied parts together underneath and secure with string. Now you have a *boulette*. Place it on a wire rack over a roasting pan filled partway with water, but do not let water touch *boulette*. (If *boulette* will not stay upright with tied parts underneath, prop up with crumbled foil.) Place reserved strips of pork fat over *boulette* and cover loosely with foil. Bake for 1½ hours. Uncover, remove fat strips, and bake 30 minutes longer to brown.

Remove crock or *boulette* from oven. Cover loosely with wax paper and refrigerate overnight. To serve, unmold from crock and slice thinly. Or, cut off tied part of *boulette* so that sausage will stand firmly, then cut a cross in top, peel back casing like a baked potato, and scoop out. Serve on crackers or rye toast rounds, accompanied by chopped onions.

Makes 2 pounds

Poultry

Up to a generation ago, poultry—chicken, turkey, game hen, pheasant, duckling, goose—was reserved for traditional holiday feasts and special Sunday dinners. But today most families enjoy poultry's mild, subtle flavor frequently because poultry is both inexpensive and readily available. Its low levels of cholesterol and calories, coupled with impressive nutritional values, add to poultry's appeal. Best of all, poultry is easy to prepare.

Buying Poultry

Except for poultry purchased directly from small farms, all fresh and frozen whole poultry on the market is ready-to-cook (dressed and plucked) and usually comes with the giblets and neck packed in the body cavity. The fresh birds are commonly sold whole, or in halves, quarters, or parts, but frozen birds are generally available only whole. Because the price per pound is generally lowest for whole poultry, consider buying whole birds and doing your own cutting (see Cutting Poultry, page 523, and Deboning Poultry Breasts, page 524). Select poultry that is most suited to your needs. Young birds are tender and best for broiling, frying, and roasting; older birds can be braised or stewed.

When you purchase fresh, chilled poultry, look for these signs of quality. There should be no odor and a minimum of coarse pinfeathers. The skin should be soft and should tear easily; it should be smooth, cream colored, and moist but

Inspection and Grading of Poultry

All poultry with a United States Department of Agriculture (USDA) inspection mark (circle) on the label, wrapper, wing tag, package insert, or giblet wrapping has been inspected for wholesomeness by the federal government or by an equivalent state inspection program. The mark indicates that the poultry came from a healthy flock, was processed under rigid sanitary conditions, contains no harmful chemicals or additives, is properly packaged, and is labeled truthfully and informatively.

A shield accompanying the circle indicates that at the packer's request the poultry has also been graded for quality. Of all the poultry grades, A and B are the ones most commonly seen in markets; other grades of poultry are usually sold for use in convenience foods such as TV dinners.

USDA Grade A—choicest, full fleshed, practically free from defects
USDA Grade B—second best, slightly less meaty and attractive than Grade A
USDA Grade C (occasionally seen on turkeys)—bruised skin, broken bones, torn skin

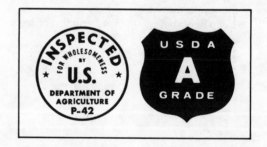

518

not wet. If you are buying a whole bird (or just breasts), the breasts should look plump and meaty. Check the breastbone and wings for clues to the age of the bird: In young poultry the breastbone should be flexible and light in color (gray is a sign of old age and indicates that the bird was frozen); the wings should offer little resistance when bent into an upright position.

Frozen poultry has slightly less flavor than fresh, but the texture is usually good. Since many frozen birds such as turkeys are prestuffed and prebasted with butter, fat, or stock, read the label to know what you are buying. Some frozen birds also have built-in thermometers that will pop up when the internal temperature reaches the well-done point.

When buying frozen poultry, check the following items. The wrap should form a complete seal. Broken wraps usually mean freezer burn, resulting in dry, unpalatable flesh. The flesh should be solidly frozen with no discoloration. There should be no evidence of pink ice around the meat, and there should be no blocks of frozen juices at the bottom of the package. These are indications that the bird has thawed and been refrozen. With repeated thawing and freezing, quality suffers—the flesh becomes stringy and tasteless.

When deciding how much fresh or frozen poultry to buy, remember that up to one-half the weight is usually lost in waste—fat, skin, bones. Use the following as a general guide: If the bird is under 12 pounds, 1 pound will serve one person; but if over 12 pounds, ¾ pound will do nicely for one. For birds over 20 pounds, allow ½ pound for one person. In boneless poultry ⅓ to ½ pound

Common Market Forms of Poultry

Poultry	Description
Chicken	
Broiler-fryer (occasionally called fryer)	young, all-purpose bird; 1½-4 pounds; available ready-to-cook in whole, halves, quarters, or parts; good broiled, fried, braised, roasted, poached
Capon	meaty, tender, juicy, castrated male; 4-7 pounds; available whole; superb roasted
Roaster	large, plump, young bird (12 weeks old); 3-5 pounds; available whole or halves; excellent roasted
Rock Cornish game hen	crossbreed of Plymouth Rock chicken and Cornish gamecock; small, tender, meaty; marketed whole; available fresh and frozen; 1-2 pounds; ideal roasted but also tasty braised, broiled, or fried
Stewing hen	large, old bird; little meat; 3-6½ pounds; good flavor; best for stocks, soups, ground chicken
Duck	
Broiler-fryer	very young bird (under 8 weeks old); less than 3 pounds; most available frozen; outstanding fried or broiled
Roaster	fatty, tender bird (8-16 weeks old); 3-6 pounds; most available frozen; best roasted or braised

[*continued*]

Common Market Forms of Poultry—*Continued*

Poultry	Description
Goose (gosling)	fatty; all meat is dark; best roasted when 4-12 pounds; good braised when over 14 pounds and older than 6 months; most available frozen
Guinea fowl	dry, delicately gamey bird; hen preferable; 2-4 pounds; ready-to-cook available at gourmet butchers; most are frozen; good roasted, braised, poached
Pheasant (farm-raised)	plump, dry bird; 2-4 pounds; most marketed frozen; ready-to-cook occasionally available at gourmet butchers; usually roasted or braised
Squab	young, domesticated pigeon; weighs less than 1 pound; usually marketed frozen but sometimes available fresh; ideal roasted but also good braised
Turkey* Fryer-roaster	small, young, tender hen or tom (16 weeks old) with smooth skin and flexible breastbone; 4-9 pounds; excellent broiled, roasted, oven-fried
Young	hen or tom (5-7 months old) with tender meat and skin; weight varies with age but usually 7-15 pounds; best roasted
Yearling	mature hen or tom (just over 1 year old); fairly tender; weight varies with age and breed but may be 20-30 pounds; usually roasted or braised

*Turkeys are sometimes categorized by weight: small, 4-10 pounds; medium, 10-19 pounds; large, 20 or more pounds.

will serve one; in prestuffed birds 1½ pounds will yield enough for one person.

Storing Poultry

Chilled, uncooked poultry is highly perishable and will keep best if the store wrap (which clings tightly and encourages spoilage) is removed and the bird is loosely rewrapped in wax paper, then refrigerated. (You can eliminate the rewrapping step if the poultry has been prepackaged in a heavy transparent wrap specially designed for storage both in the meat case and at home.) When storing a whole bird, always remove the giblets and package them separately. Never stuff the bird before storing. Use raw, refrigerated poultry within two days of purchase.

To store cooked poultry, cool it quickly, wrap it loosely, and place it in the coldest part of the refrigerator. Cutting the meat from the carcass before storing will conserve space. The bones can then be used to make a white stock, which can be reduced and frozen in ice cube trays (see Stocks, page 100).

If leftover cooked poultry has been stuffed, remove the stuffing and store it separately. Any gravy or broth should also be stored separately in a tightly closed container. You should use the stuffing and broth or gravy within two days, but you can keep the poultry itself up to four days.

For longer storage both raw and cooked poultry can be frozen. But never stuff a bird before freezing. (Commercial producers of frozen stuffed birds have access to techniques for freezing such products safely, but these methods are unavailable to cooks at home.) For top-quality poultry follow recommended wrapping procedures to prevent freezer burn (see Freezer Materials, page 753), and store no longer than the maximum length of time (see Freezer Storage table, page 756).

Thawing Poultry

As a rule thawed poultry cooks more evenly and retains better texture than frozen poultry. For safety, however, commercially stuffed and frozen turkeys should always be roasted while still frozen. Follow directions on the package for oven temperature and timing.

Poultry, whether whole or cut in parts, is easily thawed in one of three ways. Whichever method you choose, thawing will be quicker for a whole bird if the package of giblets and neck has been removed from the body cavity before freezing. Of course, parts that are wrapped in small packages thaw the quickest.

Thawing in the refrigerator is the slowest but safest way, since the outside surfaces remain cool during the entire thawing time. Keep the bird in its original wrap or cover it lightly with wax paper if unwrapped. Place poultry on a tray

Thawing Poultry

Poultry	Weight (pounds)	Time in Refrigerator	Time in Cold Water
Chicken			
Whole	3-4	12-16 hours	1-2 hours
	over 4	1-1½ days	4-6 hours
Pieces	¼-¾	3-9 hours	1 hour
Duck	3-6	1-1½ days	4-6 hours
Goose	6-12	1-2 days	4-6 hours
Guinea fowl	2-4	12-16 hours	1-2 hours
Pheasant	2-4	12-16 hours	1-2 hours
Squab	under 1	6-12 hours	1 hour
Turkey			
Whole	4-12	1-2 days	4-6 hours
	12-20	2-3 days	6-8 hours
	20-24	3-4 days	8-12 hours
Halves, breast	5-11	1-2 days	4-6 hours
Boneless roast	3-10	12-18 hours	1-3 hours
Pieces	1-3	3-9 hours	1 hour

for easy handling and to catch any drippings. Thaw until the flesh is pliable and the giblets can be taken from the body cavity. Allow from one to four days for thawing (see Thawing Poultry table, page 521).

The fastest way to thaw poultry is in cold water. (Hot water is not recommended because it warms the outer surfaces too much while the interior is still frozen.) Keep the bird sealed in the original wrap or in another watertight plastic bag, and submerge it in cold (not warm or hot) water. Change the water often and thaw until the meat is pliable and the giblets can be removed. You may also partially thaw poultry in the refrigerator and complete the thawing in cold water.

If your refrigerator is crowded with other foods, poultry can be thawed at room temperature, although the other methods are safer. Wrap the bird in a double paper bag or in several layers of newspaper. Keep tightly closed and place on a large tray to catch any drippings that escape the wrappings. Allow one hour per pound for thawing. Thaw until pliable, and remove the giblets. Cook *immediately*. If it becomes necessary to wait several hours before cooking, refrigerate the thawed poultry.

Preparing Poultry

Because most poultry on the market is ready-to-cook—it has been drawn, plucked, and cleaned—it requires very little preparation before cooking. Simply remove the giblets and excess fat from the body cavity of whole poultry, then rinse the skin with cold water or wipe with a clean, damp cloth. Also rinse the body cavity thoroughly under cold running water to remove any blood that may have accumulated. Pat dry and season the cavity with your favorite herbs and spices. Then stuff, if desired, and truss (see

Stuffing Poultry, page 524, and Trussing Poultry, page 525). Poultry parts and halves need only rinsing and drying unless you do your own cutting and deboning (see Cutting Poultry, page 523, and Deboning Poultry Breasts, page 524). Since poultry meat without skin has far less fat and fewer calories than poultry with skin attached, consider removing the skin before cooking. Simply peel back the skin and slip it off.

Since raw poultry is highly perishable, prepare well-chilled birds quickly. Always clean the countertop and all utensils thoroughly, and scrub the cutting board after preparation.

Plucking and Singeing Poultry

Most poultry on the market today has had the pinfeathers removed. However, an occasional fresh bird may need plucking and singeing. Here is how to do it:

To pluck: Use tweezers (or grasp each pinfeather between forefinger and tip of a knife) to pull out the coarse feathers. The remaining numerous smaller feathers can be removed with wax. Mix three-eighths pound of melted paraffin with seven quarts of boiling water. Brush the mixture over the bird and allow to harden. Pull off the wax. The feathers will come with it.

To singe: Hold the bird over a gas flame or candle and singe tiny pinfeathers and downy hair. Move the bird so all feathers are exposed to the heat. Avoid singeing poultry before freezing it since heat breaks down fat and hastens rancidity. Instead, singe the bird when you are ready to use it.

Preparing Giblets

Poultry giblets are exceptionally easy to prepare for cooking. Simply wash carefully in cold water and pat dry. Remove any excess fat from the gizzard, and connective tissue from the liver.

Examine the liver, and remove any greenish spots, which will impart a bitter flavor.

Cutting Poultry—Halving, Quartering, and Disjointing

You can usually save money by cutting up your own poultry. Chicken, duck, pheasant, guinea fowl, game hen, and squab are easily cut at home, but large turkeys and geese are rather cumbersome.

To halve chicken, pheasant, guinea fowl, game hen, or squab, place the bird breast-side down on a cutting board and use poultry shears or a sharp knife to cut along each side of the backbone. Remove the bone and reserve it for the stockpot. Cut the breast cartilage, flesh, and skin; then pull the halves apart and remove the keel bone.

For chicken, pheasant, and guinea fowl quarters, halve the birds, and cut diagonally along the bottom rib. (Game hens and squabs are too small to quarter.)

To cut up, or disjoint, poultry, place the bird breast-side up on a cutting board and, using a sharp knife, cut the skin between the thighs and the body. Grasp one leg of the bird in each hand and lift the bird from the board. As you lift, bend the legs back until the bones break at the hip joints. Next, turn the bird to one side and completely remove the leg and thigh by cutting from the tail toward the shoulder and cutting through the joint near the bird's back. Repeat on the other side. To separate thighs and legs (drumsticks), locate the knee joint by bending the thigh and leg together, then cut through the joint. With the bird on its back, remove the wings by cutting inside the wing over the joint. It is easiest to cut from the top down. Finally, separate the breast from the back by placing the bird on its back and cutting through the joints on either side of the rib cage. The breasts, wings, legs, and thighs are now ready for cooking. If you prefer breast halves, split the breast by cutting the wishbone at the V.

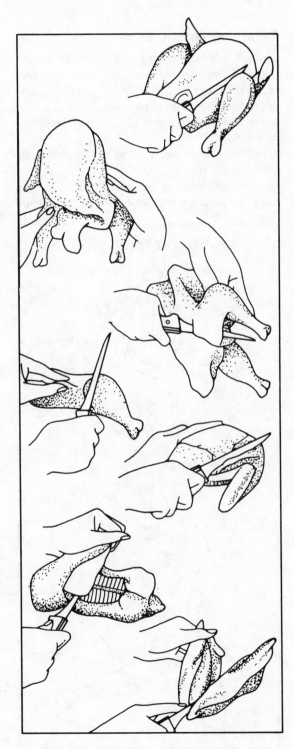

Deboning Poultry Breasts

Though whole birds, as well as legs, can be deboned, both are tedious to do. Therefore, few recipes call for them. Breasts, on the other hand, are easily deboned if you use a boning knife with a sharp, flexible blade that lets you feel the bones as you work.

Place the breast with skin-side down on your cutting board and cut the white gristle at the neck end of the keel bone. Bend the breast back and press flat to expose the bone. With your finger, loosen the bone and lift it out. On one side of the breast, insert the knife tip under the long rib bone, then slide the knife under the bone to cut the meat free. Continue to cut the flesh free of the ribs until you can lift the rib cage out. Repeat on the other side. Remove the wishbone and white tendons.

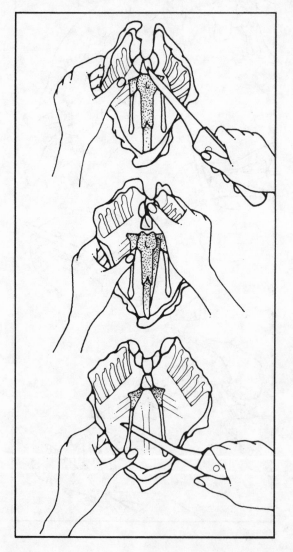

Stuffing Poultry

Well-seasoned stuffing, or dressing, makes an exceptionally delightful accompaniment for poultry. The most basic stuffing consists of bread crumbs, onions, and sage or thyme; modifications are endless. Substitute rice, bulgur, potatoes, corn bread, or chestnuts for the bread crumbs. Or, add almonds, cashews, pine nuts, currants, apples, dried fruits, celery, green peppers, mushrooms, oysters, sausage, or giblets. Simmer dried fruits, roast nuts, and cook sausage and giblets before mixing them with the other stuffing ingredients; then pack all into the bird. Since stuffing will absorb the fat of fatty birds such as ducks and geese, use a dry stuffing for these, or bake the stuffing separately.

Allow one-half to one cup of stuffing—three-quarters of a cup is a good average—for each pound of poultry (about nine cups for a 12-pound bird). Spoon stuffing lightly into the body and neck cavities. Avoid packing tightly for several reasons: During cooking, stuffing that is too compact may expand and cause the skin to burst; it may not cook thoroughly; and it tends to have an unpleasant, rubbery texture. Extra stuffing can always be wrapped in foil or packed in a baking dish and baked separately. After stuffing, truss the bird to keep the stuffing in place (see Trussing Poultry, page 525) and roast immediately. *Never* stuff poultry, then freeze at home. And *never* stuff, then cook several hours later. The warm dressing and dark, damp interior of the bird provide a perfect growing medium for microorganisms that, in large numbers, can cause serious food poisoning. Of course, the safest way to cook stuffing is to bake separately.

Trussing Poultry

Whether stuffed or not, poultry cooks more evenly, stays moister, and retains a better shape for carving if it is trussed (tied) before roasting, braising, or stewing. To truss: Pull skin flaps over the body and neck cavities and either sew the skin in place or use skewers. Tie the legs together, then fold the wings back and under the bird and tie them close to the body. During the last 30 minutes of roasting, untie the legs to permit browning of the inside of the legs.

Marinating Poultry

Marinades lend delightful, intricate flavors to poultry parts and halves. They also perform excellently as moisturizers during broiling. Use a base of lemon juice, white vinegar, cider vinegar, or white wine vinegar. Red vinegars will turn poultry flesh pink. Marinate for 3 to 24 hours—a long soak in the marinade imparts the most flavor. After marinating, reserve the sauce; it is excellent for basting the poultry as it cooks.

Preparing Wild Fowl

Wild fowl needs special cleaning—drawing and plucking—before it is cooked. Refer to a good hunting manual for a detailed description of the necessary steps.

Because wild fowl is exceptionally lean, it is tastiest when basted during roasting. And, marinating a wild bird before cooking—or placing an apple, a whole onion, celery stalk, or carrot, or some parsley sprigs in the cavity—will help lessen the gamey flavor.

Cooking Poultry

For tender, juicy meat and a uniformly cooked bird, use low to moderate heat. High temperatures toughen the protein and cause excessive shrinkage as well as a loss of juice. Dry heat—roasting or broiling—is ideal for cooking young, tender birds; but moist heat—stewing or braising—is preferable

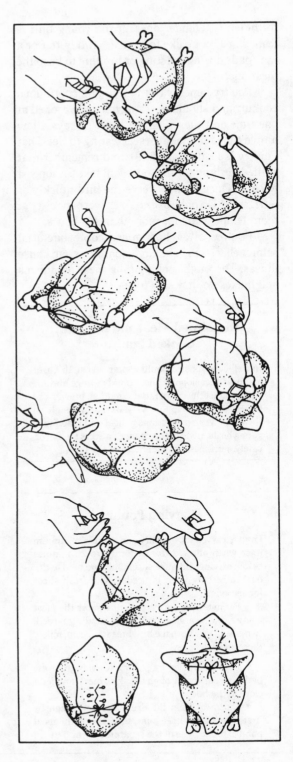

for older, less-tender ones. If the young bird is lean, some cooks like to baste it with butter or a marinade during roasting or broiling to keep the meat succulent.

Poultry benefits from thorough, continuous cooking and should never be partially cooked at one time and then finished later. Always allow ample time for cooking (see Testing to See That Poultry Is Done, page 529), and remember that stuffed birds and frozen ones will take the longest to cook. Once cooked, serve the bird quickly or refrigerate. Do not leave cooked, warm poultry at room temperature for more than 1½ hours.

Poultry often has microscopic bacteria, salmonellae, which in large quantities can cause illness. Thorough cooking kills these organisms and makes poultry safe to eat.

Discolored Meat and Bones in Cooked Poultry

In well-done roasted poultry some breast, thigh, or leg meat occasionally has a pinkish tinge and the meat nearest the bones is dark, reddish brown. The bones, too, may appear very dark. Although all these changes are reactions to heat and thawing in young birds, none of the changes affects the flavor, safety, juiciness, or tenderness of the meat.

Carving Poultry

Poultry carves most easily and retains maximum juice when allowed to rest for 15 to 20 minutes before carving. Because slices chill and tend to dry out, carve only what is needed. Cut fresh slices for seconds.

For nice even slices, patiently carve the meat using a sharp carving knife and a handle-guarded, two-tined fork. With the bird breast-side up, follow these steps:

• Remove the leg by pulling it away from the body and cutting through the skin, meat, and joint close to the body.

• Cut meat from the drumstick and thigh by first severing the knee joint, then slicing the meat parallel to the bone of the separated leg and thigh.

• Remove the wing by cutting through the joint and as close to the body as possible.

• Carve the breast meat by slicing in thin, parallel slices from the top down. Begin each slice slightly higher and end at the cut made for the wing.

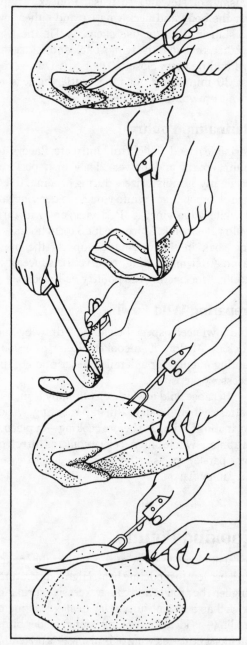

Roasting

Roasting is an exceptionally easy and tasty way of preparing all kinds of young, tender poultry—chicken, duck, goose, game hen, and turkey. Place whole poultry breast-side up, or halves or parts skin-side up, on a rack in a shallow pan. (Prick the skin of a duck or a goose with a fork to let fatty juices run out.) Roast at 325 to 350°F. Baste, if desired, every 30 to 45 minutes. During the last third of cooking time, release the trussed legs to permit the heat to circulate around them. If the bird starts to brown too quickly, place a loose tent of foil over it. Remove whole, large birds from the heat 15 to 30 minutes before serving (see Roasting table, below). A rest period will make carving easier.

Roasting Times for Poultry

Poultry	Weight* (pounds)	Approximate Cooking Time at 325°F† (hours)
Chicken		
Whole		
Broiler-fryer	2-3	2-2½
Capon	5-8½	3-4
Roaster	3-4½	2-3
Rock Cornish game hen	1-2	1-2½
Pieces	¼-¾	1-1½
Duck	4-6	2½-4
Goose	6-8	3-3½
Guinea fowl	2-4	1-2½
Pheasant	2-4	1-2
Squab	1-2	1-2
Turkey		
Whole	6-8	3-3½
	8-12	3½-4½
	12-16	4½-5½
	16-20	5½-6½
	20-24	6½-7
Halves, breast	5-11	3-5½
Boneless roast	3-10	3-4
Pieces	1-3	2-3½

*Weight of giblets and neck is included for whole poultry.
†Time is based on poultry being at refrigerator temperature at start of roasting. Times given are for stuffed poultry; unstuffed poultry may take slightly less time.

Sauces—both fruit and savory—nicely complement golden roasted poultry. Or use pan juices to make gravy (see Gravy for Meat and Poultry, page 141).

Broiling

Young, small turkeys and ducklings, as well as chickens, are excellent when broiled. Cut poultry into halves, quarters, or pieces, but leave the skin on to prevent excessive drying. Snap the wing and leg joints to help keep the pieces flat while broiling. On ducklings prick the skin to allow fatty juices to escape; on other poultry brush with oil or melted butter. Place them skin-side down on a lightly oiled broiler rack. Put the rack several inches from the heat to permit slow cooking. During broiling turn the poultry pieces two or three times. Each time you turn the pieces, brush them with the fat. Broil longest on the bone side in order to cook the interior. Allow 20 to 30 minutes to broil chicken and 1 to 1¼ hours for turkey and duckling. Extremely fatty birds such as ducks and geese may cause flaring while broiling. To reduce the chances of this happening, prick the skin and parboil first.

Broiled poultry is extremely tasty when brushed with a tomato- or soy sauce-based barbecue sauce. Serve with cold potato salad and a tray of crisp, raw carrot sticks, celery sticks, broccoli florets, radish roses, mushroom caps, and cauliflower florets.

Braising

Braising is an ideal, flavorful way of cooking mature, less-tender birds. Braise either whole or cut-up poultry in a heavy pan in a 325°F oven or over medium heat on the stove top. Place the bird in the pan and cover with a tight-fitting lid. The bird will steam in the juices released during cooking. When braising in the oven, uncover for the last 30 minutes to allow the bird to brown (if desired). When on the stove top, first brown (optional) the pieces in a small amount of hot fat (some cooks like to dredge the pieces in flour before browning); then cover and cook.

Duck benefits from braising with prunes or figs, and chicken takes well to apricots. When braising with dried fruits, add one-half cup of water as needed during cooking.

Stewing

Stewing, often called simmering, mature, less-tender poultry not only tenderizes the meat but also yields a rich, flavorful broth. Young birds can be stewed, but the resulting broth will not be full bodied. Place the poultry in enough water to cover, and season with onions, celery, and your favorite herbs. Put a tight-fitting lid on the pot and bring the water to a boil. Reduce the heat and simmer the bird, depending on its size, for 1½ to 3 hours until tender (see Testing to See That Poultry Is Done, page 529).

Stewed poultry is excellent for making salads. As a rule, you should allow one-third to one-half cup diced poultry for each person to be served. But, if you add several other ingredients, such as celery, nuts, and pineapple chunks, you can use as little as one-quarter cup per person. Blend with a flavorful homemade mayonnaise and chill thoroughly before serving.

Steaming

Steaming is a quick, moist-heat way of cooking young, tender birds. Place the bird on a rack above one inch of steaming water. Cover the pot with a tight-fitting lid, and steam poultry parts for approximately ¾ hour and whole birds for 1½ hours until well done and tender. Replenish with boiling water as necessary.

Steamed poultry, which is mild and moist, goes well with crisp, raw vegetables and whole grains. Serve hot or well chilled.

Frying

Both pan- and oven-frying are tasty methods for preparing smaller, younger birds. Before frying, cut poultry into serving-size pieces, and dredge in seasoned flour or bread crumbs, or dip in batter. If you prefer to leave poultry uncoated, be certain the pieces are thoroughly dry to prevent spattering of the hot fat.

Seasoned flour: In a clean paper bag, mix one-half cup whole wheat flour, one teaspoon paprika, and one-eighth teaspoon pepper. Shake one or two pieces of poultry in the bag at once. Repeat until all pieces are coated.

Breading: In a shallow bowl blend with a wire whisk or a fork one lightly beaten egg and three tablespoons milk or water. Dredge poultry pieces in whole wheat flour, then dip into the egg mixture, and finally roll in fine, dry bread crumbs, rolled oats, wheat germ, or wheat bran.

Batter: In a medium-size bowl blend one egg, three-quarters cup milk, and one cup whole wheat flour. Dip poultry pieces into batter; drain.

To panfry: Warm a small amount of butter or oil in a heavy skillet and brown the poultry pieces over medium heat, turning often. Reduce the heat and cook slowly, bone-side down, until well done and tender. The total cooking time for small birds will be 30 to 45 minutes. Turkey or duckling will take 45 to 60 minutes. (For turkey it is often best to finish cooking in a covered pan with two to four tablespoons of water. The moisture will hasten cooking and keep the meat juicy. Remove the lid for the last few minutes to recrisp the skin.)

To oven-fry: Dip the poultry pieces in melted fat to coat both sides. Place with the skin-side down in a greased baking pan and bake in a 350°F oven. After cooking for 30 minutes, turn and continue cooking until well done and tender (20 to 30 minutes for chickens and other small birds; 35 to 45 minutes for turkeys and other larger birds).

Served hot, fried chicken goes well with bulgur pilaf, corn on the cob, boiled brown rice, or tossed green salad.

Poultry is also good when deep fried. This method, however, noticeably increases both the fat content and the number of calories in poultry.

Pressure-cooking

Reserve your pressure cooker for cooking old, tough birds that have lots of flavor but need tenderizing. Young birds are so tender that they will fall apart if steamed or stewed under pressure. Always follow the manufacturer's directions and, for best results in appearance and taste, lower the temperature gradually.

Cooking Giblets

Place giblets in a saucepan with enough water to cover. Put a lid on the pan and simmer until the heart and liver are tender, 10 to 15 minutes. Remove the heart and liver and continue simmering until the remaining giblets are tender, one to two hours. The resulting broth and chopped, simmered giblets make flavorful additions to poultry gravies and stuffings.

A second way to cook giblets is to seal them tightly in foil and then place them in the oven with the poultry. The giblets will be done when the poultry itself is. Cooked this way, the giblets are ready to be minced for use in pâtés and other appetizers.

Cooking Frozen Poultry

Although frozen unstuffed poultry is generally best when thawed before cooking, it can be cooked while frozen. Unwrap the bird and place it on a rack in a shallow pan. Roast, uncovered, in a 325°F oven for one hour, then remove the giblets and neck from the body and neck cavities. Cook the giblets immediately and return the bird to the oven at once to complete roasting. Total roasting time will be about twice that for thawed poultry. With this method the stuffing must be cooked separately.

Birds that are commercially stuffed and frozen should always be cooked while frozen. Follow the directions on the label.

Testing to See That Poultry Is Done

For maximum flavor, as well as safety, always cook poultry until well done. The tables and discussions in this chapter are a good guide to cooking times, but also test in one of these simple ways to see that the poultry is done:

- Press the thick muscle of the drumstick. If the meat feels soft, the poultry is done. The leg should also move up and down easily (the hip joint may even break).
- Insert a fork into the breast or thick part of the thigh. When done, the fork slides in easily.
- Use a meat thermometer. The thermometer should be inserted into the fleshy inner thigh or through the carcass into the center of the stuffing—it should never touch bone. In the thigh, the thermometer should register from 180 to 185°F when the meat is done; in the stuffing, it should register 165°F when done.
- Pierce the thickest part of the thigh with a skewer or the tip of a sharp knife. The escaping juice will be clear if the meat is done.

Cooking with Leftover Poultry

Poultry leftovers readily adapt to delicious luncheon casseroles; appetizers and side dishes; hearty soups; light, elegant salads and aspics; and hot or cold sandwich fillings. Use nuts, seeds, and raw vegetables for texture and color contrast, and serve with crusty whole grain breads and crisp homemade crackers.

Since poultry leftovers are highly perishable, keep them well chilled until you are ready to make and to serve the new dish. If you are reusing the gravy, heat it to a boil before using or serving. Stuffing is easily reheated by wrapping it in foil and baking it in a 350°F oven until hot. Reheat poultry meat by the same methods as other meats (see Reheating Meat, page 474).

Chicken

Baked Chicken Cacciatore

    1 large zucchini, cut into 2-inch chunks
    3 large carrots, sliced diagonally
    4 medium-size potatoes, quartered lengthwise
    2 medium-size onions, cut into 8 pieces
    1 can (28 ounces) Italian-style tomatoes
    1 teaspoon dried oregano
    2 teaspoons dried basil
    ¼ cup chopped fresh parsley
    1 teaspoon minced garlic
       pepper, to taste
    1 chicken (broiler-fryer, 3 to 3½ pounds), cut
       into serving pieces
    ¼ cup olive oil

Preheat oven to 350°F.

Arrange zucchini, carrots, potatoes, and onions in bottom of a large roasting pan. Add tomatoes with juice. Sprinkle with oregano, basil, parsley, garlic, and pepper. Place chicken on top of vegetables, sprinkle with pepper, and drizzle olive oil over all. Bake for 1½ hours, or until meat and vegetables are fork-tender, turning meat and vegetables once or twice during cooking time.

4 to 6 servings

Baked Chicken with Spicy Barbecue Sauce

    2 chickens (broiler-fryers, 2½ to 3 pounds
       each), cut into serving pieces

    Sauce
    1 cup catsup
    ½ cup honey
    1 cup vinegar
    ¼ cup lemon juice
    1 clove garlic
    1 medium-size onion, chopped
    ¼ cup soy sauce
    ¼ teaspoon cayenne pepper
    1 tablespoon paprika

    1 tablespoon crushed bay leaves
    2 sprigs parsley
    2 teaspoons turmeric
    ½ teaspoon ground sage
    ½ tablespoon dried thyme
    2 teaspoons dry mustard

Preheat oven to 325°F.

Place chicken in a large oiled baking pan, skin-side up.

To make the sauce: Process all remaining ingredients in a blender. Pour over chicken pieces, coating each one.

Bake, uncovered, for 1½ hours, basting frequently.

6 to 8 servings

Chicken Breasts Florentine

    10 ounces fresh or frozen spinach
    ¼   cup plus 2 tablespoons butter
    ¼   cup whole wheat flour
    2   cups milk
    ¾   cup grated Parmesan cheese
    1½ teaspoons dry mustard
    1   tablespoon dried tarragon
    2   whole chicken breasts, boned, skinned, and
        halved
    3   cups cooked brown rice

Preheat oven to 400°F.

If using fresh spinach, cook for about 2 minutes, then chop and squeeze out all the water. If using frozen, just thaw, chop, and squeeze out all the water.

In a medium-size saucepan melt ¼ cup butter. When hot, add flour and stir. Add milk all at once and stir with a wire whisk until it comes to a boil. Stir in ½ cup cheese until melted. Add spinach, mustard, and tarragon.

Place chicken breasts between 2 sheets of wax paper and pound flat with a mallet.

In a large skillet melt 2 tablespoons butter until hot. Add chicken breasts and cook for about 2 minutes on each side. Remove from skillet.

Cover bottoms of 4 individual au gratin dishes or 1 large one with rice. Place chicken breasts on top of rice with space between breasts. Spoon a generous amount of sauce over each breast and sprinkle with remaining ¼ cup Parmesan. You may have some sauce and rice left over. Bake for 20 minutes.

To serve, lift out each breast with the rice underneath it.

4 servings

Chicken Breasts with Mushrooms

    1   tablespoon vegetable oil
    5½ tablespoons butter
    2   whole chicken breasts, boned, skinned, and
          halved
    1   small onion, finely chopped
    1   pound mushrooms, finely chopped
    1   teaspoon dried thyme
        pepper, to taste
    5   tablespoons whole wheat flour
    1   cup plus 3 tablespoons milk
    4   tablespoons grated Parmesan cheese
    1   teaspoon dry mustard

Preheat oven to 450°F.

In a large cast-iron skillet heat oil and 1 tablespoon butter. When hot, brown chicken breasts for 2 minutes on each side.

In a small skillet melt 1½ tablespoons butter. Add onions and sauté until translucent. Add mushrooms and cook over high heat for several minutes, drawing out their liquid. Remove skillet from heat. Place mixture in a small strainer and press down with a ladle, pressing out all the liquid. Return to skillet.

Add thyme and pepper. Sprinkle with 1½ tablespoons flour and stir until flour is completely incorporated. Add 3 tablespoons milk and cook, while stirring, until you have a thick paste. Set aside.

In a small saucepan melt 2 tablespoons butter. When hot, add remaining 3½ tablespoons flour and stir with a wire whisk for about 30 seconds. Add 1 cup milk all at once. Scrape flour off side of pan with a spoon and then stir with wire whisk until mixture comes to a boil. Stir in 2 tablespoons cheese and mustard.

Place a layer of mushroom mixture on top of each chicken breast. Cover mushrooms with about 2 tablespoons sauce. Sprinkle with remaining 2 tablespoons cheese and top with remaining 1 tablespoon butter. Bake for 15 to 20 minutes, or until hot.

4 servings

Chicken Breasts
with Pine Nuts and Lemon

    2   whole chicken breasts, boned, skinned, and
          halved
    2   tablespoons butter
    1   tablespoon vegetable oil
    1   large clove garlic, minced
    ½   cup pine nuts
        juice of 1 large lemon
    2   scallions (green tops only), chopped
    3   tablespoons orange juice
    1   tangerine, separated into segments,
          or 12 mandarin orange segments

Place chicken breasts between 2 pieces of wax paper and pound with side of a cleaver once or twice to flatten them.

In a large skillet heat butter and oil until hot. Add chicken breasts and cook over medium-high heat for about 2 minutes on each side, or until they just begin to brown slightly. Remove from skillet.

Add garlic and pine nuts to skillet and cook until pine nuts just begin to brown.

Remove skillet from heat, but while it is still hot, add lemon juice. Stir it around bottom of skillet, bringing up all the brown bits. Add scallion greens and then return chicken to skillet. Spoon pine nut mixture on top of chicken. Add orange juice. Cover skillet and cook over low heat for about 5 minutes. Add tangerine or mandarin orange segments and cook for about 3 minutes more.

To serve, place a breast on each plate and spoon pine nut mixture over it.

4 servings

Broiled Chicken with Lime Marinade

In this recipe the unusual marinade also serves as a hot sauce spooned over the chicken when it is served.

¼ cup yogurt
¼ cup cider vinegar
½ cup lime juice
2 tablespoons vegetable oil
1 teaspoon ground coriander
1 teaspoon ground ginger
¼ teaspoon crushed fresh mint
1 chicken (broiler-fryer, about 2½ pounds), quartered
½ cup cashews

In a large bowl mix together all ingredients except chicken and cashews.

Place chicken skin-side down in mixture and marinate overnight, or at least 8 hours. Turn occasionally.

Chop cashews into very small pieces. Remove chicken from marinade and place on a broiler pan. Add cashews to marinade and heat over low heat while chicken cooks.

Set broiler pan so that top of chicken is about 4 inches from the broiler unit. Broil bone-side up for 10 minutes. Lower pan about 2 inches and broil chicken skin-side up for 10 to 12 minutes. If chicken starts to burn, lower rack even more.

To serve, place chicken on a plate and spoon hot marinade sauce over it.

4 servings

Cabbage Stuffed with Chicken and Currants

This interesting version of stuffed cabbage allows for using leftover white meat for economy and introducing spices that provide a welcome surprise.

1 head cabbage
2 whole chicken breasts, boned, skinned, and chopped
1½ cups cooked long grain brown rice
1 egg
½ cup dried currants
½ teaspoon ground allspice
¼ teaspoon ground nutmeg
freshly ground pepper, to taste
2 cups tomato sauce

Preheat oven to 350°F.

Cut core out of head of cabbage. Pour boiling water over cabbage and let stand for at least 20 minutes. Carefully remove 8 outer leaves. (You may have to remove a few, then put cabbage back in the water to stand, and then remove more.)

Mix together chicken, rice, egg, currants, allspice, nutmeg, and pepper. Place about ¼ cup of chicken mixture along rib of each cabbage leaf. Roll up and then tuck ends under.

Cover bottom of a medium-size baking dish with some of the tomato sauce. Place stuffed cabbage leaves in dish seam-side down. Pour remaining tomato sauce over them. They should be just about covered. Cover dish tightly and bake for 1½ hours.

4 servings

Chicken Breasts in Yogurt Aspic

4 whole chicken breasts
4 cups rich Poultry Stock (page 110)
1 carrot, sliced
1 medium-size onion, sliced
1 stalk celery, with leaves, cut into chunks
3 sprigs parsley
1 teaspoon lemon juice
2 envelopes unflavored gelatin
⅓ cup cold water
1 cup yogurt
crisp greens
chopped fresh parsley
chopped fresh chives

In a large pot combine chicken, stock, carrots, onions, celery, parsley, and lemon juice. Cook for 30 to 45 minutes, or until chicken is tender, then turn off heat and allow chicken to cool in broth. Lift out chicken and set aside.

Strain broth and return to low heat. Simmer until liquid is reduced to 1 cup. Cool slightly and remove fat.

Meanwhile, split chicken breasts, remove bone and skin, trim off any small fragments of meat, and place breasts on a serving platter.

Sprinkle gelatin over water and allow to soften, add to reduced stock, and heat until gelatin is dissolved. Cool slightly. Fold in yogurt. Cool or chill mixture until it reaches consistency of egg whites. Then spoon aspic over each chicken breast. Chill until aspic is firm. Then coat with another layer of aspic, and chill again. Keep aspic at room temperature or slightly cooler during the coating process.

When ready to serve, garnish with greens, parsley, and chives.

4 servings

Chicken Breasts with Peaches and Paprika

     2 large whole chicken breasts, boned and
           skinned
    ½ teaspoon paprika
        freshly ground pepper, to taste
     4 tablespoons butter
     3 large firm peaches
     3 tablespoons lemon juice
     2 tablespoons lime juice
     2 tablespoons honey
     1 tablespoon water

Sprinkle tops of chicken breasts with paprika and pepper. Melt 2 tablespoons butter in a large skillet. When hot, add chicken breasts and brown for about 2 minutes on paprika side and 1 minute on the other.

Peel, pit, and cut peaches into thick slices. In a separate skillet melt remaining 2 tablespoons butter. Add peaches and sauté until just golden, turning only once. Immediately toss them with lemon juice and arrange on top of chicken.

Mix together lime juice, honey, and water and pour over all. Cover tightly and cook for 8 to 10 minutes over low heat.

4 servings

Chicken Crécy

The characteristic color and flavor of carrots in this dish make an impressive presentation and an interesting way to serve that dependable standby, chicken.

     1 chicken (broiler-fryer)
    1½ pounds carrots, cut into pieces
     1 cup cooked brown rice
    1½ teaspoons chopped fresh dill
        freshly ground pepper, to taste
    ¼ cup plus 1 tablespoon butter
    ¼ cup whole wheat pastry flour
    1½ cups milk
    ½ cup light cream
    1½ cups grated cheddar cheese
        whole grain bread crumbs

Preheat oven to 350°F.

Place chicken in a roasting pan and bake, uncovered, for about 45 minutes, or until tender.

Cover carrots with water and boil until soft.

When chicken is done, remove meat from bones and cut into large chunks. Drain carrots well. In a food processor or food mill puree carrots and rice. Add dill and pepper. Then spread puree in bottom of a shallow ovenproof casserole. Arrange chicken in a layer on top.

Melt ¼ cup butter in a medium-size saucepan. When it just starts to bubble, add flour and stir with a wire whisk. Add milk and cream all at once and stir until mixture starts to boil. Add 1¼ cups cheese and stir until melted. Spoon sauce thickly over chicken. Sprinkle with bread crumbs and then with remaining ¼ cup cheese. Dot with remaining 1 tablespoon butter.

Bake, uncovered, for 30 minutes.

4 servings

Chicken Curry

    2 medium-size onions, sliced
    2 dried chili peppers, ground (optional)
    2 cloves garlic, minced
    2 tablespoons vegetable oil
    1 stick of cinnamon
    ¼ teaspoon whole cloves
    1 tablespoon turmeric
    1 teaspoon ground ginger
    1 teaspoon ground cumin
    2 tablespoons ground coriander
    1 chicken (broiler-fryer, 3 to 4 pounds), cut into
        serving pieces
    1 cup tomato juice
    1 cup Poultry Stock (page 110)
1 to 2 tablespoons cornstarch, dissolved in
        ¼ cup cold water (optional)

In a large heavy-bottom pot, sauté onions, chilies (if used), and garlic in oil. Add cinnamon, cloves, turmeric, ginger, cumin, and coriander and sauté together until onions are translucent.

Add chicken and sauté until it is well coated with spices and slightly golden in color.

Add tomato juice and stock, cover with a tight-fitting lid, and simmer over very low heat, stirring occasionally, for 1 to 2 hours, or until chicken is tender.

If desired, thicken sauce with cornstarch just before serving.

Serve with separate small bowls of yogurt, shredded unsweetened coconut, peanuts or almonds mixed with raisins, and chutney.

    4 servings

Chicken Cutlets with Lemon

When chicken is done this way, it becomes an excellent alternative to the costly veal cutlets commonly served in this style.

    1 whole chicken breast, boned, skinned, and
        halved
    1 egg
        pinch of cayenne pepper
    ½ cup wheat germ
    1 tablespoon vegetable oil
    1 tablespoon butter
        juice of 1 lemon

    2 tablespoons chopped fresh parsley
    2 lemon wedges

Flatten each chicken cutlet by pounding with a mallet or the flat side of a meat cleaver until about ½ inch thick.

Beat egg with cayenne. Dip chicken cutlets into egg, then coat with wheat germ.

Heat oil and butter in a large skillet until foamy. Add chicken cutlets and sauté for about 3 minutes on each side. (Cut into cutlets to see if they are opaque all the way through.) Transfer to a serving platter and pour lemon juice into skillet. Cook over high heat for about 1 minute, stirring constantly. Then add parsley. Pour sauce over chicken and serve with lemon wedges.

    2 servings

Chicken Divan

    3 medium-size whole chicken breasts
    1 tablespoon minced fresh parsley
    ½ teaspoon dried thyme
    1 bay leaf
    2 cups water
    1 large head broccoli or 1 pound asparagus
    ¼ cup butter
    ¼ cup whole wheat flour
    ½ cup half-and-half
    2 tablespoons champagne vinegar
        pepper, to taste
    2 ounces Monterey Jack cheese, grated

Place chicken, parsley, thyme, bay leaf, and water in a large skillet. Cover and poach until meat is cooked through, 30 to 40 minutes. Remove chicken meat, reserving liquid. Discard bay leaf. When cool enough to handle, cut meat into bite-size pieces.

Cook broccoli or asparagus until tender, drain, and cut into bite-size pieces.

Melt butter in a medium-size skillet. Blend in flour slowly to form a paste. Gradually add 1½ cups reserved poaching liquid, stirring constantly, and cook over low heat until sauce begins to thicken. Add half-and-half, vinegar, pepper, and cheese. Continue to stir until cheese is melted and sauce is thick.

Preheat oven to 350°F.

Pour ½ cup sauce over bottom of a 9 × 13-inch baking dish. Add broccoli or asparagus, followed by another ½ cup sauce. Add chicken, top with remaining sauce, and bake for 20 minutes, or until bubbly. Serve over whole wheat noodles or brown rice.

4 servings

Chicken in Sour Cream, Paprika, and Caraway Sauce

    1 egg white
    1 tablespoon cornstarch
    2 whole chicken breasts, boned, skinned, and
         cut into bite-size pieces
    1 cup vegetable oil
    1 tablespoon butter
    1 medium-size onion, chopped
    ½ pound mushrooms, sliced
 1½ tablespoons tomato paste
 1½ tablespoons whole wheat pastry flour
    ¾ cup Poultry Stock (page 110)
    ¾ cup sour cream
    1 teaspoon paprika
    1 tablespoon caraway seeds

In a medium-size bowl mix egg white and cornstarch. Add chicken and mix well. Let stand for at least 5 minutes.

Place oil in a wok and heat slowly so that it is barely hot. Add chicken, about ⅓ at a time, and cook very slowly until it just barely turns white. Remove chicken from wok with a slotted spoon. (Save oil for another use.)

In a large saucepan melt butter. Add onions and mushrooms and sauté until onions are translucent. Remove pan from heat and stir in tomato paste and flour. Return pan to heat and add stock. Stir until mixture comes to a boil. Stir in sour cream. Add chicken and any juices that have accumulated. Stir in paprika and caraway seeds. When ready to serve, heat on top of the stove or in a 350°F oven for 20 to 30 minutes. Serve over whole wheat noodles.

4 servings

Chicken Liver Crepes

    ¼ cup plus 3 tablespoons butter
    1 medium-size onion, chopped
    1 pound chicken livers
    4 hard-cooked eggs, chopped
    ¼ cup whole wheat flour

    2 cups milk
    ⅛ teaspoon white pepper
    8 Whole Wheat Crepes (page 395)

In a large skillet melt 3 tablespoons butter over low heat. Add onions and sauté until translucent. Remove from pan with a slotted spoon. Sauté livers in same pan until just cooked through. Chop livers and place in a bowl. Mix ½ of the eggs and all the onions with livers.

Preheat oven to 350°F.

In a medium-size saucepan melt ¼ cup butter. Mix in flour to make a paste. Slowly add milk and cook, stirring constantly, over medium heat until sauce thickens and boils. Boil for at least 3 minutes. Add pepper.

Mix ½ cup sauce into liver mixture, then divide between crepes and roll up. Spread a thin layer of sauce on bottom of a shallow ovenproof casserole, and place crepes on top of sauce in a single layer. Stir remaining eggs into remaining sauce, and spoon over crepes. Bake until heated through, about 15 minutes.

Makes 8 crepes

Chicken Livers with Yogurt-Mustard Sauce

       2 tablespoons rye flour
       ¼ teaspoon dried tarragon
       ¼ teaspoon pepper
       1 pound chicken livers
 1 to 2 tablespoons butter
       2 teaspoons prepared mustard
       1 cup yogurt
          chopped fresh parsley

On a flat plate or piece of wax paper, combine flour, tarragon, and pepper. Add livers and roll and toss until livers are coated evenly.

Melt butter in a large skillet over medium heat. Add livers and cook until browned on both sides and pink in the center, about 10 minutes. Remove livers from pan and keep warm.

Remove pan from heat. Add mustard and yogurt to pan juices and stir until mixture is well blended and hot. Add livers and toss until well coated with sauce. Serve immediately, topped with parsley. Delicious served over cooked brown rice.

4 servings

Chicken Manicotti with Tomato Sauce

Manicotti is the Italian word for muffs, or hand warmers. In this recipe the "muffs" are stuffed with chicken instead of the more familiar chopped beef.

- 1 tablespoon butter
- 3 chicken breast halves, boned and skinned
- 1 cup ricotta cheese
  freshly ground pepper, to taste
- ½ cup grated Parmesan cheese
- 1 small scallion, chopped
- ¼ cup chopped fresh parsley
- 2 teaspoons chopped fresh rosemary
- 1 egg, beaten
- 2 cups tomato sauce
- 8 whole wheat manicotti shells, cooked

Preheat oven to 350°F.

Melt butter in a large skillet. Brown chicken breasts in butter for 2 minutes on each side. Remove from skillet and chop into very small pieces.

Mix chicken with ricotta. Add pepper and ¼ cup Parmesan. Add scallions, parsley, rosemary, and egg and mix well.

Cover bottom of an ovenproof baking dish with some tomato sauce. Stuff manicotti shells with chicken mixture, place in dish, and cover with remaining sauce.

Sprinkle top of manicotti with remaining ¼ cup Parmesan and bake, uncovered, for about 35 minutes, or until hot and bubbly.

4 servings

Chicken Noodle Casserole with Cheese and Dill

- 4 tablespoons butter
- 3 tablespoons whole wheat pastry flour
- 1½ cups milk
- 1¼ cups ricotta cheese
- 4 tablespoons grated Parmesan cheese
- 2½ cups large whole wheat pasta shells, cooked
- ½ cup chopped fresh dill
- ½ cup sliced almonds
- 1½ cups cubed cooked chicken
  freshly ground pepper, to taste

Preheat oven to 350°F.

In a medium-size saucepan melt 3 tablespoons butter. When hot, add flour and stir. Add milk all at once and stir with a wire whisk until mixture comes to a boil. Stir in ricotta until it melts. Add 2 tablespoons Parmesan.

Mix pasta with cheese sauce. Stir in dill and almonds. Mix in chicken and season with lots of pepper. Sprinkle remaining 2 tablespoons Parmesan over top and dot with remaining 1 tablespoon butter. Bake, uncovered, for 30 minutes, or until hot.

4 servings

Chicken Paprika

- ½ teaspoon turmeric
- 2 teaspoons paprika
- 2 whole chicken breasts, quartered
- 4 drumsticks
- 4 thighs
- 2 tablespoons vegetable oil
- ½ cup chopped onions
- 2 to 3 cups Poultry Stock (page 110)
- 1 tablespoon cornstarch, dissolved in
    2 tablespoons cold water
- 1 cup yogurt
- 2 tablespoons chopped fresh parsley
  few sprigs parsley

In a small bowl combine turmeric and paprika and coat chicken with mixture.

In a Dutch oven or large skillet brown chicken in oil. Stir in onions, sauté briefly, and then add stock. Cover, bring to a boil, reduce heat, and simmer for about 45 minutes. Remove lid and continue to simmer until stock is reduced by ½. Chicken should be fork-tender. Arrange chicken on a heated platter and keep warm.

Add cornstarch to stock, stirring constantly. Cook until sauce is thickened. Add yogurt to sauce, stirring constantly. Stir in chopped parsley. Spoon sauce over chicken and garnish with parsley sprigs.

8 servings

Chicken with Prunes, Walnuts, and Sour Cream

2 tablespoons butter
1 tablespoon vegetable oil
1 chicken (broiler-fryer), cut into serving pieces
1 tablespoon whole wheat flour
½ cup water
12 pitted dried prunes
½ cup chopped walnuts
  freshly ground pepper, to taste
½ cup sour cream

In a large heavy skillet with a tight-fitting lid, heat butter and oil until they just start to bubble. Add chicken, skin-side down, and cook over medium-high heat until skin is well browned, about 10 minutes. Turn over and cook for 5 more minutes.

Remove skillet from heat, and remove chicken from skillet.

Sprinkle flour into skillet and mix well with a wire whisk. Add water. Place skillet back on the heat and stir until mixture comes to a boil.

Return chicken to skillet. Add prunes, walnuts, and pepper. Cover and cook over low heat for about 30 minutes.

Remove chicken from skillet. Stir in sour cream. Return chicken to skillet and heat for 10 more minutes. To serve, place chicken on plate and then spoon sauce over each piece.

4 servings

Chicken Provençale

2 tablespoons butter
1 tablespoon vegetable oil
1 chicken (broiler-fryer), cut into serving pieces
1 medium-size onion, sliced
1 clove garlic, chopped
¼ pound mushrooms
1 teaspoon dried thyme
¾ teaspoon dried basil
¼ cup chopped fresh parsley
2 cups tomato sauce

In a large skillet heat butter and oil until hot. Cook chicken skin-side down over medium-high heat for 10 minutes, or until browned. Turn over and cook for 5 more minutes. Remove chicken from skillet.

Sauté onions and garlic in same skillet for 2 to 3 minutes.

Cut mushrooms in half if large, add to skillet, and sauté for 1 to 2 minutes. Return chicken to skillet and spoon mushrooms and onions over it.

Mix thyme, basil, and parsley with tomato sauce. Pour over chicken, cover, and cook over low heat for 40 minutes.

4 servings

Chicken Wings in a Hot and Spicy Tomato Sauce

16 chicken wings (about 3 pounds)
 3 tablespoons vegetable oil
 2 teaspoons chili oil
 1 large onion, chopped
 2 cloves garlic, chopped
 3 cups tomato sauce
 ¼ teaspoon cayenne pepper
 1 teaspoon chili powder
 1 teaspoon dry mustard
 1 teaspoon ground cumin
 ¼ teaspoon ground cloves
 ½ teaspoon ground coriander
 ½ teaspoon dried oregano
 1 tablespoon vinegar

Cut wings in half at the first joint so that you separate the little drumstick.

Heat vegetable and chili oils in a large heavy skillet. Add chicken and brown on both sides. (You may have to do this in 2 batches.) Remove chicken from skillet.

Sauté onions and garlic in skillet until translucent. Add tomato sauce, cayenne, chili powder, mustard, cumin, cloves, coriander, oregano, and vinegar. Return chicken to skillet. Bring to a boil, cover, and cook over low heat for 30 to 45 minutes.

4 to 6 servings

Chicken *Sevilla*

Oranges add an unusual and delightful flavor to this Spanish chicken specialty.

    2   tablespoons butter
    1   tablespoon vegetable oil
    2   whole chicken breasts, halved, or 1 chicken
        (broiler-fryer), cut into serving pieces
    1   large green pepper, chopped
    1   medium-size tomato, chopped
        freshly ground pepper, to taste
    2   navel oranges

In a large heavy skillet with a tight-fitting lid, heat butter and oil. When they just start to bubble, add chicken, skin-side down. Cook over medium-high heat until skin is browned, about 10 minutes. Turn over and cook for 5 more minutes.

Add green peppers, tomatoes, and pepper. Separate oranges into segments, remove skins, and trim the straight side of each segment. Add to chicken. Cover tightly and cook over low heat for 40 minutes.

    4 servings

Chicken with Barley
and Scallions in Light Broth

    Stock
    1   chicken (stewing hen), cut into pieces
    7½ cups cold water
    1   large onion, quartered
    1   carrot, sliced
        few sprigs parsley

    ⅓   cup barley
    1   large carrot, finely diced
    2   large scallions, white parts sliced (reserve
        green parts)
        freshly ground pepper, to taste

To make the stock: Place chicken in a 4-quart pot with water, onions, sliced carrots, and parsley. Bring to a boil, reduce heat, and simmer for 3 hours.

Remove chicken from pot and set aside. Strain stock and refrigerate overnight. The next day, remove fat from surface and pour stock into a clean pot (you should have about 6 cups).

Add barley to pot. Add diced carrots and white parts of scallions. With your fingers, pick meat from half the chicken, shred into small pieces, and add to pot. Bring to a boil and boil gently for 25 minutes. Chop scallion greens and add, along with pepper, simmer for 5 more minutes, and serve.

    4 servings

Chicken with Peanuts

    1   clove garlic, minced
    1   teaspoon minced peeled ginger root
    ¼   cup vegetable oil
    2   whole chicken breasts, boned, skinned, and
        cut into small pieces
    1   large green pepper, cut into bite-size strips
    1   large sweet red pepper, cut into bite-size strips
    ½   bunch scallions, with most of greens, sliced
    ½   cup peanuts
    1   tablespoon cornstarch
    2½ tablespoons soy sauce
    3   tablespoons water

Combine garlic and ginger. Heat oil in a large skillet. When hot, add garlic and ginger and cook until browned. Add chicken and cook, stirring constantly, until it is white. Remove from skillet with a slotted spoon. Add peppers, scallions, and peanuts to skillet. Stir-fry for a few minutes, then cover and cook until peppers are just slightly crunchy.

Mix together cornstarch, soy sauce, and water and add to vegetables. Stir in chicken, cook for a few more minutes, and serve with cooked brown rice.

    4 servings

Chicken with Vegetables and Tofu

    1   clove garlic, minced
    1   teaspoon minced peeled ginger root
    ½   large head broccoli
    ¼   pound mushrooms

1 tablespoon cornstarch
2½ tablespoons soy sauce
3 tablespoons water
¼ cup vegetable oil
2 whole chicken breasts, boned, skinned, and cut into small pieces
¼ pound snow pea pods
1 tablespoon sesame oil
½ bunch scallions, sliced
8 ounces firm tofu, drained and cut into small chunks

Combine garlic and ginger. Cut broccoli florets into small spears (stems are not needed). Cut mushrooms in half if large. In a small bowl mix together cornstarch, soy sauce, and water.

Heat vegetable oil in a wok and cook garlic and ginger until brown. Add chicken and stir-fry until it is white all over. Remove chicken from wok with a slotted spoon. Add broccoli, snow peas, and sesame oil and stir-fry until broccoli and snow peas are bright green. Stir in scallions, mushrooms, and tofu and stir-fry for 1 to 2 minutes. Return chicken to wok, add cornstarch mixture, and stir-fry for a few more minutes. Serve with cooked brown rice.

4 servings

Chilied Chicken and Corn

1 tablespoon butter
2 tablespoons vegetable oil
1 green pepper, chopped
1 large clove garlic, chopped
1 large onion, chopped
2 cups diced cooked chicken
2 cups tomato sauce
¾ teaspoon ground cumin
½ teaspoon chili powder
  freshly ground pepper, to taste
1 cup grated cheddar cheese
1 cup corn
2 cups water
½ cup cornmeal

Preheat oven to 350°F.

In a large heavy skillet heat butter and oil. Sauté green peppers, garlic, and onions until onions are translucent. Add chicken, tomato sauce, cumin, chili powder, and pepper. Simmer for 15 minutes. Stir in ¾ cup cheese, add corn, and place mixture in a 1½-quart ovenproof casserole. Let cool.

Bring 1½ cups water to a boil. Mix cornmeal with remaining ½ cup water, add to boiling water, and simmer for 10 minutes. Let cool. Then spread over chicken mixture, sprinkle with remaining ¼ cup cheese, and bake, uncovered, for 30 minutes.

4 servings

Curried Chicken and Broccoli Soufflé

5 tablespoons grated Parmesan cheese
3 tablespoons butter
¼ cup whole wheat pastry flour
½ teaspoon curry powder
½ cup Poultry Stock (page 110)
1 cup milk
7 eggs, separated
¾ cup finely chopped cooked chicken
½ cup finely chopped cooked broccoli

Preheat oven to 400°F.

Butter a 2-quart soufflé dish and sprinkle with 3 tablespoons Parmesan.

In a medium-size saucepan heat butter until hot. Add flour and curry powder and mix well. Add stock and milk all at once. Stir with a wire whisk over medium-high heat until mixture comes to a boil. Let mixture cool.

Add egg yolks to curry mixture, stirring after each yolk is added. Stir in chicken and broccoli.

Beat egg whites until stiff but not dry. Stir ¼ of the whites into chicken mixture. Then fold in the rest. Turn into prepared soufflé dish and sprinkle top with remaining 2 tablespoons Parmesan. Place in oven and immediately reduce heat to 375°F. Bake for 40 minutes without opening oven door. Serve immediately.

4 servings

Curried Chicken
with Apples and Yogurt

    2 tablespoons butter
    1 tablespoon vegetable oil
    1 chicken (broiler-fryer), cut into serving pieces
    1 cup diced apples
       juice of ½ lemon
    ½ cup finely chopped celery
    1 cup yogurt
    1 teaspoon curry powder
    1 tablespoon arrowroot (optional)

In a large heavy skillet with a tight-fitting lid, heat butter and oil until they just start to bubble. Add chicken, skin-side down, and cook over medium-high heat until skin is well browned, about 10 minutes. Turn over and cook for 5 more minutes.

Mix apples with lemon juice. Add apple mixture and celery to chicken. Cover and cook over low heat for 30 minutes.

Remove chicken from skillet. With a wire whisk stir in yogurt and curry powder. Stir in arrowroot (if used). Return chicken to skillet, cover, and cook for 10 more minutes. To serve, place chicken on plate and spoon sauce over it.

    4 servings

Florentine Chicken Sausage

    1 whole chicken (broiler-fryer, 2½ to 3 pounds),
         boned, skinned, and cubed (remove skin in 1
         piece for use as a casing, if desired)
    1 whole chicken breast, boned, skinned, and
         cubed
    2 slices whole wheat bread, crusts removed
    ¼ cup heavy cream
    ½ teaspoon crushed dried rosemary
    1 teaspoon crushed dried thyme
       few gratings of nutmeg
    1 egg
    1 sweet red pepper
10 to 12 ounces spinach, chopped, steamed until
         tender, and squeezed dry

Preheat oven to 350°F.

Grind meat from chicken and extra breast. Crumble bread into cream and allow to soak until cream is absorbed. Add to ground meat, along with rosemary, thyme, nutmeg, and egg.

Roast pepper (see Using Vegetables table, page 204), then peel and dice it. Add to meat mixture along

with spinach. This mixture will be too moist to form with hands. Mixture may be wrapped in chicken skin, stuffed into casings, or packed into an ovenproof, oiled, clay or pottery container.

If chicken skin was removed in 1 piece, roll mixture in it. Secure ends with wooden picks and wrap with string to hold together. Place on a wire rack set in a roasting pan, and bake for 40 to 50 minutes. (If other casings are used, see pages 469 and 481 for stuffing and cooking directions.)

If using an ovenproof dish, pack mixture into it and cover with chicken skin. Place dish in a pan and pour hot water into pan until it reaches halfway up the sides of the dish. Bake for 40 to 50 minutes, or until juices are clear.

After baking, cool and store in refrigerator overnight. Serve cold, thinly sliced, in sandwiches or salads.

    Makes 2½ to 3 pounds

Fried Chicken with Sesame Seeds

    ¾ cup whole wheat flour
    1 cup sesame seeds
    2 teaspoons paprika
    ¼ teaspoon pepper
    1 egg
    ½ cup milk
       vegetable oil, for frying
    1 chicken (broiler-fryer), cut into serving pieces

Place flour, sesame seeds, paprika, and pepper in a bag and shake.

Mix together egg and milk.

Fill a wide, heavy skillet ⅓ full with oil, or prepare a deep fryer. Heat over medium heat. Sprinkle chicken with additional flour, dip in milk mixture, then shake in bag with sesame seed mixture. Cook until browned. Reduce heat and cook for another 20 to 25 minutes, depending on size of chicken, turning frequently.

    4 servings

Oriental Chicken Crepes

    ¾ pound boneless white chicken meat, partially
         frozen
    2 tablespoons vegetable oil
    2 tablespoons minced onions
  1½ cups fresh or frozen baby peas
    ½ cup sliced mushrooms
    ½ teaspoon ground ginger
   12 Orange-Buckwheat Crepes (page 396)

1 navel orange
2 tablespoons cornstarch
1 cup Poultry Stock (page 110)
1 tablespoon soy sauce
1 tablespoon orange juice

Cut chicken into slivers. In a large skillet heat oil. Add chicken, onions, peas, and mushrooms, and stir-fry, adding ginger.

Preheat oven to 350°F. Butter a shallow baking dish.

Divide mixture between crepes, roll up, and arrange in prepared dish.

Section orange, remove skins, and cut each segment in half. In a jar with a tight-fitting lid, shake together cornstarch and stock. Place in a small saucepan. Add soy sauce and orange juice. Heat, stirring constantly, until mixture thickens. Add oranges. Pour or spoon over crepes, and bake until heated through, about 10 minutes.

Makes 1 dozen crepes

Sautéed Chicken Livers with Thyme and Mushrooms

¾ pound mushrooms
1½ pounds chicken livers
¼ cup plus 2 tablespoons butter
   freshly ground pepper, to taste
1 tablespoon whole wheat flour
½ cup light cream
1½ teaspoons dried thyme

Cut mushrooms in half if very large. Cut livers into halves or quarters.

Melt butter in a large skillet. When hot, add mushrooms and sauté for a minute or so over high heat. Add livers and sauté, turning, for about 5 minutes. Sprinkle pepper and flour on top. Add cream and thyme. Cook for a few more minutes and serve.

4 servings

Sautéed Chicken Strips

These are sometimes called chicken fingers and can be served as hors d'oeuvres or a snack. They also make a fine picnic food.

2 pounds chicken breasts, boned
½ cup whole wheat pastry flour
¼ cup plus 2 tablespoons olive oil

2 tablespoons butter
4 slices lemon
2 tablespoons lemon juice
   chopped fresh parsley

Cut chicken into 2-inch finger strips and lightly dust with flour. Sauté on each side in oil and butter until golden. Add lemon slices and juice and simmer for 4 minutes.

Serve on a hot platter, sprinkled with parsley.

4 servings

Southern Chicken Casserole

1 chicken (stewing hen, 3 pounds)
3¼ cups water
   few sprigs parsley
1 stalk celery, chopped
1 large onion, chopped
   pinch of dried thyme
1 package (10 ounces) frozen corn, thawed
1 package (10 ounces) frozen French-cut green
   beans, thawed
3 tablespoons cornstarch
¼ cup butter
3 cups coarse whole grain bread crumbs
1 egg, beaten
½ teaspoon ground sage
   pepper, to taste

In a large soup pot combine chicken, water, parsley, celery, ½ of the onions, and thyme. Stew chicken, covered, until very tender, about 1¼ hours. Drain, reserving stock. Cool chicken. Then skin, bone, and chop meat. Strain stock.

Spread corn and green beans in a buttered 9 × 13-inch baking pan. Add chicken. Combine cornstarch and reserved stock in a medium-size saucepan and stir until dissolved. Bring to a boil, stirring constantly. Pour sauce over chicken.

Preheat oven to 325°F.

Melt butter in a small saucepan. Add remaining onions and cook over low heat until soft. In a medium-size bowl toss bread crumbs with butter and onions, egg, sage, and pepper. Sprinkle this mixture on chicken and bake for 25 minutes, or until sauce is bubbly and top is browned.

4 to 6 servings

Southern Fried Chicken

> 2 chickens (broiler-fryers), cut into serving
>   pieces
>   juice of 1 lemon
> 2 cups milk
> ½ teaspoon pepper
> 2 cups whole wheat flour
> 3 eggs, beaten
>   corn oil, for frying

Soak chicken for 1 hour in a mixture of lemon juice and milk. Place pepper and flour in a plastic bag. Drain and dry chicken on paper towels. Discard milk. Shake each piece of chicken in bag until well coated with flour.

Place eggs in a pie plate. Dip chicken in egg and then back into bag with flour and shake again. Place pieces, not touching, on a platter lined with wax paper and chill in refrigerator for 15 minutes.

Heat corn oil to 360°F in 2 skillets with 3-inch sides so that chicken will fry in 1 layer. Fry on each side for 12 minutes, or until nicely browned.

Preheat oven to 400°F.

Drain chicken on paper towels, then place in an oven-to-table baking dish and bake for 15 minutes more, or until crisp on the outside and tender inside. Serve hot.

4 to 6 servings

Yogurt-Marinated Chicken

> ¾ cup yogurt
> ¼ teaspoon grated nutmeg
> ½ teaspoon grated lemon rind
> 2 whole chicken breasts, boned, skinned, and
>   halved (about 1 pound boneless)
> ¼ cup whole grain bread crumbs
> ½ teaspoon dried basil
> ¼ teaspoon ground sage

Combine yogurt, nutmeg, and lemon rind. Coat chicken cutlets evenly with mixture. Place in a shallow dish, cover, and refrigerate for at least 4 hours.

Preheat oven to 475°F. Lightly oil a 9-inch-square baking pan.

Combine bread crumbs, basil, and sage. Sprinkle mixture on a plate or piece of wax paper, then press cutlets into crumbs, coating each side lightly. Arrange cutlets in a single layer on bottom of prepared baking pan. Bake, uncovered, for 5 to 6 minutes on each side, or until golden and crisp.

4 servings

Variation:

Yogurt-Marinated Beef, Veal, or Lamb: Omit nutmeg and lemon rind and add 2 teaspoons prepared mustard and ¼ teaspoon garlic powder to yogurt. Proceed as for chicken, but bake 10 minutes longer.

Spanish Chicken with Almond Sauce

> 1 cup slivered almonds
> ⅓ cup whole wheat flour
>   freshly ground pepper, to taste
> 1 chicken (roaster, 4½ to 5 pounds), cut into
>   serving pieces
> 3 tablespoons olive oil
> 1 cup chopped onions
> 1 cup chopped green peppers
> 3 teaspoons minced garlic
> 2 cups chopped tomatoes
> 2 cups Poultry Stock (page 110)
> 1 tablespoon chopped fresh parsley
> 1 bay leaf
> 2 hard-cooked egg yolks
> ⅛ teaspoon crushed saffron threads

Toast almonds in a small ungreased skillet over low heat until golden, about 8 minutes. Grind ⅔ of the nuts in a food processor or nut grinder and reserve.

Combine flour and pepper in a paper bag, add 2 or 3 pieces chicken at a time, and shake to coat well. Heat oil in a large skillet and brown chicken pieces, a few at a time. Remove with tongs and place in a Dutch oven.

Pour off all but 2 tablespoons fat. Then sauté onions, peppers, and 1 teaspoon garlic until soft. Stir in tomatoes, stock, parsley, and bay leaf. Bring to a boil and then pour over chicken. Cook, partially covered, for 1 hour, or until chicken is tender. Remove bay leaf.

In a small bowl mash egg yolks, remaining 2 teaspoons garlic, and ground almonds to make a paste. Stir in saffron, then ½ cup of the liquid from chicken. Gradually stir back into chicken and simmer for 15 minutes, uncovered. Sprinkle remaining almonds over chicken and serve with cooked brown rice.

6 servings

Turkey

Braised Turkey with Apricot Stuffing

¾ pound dried apricots
½ cup butter
2 cups chopped onions
2 cups chopped celery
7½ cups cooked long grain brown rice
1 cup walnuts
½ cup sesame seeds
2 teaspoons ground cinnamon
   freshly ground pepper, to taste
1 turkey (13 to 15 pounds)

Cut apricots in half. Place in a bowl, cover with water, and let stand for 30 minutes.

Melt butter. Add onions and celery and sauté until soft. Mix together cooked rice, drained apricots, onions, and celery. Add walnuts, sesame seeds, cinnamon, and pepper.

Preheat oven to 325°F.

Stuff turkey. Place turkey in a roasting pan, cover, and cook for 3½ hours. Uncover and cook for another hour.

10 to 12 servings

Cold Turkey Salad with Tofu and Scallions

2 cups cubed cooked turkey
1 tablespoon tarragon vinegar
2 tablespoons olive oil
¼ cup plus 3 tablespoons corn oil
25 Italian green beans
8 ounces firm tofu, drained and cubed
2 scallions, sliced
1 stalk celery, chopped
½ green pepper, finely chopped
¼ cup chopped fresh parsley
15 cherry tomatoes, halved

1 teaspoon dried thyme
1 tablespoon lemon juice
2 tablespoons yogurt

Mix together turkey, vinegar, olive oil, and ¼ cup corn oil. Let stand at room temperature for several hours.

Slice green beans and steam for 7 to 10 minutes.

Then add tofu, scallions, celery, green peppers, parsley, cherry tomatoes, green beans, and thyme to turkey mixture. Stir in lemon juice, 3 tablespoons corn oil, and yogurt. Mix well and serve.

6 servings

Puffed-Up Turkey-Cheddar Cheese Sandwiches

This is a welcome idea for using up the holiday turkey in a rather impressive way. It is also a good choice for a formal luncheon dish.

2 cups chopped cooked turkey
½ cup diced celery
1 tablespoon chopped onions
1 tablespoon chopped walnuts
2 tablespoons chopped green peppers
2 tablespoons chopped apples
3 eggs, separated
1 cup grated cheddar cheese
½ cup mayonnaise
6 slices whole wheat bread, toasted on 1 side
2 tablespoons grated Parmesan cheese

Preheat oven to 350°F.

Combine turkey, celery, onions, walnuts, peppers, apples, egg yolks, ¼ cup cheddar cheese, and mayonnaise. Blend well. Place bread on a baking sheet, toasted-side down. Spread untoasted side with turkey mixture. Bake for 15 minutes.

Beat egg whites until stiff but not dry. Fold remaining ¾ cup cheddar cheese into egg whites. Remove sandwiches from oven after 15 minutes baking time and top each with a dollop of egg white mixture. Sprinkle each with Parmesan. Increase oven temperature to 450°F and bake for a few more minutes, until topping is puffy and golden brown. Serve immediately.

6 servings

Sautéed Turkey Breast with Mustard and Cream

- 1 frozen turkey breast half (about 2½ pounds)
- 2 tablespoons butter
- ½ large green pepper, sliced
- 1 tablespoon French-style mustard
- ½ cup heavy cream
  freshly ground pepper, to taste
- 1 tablespoon grated Parmesan cheese

While turkey is still slightly frozen, slice thin pieces on the diagonal, using a thin knife such as a ham knife. The pieces should resemble thin pieces of white veal. Pick out enough pieces for 4 people and dry them between paper towels.

Melt butter in a large skillet. When very hot, brown turkey slices for about 2 minutes on each side, then remove from skillet.

In same skillet sauté green pepper so that it is somewhat soft but still bright green. Remove green pepper from skillet, and remove skillet from heat. Mix in mustard. Return skillet to heat and stir in cream with a wire whisk. Season with pepper and Parmesan. Return turkey and green pepper to skillet and heat for 1 to 2 minutes. When hot, place turkey on plate and spoon sauce over it.

4 servings

Sweet and Tangy Turkey

- ⅓ cup lemon juice
- ⅓ cup honey
- 2 tablespoons prepared mustard
- 1 tablespoon sesame seeds
- 1 small whole turkey breast

Mix together lemon juice, honey, mustard, and sesame seeds. Let stand for 1 hour.

Cut turkey breast in half. Remove meat in 1 piece, with skin on, from each half. (Also remove small chunk of turkey on underside.) Place turkey in a bowl and pour marinade over it. Let stand for at least 1 hour.

Pour marinade off turkey into a small pan and heat over low heat.

Place turkey skin-side down on a broiler pan, place about 4 inches from broiling unit, and cook for 10 minutes. Turn over and cook for 5 more minutes. Lower pan 1 notch and cook for 5 minutes longer. If not done, turn over and cook for 5 more minutes. (It does not matter if skin burns.)

Remove burned skin. Slice turkey into thin pieces across grain. Place turkey on plate and spoon marinade over it.

4 to 6 servings

Turkey Breast with Asparagus and Cheese

- 1 frozen turkey breast half (about 2½ pounds)
- ½ pound asparagus, cut into bite-size pieces
- 1 medium-size tomato, chopped
  chopped fresh thyme, to taste
  freshly ground pepper, to taste
- 1 cup grated Swiss or Gruyère cheese

Preheat oven to 400°F. Lightly oil a baking sheet.

While turkey is still slightly frozen, slice on the diagonal, using a thin knife such as a ham knife. Cut pieces so that each is about ⅜ inch thick and as large as possible.

Cook asparagus in a small amount of water until barely soft.

Place 4 large or 8 smaller pieces of turkey on prepared baking sheet. Cover each piece with asparagus and tomatoes. Sprinkle with thyme and a little pepper. Cover each piece with cheese and heat for 10 minutes, or until turkey is done.

4 servings

Turkey Chili

- 3 cups dried kidney beans
- 2 tablespoons butter
- 2 tablespoons vegetable oil
- 2 large onions, chopped
- 2 large cloves garlic, chopped
- 4 cups tomato sauce
- ¼ cup tomato paste
- 1 tablespoon chili powder
- 2 teaspoons ground cumin
- ½ teaspoon crushed red pepper
- 2 cups shredded cooked turkey
- 2 cups grated cheddar cheese

Soak beans (see page 261 for soaking directions). Then add fresh water to cover and cook over low heat for 2 to 3 hours, or until soft.

In a large pot heat butter and oil. Add onions and garlic and sauté until translucent. Drain beans well and add to onions and garlic. Stir in tomato sauce, tomato paste, chili powder, cumin, red pepper, and turkey. Simmer for 1 hour or more, adding water if necessary.

Serve turkey chili over cooked brown rice and sprinkle grated cheese on top.

4 to 6 servings

Turkey Hash

 1 medium-size onion, minced
 ½ sweet red or green pepper, minced
 2 tablespoons vegetable oil
 2 cups diced cooked turkey
 2 cups diced cooked potatoes or cooked
   brown rice
 ¼ cup unsweetened applesauce
 1 tablespoon minced fresh parsley
 ⅛ teaspoon pepper
 ½ teaspoon poultry seasoning
 4 poached eggs (optional)

In a large heavy skillet stir-fry onions and peppers in oil until onions are pale golden. Add remaining ingredients, except eggs. Press down with a wide spatula and cook, uncovered, without stirring, for about 10 minutes, or until a brown crust forms on bottom. Turn hash and brown other side for about 10 minutes. Top each serving with a poached egg, if desired.

4 servings

Turkey *Misto*

 2 eggs, separated
 1 cup water
 1 tablespoon butter, melted
 1⅓ cups brown rice flour
 1 medium-size sweet potato
 1 small turkey breast half, boned and skinned
   vegetable oil, for frying
   soy sauce or Chinese Sweet and Sour Sauce
   (page 150)

In a medium-size bowl mix together egg yolks, water, and butter with a fork. Add flour, about ⅓ at a time, and mix lightly until just blended. Cover and refrigerate for at least 2 hours and no more than 12.

Cut sweet potato into slices ⅛ inch thick and 1½ inches wide. Dry on a paper towel.

Cut turkey into ¼-inch-thick cubes or strips. They should be no thicker or longer than small shrimp.

You should have about 1½ cups. Pat dry with paper towels and let air-dry.

Heat oil in a deep fryer, wok, or deep skillet to 375°F and try to maintain that temperature. Beat egg whites until stiff. Fold into batter. Dip pieces of turkey and sweet potato into batter, and then into hot oil, and cook until just slightly browned. Remove with a slotted spoon, drain on a paper towel, and keep warm in a 175°F oven. Serve with sauce for dipping.

4 servings

Turkey Pie Duchesse

 5 baking potatoes, diced
 2 eggs
 10 tablespoons butter
   pepper, to taste
 1 pound mushrooms
 1 set of turkey or chicken giblets or 4
   chicken livers
 ¼ cup whole wheat flour
 1 tablespoon tomato paste
 2 cups Poultry Stock (page 110)
 ½ cup milk or light cream
 1 teaspoon dried thyme
 4 cups diced cooked turkey
 ¼ cup grated Parmesan cheese

Cook potatoes in boiling water until soft. Drain well. Mash potatoes until smooth. Beat in eggs and 4 tablespoons butter. Season well with pepper. Set aside.

Cut mushrooms into large bite-size pieces. Melt 1 tablespoon butter in a medium-size skillet. Add mushrooms and sauté. Drain off liquid.

Melt 4 tablespoons butter in a medium-size saucepan. Brown giblets or livers very well until bottom of pan is browned but not burned. Remove from heat. With a wire whisk mix in flour and tomato paste. Cook for 1 minute. Add stock and milk or cream and stir until mixture comes to a boil. Stir in thyme.

Mix together sauce, drained mushrooms, and turkey and place mixture in a 3-quart shallow baking dish.

Preheat oven to 375°F.

With a pastry bag or your fingers, cover top of casserole with potatoes. Sprinkle with cheese, dot with remaining 1 tablespoon butter, and bake for about 30 minutes, or until top starts to brown.

4 to 6 servings

Turkey Tetrazzini

¼ pound mushrooms, sliced
4 tablespoons butter
½ pound whole wheat noodles or spaghetti, cooked
¼ cup light cream
8 tablespoons grated Parmesan cheese
2 cups cubed cooked turkey

Preheat oven to 375°F. Butter a medium-size ovenproof casserole.

Sauté mushrooms in 1 tablespoon butter for 5 minutes. Meanwhile, to cooked noodles or spaghetti add remaining 3 tablespoons butter, cream, and 6 tablespoons cheese. Toss gently until thoroughly mixed. Then place ½ of the mixture in prepared casserole. Place turkey on this and cover with mushrooms and remaining pasta. Top with remaining 2 tablespoons cheese. Bake for 20 to 25 minutes, or until browned.

6 servings

Turkey with Fettuccine and Cream

2 tablespoons chopped shallots or scallions
2 cups Poultry Stock (page 110)
2 cups heavy cream
2 tablespoons butter, softened
2 tablespoons whole wheat flour
½ cup fresh or frozen peas
¼ pound mushrooms, sliced
1 tablespoon butter
1½ cups diced cooked turkey
2 scallions (green tops only), chopped
¼ cup grated Parmesan cheese
   freshly ground pepper, to taste
1 pound uncooked spinach whole wheat fettuccine

Place shallots or scallions and stock in a medium-size saucepan. Boil over high heat until reduced to

½ cup. Add cream, bring to a slow boil, and boil until thickened, stirring constantly. It will be barely thick enough to coat the back of a metal spoon.

Mash together softened butter and flour until totally combined. Stir into cream mixture with a wire whisk.

If using fresh peas, blanch them. If using frozen, just thaw them.

Sauté mushrooms in 1 tablespoon butter.

Add turkey, peas, mushrooms, scallion greens, Parmesan, and pepper to sauce. Heat until hot.

Cook fettuccine until tender. Serve on individual plates with hot sauce spooned over top.

4 servings

Turkey with Vegetable Medley

1 large turnip, peeled
4 large stalks celery
1 green or sweet red pepper, chopped
3 large carrots
2 leeks or 1 medium-size onion
   freshly ground pepper, to taste
½ cup chopped fresh parsley
1 tablespoon dried thyme
1 tablespoon dried basil
½ cup water
1 turkey breast half
2 turkey legs, with thighs

Preheat oven to 325°F.

Cut turnip into quarters and cut each quarter into thin slices. Cut celery into 2- to 2½-inch pieces. Cut carrots on the diagonal into ¼-inch slices. Cut leeks into 2-inch pieces and then cut in half lengthwise, or coarsely chop onions.

Mix together all vegetables in bottom of a roasting pan. Add parsley, thyme, basil, and water. Place turkey pieces skin-side up on top of vegetables. Cover with foil.

Bake, covered, for 1¾ hours. Remove foil and cook for 45 more minutes, or until turkey is well browned.

4 to 6 servings

Other Fowl

Duck with Diced Pineapple

>   2   ducks (4 pounds each), with giblets
>   ½   cup water
>   1¼ cups orange juice
>   2   tablespoons butter
>   1   small onion, finely chopped
>   ½   teaspoon minced garlic
>   1½ tablespoons whole wheat pastry flour
>   1   teaspoon tomato paste
>   ¾   cup Poultry Stock (page 110)
>   1   cup diced fresh pineapple

Rinse giblets and drain. Dry with paper towels and set aside.

Prick ducks all over with a knife so that fat will run out while cooking, then place them breast-side up on a rack in a roasting pan.

Mix together water and ½ cup orange juice and pour about ¼ of the mixture over duck.

Preheat oven to 350°F.

Cook ducks for 45 minutes. Turn ducks over and cook for another 30 to 40 minutes. Then turn them breast-side up again and cook for another 45 minutes, or until sufficiently browned on top. Gradually add remaining orange juice mixture during cooking, and baste often.

Meanwhile, make the sauce. Melt butter in a small skillet. Add duck giblets and brown well so that there are brown bits on bottom of pan. Remove giblets and discard. Add onions and garlic and cook until translucent. Remove skillet from heat. Add flour and tomato paste and stir well. Add remaining ¾ cup orange juice and stock all at once and stir with a wire whisk over medium-high heat until mixture comes to a boil. Stir in pineapple and cook over low heat until pineapple is soft, about 20 minutes.

To serve ducks, cut in half along the backbone. Place a half on each plate and spoon some sauce over each. Serve extra sauce in a sauceboat.

4 servings

Goose Stuffed with Mashed Potatoes and Caraway

>   2½ pounds potatoes
>   ¼   cup butter
>   2   eggs
>   1   teaspoon caraway seeds
>   1   teaspoon ground sage
>   1   goose (about 12½ pounds)
>   3   cups water

Cut potatoes into quarters and boil in enough water to cover until tender. Drain. Mash potatoes with butter and eggs until smooth. Add caraway seeds and sage.

Remove large chunks of fat from neck of goose. Stuff goose with mashed potatoes and tie or close legs together.

Preheat oven to 450°F.

Place goose breast-side up on a rack in a roasting pan. Prick skin all over with a knife so that fat will run out while cooking. Roast for 10 minutes. Turn over and roast for 10 minutes longer. Turn again and roast for 10 more minutes.

Reduce heat to 325°F. Remove goose from rack and pour out fat. Put goose directly in roasting pan. Add water and cover pan. Cook for 3 hours, uncovering goose for the last 45 minutes.

Remove stuffing and carve as you would a turkey.

6 servings

Squab with Cinnamon and Raisins

2 tablespoons butter
1 tablespoon vegetable oil
4 squabs
¼ heaping teaspoon ground cinnamon
½ cup raisins
½ cup water

Preheat oven to 350°F.

Melt butter and oil in a Dutch oven. Brown squabs in butter and oil for about 8 minutes on each side, or until well browned. Remove pot from heat and let cool.

Turn squabs breast-side up and sprinkle lightly all over with cinnamon. Add raisins and water. Bring to a boil on top of the stove, then cover and cook in the oven for 45 minutes.

4 servings

Game Hens with Tarragon and Mushrooms

3 Rock Cornish game hens
¼ cup plus 1 tablespoon butter, softened
¼ cup minced shallots or onions
¼ cup minced fresh parsley
8 teaspoons minced fresh tarragon or
   6 teaspoons dried tarragon
2 tablespoons lemon juice
   pepper, to taste
¼ cup plus 2 tablespoons butter
¾ pound mushrooms, thickly sliced

Slip your fingers between breast meat and covering skin and gently loosen skin from meat.

Mix together softened butter, shallots or onions, parsley, 6 teaspoons fresh or 4 teaspoons dried tarragon, lemon juice, and pepper. Using ⅓ of the butter mixture for each hen, stuff between skin and breast, spreading it out as much as possible.

Preheat oven to 400°F.

Melt 2 tablespoons butter in a Dutch oven. Add mushrooms and sauté for 2 to 3 minutes. Remove mushrooms and set aside.

Add remaining ¼ cup butter to pot and put it in the oven. When butter is melted, put hens in breast-side down and brush backs with melted butter. Bake for 10 minutes. Then turn birds over, brush with butter, and bake for 10 more minutes.

Reduce heat to 350°F. Add mushrooms to pot and sprinkle remaining 2 teaspoons tarragon over all. Cover and bake for 35 more minutes. To serve, cut hens in half, if desired. Place on plates and spoon mushrooms and juices over them.

3 to 6 servings

Game Hens with Wild Rice and Macadamia Stuffing

Stuffing
1 cup uncooked wild rice
3 cups water
1 large bay leaf
½ cup chopped onions
2 tablespoons butter
6 Rock Cornish game hen livers, chopped
1 cup chopped mushrooms
1 tablespoon chopped, fresh flat-leaf parsley
¾ to 1 cup chopped macadamia nuts, pecans,
   or walnuts

Hens
6 Rock Cornish game hens (about 1¼ pounds
   each)
¼ teaspoon freshly ground pepper
3 tablespoons vegetable oil
½ cup Poultry Stock (page 110)

To make the stuffing: Wash rice several times in cold water. Drain.

In a large saucepan combine water, bay leaf, and ¼ cup onions. Bring to a boil. Add rice and cook, uncovered, for 30 minutes, or until rice is tender. Remove bay leaf. Drain if any liquid remains.

Melt butter in a large skillet. Add livers and remaining ¼ cup onions and sauté until onions are soft. Stir in mushrooms, parsley, and nuts and cook for 1 minute. Stir into rice.

Preheat oven to 400°F.

To prepare the hens: Sprinkle body cavities with pepper. Spoon stuffing into body cavities of hens. (If there is extra, place it in a small ovenproof casserole, cover, and bake for 20 minutes.)

Twist wing tips flat against backs of hens, tie legs together, rub skin with oil, and place breast-side up in a shallow baking pan. Roast for 45 minutes, basting twice. Untie legs and transfer hens to a serving platter.

Skim fat from pan drippings. Add stock to pan and heat over low heat, stirring up brown pieces from pan. Spoon over hens.

6 servings

Stuffings

Bread Stuffing

    4 cups whole grain bread cubes
    ¼ cup butter
    1 cup chopped onions
    1 clove garlic, minced
    1 cup chopped celery
    ½ cup wheat germ
    1 teaspoon ground sage
    2 eggs, beaten
1 to 2 cups Poultry Stock (page 110) or milk

Place bread cubes in a large bowl.

Melt butter in a large skillet. Add onions, garlic, and celery and sauté until onions are translucent. Then add mixture to bread cubes. Add wheat germ, sage, and eggs and toss. Stir in enough stock or milk to moisture mixture. Mix thoroughly. Use to stuff poultry

or bake in a buttered baking dish at 325°F until lightly browned, about 45 to 60 minutes.

Yields about 8 cups

Variation:

Oyster Stuffing: Add 2 cups lightly sautéed chopped oysters and 2 tablespoons chopped fresh parsley to bread cubes.

Prune and Poppy Seed Stuffing

    ¼ cup plus 2 tablespoons butter
    1 cup chopped onions
    1 cup chopped celery
    ½ cup water
    3 cups whole grain bread cubes
    1 cup pitted dried prunes
    ½ cup poppy seeds
    1 egg, beaten

Melt butter in a large skillet. Add onions and celery and sauté until translucent. Add water. Combine with bread cubes in a large bowl. Add prunes, poppy seeds, and egg and mix.

Yields 6 cups

Corn Bread and Sunflower Seed Stuffing

    4½ cups crumbled stale corn bread
      1 cup sunflower seeds, toasted
      1 apple, chopped
    1½ large onions, chopped
      ½ green pepper, chopped
      ¼ cup butter
      ¼ cup water
      ½ cup apple butter or unsweetened applesauce
      1 egg, beaten

In a large bowl combine corn bread, sunflower seeds, and apple.

Sauté onions and green peppers in butter until just soft. Mix in water and apple butter or applesauce and add to corn bread mixture. Blend immediately. Add egg and mix.

Yields 5½ cups

Bulgur, Apple, and Almond Stuffing

¼ cup plus 1 tablespoon butter
1 large clove garlic, minced
1 cup chopped onions
1 cup chopped celery
4 cups water or Poultry Stock (page 110)
1 cup bulgur
2 cups diced apples
½ cup almonds
½ teaspoon ground nutmeg
¼ teaspoon ground allspice
    pepper, to taste

Melt butter in a medium-size saucepan. Add garlic, onions, and celery and sauté slightly. Add water or stock. Stir in bulgur. Bring to a boil, reduce heat, and simmer, covered, for about 25 minutes.

Add apples, almonds, and spices to bulgur and mix well.

Yields about 4½ cups

Mushroom-Chestnut Stuffing

1 pound chestnuts
2 medium-size onions, chopped
2 stalks celery, sliced
½ pound mushrooms, sliced
¼ cup chopped fresh parsley
2 tablespoons safflower oil
2 cups Poultry Stock (page 110) or Vegetable
    Stock (page 111)
¼ teaspoon celery seeds
1 teaspoon ground sage
¼ teaspoon pepper
2 tablespoons soy sauce, or to taste
1 pound whole grain bread, cubed
1 egg, beaten

Slash chestnuts on the flat side and simmer, covered, in just enough water to barely cover for 20 minutes. Cool, remove shells and inner skins, and quarter chestnuts.

In a large skillet sauté onions, celery, mushrooms, and parsley in oil until almost soft. Add stock and seasonings. Stir in bread cubes, chestnuts, and egg. Mix well. Fill poultry cavity or bake in an ovenproof casserole, covered, at 350°F for 40 minutes, then remove cover, and bake for another 15 minutes to brown top.

Yields 10 to 12 cups

Victorian or Old-fashioned Dressing for Turkey

1 pound chestnuts
10 cups whole grain bread cubes
1 cup chopped fresh parsley
1½ teaspoons dried thyme
1 teaspoon ground sage
½ teaspoon ground nutmeg
½ teaspoon pepper
¾ cup butter
1½ cups chopped celery
1 cup sliced mushrooms
¾ cup sliced scallions
½ cup Poultry Stock (page 110), or more
    as needed
2 cups nuts (Brazil nuts, pecans, walnuts, or a
    combination), coarsely cut, not chopped

Preheat oven to 400°F.

To cook chestnuts: Make 1 or 2 slits in each chestnut. Roast in a shallow baking pan for 20 minutes. Cool, then remove shells and inner skins from chestnuts. Cook chestnuts in boiling water for 15 to 20 minutes, or until tender. Cool. Cut or break into halves and set aside.

In a large bowl combine bread cubes, parsley, thyme, sage, nutmeg, and pepper.

Melt butter in a large skillet. Add celery, mushrooms, and scallions and sauté, stirring often, for 5 minutes, or until tender but not brown. Add to bread mixture and toss to mix. Gradually add stock to moisten. (Depending on bread, add more stock to moisten, if desired.) Lightly toss in nuts and chestnuts.

Yields about 12 cups

Fish and Shellfish

Fish is one of our most accessible foods; our oceans, rivers, lakes, and streams teem with them. The types are so numerous that only a small percentage of the actual number of edible species is represented among commercial sources. Best of all, even the most common varieties of fish provide noteworthy dining—if the fish is fresh and properly cooked.

In terms of nutrition, fish is remarkably attractive. Several low-fat varieties such as cod, haddock, and flounder are ideal protein sources for those who wish to reduce their calorie intake, since those varieties have fewer calories than beef or pork. A four-ounce serving of fish satisfies almost one-half of an adult's daily protein requirement, and fish protein is highly digestible. The fats in many fish are 60 to 80 percent polyunsaturated, and most are recommended for maintaining a healthy cholesterol level. Fish-liver oils are rich in vitamins A and D; the flesh and skin contain various elements of the B complex. Many fish are also mineral rich: Sardines and

Nutritional Values in Selected Fish
(based on 100 grams edible portion)

Fish	Calories	Protein (grams)	Fat (grams)	Carbo-hydrates (grams)	Calcium (milli-grams)
Bluefish, broiled	159	26.2	5.2	0	29
Cod, broiled	170	28.5	5.3	0	31
Crab, steamed	93	17.3	1.9	0.5	43
Croaker, Atlantic, baked	133	24.3	3.2	0	. . .
Cusk, steamed	106	23.4	0.7	0	27
Haddock, fried	165	19.6	6.4	5.8	40
Halibut, broiled	171	25.2	7.0	0	16
Lobster, northern, canned or cooked	95	18.7	1.5	0.3	65
Mackerel, Atlantic, broiled with butter	236	21.8	15.8	0	6
Ocean perch, Atlantic, fried	227	19.0	13.3	6.8	33
Rockfish, oven-steamed	107	18.1	2.5	1.9	. . .
Roe, baked, broiled	126	22.0	2.8	1.9	13
Salmon, baked, broiled	182	27.0	7.4	0	. . .
Shad, baked	201	23.2	11.3	0	24
Shrimp, french-fried	225	20.3	10.8	10.0	72
Swordfish, broiled	174	28.0	6.0	0	27
Weakfish, broiled	208	24.6	11.4	0	. . .

salmon are known suppliers of calcium and salt-water fish are rich in iodine. Most fresh and salt-water fish (except those frozen or canned with brine) are relatively low in sodium. (See Nutritional Values in Fish table, below.)

Fish cooked in the simplest manner, lightly flavored with butter and lemon, is a gustatory treat. But fish can be, and often is, prepared more elaborately. Classic fish and seafood recipes include numerous sauces, stuffings, and seasoned butters that offer variations on the basic goodness of fine fish. For different zesty sauces and butters to use when cooking fish, see Sauces chapter. For seasonings that are good for fish, see Herb and Spice Reference Table, page 54.

Besides the wide variety of finfish, the kingdom of the sea provides another category of food that is, for some, the most highly coveted of all seafood. Referred to collectively as shellfish, these creatures are invertebrates covered by some type of outer shell—unlike finfish which are vertebrates covered with scales. Shellfish are divided into two groups—crustaceans and mollusks. Crustaceans have crustlike shells with segmented bodies. They include crabs, lobsters, and shrimp. Mollusks have soft structures partially or totally enclosed in a hard shell. They include the bivalves: clams, oysters, scallops, mussels, and abalones. Although bivalves are among the most savory delicacies the sea has to offer, it is important to know that the shallow waters these shellfish inhabit have become increasingly polluted over the years; bivalves have been implicated frequently in outbreaks of hepatitis and paralytic shellfish poisoning. Buy your supply from reliable dealers who know and can control their sources. It is not wise to patronize free-lancers for bivalves, nor is it good to harvest your own unless you are sure that the waters are free of pollutants. In any case, though often eaten in the raw state, bivalves should be well cooked before serving. High temperatures destroy most of the life-threatening organisms they harbor. Eating raw clams, oysters, or mussels is very chancy.

Phosphorus (milligrams)	Iron (milligrams)	Sodium (milligrams)	Potassium (milligrams)	Vitamin A (international units)	Thiamine (milligrams)	Riboflavin (milligrams)	Niacin (milligrams)	Ascorbic Acid (milligrams)
287	0.7	104	. . .	50	0.11	0.10	1.9	. . .
274	1.0	110	407	180	0.08	0.11	3.0	. . .
175	0.8	. . .	. . .	2,170	0.16	0.08	2.8	2
. . .	. . .	120	323	70	0.13	0.10	6.5	. . .
283	1.0	74	386	. . .	0.03	0.10	2.7	. . .
247	1.2	177	348	. . .	0.04	0.07	3.2	2
248	0.8	134	525	680	0.05	0.07	8.3	. . .
192	0.8	210	180	. . .	0.10	0.07	. . .	. . .
280	1.2	. . .	. . .	530	0.15	0.27	7.6	. . .
226	1.3	153	284	. . .	0.10	0.11	1.8	. . .
. . .	. . .	68	446	. . .	0.05	0.12	. . .	1
402	2.3	73	132	. . .	. . .	. . .	. . .	. . .
414	1.2	116	443	160	0.16	0.06	9.8	. . .
313	0.6	79	377	30	0.13	0.26	8.6	. . .
191	2.0	186	229	. . .	0.04	0.08	2.7	. . .
275	1.3	. . .	. . .	2,050	0.04	0.05	10.9	. . .
. . .	. . .	560	465	. . .	0.10	0.08	3.5	. . .

The other shellfish, the crustaceans, are found in deeper waters that are less likely to be polluted. Further, they do not tend to retain pollutants in high concentrations as bivalves do.

NOTE: Shellfish such as crabs, lobsters, and shrimp have a higher cholesterol content than low-fat finfish. If you are concerned about your intake of cholesterol, eat these fish in moderation.

Availability of Fish

The type of fish most readily available commercially depends on where you live. However, many types of fish are shipped to markets all over the country, and professional fishermen are generally careful about keeping the fresh catch on ice and well preserved for optimal freshness. Some of the most commonly marketed finfish in this country are tuna, salmon, haddock, codfish, mackerel, herring, whiting, pollack, sole, and flounder. Supplies of halibut, trout, swordfish, carp, bluefish, catfish, shad, bass, and red snapper are more dependent on the season, but they are usually available fresh or frozen.

The varieties of fish include both saltwater and freshwater fish. Differences in flavor and quality depend on their native waters. Most of the best-quality fish come from cold, clear, deep waters. The flavor of saltwater fish is usually more distinctive than that of freshwater fish.

Both freshwater and saltwater fish are classified according to their fat content: Less than 2 percent fat in the edible flesh means a lean fish; 2 to 6 percent, moderately fatty; fatty fish have over 6 percent fat. Fatty or oily fish have a more pronounced flavor than lean fish and usually have more pigmented flesh. As a rule, white-fleshed fish are lean.

It is helpful to know the fat content of the fish before you begin to prepare it. Fish with a moderate or high fat content is easily broiled without drying out and needs few, if any, additions to keep it moist. Citrus juices or vinegar are popular for mellowing the stronger taste of fatty fish. Moderately fatty fish takes well to mayonnaise-based sauces and light sauces. Rich,

buttery sauces and other liquids are nice enhancements for lean fish. Moist-heat cooking methods, such as poaching or steaming, that retain or contribute to whatever moisture the fish

Fat Content of Selected Fish

Lean (under 2 percent fat)	Moderately Fatty (2-6 percent fat)	Fatty (over 6 percent fat)
Barracuda	Buffalo	Bluefish
Blackfish (or tautog)	Carp	Butterfish
	Catfish	Eel
Black Drum	Crevalle	Herring
Black sea bass	Grunt	Mackerel
Blowfish tails	Hake (or whiting)	Mullet
Burbot (or freshwater cod)	Kingfish	Pompano
	Muskellunge	Sablefish
Clams	Oysters	Salmon,
Cod	Perch, white	Atlantic and
Crab	Porgy (or scup)	Pacific
Crappie	Roe	Sardines
Croaker	Smelts	Shad
Cusk	Striped bass	Whitefish
Dabs	Swordfish	
Flounder	Tuna	
Fluke		
Frogs' legs		
Gray sole		
Grouper		
Haddock		
Halibut		
Lemon sole		
Lingcod		
Lobster		
Monkfish		
Perch, ocean		
Perch, yellow		
Pollack		
Red snapper		
Rockfish		
Scallops		
Scrod		
Shark		
Shrimp		
Skate		
Squid		
Tilefish		

NOTE: The fat content of individual fish varies widely during different seasons of the year, in various stages of maturity, and in different locales.

has, are ideal for low-fat fish. Lean fish may also be cooked using dry-heat methods such as broiling or baking, but the fish must then be basted with enough butter or oil to prevent it from drying out. Most fish recipes (whether for saltwater or freshwater varieties) are interchangeable, but you must know the fish's particular properties.

What to Look For When Buying Fish

Ask your local fish dealer what fish is in season, consequently plentiful, and usually less expensive. Examine fish carefully before buying. Fresh fish has firm flesh, a stiff body, and tight scales. If you poke the flesh, it should spring back leaving no indentation. It should not separate easily from the bones, and the surface should be free of dirt or slime. The gills are normally a reddish pink—with age they fade to pink, then gray, then brownish green. Look for bright, clear, bulging eyes—on stale fish the eyes cloud over and become sunken. Fresh fish should have the mild, characteristically briny smell of the sea, not a strong fishy odor. Fish fillets should show no trace of browning or drying around the edges.

Frozen fish may be purchased whole or dressed, and as steaks, fillets, or chunks. Frozen fish should have little or no odor, and it should be wrapped in moistureproof and vaporproof material. When buying frozen fish, choose packages that feel solid.

Most Common Market Forms of Fresh Fish

Market Forms	Description	Amount to Allow per Person (pounds)	Common Cooking Methods
Whole or round fish	fish exactly as it comes from the water	¾ – 1	steam, poach, bake (stuffed or unstuffed)
Whole-dressed fish	fish that has been gutted, scaled, with fins removed	¾ – 1	steam, poach, bake (stuffed or unstuffed)
Drawn fish	fish that has been gutted only	¾ – 1	steam, poach, bake (stuffed or unstuffed)
Pan-dressed fish	usually small fish, gutted, with head, tail, fins removed	½ – ¾	bake (stuffed or unstuffed); if small, panfry or oven-fry
Steaks	crosscut sections of the dressed fish (generally larger sizes of firm-fleshed ones such as halibut, salmon, cod, or swordfish)	$1/3 - 1/2$	bake, broil, steam
Fillets	sides of the fish cut lengthwise away from backbone; may be skinned or unskinned, but are always boned	¼ – $1/3$	panfry, oven-fry, deep fry, bake, broil
Butterfly fillets	the two sides of the fish cut away from the backbone and held together by the belly skin of the fish	$1/3 - 1/2$	panfry, oven-fry, bake, broil
Chunks	cross sections of fish after it has been dressed; portions of the backbone left in	½ – ¾	bake, broil, steam, poach
Sticks	uniform pieces of fish, cut lengthwise or crosswise from fillets or steaks	¼ – $1/3$	panfry, oven-fry, deep fry, bake, broil

Cured Fish

Curing fish by pickling, salting, drying, or smoking is a common commercial practice for several varieties of fish, including codfish, salmon, mackerel, haddock (finnan haddie), and kippered herring. These curing methods result in highly salted products, and the fish are sometimes injected with pigment and other additives as well. In the case of smoked fish, the polycyclic hydrocarbons of wood smoking may be carcinogenic. For these reasons cured forms of fish are best avoided by those concerned about good health.

Canned Fish

Canned fish can be an acceptable alternative to fresh fish, provided it is not loaded with salt and/or oil. Tuna and salmon are the most commonly consumed canned fish in this country, but sardines, mackerel, lobster, crabs, and shrimp can also be found packaged this way.

There are actually several species of tuna that may be labeled *tuna*. Only the albacore species may be labeled *white meat*. *Light meat* tuna refers to all other species. *Bonito* is also a variety of canned fish (related to the tuna species) that is becoming more popular. It usually costs less than fish labeled *tuna* and has a similar taste. Tuna comes packed in three different styles: fancy or solid pack, chunk style, and flaked or grated style. All represent good-quality tuna. When purchasing tuna or any other canned fish, check the label to see whether it is packed in water or oil. Naturally, water-packed fish is more desirable—it is lower in calories, and you can season it to satisfy your own taste.

As with tuna, several species of salmon may be labeled *salmon* when canned. The deep-colored, red-fleshed varieties are usually more expensive and are higher in oil and vitamin A.

Preparing Fish

You can purchase fish cut in just about any style desired (see Market Forms of Fresh Fish table, page 555). However, if you catch your own fish or just prefer to buy it whole, you will find it surprisingly simple to prepare the fish yourself.

With a little practice, almost anyone can learn to clean and fillet a whole fish. Turning out cleanly cut fillets with a maximum amount of flesh retained may be awkward at first, but you will soon discover the most comfortable way to do the job. Here are some tips for making things easier:

- Have the proper tools at hand: a fish scaler (a rigid, sharp knife blade held at an angle may also be used); a very sharp knife, especially important for filleting; strong scissors, helpful for cutting away the gills and fins; a strong cleaver or a saw, essential for cutting through the spine if the fish is large enough to make into fish steaks.
- Put several layers of newspaper on the cutting surface to catch the scales. Remove the top layers of the newspaper after scaling each side of the fish.
- If the fish is extremely slippery, hold the tail with a cloth or with a large-pronged serving fork when scaling and cutting.
- When filleting the fish, you should feel the bones just touching the knife blade as you cut flesh from bone.
- When removing the fillet from the skin, remove all paper from the work surface and lay the fish flat, skin-side down, on the cutting board or surface.

Whole Fish

The following steps are necessary to prepare any freshly caught or bought whole fish for cooking:

1. *Remove the scales.* Hold the fish firmly by the tail and, with a scaler or sharp knife,

remove the scales using a brushing motion from the tail end toward the head.

2. *Eviscerate the fish.* (This preliminary step is often done by fishermen where the fish is caught so that it can be washed as it is gutted.) Cut the belly from the level of the gills down to the anal opening. Inside the belly look for the roe in the form of two long sacs, and cut them away carefully. Wash and reserve (see Fish Roe, page 562).

3. *Remove the gills.* Hold them firmly in your hand and cut around the membrane with a knife, then with scissors cut them off where they join the body.

4. *Remove the fins.* Fins may be cut from the fish with large scissors or with a sharp knife. If using a knife, make a V-shaped incision around the fin and lift it out.

5. *Wash the fish thoroughly* under running water, making sure all blood spots and entrails are removed. Wipe the fish dry with paper towels.

At this point you have a whole-dressed fish ready to be cooked, using any of several methods including stuffing and baking. If you do not intend to cook the fish right away, wrap it in foil or plastic wrap and refrigerate immediately (see Storing Fish, page 558).

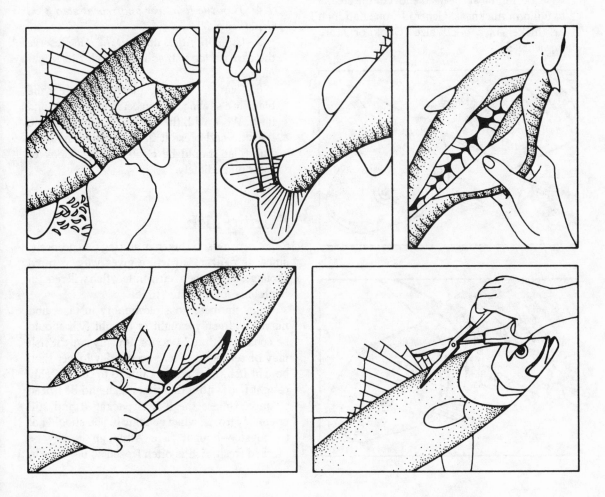

Fish Steaks

If your whole fish is large enough in circumference to make into fish steaks, you may do so after following directions for whole fish (see Preparing Fish, page 556). Then:

1. *Remove the head.* Make the incision right behind the gills, slicing through the flesh with a sharp knife. If the fish is exceptionally large, you may need a cleaver to cut through the spine. Save the head and discarded bones for making fish soups or Fish Stock (see page 111).

2. *Slice the fish into steaks.* Cutting width-wise, beginning at the head end, cut the steaks to uniform thickness. Generally, one-half inch or thicker is a good size. Cook or store immediately.

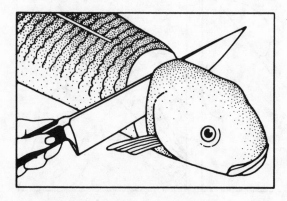

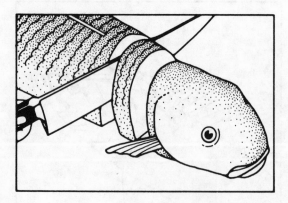

Fish Fillets

1. *Make an incision behind the gills.* Lay the fish on its side and cut from the top of the fish diagonally down to the belly.

2. *Make a cut from the head down to the tail,* holding the fish's backbone toward you, with the fish still on its side. The cut should be about an inch deep—you should feel the backbone with the knife.

3. *Slice the flesh from the center bone,* following the plane of the backbone but not breaking the structure. With your free hand pull back the flesh as you slice. Do not cut fillet off at the tail end; leave the tail attached.

4. *Turn the fish over and repeat step 3 on the other side.*

5. *Cut both fillets away at the tail.* Reserve the carcass for fish soups or Fish Stock (see page 111).

6. *Skin the fillet* by moving a large knife blade in a sawing motion between the skin and flesh. Work with the blade at a slight angle to the skin and press it firmly against the skin. The fillet should be clean looking. Cook or store immediately.

Storing Fish

Great care must be taken in storing fish properly, since its delicate structure gives way to rapid spoilage. Even when refrigerated, fish will remain fresh only for a limited time.

For the best possible quality in taste and nutrition, freshly caught or bought fish should be cooked within 24 hours. Freshly caught fish may be refrigerated for about a day longer than bought fish. If you do not intend to cook freshly caught fish within this time, it should be frozen at once. Unless the fish is packaged and still obviously frozen when you buy it, you should not freeze store-bought fish. Although it may be marked fresh, fish is often frozen somewhere in

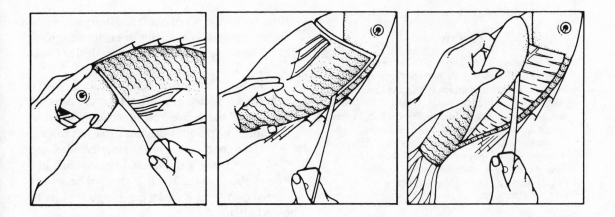

transit from its source to the market. (Once cooked, it may, of course, be frozen again.)

If wrapped properly, most fish can be frozen for up to three months. Before freezing fresh fish, clean it well and cut it to the desired form and recipe-size portions. Wrap the whole fish or the cut portions individually in moistureproof freezer paper or heavy-duty foil. Freezing fish as wet as possible helps prolong its storage life. Be sure to squeeze all air out of the package and tape it securely. Label the package with the type of fish, how it is cut, and the date it is frozen.

Whole fatty fish (see Fat Content of Fish table, page 554) will be preserved longer if dipped for one minute in a solution of ascorbic acid or lemon juice and water before being frozen. Mix 1½ tablespoons of ascorbic acid crystals (vitamin C, which you can buy at a drugstore) or lemon juice with one quart of very cold water.

Whole lean fish may be preserved by "ice-glazing," which prevents dehydration and thus increases its storage life. Dip the fish in ice cold water, then wrap it while wet, and freeze until an ice crust forms. Unwrap and repeat once more.

Thawing Fish

It is best not to thaw frozen fish completely before cooking it. The fish will keep more of its juices and thus be moister if you cook it just before it is thoroughly thawed.

Cooking Fish

Fish is cooked to develop its flavor, not to tenderize it. Unlike meat, which contains a great deal of connective tissue, fish flesh is already tender. It should not be cooked at a high temperature for very long or it will shrivel and dry out. For best results fish is cooked briefly at moderate temperatures that allow it to retain its moistness. (Some fish fillets may cook in as little as five minutes.)

Generally the method chosen for cooking fish is the one that will best bring out its delicate flavor. The choice usually involves several factors: the size of the fish, the style of the cut, and the fat content of the fish. A quick-cooking method such as sautéing is quite suitable for small fillets but would never do for a large, thick-fleshed fish that must be cooked through slowly. If the fish is lean—bass, codfish, or halibut, for example—a cooking method such as steaming or sautéing that supplies some moisture and lubricating butter or cooking oil is best. Fatty fish, such as salmon, trout, or bluefish, is less likely to dry out; baking or broiling are the methods most suited to their texture.

Fish Heads

In this country whole fish is often served without the head. However, fish may be prepared and served with the head intact. If it is, the fish is less likely to dry out during cooking, because the head helps to keep the body fluids inside the fish. In the larger species the head often carries a significant amount of edible flesh. When serving fish large enough to have fleshy cheeks, scoop them out with your fingers or a knife and savor this delicacy, highly prized among regular fish eaters.

Broiling

Broiling is a good way to develop flavor in fatty fish. It is also a suitable cooking method for large fish cut into chunks, small fish left whole after dressing, whole fish that are butterflied so that they lie flat, as well as fillets and steaks. Fish to be broiled should range in thickness from ½ to 1½ inches; if thicker, it will dry out before being fully cooked. (Baking is a more effective method for thicker fish.) Place the fish on an oiled or buttered perforated rack that fits over a pan. Broil 3 to 4 inches below the source of heat. Whole split fish and thicker steaks should be carefully turned over with a wide spatula.

Baking

Baking is a suitable cooking method for any type of fish. It is the most expedient means of cooking large whole stuffed fish. But smaller fillets and steaks may also be baked. Place the fish in an oiled or buttered baking dish and bake in a preheated oven (anywhere from 325 to 400°F, depending on the size and style of the fish). Allow more time for fish that is stuffed or baked in sauce. Test often to see whether fish is done. Fish is usually baked in an uncovered dish, but if keeping fish moist is a concern, a cover may be used and the cooking time extended slightly.

Frying

Frying or sautéing is a quick cooking method that works best for small fillets, small whole fish, or thinly sliced steaks. *Panfrying, oven-frying,* and *deep frying* are three different ways of frying that all contribute a great deal of flavor to fish.

Panfried fish is first lightly breaded. Then it is fried in a skillet with a thin layer of heated oil or clarified butter over medium heat. The fish is fried briefly on both sides until golden brown.

Oven-fried fish is also lightly breaded and then placed in a well-buttered baking dish in a 450 to 500°F oven. The fish does not have to be turned over, and it cooks quickly so it must be tested often.

Deep-fried fish is dipped in a batter, then cooked in very hot oil (370°F) in a deep skillet until crisp and golden brown. The batter seals in moisture and keeps the outside dry. Use only fresh vegetable oil for deep frying and drain the fish on absorbent paper.

Poaching and Steaming

Poaching and steaming are most effective in protecting the delicate flavor of lean fish, but these cooking methods should only be used for the larger firm-fleshed varieties that are less apt to fall apart.

Poaching liquids are usually aromatic broths such as court bouillon, fish stock, or *fumet; mirepoix* also may be used. (See Index.) The fish should be wrapped in a double layer of moistened cheesecloth, immersed in the boiling liquid, and then simmered, *not boiled,* over low heat until cooked. When done, allow the fish to cool and drain over the poaching liquid before removing the cheesecloth. The poaching liquid may be strained, frozen, and reused for poaching or as a base for soups or sauces.

Steaming may be done in a covered pot or fish poacher. The fish is placed on a rack raised above a simmering liquid—usually water, but sometimes flavored broth. Cooking time will vary with the fish so test often to avoid overcooking. Steamed fish are often served with light sauces.

Handling Cooked Fish

A major concern with cooked fish is preserving its form after it is cooked. Its fragile structure will crumble quickly, so handle it very carefully. When possible, serve fish in the vessel it was cooked in. If cooked fish must be moved, use two long spatulas to support its weight. Fish which is to be poached or steamed may be tied in a cheesecloth and cooked, then cooled that way to keep it from breaking. Fish less than one-half inch thick is too fragile to turn over during broiling, so use a lower temperature (about 400 to 450°F) and cook on only one side, testing often. Baste the top with butter or oil to keep it from drying out.

Leftover Fish

Leftover cooked fish may be stored in the refrigerator for two to three days. Be sure to wrap it securely in moistureproof wrapping. Leftover fish (without bones) can often be used in the same way as most canned fish. Use it in a cold salad with a mayonnaise or vinegar-oil dressing along with cut-up vegetables. It may serve as an ingredient in a seafood quiche or be mixed with bread crumbs and seasonings and fried to make fish cakes. Toss chunks of leftover fish with steamed rice and seasoning for a hot salad. If it is to be recooked, be sure enough moisture is provided by other ingredients in the recipe or the fish may dry out.

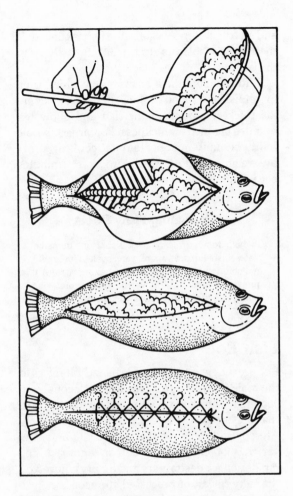

Stuffing

Stuffing fish, like serving it with a light sauce, is an embellishment, not a necessity, for good-tasting fish. It is a way to add variety to a whole fish. The fish's natural flavor mingles with the stuffing's seasonings, providing a delicious, filling treat. Stuffings can consist of well-seasoned mixtures of many different ingredients—nuts, grains, bread crumbs, chopped vegetables, or shellfish meat.

Before stuffing a gutted fish, be sure it has been washed and dried. Then cut the opening as deeply as possible without piercing through the other side or the tail. Coat the inside of the fish with lemon juice, then fill with the prepared stuffing. To keep the stuffing from leaking out, skewer the fish closed, then lace the skewers with a cord and tie it firmly. Butter both sides of the fish and cook according to the recipe.

Testing to See That Fish Is Done

Fish is fully cooked as soon as its translucent flesh turns snowy white and slips easily into tender flakes when prodded. Cooking past this optimal time will result in dry, tough, tasteless fish. So, test fish often during cooking, beginning about halfway through its recommended cooking time. With a fork or metal skewer gently prod the fish in its thickest section (usually near the center backbone). If the flakes separate easily and all translucence is gone, the fish is cooked. If the fish is whole, its flesh will fall easily from the bones.

To calculate the approximate cooking time for all fish and for all cooking methods, measure the thickest portion of the fish and allow ten minutes per inch of thickness. For large or whole fish you may also calculate cooking time by weighing it. Allow five to seven minutes per pound.

Eliminating Fishy Odors

To help remove the odor of fish from utensils, plates, dishcloths, and cookware, soak them briefly in a solution of 1½ teaspoons of baking soda to 1 quart of water. To remove the smell from your hands, rub them with lemon juice before washing.

Fish Roe

Roe are the eggs of the female fish. (Milt refers to the male fish's sperm, also used occasionally in cooking.) They are contained in two ovarian sacs that are encased in a delicate membrane pouch. Although all contain minerals and vitamins, few varieties of edible fish roe can approach the reputation for desirability and luxury enjoyed by the salty caviar, or processed sturgeon roe.

Fishing devotees know that the roe of several fish species are equally savory, and without all that salt and high cost. Shad roe is the best-known variety, but flounder, carp, pike, codfish, salmon, whitefish, mullet, tuna, alewife, herring, mackerel, sea trout, lumpfish, and haddock all offer tasty, edible roe. The roe of freshwater gar and saltwater puffer or blowfish contain toxic substances.

The best way to prepare roe is to poach it first. This may be done by simmering it for two to five minutes in water seasoned with lemon juice (one tablespoon of lemon juice per quart of water). Remove the roe from the water as soon as it turns from translucent to opaque. After cooling, it may be used in any recipe.

Squid and Octopus

Squid and octopus are high-protein, low-calorie mollusks very similar in taste and appearance. Breaded or simply sautéed and served with a sauce, both have mild, delicate flavors. An octopus may grow to be very large, but it becomes tough if over two pounds. Squid (often called *calamari* in continental-style restaurants) that are longer than six inches are also tough, and their flesh needs to be tenderized by pounding it with a mallet before cooking. Squid and octopus cook quickly and may be easily marinated, then served in cold salads. You can find both these sea animals in fish markets and sometimes in regular supermarkets, either fresh or frozen.

Frogs' Legs

The French name *grenouilles* may sound more appetizing than frogs' legs, but whatever this delicate meat is called, you will find the flavor mild—often described as similar to that of chicken. Generally, frogs' legs are sold skinned and ready to cook. You can find them in the freezer compartment of fish stores or supermarkets. The small to medium-size frogs' legs offer the best quality in taste and tenderness. The larger ones tend to be tough and bland. Allow four to six small legs per serving.

Whole Crabs

People who do their own crabbing know the pleasure of dining on freshly caught crabs. However, this culinary delight is limited to those who live near the sea habitat of this crustacean. Because whole crabs in the shell must be kept alive until cooked, it is not likely they will be found very far inland. People who live inland must rely on the efficiency of fish marketers to transport crab meat in its various commercial forms to their region. Fortunately, there are numerous recipes that are easily adapted to frozen or canned crab meat.

Buying Crabs

If you live fairly close to the ocean, you can probably purchase live crabs from a seafood market. Keep them in a cool place or refrigerated. A crab that dies before cooking should be thrown away because it may be unsafe to eat.

Crab meat is available in most areas frozen or canned, usually fully cooked. As with all seafood, it should have a fresh, mild smell. Whole hard-shell crabs should be bought live or fully cooked. Whole soft-shell crabs should only be bought live. Crabs are never frozen uncooked in the shell because the meat takes on a limp and watery texture.

Fresh, packed crab meat comes in several styles: lump, backfin, or flaked. Lump meat, the large white chunks of body meat, is considered the choicest. Backfin meat comes in smaller chunks than lump meat and may be used the same way in most recipes. Flaked meat comes from various parts of the crab. It is less expensive than lump and backfin meat and may be mixed with them in recipes. One pound of lump, backfin, or flaked meat will serve four to six, depending on the recipe.

Fresh crab meat is sometimes pasteurized, then packed in hermetically sealed cans. The meat will remain fresh as long as the can is not opened. Keep it refrigerated, and freeze only if necessary as its taste and texture will suffer somewhat.

In using canned crab meat, be sure to pick it over for small bits of shell and bone.

Cooking Crabs

Hard-Shell Crabs: Whole hard-shell crabs should be cooked in a large pot of boiling water. (Use sea water if possible.) Slide in the live crabs one at a time with tongs to avoid disrupting the boil. Allow them to cook for 10 to 15 minutes or until their shells are slightly risen. The water may be seasoned with "crab boil" or with any desired combination of herbs and spices.

Soft-Shell Crabs: To prepare soft-shell crabs for cooking, first make sure they are still alive. Then find the apron or carapace that folds under the rear of the body. With a sharp knife, cut it off. Turn the crab and cut off the face at the point just behind the back of the eyes. Lift each point of the crab at the sides and, using your finger, scrape away and discard the soft porous "lungs" underneath the shell. All of the remaining parts are edible.

The most common cooking methods for soft-shell crabs are breading and sautéing or deep frying. Depending on their size, one or two soft-shell crabs is sufficient per serving.

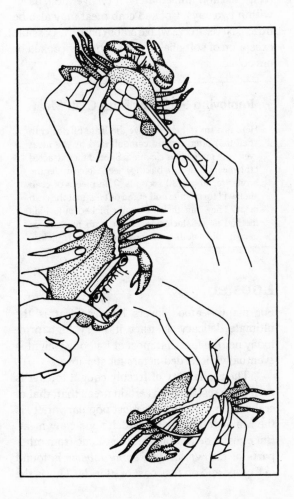

Removing Meat from Cooked Hard-Shell Crabs

Removing the meat from cooked crabs is best done by hand, using a nutcracker for the claw meat. Begin by removing the claws from the body. Remove the apron or carapace on the bottom side of the crab, taking with it the top shell. Remove and discard the inedible, spongy white gills, sand bags, and intestines. Break the body in half and extract the white meat from the segmented sections. Crack the claws with a nutcracker to remove the meat.

A 6-ounce crab will yield about 1½ to 2 ounces of meat. Reserve the extracted meat for a recipe or eat it immediately. If refrigerated, use it within two days. Cooked crab meat may also be frozen. Never freeze whole crabs (with the possible exception of soft-shell crabs), whether cooked or uncooked.

Removing Shell Bits from Crab Meat

Here is a tip to help remove the little bits of crab shell that often remain camouflaged by the meat even with meticulous cleaning: Spread the extracted crab meat thinly on a baking sheet. Place under the broiler for about 30 seconds. The pieces of crab shell will turn white and stand out against the crab meat. They can then be easily picked out. This method is satisfactory even for crab meat to be used in cold salads since it can be rechilled quickly.

Lobster

For many seafood lovers lobster meat is the ultimate delicacy. Neither its very high price today nor the fact that most of its body weight is eventually discarded deters lobster lovers.

The availability of freshly caught lobster is even more restricted to certain areas than that of crabs. In this country the most popular variety is the Maine lobster with its delicious claw meat. But equally delectable varieties come from other parts of the world. The *spiny lobster* is found in Europe and off the coast of Florida. This is the variety sold here as *rock lobster tail*. The *langoustino* or *scampo* (as it is called in Italy) is also available here but is less popular than the Maine and spiny lobsters. It is found exclusively in European waters.

Buying Lobster

When buying live lobster, make sure it is fairly active. The greener the lobster, the healthier it is. Store live lobster in the refrigerator until you are ready to cook it. If buying cooked lobster, use this test to make sure it was alive when cooked: Pull the lobster's tail straight out, then release; it should snap back to a coil.

Lobster meat is also available in the form of frozen, uncooked tails (rock lobster). Cooked lobster meat is available fresh, frozen, or canned. Edible meat usually equals about one-quarter of the lobster's weight, so a two-pound lobster will yield about one-half pound of meat. A large or jumbo one will often supply enough meat for 1½ to 2 servings, depending on how it is prepared.

Lobster is graded according to weight: chicken—¾ to 1 pound; quarter—1¼ to 1½ pounds; large—1½ to 2½ pounds; and jumbo—over 2½ pounds. Some cooks claim that the larger the lobster, the tougher the meat. Others feel there is no quality difference between large and small lobsters if they have been treated and prepared properly.

Cooking Lobster

Lobster cooks quickly. The most common cooking methods are boiling, steaming, or broiling.

Boiling

Bring a pot of water to a rapid boil—make sure there is enough water to cover the lobster when it is plunged in. Slip the live lobster into the boiling water and bring to a boil again. Time the cooking from this point—12 minutes for a 1¼-pound lobster. Add 3 minutes cooking time for each additional pound.

Steaming

To steam lobster, place a steaming rack in a pot large enough to hold the lobster. Fill with water to just below the steaming rack. Cover and bring to a boil. Then place the lobster on the rack and cover tightly. Calculate cooking time as for boiling.

Broiling

Broil only the chicken-size lobster—the larger ones tend to dry out before cooking through. Have the fishmonger split the lobster for you. To split it yourself, hold the lobster on its back. Make a vertical cut from the top down through the tail section. Remove the stomach and intestinal vein in the tail section close to the shell. Baste the lobster with butter and place it flesh-side up under the broiler for about 12 minutes. Baste often during the cooking period.

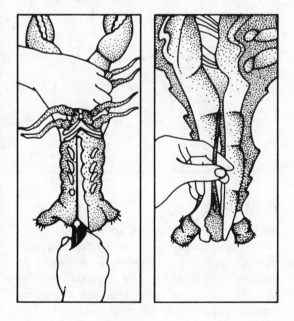

Removing Meat from Cooked Lobster

The classic way to enjoy whole cooked lobster meat is with a simple dipping sauce of drawn butter and lemon juice. The precious meat is deftly removed and slowly savored this way. Its delicately sweet taste really needs little else to enhance it. You may also wish to save the meat for use in other recipes—salads, omelets, casseroles, or quiches.

To remove the meat, begin by twisting the claws off. Then, cut through the entire length of the lobster's underside from head to tail, and break apart. Remove the intestinal vein and the stomach. The exposed tail meat can be easily extracted. Morsels of meat can then be removed from the segmented body section. Take off the legs; break them to expose the meat and suck it out. Finally, crack the claws with a nutcracker and remove the meat with your fingers.

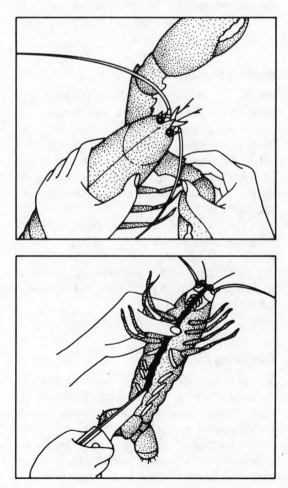

Tomalley and Coral

The tomalley, or liver, is the green substance you will find when you open a cooked lobster. It is edible and delicious. In cooked female lobsters you will also find the bright red roe, or coral, which is also edible and good tasting. Both the tomalley and coral may be used to flavor and color sauces.

Shrimp

Whether breaded, stuffed, or cold in salads, shrimp are rich-tasting, versatile shellfish. Their ease of preparation makes them accessible to scores of recipes, both hot and cold.

Buying Shrimp

Shrimp are available in two forms—fresh and uncooked or peeled, deveined, and frozen.

Fresh, uncooked shrimp, also called "green" shrimp, should be firm and dry in the shell, not soft and mushy. Frozen shrimp adapt just as well as fresh shrimp to many recipes. However, be sure not to thaw frozen shrimp before cooking them.

The number of shrimp in a pound will vary with size: tiny (Alaskan)—up to 160 per pound; small—31 to 35 per pound; medium—25 to 30 per pound; large—16 to 20 per pound; jumbo or extra large—10 to 15 per pound; and colossal—under 10 per pound.

Cleaning Shrimp

The shrimp's shell or outer covering may be removed before or after cooking. However, the shell contributes a great deal of flavor to the cooking liquid, so it is more desirable to remove it after cooking. (The shells may also be ground in a food processor and blended with butter to make a delicious seafood seasoning sauce.)

Allow shrimp to cool if you will be removing the shell after cooking them. A slight tug will release the shrimp from its covering. Deveining may also be done before or after cooking. Simply hold the shrimp's underside between your fingers and with the point of a knife remove the narrow strip of flesh on the back, exposing a dark vein or intestine that can then be easily removed.

One pound of fresh shrimp is enough for three to four servings.

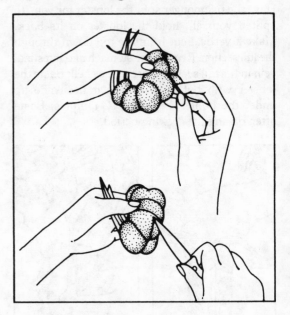

Cooking Shrimp

Shrimp cook quickly and are therefore easily overcooked. Cooked shrimp should remain juicy, delicate, but firm in texture. They should be cooked just to the point where their translucence is gone and their color becomes a pinkish orange—not a moment longer or they may become tough and rubbery. Shrimp may be cooked by either of the following methods:

Boiling
Method One: Fill a pot with enough water to cover the shrimp and bring to a boil. You may season the water, if desired, with any seafood

seasonings. Add the shrimp to the boiling water and allow them to simmer uncovered for about seven to ten minutes, or until their color turns rosy. Drain the shrimp immediately and allow them to cool for use in any recipe.

Method Two: In a pot that has a tight-fitting lid, cover shrimp with water. First bring to a boil uncovered. Then drain the water from the shrimp and cover the pot tightly. Remove the pot from the heat and allow the shrimp to remain in it for ten minutes, cooking in the steam.

Butterflying

Butterflying shrimp adds a decorative touch and is useful for shrimp that are to be stuffed. You may butterfly shrimp shelled or unshelled, but be sure to use shrimp that are medium-size or larger. Insert the tip of a sharp knife at the top part of the shrimp, and cut through the outer shell, cutting down toward the tail. Gently pull off the outer shell but do not remove the tail fan and do not cut through the shrimp. Open the shrimp and lay it flat for stuffing, baking, or broiling.

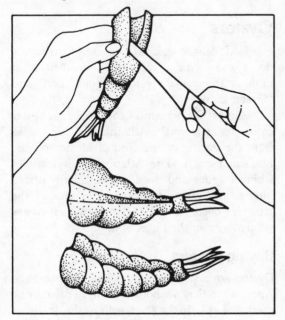

Clams

Clams, a highly favored shellfish delicacy, often appear as the appetizer at meals, but they are also good main dish ingredients. They may be of the hard- or soft-shell (surf) variety. Hard-shell clams, found embedded along the coasts (some as deep as 50 feet), include butter clams, quahogs (also called cherrystones or littlenecks), Pacific butter clams (smaller than the eastern variety), razor clams, and pizmo clams. Soft-shell clams, or longnecks, are found mostly north of Cape Cod along the coast and in the Chesapeake Bay, buried only a few inches deep in the sand.

Buying Clams

East Coast clams and those found in the Pacific Northwest are available year-round. In California clams are in season from November to April. Clams may be sold alive in the shell by the pound or by the dozen. When shucked, they are sold by the quart. Clams sold in the shell should be alive when bought. Hard-shell clams will be tightly closed. If slightly open, they should close tightly when tapped. Soft-shell clams may be partially open because of the long siphon or neck extending from inside their shells.

When buying shucked clams, look for plump ones with a fresh clear surface, packed in their liquor. Store all fresh clams, shucked or unshucked, in the refrigerator until you are ready to prepare them. Do not store fresh clams for longer than 24 hours. You can freeze shucked clams, in well-sealed containers, cooked or uncooked, for up to three months. If uncooked, cover them in their liquor first. If cooked, add some stock or other liquid before freezing.

Cleaning and Opening Clams

Clams in the shell may be very sandy, so it is best to soak them a short while in cold water, then scrub and rinse them well before cooking. Discard any clams that float or have broken shells.

Soft-shell clams may be pried open easily with a short, sharp knife or a shucking knife. The meat can then be cut from the shell. The neck meat on longnecks is too tough to eat, but may be added to stocks for flavoring, then strained out with the other ingredients. To open hard-shell clams, soak them in ice cold water for 5 to 10 minutes until they open slightly. Gently remove one at a time and quickly insert a short, rigid clam knife to pry it open. You can also place hard-shell clams in the freezer for about 30 minutes or in a moderate oven (225 to 250°F) until they open—5 to 10 minutes.

Open clams over a bowl so that you can catch the flavorful clam liquor to add to the dish you are cooking or to fish soups or sauces.

Cooking Clams

Although hard-shell clams are often eaten raw on the half shell, we recommend thoroughly cooking them (and all shellfish) to kill any dangerous organisms. Clams lend themselves to many easy ways of cooking. Large hard-shell clams, more strongly flavored than the soft-shell varieties, are a good choice for chowders, but the sweeter (and sandier) surf clams may also be used. The larger clams are good steamed and dressed, as well as cooked in soups and chowders.

Four quarts of clams in the shell will reduce to about a pint when shucked. Allow seven to eight medium-size clams per person for a recipe. One pint of shucked clams should yield three to four servings—more if combined with other ingredients in a recipe.

Steaming

Steaming is one of the easiest ways to prepare clams. It eliminates the tedious job of opening them by hand. However, to ensure that infectious organisms are destroyed, further cooking is required. Steamed clams should be added to recipes where they will be cooked slightly more.

To steam clams, place them in a steamer in a covered pot with an inch or two of water. Add one to two tablespoons of minced fresh herbs such as oregano, thyme, and parsley, if desired. Simmer over medium heat for eight to ten minutes, or until shells have opened. Discard any that do not open. If you do not have a steamer large enough to hold the clams, place them directly in the water and cook for the same amount of time.

Frying, Baking, and Broiling

Other popular methods of preparing this versatile bivalve are frying, baking, and broiling.

To panfry clams: Pat shucked clams dry, then sauté in a little butter for five to seven minutes, turning once or twice until golden brown.

To make breaded fried clams: Pat shucked clams dry; dip in beaten egg and then in seasoned bread crumbs. Fry in butter until golden brown.

To deep fry clams: Bread clams as above or dip in a batter (see Basic Batter for Frying Fish recipe, page 570). Cook for about two minutes in oil heated to 375°F.

To bake or broil clams: Season clams on the half shell with bread crumbs, garlic, and olive oil or butter. Bake at 450°F for eight to ten minutes or broil for about five minutes.

Oysters

Few foods delight seafood lovers more than oysters do. These flavorful mollusks play their most famous roles as "Oysters Rockefeller" and "Oyster Stew."

Almost 90 percent of the American oyster catch comes from the Atlantic. The rest comes from the Pacific or the Gulf of Mexico off the Louisiana coast. The Atlantic catch includes Chincoteagues and the small but highly prized blue points. The Pacific varieties include the Japanese oyster and the Olympia which comes primarily from the Puget Sound.

Buying Oysters

Oysters are best in flavor from September through April, when they are not spawning. They may be marketed alive in the shell, sold by the dozen, or shucked and sold by the quart. Shucked oysters may also be found packed in bottles and jars, frozen, or canned.

When buying oysters in the shell, make sure they are alive—the shells will be tightly closed. Shucked oysters should be plump and sold in a clear, clean liquor, free of sand, that has a fresh-water aroma. This tasty liquor adds flavor to soups and sauces.

Fresh oysters should be eaten as soon as possible after being caught, as they spoil quickly. They can be stored in the refrigerator overnight if necessary, but not much longer. Oysters may be stored in the freezer in the same way as clams (see Buying Clams, page 567).

Shucking Oysters

When opening fresh oysters in the shell, work over a strainer set above a bowl to catch the liquor. Use an oyster shucking knife or a short, strong, rigid one. Hold the oyster shell deep down in the palm of one hand. Insert the point of the knife into the hinge area of the two shells. Twist the knife until the hinge breaks. Slide the knife around the whole rim, cutting through the hinge muscle attached to one shell. When finished shucking the oysters, strain the liquor through a double thickness of cheesecloth. If the oysters are not to be cooked immediately, refrigerate them packed in their liquor in a sealed container.

Cooking Oysters

Oysters may be cooked in much the same way as clams (see page 568). Allow six to eight un-shucked oysters per person, a dozen if small. One pint of shucked oysters will serve three or four persons, depending on the recipe.

Scallops

Scallops, with their buttery texture and delicately sweet flavor, need little embellishment. There are two kinds of scallops sold in this country, both available fresh or frozen. The tiny cream-colored bay scallops come from shallow waters. The larger white sea scallops are dredged from deep waters.

Scallops should be fresh, sweet smelling, and plump. They should have a moist appearance but should be sold without any liquid. To appreciate their delicate flavor, you should eat them soon after they are caught. Purchase fresh, and keep for no longer than 24 hours after purchasing. Scallops may be stored in the freezer in the same manner as clams (see Buying Clams, page 567).

Scallops cook quickly and will become tough if overcooked. Small ones may cook in under a minute. Scallops are done as soon as they lose their translucence.

Popular treatments for scallops are broiling, sautéing, or baking with butter, garlic, and lemon juice; they are also poached and served with a cream sauce (Coquilles St. Jacques) or breaded and deep fried. Allow one-quarter to one-third pound bay or sea scallops per serving.

Mussels

Mussels are mollusks similar to clams and oysters but not quite as easy to find in all parts of the country. They are most in demand in the rocky coastal areas where they thrive. Considered the "oysters of the poor," these savory shellfish are excellent in pasta sauces, in shellfish soups, or served alone with simple seasonings. They may be cooked and served in much the same way as oysters and clams.

Fresh mussels in the shell should be cleaned well with a scrub brush. They have a "beard," which may be clipped with scissors. Discard mussels that gape and do not close when tapped, or those whose shells slide easily across each other.

Allow 10 to 12 mussels per serving—about half that if they are to be combined with other ingredients in a recipe.

Sole, Flounder, Haddock, Codfish, and Other White Fish

Basic Batter for Frying Fish

½ cup whole wheat flour
½ cup cornmeal
2 tablespoons nonfat dry milk
½ teaspoon baking powder
1 teaspoon any combination minced fresh or
    dried herbs (optional)
½ to 1 cup carbonated mineral water
    vegetable oil, for deep frying

Combine flour, cornmeal, dry milk, baking powder, and herbs (if used) in a shallow bowl or baking dish. Dip each fillet into mixture, coating evenly on both sides.

After all fillets have been coated, add ½ cup mineral water to remaining flour mixture, stirring just enough to blend. Add additional mineral water if mixture is too thick.

Place oil in a deep skillet and heat to 370°F.

Dip and coat each fillet with batter, place in hot oil, and cook until crisp and golden on both sides. Remove from pan and drain on paper towels.

Yields enough batter for 1½ pounds of fish

Fish Cakes

1 small onion, minced
1 to 2 tablespoons butter or vegetable oil
1 cup flaked cooked fillet of sole, flounder, or
    salmon
⅓ cup whole grain bread crumbs
1 egg, beaten
1½ teaspoons minced fresh dill or ½ teaspoon
    dillweed
¼ cup chopped fresh parsley
1 lemon, cut into wedges

In a large skillet sauté onions in 2 teaspoons butter or oil. Remove from heat and combine with fish, bread crumbs, egg, and dill or dillweed. Form into 4 patties.

Panbroil patties in remaining butter or oil until golden on both sides. Serve garnished with parsley and lemon wedges.

Makes 4

Flatfish Fillets in Herb Butter

6 fillets of sole, flounder fillets, or other flatfish
    fillets
1 tablespoon lemon juice
    pepper, to taste
¼ cup plus 2 tablespoons butter, softened
2 tablespoons minced fresh chives
1 tablespoon minced fresh parsley
1 teaspoon minced fresh tarragon
1 teaspoon minced fresh dill
1 cup water or Fish Stock (page 111)

Lay fillets out individually on a sheet of wax paper and sprinkle with lemon juice and pepper. Mix butter with herbs and beat with a wooden spoon until smooth. Spread on fish with a spatula and then fold fish in half and fasten with a wooden pick. Place fish in a single layer in a shallow, heavy, medium-size baking dish. Pour water or stock around fish. Butter a piece of wax paper to fit the dish and place it butter-side down over fish. Pierce paper once in center to allow steam to escape. Cover all with a heavy piece of foil and cook on top of range over low heat for 10 to 15 minutes, or until fish flakes easily. Remove wax paper and foil, place fillets on a serving platter, spoon some of the herb sauce over fish, and serve hot.

4 to 6 servings

Fresh Fish Sauce with Noodles

1 pound uncooked whole wheat spaghetti
¾ cup olive oil
1 teaspoon minced garlic
1 pound fillet of sole
1 teaspoon minced fresh oregano or ½ teaspoon
    dried oregano
⅓ cup chopped, fresh, flat-leaf parsley
¼ teaspoon freshly ground pepper

⅛ teaspoon crushed red pepper
2 tomatoes, peeled, seeded, and chopped
    grated Parmesan cheese (optional)

Cook spaghetti. Drain and keep hot.

In a 10-inch skillet heat oil to medium-hot (not sizzling). Add garlic and cook for 1 minute. Then place fish fillets in pan and sauté over medium heat, breaking into pieces as they cook. Neither garlic nor fish should brown. Cook fish until it turns white and can be flaked, 5 to 8 minutes. Just before it is done, add oregano. Remove from heat and stir in remaining ingredients. Toss with spaghetti. May serve with cheese.

4 to 6 servings

Elegant Poached Fillet of Sole

½ cup pineapple juice
1 cup white grape juice, or more as needed
½ teaspoon ground ginger
2 teaspoons lemon juice
2 pounds fillet of sole
1 cup purple grapes, halved and seeded
1 kiwi fruit, peeled and sliced
1 cup unsweetened pineapple chunks

In a large skillet bring pineapple juice, grape juice, ginger, and lemon juice to a boil. Add sole, reduce heat, and poach fish until it flakes, about 8 minutes. If liquid doesn't cover fish, add more grape juice. Remove fish from poaching liquid carefully with two spatulas to avoid breaking fillets. Garnish with grapes, kiwi fruit, and pineapple.

4 servings

Hawaiian Fillets

1 pound fillet of sole
1 cup white grape juice
1 cup yogurt
½ cup finely chopped unsweetened pineapple
2 tablespoons lime juice
¼ teaspoon ground cardamom
¼ teaspoon ground nutmeg
¼ cup chopped macadamia nuts

1 cup honeydew melon balls
1 cup seedless green grapes
    lime wedges
    mint leaves (optional)

Place fillets in a large skillet. Add grape juice and bring to a boil. Reduce heat, cover, and simmer for 5 minutes, or until cooked through. Remove from heat. Cool fillets slightly, then refrigerate until chilled or overnight.

Arrange fillets on a platter. In a small bowl, mix together yogurt, pineapple, lime juice, cardamom, and nutmeg. Spoon mixture over fillets. Top with nuts. Arrange melon balls, grapes, lime wedges, and mint leaves (if used), around edges of platter.

4 servings

Fillets of the Sea with Cream

4 cups white grape juice
1 tablespoon minced scallions
1½ cups heavy cream
6 tablespoons butter, softened
3 tablespoons lemon juice
2 pounds fillet of sole or flounder, cut into
    2-inch cubes
⅛ teaspoon white pepper
    parsley sprigs

In a medium-size saucepan bring 2 cups grape juice and scallions to a boil. Reduce heat and simmer for 5 minutes. With a wire whisk stir cream into hot mixture a little at a time, cooking until liquid is reduced to 1½ to 2 cups. Cover and keep warm.

In a large skillet heat remaining 2 cups grape juice. Add 3 tablespoons butter and 1 tablespoon lemon juice and bring to a boil. Reduce heat and poach fish in this liquid until cooked through, about 7 minutes.

While fish is poaching, simmer cream sauce. Remove sauce from heat and stir in 3 tablespoons butter, a little at a time, 2 tablespoons lemon juice, and pepper. Remove fish from skillet and arrange on a heated platter. Pour sauce over fish and garnish with parsley.

4 servings

Fish-and-Cheese Puffs

¾ cup soft whole grain bread crumbs
1 tablespoon butter, melted
¾ cup grated Swiss cheese
1 pound fillet of sole or other white fish fillets
2 medium-size potatoes, quartered
½ cup grated Parmesan cheese
1 tablespoon butter
  dash of pepper
¼ teaspoon dry mustard
½ teaspoon paprika
¼ cup grated onions
1 tablespoon chopped fresh parsley
1 egg, separated

Combine bread crumbs and melted butter. Then mix in ¼ cup Swiss cheese. Set aside.

Steam fish for 5 to 6 minutes, or just until flesh is cooked through. Cool slightly. Break into small pieces. Reserve.

Boil potatoes until tender. Drain and place in a large bowl. Add remaining Swiss cheese, Parmesan, butter, pepper, mustard, and paprika. Mash or whip until cheese is melted and potatoes are smooth and fluffy. Beat in onions, parsley, and egg yolk. In a separate bowl beat egg white until stiff but not dry. Fold egg white and reserved fish into potato mixture.

Preheat oven to 400°F. Generously butter 2 12-cup muffin tins.

Shape spoonfuls of potato-fish mixture into 24 balls about 1¼ inches in diameter, or the size of a golf ball. Roll balls in crumb mixture and place in muffin tins. Bake for 30 minutes, or until toasty brown.

Loosen with a paring knife, paying special attention to the bottoms, which tend to stick. Serve hot as appetizers or snacks, or as bite-size accompaniments to a hot soup luncheon.

Makes 2 dozen

NOTE: The potato mixture minus the egg white can be prepared in advance and refrigerated. Remove from refrigerator about an hour before you are ready to bake the puffs. Fold in the egg white and proceed according to directions.

Variation:

Baked Fish 'n Cheese Potato Boats: Bake 2 large potatoes until tender. Halve potatoes and scoop out insides, leaving a layer of potato on the skin so it retains its shape. Prepare potato mixture as for puffs. Pile mixture back into shells and sprinkle with half the amount of crumbs used for puffs. Bake at 400°F in a buttered pan on top rack of oven for about 30 minutes, or until toasty brown on top.

Perfect Pâté

1 pound fillet of sole, pike, or turbot
1 pound salmon fillets
4 cups Court Bouillon (page 111) or water
1 envelope unflavored gelatin
½ cup boiling water
½ cup cold water
1 scallion
2 hard-cooked eggs, sieved
1 cup heavy cream
1 cup mayonnaise
1 tablespoon chopped fresh dill or ½ teaspoon dillweed
1 tablespoon chopped fresh chives
1 teaspoon lemon juice

Place sole, pike, or turbot and salmon in separate saucepans and cover with boiling court bouillon or water. Poach until fish flakes, about 8 minutes for white fish and 12 minutes for salmon.

While fish is poaching, dissolve gelatin in ½ cup boiling water. Add cold water and put aside to cool but do not allow to set.

In a food processor puree fish together with scallion. Mix hard-cooked eggs into fish. When gelatin has cooled, blend it into fish.

Whip cream until stiff and fold it into fish mixture. Grease an 8-cup mold or oblong pan, pour pâté mixture into it, and chill in refrigerator until well set.

In a blender or food processor mix mayonnaise, dill or dillweed, chives, and lemon juice. To serve, turn pâté out of mold, slice, and serve topped with dressing.

6 to 8 servings

Scandinavian Fish Mold with Pink Sauce

1½ pounds fillet of sole, flounder fillets, or other
    skinless white fish fillets, slightly frozen
¼ teaspoon white pepper
¼ teaspoon ground nutmeg
¼ cup butter, softened
1 tablespoon whole wheat flour
1 cup heavy cream, whipped
    Pink Sauce (see below)

Place pieces of slightly frozen fish into a food processor or blender. In several batches, puree until smooth, adding pepper and nutmeg. Remove to a bowl. In food processor or blender, cream butter with flour and then add a small amount of fish puree. Transfer mixture to a large bowl and add remaining fish puree. Slowly add whipped cream, a bit at a time, to puree, beating with a mixer until light and airy.

Preheat oven to 325°F.

Spoon mixture into a well-buttered, ovenproof, fish-shaped mold, or any other shape mold. Cover tightly with a piece of buttered foil and place in a larger pan half filled with boiling water. Bake for 1 hour.

When mold is finished baking, let rest for 10 minutes before unmolding. Serve warm with some sauce spooned over the pudding and the rest passed at the table.

4 servings

Pink Sauce

3 tablespoons butter
3 tablespoons whole wheat flour
2 cups hot Fish Stock (page 111) or milk
1 mushroom, chopped
1 medium-size tomato, peeled and chopped
    pepper, to taste
1 egg yolk
2 tablespoons heavy cream

In top of a double boiler, melt butter. Add flour and stir and cook 5 minutes. Slowly add stock or milk, stirring constantly. Then add mushrooms, tomatoes, and pepper, and simmer over hot water for 30 minutes, stirring occasionally. Strain, pressing solids against strainer. Discard solids. Return sauce to double boiler. Add a little sauce to egg yolk, stir, and add to double boiler. Stir and cook a few minutes. Then add cream. Cook until slightly thickened.

Yields about 2 cups

Spinach-Stuffed Fish Roll

Stuffing
¼ cup plus 2 tablespoons butter
½ cup chopped celery
½ cup chopped scallions
¼ teaspoon dried thyme
¼ teaspoon ground sage
¼ teaspoon pepper
2 cups soft whole grain bread crumbs
⅓ cup Fish Stock (page 111) or light cream

Fillets
6 fillets of sole or flounder fillets, not more than
    ½ inch thick, skinned
¼ cup plus 2 tablespoons butter, melted
    pepper, to taste
6 tablespoons chopped fresh spinach
1 tablespoon lemon juice
6 small basil leaves
6 strips pimiento

To make the stuffing: Melt butter in a medium-size skillet. Add celery and scallions and sauté until soft. Add thyme, sage, and pepper and mix.

In a medium-size bowl, combine celery-herb mixture with bread crumbs. Moisten slightly with cream or stock.

Preheat oven to 375°F. Butter a medium-size baking dish.

To prepare the fillets: Brush each fillet with melted butter and sprinkle with pepper. With a spatula, spread a layer of bread stuffing on each fillet, then over that, 1 tablespoon spinach. Roll and fasten each with a wooden pick and place them close together in 1 layer in a baking dish. Mix rest of butter with lemon juice, pour over rolled fillets, and bake for 15 to 20 minutes, or until fish flakes when tested with point of a knife. Top each roll with a basil leaf and a strip of pimiento.

2 to 3 servings

Almond-Stuffed Flounder in Orange Sauce

Stuffing

2 tablespoons butter
1 clove garlic, minced
1 small onion, finely chopped
1 stalk celery, finely chopped
½ teaspoon grated orange rind
1½ cups soft whole grain bread crumbs
½ cup finely ground almonds
¼ cup chopped golden raisins
⅛ teaspoon pepper
2 tablespoons orange juice

2 pounds flounder fillets

Sauce

¼ cup slivered almonds
¼ cup butter
¼ cup plus 2 tablespoons orange juice

Preheat oven to 400°F. Butter a baking pan.

To make the stuffing: Melt butter in a large skillet. Sauté garlic, onions, and celery until tender. Add orange rind, bread crumbs, ground almonds, raisins, pepper, and orange juice and mix.

Place stuffing in pan, arrange fish fillets on top of stuffing, and bake, uncovered, for 20 minutes.

To make the sauce: Sauté almonds in butter until golden brown. Add juice and simmer for 1 minute. Pour sauce over fish and bake 5 to 10 minutes more, or until fish flakes when tested with a fork.

4 servings

Baked Flounder in a Bed of Vegetables

1 cup shredded carrots
2 stalks celery, very thinly sliced
2 medium-size onions, thinly sliced
½ cup shredded cabbage
1 medium-size potato, shredded
2 tablespoons chopped fresh parsley
1½ tablespoons chopped fresh dill or 2 teaspoons dillweed
2 tablespoons water
¼ cup lemon juice
¼ cup plus 2 tablespoons butter, melted
2 cups shredded cheddar cheese
1½ pounds flounder fillets

Combine carrots, celery, onions, cabbage, potatoes, parsley, dill, water, lemon juice, and 2 tablespoons butter in a large saucepan. Cover and steam for 5 minutes over medium-low heat. Stir to prevent sticking. Remove from heat and stir in 1½ cups cheese.

Preheat oven to 400°F. Butter a baking dish.

Place about ⅔ of the vegetable-cheese mixture in baking dish. Arrange fish on top. Brush fish with remaining butter. Spoon rest of vegetable-cheese mixture over all. Sprinkle with remaining cheese and bake, uncovered, for 20 minutes, or until fish is baked through.

4 to 6 servings

Creole Flounder

2 pounds flounder fillets
1 cup uncooked brown rice
2 cups Poultry Stock (page 110)
1 bay leaf
2 tablespoons vegetable oil
1 medium-size onion, chopped
2 cloves garlic, minced
1 large green pepper, chopped
½ teaspoon minced fresh thyme or ¼ teaspoon dried thyme
⅛ teaspoon cayenne pepper
2 cups crushed stewed tomatoes
2 teaspoons soy sauce
¼ pound medium-size shrimp, cooked, peeled, and deveined (optional)

Steam fish for about 10 minutes, or until it is just cooked but flesh remains firm. Break fish into pieces and set aside.

In a medium-size saucepan bring rice, stock, and bay leaf to a boil. Reduce heat, cover pan, and simmer for about 40 minutes, or until rice is tender. Meanwhile, heat oil in a large skillet. Add onions, garlic, and pepper and sauté until onions are translucent and pepper loses its crunch. Stir in thyme, cayenne, tomatoes, and soy sauce. Cook mixture until it begins to boil.

Remove bay leaf from rice and stir in all but 1 cup of the sauce. Add shrimp (if used) and fish to sauce left in skillet and cook about 1 minute, or just until fish is heated through. Spoon rice onto a serving dish and arrange fish on top.

4 to 6 servings

Curry of the Sea

1 large banana, sliced
lemon juice or acidulated water (page 468)
2 cups orange juice, or more as needed

½ teaspoon ground cinnamon
¼ teaspoon ground ginger
1 teaspoon curry powder, or to taste
¼ cup raisins (optional)
4 medium-size sweet potatoes, cut into
    ½-inch slices
2 pounds flounder or haddock fillets
½ cup unsweetened grated coconut

Dip banana slices in lemon juice or acidulated water and set aside in a small bowl.

In a large Dutch oven, bring orange juice to a boil. Add cinnamon, ginger, curry powder, raisins (if used), and sweet potatoes. Reduce heat to simmer, cover, and cook until sweet potatoes are barely fork-tender, about 15 minutes. Push sweet potatoes to sides of pan and add fish fillets. Fillets should be covered by juice—add more juice if necessary. Cover and simmer until fish flakes, 6 to 10 minutes. Remove fish and potatoes to heated platter and spoon some liquid over all. Garnish with banana slices and sprinkle with coconut. Serve remaining liquid in a gravy boat.

4 servings

Fish Fillets with Fruit and Nuts

2 tablespoons butter, softened
1 teaspoon raisins
3 tablespoons lemon juice
1½ pounds flounder, sole, weakfish, or bluefish
    fillets
¼ teaspoon cayenne pepper
1 small clove garlic, minced
3 tablespoons peanut butter
3 tablespoons mayonnaise
½ cup milk
1 teaspoon curry powder
¼ teaspoon ground cumin
¼ cup unsweetened grated coconut
½ red crisp apple, chopped
¼ cup coarsely chopped peanuts

Preheat oven to 425°F. Grease a medium-size baking pan with softened butter.

Soak raisins in 1 tablespoon lemon juice for about 10 minutes.

Arrange fillets side by side in pan and sprinkle with cayenne pepper.

In a small bowl combine garlic, peanut butter, remaining lemon juice, mayonnaise, milk, curry powder, and cumin. Beat until smooth with a wooden spoon. Pour over and around fish and bake for 4 minutes.

In another bowl combine raisins, coconut, apple, and peanuts; sprinkle over fish. Continue baking for 3 to 4 minutes more, or until fish flakes easily. Place under broiler for a few seconds to toast nuts. Serve hot with rice.

4 servings

Fish Rolled in Swiss Chard, Chinese Style

6 flounder or fluke fillets or fillets of sole
    white pepper, to taste
2 scallions (green parts only), minced
3 mushrooms, minced
1 pimiento, minced
1/3 cup cooked brown rice
3 drops hot pepper sauce
2 tablespoons lemon juice
2 tablespoons soy sauce
1 teaspoon sesame seed oil
½ teaspoon honey
½ teaspoon grated peeled ginger root
6 large leaves Swiss chard
1 tablespoon sesame seeds, toasted

Place each fish fillet between 2 sheets of wax paper and, with the side of a heavy knife, flatten it so it is 4 inches across widest part. Form 6 pieces of foil into 12-inch squares and set aside. Sprinkle fish with pepper.

Preheat oven to 450°F.

In a small bowl mix scallions, mushrooms, pimientos, and rice. In a cup mix hot pepper sauce, lemon juice, soy sauce, oil, honey, and ginger. Add sauce to rice mixture and toss.

Trim stems from Swiss chard and place 1 large leaf on each piece of foil. Place 1 fish fillet over each leaf and spread 1½ tablespoons rice filling over fish. Roll chard and fish, enclosing filling, to one end of foil. Start at that end and roll foil in opposite direction to encase fish roll. Repeat until all are rolled. Tighten ends and place the 6 bundles in a shallow, heavy, medium-size baking pan. Bake for 10 to 15 minutes. Then let rest to allow foil to cool slightly. Remove foil and place rolls on a warm platter. Pour accumulated juices over rolls and sprinkle with toasted sesame seeds.

4 servings

Flounder-Crab Roulades with Lobster Sauce

4 medium-size flounder fillets, cut into halves
    lengthwise
1 teaspoon lemon juice
½ pound cooked king crab meat, shredded
1 egg, beaten
¼ cup whole grain bread crumbs
    Lobster Sauce (see below)

Preheat oven to 350°F.

Brush fillets with lemon juice. Mix crab meat, egg, and bread crumbs. Divide among fillets, placing most on large ends, and roll up around stuffing. Place roulades in a medium-size buttered ovenproof casserole, seam-side down. Pour sauce over all, cover, and bake for about 30 minutes, or until fish is cooked through. Sprinkle with paprika and serve immediately.

4 servings

Lobster Sauce

¼ cup white grape juice
¼ teaspoon lemon juice
2 tablespoons cornstarch
1 cup heavy cream
1 lobster tail, cooked and chopped
⅛ teaspoon paprika

In a jar with a tight-fitting lid, shake grape juice, lemon juice, and cornstarch together. Heat cream in a small saucepan, stir in cornstarch mixture, and cook until thickened. Stir in lobster and paprika.

Yields about 1½ cups

Oven-Fried Tarragon Fish

1 egg
1 cup whole grain bread crumbs
1 scallion, minced
    pepper, to taste
2 tablespoons minced fresh tarragon or
    1 teaspoon dried tarragon
2 pounds flounder or other flatfish fillets
3 tablespoons olive oil
3 tablespoons butter, melted
    lemon wedges

Preheat oven to 500°F.

Beat egg in a small bowl. In a shallow pie plate mix together bread crumbs, scallions, pepper, and tarragon.

Dip fish in egg and then coat with crumb mixture. Arrange in a medium-size, oiled, ovenproof baking pan. Pour oil and butter over fish, place in topmost part of oven, and bake for 3 to 8 minutes, depending on thickness of fish, or until fish flakes easily when tested with a metal skewer and crust is golden. Serve with lemon wedges.

4 to 6 servings

Fresh Fish Hash
with Poached Eggs and Sautéed Vegetables

2 scallions, chopped
1 stalk celery, with leaves, chopped
6 to 7 tablespoons butter
4 medium-size potatoes, halved
4 carrots, cut diagonally into 1½-inch pieces
1 tablespoon cider vinegar
½ teaspoon minced fresh thyme or ¼ teaspoon
    dried thyme
¼ teaspoon white pepper
1 bay leaf
4 cups water
¾ pound haddock or codfish fillets
2 tablespoons minced onions or chives
2 tablespoons minced fresh parsley
1 egg, beaten
1 large cucumber, quartered lengthwise, seeded,
    and cut diagonally into 1½-inch pieces
½ teaspoon minced fresh basil or ¼ teaspoon
    dried basil
½ teaspoon chopped fresh mint or ⅛ teaspoon
    dried mint
4 poached eggs

In a 4-quart saucepan sauté scallions and celery in 2 tablespoons butter for 3 minutes. Add potatoes, carrots, vinegar, thyme, pepper, bay leaf, and water. Cover, bring to a boil, reduce heat, and simmer for 15 minutes, or until potatoes and carrots are tender. Remove potatoes and carrots and let them cool. Add fish to stock. Cover saucepan, bring to a boil, reduce heat, and barely simmer for 8 to 10 minutes, or until fish flakes apart easily. Cool fish in stock. Discard bay leaf and refrigerate vegetables and fish until ready to make hash.

Flake fish into a large bowl. Peel potatoes and chop into very small pieces. Add potatoes, onions or chives, and parsley to fish. Mix well. (It is better not to use a food processor for this hash.) Blend in beaten egg and about ¼ cup of fish stock, just enough to moisten mixture (it should not be mushy). Form into 8 flat cakes. Heat 2 tablespoons butter in a large skillet and sauté cakes slowly in 2 batches until golden brown on both sides, adding more butter if needed. Keep cakes warm until all are cooked.

In another skillet, melt 2 tablespoons butter and stir-fry cucumber pieces for 5 minutes. Add carrots and heat through. Sprinkle with basil and mint. Serve fish cakes with poached eggs on top and sautéed vegetables on the side.

4 servings

Haddock Ceviche

This is a delicate and flavorful preparation commonly used in Latin countries. The citrus marinade "cooks" the fish without using heat. It will take two to four hours, so plan to start the process early.

1½ pounds haddock fillets, cut into ½-inch pieces*
1 cup lemon juice
1 large navel orange
½ cup raisins
¾ cup unsweetened shredded coconut
2 tablespoons orange juice

In a glass bowl, combine fish and lemon juice. (This will "cook" fish.) Let stand for 2 to 4 hours, stirring frequently. Drain and discard lemon juice.

Separate orange into segments. Quarter segments and mix with raisins; then add to drained fish. Add coconut and orange juice and toss. Chill well before serving.

4 servings

*It is essential that only the freshest fish be used for this recipe.

Haddock with Tomato Stuffing

Stuffing
1 small onion, minced
1 tablespoon butter
½ teaspoon dried oregano
1 clove garlic, minced
2 large tomatoes, peeled, seeded, and chopped
2 cups soft whole grain bread crumbs

1 egg, beaten
2 ounces mozzarella cheese, shredded

2 pounds haddock fillets

Preheat oven to 350°F. Lightly butter a medium-size ovenproof casserole with cover.

To make the stuffing: In a large skillet, sauté onions in butter until translucent but not brown. Remove from heat and add oregano, garlic, tomatoes, and bread crumbs. Mix in egg and cheese.

To prepare the fillets: Cut fillets into halves, crosswise. Lay half of each fillet in casserole and top with stuffing. Put remaining fillets over stuffing. Dot with butter, cover casserole, and bake for 15 minutes. Remove cover and continue to cook until fish flakes, about 10 minutes.

4 servings

Scalloped Spuds and Haddock

3 tablespoons vegetable oil
2 pounds haddock fillets, cut into serving pieces
2 large onions, sliced and separated into rings
2 cups cold milk
¼ cup butter
¼ teaspoon white pepper
¼ cup whole wheat flour
½ cup water
1 tablespoon champagne vinegar
4 large potatoes, cooked and sliced
1 cup whole grain bread crumbs

In a large skillet, heat oil. Add haddock and sauté 3 to 5 minutes on both sides. Remove fish and set aside. In same skillet, sauté onion rings until they are soft. Remove with a slotted spoon and set aside.

In a medium-size saucepan, combine 1½ cups milk, 2 tablespoons butter, and pepper. Bring mixture just to the scalding point. Pour remaining ½ cup milk into a jar. Add flour, and shake until smooth. Add flour mixture to hot milk, stirring constantly. Cook until mixture thickens and bubbles. Add water and vinegar and continue to stir until sauce thickens again.

Preheat oven to 350°F.

In a 3-quart ovenproof casserole, layer fish, onions, potatoes, and sauce, beginning and ending with sauce. Sprinkle with bread crumbs and dot with the remaining 2 tablespoons butter. Bake for 20 minutes, or until brown and bubbly.

4 servings

Terrific Tricorns

pastry for 2 Basic Rolled Piecrusts (page 718)
¾ pound flaked cooked haddock, halibut, codfish, or flounder
¼ cup whole grain bread crumbs
1 tablespoon minced onions
1 teaspoon grated horseradish
¼ cup tomato sauce
⅛ teaspoon pepper
1 cup shredded cheddar cheese
1 egg, beaten

Roll out pastry on floured surface, and cut into about 14 squares, 4 inches on a side. Combine fish, bread crumbs, onions, horseradish, tomato sauce, and pepper.

Preheat oven to 400°F.

Place about 1 tablespoon of fish mixture in center of each pastry square. Sprinkle cheese over fish mixture. Fold pastry squares to form triangles, sealing edges with beaten egg. Make a small slit in top of each tricorn and brush with remaining egg. Place on a baking sheet and bake until golden, about 15 minutes.

4 to 6 servings

Broiled Codfish

½ cup plus 2 tablespoons wine vinegar
4 tablespoons olive oil
4 cloves garlic, crushed
2 teaspoons dried thyme
2 to 2½ pounds codfish fillets
2 tablespoons butter
2 large onions, thinly sliced
4 cloves garlic, minced
3 cups sliced mushrooms
1 tablespoon plus 1 teaspoon dried basil
½ cup grated Parmesan or Romano cheese
½ pound uncooked whole wheat spaghetti

Combine ½ cup wine vinegar, 2 tablespoons olive oil, crushed garlic, and 1 teaspoon thyme and blend well. Add fillets, cover, and refrigerate for 1 hour.

Heat butter and 2 tablespoons oil in a large skillet. Sauté onions, minced garlic, and mushrooms until onions are translucent and mushrooms are wilted. Stir in basil, remaining thyme, and 2 tablespoons vinegar and cook 1 minute more. Remove from heat and add cheese.

Cook spaghetti. Drain and keep hot.

Remove fish from marinade. Place on a rack about 6 inches from broiler and broil 5 minutes on each side, or until done. Place spaghetti in an oven-proof serving dish. Layer fish on top, cover with sautéed mixture, and place under broiler for 1 to 2 minutes, or until lightly browned.

4 to 6 servings

Codfish with Cheese Sauce

3 tablespoons butter
3 tablespoons cornstarch
2 cups milk
5 ounces mild white cheddar cheese
1 large tomato, seeded and finely chopped
1 teaspoon chopped fresh basil
1½ pounds codfish fillets
3 cups hot cooked brown rice

In a medium-size saucepan, melt butter. Mix in cornstarch to make a paste. Gradually add milk, stirring constantly, and bring to a boil. Boil, while stirring, for 5 minutes. Mix in cheese. When cheese has melted, add tomatoes and basil. Remove from heat.

Poach codfish fillets in water for about 8 minutes, or until just cooked through.

Divide rice among 4 plates. Break fish into chunks and place on top of rice. Pour sauce over all and serve immediately.

4 servings

Codfish Kabobs

Any large, firm-fleshed fish, such as shark or salmon, will serve for this recipe if codfish is not available. An interesting choice for a cookout in place of the usual fare.

¼ cup lemon juice
¼ cup orange juice
¼ cup vegetable oil
⅛ teaspoon pepper
¼ teaspoon dillweed
1 clove garlic
½ cup unsweetened pineapple chunks

1 green pepper, seeded and cut into 1-inch pieces
1 orange, separated into segments
1 large tomato, cut into 1-inch pieces
1½ pounds codfish, 1½ inches thick, cut into
    1-inch pieces

Combine lemon juice, orange juice, oil, pepper, dillweed, and garlic. Allow to stand at room temperature for 2 hours. Remove garlic.

Alternate pineapple, green pepper, orange segments, tomatoes, and fish pieces on 6 skewers. Place skewers on a broiling rack set in a baking pan containing a little water. Brush kabobs with juice mixture and broil for about 8 minutes, or until fish is firm and no longer translucent. Turn skewers. Baste with juice, and broil about 5 minutes more.

6 servings

Codfish Steak Supreme

2 tablespoons vegetable oil
1 small onion, finely chopped
1 can (16 ounces) tomatoes, chopped
1 tablespoon chopped fresh parsley
⅛ teaspoon garlic powder
½ teaspoon ground thyme
½ cup water
1 tablespoon champagne vinegar
1 tablespoon lemon juice
    pepper, to taste
1 tablespoon cornstarch
1½ pounds codfish fillets
4 medium-size potatoes, cooked and sliced
½ cup wheat germ

In a medium-size saucepan, heat oil. Add onions and sauté until soft. Add tomatoes, parsley, garlic powder, thyme, water, vinegar, lemon juice, and pepper. Stir in cornstarch until mixture is smooth. Cook, stirring constantly, until sauce thickens slightly.

Preheat oven to 400°F.

Place about ⅓ of the sauce in the bottom of an 8 × 11-inch ovenproof casserole. Arrange fish in a layer over sauce, with potato slices around and between fillets. Top with remaining sauce and sprinkle with wheat germ. Bake for 20 minutes, or until fish flakes apart easily.

4 servings

Red Snapper with Black Butter

½ cup butter
2 tablespoons olive oil
1 whole red snapper (5 to 6 pounds), gutted
1 tablespoon whole wheat flour
    pepper, to taste
    juice of 1 lemon or lime
2 tablespoons minced fresh parsley

Heat butter slowly in a small, heavy saucepan for 20 to 25 minutes, or until dark brown.

Preheat oven to 400°F. Grease a shallow, heavy baking pan with 1 tablespoon of the oil.

Place fish in baking pan, sprinkle with flour and pepper, and drizzle remaining oil over top of fish. Bake on top shelf of oven, about 8 inches below broiler, for 30 minutes. Then turn oven to broil setting and broil fish 5 minutes on each side to brown. Test fish with a fork or skewer to see if fish flakes easily and continue broiling if not completely cooked. Remove fish to a warm platter. Add lemon or lime juice to butter and pour over fish. Sprinkle with parsley and serve.

6 servings

Red Snapper with Ginger Sauce

3 cups Fish Stock (page 111)
2 tablespoons soy sauce
1 clove garlic, crushed
1 cup heavy cream
1 slice peeled ginger root, minced
4 tablespoons butter
1 tablespoon vegetable oil
6 red snapper fillets (about 1½ pounds)
⅓ cup slivered almonds, lightly toasted
    (optional)

In a saucepan, combine stock, soy sauce, and garlic. Boil, uncovered, until reduced to 1 cup. Remove garlic. Add cream and simmer until reduced to 1½ cups sauce. Strain through a sieve. Add ginger, and keep sauce warm. Just before serving, swirl in 2 tablespoons butter.

Melt 2 tablespoons butter in a large skillet, add oil, and sauté fillets until lightly browned on both sides and cooked through. Place them on a heated platter or individual dishes. Top with sauce and sprinkle with almonds (if used).

6 servings

Baked Fish in Foil, Mediterranean Style

6 tablespoons butter, softened
3 tablespoons lemon juice
¼ cup olive oil
    pepper, to taste
6 whole fish (¾ pound each), gutted, or 6 fish
    fillets (use any freshwater or saltwater fish)
6 slices red onion
6 thick slices tomato
6 green pepper rings
6 thin slices lemon
6 small sprigs rosemary

Cut 6 large pieces of heavy foil. Rub center of each with 1 tablespoon butter.

Combine lemon juice, olive oil, and pepper. Put a teaspoon of this mixture on bottom of each piece of foil, turning up edges so liquid will not run out. Lay 1 whole fish or fillet in center and distribute rest of liquid equally on outside and inside of fish cavity. Place over each, 1 slice onion, 1 slice tomato, and 1 green pepper ring. Top each with 1 slice lemon and 1 sprig rosemary. Double-fold foil into tight packages.

Preheat oven to 375°F.

Place fish packets in a shallow baking pan and bake for 12 to 18 minutes. Open 1 packet after 15 minutes and test fish with tines of a fork. If fish flakes and is not translucent, it is done. Serve 1 foil packet to each person.

6 servings

Summer Sea Salad

1½ cups flaked poached perch or flounder
½ cup sliced radishes
½ cup peeled, seeded, and chopped zucchini
2 medium-size tomatoes, peeled and chopped
¼ cup raisins (optional)
2 tablespoons natural dill relish
2 tablespoons minced scallions
½ cup mayonnaise
1/3 cup sour cream
2 teaspoons French-style mustard

3 hard-cooked eggs, chopped
    lettuce leaves

Mix together fish, radishes, zucchini, tomatoes, raisins (if used), relish, and scallions. Combine mayonnaise, sour cream, mustard, and eggs. Line a salad bowl with lettuce leaves. Toss fish mixture with dressing and serve in bowl on top of lettuce leaves.

4 servings

Bass Latino

This spicy dish is an intriguing change from the more common treatments of bass and similar white fish.

2 pounds striped bass fillets or other firm-
    fleshed white fish fillets
½ to ¾ cup whole wheat flour
    freshly ground pepper
3 tablespoons butter
½ cup olive oil
3 large onions, sliced
4 chili peppers, seeded and sliced into strips
½ teaspoon dried oregano
¼ cup cider vinegar

Cut fillets into 4 to 6 chunks, coat them with flour, and season with pepper. Melt butter in a large heavy skillet and fry fish over medium heat until golden on both sides. Remove and keep warm.

Add oil to skillet and fry onions and chilies until they are tender. Add oregano and cook 2 minutes longer. Add vinegar and turn off heat. Spoon onion-chili mixture over fish and serve.

4 to 6 servings

Vegetable-Stuffed Bass

1 whole striped bass (3 pounds), dressed (with
    head on)
¼ cup lemon juice
2 tablespoons butter

1 carrot, diced
1 small onion, diced
1 medium-size green pepper, diced
1 stalk celery, diced
4 large mushrooms, diced
1 teaspoon dried tarragon
    pepper, to taste
2 tablespoons butter, melted

Preheat oven to 400°F. Butter a medium-size roasting pan.

Rub inside of fish with lemon juice. Melt 2 tablespoons butter in a medium-size skillet. Add carrots, onions, peppers, celery, and mushrooms and lightly sauté. Add tarragon and pepper. Drain. Stuff fish with vegetables and truss. Place in roasting pan and brush with melted butter. Cover head and tail with foil and bake for 40 minutes, basting frequently with pan juices.

6 servings

Tilefish Quenelles with Crab Meat Sauce

   ½ cup milk
   6 tablespoons butter, softened
   ¾ cup whole wheat flour
½ to ⅔ pound cooked, boned, and flaked tilefish
      (or other white fish)
   2 egg whites
   2 eggs, beaten
   ¼ teaspoon ground nutmeg
   ¼ teaspoon white pepper
   Crab Meat Sauce (see opposite)
10 to 12 small mushroom caps

Combine milk and 1½ tablespoons butter in a deep, medium-size saucepan and bring to a boil. Watch carefully, and remove from heat before it boils over. Return pan to low heat, stir in flour all at once, and continue stirring until mixture clears sides of pan, about 3 minutes. Put mixture on a plate, flatten to a cake, and chill in refrigerator for 1 hour.

In a food processor puree fish until fine. With motor running, add egg whites through tube. Incorporate chilled flour-milk mixture by breaking into pieces and adding a few at a time, blending after each. Add whole eggs, 4 tablespoons butter, nutmeg, and pepper. Blend well. (Alternate method: Fish can be pureed by forcing it through a sieve or food mill; quenelle mixture can be blended in using an electric mixer or by hand.) Chill mixture until firm enough to hold its shape.

Fill an 8- to 10-quart pan ¾ full of water and bring it to a boil. Reduce heat so that water gently bubbles. Form quenelles into ovals using 2 large tablespoons (serving size) and drop into simmering water, or spoon up mixture with a serving spoon and release from spoon with a rubber spatula, making 8 to 10 dumplings. When they are all in the water, poach for 7 minutes. Remove with a slotted spoon, and place in an 8 × 12-inch buttered ovenproof casserole.

Preheat oven to 350°F.

Pour sauce over quenelles and bake for 25 to 30 minutes, or until bubbly throughout.

Sauté mushroom caps in remaining butter, and use them as a garnish.

4 to 5 servings

Crab Meat Sauce

1¾ cups Fish Stock (page 111) or clam juice
  1 cup heavy cream
  ¼ teaspoon paprika
  ¼ teaspoon white pepper
  3 tablespoons cornstarch
  6 ounces fresh or frozen crab meat, with
      cartilage removed, cut into chunks

In a medium-size saucepan combine stock or clam juice with ½ cup cream. Boil gently for 5 minutes, reducing mixture to 1½ cups. Add paprika and pepper. Keep sauce at a gentle boil. Pour remaining ½ cup cream into a cup and stir in cornstarch until smooth. Pour all at once into hot sauce, stirring constantly until thickened. Stir in crab meat.

Yields about 2½ cups

Perch Fillets Florentine

1 pound spinach
1 cup cold milk
2 tablespoons butter
   pepper, to taste
2 tablespoons whole wheat flour
¼ cup Poultry Stock (page 110)
1 teaspoon minced fresh tarragon or ½ teaspoon
   dried tarragon
1 pound perch fillets
¼ cup freshly grated Parmesan cheese
   paprika

Cook spinach (in just the water that clings to the leaves) until wilted. Drain and chop.

Scald ½ cup milk with butter and pepper in a small saucepan. Pour remaining ½ cup cold milk into a jar. Add flour, cover, and shake until smooth. Add flour mixture to scalded milk, stirring constantly, and cook until sauce bubbles and thickens. Add stock and tarragon, stirring until sauce thickens again.

Preheat oven to 375°F.

Spread a little sauce in a 3-quart ovenproof casserole. Add spinach, ½ of the remaining sauce, perch fillets, and rest of sauce. Top with Parmesan and a light sprinkling of paprika. Bake for 20 minutes, or until fish is cooked through.

4 servings

Combination Quiche

The strawberries add a light and surprising touch to this rich and versatile dish.

1 cup flaked cooked whitefish
½ cup flaked fresh or frozen crab meat, with
   cartilage removed
1 baked Basic Rolled Piecrust (page 718)
½ cup halved fresh strawberries
6 ounces Gruyère cheese, grated
2 eggs, beaten
1 cup half-and-half or light cream
½ teaspoon ground nutmeg

Preheat oven to 350°F.

Mix together whitefish and crab meat and place on bottom of cooled piecrust. Top with strawberry halves and sprinkle with cheese.

Mix together eggs, half-and-half or cream, and nutmeg and pour over contents of piecrust. Bake on a baking sheet for 35 minutes, or until knife inserted in center comes out clean. Allow quiche to rest for 10 minutes before cutting.

6 servings

Crepes *de Mer* with Curry Sauce

½ tablespoon chopped fresh tarragon or ½
   teaspoon dried tarragon
1 tablespoon finely chopped fresh chives
   batter for 12 Whole Wheat Crepes (page 395)
3 tablespoons butter
1 tablespoon minced scallions
¼ cup chopped mushrooms
1 tablespoon chopped fresh parsley
1 cup cooked king crab meat, cut into chunks
1½ cups flaked cooked whitefish
½ cup sour cream
   Curry Sauce (see below)

Mix tarragon and chives into crepe batter, and make crepes according to recipe instructions.

In a large skillet melt butter. Add scallions and mushrooms and sauté until they begin to soften. Add parsley, crab meat, and whitefish, stirring until lightly sautéed and heated through. Mix in sour cream and cook until just heated. (Do not allow to boil.) Divide among crepes.

Preheat oven to 375°F.

Roll crepes and place, seam-side down, in a large buttered ovenproof casserole. Top with sauce. Bake for about 10 minutes, or until sauce is bubbly and crepes are heated through.

6 servings

Curry Sauce

3 tablespoons butter
1 teaspoon minced scallions
3 tablespoons cornstarch
1½ cups milk
1 teaspoon curry powder, or to taste
¼ teaspoon ground ginger
1 teaspoon honey
1 teaspoon lemon juice

In a medium-size saucepan, melt butter. Add scallions and sauté until translucent but not browned. Work in cornstarch to make a paste. Gradually mix in milk, stirring constantly over medium heat. Add curry powder, ginger, and honey. Bring to a boil and boil for 3 minutes, stirring constantly. Remove from heat and mix in lemon juice.

Yields about 1½ cups

Fish Balls in Broth with Spinach *Pistou*

This recipe tops off the fish balls and soup with a hearty cheese and spinach sauce that is a refreshing change from bland cream sauces commonly served with such dishes.

Fish Balls
6 medium-size potatoes
1½ cups cooked, boned, and flaked fish
1 egg, beaten
2 tablespoons minced onions
1 tablespoon minced fresh parsley
¼ teaspoon white pepper
1 to 1½ cups whole grain bread crumbs
3 tablespoons olive oil

Soup
7½ cups rich Fish Stock (page 111) or Poultry
　　Stock (page 110)
2 large carrots, thinly sliced
2 stalks celery, thinly sliced
3 medium-size tomatoes, peeled and chopped
⅛ pound uncooked whole wheat spaghetti,
　　broken into 2-inch lengths

Pistou
1 cup cooked spinach, drained
½ cup rich Fish Stock (page 111) or Poultry
　　Stock (page 110), or more as needed
4 ounces Gruyère cheese, cubed
1 clove garlic, sliced
¼ teaspoon pepper
¼ cup olive oil

To make the fish balls: Cook potatoes in enough water to cover. Drain and mash. (Do not add milk.) Thoroughly blend fish, 2 cups mashed potatoes, egg, onions, parsley, and pepper by hand. Using 2 table-spoons, form mixture into ovals and dip into crumbs. Heat oil in a large skillet, and fry fish balls until brown on all sides. Set them aside.

To make the soup: In a 4-quart soup pot combine stock, carrots, celery, and tomatoes. Bring to a boil, and cook, uncovered, for 10 minutes. Add spaghetti, and continue cooking at a medium boil until tender, about 8 minutes, stirring occasionally.

To make the *pistou*: In a blender or food processor combine spinach, stock, cheese, garlic, pepper, and oil, and blend to a puree, adding more stock if needed.

Just before serving, heat fish balls in soup. Place a rounded tablespoon of the *pistou* in the center of each serving.

6 servings

Fish Fillets
with Almonds and Mustard Sauce

1 pound mild-flavored fish fillets, skinned
　　pepper, to taste
2 tablespoons French-style mustard
3 tablespoons butter, softened
1 cup soft whole grain bread crumbs, toasted
½ cup sliced or slivered almonds, toasted
½ cup sour cream
1 tablespoon mayonnaise
　　parsley sprigs

Preheat oven to 425°F. Oil a shallow medium-size ovenproof casserole.

Place fish in 1 layer in casserole and sprinkle with pepper. Mix mustard with 2 tablespoons butter and spread on surface of fish with a small spatula. Bake for 5 to 8 minutes, or until fish flakes.

Meanwhile, melt remaining 1 tablespoon butter and toss with bread crumbs. Set aside. Combine almonds with sour cream and mayonnaise. Remove fish and spread almond-sour cream mixture over it. Broil for 2 minutes. Remove and pile toasted bread crumbs on top. Return to broiler for a few seconds more. Serve garnished with parsley sprigs.

2 to 4 servings

Fish Soufflé

½ cup fine whole grain bread crumbs, toasted
1 tablespoon butter
2 tablespoons flour
⅔ cup milk
¾ cup chopped spinach
¼ cup minced chives
1 teaspoon lemon juice
    pepper, to taste
¼ teaspoon ground nutmeg
4 egg yolks, lightly beaten
2 cups cooked fish, pureed in a blender
5 egg whites, at room temperature

Generously butter a 6-cup soufflé dish with deep sides. Add bread crumbs. Shake and rotate dish until completely covered with crumbs. Shake out excess.

Preheat oven to 375°F.

In top of a double boiler melt butter. Add flour and beat with a wire whisk. Cook for 1 to 2 minutes. Gradually add milk, whisking constantly. Cook and stir for 5 minutes. Then cover pot and cool to lukewarm. When cooled, add spinach, chives, lemon juice, pepper, and nutmeg. Beat with a whisk. Add the yolks and fish puree and beat again.

In a separate bowl, beat egg whites until stiff. Fold into fish mixture, ⅓ at a time. Spoon into soufflé dish and place dish in a pan of hot water. Bake on bottom shelf of oven for 45 minutes. (Do not open oven door while baking.) Serve immediately.

4 servings

Marinated Whitefish with Fruit

1 cup white grape juice
    juice of 3 limes
¼ cup soy sauce
½ teaspoon ground ginger
1½ to 2 pounds thick firm whitefish fillets
2 firm pears
12 unsweetened pineapple chunks
3 tablespoons butter, melted
    ground ginger, to taste

Mix together fruit juices, soy sauce, and ginger in a shallow glass or ceramic dish. Add fish to mixture and marinate in refrigerator for 6 hours or overnight, turning once. Drain and discard marinade.

Cut fish into 1½-inch pieces. Cut pears into chunks. (If not to be used immediately, pear chunks should be dipped in lemon or lime juice.) Thread fish on 4 skewers, alternating with pears and pineapple, and lay them on a foil-covered broiler pan. Preheat broiler. Brush fish and fruit with butter. If desired, sprinkle fruit with additional ginger. Broil 5 minutes on each side. Place skewers on large platter. To serve, gently remove from skewers onto individual plates.

4 servings

Gefilte Fish

Poaching Stock
fish trimmings, bones, skin, and heads (with eyes and gills removed) from pike and carp used for fish balls
2 medium-size onions, diced
1 onion skin (for color)
2 carrots, sliced diagonally ¼ inch thick
½ teaspoon pepper
8 cups water, or more as needed

Fish Balls
1 pound whitefish fillets
1½ pounds yellow pike
½ pound carp
1 whole onion
¼ cup cold water
2 eggs, lightly beaten
½ teaspoon white pepper
2 tablespoons matzo meal

To make the poaching stock: Place trimmings, onions, onion skin, carrots, pepper, and water in a large soup pot. Cover pot and bring to a boil. Reduce heat to a simmer and cook for 1 hour. Remove carrots and reserve for garnish. Strain stock and discard solids. There should be about 6 cups of stock. If not, add enough water to equal 6 cups. Return stock to a boil and simmer while preparing fish.

To make the fish balls: Put fish and onion through a meat grinder or process in a food processor. Then turn out into a wooden chopping bowl and chop for 10 minutes, or until mixture gets very sticky and gelatinous. While chopping, slowly add the cold water, eggs, pepper, and matzo meal, a bit at a time. Dip hands in cold water and form mixture into ovals. Pour simmering stock into a fish poacher or small turkey roaster with a cover. Place fish in liquid, side by side. Cover pot and simmer slowly for 2½ hours. Baste occasionally with liquid or add more water, if necessary. Let fish cool in broth; then lift out with slotted spoon. Garnish with reserved carrot slices. Chill stock until jelled and spoon over fish. Serve cold with horseradish passed at the table.

4 servings

Ocean Tabbouleh

Add fish to this bulgur favorite, and you add new interest to a wonderful buffet standby.

    1 cup bulgur
    2 cups boiling Court Bouillon (page 111)
       or water
¾ to 1 pound cooked, boned, and flaked whitefish
    2 large tomatoes, peeled and chopped
    1 large sweet onion, chopped
  1/3 cup chopped, fresh, flat-leaf parsley
    2 tablespoons chopped fresh mint
    ½ cup vegetable oil
    ¼ cup lemon juice, or more to taste
       pepper, to taste
       lettuce leaves

Place bulgur in a medium-size bowl. Pour boiling bouillon or water over it. Stir and let stand for 1 hour. Drain in a sieve, pressing out excess liquid with the back of a wooden spoon.

In a large bowl combine bulgur with remaining ingredients, except lettuce leaves. Cover and chill in refrigerator for several hours or overnight. Serve over lettuce leaves.

4 to 6 servings

Mackerel, Herring, Pompano, and Smelts

Baked Mackerel with Chick-peas and Hot Chili

    2 tablespoons olive oil
 1½ pounds whole mackerel, dressed, or fillets
    1 large clove garlic, crushed
    1 hot chili pepper, cut in half lengthwise, 1 dried
       hot chili pepper, or ½ teaspoon crushed
       red pepper
    1 can (14 ounces) Italian-style tomatoes, crushed
    ¼ teaspoon ground cumin
    ¼ teaspoon chili powder
    ⅛ teaspoon dried oregano
    1 cup cooked chick-peas, drained
    ½ cup shredded sharp cheddar cheese
    ¼ head iceberg lettuce, shredded
    1 small onion, minced
    1 tablespoon minced fresh parsley

Preheat oven to 425°F. Grease a shallow baking pan with 1 tablespoon oil and place fish in pan.

Heat remaining 1 tablespoon oil in a large skillet. Add garlic and pepper, reduce heat, and sauté slowly until garlic starts to turn tan. Remove with a slotted spoon. Add tomatoes, cumin, chili powder, and oregano and simmer for 5 minutes. Stir in chick-peas. Pour this sauce over and around fish. Bake for 15 to 20 minutes, or until fish flakes when tested with a fork. Sprinkle with cheese and broil until cheese melts and bubbles. Serve immediately. Pass bowl of shredded lettuce and another bowl of onions and parsley mixed together to sprinkle on top of fish at the table.

4 servings

Herring Puff with Sour Cream Sauce

1 pound herring fillets, skinned
3 eggs, beaten
1 tablespoon grated onions
   pepper, to taste
2 cups fresh whole grain bread crumbs
½ teaspoon dillweed
2 cups milk
   Sour Cream Sauce (see below)

Preheat oven to 350°F. Butter a 1½-quart ovenproof casserole.

In a food mill or food processor, grind herring. Add eggs, onions, and pepper, mixing well. Stir in bread crumbs and dillweed, and then gradually add milk. Turn into casserole and bake, uncovered, for 45 to 50 minutes, or until a knife inserted in center comes out clean.

Slice and serve hot as an appetizer, topped with sauce.

6 to 8 servings

Sour Cream Sauce

1½ cups sour cream
1 teaspoon Worcestershire sauce (optional)
½ cup chopped Bermuda onions
1 tablespoon grated horseradish
1 medium-size cucumber, peeled, seeded, and
   finely chopped, or ½ cup finely chopped
   radishes (optional)

Mix together all ingredients and chill for 2 hours to blend flavors.

Yields about 2 cups

Lime-Baked Pompano

1 tablespoon French-style mustard
¼ cup lime juice
½ teaspoon dried tarragon
1 teaspoon onion juice
2 pounds pompano or red snapper fillets, about
   1½ inches thick
1 lime, sliced
   parsley sprigs

Preheat oven to 350°F. Lightly butter a medium-size ovenproof casserole.

Mix together mustard, lime juice, tarragon, and onion juice. Place fish in casserole. Using a pastry brush, coat all sides with lime mixture. Arrange lime slices on top and bake for 15 minutes, or until fish flakes. Serve garnished with parsley.

4 servings

Panfried Smelts with Herb Butter

Herb Butter
¼ cup plus 2 tablespoons butter, softened
1 tablespoon chopped fresh parsley
½ teaspoon paprika
½ teaspoon grated lemon rind
¼ teaspoon dillweed
¼ teaspoon dried basil
¼ teaspoon dried thyme
¼ teaspoon cayenne pepper

Smelts
1 pound small smelts, pan-dressed
3 tablespoons whole wheat flour
3 tablespoons cornmeal
½ teaspoon paprika
¼ teaspoon pepper
½ cup olive oil or vegetable oil
3 or 4 cloves garlic, crushed
   lemon wedges

To make the herb butter: Mix ingredients together until well blended. Lay a piece of plastic wrap on a plate. Spoon butter onto wrap and pat it into about a 6-inch cylinder with the back of a spoon. Pick up the 2 ends of wrap and fold over cylinder to complete shaping. Chill for at least 1 hour.

To prepare the smelts: Remove backbones. Rinse fish and shake so that they are damp but not wet. Measure flour, cornmeal, paprika, and pepper into a bag. Add half the smelts, hold closed, and shake to coat fish evenly. Repeat with second half.

Heat oil in a large heavy skillet. Fry smelts in batches until golden on both sides, adding a clove of garlic to each batch. Do not crowd pan. Remove garlic if it gets too brown and discard after frying each batch. When all the smelts are cooked, cut "coins" of herb butter to place in the cavity of each smelt. Serve with lemon wedges.

4 servings

Salmon, Swordfish, Trout, and Tuna

Broiled Fish Steak with Cucumber-Dill Butter

2 pounds salmon or halibut steaks
¼ cup butter, softened
½ cup finely chopped and drained cucumber
2 tablespoons minced fresh dill
    pepper, to taste
    dill sprigs
    lemon wedges

Arrange fish in broiler pan.

In a small bowl, combine butter, cucumbers, dill, and pepper. Beat well with a wooden spoon and spread evenly on fish. Place under broiler and broil about 5 to 8 minutes, or until fish flakes when tested with a fork. While broiling, baste with some of the butter in the pan. Remove to hot platter and pour sauce over fish. Garnish with dill sprigs and lemon wedges.

4 servings

Salmon-Cannellini Salad

2 cups cooked white kidney beans (cannellini), drained
1 pound cold poached salmon, cut into chunks
2 tablespoons chopped pimientos
1 tablespoon lemon juice
½ cup mayonnaise
2 tablespoons tomato paste
¼ teaspoon dried basil
1 teaspoon grated Parmesan cheese
    white pepper, to taste
4 lettuce cups
1 small onion, sliced and separated into rings

Toss together beans, salmon, and pimiento. Mix lemon juice, mayonnaise, tomato paste, basil, Parmesan, and pepper and stir into bean-salmon mixture. Put 1 lettuce cup in each of 4 salad bowls. Divide salad among bowls. Garnish with onion rings.

4 servings

Salmon with Basil Sauce

½ cup olive oil
1 cup chopped spinach
½ cup fresh basil
¼ teaspoon garlic powder
¼ cup grated Romano cheese
2 tablespoons Court Bouillon (page 111) or water
    pepper, to taste
3 tablespoons butter, melted
1 teaspoon lemon juice
2 pounds salmon fillets, about ½ inch thick
2 hard-cooked eggs, sliced

Place olive oil, spinach, basil, garlic powder, cheese, stock or water, and pepper in a food processor. Process until pureed, about 15 seconds. Heat puree in a medium-size saucepan. Keep warm.

Combine butter and lemon juice, then brush salmon on both sides with the mixture. Broil about 3 minutes. Turn and baste with lemon butter. Broil another 3 minutes, or until salmon flakes when tested with a fork. Place on heated platter, pour on sauce, and garnish with egg slices.

4 servings

Salmon Salad

1½ pounds salmon fillets (tail section is best), steamed or poached, then cut into chunks
8 medium-size potatoes, cooked and cut into chunks (about 3 cups)
¼ cup minced scallions
½ cup finely chopped cucumbers
2 teaspoons honey
3 hard-cooked eggs, chopped
1 cup coarsely chopped seeded zucchini
1 tablespoon olive oil
1 tablespoon cider vinegar
1½ cups mayonnaise
2 teaspoons fresh dill (optional)
½ head lettuce

In a large bowl, mix salmon, potatoes, scallions, cucumbers, honey, eggs, and zucchini. Combine oil, vinegar, 1 cup mayonnaise, and dill (if used). Add to salad and toss. Chill well. Serve on bed of lettuce, and top with ½ cup mayonnaise.

4 servings

Solianka
(Russian Fish Stew)

¼ cup butter
1 large onion, chopped
6 medium-size tomatoes, peeled and chopped
1¼ pounds salmon, cut into 2-inch chunks
4 cups Fish Stock (page 111) or water
1 large cucumber, seeded and chopped
2 tablespoons chopped fresh parsley
1 tablespoon chopped fresh dill or 1 teaspoon
    dillweed
¼ teaspoon white pepper
1 bay leaf
1 thick slice lemon, quartered
    juice of 1 lemon

In a 4-quart saucepan, melt butter. Add onions and sauté until translucent. Stir in tomatoes and cook 5 minutes longer. Add remaining ingredients. Bring to a boil, reduce heat, and simmer for 15 minutes. Remove bay leaf. Serve in deep bowls. Rye bread is a good accompaniment.

4 servings

Deviled Swordfish

2 pounds swordfish steaks, about 1 inch thick
2 tablespoons soy sauce
1 tablespoon Worcestershire sauce
¾ cup tomato juice
2 tablespoons lemon juice
½ teaspoon dry mustard
½ cup chili sauce
1 teaspoon grated horseradish
1 teaspoon French-style mustard

Place swordfish in glass dish. Mix together soy sauce, Worcestershire sauce, tomato juice, lemon juice, and dry mustard. Pour over fish. Cover and marinate in refrigerator for 2 to 4 hours, turning twice.

Remove fish from marinade and broil for 5 to 7 minutes on each side. While fish is broiling, mix together chili sauce, horseradish, and French-style mustard. Serve on top of fish.

4 servings

Hawaiian Fish with Coconut and Pineapple

¼ cup plus 2 tablespoons whole grain bread
    crumbs
8 tablespoons unsweetened shredded coconut
1½ pounds firm swordfish or halibut steaks,
    boned and cut into chunks
    pepper, to taste
1 can (15 ounces) unsweetened pineapple
    chunks, drained
1 tablespoon honey

Combine bread crumbs with 6 tablespoons coconut. Sprinkle fish with pepper, then dip in bread crumb mixture until well coated. Place fish on a wire rack resting on a pan of boiling water to create moisture. Broil fish for 5 to 7 minutes on each side, or until it flakes when tested with a fork. If coconut becomes too brown, turn off oven and let fish steam. Meanwhile place pineapple in a separate baking pan. Add honey and mix. Sprinkle with remaining coconut and heat in oven while fish is broiling. Serve with pineapple spooned over the fish.

4 servings

Oriental Swordfish

¼ cup soy sauce
¼ cup water
1 tablespoon cornstarch
1 tablespoon honey
5 or 6 thin slices peeled ginger root
3 cloves garlic, crushed
2 tablespoons white vinegar
1 to 1½ pounds swordfish

Mix all ingredients, except swordfish, in a shallow glass or ceramic dish. Add swordfish to mixture and marinate for 6 hours in refrigerator, turning fish 3 or 4 times.

Discard marinade. Place fish in an oiled pan and broil without turning for 15 to 20 minutes, or until fish is cooked through and flakes easily at its thickest part.

2 to 3 servings

Swordfish Kabobs with Basil and Garlic

½ cup corn oil
½ cup olive oil
1 cup white wine vinegar
1 large clove garlic, crushed
1 tablespoon minced fresh basil
1 teaspoon soy sauce
¼ teaspoon pepper
2 pounds swordfish, cut into ¾-inch-thick
   chunks
   parsley sprigs

In a medium-size bowl, mix together all ingredients except fish and parsley. Add fish and marinate for several hours in refrigerator. Stir occasionally.

Remove fish and reserve marinade for basting. Skewer fish, leaving space between chunks. Place a pan under skewers to catch drippings and broil for about 8 to 10 minutes, basting and turning several times. Serve on skewers with some of the pan drippings poured over kabobs. Garnish with parsley.

4 servings

Swordfish with Mushroom Dressing and Sauce Roquefort

1 tablespoon vegetable oil
6 tablespoons butter
1/3 pound mushrooms, sliced
1 large onion, chopped
   juice of 1 large lemon
1/3 cup whole grain bread crumbs
1 tablespoon minced fresh parsley
1½ pounds swordfish
4 ounces Roquefort cheese, crumbled

Heat oil and 2 tablespoons butter in a 10-inch skillet (the same skillet can be used for each step of this recipe, without washing). Sauté mushrooms and onions until moisture evaporates and mushrooms brown. Stir in lemon juice. Cook about 30 seconds longer and remove from heat. Stir in bread crumbs and parsley. Spoon dressing onto serving platter and keep warm. Add 2 tablespoons butter to skillet. Fry swordfish over medium heat for about 10 minutes, or until cooked through, turning it gently halfway through cooking time. Place swordfish on dressing. Melt remaining 2 tablespoons butter in skillet. Add Roquefort, and cook, stirring, until cheese melts, about 2 minutes. Pour sauce over swordfish.

4 servings

Chilled Trout with Dill-Radish Sauce

2 tablespoons butter
1 stalk celery, with leaves, chopped
1 onion, chopped
1 cup water
   juice of 2 lemons
1 tablespoon chopped fresh parsley
¼ teaspoon dried thyme leaves
¼ teaspoon pepper
2 bay leaves
2 large whole trout (10 to 12 ounces each),
   dressed
   whole red radishes
   parsley sprigs
   Dill-Radish Sauce (see below)

In a 12-inch skillet melt butter. Add celery and onions and sauté until tender but not brown. Add water, lemon juice, parsley, thyme, pepper, and bay leaves and stir. Lay trout in pan, bring to a boil, cover, and simmer until trout are tender in thickest part and flesh has lost its translucence, 10 to 15 minutes. When done, gently pick up each trout, using 2 spatulas, and lay them on a serving platter. Discard liquid. Chill trout for several hours in refrigerator.

Before serving, garnish trout with whole radishes and parsley sprigs. Serve with the sauce.

4 servings

Dill-Radish Sauce

1 cup yogurt
¼ cup mayonnaise
¼ cup chopped radishes
1 tablespoon chopped fresh dill or 1 teaspoon
   dillweed

In a small bowl mix together yogurt, mayonnaise, radishes, and dill or dillweed.

Yields about 1½ cups

Golden Tuna Turnovers

½ cup mayonnaise
1½ teaspoons curry powder
1 can (6 to 7 ounces) water-packed tuna, flaked
¼ cup golden raisins
pastry for 2 Basic Rolled Piecrusts (page 718)

Mix together mayonnaise and curry powder until well blended. Add tuna and mix well. (This can be done in a food processor if you wish.) Stir in raisins.

Preheat oven to 400°F. Oil a baking sheet.

Roll out half the pastry at a time on a floured surface, keeping the rest chilled. Form it into an oblong shape, 12 × 8 inches. Trim edges, and cut the pastry into 6 4-inch squares. Place a rounded tablespoon of tuna filling into the center of each square, and fold squares to make triangles. Press edges together with tines of a floured fork. Cut a slit in the top of each turnover. Repeat process with second half of pastry. Bake for 15 to 20 minutes, or until golden brown.

Makes 1 dozen

Tuna Mousse with Mustard Dressing

Use this dish as a dazzling first course for a formal dinner or a delightful main course for a luncheon.

1½ cups Fish Stock (page 111), or 1 cup clam juice and ½ cup water
2 envelopes unflavored gelatin
1 can (12½ to 13 ounces) water-packed tuna, flaked
8 ounces cream cheese, softened
¼ cup mayonnaise
1 tablespoon minced fresh chives
1 tablespoon minced fresh parsley
1 tablespoon minced fresh dill or 1 teaspoon dillweed
2 tablespoons lemon juice
¼ teaspoon white pepper

Mustard Dressing
5 tablespoons olive oil or vegetable oil
3 tablespoons cider vinegar
1 tablespoon minced onions
1 tablespoon prepared mustard
1 teaspoon dry mustard

dill sprigs
carrot slices

In a small saucepan, combine stock or clam juice and water with gelatin. Stir over low heat until gelatin is dissolved, about 3 minutes. Refrigerate mixture in pan until cool and slightly thickened, about 1 hour.

Combine tuna, cheese, mayonnaise, herbs, lemon juice, and pepper. (This can be done in a food processor.) Gradually add gelatin mixture. Pour into a 6-cup mold. Chill until firm, at least 6 hours.

To make the dressing: Combine oil, vinegar, onions, prepared mustard, and dry mustard in a jar, cover, and shake to blend. Shake again before using.

Invert mousse onto plate. Garnish with dill sprigs and carrot slices. Cut small V's around edges of carrot slices to make them resemble flowers.

To serve, pour dressing around wedge of mousse on individual plate.

6 servings

Tuna Frittata

2 tablespoons vegetable oil
1 large shallot, finely chopped
1 large green pepper, chopped
1 can (6 to 7 ounces) water-packed tuna, flaked
5 eggs
1 tablespoon water
2 tablespoons grated Romano cheese
freshly ground pepper

Heat oil in a 10-inch skillet with an ovenproof handle. Add shallots and sauté until sizzling. Add green pepper and continue to cook until pepper is soft. Add tuna. Beat eggs and water together, pour into hot vegetables and fish, and cook over medium to low heat. As eggs set at edges, lift edges up with a spatula and allow unset portion to run underneath. Repeat until unset portion is used up, about 8 minutes. The top of the eggs will still be soft. Place pan under a preheated broiler until top is set. Slide onto serving dish. Season with cheese and pepper. Serve cut into wedges.

4 servings

Tuna Soufflé

4 eggs, separated
2 tablespoons butter
1 stalk celery, finely chopped
2 scallions, finely chopped
8 to 10 large mushrooms, thinly sliced
1½ cups milk
1½ cups soft whole grain bread crumbs (about 2 slices bread)
⅛ teaspoon pepper
4 ounces Gruyère cheese, coarsely grated
1 can (6 to 7 ounces) water-packed tuna, flaked

Preheat oven to 325°F. Butter bottom and sides of a 9-inch-square baking dish and dust with flour.

Beat egg whites until stiff but not dry. Set aside. In a large saucepan, melt butter. Add vegetables and sauté until tender but not brown. Add milk, and heat until scalded. Stir in bread crumbs and pepper. Cook over low heat, stirring, for 3 minutes. Pour into a medium-size bowl.

Beat egg yolks well, and stir into hot mixture, a little at a time, until all has been blended. Return mixture to saucepan and cook 3 minutes over low heat, stirring. Remove from heat. Fold in cheese, then tuna, and then egg whites. Spoon into baking dish and bake for 50 minutes, or until risen, golden brown, and set at the center. (A table knife inserted 1 inch from the center should come out clean.) Serve immediately.

4 to 6 servings

Tuna Tostada

1 cup yogurt
2 teaspoons chili powder
4 chapati, split pita bread pockets, or flour tortillas, buttered and grilled until almost crisp
1 can (12½ to 13 ounces) water-packed tuna, flaked
1 cup grated Monterey Jack or colby cheese
1 cup shredded salad greens
½ cup chopped tomatoes

Combine yogurt and chili powder and allow to set at least 30 minutes to mellow flavors.

Brush grilled chapati, pita bread, or tortillas lightly with yogurt mixture. Spoon ¼ of the tuna onto each serving. Sprinkle each portion with ¼ of the cheese and broil until cheese is melted. Top each with salad greens and tomatoes. Drizzle with remaining yogurt mixture.

4 servings

Frogs' Legs, Shad Roe, and Squid

Shrimp and Frogs' Legs Oriental

1 cup pineapple juice
2 tablespoons soy sauce
1 tablespoon lemon juice
1 tablespoon honey
1 clove garlic, quartered
2 pounds frogs' legs, skinned, boned, and cut into pieces
1 pound uncooked small shrimp, peeled and deveined
¼ to ½ cup vegetable oil
2 cups thinly sliced broccoli
½ cup Poultry Stock (page 110)
2 tablespoons cornstarch
¼ cup slivered almonds

Mix together pineapple juice, soy sauce, lemon juice, honey, and garlic, stirring until honey is dissolved. Pour ½ of the mixture over frogs' legs, and the rest over shrimp, in separate containers. (Be sure garlic is divided.) Cover and refrigerate for 2 to 4 hours. Remove garlic and drain, reserving marinade.

Heat ¼ cup oil in a Dutch oven. Stir-fry frogs' legs until cooked through, about 4 minutes. Remove and keep hot. Stir-fry shrimp until pink and no longer translucent, 3 to 5 minutes, adding more oil if needed. Remove and keep hot. Wipe out Dutch oven with paper towels. Add more oil and stir-fry broccoli for about 2 minutes. Remove broccoli and wipe out Dutch oven. Return frogs' legs, shrimp, and broccoli to Dutch oven. Add reserved marinade and heat. In a jar with a tight-fitting lid, shake stock and cornstarch. Mix into marinade, stirring over medium heat until thickened. Serve on a platter, garnished with almonds.

4 servings

Shad Roe and Asparagus Soufflé

    3 tablespoons butter
½ to ¾ pound shad roe
    1 cup cooked chopped asparagus
    2 tablespoons grated Parmesan cheese
    8 egg whites
    6 egg yolks
 1½ cups Béchamel Sauce (page 141)
    1 tablespoon lemon juice
    ¼ teaspoon dried thyme
    ¼ teaspoon white pepper

Melt 2 tablespoons butter in a medium-size skillet. Add roe and sauté for 6 minutes, turning once. Break up roe into very small pieces, discarding any membrane. Further chop asparagus into very small pieces, but do not puree.

Set oven rack to middle level, and preheat oven to 375°F. Butter all surfaces of a 2-quart soufflé dish or ovenproof bowl with remaining butter. Sprinkle bottom and sides of dish with 1 tablespoon Parmesan.

In a medium-size bowl beat egg whites until stiff and set aside. In a large bowl beat egg yolks. Beat in white sauce, lemon juice, thyme, and pepper. Stir ¼ of the beaten egg whites into yolk mixture to lighten it. Then fold in rest of egg whites. Fold in roe and asparagus. Sprinkle top of soufflé with remaining Parmesan and bake for 40 to 45 minutes, or until richly brown and well puffed. Serve immediately.

    4 to 6 servings

Squid and Scallion Salad

    4 cloves garlic
2½ to 3 pounds squid, cleaned
    3 bay leaves
    2 bunches scallions, with tops, chopped
    3 stalks celery, with leaves, chopped
    2 sweet red peppers, sliced into rings
   12 thin slices lemon, seeded
    ¼ cup chopped fresh parsley
    ¾ cup olive oil
    ½ cup white vinegar
    1 teaspoon dried oregano
    ½ teaspoon freshly ground pepper
    ¼ teaspoon crushed fennel seeds
   24 whole grain toast triangles (6 slices bread)

Crush 3 cloves garlic and mince 1 clove. Place squid in an 8-quart pan with crushed garlic, bay leaves, and water to two-thirds the depth of the pan. Bring to a boil and cook until tender, about 15 minutes. Drain, rinse, and cool squid. Discard bay leaves. Cut meat and tentacles into ½-inch pieces, removing and discarding any cartilage.

In a large bowl, combine squid with minced garlic and all remaining ingredients except toast. Cover and marinate overnight in refrigerator. Serve with toast.

    6 servings

Crabs

Chinese-Style King Crab with Mushrooms and Snow Peas

    ¼ pound snow pea pods
    3 tablespoons peanut oil
    1 clove garlic, crushed
    ¾ pound fresh or frozen king crab meat
    ¾ pound mushrooms, thinly sliced
    1 cup Poultry Stock (page 110)
    ½ teaspoon white pepper or 3 drops hot
       pepper sauce
    1 tablespoon cornstarch, dissolved in ½ cup
       cold water
    ½ teaspoon ground ginger
    2 scallions (green parts only), minced

Steam snow pea pods for 5 minutes. Place in bottom of serving dish and keep warm.

In a large skillet, heat oil until very hot but not smoking. Add garlic and sauté until golden. Remove. Add crab meat and toss, cooking for 1 minute. Stir in mushrooms and cook for 1 minute more. Add stock and pepper or hot pepper sauce and bring to a boil. Add cornstarch mixture and cook, stirring, until sauce thickens. Pour over snow pea pods, sprinkle with ginger, and toss to mix. Sprinkle with scallions and serve hot with cooked brown rice.

    4 to 6 servings

Crab Cakes, Southern Style

In the South crab cakes are on the spicy side, and you will see that that is all to the good.

    2 tablespoons butter
    3 scallions, minced

½ sweet red pepper, minced
½ green pepper, minced
2 pounds fresh or frozen crab meat, with
    cartilage removed
¾ cup soft whole grain bread crumbs
2 teaspoons French-style mustard
½ teaspoon Worcestershire sauce
4 drops hot pepper sauce
2 eggs
⅛ teaspoon paprika
¾ cup fine whole grain bread crumbs
    corn oil, for frying
    lemon wedges
    minced fresh parsley

In a large heavy skillet, melt butter. Add scallions and peppers and sauté until soft. Stir in crab meat, then add soft bread crumbs. (If mixture is too dry, add water.) Cool slightly. Beat together mustard, Worcestershire, pepper sauce, 1 egg, and paprika; add to skillet. Wet hands and form mixture into 1½-inch balls, then flatten slightly with palm of hand. Chill on wax paper in refrigerator for 15 minutes.

Beat remaining egg in a pie plate. Have another pie plate ready with fine bread crumbs. Gently dip cakes on both sides in egg, then in bread crumbs. Chill again for 30 minutes.

Heat about 2 inches of oil in a large deep-sided skillet to 370°F. Lift cakes with a spatula and fry a few at a time, turning gently, until brown on both sides. Drain on paper towels. Keep hot in 400°F oven until all are fried. Serve with lemon wedges dipped in parsley.

Makes about 14

Crab Meat and Artichoke Casserole

¼ cup butter
3 tablespoons minced scallions
1 clove garlic, minced
3 tablespoons whole wheat flour
1 cup milk
3 tablespoons lemon juice
1 pound fresh or frozen crab meat, with
    cartilage removed
¾ cup coarsely chopped frozen artichoke hearts
1 teaspoon dried oregano
    cayenne pepper, to taste
⅓ cup grated Parmesan cheese
3 tablespoons whole grain bread crumbs

Preheat oven to 375°F.

Melt butter in a medium-size saucepan. Sauté scallions and garlic until soft. Add flour. Gradually add milk, stirring continuously, until thickened. Add lemon juice, crab meat, and artichoke hearts. Season with oregano and cayenne. Pour into a large buttered casserole and sprinkle with Parmesan and bread crumbs. Bake until brown, about 15 to 20 minutes.

4 servings

Crab Meat au Gratin in Ramekins

¼ cup plus 1 tablespoon butter
3 tablespoons chopped scallions
2 tablespoons chopped celery
2 tablespoons minced almonds
2 tablespoons whole wheat flour
1 cup milk
2 tablespoons lemon juice
2 teaspoons dry mustard
¼ teaspoon ground ginger
1 egg yolk
1 cup heavy cream
½ cup grated Gruyère cheese
½ cup grated Parmesan cheese
1½ pounds fresh or frozen crab meat, with
    cartilage removed
    cayenne pepper, to taste
1 tablespoon chopped fresh parsley
¼ cup whole grain bread crumbs

In a large saucepan melt ¼ cup butter. Add scallions and celery and sauté until soft. Add almonds and sauté another 2 minutes. Over medium heat, stir in flour. Gradually add milk, stirring continuously, until mixture has thickened. Add lemon juice, mustard, and ginger, while stirring.

In a small bowl beat egg yolk, then combine with heavy cream. Pour into flour-milk mixture and reduce heat to low. Add Gruyère and Parmesan and stir until cheeses have melted. Make sure mixture does not boil. Blend in crab meat, cayenne, and parsley. If possible, allow mixture to stand for a while so that crab meat may fully absorb seasonings. Reheat if necessary. Spoon into ramekins, sprinkle with bread crumbs, and dot with remaining butter. Place in a shallow baking pan under broiler to brown bread crumbs, or bake in oven at 450°F.

4 to 6 servings

Marinated Crab

This is a recipe that takes care of itself while you do other things. Just mix the ingredients, allow two to three hours for the magic to work, and serve as a luncheon or buffet centerpiece, or as a summer supper dish.

2/3 cup olive oil
1 or 2 cloves garlic, minced
3 tablespoons lemon juice
1 tablespoon minced fresh parsley
½ tablespoon minced lemon rind
1 stalk celery, minced
1 teaspoon dried thyme
2 dashes of cayenne pepper
2 pounds fresh or frozen crab meat, with
    cartilage removed

Combine oil, garlic, and lemon juice. Add parsley, lemon rind, celery, thyme, and cayenne, and stir until all seasonings are well blended. Stir in crab meat, cover, and marinate in refrigerator for 2 to 3 hours.

Serve crab and marinade on a bed of lettuce.

4 to 6 servings

Soft-Shell Crab
Sautéed with Herbs and Almonds

4 to 6 soft-shell crabs
¾ cup whole wheat flour
1 tablespoon plus 1 teaspoon minced fresh
    tarragon
1 tablespoon plus 1 teaspoon minced fresh thyme
½ cup butter
½ cup slivered blanched almonds
    juice of ½ lemon
    lemon wedges
    parsley sprigs

Prepare soft-shell crabs (see page 563).
Place flour on a plate. Add 1 tablespoon tarragon and 1 tablespoon thyme and blend.
In a large skillet melt butter. Coat crabs with flour mixture and sauté in butter about 4 minutes on each side, keeping heat at medium temperature so that butter does not burn before crabs have cooked through. Remove crabs to serving dish.

Add almonds to butter in skillet. Add lemon juice, 1 teaspoon tarragon, and 1 teaspoon thyme to almond-butter mixture and stir. Pour over crabs and garnish with lemon wedges and parsley sprigs.

2 to 3 servings

Soft-Shell Crab in Light Batter
with Garlic and Ginger Mayonnaise

4 to 6 soft-shell crabs
¾ cup whole wheat flour
    cayenne pepper, to taste
    vegetable oil, for frying
½ cup mayonnaise
1 teaspoon minced garlic
1 teaspoon ground ginger
    lemon wedges
    parsley sprigs

Prepare soft-shell crabs (see page 563).
Combine flour and cayenne on a plate.
In a large skillet heat oil to 350 to 375°F. Coat crabs with flour mixture and sauté in oil 4 to 5 minutes on each side, or until brown.
While crabs are frying, mix mayonnaise, garlic, and ginger in a small bowl.
Remove crabs from skillet and place on paper towels to absorb oil. To serve, place crabs on individual plates and garnish with spiced mayonnaise, lemon wedges, and parsley sprigs.

2 to 3 servings

Lobster

Baked Lobster Tails in Hot Sauce

6 uncooked lobster tails (about 1/3 pound each)
¼ cup olive oil
2 cloves garlic, minced
3 scallions, minced
1 can (6 ounces) tomato paste
¼ cup champagne vinegar
¾ cup water
½ teaspoon dried oregano

2 leaves fresh basil, minced, or ¼ teaspoon
   dried basil
¼ teaspoon aniseed. crushed
½ teaspoon crushed red pepper
3 tablespoons minced fresh parsley

Remove lobster meat from shells and, with a sharp knife, remove thin membrane on each side of meat. Cut into bite-size chunks. Place shells in a large shallow ovenproof casserole and set both shells and lobster aside while preparing sauce.

In a heavy medium-size skillet heat oil. Add garlic and scallions, stir, and cook for 1 minute. Mix tomato paste with vinegar and water and add to skillet. Stir in oregano, basil, aniseed, and pepper and bring to a boil. Reduce heat, cover pan, and simmer for 10 minutes, stirring occasionally.

Preheat oven to 375°F.

Pour ½ of the sauce over and around empty shells in casserole. Add chunks of lobster to shells, mounding evenly. Spoon rest of sauce over lobster meat and bake for 15 to 20 minutes, basting once or twice. Sprinkle with parsley before serving.

6 servings

Garlic Lobster with Sautéed Vegetables

With this dish you can enjoy the luxury of serving lobster and still not go into heavy debt. It takes only one pound to treat four to six diners.

½ cup fresh or frozen peas
2 tablespoons soy sauce
1 tablespoon white grape juice
1½ teaspoons cider vinegar
1 small slice peeled ginger root
2 tablespoons peanut oil
½ cup diced carrots
1 cup sliced mushrooms
2½ tablespoons minced garlic
2 tablespoons chopped scallions
1 cup chopped bok choy (Chinese celery)
1 cup shredded Chinese cabbage
1 cup bean sprouts
1 pound cooked lobster meat, diced

1 cup Poultry Stock (page 110)
1 tablespoon cornstarch

Cook peas, covered, in a small amount of water for 4 to 5 minutes or until barely tender. Drain and set aside.

Prepare seasoning mixture in a cup by combining 1 tablespoon soy sauce, grape juice, vinegar, and ginger. Set aside.

Heat oil in a wok or large heavy skillet. Add carrots and sauté for 3 minutes. Add mushrooms and sauté for 2 minutes. Reduce heat if oil becomes too hot. Add garlic, scallions, bok choy, cabbage, and bean sprouts, and sauté for 1 minute. Stir in lobster and sauté for 1 minute. Stir in seasoning mixture, blending thoroughly with vegetables. Add peas and ½ cup stock, cover, and bring to a boil.

In a cup combine cornstarch, ½ cup stock, and 1 tablespoon soy sauce. As soon as vegetables and stock come to a boil, add cornstarch mixture, stirring constantly. Serve with steamed brown rice.

4 to 6 servings

Lobster Salad with Exotic Fruit

1 cup mayonnaise
1½ teaspoons minced peeled ginger root
2 cooked lobster tails or 1 cup cooked lobster
   meat
lettuce leaves
2 kiwi fruit, sliced
1 avocado, sliced
1 mango, sliced
3 slices fresh pineapple
juice of ¼ lemon

In a bowl mix mayonnaise and ginger. If using lobster tails, remove meat from shells. With a sharp knife, remove thin membrane covering meat. Dice lobster meat and stir into mayonnaise mixture. Place torn lettuce leaves on plates and scoop lobster salad onto center of each. Arrange slices of fruit around lobster. Squeeze lemon juice over all.

2 to 3 servings

NOTE: Other fruits may be substituted according to availability.

Lobster Thermidor

2 uncooked whole lobsters or lobster tails
1 cup Fish Stock (page 111)
2 tablespoons finely chopped shallots or scallions
1 tablespoon minced fresh tarragon
1 tablespoon olive oil
¾ cup chopped mushrooms
4 tablespoons butter
1 tablespoon soy sauce
¼ cup plus 1 tablespoon lemon juice
1 cup Béchamel Sauce (page 141)
2 egg yolks
½ cup heavy cream
   cayenne pepper, to taste
⅓ cup grated Parmesan cheese
   dash of paprika

Poach lobsters or lobster tails. If using whole lobsters, remove meat from body and claws. If using lobster tails, remove meat from shells and remove membrane covering meat with a sharp knife. Dice meat. Clean and reserve shells.

Bring stock to a boil. Add shallots or scallions, tarragon, and oil. Cook until mixture is reduced to one-quarter.

Sauté mushrooms in 3 tablespoons butter for 3 minutes. Add reduced broth, soy sauce, and lemon juice to mushrooms. Then add white sauce to mixture. Preheat oven to 375°F.

Beat egg yolks in a small bowl. Add cream and then pour into mushroom mixture. Heat until thickened, but do not boil. Add diced lobster and sprinkle with cayenne. Fill lobster shells with mixture. Top with Parmesan, dot with butter, and sprinkle with paprika. Bake until brown, about 15 minutes.

2 servings

Shrimp

Italian-Style Broiled Garlic Shrimp

2 tablespoons lemon juice
2 tablespoons olive oil
3 tablespoons butter, melted
1 large clove garlic, minced
¼ teaspoon pepper
1½ to 2 pounds uncooked large shrimp, peeled and deveined, but with tails left intact
2 tablespoons minced fresh parsley

Combine lemon juice, oil, butter, garlic, and pepper in a bowl. Add shrimp and stir until completely coated. In a broiling pan arrange shrimp in a single layer facing one direction and pour remaining garlic sauce over all. Broil about 3 minutes. Turn with tongs and broil for 3 to 4 minutes more or until shrimp are pink. Transfer, with sauce, to warm serving platter and sprinkle with parsley.

4 to 6 servings

Shrimp Creole

⅔ cup corn oil
⅓ cup whole wheat flour
⅓ cup chopped celery
1 cup chopped onions
1 cup minced green peppers
3 cloves garlic, minced
1 can (28 ounces) Italian-style tomatoes
1 can (12 ounces) tomato paste
1 bay leaf
3 whole allspice
2 whole cloves
½ teaspoon pepper
¼ teaspoon cayenne pepper
¼ teaspoon chili powder
½ teaspoon dried thyme
2 cups water
2 pounds uncooked medium-size shrimp, peeled and deveined
1 tablespoon lemon juice
1 cup minced scallions with tops
2 tablespoons minced fresh parsley

In a heavy 6-quart pot, heat oil. Gradually add flour and stir over low heat with a wooden spoon until it begins to bubble, about 2 to 3 minutes. Remove from heat and add all vegetables except tomatoes. Stir and return to heat. Stir in tomatoes and tomato paste.

Place bay leaf, allspice, and cloves in a cheesecloth bag, tie shut, and add to pot. Stir in remaining spices and thyme. Add water and simmer 20 to 30 minutes with pot lid ajar. Add shrimp and cook for 10 minutes more. Remove from heat, lift out cheesecloth bag, and stir in lemon juice. Sprinkle with scallions and parsley. Serve over cooked brown rice.

8 servings

Coconut Fried Shrimp with Mustard Dip

16 uncooked large shrimp (about 1 pound)
½ cup cornstarch
1 cup unsweetened grated coconut
2 egg whites
1 teaspoon soy sauce
   vegetable oil, for deep frying
   lime or lemon wedges
   Mustard Dip (see below)

Peel and devein shrimp, leaving tails on.

Measure about ¼ cup cornstarch into a deep plate. Place coconut in another deep plate.

In a small bowl combine egg whites with ¼ cup cornstarch and stir with a wooden spoon to make a smooth batter. Stir in soy sauce. Dredge shrimp in cornstarch, shaking and tapping off excess. Holding by tails, dip shrimp, one at a time, in egg white batter, and then in coconut to coat evenly. Place in single layer on a baking sheet.

Heat oil (at least 2 inches deep) to 300°F in a deep fryer or small Dutch oven. Deep fry shrimp, 4 at a time, for 3 to 4 minutes, or until golden brown and cooked through. Drain on paper towels. Serve hot with lime or lemon wedges and mustard dip.

4 servings

Mustard Dip

1 cup mayonnaise
1 tablespoon prepared mustard
½ teaspoon dry mustard
¼ teaspoon turmeric
1 teaspoon honey

Combine all ingredients and blend well.

Yields about 1 cup

Shrimp Curry with Pineapple and Coconut

¼ cup plus 2 tablespoons butter or vegetable oil
2 medium-size onions, chopped
2 tablespoons finely chopped garlic
2 green chili peppers
1 tablespoon grated peeled ginger root or ½ teaspoon ground ginger
1 to 2 tablespoons curry powder
1 cup coconut milk
2 cups milk
1 cup cubed fresh pineapple
2 tablespoons lemon juice
1 tablespoon unsweetened grated coconut
1½ pounds uncooked medium-size shrimp, peeled and deveined
1 cup heavy cream or yogurt

In a large skillet heat butter or oil. Add onions, garlic, and chilies and sauté until onions are slightly browned. Add ginger and curry powder and stir. Add coconut milk, milk, pineapple, lemon juice, and coconut. Cook for 20 minutes over low to medium heat, making sure mixture does not boil. Stir occasionally. Add shrimp and cook for 5 minutes. Stir in heavy cream or yogurt. Adjust seasonings if necessary and serve on mound of cooked brown rice.

4 to 6 servings

Shrimp Remoulade, New Orleans Style

Plan on allowing the shrimp and sauce to marry for several hours, or overnight, when serving this dish.

½ cup catsup
3 tablespoons olive oil
1 tablespoon minced scallions
2 tablespoons horseradish, drained
2 tablespoons minced celery
1 tablespoon minced fresh parsley
1 pound medium-size shrimp, cooked, peeled, and deveined
   juice of 1 lemon
   shredded lettuce

Combine catsup, oil, scallions, horseradish, celery, and parsley and mix thoroughly. Stir in shrimp and lemon juice. Marinate in refrigerator for at least 2 to 3 hours, or overnight. Adjust seasoning if necessary and spoon shrimp and sauce on bed of shredded lettuce.

4 servings

Clams

Sautéed Clams over Parsley Rice

6 to 7 dozen clams in shells
   6 cups water
   1 medium-size onion, chopped
   8 tablespoons butter
1½ cups uncooked brown rice
   3 tablespoons chopped fresh parsley
   ½ teaspoon dried thyme
   2 tablespoons lemon juice
     cayenne pepper, to taste
   2 cloves garlic
     pepper, to taste

Wash clams. Steam in 3 cups of water for 8 to 10 minutes, or until shells open. Remove clams from pot, strain broth through doubled cheesecloth, and return broth and clams to pot. Discard any clams that have not opened.

In a large saucepan, sauté onions in 2 tablespoons butter until translucent. Add 3 cups water and bring to a boil. Add rice, 2 tablespoons parsley, thyme, 1 tablespoon lemon juice, and cayenne. When mixture returns to a boil, cover, reduce heat, and cook for 45 minutes, or until rice is tender and liquid is absorbed.

While rice is cooking, remove clams from shells. Melt remaining butter in a large skillet. Add garlic and clams and sauté for 1 to 2 minutes. Stir in 1 tablespoon lemon juice, 1 tablespoon parsley, and pepper. Add ¾ cup of reserved clam broth, and correct seasoning, if necessary. Serve clams over rice.

   4 servings

Baked Stuffed Clams with Pine Nuts

Serve these as a main course (six to a person), or as an appetizer (three or four to a person).

   2 dozen clams in shells
1½ cups water
   ½ cup finely chopped onions
   2 cloves garlic, finely chopped
   2 tablespoons butter
   ¾ cup whole grain bread crumbs, toasted
   2 tablespoons minced fresh parsley
   1 teaspoon dried tarragon
     pepper, to taste

   2 tablespoons ground pine nuts
   2 tablespoons grated Parmesan cheese

Wash clams. Steam in water for 8 to 10 minutes, or until shells open. Remove from pot and strain broth through doubled cheesecloth. Reserve broth. Remove clams from shells, discarding any that have not opened. Mince clams and reserve shells.

Preheat oven to 425°F.

Sauté chopped onions and garlic in butter until soft. Add clams, bread crumbs, 1 cup of reserved broth, parsley, tarragon, and pepper and cook for 3 minutes over medium heat. Fill clam shells with mixture, sprinkle with pine nuts and Parmesan, and bake until lightly browned.

   4 servings

Clam Frittata

   1 cup minced clams
   ½ pound spinach, chopped
   2 tablespoons olive oil
   1 cup chopped mushrooms
   2 tablespoons chopped scallions
   2 tablespoons lemon juice
   1 tablespoon finely chopped fresh parsley
     pepper, to taste
   8 eggs
   2 tablespoons light cream
   1 tablespoon soy sauce
   1 tablespoon chopped fresh basil or ¼ teaspoon
     dried basil
   5 tablespoons grated Parmesan cheese

If using fresh clams, steam and mince, reserving cooking liquid. If using canned clams, drain, reserving liquid, and mince.

Chop and cook spinach. Drain in colander.

In a medium-size skillet heat 1 tablespoon oil, then sauté mushrooms and scallions for 2 to 3 minutes. Add mushrooms and scallions to spinach in colander and make sure all excess liquid is removed. Place mixture in a large bowl and stir in clams, lemon juice, parsley, and pepper.

Beat eggs. Add cream, 2 tablespoons reserved clam liquid, soy sauce, basil, and 2 tablespoons Parmesan.

Preheat oven to 425°F.

In a large omelet pan or heavy skillet, heat 1 tablespoon oil. Spread clam and spinach mixture in pan. Pour beaten eggs over mixture, cover, and cook over medium heat until eggs are set on bottom. Remove from heat. Sprinkle remaining Parmesan cheese over eggs. Place in oven or under broiler until eggs have set on top and are light golden in color. Slide frittata onto large plate and serve immediately.

4 servings

Oysters

Marinated Vegetables and Oysters en Brochette

A delicious way to serve oysters. This recipe also ensures thorough cooking, thus avoiding concern about the infectious organisms bivalves can carry.

3 to 4 dozen small to medium-size oysters
  ½ cup olive oil
  1 tablespoon lemon juice
  2 cloves garlic, minced
  3 tablespoons chopped fresh parsley
  ⅛ teaspoon dried thyme
  1 thin slice peeled ginger root
    dash of cayenne pepper
  2 tablespoons butter
  1 medium-size onion, chopped
  ½ cup chopped celery
  2 cups chopped mushrooms
  1 tablespoon soy sauce
    dash of black pepper
  1 large green pepper, halved
  1 pint cherry tomatoes

Shuck oysters and set aside.

In a large bowl combine oil, lemon juice, garlic, parsley, thyme, ginger, and cayenne. Add oysters and marinate in refrigerator for 1 hour.

In a medium-size skillet melt butter. Add onions and celery and sauté until soft. Add mushrooms, soy sauce, and black pepper and sauté for another 2 minutes. Toss and remove from heat.

While oysters are marinating, plunge green pepper into boiling water for about 3 minutes, or just until it begins to soften. Remove from boiling water and rinse with cold water to prevent further cooking. Cut pepper into 1 to 1½-inch squares.

Preheat oven to 425°F.

On skewers place cherry tomatoes, oysters, and green pepper squares until all have been used. Spread marinade over each skewer and place in oven or under broiler until heated through, about 10 minutes. If using broiler, place on lower rack to prevent burning.

Heat mushroom and onion mixture. Place skewers on platter or individual plates and spoon mushroom and onion mixture over top.

4 servings

Oysters Rockefeller

The rock salt traditionally used with this dish is present only to hold the heat. If you do not have it, go ahead with the recipe anyway, since the flavor is not affected by the salt.

  4 cups rock salt
  2 dozen oysters on the half shell
  ¼ cup plus 2 tablespoons butter
  2 cloves garlic, finely chopped
  ½ cup chopped celery
  ¼ cup chopped scallions
    cayenne pepper, to taste
  3 cups chopped watercress
  ¼ cup chopped fresh parsley
  1 teaspoon fennel seeds
  1 teaspoon lemon juice
  ½ cup soft whole grain bread crumbs
  ⅛ teaspoon black pepper

Preheat oven to 450°F.

Fill 4 individual pie plates with 1 cup each of rock salt and place oysters on top. (If rock salt is not used, place oysters in shells directly in pie plates.)

In a large skillet melt butter. Add garlic, celery, and scallions, and sauté for 2 minutes. Add cayenne, watercress, and parsley. Remove from heat and toss. Crush fennel seeds with a mortar and pestle and add to mixture. Add lemon juice and bread crumbs. Process all ingredients in a blender, or push through a fine sieve. Sprinkle mixture with black pepper and blend. Spread sauce on tops of oysters to edges of shells and bake for 5 to 7 minutes.

4 servings

Oyster Stew

    5 tablespoons butter
    2 tablespoons finely chopped onions
    1 dozen small oysters, shucked
    1 cup milk
    1 cup light cream
      pepper, to taste
      parsley sprigs

Melt 2 tablespoons butter in a small skillet. Add onions and sauté over very low heat until onions are soft but not brown.

In a double boiler or in a large saucepan, melt remaining butter over very low heat. Stir in onions, oysters, milk, cream, and pepper and cook for 10 minutes. If cooking in a saucepan, make sure stew does not boil. Serve in individual bowls and garnish with parsley.

    4 servings

Scallops

Creamy Scallops Florentine

A very impressive and unusual treatment of scallops, with a lively cream sauce.

    1 pound spinach
    ½ cup butter
    ¼ cup whole wheat pastry flour
    2 cups milk
    4 tablespoons lemon juice
  1½ tablespoons soy sauce
    1 teaspoon dry mustard
      several pinches of dried tarragon
    ¼ cup chopped fresh parsley
      black pepper, to taste
      cayenne pepper, to taste
    3 cloves garlic, finely chopped
1½ to 2 pounds scallops
    1 cup shredded Swiss cheese
    2 tablespoons whole grain bread crumbs

Steam spinach over low heat in just the water that clings to the leaves after washing, about 5 minutes. Drain. Chop, drain again, and set aside.

In a large saucepan, melt ¼ cup butter. Add flour and stir into a paste. Gradually add milk and stir continuously with a wire whisk until mixture has thickened. Add 2 tablespoons lemon juice, soy sauce, mustard, and tarragon. Stir in spinach, parsley, black pepper, and cayenne.

Preheat oven to 425°F.

In a large skillet, melt remaining butter over medium heat. Add garlic and 2 tablespoons lemon juice and stir. Add scallops and sauté for 1 minute over medium to low heat. If large scallops are used, cut them in half before sautéing.

Spoon spinach mixture into individual casseroles. Place scallops and butter sauce on top, sprinkle with cheese and bread crumbs, dot with butter, and bake for about 10 minutes, or until cheese and bread crumbs have turned a golden color. Serve immediately.

    4 to 5 servings

Scallops Mornay with Asparagus Tips

Scallops and asparagus, coupled with a rich cream sauce, add up to a special-occasion dish.

    ½ cup butter
    3 tablespoons whole wheat pastry flour
  1½ cups milk
    ½ cup light cream
    2 egg yolks
    ½ cup grated Gruyère cheese
    ½ cup grated Parmesan cheese
    2 tablespoons lemon juice
      dash of cayenne pepper
      several pinches of dried tarragon
    1 medium to large bunch fresh asparagus or
      2 packages (10 ounces) frozen asparagus
      spears
2 to 2½ pounds scallops
      several dashes of paprika

In a large heavy saucepan melt ¼ cup butter over medium heat. Add flour and stir into a paste. Gradually add milk, stirring continuously with a wire whisk until mixture has thickened.

Beat cream and egg yolks together. Stir 2 tablespoons of sauce into egg yolk mixture, then pour egg yolk mixture into saucepan. Make sure mixture does not boil, as it will curdle. Add Gruyère, ⅓ cup Parmesan, 1 tablespoon lemon juice, cayenne, and tarragon. Remove from heat.

Preheat oven to 450°F.

Steam asparagus until crisp-tender. Remove from heat and set aside.

If using large scallops, cut in half. Sauté scallops in ¼ cup butter for 2 to 3 minutes, or until no longer translucent. Add 1 tablespoon lemon juice.

Place asparagus in an oblong ovenproof casserole or in individual casseroles, top with scallops, and pour sauce over all. Sprinkle with remaining Parmesan and paprika. Bake for about 10 minutes, or until casserole begins to bubble.

6 servings

Indian-Curried Scallops

2 tablespoons vegetable oil
1 medium-size onion, chopped
1 tablespoon chopped garlic
6 to 8 medium-size tomatoes, chopped
1 teaspoon turmeric
2 teaspoons ground cumin
2 teaspoons ground coriander
2 teaspoons vinegar
2 teaspoons soy sauce
¼ to ½ teaspoon cayenne pepper
1 to 1½ pounds scallops
1 cup sour cream
1 green pepper, finely chopped
3 tablespoons minced fresh coriander

In a large skillet, heat oil. Add onions and sauté until soft. Add garlic and sauté for 1 minute. Then add tomatoes, turmeric, cumin, ground coriander, vinegar, soy sauce, and cayenne. Cover and cook for 35 minutes. Add scallops, cover, and cook for 3 minutes, or until scallops are no longer translucent. Do not overcook. Serve over brown rice and place sour cream, green peppers, and fresh coriander in separate bowls to be used as condiments.

4 to 6 servings

Scallops Vinaigrette

6 cups water
1½ pounds scallops
2 tablespoons vinegar
1 tablespoon finely chopped scallions
1 teaspoon French-style mustard
juice of 3 lemons
½ teaspoon ground cumin
½ teaspoon dillweed
½ tablespoon minced fresh parsley
pepper, to taste
⅓ cup olive oil
6 to 8 cups romaine lettuce, torn into pieces
1 medium-size green pepper, cut into thin strips
3 carrots, cut into thin strips
2 or 3 avocados, quartered

Bring water to a boil. Add scallops and poach for 30 to 60 seconds, depending on size of scallops. Do not overcook. Remove from water. If using larger scallops, cut in halves or quarters and set aside.

In top of a double boiler or in a small saucepan placed over very low heat, blend together with a wire whisk the vinegar, scallions, mustard, lemon juice, cumin, dillweed, parsley, and pepper. Gradually add oil. Keep dressing warm.

Place lettuce on individual plates. Mound scallops in center and arrange green pepper, carrots, and avocados around scallops. Pour heated dressing on top and serve immediately.

4 to 6 servings

Hot and Spicy Scallops

        2 pounds scallops
        2 cups dried mushrooms
        1 cup frozen peas
        3 tablespoons sesame oil
        2 cups diced carrots
        1 small slice peeled ginger root
1 to 2 teaspoons crushed red pepper
        2 tablespoons chopped garlic
        2 cups Fish Stock (page 111) or clam juice
        3 tablespoons soy sauce
     1½ tablespoons white grape juice
        1 tablespoon rice vinegar
        6 scallions, cut lengthwise into quarters
        2 tablespoons cornstarch, dissolved in
           2 tablespoons water

If using large scallops, cut in halves or quarters. Soak mushrooms in cold water for 30 minutes.

In a small saucepan add peas to small amount of boiling water and cook only until thawed. Drain and set aside.

In a wok or large skillet heat sesame oil. Add carrots, ginger, and pepper and sauté for 5 minutes. Add garlic and cook for another 2 minutes. (Reduce heat to avoid burning garlic.) Add peas, stock or clam juice, soy sauce, grape juice, and rice vinegar. Add scallions to wok. Bring liquid to a slow boil and then add scallops and mushrooms. Cover and cook for 2 to 3 minutes, or until scallops turn opaque. Do not overcook.

Stir cornstarch mixture into wok and cook for another minute. Adjust seasoning for hotter flavor if desired. Serve over steamed brown rice.

        4 to 6 servings

Mussels

Hot or Cold Mussels Pesto

        3 dozen mussels
        2 cups water
        ¾ cup chopped fresh basil
        ¼ cup chopped pine nuts
        2 cloves garlic, chopped
        ½ cup olive oil
        3 tablespoons lemon juice
        ⅓ cup grated Parmesan cheese
           pepper, to taste

Wash mussels, and remove beards. Place mussels in a pot with water and steam until shells open, about 3 to 5 minutes. Remove from pot and discard any mussels which have not opened. Remove top shells from mussels and discard. Reserve mussels in lower shells, loosening meat from shells.

Process basil, pine nuts, and garlic in a blender or pound into a paste in a mortar. Add oil, lemon juice, Parmesan, and pepper and again process to a paste.

Serve heated or slightly chilled. If serving hot, preheat oven to 425°F. Spoon pesto on top of each mussel in shell and bake for about 5 minutes. If serving slightly chilled, place in refrigerator for 10 minutes before serving.

        4 to 6 servings

Mussels in Tomato Sauce

3½ to 4 dozen mussels
        2 tablespoons olive oil
        1 medium-size onion, chopped
        1 tablespoon chopped garlic
        8 medium-size tomatoes, chopped
        2 tablespoons lemon juice
        2 cups water
        2 bay leaves
        1 tablespoon chopped fresh basil or 1 teaspoon
           dried basil
           several pinches of fresh or dried rosemary
           several pinches of fresh or dried thyme
           pepper, to taste
1 to 1½ pounds uncooked whole wheat spaghetti
           or toasted garlic bread rounds

Wash mussels and remove beards. Place mussels in a bowl of water for 10 minutes so that any sand may settle to bottom of bowl. Rinse.

In a large pot, heat oil. Add onions and sauté until soft. Add garlic and sauté for 1 minute. Stir in tomatoes, and add lemon juice, water, bay leaves, basil, rosemary, thyme, and pepper. Cover and simmer for 40 minutes over medium to low heat, stirring occasionally. Add a bit of water if necessary.

If serving mussels with spaghetti, cook pasta when tomato sauce is almost done. Drain and keep hot.

When sauce has cooked for 40 minutes, add mussels and cook only until shells open, about 3 to 5 minutes. Discard any mussels which have not opened. Serve immediately. Pour sauce over hot spaghetti (if serving this way), and arrange mussels in shells on the top. Or serve in a bowl and spoon over toasted garlic bread rounds.

4 servings

Mussels with Egg and Lemon Sauce

4 to 5 dozen mussels
 2 cups water
 2 tablespoons butter
 2 tablespoons whole wheat flour
 1 cup milk
 3 egg yolks
 2 tablespoons lemon juice
 1 tablespoon chopped fresh chervil or parsley
 2 tablespoons grated Parmesan cheese
  cayenne pepper, to taste

Wash mussels and remove beards. Place mussels in a pot with water and steam until shells open, about 3 to 5 minutes. Remove from pot and discard any mussels which have not opened. Remove top shells from mussels and discard.

In a medium-size saucepan, melt butter. Add flour and stir into a paste. Gradually add milk, stirring continuously with a wire whisk. Beat egg yolks. Add a bit of white sauce to egg yolks and then pour egg yolk mixture back into white sauce, making sure sauce does not boil. Add remaining ingredients and cook over medium heat, stirring constantly, until hot and slightly thickened.

Place mussels in half shells in a large serving bowl and pour heated sauce over them. Serve with French bread.

4 servings

Mussels with Fresh Basil and Walnuts in Cheese Sauce

4 to 5 dozen mussels
 2 cups water
 2 tablespoons butter
 2 cloves garlic, finely chopped
 2 tablespoons lemon juice
 2 cups milk
 4 cups shredded medium-sharp cheddar cheese
 1/3 cup chopped fresh basil
 1/3 cup finely chopped walnuts
 2 tablespoons whole grain bread crumbs

Wash mussels and remove beards. Place mussels in a pot with water and steam until shells open, about 3 to 5 minutes. Remove from pot and discard any mussels which have not opened. Remove mussels from shells.

Melt butter in a large skillet. Add garlic, lemon juice, and mussels and sauté for 1 minute. Set aside.

Preheat oven to 425°F.

Heat milk in a large saucepan. Add cheese, basil, and walnuts. Stir until cheese melts. Do not let mixture boil.

Spoon mussels into ramekins or a medium-size ovenproof casserole and pour cheese sauce over all. Sprinkle with bread crumbs and bake for 5 minutes, or until bread crumbs are lightly browned. If using small ramekins, allow 2 per person.

4 servings

Mixed Shellfish

Paella

This is a grand presentation–a true company dish that cannot fail to impress even the most sophisticated guest.

> 6 tablespoons olive oil
> 3 cloves garlic
> 1 chicken (broiler-fryer)
> 1 tablespoon minced fresh thyme or 1 teaspoon dried thyme
> 1 pound fresh spicy Spanish or Italian sausage
> 1 cup chopped onions
> 1 green pepper, chopped
> 2¼ cups uncooked brown rice
> 4 cups Poultry Stock (page 110)
> 1 to 2 teaspoons saffron
> ½ teaspoon ground coriander
> 1 teaspoon minced fresh oregano or ½ teaspoon dried oregano
> 1 teaspoon paprika
> ¼ cup lemon juice
> 1 tablespoon chopped pimientos
> ⅛ to ¼ teaspoon cayenne pepper
> 1½ dozen clams in shells
> 1½ pounds cooked lobster meat or uncooked lobster tails
> 1 pound uncooked medium-size shrimp, peeled and deveined

Slowly heat 3 tablespoons oil in a large skillet. Halve and add 1 clove garlic. Rub garlic in oil and around skillet.

Cut chicken breast and thighs in half. Rub pieces of chicken with thyme.

Remove garlic from pan, add chicken, and increase heat to medium. Brown chicken and set aside.

Cut sausage into pieces, brown, and set aside.

In a wok or large deep pot, sauté onions in remaining oil until soft. Chop 2 cloves garlic and add. Stir in green peppers and continue to sauté for 2 minutes. Stir in rice, stock, saffron, coriander, oregano, paprika, lemon juice, pimientos, and cayenne and bring to a boil. Then add chicken, cover, and cook over low heat for 20 minutes.

Wash clams. Set in water for a few minutes to allow any sand to sink to the bottom of the bowl.

Add sausage to wok or pot and cook for 15 minutes. Add lobster meat or lobster tails (it is not necessary to remove shell) and cook for 10 minutes. Add shrimp and clams. (If clams cannot fit in wok or pot, they may be steamed separately.) Cook for 10 to 15 minutes. Remove shell from lobster tails, if used. Cut lobster meat into pieces and arrange in wok along with clams, if clams have been steamed separately. Serve immediately.

6 to 8 servings

Seafood Gumbo

> 3 tablespoons vegetable oil
> 1 medium-size onion, chopped
> ½ cup chopped celery
> 1½ pounds okra, chopped
> 2 cups chopped tomatoes
> 3 bay leaves
> 2 tablespoons chopped fresh parsley
> 2 tablespoons lemon juice
> pepper, to taste
> 6 cups water
> 1 tablespoon soy sauce
> cayenne pepper, to taste
> 3 cups fresh or frozen crab meat or 6 to 12 small to medium-size hard-shell crabs, cracked into quarters, with cartilage removed
> 3 cups uncooked medium-size shrimp, peeled and deveined
> 1 dozen small oysters, shucked

In a large skillet, heat oil. Add onions and celery and sauté for 2 to 3 minutes over low to medium heat. Add okra, cover, and cook for 30 minutes, stirring frequently. If okra begins to stick to the bottom of pan, add a little water and continue to cook. Add tomatoes, bay leaves, parsley, lemon juice, and pepper. Cover and cook for 20 minutes, stirring occasionally.

Transfer ingredients to a large pot and add water, soy sauce, and cayenne. Cover and cook for 1 hour. Add a bit of water if evaporation takes place during cooking. Stir in seafood and allow to cook over medium heat for 30 minutes. Discard bay leaves. Adjust seasoning for desired hotness. Serve over cooked brown rice in individual bowls.

8 to 10 servings

Seafood Quiche

    pastry for 1 Basic Rolled Piecrust (page 718)
    2 tablespoons butter
    2 tablespoons chopped scallions
    2 tablespoons chopped celery
    ¾ cup chopped uncooked shrimp
    ½ teaspoon soy sauce
    ¾ cup fresh or frozen crab meat, with cartilage
        removed
    4 eggs
    1 cup milk
    ½ cup heavy cream
    ⅛ teaspoon ground nutmeg
    2 pinches of dried tarragon
        pepper, to taste
    1 cup shredded Swiss cheese

Preheat oven to 425°F.

Roll out pastry and line a 9-inch deep-dish pie plate. Prick pastry with a fork and bake for 8 minutes, or until lightly browned. Remove from oven and set aside.

Melt butter in a large skillet. Add scallions, celery, and shrimp and sauté for 3 minutes. Add soy sauce and crab meat. Toss ingredients and set aside.

Beat eggs in a medium-size bowl. Add milk, cream, nutmeg, tarragon, and pepper.

Sprinkle cheese on bottom of piecrust. Then add crab meat and shrimp mixture. Pour in egg mixture and bake in 425°F oven for 10 minutes. Reduce heat to 350°F and continue to bake for about 25 minutes, or until quiche is set.

6 to 8 servings

Yosenabe

"A gathering of everything." A Japanese-style bouillabaisse containing several types of shellfish, fish, and vegetables.

    6 dried mushrooms
    1 dozen clams in shells
    ½ pound spinach
    6 cups Fish Stock (page 111) or clam juice (or
        3 cups stock or juice and 3 cups water)
    3 tablespoons soy sauce
    4 scallions, cut lengthwise and in quarters
    1 tablespoon rice vinegar
    1½ tablespoons white grape juice
    ¼ cup crumbled dried seaweed* (optional)
    ⅓ pound red snapper or rock cod fillets
    6 uncooked large shrimp, peeled and deveined
    6 scallops
    ¾ cup small to medium-size shucked oysters
    2 cups chopped bok choy (Chinese cabbage)
    4 ounces tofu, drained
    3 ounces bean threads*

Soak mushrooms in a small bowl of cold water for 30 minutes. Drain. Discard water and tough stems. Set mushroom caps aside.

Wash clams. Set in water for a few minutes to allow any sand to sink to bottom of bowl.

Plunge spinach into boiling water for 1 to 2 minutes. Drain and set aside.

In a wok or large pot bring stock or clam juice (and water, if used) to a boil. Add soy sauce, scallions, vinegar, grape juice, and seaweed (if used).

Place all seafood in wok or pot. Cook for 2 minutes, or until scallops are opaque. Remove scallops and set aside. Cook remaining seafood for another 8 minutes, or until fish flakes, shrimp is pink, and clams have opened their shells. Remove seafood from wok or pot and set aside.

Add spinach, mushrooms, cabbage, tofu, and bean threads and cook for 10 minutes. Return seafood to wok or pot, heat through, and serve immediately.

6 to 8 servings

*Available in oriental grocery stores.

Fruits

Light yet satisfying, fruits are ideal by themselves as snacks, appetizers, and desserts. They can also add distinctive flavors to poultry, meat, and fish dishes, grain and vegetable dishes, salads, pastries, and cakes. Finally, fruits are easily juiced (average water content is 85 percent), and their juices serve well as beverages, in ices, and in cold soups.

Although the calorie contents of most fruits are higher than those of vegetables, fruits still find a welcome place in nearly all weight control diets. Most fruits have fewer than 100 calories per one-half-cup serving, very little fat (avocados are the exception), and lots of fiber, or pectin. (Many fruits jell nicely thanks to that abundance of pectin.) Of course, the vitamin and mineral values of fruits are commonly admired: Citrus fruits are noted for vitamin C, apricots for vitamin A, bananas for potassium, and raisins and prunes for iron.

Some of the foods we use as nuts and grains, and vegetables such as tomatoes, cucumbers, and eggplants, are actually fruits in strict botanical terms. (Walnuts are the fruit of the walnut tree, just as lettuce is the leaf of the lettuce plant, broccoli the flower of the broccoli plant, and carrots the roots of the carrot plant.) Custom, fleshiness, juiciness, and sweetness determine which foods we consider fruits.

Use fruits to bring color and change to familiar dishes. Grain and meat dishes benefit from the textures and flavors of fruits. Eaten plain, fresh fruits are among the original fast foods, yet they are unspoiled by processing and are exceedingly wholesome. (See Fruits table, page 610, for guidelines on selection, storage, preparation, and popular uses of the many varieties available.)

Selecting Fruits

Fresh: Fruits at the peak of their growing season boast the highest quality and often the most reasonable price. Look for firm, plump fruits with bright, full colors and no dark, soft, bruised areas or other signs of aging or decay. A fruit that feels heavy for its size is often the juiciest. But be wary of oversize specimens; they can be fibrous and pithy. Look for fruits that are just ripe. Refrigerated, they will keep for several days, whereas unripe fruits may never ripen and, of course, overripe fruits spoil rapidly. Since ripe fruits do deteriorate quickly, buy only the quantity you can use within a few days.

Purchase fresh fruits directly from the grower whenever you can. A pick-your-own operation is the best buy, where you can select the choicest fruits and pick them yourself. What could be fresher? Otherwise, shop in a market that has a fast turnover of fresh produce that is displayed in chilled cases, or at least not in direct sunlight.

Frozen: Fruits purchased frozen have most of the full flavor of fresh fruits but usually lack optimum texture. They generally cost more than fruits in season or canned fruits.

Choose clean, firm packages whose pieces of fruit rattle around inside. If the pieces are not loose, they have probably thawed and refrozen into a solid block. Each time thawing and refreezing take place, ice crystals form, breaking down some of the fruits' cell walls. Eventually, the fruits take on the texture of a watery puree.

If the packages are transparent, observe the fruits for color and defects. The color should be the same as that for the fresh fruit: bright and clear. Avoid fruits that appear dark, dull, or

606

Which Apple Is Best?

Variety of Apple	Best for Eating	Best for Cooking
Baldwin	●	●
Cortland	●	●
Crabapple		●
Delicious, Golden	●	
Delicious, Red	●	
Granny Smith	●	●
Gravenstein	●	●
Jonathan	●	●
McIntosh	●	●
Northern Spy	●	
Rhode Island Greening		●
Rome Beauty (Red Rome)		●
Stayman		●
Winesap	●	●
York Imperial		●

artificial because that is a good indication of poor quality.

Check the package label for additional information. It will indicate if sugar has been added and whether the fruit has been sliced or left whole.

Canned: Select canned fruits by the information found on the label. It tells you whether the fruit is packed in natural juice or in a sugar syrup; whether the fruit is whole or has been cut into halves, slices, or odd-shaped pieces; and whether the fruit is Grade A (U.S. Fancy), Grade B (U.S. Choice), or Grade C (U.S. Standard).

Grades are based on color, texture, flavor, shape, and freedom from defects. Since the nutritional values of all grades are the same, you may want to use Grades B and C, which are lower in price than Grade A, for making cobblers and other dishes in which flavor is more important than appearance.

Dried: There are several advantages to using dried fruits. You can store them in any cool, dry place, they take up little space, and they travel well to picnics and lunches.

When dried fruits are in transparent packages, look for bright colors and freedom from defects and insect damage. Pick up a package and squeeze it gently. Quality dried fruits are pliable.

Check the package label for information about preservatives. Fruits sold in large markets often have been treated with sulfur dioxide, lye, and metal bromide to keep the colors exceptionally bright. Dried fruits available in natural foods stores are usually slightly darker in color since they contain no preservatives.

Storing Fruits

Fresh: Unripe fruits ripen nicely at room temperature and out of direct sunlight. If you are in a hurry, put them in a paper bag to ripen. Twist the top of the bag to lock in the air. Check them every 24 hours.

Once ripe, fruits should be stored in the refrigerator. You can wash and dry them either before or after chilling. (Berries, strawberries, and cherries are the exception; they should always be stored unwashed.) Avoid crowding the pieces, and put them in the crisper section or in plastic bags. There most fruits will remain plump and firm for two to five days. For longer storage, fruit should be frozen, canned, or dried (see Preservation chapter).

Frozen: Store frozen fruits at 0°F or lower, a temperature at which they will retain high quality for 8 to 12 months. Never refreeze a fruit once it has thawed; the fruit's firm texture will surely deteriorate.

Canned: Stored in a cool, dry place, canned fruits will maintain their quality for as long as a year after you put them up or purchase them. If you keep them longer than that (or keep them in a warm place), quality will suffer even though the contents will still be safe to eat.

After opening a can of fruit, you can leave the remaining portion in the open can if you cover and refrigerate it. Stored that way, however, some fruits acquire an unpleasant, if harmless, metallic taste; so a fruit removed from the can and stored in a jar or dish is preferable. Use the fruit within three days.

Dried: In hot, humid weather refrigerate dried fruits. During the rest of the year, they keep well at room temperature in a tightly covered container.

Preparing Fruits

Fresh: Ripened to perfection, the vast majority of fruits need only a quick wash and pat dry. Berries, grapes, cherries, and strawberries should be quickly rinsed in a colander and drained. Avoid soaking fruits. They become waterlogged easily and shed precious vitamins and minerals in that state.

Fruits are superb when eaten out of hand, and most can be served whole with the skin intact. Preserving the skin maximizes taste, texture, fiber, and nutrients.

When you do peel fruits for special recipes, peel as thin as possible and use a stainless steel knife or peeler, instead of a carbon steel one, to help prevent darkening. Keep pieces large and dip them in lemon, lime, orange, or pineapple juice to slow oxidation, which causes fruits to brown. The fruits will remain bright until the juice itself has oxidized. When prepared as needed, not ahead of time, the classic beauty of a fruit is at its best.

Frozen: For tasty frozen fruits with nice texture and shape, thaw them in the refrigerator and serve them while they are still partially frozen.

Canned: Fruits canned in water or in their own juice need no special preparation.

Dried: Dried fruits are delicious and satisfying simply eaten plain, with no preparation. But they also may be reconstituted for use in salads, soups, compotes, and baked dishes. When possible, use the soaking water in further preparation of the recipe.

Tips for Cutting Dried Fruits

- Flour each piece of fruit to reduce stickiness.
- Cut small quantities with a warm knife or scissors.
- Use a meat grinder or a food processor for large quantities.

To plump dried fruits: Place them in a large saucepan with enough water to cover, then bring the water to a gentle boil and simmer the fruits just until they are puffed up and tender (see Simmering Fruits table, page 609, for approximate cooking time). Or, pour one cup of boiling water over one cup of dried fruits and set aside to steep for 5 to 15 minutes. The amount of time needed to tenderize depends on the variety of the fruit.

Leftover Fruits: Since the brightness and texture of cut fruits—fresh, frozen, or canned—deteriorate within a few hours, the most desirable way to use leftover fruits is in sauces, gelatin salads, puddings, pies, and cakes.

Cooking Fruits

While fresh fruits yield optimum results when cooked, canned and frozen fruits may be simmered, baked, broiled, or sautéed using the same procedures.

The best-known cooked fresh fruits include baked apples, broiled grapefruit halves, poached pears, sautéed pineapple rings, and simmered rhubarb. Any one of them will bring a delicate touch to a heavy meal.

Though a sweetener is generally added to bring out the flavor of cooked fruits, the quantity must be minimal. Too much sweetener will overpower the flavor of the fruit.

Cooking time also should be minimized. Cook fruits just until tender. Overcooking results in mushiness, washed-out color, and flat flavor. Strawberries and cherries actually develop off-flavors.

Simmering (Poaching)

Mix the appropriate amount of sweetener and water in a large saucepan (see Simmering Fruits table, below). For special flavor add fresh mint, grated orange or lemon rind, a stick of cinnamon, or whole cloves to the syrup; or, replace the water with a complementary fruit juice. Bring the syrup mixture to a boil and add the fruit of your choice. Cover the pan and return the liquid to a boil, then reduce the heat and simmer until the fruit is barely tender. Stir only enough to keep the fruit from sticking to the pan. When done, remove the

Simmering Fresh and Dried Fruits

Kind of Fruit	Amount of Fruit	Amount of Water (cups)	Amount of Honey (tablespoons)	Cooking Time (minutes)	Number of Servings (½ cup)
Apples					
Fresh	2 pounds	½	2	8-10	6
Dried	8 ounces (about 3 cups)	3½	. . .	10	8
Apricots					
Fresh	1½ pounds	½	8	5	6
Dried	8 ounces (about 1¼ cups)	2¼	1	10	4
	11 ounces (about 2 cups)	3	2	10	6
Mixed dried fruits	8 ounces (about 2 cups)	2¼	. . .	20	5
	11 ounces (about 2½ cups)	3	. . .	20	7
Peaches					
Fresh*	1½ pounds	¾	6	5	6
Dried	8 ounces (about 2 cups)	3	3	25	6
	11 ounces (about 3 cups)	4	5	25	8
Pears					
Fresh					
Firm varieties†	2 pounds	⅔	3	25	6
Soft varieties	2 pounds	⅔	3	15	6
Dried	8 ounces (about 2 cups)	2	. . .	25	4
	11 ounces (about 3 cups)	3	. . .	30	7
Plums					
Fresh	1 pound	½	4	5	5
Dried (unpitted prunes)	1 pound (about 2½ cups)	4	3	25	8

NOTE: If more honey is desired, add it at the end of the cooking period. Adding honey at the beginning makes fruits less able to absorb moisture and become tender.

*Fresh peaches need not be peeled before simmering. Their skins will slip off easily after cooking.
†When cooking firm varieties of pears, do not add honey until the final 10 minutes of cooking.

fruit from the pan and drain immediately. The fruit will retain enough heat to continue cooking for several seconds after being taken from the hot liquid.

Making Fruit Sauce

A fruit sauce is made by simmering chopped or whole small fruits in a small amount of water or juice until fully tender. The liquid may be retained and mixed in with the fruit, to thin the sauce. Or, if the sauce is thinner than desired, cornstarch or arrowroot—which does not intrude on clarity or color—can be used to thicken it. Honey should be added after rather than

Making Fresh Fruit Sauces

Kind of Fruit	Amount of Fruit (pounds)	Amount of Water (cups)	Cooking Time (minutes)	Amount of Honey	Yield (cups)
Apples	2	1/3	12-15	2 tablespoons	2½-3
Cherries					
Sour	1	2/3	5	2-3 tablespoons	2
Sweet (Bing)	1	2/3	5	1 tablespoon	2
Cranberries	1	2	15	1 cup	4 (whole) 3 (strained)
Peaches	1½	1	6-8	6 tablespoons	3
Rhubarb	1½	¾	2-5	1/3 cup	3

NOTE: Add honey after the fruit has been cooked.

Selecting and Using Fruits

Fruit	Quantity for 4	Peak Season	Look For
Apples*	4 medium (about 1 pound)	September-May	Firm; unblemished skin; bright color for variety.
Apricots	12-16 medium (about 1 pound)	June-July	Plump, juicy looking; smooth skin; bright golden orange color; yield to gentle pressure.
Avocados	2 medium	year-round	Smooth, green skin or pebbly, purple black skin; feel slightly soft.

*The table on page 607 lists the common varieties of apples and notes which are best for eating and which are best for cooking.

before simmering; adding the sweetener before cooking makes the fruit less able to absorb moisture and become fully tender. (See Fruit Sauces table, page 610, for cooking times and ingredients for some basic sauces.)

Larger fruits such as apples and peaches may be put through a strainer or a food mill before the honey is added. Berries and pitted cherries can be left intact for a chunky sauce or strained for a smooth one. (See Dessert Sauces and Glazes, page 639, for additional guidelines.)

Baking

Baking is an attractive, simple way to prepare fresh apples, apricots, bananas, peaches, pears, and plums. Heat the oven to 400°F. Pit or core the fruit and arrange the pieces in a baking dish. Pour one-half to one cup water mixed with two teaspoons lemon juice and two tablespoons honey into the dish. Bake, uncovered, until the fruit is softened, 20 to 60 minutes.

Broiling

Place slices of fruits—apples, bananas, peaches, pears, and pineapples are delicious when broiled—on the broiler rack, three to six inches below the heat. Broil them on one side; then turn them over and heat until warm and slightly browned. Watch closely; under the intense heat fruits will scorch in a matter of seconds.

Sautéing

Hot, bubbly, and lightly browned in sweet butter, sautéed fruits are a tasty accompaniment to poultry, meat, or fish. Moderately thick slices of fruit work best. Sauté the fruit in melted butter until hot and just tender, 10 to 15 minutes. Drizzle the slices with honey or sprinkle them with ground cinnamon, nutmeg, mace, or allspice.

Storage	Preparation	Popular Uses
Refrigerate in perforated plastic bags; will keep 2 weeks.	Wash. Core and peel for some recipes. Dip in lemon juice to slow browning. (Exception—Cortland apples do not brown when cut.)	Cooked or raw: cakes, cookies, jams jellies, pies, puddings, salads, sauces. Crabapples are usually cooked. Available: canned, dried, fresh, frozen, juice.
Ripen at room temperature. Refrigerate ripe apricots; will keep 3-5 days.	Wash. Pit and peel for some recipes. To peel, plunge in boiling water for 45 seconds; slip skin off. Dip in lemon juice to slow browning.	Cooked or raw: compotes, pies, preserves, salads. Available: canned, dried, fresh, juice.
Ripen at room temperature. Refrigerate ripe avocados; will keep 3-5 days.	Wash. Cut in half lengthwise and twist to remove pit. Peel for some recipes. Dip in lemon juice to slow browning.	Cooked or raw: dips, salads, stuffed. Available: fresh.

[*continued*]

Selecting and Using Fruits—*Continued*

Fruit	Quantity for 4	Peak Season	Look For
Bananas	4 medium (about 1 pound)	year-round	Unblemished skin with or without brown speckles; yellow color.
Berries Blackberries Boysenberries Dewberries Loganberries Raspberries Youngberries	2 cups (1 pint)	June–July	Plump; bright color for variety.
Blueberries	2 cups (1 pint)	May–August	Firm; dry; well-rounded shape; bright, purple blue color with slightly frosted appearance.
Cranberries	2 cups	September–January	Firm; plump; high luster. (Good berries will bounce like rubber balls.)
Currants (fresh)	2 cups	midsummer	Firm; plump; bright red, almost translucent color.
Strawberries	4 cups (1 quart)	May–June	Firm; dry; clear red color with bright green caps.

Cherries
Sour cherries
Sweet cherries
    Bing
    Lambert
    Royal Ann
	1 pound	May–August	Firm; stems attached; good color for variety.

Citrons	4 slices	year-round (packaged)	Resembles lemon but is as large as an avocado; thick skin.

Storage	Preparation	Popular Uses
Ripen at room temperature. Refrigerate ripe bananas (skin will blacken); will keep 2-3 days.	Peel skin, starting at stem end. Dip in lemon juice to slow browning.	Cooked or raw: baked, fritters, ice cream, milk shakes, pies, salads, sautéed. Available: dried, fresh.
Refrigerate, unwashed and uncovered; will keep 1-2 days.	Immediately before using, rinse and drain in a colander. Remove stems and any damaged berries. Pit for some recipes.	Cooked or raw: cakes, jams, muffins, pies, salads, sauces. Available: canned, fresh, frozen.
Refrigerate, unwashed and uncovered; will keep 1-2 days.	Immediately before using, rinse and drain in a colander. Remove stems and any damaged berries.	Cooked or raw: cakes, jams, muffins, pancakes, pies, puddings, salads, sauces. Available: canned, fresh, frozen.
Refrigerate, unwashed and uncovered; will keep 2 weeks.	Immediately before using, rinse and drain in a colander. Remove any damaged berries.	Cooked or raw: cakes, muffins, puddings, punch, sauces, stuffings, relishes. Available: fresh, frozen, juice.
Refrigerate, unwashed and uncovered; will keep 1-3 days.	Immediately before using, rinse and drain in a colander. Remove any damaged berries.	Cooked or raw: cakes, jams, jellies, salads, sauces. Available: Fresh. (Dried currants are usually dried Zantes grapes; they are no relation to fresh currants.)
Refrigerate, unwashed and uncovered; will keep 1-2 days.	Immediately before using, rinse and drain in a colander. Remove stems and caps. Serve at room temperature for full flavor.	Cooked or raw: compotes, ice cream, pies, preserves, salads, sauces, shortcakes. Available: fresh, frozen.
Refrigerate, unwashed and uncovered; will keep 1-2 days.	Immediately before using, rinse and drain in a colander. Remove stems, then scoop out pits with tip of vegetable peeler.	Cooked or raw: cakes, ice cream, jams, pies, puddings, salads, sauces. Sour cherries are usually cooked. Available: canned, fresh, frozen.
Usually preserved by candying. Refrigerate candied peel in tightly covered jar.	Wash. Peel and candy rind.	Cooked: cakes, candied, puddings. Available: candied (peel), fresh.

[continued]

Selecting and Using Fruits—*Continued*

Fruit	Quantity for 4	Peak Season	Look For
Dates	12 medium (about 1 pound)	year-round (packaged)	Shiny skin; gold brown color.
Figs	4 medium (about 1 pound)	midsummer	Slightly firm; light yellow, reddish brown, or black color.
Grapefruits	2 medium	October-April	Heavy for size; well-rounded shape; smooth, thin skin.
Grapes	1-1½ pounds	July-November	Plump; firmly attached to green, pliable stems; good color for variety.
Guavas	1 pound	September-December	Depending on variety: pear or fig shape, red or yellow color.
Kiwi fruits	4 medium	June-December	Firm; fuzzy, brown skin.
Kumquats	10-12 medium	November-February	Heavy for size; firm; bright, orange yellow color.
Lemons	2 medium	April-August	Heavy for size; firm; glossy, thin skin; light yellow color.
Limes	2 medium	April-August	Heavy for size; firm; glossy, thin skin; bright green color.
Mangoes	4 medium	midsummer	Deep green color with tinges of yellow and red; yield to gentle pressure.

Storage	Preparation	Popular Uses
Refrigerate, tightly wrapped; will keep several months.	Wash. Pit for some recipes.	Cooked or raw: baked, cakes, confections, muffins, salads, stuffed. Available: dried, fresh.
Ripen in refrigerator; ripe figs will keep 1-2 days.	Wash. Peel for some recipes. Use only cooked or canned figs in gelatin dishes; an enzyme in raw figs inhibits jelling.	Cooked or raw: cakes, pies, puddings, stewed, stuffed. Available: canned, dried, fresh.
Refrigerate; will keep 1-2 weeks.	Wash. Cut in half perpendicular to core. With a grapefruit knife loosen each segment. Or, peel skin off in a spiral; separate and skin segments.	Cooked or raw: baked, broiled, compotes, marmalades, salads. Available: canned, fresh, juice.
Refrigerate; will keep 4-6 days.	Rinse and drain in a colander. Remove stems.	Cooked or raw: jellies, salads. Available: dried—as raisins (dried Zantes grapes are commonly called dried currants), fresh, juice.
Ripen at room temperature. Refrigerate ripe guavas; will keep 2-3 days.	Wash. Cut out seeds. Peel for some recipes. Slice.	Cooked or raw: creamed, salads. Available: fresh.
Ripen at room temperature. Refrigerate ripe kiwi fruits; will keep 3-6 weeks.	Wash. Peel and slice. Use only cooked kiwi fruit in gelatin dishes; an enzyme in raw kiwi fruit inhibits jelling.	Cooked or raw: garnishes, pies, salads. Available: fresh.
Refrigerate; will keep several days.	Wash. Skin and seeds are edible.	Cooked or raw: garnishes, marmalades, salads. Available: fresh.
Refrigerate; will keep 2 weeks.	Wash. Peel or grate rind (but not white membrane, which is bitter), juice, slice, or cut into wedges. Remove seeds.	Cooked or raw: beverages, garnishes, marinades, pies, sherbets. Available: fresh, juice.
Refrigerate; will keep 2 weeks.	Wash. Peel or grate rind (but not white membrane, which is bitter), juice, slice, or cut into wedges. Remove seeds.	Cooked or raw: beverages, garnishes, marinades, pies, sherbets. Good substitute for lemons. Available: fresh, juice.
Ripen at room temperature. Refrigerate ripe mangoes; will keep 2-3 days.	Wash. Cut lengthwise slices and pull away from pit. Pull skin down as with bananas.	Cooked or raw: baked, curries, ice cream, poached, relishes. Available: fresh.

[*continued*]

Selecting and Using Fruits—*Continued*

Fruit	Quantity for 4	Peak Season	Look For

Melons
  Muskmelons
    Cantaloupe
    Casaba
    Crenshaw
    Honeyball
    Honeydew
    Persian
	1-2 medium	May-October	Heavy for size; pleasant, fruity aroma; color varies with variety; yield to slight pressure at blossom end.

Watermelons	¼ large	May-September	Smooth, velvety skin; creamy, not white or pale green, underside; firm, juicy flesh with good red or cream color; shiny, brown or black seeds.
Nectarines	4 medium	June-September	Firm; plump; smooth skin; reddish yellow color; slight softening along seam edge.

Oranges
  Sweet or juice oranges
    Hamlin
    Indian River
    Jaffa
    Navel (seedless)
    Valencia
	4 medium	winter-spring	Heavy for size; firm; bright, smooth skin.

Mandarin oranges
  (slip skin)
    Tangelo
    Tangerine
    Temple
	4 medium	October-January	Heavy for size; firm; loose skin; tangerines—glossy skin.

Papayas	4 medium	year-round	Green (unripe) to bright orange or yellow (ripe) color; yield to gentle pressure.

Peaches
  Clingstone
  Freestone
	4 medium
	(about 1 pound)
		May-October	Firm; plump; slightly fuzzy skin; white to yellow color with red blush; yield to gentle pressure.

Storage	Preparation	Popular Uses
Ripen at room temperature. Refrigerate ripe muskmelons, tightly wrapped; will keep 2-3 days.	Wash. Cut into halves or quarters. Remove seeds and membranes.	Cooked or raw: beverages, salads, soups. Available: fresh, frozen.
Refrigerate. Once cut, wrap exposed surface; will keep 1 week.	Wipe outer surfaces. Slice or cut into wedges.	Raw: compotes, pickled (rind), salads. Available: fresh.
Ripen at room temperature. Refrigerate ripe nectarines; will keep 3-5 days.	Wash. Pit and peel for some recipes. To peel, plunge in boiling water for 45-60 seconds; slip skin off. Dip in lemon juice to slow browning.	Cooked or raw: puddings, pies, salads. Available: fresh.
Refrigerate; will keep 2 weeks.	Wash. Peel skin off in a spiral. Slice thin or separate segments. Skin segments for some recipes.	Cooked or raw: cakes, compotes, confections, marmalades, pies, salads, sauces, sherbets. Available: canned, fresh, juice.
Refrigerate; will keep 1-2 weeks.	Wash. Peel. Separate segments. Skin segments for some recipes.	Raw: compotes, gelatins, salads. Available: fresh, canned (tangerines, as mandarin oranges), juice.
Ripen at room temperature. Refrigerate ripe papayas; will keep 3-4 days.	Wash. Cut in half lengthwise. Remove seeds and peel. Dip in lemon or lime juice to slow browning. Use only cooked papaya in gelatin dishes; an enzyme in raw papaya inhibits jelling. Papaya juice makes an excellent meat tenderizer.	Cooked or raw: baked, salads. Available: fresh, juice.
Ripen at room temperature. Refrigerate ripe peaches; will keep 3-4 days.	Wash. Pit and peel for some recipes. To peel, plunge in boiling water for 45 seconds; slip skin off. Dip in lemon juice to slow browning. Discard pits.	Cooked or raw: broiled, cobblers, compotes, pies, preserves, salads. Available: canned, dried, fresh, frozen.

[continued]

Selecting and Using Fruits—*Continued*

Fruit	Quantity for 4	Peak Season	Look For	

Pears
  Anjou
  Bartlett
  Bosc
  Comice
  Kieffer
  Seckel
	4 medium
	(about 1 pound)
		fall-winter	Firm but starting to soften; plump; color varies with variety.	

Persimmons	4 medium	October-December	Resembles tomato in shape; firm (unripe) to soft (ripe); plump; deep orange or red color; green stem caps attached.	
Pineapples	1 large	year-round	Large; heavy; sweet aroma; depending on variety, green or golden yellow color; fresh, deep green crown leaves; nearly all eyes at base are yellow. Avoid pineapples with soft or discolored spots, watery or dark eyes, or brown leaves.	
Plums	4 medium (about 1 pound)	June-September	Plump; good color for variety; yield to gentle pressure.	
Pomegranates	4 medium	September-December	Heavy for size; thin skin; light yellow to purple red color.	
Rhubarb	1 pound	January-June	Crisp, reddish green stalks.	

Storage	Preparation	Popular Uses
Ripen at room temperature. Refrigerate ripe pears; will keep 3-5 days.	Wash. Cut in half, core, and peel for some recipes. Dip in lemon juice to slow browning.	Cooked or raw: baked, compotes, pies, salads, stewed. Available: canned, dried, fresh, juice.
Ripen at room temperature in a bag containing an apple. Refrigerate ripe persimmons; will keep 1-2 days.	Wash and remove cap. For some recipes, peel and press through strainer or food mill to eliminate seeds. Dip or mix in lemon or lime juice to slow browning.	Cooked or raw: cakes, custards, pureed, salads. Available: fresh, frozen.
Refrigerate; will keep 1-2 days.	Wash. For rings and cubes: Slice off crown and then cut into 1-inch slices; trim away rind, eyes, and core; serve as rings or cut into cubes. For half shells: Slice in half lengthwise through crown; using a curved knife, scoop out core and flesh. Use only cooked or canned pineapple in gelatin dishes; an enzyme in raw pineapple inhibits jelling. Pineapple juice makes an excellent meat tenderizer.	Cooked or raw: cakes, cookies, garnishes, meat tenderizer, pies, punch, salads. Available: canned, dried, fresh, juice.
Refrigerate; will keep 3-5 days.	Wash. Pit for some recipes.	Cooked or raw: jams, salads, sauces. Available: canned, dried (unpitted, as prunes), fresh.
Refrigerate; will keep 1 week.	Wash. Cut into wedges and carefully remove juicy kernels.	Cooked or raw: beverages, garnishes, salads. Juice makes grenadine. Available: fresh.
Refrigerate; will keep 3-5 days.	Scrub under cold running water. Discard leaves; they are poisonous. Cook in very small amount of simmering water.	Cooked: pies, preserves, stewed. Available: fresh, frozen.

Medley of Fruits

Fruits are used abundantly in recipes throughout this book. A cross section of fruit types and meal categories is presented here; consult the Index and individual chapters for additional recipes and suggestions about using these versatile foods.

Applesauce

    3 medium-size apples, peeled and cored (about
        1 pound)
⅓ to ⅔ cup apple juice
    ½ teaspoon ground cinnamon

Cut apples into chunks. Place in a medium-size saucepan, add juice, cover pan with a tight-fitting lid, and simmer for 5 to 10 minutes, or until apples are tender. Add cinnamon. Cool and serve.

    Yields about 2 cups

Honey-Baked Apples

    6 large apples
    3 tablespoons chopped walnuts
    3 tablespoons raisins
    1 cup water
    ⅓ cup honey
    1 stick of cinnamon, 2 inches long
    1 tablespoon lemon juice

Scoop out core of apples to within ½ inch of bottom.

Mix chopped walnuts and raisins together. Fill apple cavities with mixture and place in a baking dish.

In a small saucepan combine water, honey, and cinnamon. Place over medium heat and bring to a boil. Simmer for 5 minutes. Remove from heat and stir in lemon juice. Remove cinnamon and pour syrup over apples.

Bake, uncovered, for 45 minutes, or until apples are tender. Baste occasionally. Remove from oven and cool to room temperature before serving.

    6 servings

Kefir-Avocado Dip

    1 ripe avocado, peeled and pitted
    ½ cup finely chopped tomatoes
    2 tablespoons finely chopped onions
    1 clove garlic, minced
    1 tablespoon lemon juice
        dash of pepper
    ½ teaspoon soy sauce
    ¾ cup kefir (page 448)

Mash avocado in a medium-size bowl. Add tomatoes, onions, garlic, lemon juice, pepper, and soy sauce. Mix well, then fold in kefir and chill for 30 minutes. Serve as a dip with crisp raw vegetables.

    Yields 2½ cups

Blini with Raspberries

Blini, the buckwheat crepes that originated in eastern Europe, work best with assertive-flavored fruits.

    Batter
    ½ tablespoon dry yeast
    1 teaspoon light honey
    ¼ cup warm water
    1½ cups sifted buckwheat flour
    1 egg
    1 egg yolk
    2 tablespoons sweet butter, melted and cooled
    ¼ cup milk, or more as needed

    Filling
    ¼ cup light honey
    2 cups fresh raspberries
    ½ cup Clarified Butter (page 148), melted
    1 cup sour cream or crème fraîche (page 450)

To make the batter: Dissolve yeast and honey in water and set aside to proof. In a large mixing bowl combine flour, egg, egg yolk, cooled butter, dissolved yeast, and milk. Mix with a wire whisk until smooth. Add more warm milk if necessary to bring batter to consistency of heavy cream. Cover bowl with a cloth and let stand in a warm place for about 30 minutes, or until batter rises and becomes puffy.

To make the filling: Just before blini are ready to cook, heat honey in a 3-cup saucepan until dissolved.

Remove from heat. Add raspberries and gently fold into honey. (Do not reheat after adding raspberries.) Transfer to a serving bowl and set aside. Place clarified butter and sour cream or crème fraîche in separate serving bowls.

To cook the blini: Heat an omelet pan or small skillet until a speck of butter instantly sizzles and browns. Butter pan. Pour about 2 tablespoons batter into pan and spread it thin, to about 4 inches in diameter. Brown on one side and then the other. When done, stack in a warmed napkin placed on a serving platter. Prepare all blini in this manner.

When blini are ready, serve immediately, accompanied with bowls of clarified butter, raspberries, and sour cream or crème fraîche. To eat, spread a few drops of butter on blini, top with raspberries and cream, and roll up.

4 to 6 servings

NOTE: The batter can be made 1 to 2 hours ahead of time and refrigerated. Blini should be cooked just before serving.

Cranberry *Kisel*

Kisel is a light, tart fruit puree served chilled, with sour cream or heavy cream. It has long been popular in northern Europe, where it is commonly prepared with lingonberries, cousins of the cranberry.

3 cups fresh cranberries (12 ounces)
2 cups water
½ cup light honey, or more to taste
1 tablespoon cornstarch or arrowroot, dissolved in 1 tablespoon water
1 cup sour cream or heavy cream

Combine cranberries and water in a 2-quart heavy-bottom pot, and bring to a boil over high heat. Reduce heat and simmer, uncovered, until fruit is tender and skins break, 10 to 15 minutes.

Rub mixture through a fine strainer or food mill. Return pureed cranberries to pot, add honey, and bring to a boil over high heat. Remove from heat and taste for sweetness. Add more honey if desired.

Stir dissolved cornstarch or arrowroot into pureed cranberries. Return mixture to moderate heat and stir until it comes to a boil and thickens slightly. Remove from heat and cool to room temperature.

Pour cooled puree into a serving bowl or individual dessert glasses. Refrigerate until thoroughly chilled. Serve with a separate bowl of sour cream or heavy cream (unwhipped) to use as a topping.

6 servings

NOTE: *Kisel* can be prepared as much as 2 days in advance and refrigerated.

Hot Blueberry Sauce over Lemon Ice Cream

¾ cup blueberry jam
2 teaspoons lemon juice
2 to 3 cups fresh blueberries
Lemon Ice Cream (see below)

Rub jam through a fine strainer. Combine with lemon juice in a 4-cup saucepan and stir over low heat until it comes to a boil. Add blueberries and continue to stir until mixture is warm. (Do not cook berries too long; they should not disintegrate.)

Serve hot over scoops of lemon ice cream placed in individual dessert glasses. Refrigerated, sauce keeps well up to 2 days.

6 to 8 servings

Lemon Ice Cream

¾ cup light honey
½ cup lemon juice
grated rind of 3 lemons
6 egg yolks
2 cups heavy cream
2 cups light cream or half-and-half

Combine honey, lemon juice, and lemon rind in a small saucepan and stir over low heat until blended. Set aside.

In a large bowl beat egg yolks until light and thick. Continue beating while slowly adding honey and lemon mixture. Beat until mixture is thick and thoroughly cooled. Add heavy cream and light cream or half-and-half. Pour mixture into the can of an ice cream maker. Process until ice cream is firm. Remove paddle and pack down ice cream in can or transfer to a freezer container. Place ice cream in freezer at 0°F to harden.

Makes 1½ quarts

Savarin with Berries in Pastry Cream

This classic sweet bread baked in a ring mold becomes a glorious dessert presentation when its center overflows with fresh berries in rich pastry cream.

Savarin Ring
1 tablespoon dry yeast
¼ cup warm water
1 cup plus 2 tablespoons sifted whole wheat pastry flour
3 eggs, beaten
2 tablespoons sweet butter, softened
1 tablespoon light honey
2 tablespoons dried currants (optional)
2 tablespoons sweet butter, melted and cooled

Syrup
¾ cup light honey
1 cup water
6 whole cloves
    finely grated rind of 1 large orange

Glaze
¾ cup apricot jam
1 tablespoon lemon juice

Topping
2 cups fresh blackberries, blueberries, raspberries, or strawberries
2 cups Vanilla Pastry Cream (page 699)

To make the savarin ring: Dissolve yeast in water and set aside to proof. Place flour in a medium-size bowl. Add eggs and dissolved yeast. Beat with your fingers (slightly cup your hand and use it like a wire whisk) until mixture is light and elastic. Cover bowl with plastic wrap and a cloth, and let dough rise in a warm place (ideally about 80°F) for 45 minutes.

In a large bowl beat softened butter until creamy. Add honey and beat again until light and creamy. After dough has risen, add butter mixture to dough and mix well, using a rubber spatula. Mix in currants (if used).

Brush an 8-inch ring mold with cooled melted butter. Spread dough in mold. (It will be about ¼ full.) Cover mold with a cloth and let stand in a warm place until dough rises to top of mold.

Preheat oven to 375°F.

Bake savarin for 35 minutes, or until well risen and lightly browned. Turn out onto a wire rack.

To make the syrup: Combine honey, water, cloves, and orange rind in a 3-cup saucepan and bring to a boil. Simmer for 5 minutes. Place wire rack holding savarin ring on a jelly-roll pan. Spoon hot honey syrup over savarin. Pour syrup that collects in jelly-roll pan back into saucepan, and continue spooning syrup over still-warm savarin ring until it has absorbed all the syrup.

To make the glaze: Combine apricot jam and lemon juice in a small saucepan and stir over low heat until jam is dissolved. Rub mixture through a fine strainer. Brush savarin ring all over with glaze. Set aside.

To make the topping: At serving time carefully transfer savarin ring to a serving platter. Fold berries into pastry cream and pile mixture in middle of ring.

6 to 8 servings

NOTE: The savarin ring and pastry cream may be prepared up to 1 day in advance, then assembled with berries just before serving.

Strawberry Fritters with Raspberry Sauce

Marinated Strawberries
¼ cup light honey
½ cup water
    shredded rind of 1 orange
24 large fresh strawberries

Batter

2 eggs, separated
1 cup whole wheat pastry flour
1 tablespoon sweet butter, melted and cooled
2 tablespoons orange juice
⅔ to 1 cup cold water

Sauce

1 cup seedless raspberry jam
1 tablespoon lemon juice

vegetable oil, for deep frying

To make the marinated strawberries: In a small heavy-bottom pot combine honey, water, and orange rind. Stir over moderate heat until it comes to a boil. Reduce heat and simmer for 5 minutes. Chill syrup thoroughly. Pour cold syrup over whole strawberries and allow to marinate for 1 to 2 hours.

To make the batter: Place egg yolks in a medium-size bowl and beat with a wire whisk until frothy. Add flour and mix well. Add butter and orange juice and mix again. Thin with cold water to consistency of thick cream. Let batter rest in refrigerator for at least 30 minutes.

To make the sauce: Combine jam and lemon juice in a small saucepan. Stir over low heat until jam is dissolved. Rub through a fine strainer and cool to room temperature.

Heat oil in a deep fryer to 375°F (use a deep frying thermometer).

Beat egg whites until they form soft peaks, then gently fold them into batter. Drain syrup from strawberries. Add ¼ of the strawberries to batter, and make sure they are coated all over. Using a spoon, drop them one at a time into hot oil. When fritters are golden and crisp, remove with a slotted spoon and drain on paper toweling. Keep fritters warm while remaining batches are fried.

Place fritters on a warmed napkin on a serving platter, or divide onto warmed individual serving plates. Serve raspberry sauce in a separate bowl. Fritters also go well served with ice cream.

4 to 6 servings

NOTE: The batter and sauce may be prepared a few hours ahead. Coat and fry fritters at serving time.

Hungarian Cold Sour Cherry Soup

This is a marvelous way to take advantage of a bounty of sour cherries, but remember to prepare this dessert soup several hours to a day ahead to allow for chilling thoroughly.

¾ cup light honey
2½ cups water
2 strips orange rind, 4 inches long
1 stick of cinnamon
3 cups pitted fresh sour cherries (1½ pounds, with pits)
1 tablespoon arrowroot, dissolved in 2 tablespoons water
1 cup sour cream

Combine honey, water, orange rind, and cinnamon in a 2-quart saucepan and stir over moderate heat until it comes to a boil. Add cherries and bring to a boil again. Reduce heat, partially cover pot, and simmer for 30 to 35 minutes.

Remove orange rind and cinnamon. In a small bowl combine dissolved arrowroot with about ½ cup hot soup and mix well. Add this mixture to soup in pot. Stir soup over low heat until it comes to a simmer. Cook for another 2 to 3 minutes, or until it is clear and slightly thickened. Chill mixture for several hours or overnight.

To serve, stir sour cream into chilled soup. Transfer soup to a large crystal serving bowl embedded in cracked ice. Serve in small well-chilled serving bowls.

4 to 6 servings

Individual Hot *Clafouti*

Clafouti, *a home specialty from the Limousin region of France, is a dessert which is gaining popularity in America because it is so easy to prepare and so good to eat. Traditionally, it is a preparation of crepe batter poured over sweet cherries in a shallow dish, baked, and served at room temperature or cold. But it looks so tempting while still hot and puffy, this recipe suggests serving it that way.*

    ½ cup whole grain bread crumbs
    ½ teaspoon ground cardamom
2 to 3 cups fresh sweet cherries, pitted
    3 eggs, beaten
    ¼ cup plus 1 tablespoon sifted whole wheat pastry flour
    2 cups milk or light cream
    ¼ cup light honey
    1 cup crème fraîche (page 450) or whipped cream (optional)

Butter 4 to 6 custard cups. Mix bread crumbs and cardamom, and dust inside of each cup with this mixture. Divide cherries evenly among cups and place cups on a jelly-roll pan.

Preheat oven to 375°F.

In a large bowl combine eggs and flour and mix well. Add milk or light cream and beat for 3 minutes. Add honey and beat for 2 minutes. Pour batter into custard cups. Bake for 30 minutes, or until tops are lightly browned and puffy. Serve hot, accompanied with a separate bowl of crème fraîche or whipped cream if a topping is desired.

    4 to 6 servings

Lemon Bavarian Cream with Candied Lemon Slices

This beautiful dessert should be prepared a day ahead to set. It may be unmolded or served from the same bowl in which it has chilled.

    6 eggs, separated
    ¼ cup plus 2 tablespoons light honey
    3 envelopes unflavored gelatin
1½ cups light cream
    grated rind of 3 lemons
    1 cup lemon juice
    1 cup heavy cream, whipped
    Candied Lemon Slices (see below)
    mint sprig

Use an electric mixer to beat egg yolks and honey together in a large bowl until light and thick. Reduce mixer speed and mix in gelatin.

Heat cream in a medium-size saucepan over low heat until it comes to a boil. Very slowly add hot cream to egg yolk mixture, beating constantly. Transfer mixture to saucepan and stir over low heat until this custard mixture coats the back of a spoon. Remove from heat and stir in lemon rind and juice. Cover saucepan and let stand in refrigerator or freezer until mixture is completely cool and at point of setting.

Beat egg whites until they form soft peaks, then fold them into cooled custard, using a rubber spatula. Fold in whipped cream gently and evenly. Spoon mixture into a 1½-quart mold (if it is to be later unmolded) or a large serving bowl, and refrigerate for at least 6 hours or overnight to set.

Prepare candied lemon slices and set aside.

When well set, unmold Bavarian cream, if desired. Arrange a border of candied lemon slices, slightly overlapping, on top of Bavarian cream. Place mint sprig in center. Refrigerate until serving time.

    6 to 8 servings

Candied Lemon Slices

    2 lemons
    ⅓ cup light honey
    ⅔ cup water

Cut lemons neatly into paper-thin slices. Use a very sharp knife. In a small heavy-bottom pot combine honey and water and stir over moderate heat until it comes to a boil. Place lemon slices in syrup and poach them over low heat until rind is translucent, about 15 minutes. Remove slices carefully with tongs and place on a lightly greased baking sheet to cool.

Makes about 5 dozen

Orange-Almond Bavarian Cream

    1 envelope unflavored gelatin
1¾ cups milk
    2 tablespoons honey
    2 tablespoons orange juice
    1 teaspoon grated orange rind
    ⅛ teaspoon almond extract
    2 egg whites

Combine gelatin and milk in a medium-size saucepan. Place over low heat and stir until gelatin is dissolved. Remove from heat and gradually stir in honey, orange juice, orange rind, and almond extract. Mix well, then cover and refrigerate until mixture begins to set.

Beat egg whites until soft peaks form, then fold them into gelatin mixture, using a rubber spatula. Pour into a serving dish or a 1-quart mold and chill for several hours, until firm.

4 servings

Orange Mousse

This elegant dessert is simple to prepare, even for an amateur cook. Just be sure to allow for chilling-setting time—at least six hours.

    2 large oranges
    3 eggs
    2 egg yolks
    3 tablespoons light honey
    ¾ cup orange juice
1½ tablespoons unflavored gelatin
    ½ cup heavy cream, whipped
    ¼ cup red currant jelly
    1 tablespoon lemon juice

Grate rind of 1 orange and reserve. Skin segments of both oranges and set aside in refrigerator, in a covered container, until ready to use.

Use an electric mixer to combine eggs, egg yolks, and honey in a large bowl. Beat until mixture is thick and almost holds its shape. Add orange rind and mix.

Combine orange juice and gelatin in a small saucepan and stir over low heat until gelatin is dissolved. Cool to room temperature, then sprinkle it over beaten egg mixture. Fold in carefully, using a rubber spatula. Add whipped cream, folding it in gently and evenly. Transfer mousse to a serving bowl and place in refrigerator at least 6 hours or overnight to chill and set.

When mousse has set, combine jelly and lemon juice in a small saucepan and stir over low heat until jelly is dissolved. Set aside to cool to room temperature. Arrange orange segments in a border on top of mousse. Brush each section with dissolved jelly. Return to refrigerator until serving time.

4 servings

NOTE: This mousse can also be served in star-cut orange shells. Allow mousse to chill and set. Before decorating, spoon mousse into orange shells. Then poke 3 orange segments partway into mousse, and gently brush each with a little dissolved jelly.

Stuffed Figs

25 dried figs or 1 package string figs
25 whole walnuts or almonds, roasted
    1 cup orange juice

Slice figs ¾ of the way around without disturbing stems. Open each fig, insert a nut, and squeeze together to seal. Place figs in a medium-size bowl. Pour orange juice over them and soak for 30 minutes.

Preheat oven to 350°F.

Drain off orange juice, place figs on a lightly greased baking sheet, and bake for 10 minutes.

Makes 25

Kiwi Eggcup

A dramatic yet simple brunch treat that is sure to cause favorable comment.

    1 kiwi fruit
    1 egg
    1 teaspoon light cream
    1 teaspoon butter
    freshly ground pepper, to taste

Cut unpeeled kiwi fruit in half around its waist. Slide a paring knife around inside, about ⅛ inch away from skin, to loosen pulp. Remove pulp in a whole section, without injuring skin. You want 1 good empty half shell left intact. Place half shell in an eggcup on a serving plate. (Remaining skin can be discarded.) Slice kiwi fruit pulp and arrange overlapping slices on plate next to eggcup.

Beat egg and cream in a small bowl. Heat butter in a small skillet, add egg mixture, and scramble over moderate heat just until egg begins to set. Remove from heat at once. Sprinkle with pepper. Carefully fill kiwi shell with scrambled egg and serve immediately.

    1 serving

Grape Granita Violetta

Granita, a European fruit-flavored ice, can be made with a variety of juicy fruits, particularly citrus. For this grape granita, the fresh flower garnish is an eye-catching touch.

    5 cups Concord or purple Ribier grapes
    ½ cup light honey, or more to taste
    1 tablespoon grated orange rind
    2 teaspoons unflavored gelatin
    1 tablespoon lemon juice
    1 tablespoon water
    1 egg white
    2 cups Crème Chantilly (page 695)
    4 to 6 violets (purple grapes may be substituted)

If Concord grapes are used, slip skins from grapes. Combine both grape pulp (with seeds) and skins in a medium-size saucepan. If Ribier grapes are used, cut each grape in half. Place grapes (with seeds) in a medium-size saucepan.

Place saucepan with grapes (no water) over moderate heat and bring to a rolling boil. Rub hot grapes through a fine strainer into a large bowl to remove seeds and skins. Return pureed grapes to

saucepan and add honey and orange rind. Combine gelatin with lemon juice and water and add to grape mixture. Stir over moderate heat until mixture comes to a boil, then reduce heat and simmer for 2 minutes. Add more honey, if desired. Refrigerate mixture until chilled.

Place chilled mixture in the can of an ice cream maker and process until almost firm.

Beat egg white until it forms soft peaks, then add to half-frozen granita. Continue processing until granita is firm; then remove from can and use immediately or pack granita down and place in freezer to harden.

Thoroughly chill individual dessert glasses. Place a large scoop of grape granita in each. Put Crème Chantilly in a pastry bag fitted with a small star tube, and pipe little rosettes all over granita. Return to freezer until serving time. When ready to serve, decorate each with a fresh violet.

    4 to 6 servings

NOTE: Granita keeps well in the freezer for 2 to 3 days. If it is too hard at serving time, soften by crushing it in a food processor.

Ginger-Melon Chicken with Parsley Rice

    1½ cups rich Poultry Stock (page 110)
      6 slices peeled ginger root or 1 teaspoon ground ginger
    4 to 6 chicken breast halves or whole legs, skinned
      2 cups cubed cantaloupe
      2 cups cubed honeydew melon
      ¼ cup sweet butter, cut into bits
    3 to 4 cups hot cooked brown rice
      ½ cup minced fresh parsley

Pour stock into a steamer or medium-size heavy-bottom pot. Add ginger to stock. Place chicken on steamer platform or on bottom of pot. Bring stock to a boil, then reduce heat, cover, and simmer until chicken is tender, about 30 minutes.

Arrange chicken on a serving platter and keep it warm. Transfer remaining stock to a large skillet and remove ginger slices (if used). Add cantaloupe and honeydew cubes and warm over moderate heat. (Do not cook melon for any length of time; it should remain firm.) Using a slotted spoon, transfer melon cubes to serving platter and arrange them along one side. Keep chicken and melon warm while preparing sauce.

Cook stock in skillet, uncovered, until it is reduced to about ½ cup. Using a wire whisk, beat butter into stock, bit by bit.

Toss hot rice with ½ of the parsley and place in a serving bowl.

To serve, spoon sauce over chicken and sprinkle chicken (not melon) with remaining parsley. Serve with rice.

Or, to make individual servings, generously oil 4 to 6 small molds and pack each with rice mixture. Invert rice molds onto individual serving plates. Place chicken on each plate, cover with sauce, and sprinkle with parsley. Arrange generous servings of melon cubes next to chicken.

4 to 6 servings

NOTE: The chicken can be poached the day before and refrigerated in the broth. At serving time, rewarm, and prepare melon, sauce, and rice.

Baked Papaya Stuffed with Chili Beef

A truly unusual main dish idea featuring a delicious flavor combination.

    3 firm ripe papayas, 6 inches long
    3 tablespoons sweet butter
    1 medium-size onion, finely chopped
    ½ teaspoon minced garlic
    ½ cup finely chopped green peppers
    1 pound lean ground beef
    2 tablespoons soy sauce
    1 teaspoon chili powder
    1 large tomato, peeled, seeded, and chopped
    6 tablespoons grated Parmesan cheese

Cut papayas in half lengthwise and remove seeds. Pulverize seeds in a blender or food processor and set aside. Cut a thin slice from bottom of each papaya half so it will stand steadily. Place papayas on a baking sheet.

Heat 1 tablespoon butter in a large skillet. Add onions and garlic and stir over moderate heat until onions are translucent. Add peppers, 3 tablespoons pulverized papaya seeds, and ground beef, and stir over high heat until meat is no longer pink. Add soy sauce and chili powder and stir mixture. Add tomatoes and stir over high heat for 1 minute.

Preheat oven to 350°F.

Fill hollow of each papaya half with meat mixture. Sprinkle 1 tablespoon cheese and a few drops of melted butter over top of each. Bake for 30 minutes, or until papayas are tender and topping is lightly browned. Carefully transfer stuffed papayas to a warmed serving platter. Serve hot.

6 servings

NOTE: Papaya halves can be stuffed several hours to 1 day ahead, then baked just before serving.

Spicy Peaches with Strawberry Hearts

    4 to 6 large or 8 to 12 small ripe peaches
    2 tablespoons lemon juice
    ¾ cup light honey
    ¾ cup water
    6 whole cloves
      shredded rind of 1 large orange
16 to 20 fresh strawberries
    1 cup crème fraîche (page 450) or whipped
      cream (optional)

Immerse peaches in boiling water for 20 to 30 seconds, then immediately plunge them into cold water and slip off skins. Sprinkle peeled peaches with lemon juice to retard discoloration.

In a heavy-bottom pot large enough for all peaches to fit on the bottom, combine honey, water, cloves, and orange rind. Stir mixture over moderate heat until it comes to a boil. Reduce heat and simmer syrup for 5 minutes. Add peaches, bathe them with syrup, and cover pot. Simmer large peaches for about 10 minutes, or small peaches for 5 to 7 minutes, turning them occasionally. (They should still seem raw after poaching because they will continue to soften in the hot syrup.) Remove pot from heat and allow to cool somewhat. Then place peaches and syrup in refrigerator to chill thoroughly.

When chilled, drain syrup from peaches and remove cloves. Add strawberries to syrup and set aside for 1 to 2 hours.

Insert a strawberry in each peach as follows: Make a single cut down side of peach. Carefully remove pit without breaking peach. Replace pit with a strawberry. Close peach. Place it cut-side down in a chilled shallow serving bowl. Prepare and arrange all peaches in this manner. Spoon remaining strawberries and syrup around peaches. Serve with a separate bowl of crème fraîche or whipped cream, if desired.

4 to 6 servings

Baked Pears with Almonds and Yogurt

6 firm ripe pears, cored and sliced
¼ to ⅓ cup honey
1 teaspoon vanilla extract
½ cup slivered almonds
2 tablespoons butter
1 cup yogurt

Preheat oven to 350°F. Butter a 9-inch-square baking dish.

Arrange pears in attractive rows in prepared dish. Mix honey and vanilla and drizzle over pears. Top with almonds, dot with butter, and bake for 10 to 15 minutes, or until pears are tender. Baste frequently during baking, using accumulated juice. Serve hot or cold, topped with yogurt.

6 servings

Maple-Baked Pears

6 firm pears (apples may be substituted)
¼ cup raisins
⅓ cup chopped walnuts or pecans
4 tablespoons maple syrup
¼ teaspoon ground cinnamon
½ cup hot water

Preheat oven to 350°F.
Core pears to within ¼ inch of bottom.
Combine raisins, nuts, 2 tablespoons maple syrup, and cinnamon in a small cup. Divide among pears, pushing filling into cavities with a spoon handle. Place in a shallow baking dish just large enough to hold pears without crowding.

Pour remaining 2 tablespoons maple syrup over pears. Pour hot water into baking dish, cover with foil, and bake for 40 minutes, or until pears are tender when pierced with a fork. Baste pears several times during baking.

Serve warm or cool with heavy cream.

6 servings

Poached Pears

8 ripe pears*
1½ cups water
¼ cup honey

1 vanilla bean, 2 inches long, or 2 teaspoons vanilla extract

Core pears to ½ inch of bottom. Cut a thin slice from bottom of each pear so it will stand upright.

In a saucepan large enough for all pears to fit on bottom, heat water and then add honey. Stir until completely dissolved, to make a syrup. Cut vanilla bean lengthwise, scrape seeds into syrup, and then add pod; or, add vanilla extract to syrup. Stand pears in syrup, cover pan, and simmer until pears are barely tender, basting occasionally. Cook for 5 to 25 minutes, depending on ripeness and variety of pears. Do not overcook. Remove from heat and cool pears slightly in syrup.

To serve, cut pears in half and place 2 halves in each of 8 individual fruit dishes.

8 servings

*If a firm variety of pear is used, the longer cooking time will be needed. Add honey after 10 minutes, rather than at the beginning, of simmering.

Variations:
■ Whip 4 cups ricotta cheese with a rotary beater. Blend in 3 tablespoons honey, or more to taste. Spoon over poached pears.
■ Garnish poached pears with a sprinkle of fresh raspberries.

Old-fashioned Rhubarb Tapioca Cream

Rhubarb Puree
2 pounds rhubarb, cut into 1-inch pieces
¾ cup light honey
grated rind of 1 lemon

Tapioca Cream
3 tablespoons quick-cooking tapioca
¼ cup light honey
2 cups milk
2 eggs, separated
1 teaspoon vanilla extract

Candied Lemon Shreds
1 lemon
¼ cup light honey
¼ cup water

1 cup cold English Custard Sauce (page 663)
or whipped cream

To make the rhubarb puree: In a deep heavy-bottom pot combine rhubarb, honey, and lemon rind. Cover and cook for several minutes over low heat until rhubarb is soft. Stir occasionally to prevent scorching. Puree mixture in a blender or food processor. (You should have about 2 cups puree.) Chill thoroughly.

To make the tapioca cream: In a 1-quart heavy-bottom pot combine tapioca, honey, milk, and slightly beaten egg yolks. Let mixture stand for 5 minutes. Then cook over moderate heat, stirring constantly, until mixture comes to a full boil, about 5 minutes. Remove from heat and cool to room temperature. Blend in vanilla. Beat egg whites until they form soft peaks, and fold them evenly into mixture, using a rubber spatula. Chill thoroughly.

To make the candied lemon shreds: Using a vegetable peeler, peel strips of rind from lemon. Then, using a sharp French knife, cut rind on the diagonal into long hair-thin shreds. Combine honey and water in a small saucepan and bring to a boil. Add lemon shreds and simmer for 5 minutes. Drain lemon shreds in a strainer and set aside.

Combine rhubarb puree and tapioca cream and fold together until smooth. Transfer mixture to a serving bowl and scatter lemon shreds on top. Chill until serving time. Serve in dessert glasses, accompanied with a separate bowl of custard sauce or whipped cream.

4 to 6 servings

NOTE: This dessert may be prepared the day before serving.

Prune Plum and Bread Pudding

Fried Bread
10 slices whole grain bread
6 tablespoons sweet butter
2 tablespoons light honey

Poached Plums
½ cup light honey
½ cup water
2 strips of orange rind, 4 inches long

1½ pounds Italian prune plums (10 to 15), halved
and pitted

Custard
2 eggs
2 egg yolks
¼ cup reserved poaching syrup
1¼ cups milk
1 teaspoon vanilla extract
light honey, to taste

1 cup crème fraîche (page 450) or
whipped cream

To make the fried bread: Trim crusts neatly from bread slices. Melt 3 tablespoons butter in a 10-inch skillet, then blend in 1 tablespoon honey. Add bread slices to skillet, a few at a time, and sauté on each side, adding remaining butter and honey as necessary. Place slices on a baking sheet to cool. Cut each slice neatly into 4 squares and set aside.

To make the poached plums: In a deep heavy-bottom pot combine honey, water, and orange rind. Stir over moderate heat until mixture comes to a boil, then reduce heat and simmer syrup for 3 minutes. Add plums, cover, and simmer for 5 to 8 minutes, or until plums are tender but still firm. (They should not become mushy or disintegrate.)

Preheat oven to 350°F. Butter a 5-cup shallow baking dish.

Arrange ½ of the fried bread squares on bottom of prepared baking dish. Using a slotted spoon, remove plums from syrup and place them on top of bread. (Reserve poaching syrup.) Cover plums with remaining squares of bread in rows, slightly overlapping.

To make the custard: Combine eggs, egg yolks, ¼ cup reserved poaching syrup, milk, and vanilla in a large bowl and beat until well mixed. Blend in honey.

Pour custard mixture over bread-plum assembly, then place baking dish in a roasting pan. Fill roasting pan halfway with hot water. Place in oven and bake for 30 minutes. While pudding is cooking, press down top with a wide spatula once or twice to keep it moist and in place. After 30 minutes increase oven temperature to 425°F. Remove pudding as soon as top is nicely browned. Serve warm or cold, accompanied with a separate bowl of crème fraîche or whipped cream.

6 servings

Pineapple and Curried Seafood Salad in Pineapple Shells

Salad

2 ripe pineapples
1 can (6 to 7 ounces) water-packed chunk tuna, flaked
½ pound medium-size shrimp, cooked, peeled, and deveined
1 tablespoon curry powder

Dressing

½ cup mayonnaise
½ teaspoon dry mustard
1 teaspoon catsup
¼ teaspoon soy sauce
1 teaspoon chopped pimientos
2 teaspoons minced chives
2 teaspoons minced green peppers
1 teaspoon minced fresh parsley
½ hard-cooked egg, finely chopped
1 teaspoon grated horseradish

To make the salad: Cut off top of each pineapple. Cut each pineapple in half lengthwise. Using a small sharp knife, cut along both sides of core at an angle, then pull out core and discard it. Carefully cut out pineapple pulp, leaving ⅜-inch-thick shell. Cut pineapple pulp into thin strips and place in a large bowl.

In a medium-size bowl combine tuna and shrimp. Sprinkle with curry powder and toss lightly. Add seafood to bowl of pineapple strips. (Do not toss yet.)

To make the dressing: In a large bowl combine mayonnaise, dry mustard, catsup, and soy sauce and beat well. Add pimiento, chives, green peppers, parsley, egg, and horseradish and beat again.

Pour dressing over seafood and pineapple and toss lightly. Chill mixture and pineapple shells separately until serving time. Then fill each pineapple shell with salad mixture. Garnish with watercress and lemon wedges.

4 servings

NOTE: The salad may be prepared up to 1 day in advance of assembling and serving.

Piima Fruit Cup

2 cups undrained chopped fresh pineapple
1 cup chopped bananas, mashed fresh strawberries or raspberries, or whole seedless grapes
¼ cup chopped pecans
1 teaspoon maple syrup
1 cup piima (page 448)
4 sprigs mint

Combine pineapple, pineapple juice, bananas or berries or grapes, nuts, and maple syrup. Chill. At serving time fold in piima and garnish with mint. Serve immediately.

4 servings

Desserts

Elegant mousses and soufflés, as well as simple custards, pies, cakes, cookies, and confections—in fact, most of the classic desserts that have charmed cooks for ages—can be made with natural ingredients and turn out as tempting and delicious as ever. Our great grandparents did it all the time. The traditional favorites were created in an era when few processed ingredients were available. We believe that natural ingredients still have the most to offer. Use them in making the rich desserts that are a wonderful occasional treat and for the broad range of delectable low-calorie, low-fat desserts that are so popular today.

Natural Ingredients

No sweetener is healthful when used excessively, so we have minimized the sweetening for the recipes that appear in this book. Honey is frequently used to replace refined white sugar, because unrefined, uncooked honey, unlike sugar, retains its natural nutrients (see A Guide to Sugars and Liquid Sweeteners, page 633). A mild honey can be used to add a pleasant flavor to foods, or it can be used so discreetly that the final product has the desired sweetness, with no honey flavor at all.

Honey is usually classified according to its flower source. Orange blossom and clover blossom honeys are noted for their pleasing mild flavor. Buckwheat honey is dark and has a pleasantly pronounced flavor. In general, the darker the honey is, the more sweetness it imparts. When you substitute honey for sugar, the object is to add enough honey for sweetness without an overwhelming honey flavor. The recipes in this book achieve that aim. Honey has about twice the sweetening power of sugar, so use only half as much honey, or less, as a substitute for sugar in a recipe. Compensate for the semiliquid state of honey by adding less liquid or more dry ingredients in the recipe.

Cakes and cookies in which honey has replaced sugar will be a little coarser in texture, and they will be moist and soft. Honey enhances the keeping qualities of most baked goods because of its ability to retain water. So cakes, cookies, frostings, and all confections made with honey remain moist for a longer time than desserts made with sugar.

Maple syrup and molasses are also used as sweeteners in dessert recipes. Maple syrup, used in about the same proportion as honey, has a mild, distinctive flavor that is welcome in some desserts. It is especially good as a sweetener for certain sauces, fillings, and frostings. Both unsulfured and blackstrap molasses (sulfured molasses is not used here) blend well with spices and are generally used for gingerbread and other spice cakes. Some recipes call for a combination of honey and molasses.

632

Syrups made from grains may be used as sweeteners in baking (see Grain Sweeteners, page 634). Natural fruit juices also serve well as sweeteners in recipes. Orange, apple, prune, and pineapple juices all add a significant sweetness to recipes where their flavors will not intrude on the intended taste.

There is no question that desserts made with whole wheat are more wholesome than those made with refined white flour. The baked goods will be slightly heavier and richer tasting than those baked with white flour. They will also be moister because of the higher oil content of whole wheat flour.

To lighten whole grain flour, stir it with a wire whisk or sift it. Return the bran that remains in the sifter to the flour or add it to another recipe.

Cakes, cookies, pies, and pastries adapt very nicely to the use of whole wheat flour. The final products often have the rich, golden brown color of the flour.

Whole wheat *pastry* flour is a much finer grind of whole wheat and is lighter than regular whole wheat flour. It should also be sifted or whisked to fluff it before it is added to a dough mixture. Because of its lightness, whole wheat pastry flour is most often used for cakes, pies, and delicate cookies.

Carob has become popular as a substitute for chocolate and cocoa in desserts, as well as in beverages (see Carob-Flavored Drinks, page 736). Most cooks prefer the texture that results when powdered carob is made into a syrup (see Basic Carob Syrup, page 737) before adding it to a recipe. One-quarter cup of this syrup may be

A Guide to Sugars and Liquid Sweeteners

Sucrose, refined from sugar cane or sugar beets, is ordinary table sugar. The refining process leaves it devoid of just about all nutrients. *Confectioner's sugar,* or *powdered sugar,* is made by processing this white sugar with cornstarch.

Fructose, or fruit sugar, is found in fruits and honey. It is about twice as sweet as table sugar and more easily absorbed into the body. Fructose has been suggested as a healthful alternative to sucrose, but it has been implicated in the rise of levels of triglycerides and other fats associated with heart disease.

Brown sugar, supposedly a less refined product than table sugar, is actually white sugar mixed with a small amount of molasses, which gives it its characteristic flavor and color. Nutritional differences between this and white sugar are negligible.

Raw sugar is actually the first batch of crystals separated from cane syrup in the refining process. In this form raw sugar is banned from sale in this country because it contains many impurities. It is sometimes sanitized, then sold as *turbinado* sugar. It does not differ greatly in nutritional value from white sugar.

Honey is about twice as sweet as white sugar.

Honey contains small quantities of minerals such as potassium, calcium, and phosphorus (but should not be considered as a source for any of these). The type of sugar found in honey varies, depending on the type and batch of honey. Sucrose is the dominant sugar found in clover honey; orange blossom honey contains mostly fructose. All honey, even raw honey, is heated to some extent during the necessary processing. However, some honey found in supermarkets is heated for unnecessarily long periods and at high temperatures, simply to keep it clear for a long shelf life.

Maple syrup, the sap of maple trees, boiled down, has a distinct flavor, popular for sweetening desserts. It is sweeter than white sugar but not quite as sweet as honey, and contains about 65 percent sucrose.

Molasses, a by-product of sugar refining, contains vitamins and minerals such as thiamine, riboflavin, iron, and calcium that are refined from white sugar. Molasses is about 50 to 70 percent sucrose. Blackstrap molasses contains even more nutrients because more sucrose is refined from it. Its sweetening power is about half that of white sugar, and its flavor is strong and distinct.

substituted for every two squares of melted bitter chocolate. The carob syrup sold commercially cannot be substituted for this ingredient.

The only other major differences between natural desserts recipes and those for traditional recipes are in the choice of fat and the use of salt. Vegetable oil and butter are favored over processed shortening, margarine, and hydrogenated oils. Butter—unsalted is the tastiest—imparts a great deal of its own rich flavor to baked goods and other desserts. When the butter flavor might interfere in a recipe, mild-flavored vegetable oil may be used instead.

In most dessert recipes salt is merely an added flavor. It is very easily dispensed with in foods such as these, which are primarily sweet.

Grain Sweeteners

Barley malt, corn, rice, and sorghum syrups are several grain sweeteners that can be used for some baked goods. These grain syrups are products of malting techniques (except for corn syrup, which is produced by the hydrolysis of cornstarch). Several of these sweeteners have been used commercially for years. All are available at natural foods stores for household use.

They impart flavor, color, and sweetness to baked goods. They can be used in baking in the same way honey is used. There are slight variations in the amount of sweetness and color each syrup contributes, but in general they are much less sweet than honey. Corn and rice syrups, with sweetening power equal to that of white sugar, are about the sweetest; dark corn syrup is less refined than light. Barley contributes the richest color. Made from maltose (fermented grain sugar), it has less than half the sweetening power of sugar. Rice is the lightest-colored syrup. Sorghum has a taste close to that of molasses.

These sweeteners enhance the moistness and keeping quality of baked goods as honey does. However, if used as the sole sweetener, too much may be needed to get the desired effect and the volume of the product may be affected adversely. For best results in volume and texture, grain sweeteners should be used in conjunction with another sweetener.

Choosing Desserts

When you start thinking of desserts in terms of natural food, you will soon realize how wide your choice really is—from a simple but elegant plate of fruit and cheese, to unadorned tea cookies, to a lavish nut torte laden with whipped cream. Of course, the kind of dessert you serve should complement the meal that precedes it. A simple rule is to use light desserts to end rich meals and richer desserts after light meals. At the same time, try to select desserts that will enhance the overall nutrition of the meal. For example, one might round out a light meal, such as a vegetable soup and a salad, with a dessert based on milk, eggs, or cheese, such as a custard, a cream pie, or cheesecake. Such dairy desserts are filling and rich in protein.

Try to avoid serving desserts that repeat part of the meal. For example, if fruit is an accent to the main course, it is redundant to serve a fruit-based dessert. Likewise, a custard or a milk-based pudding would be a poor choice to follow a meal that features dairy ingredients in cream soups or sauces, a quiche, or any egg and cheese dish. A fruit dessert would be much more effective.

Meals that include meat, fish, or fowl are usually quite substantial and are best topped off by a light, refreshing dessert such as fruit, fruit custard, or a light sponge cake.

Fruit Desserts

The most satisfying desserts are often the simplest. Fresh and dried fruits, cheese, and nuts are the rudiments of such desserts. For nutrition-conscious cooks, the generous food values in all these ingredients make them even more appealing.

Fresh, sliced fruit, sometimes enhanced by a touch of honey or maple syrup, is a fundamental pleasure. Dieters who must shun all other desserts often take refuge in a fruit-based one because, as desserts go, fruits are low in calories, yet provide a satisfying sweet. Fresh fruit eaten at the end of a meal to aid digestion is also an age-old tradition.

A beautiful bowl of fresh fruits, carefully combined, makes a very attractive and nutritious dessert. Skewered fruit chunks or fruit cups are equally handsome and appetizing (see Fruits chapter).

Fresh fruit served with cheese at the end of a meal is a popular European custom that can also be enjoyed as a snack between meals. Fruit may be served with any cheese but is most often paired with the semihard ones. Serve a variety of cheeses on a tray with different kinds of fruits.

Fruit desserts usually require less time and work than others. You can parboil or poach fruits, or bake, sauté, or broil them. Because they are naturally sweet, many fruits fit very well into baked desserts. Any kind of cooking only intensifies their natural sugar, lessening the need for additional sweetener. Fruit dumplings, cobblers, pies, and tarts are all favorites with dessert lovers.

Frozen and Chilled Desserts

Ice cream is the universal favorite among desserts. Based on carefully prepared, well-chilled syrups, rich custards, and heavy creams, it has a texture that is hard to resist—a most refreshing way to end any meal.

If you can afford the time, it is easy and fun to make ice cream at home with a hand-crank freezer, as in olden days. You can also speed things up by using an electrically powered freezer, or just make your ice cream in an ice cube tray without the divider. When you make ice cream at home, you can season it with any of your favorite flavors, using only natural ingredients. You will not have to concern yourself about the huge amounts of sugar, additives, or thickeners that characterize so many commercial brands.

In homemade ice cream the freezing process is what dictates the consistency of the final product. Ice cream, properly frozen and churned, will be smooth and not grainy. During the freezing process the water in the ice cream mixture begins to form ice crystals. Stirring this mixture as it freezes is what prevents those crystals from becoming too large and keeps the mixture pleasantly smooth. The stirring also aerates, therefore lightens, the mixture. In a home ice cream maker the churning does this job. When using the still-freeze, or refrigerator-tray, method, it is necessary to stir the mixture with a chilled rotary beater.

There are two basic types of ice cream: plain ice cream, which is made without eggs, and French ice cream, which uses whole eggs or egg yolks as a major ingredient. The eggs, which usually require some precooking, give the French ice cream a custard quality and make it the richest of all frozen desserts.

The water-based frozen desserts, such as ices, sherbets, sorbets, and granitas, are less extravagant. Unlike for ice cream, a grainy texture is desirable for some of these frozen desserts. That means they may be made in ice cube trays with only occasional blending to break down the ice crystals.

All of the following belong to the family of frozen and chilled desserts, including those that are completely frozen and those that must be thoroughly chilled but not frozen.

Ice milk can be made from the same recipes as ice cream, substituting milk for the cream. Whole milk or fat-free milk may be used. The texture and taste of the product will be different, but the result is quite satisfactory. For a softer, creamier ice milk, substitute milk for cream in a custard ice cream recipe.

Frozen yogurt is a popular variation on ice milk or sherbet, in which most or all of the milk is replaced by yogurt, producing a tangy flavor. Frozen yogurts are most often flavored with fruits, but they readily accept the same flavorings as ice cream. Low in calories and high in nutrition and flavor, frozen yogurt is a refreshing change from richer ice cream desserts.

Frozen soy desserts are somewhat lighter than frozen dairy desserts. They can be made by using most of the same methods used in making other frozen desserts. Soymilk and tofu readily lend themselves to most of the same recipes as frozen dairy desserts. Much lower in calories and fat, soy desserts provide a tasty alternative for those who must avoid dairy products and for anyone else who likes tasty desserts.

For a richer dessert, some cream or milk may be substituted for the soymilk called for in a recipe. Conversely, in richer recipes soymilk can substitute for some of the milk or cream.

Ices contain neither eggs nor milk; they are made with pure fruit juice, perhaps some honey, and crushed ice—all blended together, then frozen in an ice cream freezer or ice cube tray. To attain the same smooth texture in the ice cube tray as in an ice cream freezer, the ice must be beaten well and often during the freezing process. Starting one hour after the mixture has been put into the freezer, when the ice is set around the sides but still mushy in the center, the beating should take place every half hour until the ice is frozen solid.

Granitas are Italian ices with a snowlike texture.

Sherbet is made from mixtures of light syrups. It is a fine-textured fruit dessert generally water based. Traditionally, sherbets are seasoned with fruits, liqueurs, or heavy wines. Gelatin or egg white may be added to make sherbet smoother. If you use an ice cream maker, scrape the inside of the container from time to time to loosen any sherbet sticking to the sides of the can, but do not stir.

Sorbet is the French version of sherbet, made in the same way.

Frappés are similar to sherbet, but they have a mushier texture. Frappé may also refer to a combination of fruit or fruit puree and yogurt or milk pureed in a blender to form a thick beverage.

Parfaits consist of ice cream or whipped cream alternately layered with a topping in a tall glass. The topping is based on a boiled syrup to which flavoring is added, often in the form of crushed fruit or nuts. Parfaits should be frozen without being stirred.

Bombe, as its French name denotes, was originally a spherical-shaped frozen dessert. Today this layered frozen dessert, which may consist of ice cream and/or sherbet or ice, may be molded into any desired shape, provided the mold can be covered. The various layers are most often of contrasting flavors and colors. Sometimes the bombe mold is lined with cake or crushed cookies.

Mousses can be made with eggs or whipped cream or both. They are light and usually delicate, and almost any flavor works well. They may be set into a large mold, but more often they are set into individual molds such as sherbet glasses and chilled for about four hours before serving.

A *cold soufflé* is very similar in its light airy appearance to a hot soufflé. Instead of taking its volume from beaten egg whites alone, a cold soufflé relies on gelatin as well. The height of the soufflé may be extended with a collar of paper (see Procedure for Making a Soufflé Collar, below) that allows you to fill the mold above the original rim. In a layered frozen soufflé each layer must be thoroughly frozen before the next is added.

Procedure for Making a Soufflé Collar

For cold soufflés the wax paper collar and the soufflé dish should be oiled before the collar is positioned on the soufflé dish, to permit easy unmolding. (For a hot soufflé the dish and collar can be oiled or buttered.) The paper collar is made from a length of wax paper long enough to go around the dish with some overlap, and wide enough to extend two to three inches above the rim of the dish when folded in half. Fold the paper in half lengthwise and brush the inside of the collar with oil or butter. Position the collar around the outside of the dish, securing it with string or with paper clips.

Method for Churned Ice Cream

Chill the cream mixture and pour it into the freezer can, filling it no more than two-thirds full—to allow for expansion. Cover securely.

Fill the tub one-third full of crushed ice cubes, then layer ice and rock salt (or regular household salt) to a level slightly above the level of the mixture in the can.

Process (work the churn) until the ice cream is smooth and thick. If you use an electric freezer, the freezer turns off automatically when this point is reached.

Remove the dasher from the can and pack the ice cream down solidly with a wooden spoon.

The ice cream is now ready to be hardened. This can be done by repacking the tub of the freezer, surrounding the can with more ice and salt, and then covering the whole machine with burlap or newspapers; by removing the container from the tub, covering it, and placing it in a freezer to harden; or by spooning ice cream into a plastic container with a tight-fitting lid and placing it in the freezer. Whatever system you use, the finished ice cream should be allowed to mellow and harden for two to three hours before serving.

If you mix the ice cream ingredients well ahead of time and chill them for an hour or two in the refrigerator, the subsequent processing time will be reduced.

The texture of the finished product depends largely on how fast it is processed. The slower the freezing process, the smoother the texture. You can easily control the processing rate, and hence the finished texture, by varying the amount of salt you use. Using about three-quarters of a standard 26-ounce box of salt will result in a reasonably fast freezing action and produce a relatively smooth-textured finished product. Using up to a full box of salt will shorten the processing time and produce a coarser, more granular texture.

Method for Still-Freeze, or Refrigerator-Tray, Ice Cream

Prepare the mixture as directed and pour it into an ice cube tray without the dividers. Place the tray in the freezer compartment of your refrigerator (or a separate freezer if you have one) for about an hour, or until the mixture is mushy but not solid.

Transfer the ice cream from the tray to a chilled bowl and beat it rapidly (with a chilled

rotary beater) until the mixture is smooth. Work as quickly as possible to prevent melting.

Return the mixture to the tray, and when it has frozen almost solid, remove and beat again until smooth.

Cover the tray with plastic wrap to prevent ice crystals from forming on the top of the cream. Place in the freezer again to complete setting.

Custards, Puddings, and Hot Soufflés

Scores of desserts are based on various treatments of the milk-and-egg combination. Puddings, custards, and hot soufflés all take their character from this common foundation.

Although there is very little mystery involved in making these desserts, some basic precautions should be observed whenever cooking with eggs.

All egg dishes must be cooked gently and slowly. If a silky smooth custard is desired, it cannot be hurried. Too much heat or overcooking will cause it to curdle or weep.

Puddings enriched with eggs or egg yolks are essentially thick, sweet sauces and must be treated with the same care as savory sauces.

For successful soufflés it is essential that egg whites be properly beaten. They must be soft, billowing peaks, not firm or stiff, if the soufflé is to achieve its greatest volume and height.

Custards

Custards should be smooth, tender, and light. The techniques to achieve this are explained in detail in the Eggs chapter (see Custards, page 426).

The greatest danger with custards is curdling, and this is easily avoided by slow, gentle cooking. Stirred custards, or soft custards, are cooked in the top of a double boiler over simmering (never boiling) water, or in a heavy-bottom stainless steel saucepan. Whichever vessel you use, you must be careful to keep the heat low and stir constantly.

A hot water bath, or a *bain marie,* is a safeguard against curdling for baked custards.

Puddings

The consistency of puddings varies from soft and springy to thick and creamy. Their texture depends on the type of thickening agent used. Gelatin, whole wheat flour, arrowroot, or cornstarch may be used in addition to egg yolks to thicken puddings. Those puddings based on bread or whole grains such as rice, barley, wheat, or cornmeal have a natural viscosity and need no added thickening agent.

Like custards, puddings are usually prepared in the top of a double boiler or in a heavy-bottom saucepan. The slow cooking in this case is important to prevent scorching, and constant stirring is necessary to prevent lumping.

Steamed Puddings

Steamed pudding, an age-old preparation, is still very popular during winter holidays. This dessert is most often very dense and filling, but it may be made light and delicate.

The old English tradition uses suet, the hard fat around the kidneys and loins in beef, to bind and enrich these puddings. You can purchase suet from a supermarket or from a butcher.

The long cooking in humid heat keeps the pudding moist and permits the flavors of the ingredients to mellow and blend together. If you do not have a proper pudding mold, metal, ceramic, or ovenproof bowls can also be used. Coffee cans also work fine. If the mold does not have a lid, it may be covered with parchment paper or foil, secured snugly with a string. Butter the inside of the mold or container lightly and fill it only about two-thirds full to allow for rising and expansion. If using parchment paper or foil to cover the mold, butter the inside of that as well.

For steaming, select a pot at least four inches larger than your pudding containers so you will have about two inches of space on each side of the mold. Place a rack or steaming basket in the pot, and then place the mold or molds on the rack. Pour boiling water into the pot, around the mold, until it comes halfway up the sides of the mold. Cover the large pot and adjust the heat so that the water remains at the boiling point throughout the steaming period. Steam for the length of time suggested in the recipe.

Hot Soufflés

Hot soufflés, the lightest of fancy desserts, have an airiness that is remarkable, but fleeting. Soufflés are so delicate that they must be served almost immediately, or their fragile structure will begin to give way and set. Dessert soufflés are based on the same principle as savory ones. (See Soufflés, page 424.)

The base of a soufflé may be made in advance and stored in the refrigerator in a well-covered container. When you are ready to prepare the soufflé for serving, bring the mixture to room temperature before adding the beaten egg whites. Then bake immediately. To make an even, fairly firm soufflé, bake at 325°F for 30 to 40 minutes. To make a soufflé with a crusty top and soft center, bake at 375°F for 20 minutes.

International Specialties

The wide variety of desserts from around the world attest to the fact that an appetite for sweets is universal. Every culture seems to have developed several specialties. Some are as flamboyant and dazzling as Coeur à la Crème, while others are as modest as Crème Caramel. Many already incorporate all-natural ingredients or adapt very well to their use. After all, these recipes originated in Europe and other parts of the old world where honey and whole grain flours preceded refined white sugar and flour by several centuries.

Assembling most of these desserts requires no special skill. Where necessary, refer to information given in other sections such as for omelets, crepes, custards, or cakes.

Dessert Sauces and Glazes

Some desserts are perfect without further embellishment, but for many a sauce is just the thing needed to accent their goodness. Choose a sauce that will complement the dessert, not merely repeat the same texture and flavor. For example, a light fruit sauce provides an effective contrast of flavor, texture, and color for a creamy custard or a plain light cake. Tangy fruit sauces for cheesecakes and bread puddings are a traditional pairing. Sauces are also a perfect way to perk up leftover cakes or puddings.

Sweet sauces are very similar in nature to their savory counterparts, and the same precautions should be taken to avoid curdling or lumping when cooking them. The thickening agent may be whole egg, egg yolk, flour, cornstarch, or arrowroot. Milk, cream, or fruit juice may form the body of cooked sweet sauces. Flavorings for hot sauces should be added after the sauce has been removed from the heat; this avoids having their aromatic essences dissipate during cooking. Serve these sauces hot with desserts that are served hot, and well chilled with cold desserts. Most of these sauces can be made in advance and stored in the refrigerator in tightly sealed containers.

One cup of sauce is usually sufficient for four to six servings of desserts.

Glazes

Since they are thickened differently, glazes are somewhat lighter than sauces. Like sauces they may be made from any kind of fruit. The mixture of fruit and honey is cooked until it becomes syrupy, sweet, and brightly colored, almost like a jam but not as thick.

Glazes are usually used in smaller proportions than sauces. Their purpose is to enhance flavor and appearance and to add color. Glazes last about as long as jams. Store them the same way in the refrigerator.

Fruit-Based Desserts

Apple Crisp

> 4 large tart apples, sliced
> ½ cup raisins
> 1½ teaspoons ground cinnamon
> 1 cup corn germ
> ½ cup rolled oats
> 2 tablespoons honey
> ¼ cup butter, melted

Preheat oven to 350°F. Butter an 8-inch-square baking dish.

In a medium-size bowl combine apples, raisins, and ½ teaspoon cinnamon and place in prepared baking dish.

In another medium-size bowl combine corn germ, rolled oats, and remaining 1 teaspoon cinnamon.

Mix honey with butter in a small bowl, then combine with corn germ mixture. Spoon this mixture over fruit and bake for 30 minutes, or until apples are tender and topping is browned.

6 to 8 servings

Apple Pandowdy

This dish is even more American than apple pie, since it was an early New England favorite before the idea of putting the crust on the bottom took over.

> 6 medium-size tart green apples, peeled, cored, and thinly sliced
> ½ cup molasses
>   juice of 1 lemon
> 1 teaspoon ground cinnamon
> ¼ cup butter, cut into small pieces
>   pastry for 1 Rich Piecrust (page 719)

Preheat oven to 300°F.

In a deep baking dish or ovenproof casserole, combine apples, molasses, lemon juice, cinnamon, and butter. Blend well and bake for 1½ hours. Remove from oven to stir occasionally during baking.

Transfer to a buttered 9-inch pie plate and cover with crust. Make small slits in crust to allow steam to escape, increase heat to 375°F, and bake for 30 to 40 minutes longer, or until crust is golden. Serve warm.

6 to 8 servings

Apple Fritters

2 eggs, separated
½ cup honey, warmed
1 cup yogurt
2 cups whole wheat pastry flour
½ teaspoon ground nutmeg
½ teaspoon baking soda
1 tablespoon butter, melted
½ cup vegetable oil
4 tart apples, cored and cut into ¼-inch slices

In a medium-size bowl beat egg yolks with honey until smooth and light. Add yogurt and stir until smooth.

Sift together flour, nutmeg, and baking soda. Add to egg mixture, then stir in butter.

In a small bowl beat egg whites until stiff but not dry, then fold into mixture.

In a heavy iron skillet heat oil to 370°F, or until oil starts to smoke. Dip apple rings into batter and then fry in hot oil until golden brown on both sides. Keep fritters warm until all apples and batter have been used.

Serve hot with a small pitcher of maple syrup on the side.

Makes about 2 dozen

NOTE: Fresh peaches, pears, pineapple, or bananas may be substituted for apples in this recipe.

Baked Banana Dream

A hot banana dessert that brings citrus and cinnamon into the picture for an appetizing contrast.

2 tablespoons butter
6 bananas, split lengthwise
2 tablespoons butter, cut into slivers or cubes
    grated rind of 2 oranges
½ cup orange juice
3 tablespoons lime juice
½ teaspoon ground cinnamon or ginger
¼ cup honey
1½ cups crème fraîche (page 450)

Preheat oven to 375°F.

Melt 2 tablespoons butter in a large shallow baking dish. Roll banana halves in the melted butter

and coat well. Arrange them in a single layer on bottom of baking dish. Top evenly with 2 tablespoons slivered or cubed butter, orange rind, orange juice, lime juice, cinnamon or ginger, and honey. Bake for 15 minutes.

Serve hot, topped with crème fraîche.

6 servings

Blueberry Buckle

¼ cup butter
¼ cup honey
1 egg
1 cup whole wheat pastry flour
1 teaspoon baking soda
1/3 cup buttermilk or yogurt
2 cups fresh or frozen blueberries

Topping
¼ cup butter
2 tablespoons honey
1/3 cup whole wheat pastry flour
½ teaspoon ground cinnamon

Preheat oven to 350°F. Butter an 8-inch-square baking dish.

In a medium-size bowl cream together butter, honey, and egg. Add flour, baking soda, and buttermilk or yogurt. Mix well. Spread in prepared baking dish and cover with blueberries.

To make the topping: In a small bowl combine butter, honey, flour, and cinnamon until mixture resembles coarse crumbs. Spread over blueberries and bake for about 40 minutes. Cut into squares.

6 to 8 servings

Blueberry Supreme

2 egg yolks
½ cup nonfat dry milk
½ cup warm water
¼ cup honey
3¼ cups fresh blueberries
1½ cups yogurt
¼ cup pecans

Place egg yolks, dry milk, water, and honey in a medium-size saucepan. Cook over low heat, stirring constantly, for 20 to 30 minutes, or until thickened. Remove from heat.

Stir in 3 cups blueberries, fold in yogurt, and transfer to individual serving dishes. Top with pecans and remaining blueberries. Chill for 2 to 3 hours.

6 servings

Crusty Prune Delight

2 cups pitted prunes
2 cups apple juice
1 cup wheat germ
½ cup butter
¼ teaspoon ground cloves

Preheat oven to 350°F. Butter an 8-inch-square baking pan.

In a medium-size bowl soak prunes in apple juice until juice is absorbed, for several hours or overnight.

In a small bowl mix wheat germ with ¼ cup butter, then stir in cloves. Place ½ of mixture in prepared baking pan. Pour prune mixture over top, sprinkle with remaining wheat germ mixture, and dot with remaining butter. Bake for 35 minutes.

Serve topped with yogurt, if desired.

6 to 8 servings

Grapefruit Treat

A good choice for dessert after a heavy or too-rich meal, simple and original.

4 grapefruits
2 navel oranges
½ cup honey
½ cup unsweetened shredded coconut
½ cup almonds, grated
1 teaspoon grated nutmeg

Peel grapefruits and oranges and separate into segments. Arrange grapefruit segments on a large platter, inserting orange segments between grapefruit segments. Brush completely with honey.

In a small bowl mix coconut, almonds, and nutmeg together. Sprinkle mixture over grapefruit and oranges. Chill for several hours before serving.

8 servings

Fresh Fruit Ambrosia

4 navel oranges
3 ripe pears
6 slices fresh pineapple, ½ inch thick
3 bananas
1 cup orange juice
¼ teaspoon almond extract
1 cup grated fresh coconut

Peel oranges and slice crosswise into very thin slices. Peel and core pears, and cut into slices about ¼ inch thick. Peel and core pineapple slices, and cut into pieces about 1½ inches wide. Peel and cut bananas into slices about ¼ inch thick.

In a large serving bowl layer fruit, ending with oranges. In a small bowl mix orange juice and almond extract, pour over fruit, and chill for several hours to allow flavors to blend.

When ready to serve, top with a layer of coconut.

6 to 8 servings

Maple-Nut Cranberry Mold

3 cups fresh or frozen cranberries (12 ounces)
¾ cup maple syrup
1 envelope unflavored gelatin
1 cup apple juice
1¼ cups chopped celery
1 to 1½ cups chopped walnuts or pecans
endive
apple wedges

Put cranberries through a food chopper, using the coarse blade. Add maple syrup and let stand for 30 minutes, stirring occasionally.

In a small bowl sprinkle gelatin over ½ cup apple juice and let soften for 5 minutes. Heat over low heat, stirring until gelatin is dissolved.

Add gelatin, remaining apple juice, celery, and nuts to cranberries. Stir to mix and turn into a 4- or 5-cup mold. Chill until firm, 6 hours or overnight.

When ready to serve, unmold onto a serving plate and garnish with endive and apple wedges.

8 servings

Orange Custard

The orange slices are a pleasant surprise under the tasty topping and smooth custard of this dessert—good hot or cold.

5 navel oranges
¼ teaspoon ground cinnamon
¼ teaspoon ground nutmeg

Custard
1 cup butter
6 eggs
1 cup nonfat dry milk
1 teaspoon vanilla extract
½ cup honey

Topping
½ cup whole wheat pastry flour
½ cup date sugar
¼ cup butter
¼ teaspoon ground cinnamon

Preheat oven to 350°F.

Peel and slice oranges. Arrange in individual serving dishes or in a 1½-quart baking dish. Sprinkle oranges with cinnamon and nutmeg.

To make the custard: Place butter and eggs in a 2-quart saucepan. Blend well. Add dry milk, vanilla, and honey and cook over low heat, stirring constantly, until thickened. Pour custard over orange slices.

To make the topping: In a small bowl mix together flour, sugar, butter, and cinnamon until mixture resembles coarse crumbs. Sprinkle over custard and bake for 45 minutes. Serve hot or cold.

6 servings

Peach Cloud

This heavenly dessert sounds (and is!) too good to pass up if you have peaches and eggs on hand and need a show stopper in a hurry.

4 cups sliced peeled peaches
2 tablespoons lemon juice
2 tablespoons quick-cooking tapioca
¼ cup toasted sliced almonds
5 large egg whites
2 tablespoons maple syrup
¼ teaspoon ground cinnamon

Preheat oven to 375°F. Butter a 9-inch pie plate.

Arrange peaches in prepared pie plate. Sprinkle with lemon juice to prevent discoloration. Sprinkle with tapioca and almonds. (Save a few almonds to decorate top.) Bake, covered with foil, for 20 minutes.

Meanwhile, in a medium-size bowl beat egg whites until stiff but not dry. Add maple syrup and continue beating for a few minutes.

When peaches are softened, remove from oven and completely cover fruit with beaten egg whites. Pull egg whites into peaks with a spatula. Sprinkle cinnamon and a few almonds on top. Return to oven and bake for 10 minutes, or until lightly browned.

6 to 8 servings

Peach Cobbler

4 cups sliced peeled peaches
2 tablespoons honey
1 egg, well beaten
1 tablespoon tapioca
1 cup whole wheat pastry flour
1 teaspoon baking soda
1 tablespoon butter, softened
⅓ cup buttermilk
1 cup English Custard Sauce (page 663)

Preheat oven to 425°F. Butter a 9-inch-round baking dish.

Combine peaches, honey, egg, and tapioca in a medium-size bowl, then spread evenly over bottom of prepared baking dish.

In another medium-size bowl combine flour, baking soda, butter, and buttermilk. On a well-floured surface roll dough to ½-inch thickness. Prick dough with a fork and place loosely over peaches. Bake for 20 to 30 minutes.

Serve warm, topped with English Custard Sauce.

6 servings

Peachy Parfaits

8 unpeeled peaches, pitted
2 tablespoons lemon juice
¼ cup honey (optional)
1 cup nonfat dry milk
1 cup warm water
2 eggs, separated
fresh mint leaves

Place peaches in a blender and process until pureed. Stir in lemon juice and honey (if using).

In a medium-size saucepan mix dry milk with water. In a small bowl beat egg yolks slightly and add to milk. Cook over low heat until mixture is slightly thickened. Remove from heat and cool. Add pureed peaches to egg mixture.

In another small bowl beat egg whites until stiff but not dry, and fold into peaches. Spoon into parfait glasses and chill. Decorate with mint leaves before serving.

6 servings

Summer Dessert Omelet

This marvelous surprise works equally well as a brunch feature whenever the season provides the bounty of fruit for the perfect filling.

6 seedless white grapes, halved
8 fresh strawberries, quartered
1 banana, sliced
1 cup sour cream
4 eggs
2 tablespoons orange juice
½ teaspoon orange rind
1 teaspoon ground cinnamon
2 tablespoons butter

Mix together grapes, strawberries, bananas, and sour cream.

Lightly beat eggs, adding orange juice, orange rind, and cinnamon.

Melt butter in a medium-size skillet or omelet pan. Pour in eggs and cook over medium heat, lifting edges and allowing liquid on top to run off onto bottom of pan. Cook for about 6 minutes, or until omelet is firm. Place sour cream and fruit on one side of omelet, fold other side over it, and serve immediately.

4 servings

Frozen and Chilled Desserts

Basic Custard Ice Cream

1 tablespoon cornstarch
⅓ cup honey
2 cups cold milk
2 egg yolks, lightly beaten
2 cups heavy cream
1 tablespoon vanilla extract

In a small bowl combine cornstarch, honey, and ½ cup cold milk. Stir until smooth.

In the top of a double boiler, scald remaining 1½ cups milk. Stir in cornstarch mixture very slowly. Cook over hot water for 8 minutes. Add egg yolks and cook for 2 more minutes. Mixture should be thick and smooth. Remove from heat and cool.

Stir cream and vanilla into mixture and pour into the can of an ice cream maker. Process until mixture begins to freeze and thicken.

Spoon into a plastic container, cover, and place in freezer to harden.

Yields 3 pints

Variations:

Prune Custard Ice Cream: Add 1 cup pureed cooked prunes to mixture before or after processing.

Pumpkin Custard Ice Cream: Add 1 cup pumpkin puree, sweetened with ⅓ cup honey and seasoned with ½ teaspoon ground cinnamon, ⅛ teaspoon ground ginger, and ⅛ teaspoon ground cloves, to mixture before processing.

Basic Vanilla Ice Cream

½ cup honey
2 cups light cream
2 cups heavy cream
1½ teaspoons vanilla extract

In a small saucepan dissolve honey in ½ cup light cream over very low heat, stirring until well blended. Remove from heat and cool.

Pour remaining cream into the can of an ice cream maker. Add honey mixture and vanilla. Stir with a wooden spoon until well mixed and smooth. Process for 30 to 40 minutes, or until mixture begins to freeze and thicken.

Spoon into a plastic container, cover, and place in freezer to harden.

Yields 2 quarts

Variations:

Apple Ice Cream: Add 1 cup coarsely mashed applesauce to mixture after processing.

Bisque Ice Cream: Add 1 cup toasted, finely chopped almonds or hazelnuts to mixture before or after processing.

Mint Ice Cream: Add ½ teaspoon mint extract to mixture before processing.

French Carob Ice Cream

½ cup honey
½ cup Basic Carob Syrup (page 737)
2 tablespoons whole wheat flour
2 cups half-and-half
2 eggs
2 cups light cream
1½ teaspoons vanilla extract

In a medium-size saucepan combine honey, carob syrup, and flour. Place over low heat and gradually add half-and-half. Cook and stir until mixture begins to thicken.

In a small bowl beat eggs until fluffy. Add slowly to hot mixture and cook for 1 more minute. Remove from heat, cool, and chill.

Stir in cream and vanilla. Pour mixture into the can of an ice cream maker, chill thoroughly, then process until thick and smooth.

Spoon into a plastic container, cover, and place in freezer to harden.

Yields about 3 pints

Old-fashioned Vanilla Custard Ice Cream

4 eggs, separated
½ cup honey
1 teaspoon arrowroot
4 cups milk, scalded
2 teaspoons vanilla extract

In a medium-size bowl beat egg yolks lightly. Gradually add honey and arrowroot. Slowly stir hot milk into egg mixture. Pour mixture into a heavy-bottom saucepan and cook over medium heat until thick. Remove from heat, cool, and chill for several hours.

When ready to freeze, stir in vanilla. In a small bowl beat egg whites until soft peaks form, and fold into mixture. Pour into the can of an ice cream maker and process until thick and creamy.

Spoon into a plastic container, cover, and place in freezer to harden.

Yields about 1 quart

Peach Ice Cream

4 cups sliced peeled peaches
3 tablespoons honey
1 tablespoon lemon juice
½ teaspoon unflavored gelatin
1 cup heavy cream, whipped

Place peaches in a medium-size bowl. Mix honey and lemon juice in a small bowl and drizzle over peaches. Cover and set aside for 2 hours.

Drain fruit, reserving ¾ cup of juice. In a small saucepan combine reserved juice with gelatin and cook over low heat until gelatin is completely dissolved.

Place peaches in a blender. Add gelatin mixture and process at medium speed until peaches are finely chopped. Refrigerate.

When mixture begins to thicken, fold in whipped cream. Pour into the can of an ice cream maker and process until thick and creamy.

Spoon into a plastic container, cover, and place in freezer to harden.

Yields about 1 quart

Basic Vanilla Ice Milk

4 cups milk
⅓ cup honey
1 teaspoon vanilla extract

Pour milk into the can of an ice cream maker. Add honey and vanilla. Stir with a wooden spoon to dissolve honey, then process until thick and creamy.

Spoon into a plastic container, cover, and place in freezer to harden.

Yields 1 quart

Variations:

Tutti-Frutti Ice Milk: Add ¼ cup unsweetened shredded coconut and 1 cup mashed or pureed seasonal fruits such as strawberries, raspberries, apricots, peaches, and oranges to mixture after processing but before hardening.

Butterscotch Ice Milk: Boil ½ cup honey over low heat for 4 to 5 minutes until it is thick and dark golden in color. Remove from heat and beat in ¼ cup butter and ¼ cup milk or cream. When mixture is cool, add to basic ice milk mixture and process.

Fruited Milk Freeze

⅓ cup honey
2 teaspoons grated lemon rind
1 tablespoon lemon juice
2 cups milk
1 cup combined crushed unsweetened
    pineapple, mashed banana, and chopped
    orange sections

In a small bowl combine honey, lemon rind, and lemon juice. Mix well.

Pour milk into a large bowl and add honey-lemon mixture very slowly. Stir in fruit and pour mixture into 2 ice cube trays. Freeze until almost firm.

Return mixture to bowl and beat until light. Pour back into tray and freeze until firm.

Yields 1 quart

Peach-Almond Frozen Yogurt

1 envelope unflavored gelatin
¼ cup water or fruit juice
2 cups yogurt
1 cup mashed peaches
¼ to ½ cup honey
¼ cup chopped toasted almonds

In a small saucepan combine gelatin and water or juice. Place over low heat and stir until gelatin is completely dissolved, about 3 minutes.

In a medium-size bowl beat yogurt with a wire whisk until smooth. Stir in peaches, honey, and nuts, then fold in gelatin mixture. Whisk lightly until well blended.

Pour into 2 ice cube trays, cover, and place in freezer for 2 hours or longer.

Remove from freezer 20 minutes before serving.

Yields 1½ pints

Variation:

Pineapple-Pecan Frozen Yogurt: Substitute crushed unsweetened pineapple for peaches and pecans for almonds. Follow same procedure.

Maple-Banana Soy Freeze

3 cups soymilk
¾ cup maple syrup
2 teaspoons vanilla extract
½ cup heavy cream
1½ cups very ripe banana slices

Combine all ingredients in a blender and process until well blended. Pour into the can of an ice cream maker and process until thick and creamy.

Spoon into a plastic container, cover, and place in freezer to harden.

Yields 1 quart

Lemon Granita

½ cup honey
2 cups water
    grated rind of 1 lemon
1 cup lemon juice
    lemon slices

In a medium-size saucepan dissolve honey in water over high heat, stirring constantly. Boil for 2 to 3 minutes, while stirring. Remove from heat, stir in lemon rind and lemon juice, and pour into 2 ice cube trays.

Freeze until mixture begins to thicken. Stir with fork. Repeat this method until ice pellets form.

Spoon granita into parfait glasses and serve with lemon slices.

Yields about 1½ pints

Grape Ice

1 cup grape juice
1 tablespoon chopped lemon, with rind
1 teaspoon honey
1 cup ice cubes (about 6)

Place grape juice, lemon, and honey in a blender and process at medium speed until lemon is pureed. Then add ice cubes and process at high speed until mixture is a snowy consistency. Serve at once.

Yields about 1 pint

Grapefruit Ice

3 cups water
1 cup honey
2 cups grapefruit juice
1 tablespoon grated grapefruit rind
½ cup lemon juice

In a medium-size saucepan combine water and honey. Bring to a boil and simmer for 5 minutes. Add grapefruit juice, grapefruit rind, and lemon juice. Mix thoroughly.

Pour into the can of an ice cream maker and process until thick and smooth.

Spoon into a plastic container, cover, and place in freezer to harden.

Yields about 3 pints

Raspberry Ice

3 cups raspberries
½ cup honey
1½ cups water
2 tablespoons lemon juice

In a medium-size bowl combine raspberries and honey and allow to stand for 1 to 2 hours. Mash and strain through a fine sieve. (This should yield 1 cup puree.)

Add water and lemon juice. Stir well, then pour into the can of an ice cream maker and process until thick and smooth.

Spoon into a plastic container, cover, and place in freezer to harden.

Yields 1 quart

Orange-Banana Sherbet

1 cup honey
1 cup orange juice
½ cup lemon juice
2 ripe bananas, mashed (about 1¼ cups)
1 cup heavy cream, whipped
2 egg whites

In a medium-size bowl combine honey, orange juice, lemon juice, and banana. Mix well, and then chill.

Fold cream into chilled mixture. In a small bowl beat egg whites until stiff but not dry, then fold into mixture. Pour mixture into an 8-inch-square baking dish. Place in freezer until mixture is partially frozen, stirring occasionally to blend well.

Remove from freezer and beat with a wire whisk or electric mixer until slightly soft but not melted. Return to freezer and freeze until firm, 6 to 8 hours or overnight.

When ready to serve, dip baking dish briefly in hot water and invert onto a serving plate. Decorate with mint leaves and orange segments, if desired.

6 servings

Pineapple-Buttermilk Sherbet

3 cups buttermilk
1 cup crushed unsweetened pineapple
⅓ cup honey
3 tablespoons lime juice
1 teaspoon grated lime rind
1 egg white

In a medium-size bowl combine buttermilk, pineapple, honey, lime juice, and lime rind and mix well. In a small bowl beat egg white until stiff but not dry, then fold into mixture.

Pour into the can of an ice cream maker and process until thick and smooth, about 30 minutes.

Spoon into a plastic container, cover, and place in freezer to harden.

Yields about 1 quart

Raspberry Sherbet

2 cups fresh raspberries, mashed, or 2 cups frozen unsweetened raspberries, thawed, drained, and mashed
2 tablespoons honey
½ cup orange juice
4 cups milk
2 egg whites

In a large bowl combine raspberries, honey, orange juice, and milk and pour into the can of an ice cream maker. Process until partly frozen.

In a small bowl beat egg whites until stiff but not dry, fold into mixture, and continue to process until thick and smooth.

Spoon into a plastic container, cover, and place in freezer to harden.

Yields about 1 quart

Strawberry Sorbet

    1 tablespoon finely grated lemon rind
$1/3$ to ½ cup honey
    ¼ cup lemon juice
    3 cups pureed strawberries
    2 egg whites

In a medium-size bowl combine lemon rind, honey, lemon juice, and strawberries. Mix well, pour into ice cube trays, then place in freezer until partly frozen but still mushy.

In a separate bowl beat egg whites until stiff but not dry.

Beat partly frozen strawberry mixture until fluffy and then fold in egg whites. Return to freezer for at least 2 hours.

Yields about 1 quart

Melon Melba

    ¾ cup seedless red raspberry jam
    2 teaspoons lemon juice
    2 small cantaloupes or honeyball melons
    1 quart Basic Vanilla Ice Cream (page 643)
    1 cup heavy cream, whipped
    ¼ cup slivered almonds, toasted

Combine raspberry jam and lemon juice in a small saucepan and stir over low heat until dissolved and blended. Remove from heat, rub through a fine strainer, and cool to room temperature.

Cut melons in half and remove seeds and membranes. Cut a thin slice off bottom of each melon half so it will stand steadily. Line 4 individual serving plates with paper doilies and place melon half on each. Place scoop of ice cream in each melon half and spoon raspberry sauce on top. Place whipped cream in a

pastry bag fitted with a medium star tube and pipe decorative border around ice cream. Sprinkle with almonds.

4 servings

Brownie Bombe

For guests you want to impress with a dessert that is beautiful and delicious, try this. It can be prepared days in advance.

    1½ cups Raspberry Ice (page 646)
    1½ cups Basic Vanilla Ice Cream (page 643)
    1½ cups Tutti-Frutti Ice Milk (page 644)
    2 cups Carob Brownie (page 709) crumbs

Chill a 6-cup mold thoroughly.

Remove ice, ice cream, and ice milk from freezer and allow to soften slightly.

Spread ice in bottom of mold. Top with $1/3$ of the crumbs. Press to pack tightly. Add layer of ice cream. Spread evenly, then cover with ½ of the remaining crumbs. Press again. Spread with ice milk and add remaining crumbs. Press very firmly. Cover and freeze overnight, or until firm.

When ready to serve, invert onto a serving plate and cut into wedges.

6 to 8 servings

Variation:
    Granola Bombe: Substitute Granola (page 307) for crumbs.

Rainbow Parfait

    1½ cups Raspberry Ice (page 646)
    1½ cups Basic Vanilla Ice Cream (page 643)
    $2/3$ cup pureed peaches, sweetened to taste
        with honey
    $2/3$ cup pureed strawberries or blueberries,
        sweetened to taste with honey
    ½ cup heavy cream, whipped

Remove ice and ice cream from freezer and allow to soften slightly.

Divide ice into bottoms of 8 parfait glasses. Cover with peaches. Layer ice cream over peaches, and then cover with berries. Freeze for 1 hour.

When ready to serve, top each parfait with whipped cream.

8 servings

Vanilla-Grape Parfait

3 cups Basic Vanilla Ice Cream (page 643)
1 can (6 ounces) unsweetened grape juice
    concentrate
½ cup heavy cream, whipped

Remove ice cream and grape juice from freezer and allow to soften slightly.

Divide 1 cup ice cream into bottoms of 6 parfait glasses. Spoon ⅓ of grape juice over ice cream. Cover with remaining ice cream, then cover with remaining grape juice. Freeze for 1 hour.

When ready to serve, top each parfait with whipped cream.

6 servings

Spanish Cream

3 cups milk
1½ envelopes unflavored gelatin
¼ cup honey
3 eggs, separated
1 teaspoon vanilla extract

In the top of a double boiler, scald milk. Slowly add gelatin and honey. Lightly beat egg yolks. Pour a few tablespoons of milk mixture over yolks, then add egg mixture to milk mixture. Place over hot water and cook until thick and smooth. Remove from heat and add vanilla. In a small bowl beat egg whites until stiff but not dry, then fold into mixture. Pour into a 1½-quart mold and chill. Mixture will form 2 layers as it sets.

When ready to serve, invert mold onto a large serving plate and cover mold with a cloth dipped in hot water and wrung out. Allow to stand until molded cream drops onto plate.

6 to 8 servings

Carob Mousse

¼ cup water
¼ cup sifted powdered carob
¼ cup honey

2 tablespoons butter
2 eggs, separated
1 teaspoon vanilla extract

Combine water, carob, and honey in a small saucepan. Place over low heat, bring to a boil, and simmer for 5 minutes, stirring constantly. Remove from heat and cool for 2 minutes. Gradually add butter and egg yolks and stir briskly over low heat until mixture thickens. Stir in vanilla.

In a small bowl beat egg whites until stiff but not dry. Stir a spoonful of whites into carob mixture, then fold in remainder. When thoroughly combined, pour mixture into 4 individual serving dishes and freeze for 15 to 20 minutes.

4 servings

Maple Mousse

4 eggs
⅔ cup maple syrup
2 cups heavy cream, whipped
⅓ cup finely chopped nuts (optional)

In the top of a double boiler, beat eggs lightly, then gradually add syrup. Set over hot water and cook until thick and smooth, about 8 minutes, stirring with a wire whisk or wooden spoon. Remove from heat and cool.

Fold in whipped cream and spoon into individual soufflé dishes or parfait glasses. Freeze for several hours.

When ready to serve, top with chopped nuts (if used).

6 to 8 servings

Strawberry-Topped Brown Bread Mousse

Brown bread mousse, an old yet unsung delight, is a flattering accompaniment to the season's best berries. The mousse should be prepared a few hours to a day ahead to chill and set.

Mousse
5 slices whole wheat bread
5 eggs
4 egg yolks

¼ cup light honey
2 envelopes unflavored gelatin
½ cup orange juice
3 tablespoons water
¼ cup heavy cream, whipped
2 teaspoons vanilla extract

Topping
½ cup red currant jelly
2 teaspoons lemon juice
3 cups small fresh strawberries

Preheat oven to 350°F.

To make the mousse: Place bread on a baking sheet and toast lightly in oven on both sides until crisp. Then break into pieces and place in a food processor or blender. Process until you have coarse crumbs. Set aside.

In a large bowl combine eggs, egg yolks, and honey and beat until mixture is light and thick.

In a small saucepan combine gelatin with orange juice and water. Stir over low heat until gelatin is dissolved. Cool to room temperature.

Slowly add gelatin to egg mixture, beating constantly. Using a rubber spatula, fold in whipped cream, then bread crumbs, and finally vanilla. Pour mousse into a serving bowl and let stand in refrigerator for several hours or overnight, until thoroughly chilled and set.

To make the topping: Combine jelly and lemon juice in a small saucepan and stir over low heat until jelly is dissolved. Cool to room temperature. Cover top of mousse with whole strawberries, standing them bottom-side up. Brush each berry lightly with jelly glaze. Refrigerate preparation until serving time.

6 servings

Fruit Soufflé

1 envelope unflavored gelatin
2 tablespoons lemon juice
6 eggs, separated
⅓ cup honey
1 cup pureed fruit (strawberries, raspberries, peaches, apricots, or any seasonal fruit)
1 cup heavy cream, whipped

Prepare a 1-quart soufflé dish with a collar (see page 636 for directions for making a soufflé collar).

Soften gelatin in lemon juice.

In the top of a double boiler, beat egg yolks and honey until smooth and thick. Place over hot water, add gelatin, and continue to beat. Add fruit puree and stir until mixture thickens. Remove from heat and cool.

In a small bowl beat egg whites until stiff but not dry, then fold into mixture. Fold in whipped cream, spoon into prepared soufflé dish, and chill for at least 4 hours.

When ready to serve, remove collar and decorate with fresh fruit.

6 servings

Lemon Soufflé

1 envelope unflavored gelatin, dissolved in 2
    tablespoons water
    grated rind of 4 lemons (about ½ cup)
½ cup lemon juice, strained (juice of 2 lemons)
½ cup honey
7 egg whites
1 cup heavy cream, whipped
    mint leaves
2 tablespoons cookie crumbs
7 or 8 very thin lemon slices

In a small saucepan combine gelatin with lemon rind and juice, then add honey. Stir over low heat until gelatin is dissolved. Chill until mixture starts to jell.

Prepare a 1-quart soufflé dish with a collar (see page 636 for directions for making a soufflé collar).

In a small bowl beat egg whites until stiff but not dry. Fold into gelatin mixture, stirring carefully but thoroughly. Fold whipped cream into mixture, reserving about ⅓ cup for decoration. Spoon mixture into prepared soufflé dish and chill.

When ready to serve, remove paper collar and decorate with a border of whipped cream, mint leaves, a sprinkling of crumbs, and lemon slices.

6 servings

Piima Soufflé

The tang of piima imparts a fresh dimension to this handsome dessert.

2 envelopes unflavored gelatin, dissolved in 2 tablespoons cold water
2 tablespoons grated lemon or orange rind
¼ cup lemon or orange juice
⅓ cup honey
7 egg whites
1 cup pureed strawberries
1 cup piima (page 448)
fresh strawberries, sliced or halved

Prepare a 1-quart soufflé dish with a collar (see page 636 for directions for making a soufflé collar).

In a small saucepan combine gelatin with lemon or orange rind, juice, and honey. Stir over low heat until gelatin is dissolved. Remove from heat, transfer to a medium-size bowl, and cool.

In a separate bowl beat egg whites until stiff but not dry, and fold into cooled mixture. Then fold in pureed strawberries and piima. Spoon into prepared soufflé dish and chill.

When ready to serve, remove collar and decorate with strawberries.

6 servings

Custards, Puddings, and Hot Soufflés

Apricot-Currant Molded Custard

⅔ cup sliced peeled apricots
½ cup currants
¼ cup honey
4 egg yolks
1 teaspoon cornstarch
2 cups milk, scalded
1 teaspoon vanilla extract
1 envelope unflavored gelatin, dissolved in 3 tablespoons cold water

Lightly oil a 3-cup mold.

Puree apricots in a blender or food processor. Place in a small bowl with currants and set aside for several hours, or until currants are soft.

In a medium-size bowl gradually beat honey into egg yolks and continue beating for 2 to 3 minutes, or until well mixed and foamy. Beat in cornstarch. While still beating, slowly add milk.

Transfer mixture to a heavy-bottom saucepan and place over medium heat. Stirring slowly and constantly, cook just until sauce thickens enough to coat a spoon with a thin layer. Remove from heat and stir for several minutes. Stir in vanilla.

Stir gelatin into custard sauce, mixing until well combined, and refrigerate until mixture has thickened enough to form soft mounds when dropped from a spoon. Then stir in apricot-currant mixture. Pour into prepared mold and chill until firm.

Unmold and serve with warmed Apricot Glaze (page 664).

6 servings

Coconut Mounds

2 tablespoons cornstarch
1¾ cups milk
⅓ cup honey
½ cup brown rice, cooked
½ cup chopped pecans
1 teaspoon vanilla extract
3 eggs, separated
½ cup unsweetened shredded coconut
¼ cup very finely ground pecans

Preheat oven to 350°F. Butter 6 individual custard cups.

In a medium-size saucepan combine cornstarch, milk, and honey and cook over low heat until thickened, stirring occasionally. Remove from heat and stir in rice, chopped nuts, and vanilla. Beat egg yolks in a small bowl and stir in slowly, then pour mixture into prepared cups.

Place cups in a pan and pour hot water into the pan until it reaches halfway up the sides of the cups. Bake for 30 minutes, or until firm. Cool slightly, then unmold onto a buttered baking sheet.

In a small bowl beat egg whites until stiff but not dry. Spread on tops and sides of custards. Combine coconut and ground nuts and sprinkle over egg whites.

Return to oven and bake 5 minutes longer, or until mounds are lightly browned.

6 servings

Crumb-Pecan Molds

4 eggs, separated
¼ teaspoon cream of tartar
½ cup plus 2 tablespoons honey
1 cup whole wheat bread crumbs
¾ cup finely ground pecans
1 tablespoon lemon juice
½ teaspoon ground cinnamon
½ teaspoon ground nutmeg
½ teaspoon ground cloves
¾ cup apple cider or apple juice

Preheat oven to 350°F. Butter 8 individual custard cups.

In a small bowl beat egg whites until foamy, then add cream of tartar. Continue beating until whites are stiff but not dry. Set aside.

In a medium-size bowl beat egg yolks until thick and lemon colored. Add ¼ cup honey gradually and beat until light and fluffy. Beat in bread crumbs, nuts, lemon juice, and spices. Fold in egg whites. Pour batter into prepared cups and bake for 30 to 40 minutes, or until firm. Remove from oven and set on a wire rack.

Combine cider or apple juice and remaining honey in a small saucepan and bring to a boil. Pour some of this sauce on each custard. Serve warm with whipped cream.

8 servings

Rice Custard

This homey, traditional treat is a welcome reminder of the good old days, a change of pace from trendy dessert ideas that can become tiresome.

3 eggs, lightly beaten
⅓ cup honey
3 cups milk, scalded
½ teaspoon vanilla extract
1 cup cooked brown rice

½ teaspoon grated lemon rind
½ cup raisins
    ground nutmeg

Preheat oven to 350°F. Butter 6 individual custard cups.

In a medium-size bowl combine eggs and honey. Add milk slowly, stirring constantly, until mixture is smooth. Add vanilla, rice, lemon rind, and raisins. Pour into prepared cups and sprinkle nutmeg on top of each.

Place cups in a pan and pour hot water into the pan until it reaches halfway up the sides of the cups. Bake for 30 to 40 minutes, or until a knife inserted in center of custards comes out clean.

6 servings

Almond Cream Pudding

2 eggs, separated
½ cup heavy cream
¼ cup honey
¼ cup whole wheat flour
1 cup boiling milk
1 teaspoon almond extract
½ cup blanched almonds, lightly toasted and
    finely ground

Preheat oven to 350°F. Butter a 1-quart oven-proof casserole.

In a small bowl beat egg whites until stiff but not dry. Set aside. Whip cream in a separate bowl. Set aside.

In a medium-size bowl beat egg yolks until frothy, then gradually beat in honey. Continue beating until yolks are thick and lemon colored. Beat in flour. While still beating, very slowly pour in boiling milk in a thin stream.

Pour mixture into a 2-quart saucepan and bring to a boil over medium heat, stirring constantly. Cook until thick and smooth. Remove from heat and stir in almond extract and almonds. Fold in egg whites and whipped cream. Pour into prepared dish and bake for 35 minutes, or until golden and firm. Remove from oven and cool slightly. Serve while still warm.

4 servings

Carob Bread Pudding

3¾ cups milk
3 tablespoons sifted powdered carob
1 egg
2 eggs, separated
⅓ cup honey
1 teaspoon vanilla extract
4½ cups whole grain bread cubes
½ teaspoon honey, warmed

Preheat oven to 400°F.

Place milk in a medium-size saucepan. Add carob. Heat over low heat and beat with a rotary beater or wire whisk until well blended.

In a large bowl lightly beat 1 whole egg and 2 yolks, then beat in honey. Gradually beat in carob mixture and vanilla. Stir in bread cubes and let stand for about 10 minutes, then turn mixture into a 1½-quart ovenproof casserole.

Place casserole in a pan and pour hot water into the pan until water reaches halfway up the sides of the casserole. Bake for 1 hour.

Beat egg whites until foamy. Add warmed honey very slowly and continue to beat until stiff but not dry. Pile meringue in mounds on top of pudding. Return to oven and bake for 5 to 10 more minutes, or until lightly browned. Serve warm or cold.

4 to 6 servings

Cherry Bread Pudding
with English Custard Sauce

Cherries are an admirable addition to an old favorite.

4 slices whole wheat bread
2 tablespoons butter
2 cups tart cherries
⅓ cup honey
3 eggs
1 cup milk, scalded
1 teaspoon vanilla or almond extract
¼ teaspoon ground cinnamon
¼ teaspoon ground cloves
grated nutmeg
1½ cups English Custard Sauce (page 663)

Preheat oven to 325°F. Butter an 8½ × 4½-inch loaf pan.

Lightly spread both sides of bread slices with butter. Place 2 slices of bread in bottom of loaf pan, trimming to fit if necessary. Cover with cherries and place remaining 2 slices of bread on top.

In a medium-size bowl gradually beat honey into eggs and continue beating for 2 to 3 minutes, or until pale yellow. Gradually pour in milk, beating constantly. Stir in extract and spices. Pour mixture over bread and cherries. Sprinkle with grated nutmeg and let stand for 10 minutes.

Cover with foil and bake for 30 minutes. Remove foil and bake for 30 more minutes.

Remove from oven and let cool slightly before serving with English Custard Sauce.

6 to 8 servings

Cornstarch Milk Pudding with Pistachio Nuts

¼ cup plus 2 tablespoons cornstarch
4 cups milk
½ cup mild honey
2 tablespoons orange flower water*
2 tablespoons chopped pistachios, lightly toasted

In a small bowl dissolve cornstarch in 1 cup milk, stirring until smooth.

Place remaining milk and honey in a medium-size saucepan and add dissolved cornstarch. Slowly bring mixture to a boil, then lower heat and simmer, while stirring, for 3 minutes. Stir in orange flower water.

Rinse a 1-quart mold or 6 individual custard cups and pour in pudding mixture. Chill in refrigerator for several hours. Serve pudding unmolded on a serving plate or in individual cups, topped with toasted pistachios.

6 servings

*Orange flower water can be purchased in Middle Eastern grocery stores.

Crimson Classic

Use any red fruit to make this bright and light finale to a meal.

4 cups fresh red fruit (currants, raspberries, cherries, or strawberries, used alone or in combination)
3⅓ cups water

1/3 cup honey
1/3 cup arrowroot
1/2 teaspoon vanilla extract

Combine fruit and water in a stainless steel or enameled 2- or 3-quart saucepan. Bring to a boil, reduce heat, and simmer for 20 minutes.

Strain juice through a muslin cloth or bag.

Rinse saucepan and combine honey and arrowroot in it. Gradually add juice, stirring to combine well. Cook over low heat until thickened and clear, stirring constantly. Remove from heat and stir in vanilla. Pour into a bowl and chill. Serve with cream, plain or whipped.

4 to 6 servings

Custard-Crumb Pudding with Fruit and Meringue Topping

1 cup whole wheat bread crumbs
1½ cups milk
3 tablespoons butter
1/3 cup plus 2 tablespoons honey
3 eggs, separated
½ teaspoon vanilla extract
¼ teaspoon cream of tartar
2 cups fresh fruit (strawberries, raspberries, peaches, apricots, blackberries, currants, or gooseberries)

Preheat oven to 350°F. Butter a 1½-quart ovenproof casserole.

Soak bread crumbs in milk for 5 minutes.

Cream butter, then gradually beat in 1/3 cup honey. Add egg yolks, one at a time, and beat well after each addition. Beat in vanilla, then soaked bread crumbs. Pour batter into prepared casserole.

Place casserole in a pan and pour 1 inch of hot water into pan. Bake for 1¼ hours, or until firm.

Beat egg whites until foamy, then add cream of tartar. While still beating, gradually add remaining honey. Continue beating until stiff but not dry.

Remove pudding from oven and spread fruit on top. Cover with meringue, sealing edges, and bake for 10 more minutes, or until meringue is golden. Remove from oven and let cool. Serve at room temperature.

6 servings

Date-Nut Pudding

¼ cup butter
¼ cup honey
1 egg
1 cup sifted whole wheat flour
½ teaspoon baking soda
1/3 cup buttermilk
1 cup coarsely chopped dates
1 cup coarsely chopped pecans or walnuts

Preheat oven to 350°F. Butter an 8-inch-square baking pan.

In a medium-size bowl cream butter until light and fluffy. Gradually pour in honey and continue beating at medium speed of electric mixer for 1 minute. Add egg and blend well.

Combine flour and baking soda and add to creamed mixture, along with buttermilk. Blend and then add dates and nuts. Pour batter into prepared pan and bake for 30 minutes, or until it is light brown and springs back when touched. Remove from oven and let cool slightly. Serve warm with whipped cream or ice cream.

9 servings

Fruited Tapioca

One of those old reliables that benefits greatly from the simple addition of fruit.

1/3 cup quick-cooking tapioca
2 cups fruit juice or water
2 cups fresh fruit (peaches, apricots, strawberries, or cherries), cut into bite-size pieces
1/3 cup honey
1 tablespoon lemon juice

Combine tapioca and fruit juice or water in a stainless steel or enameled 2-quart saucepan. Let stand for 5 minutes.

Bring to a boil, stirring often. Remove from heat and stir in fruit, honey, and lemon juice. Pour into a bowl and chill. Serve plain or decorated with whipped cream.

6 to 8 servings

Variation:

Cranberry-Orange Tapioca: Use fresh whole cranberries and orange juice. Add cranberries with juice and tapioca. Increase honey to ½ cup.

Orange Bread Pudding

> 4 slices whole wheat bread
> 1¼ cups orange juice
> ¼ cup lemon juice
> 2 eggs, separated
> ¼ cup plus 2 tablespoons butter
> ¼ cup honey

Preheat oven to 325°F. Butter a 1-quart ovenproof casserole.

Tear bread into small pieces and place in a small bowl. Pour orange and lemon juices over bread. Set aside.

Beat egg whites in a separate bowl until stiff but not dry. Set aside.

In a medium-size bowl cream butter until light and fluffy. Gradually add honey and beat at medium speed of electric mixer for 2 minutes. Add egg yolks, one at a time, and beat just enough to incorporate after each addition. Stir in soaked bread. Fold in egg whites. Pour into prepared casserole and bake for 1 hour. Serve warm with whipped cream or ice cream.

> 4 servings

Variation:

Orange-Raisin Bread Pudding: Stir in ¼ cup raisins just before adding egg whites.

Maple-Walnut Tapioca Pudding

> 2 cups milk
> ¼ cup tapioca
> ⅓ to ½ cup maple syrup
> 1 egg, separated
> ½ cup chopped walnuts

In the top of a double boiler, combine milk, tapioca, and maple syrup. Cook over hot water for 15 minutes, stirring frequently.

Beat egg yolk, then stir a few spoonfuls of hot mixture into egg yolk. Mix well, then add to rest of hot pudding. Cook and stir for about 3 minutes. Then remove from hot water and cool.

Stir in nuts. Beat egg white until stiff but not dry and fold in, then refrigerate. Top with whipped cream, sour cream, or yogurt, if desired.

> 6 servings

Jam and Cake-Crumb Pudding

> ¾ cup Pound Cake (page 682) crumbs
> ⅓ cup milk
> ¼ cup plus 1 tablespoon butter
> ⅓ cup honey
> 3 eggs
> ½ teaspoon vanilla extract
> ¾ cup fruit jam or preserves (apricot, peach, strawberry, or blackberry)
> ¾ cup coarsely chopped nuts (pecans, walnuts, almonds, or hazelnuts)

Preheat oven to 300°F. Butter a 1-quart ovenproof casserole.

Soak cake crumbs in milk for 5 minutes.

Cream butter, then gradually beat in honey and continue beating for 2 minutes, or until thick and fluffy. Add eggs, one at a time, and beat well after each addition. Beat in vanilla and soaked cake crumbs, then jam or preserves and nuts. Pour batter into prepared dish and bake for 1¼ hours, or until firm. Remove from oven and let cool slightly. Serve while still warm, topped with whipped cream or ice cream, if desired.

> 4 to 6 servings

Pumpkin Custard Pudding

> ½ cup buttermilk
> ½ cup orange juice
> 1 cup pumpkin pulp
> 2 tablespoons butter
> ¼ cup honey
> ½ teaspoon ground nutmeg
> 2 tablespoons whole wheat flour
> 2 tablespoons water
> 2 eggs, separated
> ⅛ teaspoon cream of tartar
> 1 tablespoon honey
> ½ teaspoon orange extract or orange blossom water*

Preheat oven to 325°F. Butter a 1½-quart ovenproof casserole.

Combine buttermilk, orange juice, pumpkin, butter, honey, and nutmeg in a medium-size saucepan and blend well. Heat to boiling.

In a small bowl combine flour and water and stir into pumpkin mixture. Simmer for 20 minutes, or until thick and smooth, stirring frequently. Remove from heat.

Beat egg whites in a separate bowl until foamy. Add cream of tartar and continue beating. Gradually add honey and continue beating until stiff peaks form.

In another small bowl beat egg yolks lightly, stir a little pumpkin mixture into them, and then add yolks to pumpkin mixture. Blend thoroughly. Add orange flavoring. Fold in egg whites. Pour batter into prepared dish and bake for 1 hour, or until firm. Serve warm with whipped cream.

4 to 6 servings

*Orange blossom water can be purchased in Middle Eastern grocery stores.

Steamed Cardamom Pudding

The exotic flavor and aroma of cardamom will please those on the lookout for a different kind of pudding.

$1/3$ cup butter
$1/3$ cup whole wheat flour
$1\frac{1}{4}$ cups milk, scalded
4 eggs, separated
$1/4$ cup honey
$1/4$ teaspoon ground cardamom
$1/3$ cup ground almonds, pistachios, or cashews
$1/8$ teaspoon saffron

Butter a 2-quart steamed pudding mold or ovenproof casserole. Select a pan wide enough and deep enough to hold the mold or casserole. Place a rack in bottom of pan.

Melt butter over medium heat in a 1-quart heavy-bottom saucepan. Stir in flour and cook for several minutes, but do not brown. Pour in milk and stir until well blended. Cook over low heat until very thick and smooth, stirring constantly. Remove from heat and cool to lukewarm.

Beat egg whites in a small bowl until stiff but not dry. Set aside.

In a separate bowl combine egg yolks with honey, cardamom, nuts, and saffron and beat until frothy. Combine egg yolk mixture with white sauce and transfer to a large bowl. Fold in egg whites. Pour into

pudding mold or casserole and cover tightly with a lid or 2 thicknesses of foil or parchment paper tied with string. Set mold on rack in pan, pour boiling water into pan until water reaches halfway up the sides of the mold, and cover the pan. Set over low heat so that water boils gently, and cook for 2 hours. Add more water if necessary as pudding cooks.

Let cool for 10 minutes. Unmold onto a serving plate and serve with a hot Cherry Sauce (page 663) or Raspberry Sauce (page 664).

8 to 10 servings

Steamed Fruit Pudding

1 egg, beaten
$1/4$ cup honey
3 tablespoons butter or vegetable oil
1 cup pineapple juice
$1/2$ cup chopped raisins
$1/2$ cup chopped nuts
1 cup chopped dates
1 teaspoon vanilla extract
$1\frac{1}{2}$ cups whole wheat flour
$1/4$ teaspoon ground nutmeg
1 teaspoon ground cinnamon
$3/4$ teaspoon baking soda
$1/4$ cup yogurt

Butter a 1-quart mold. Select a pan wide enough and deep enough to hold the mold. Place a rack in bottom of pan.

In a large bowl combine egg, honey, butter or oil, and pineapple juice. Stir in raisins, nuts, dates, and vanilla. Mix well.

Mix together flour, nutmeg, and cinnamon. Add to liquid ingredients.

Mix baking soda and yogurt and add to batter. Pour into mold, and cover tightly. Set mold on rack in pan, pour boiling water into pan until water reaches halfway up the sides of the mold, and cover the pan. Set over low heat so that water boils gently, and cook for 1 hour. Remove from steamer and transfer to a 250°F oven. Bake for 1 hour.

Unmold pudding by inverting mold onto a large serving plate. Serve with warmed Cherry Sauce (page 663) or Raspberry Sauce (page 664).

6 servings

Fallen Nut Soufflé

Consider this recipe when fall winds shake down the nuts in your yard, or when nuts are plentiful in the market.

> 5 eggs, separated
> ½ cup honey
> 1 cup sifted whole wheat flour
> 1 cup nuts, finely ground (walnuts, pecans, almonds, or hazelnuts)
> ½ cup milk

Preheat oven to 350°F. Butter bottom and sides of a 1½- or 2-quart ovenproof casserole.

Beat egg whites until stiff but not dry. Set aside.

Beat egg yolks until frothy, then gradually beat in honey. Beat until thick and lemon colored. Beat in flour and nuts. Add milk and blend well. Fold in egg whites. Pour into prepared dish and bake for 45 minutes. Remove from oven and let cool on a wire rack.

4 to 6 servings

Apricot Soufflé

> ½ cup finely ground blanched almonds, toasted
> 1 cup firmly packed dried apricots
> 1 tablespoon lemon juice
> ½ teaspoon almond extract
> 1 tablespoon arrowroot
> 4 eggs, separated
> ⅓ cup plus 2 tablespoons honey
> ¼ teaspoon cream of tartar
>   whipped cream
>   blanched toasted slivered almonds

Preheat oven to 375°F.

Butter bottom and sides of a 1½-quart soufflé dish or charlotte mold and dust with ¼ cup finely ground almonds.

Place apricots in a small saucepan and just cover with water. Bring to a boil, then lower heat and simmer gently for 20 minutes, or until very soft.

Puree apricots in a blender or food processor. Transfer puree to a medium-size bowl and stir in lemon juice, remaining ¼ cup finely ground almonds, almond extract, and arrowroot.

In a medium-size bowl beat egg yolks until pale. Gradually add ⅓ cup honey and continue beating until light and fluffy. Beat in puree mixture.

In a separate bowl beat egg whites until foamy. Add cream of tartar and continue beating. Gradually add remaining honey and continue beating until stiff but not dry. Fold ¼ of the egg whites into apricot mixture and blend well. Fold in remaining egg whites just enough to combine. Pour batter into prepared dish and bake for 25 to 30 minutes. Remove from oven and decorate with whipped cream rosettes and slivered almonds. Serve immediately.

4 to 6 servings

Pineapple Soufflé

> ¼ cup finely ground cake crumbs or nuts
> ¼ cup butter, melted
> ¾ cup whole wheat bread crumbs
> 1 cup unsweetened crushed pineapple, drained
> 4 eggs, separated
> ¼ cup plus 2 tablespoons honey
> ¼ teaspoon cream of tartar
>   whipped cream

Preheat oven to 350°F. Butter a 1½-quart soufflé dish or charlotte mold and dust with finely ground cake crumbs or nuts.

Combine butter and bread crumbs in a small bowl and let stand for 5 minutes. Stir in pineapple.

In a medium-size bowl beat egg yolks until pale. Gradually add ¼ cup honey and continue beating until light and fluffy. Beat in pineapple mixture.

In a separate bowl beat egg whites until foamy. Add cream of tartar and continue beating. Gradually add remaining honey and continue beating until stiff but not dry. Fold ¼ of the egg whites into pineapple mixture and blend well. Fold in remaining egg whites just enough to combine. Pour batter into prepared dish and bake for 25 to 30 minutes. Remove from oven and decorate with whipped cream rosettes. Serve immediately.

6 to 8 servings

Dessert Crepes

Carob Crepes

These are marvelous rolled up with flavored whipped cream or topped with a dessert sauce.

¼ cup plus 2 tablespoons whole wheat pastry flour
3 tablespoons sifted powdered carob
3 eggs
1 tablespoon plus 1 teaspoon honey
¼ cup vegetable oil
⅓ cup milk

In a blender combine flour, carob, eggs, honey, oil, and milk. Blend at medium speed until smooth. Chill for 45 minutes.

When ready to cook, heat a 6-inch crepe pan or small skillet, and oil it lightly. Pour in about 1½ tablespoons batter, and tip pan quickly to spread batter over entire surface of pan. Cook for about 1 minute, or until edges brown and pull away from sides of pan. Then turn and cook other side for about 30 seconds.

Makes 1 dozen

Cheesy Apple Crepes

¼ cup ricotta cheese
½ cup grated cheddar cheese
¼ to ⅓ cup light cream
10 Carob Crepes (see above) or Whole Wheat Crepes (page 395)
1 cup water
½ cup honey
¼ teaspoon ground cinnamon
6 medium-size apples, peeled, cored, and sliced
¼ cup raisins

Beat together ricotta, cheddar, and enough cream to obtain a consistency that can be spread. Spread on crepes.

In a large saucepan simmer water, honey, cinnamon, apples, and raisins until apples are soft. Drain, reserving cooking juice. Divide mixture between crepes, folding each over to make a roll. Place crepes in a chafing dish. Bring reserved cooking juice to a boil, and pour over crepes. Serve immediately.

Makes 10

Ginger Peachy Crepes

Filling
½ cup honey
1 tablespoon cornstarch, dissolved in ¼ cup water
4 cups cubed peeled peaches
½ teaspoon vanilla extract
1 teaspoon ground ginger

8 Whole Wheat Crepes (page 395), warmed

Sauce
1 tablespoon honey
1 cup milk
2 teaspoons cornstarch
1 egg, beaten
½ teaspoon vanilla extract

To make the filling: Place ½ cup honey in a large saucepan. Add cornstarch to honey, mixing well. Heat, stirring constantly, until mixture thickens. Add peaches, vanilla, and ginger. Simmer until fruit is soft.

Divide between crepes, placing fruit on half of crepe and folding other half over filling.

To make the sauce: In a small saucepan blend together honey and ¾ cup milk. In a jar with a tight-fitting lid, shake together cornstarch and ¼ cup milk. Add to milk in saucepan. Cook until mixture thickens, stirring constantly. Add 1 tablespoon thickened mixture to egg, then pour egg mixture into saucepan and cook for 2 more minutes. Remove from heat and stir in vanilla. Spoon over crepes. Serve at once.

Makes 8

Ice Cream Carob Crepes

6 ounces carob chips
⅓ cup honey
⅓ cup light cream
1 tablespoon butter
½ teaspoon vanilla extract
2 tablespoons peanut butter
½ gallon Basic Vanilla Ice Cream (page 643)
10 Carob Crepes (page 657) or Whole Wheat
    Crepes (page 395)
1 cup heavy cream, whipped
¼ cup chopped pecans

In top of a double boiler, heat carob and honey. Stir in light cream, and heat until blended. Stir in butter, vanilla, and peanut butter. Heat until melted.

Put a scoop of ice cream on one side of each crepe. Fold over. Top with warm carob mixture. Add whipped cream and garnish with nuts.

Makes 10

Orange Crepes in Orange Sauce

A natural interpretation of a classic dessert, Crepes Suzette, that will never lose its popularity.

Orange Butter
¼ cup plus 2 tablespoons butter
¼ cup light honey
    grated rind of 1 large orange
1 teaspoon grated lemon rind

16 Whole Wheat Crepes (page 395)

Sauce
3 large oranges
¼ cup plus 2 tablespoons butter
¼ cup plus 2 tablespoons light honey
    juice of 2 oranges (about 1 cup)
1 tablespoon lemon juice

To make the orange butter: Use an electric mixer to beat butter in a small bowl until creamy. Add honey and beat until mixture is thoroughly combined and creamy again. Add orange and lemon rinds and beat again.

Spread orange butter on underside of each crepe (side cooked after crepe was turned in pan). Fold crepes in half and then in half again.

To make the sauce: Finely grate rind of 1 orange. Finely shred rind of another. Skin segments of both oranges and remaining orange. Set aside.

In a large skillet combine butter, honey, orange juice, lemon juice, and grated and shredded orange rind. Stir mixture over low heat until rind becomes translucent. Let sauce barely simmer for 5 minutes. Add orange segments and warm them briefly in sauce over low heat.

To serve, carefully place folded crepes in skillet of warm sauce and heat briefly until they are warmed. Use a large spoon to transfer individual portions of crepes and sauce to serving plates.

Makes 16

NOTE: The crepes, orange butter, and sauce may be prepared up to 1 day in advance, then combined at serving time.

Raspberry Cream Stacks

¼ cup plus 1 teaspoon honey
2 cups milk
3½ tablespoons cornstarch
1 tablespoon whole wheat flour
3 egg yolks, lightly beaten
¼ teaspoon vanilla extract
2 cups frozen raspberries, thawed and drained
    with liquid reserved
1 teaspoon lemon juice
12 Whole Wheat Crepes (page 395)
1 cup heavy cream

Place ¼ cup honey in a medium-size saucepan. In a jar with a tight-fitting lid, shake together ½ cup milk, 2 tablespoons cornstarch, and flour. Stir into honey. Slowly mix in remaining milk. Cook, stirring constantly, until mixture thickens. Stir 2 tablespoons hot mixture into egg yolks, then pour egg yolk mixture into saucepan. Cook, stirring constantly, for 2 more minutes. Add vanilla and set aside to cool.

Place raspberries in another medium-size saucepan. Shake ⅓ cup reserved juice and 1½ tablespoons cornstarch in a jar with a tight-fitting lid. Add to raspberries, along with lemon juice. Cook, stirring constantly, until mixture thickens. Cool slightly.

Spread cooled vanilla cream on 5 crepes. Stack them, one on top of the other, cream-side up. Top with a 6th crepe. Stack remaining crepes in the same manner. Spoon raspberry mixture on top of each stack. Cut each stack in 4. Whip cream with 1 teaspoon honey, and spoon onto top of individual servings.

8 servings

Tropical Crepes

1½ cups unsweetened crushed pineapple
1½ cups navel orange segments, skinned and cut in 3
¾ cup unsweetened flaked coconut
1½ cups yogurt
8 Whole Wheat Crepes (page 395)
yogurt, for topping

Mix together pineapple, oranges, coconut, and 1½ cups yogurt. Divide mixture between crepes and roll up. Serve with dollop of yogurt on top.

Makes 8

International Desserts

Baked Alaska

Success in producing this famous dessert lies in the timing. Get the meringue on quickly and completely, watch it carefully in the oven, and serve it fast.

½ gallon ice cream, any flavor, softened
1 Basic Sponge Cake (page 673)
10 egg whites, at room temperature
½ teaspoon cream of tartar
2 tablespoons honey, warmed
1 teaspoon vanilla extract

Line a 2-quart mold with plastic wrap. Pack ice cream into it, cover with plastic wrap, and place in freezer.

Cut cake so that it is 1½ inches larger than the opening of the mold on all sides. When ice cream is

very firm, unmold it on top of cake. Cover with wrap and return to freezer.

Preheat oven to 450°F.

Just before serving, beat egg whites until foamy. Add cream of tartar and then add honey, 1 teaspoon at a time, beating until egg whites are stiff but not dry. Fold in vanilla. Completely cover ice cream and sides of cake with thick layer of meringue. Make peaks in the meringue with a knife or spatula. Bake on baking sheet on middle shelf of oven for 3 to 4 minutes, or until peaks of meringue have browned and the rest is golden. Serve immediately.

6 servings

Cannolis

Italians serve these golden tubes of pastry stuffed with a sweet ricotta cheese mixture to their most honored guests. You will too.

1 cup whole wheat pastry flour
1 tablespoon honey
1 tablespoon butter, softened and cut into pieces
¼ cup white grape juice
oil, for frying
2½ cups ricotta cheese
2 tablespoons Basic Carob Syrup (page 737), or 1½ tablespoons honey and ½ cup finely chopped dried apricots or currants

Place flour in a medium-size bowl and make a well in center. Place 1 tablespoon honey and butter in well. Add grape juice and work into flour to form dough. On a floured surface roll out dough to ⅛-inch thickness. Cut into 3½-inch squares. Roll around cannoli forms (or similar cylinders) so that 2 corners overlap in center. Wet and press corners together.

Pour oil into a Dutch oven to a depth of ¾ inch and heat to 370°F. Fry pastries a few at a time, turning occasionally, until they are golden, about 8 minutes. Slip cannoli shells off forms by holding forms with tongs and pushing shells. Drain on paper toweling.

Mix together ricotta and carob syrup or honey and fruit. Stuff shells carefully not more than 2 hours before serving.

Makes about 1 dozen

Charlotte Russe

Ladyfingers encase a rich mousse in this justly famous dessert. You can serve slim slices since it is so satisfying.

> 20 single Ladyfingers (page 673)
> 4 egg yolks
> 3 tablespoons honey
> 1 cup milk
> 1 piece vanilla bean, 1 inch long
> 1 envelope unflavored gelatin, dissolved in 2
>   tablespoons cold water
> 1 cup heavy cream, whipped

Line a 1-pint charlotte mold or small casserole with ladyfingers. Cut ladyfingers to fit together as tightly as possible along bottom and sides of mold.

In a small bowl combine egg yolks and honey. Stir until smooth and creamy.

In top of a double boiler, scald milk with vanilla bean and gradually pour it over egg mixture, stirring briskly. Return mixture to double boiler and place over hot water. Cook, stirring constantly, until smooth and thick. Remove from heat and discard vanilla bean. Add gelatin and stir until dissolved. Cool.

Fold in whipped cream (reserving ½ cup for decoration) and pour pudding into prepared mold. Chill.

When ready to serve, unmold onto a serving plate and decorate lightly with whipped cream.

> 4 to 6 servings

Cherry Bakewell Tart

This starts where other cherry tarts leave off, since the delectable cherry filling is topped with a fluffy nutty batter and whipped cream.

> 1 baked Basic Rolled Piecrust (page 718)
> 1 cup cherry preserves or chopped sweet
>   cherries
> ¼ cup honey, if using pitted cherries (optional)
> ½ teaspoon grated lemon rind
> 1 tablespoon lemon juice
> 4 egg whites, at room temperature
> 4 egg yolks

> ⅓ cup honey
> ½ cup whole wheat flour
> ⅓ cup chopped hazelnuts, toasted
> ½ cup heavy cream

Set piecrust aside to cool. Reduce heat to 350°F.

Mix cherries, ¼ cup honey (if used), lemon rind, and lemon juice.

Beat egg whites until stiff but not dry.

Beat egg yolks until thick and lemon colored, adding ⅓ cup honey. Mix flour and nuts into egg yolks. Fold in beaten egg whites. Spread cherry mixture on bottom of pie shell. Turn batter into pie shell over cherries, and bake until a wooden pick inserted in center comes out clean, about 25 minutes. Cool well. Whip cream until it stands in peaks and mound in middle of tart.

> 6 servings

Coeur à la Crème

Beautiful, extravagant, and perfect for a real occasion, this dish is easy to prepare and sure to please. Of course, the classic molds are heart shaped and nice to have, but not necessary.

> 1½ cups cottage cheese
> 1 cup heavy cream
> 1 teaspoon honey
> 2 cups fresh strawberries, raspberries, peaches,
>   or currants
> 1 teaspoon lemon juice
> 1 teaspoon grated lemon rind
> 1 tablespoon honey, or to taste

Rub cottage cheese through a sieve into a mixing bowl. Stir in cream and honey, and beat with an electric mixer at medium speed until mixture is thick.

Press cheese mixture into 6 individual *coeur à la crème* molds or a muslin-lined bowl-shaped sieve. (The container you use must have holes or perforations to allow liquid to drain.) Place molds or sieve over a pan or bowl, cover with plastic wrap, and allow to drain overnight in refrigerator.

When ready to serve, combine fruit, lemon juice, lemon rind, and honey.

If using molds, unmold cream onto individual serving plates, surround with fruit, and serve immediately. If using sieve, unmold mound of cream onto center of a large serving plate and surround with fruit. Cut into 6 wedges, and serve immediately on individual serving plates.

6 servings

Crème Caramel

Every French restaurant has this light and refreshing dessert engraved on the menu. Just a simple custard with a thin, flavorful sauce that is a perfect ending for a meal.

¼ cup plus 1 tablespoon honey
2 tablespoons water
2 eggs
2 egg yolks
2 cups milk
1 teaspoon vanilla extract

Preheat oven to 325°F.

In a small saucepan heat ¼ cup honey and water, stirring until honey is dissolved. Boil rapidly until syrup is golden brown. Do not stir. Remove from heat and pour into 5 individual custard cups. Allow caramel to cool and set.

In a medium-size bowl combine eggs and egg yolks. Beat very lightly with a wire whisk, then add milk and 1 tablespoon honey. Stir until mixed evenly. Add vanilla. Strain.

Pour custard into cups on top of caramel. Place cups in a pan and pour hot water into the pan until water reaches halfway up the sides of the custard cups. Bake for about 25 minutes, or until center of custard is set.

5 servings

Greek Walnut Cake

½ cup butter, softened
½ cup honey, warmed
8 egg yolks
8 egg whites, at room temperature
½ teaspoon cream of tartar
2½ cups whole wheat pastry flour, sifted
2 teaspoons baking powder
2 teaspoons ground allspice
2½ cups chopped walnuts
1/3 cup yogurt
1 cup honey

¾ cup water
½ cup date sugar

Preheat oven to 350°F. Butter 2 9-inch-round baking pans.

In a large bowl cream together butter and warmed honey. Beat egg yolks in a small bowl and add to butter, beating until well mixed.

In a separate bowl beat egg whites and cream of tartar until soft peaks form. Fold into butter mixture.

Sift together flour, baking powder, and allspice. Add to butter mixture. Stir in 2 cups walnuts, and then yogurt. Bake in prepared pans for 25 minutes, or until a wooden pick inserted in center comes out clean. Cool on wire racks.

Boil together honey, water, and date sugar for about 2 minutes. Add remaining ½ cup walnuts. Pour ½ of the syrup over one layer, top with second layer, and pour remaining syrup over top of cake. Allow to set for 1 hour before serving.

10 servings

Halva

Featherlight and rich as satin, this classic cake is drenched in honey syrup in the style of the Middle East.

½ cup butter
1/3 cup honey, warmed
2 eggs
1 cup farina, uncooked
½ teaspoon ground cinnamon
½ cup finely chopped almonds
¼ cup honey
¼ cup water

Preheat oven to 350°F. Butter an 8-inch-square baking pan.

In a medium-size bowl cream butter. Add warmed honey and mix well. Beat in eggs, one at a time. Gradually fold in farina, cinnamon, and almonds. Pour into prepared pan and bake for 30 minutes.

Remove from oven and cool for 15 minutes.

Simmer honey and water for 10 minutes and pour over *halva*. Cool and cut into squares or diamonds.

8 servings

Trifle

Though the English christened this dish trifle, it is anything but that—rich, flavorful, and fancy, it is a major attraction whenever it is served.

1 piece Pound Cake (page 682) about
8 × 8 × 1 inch
1/3 cup Raspberry Sauce (page 664)
1/2 cup slivered almonds
2 cups fresh fruit (raspberries, strawberries, sliced peaches, blueberries, or cherries) or unsweetened frozen fruit, defrosted and drained
2 cups English Custard Sauce (page 663)
1 cup heavy cream, whipped

Select a glass serving bowl about 7 inches in diameter and 3 inches deep.

Cut several pieces of cake (enough to line the bottom of the dish), and coat them with raspberry sauce. Arrange coated pieces in the bottom of the bowl. Cover with remaining sauce.

Cut rest of cake into cubes, and scatter over cake slices. Sprinkle 1/2 of the almonds over cubes.

Spread 1/2 of the fruit over cake, then spoon custard over fruit. Next, add whipped cream, smoothing over the surface. Decorate cream with remaining fruit and almonds.

6 to 8 servings

Oeufs à la Neige

Many remember this perennial favorite as Floating Island dessert, a childhood treat that retains its appeal at any age. The raspberry sauce adds a touch of sophistication.

8 egg yolks
1/4 cup plus 1 tablespoon honey, warmed
2 cups milk, scalded
1 teaspoon vanilla extract
5 egg whites
1/4 cup Raspberry Sauce (page 664)

In top of a double boiler, beat egg yolks until foamy. Then add 1/4 cup honey and beat until smooth. Place over hot water, add milk, and cook, without boiling, until custard is thick. Add vanilla and strain into a serving dish.

Beat egg whites until foamy. Continue to beat while adding remaining honey very slowly. Beat until mixture is stiff but not dry.

Pour water into a deep open skillet to a depth of about 1 1/2 inches and heat to simmering. Using 2 dessert spoons, shape egg whites into egg-shaped mounds and slide them into simmering water. Be sure they do not touch bottom.

Poach "eggs" for about 1 1/2 minutes on each side. Carefully remove from pan with a slotted spoon and place on paper towels to drain. When all "eggs" have been poached, set them to float on the custard and chill for several hours, uncovered. Do not store for a long period or "eggs" might begin to weep. When ready to serve, decorate with raspberry sauce.

6 servings

NOTE: Most recipes for *Oeufs à la Neige* recommend poaching the egg whites in milk, which tends to produce a gummy, sticky meringue. Poaching in water yields a light, tender meringue, which holds up very well and is easy to prepare.

Mont-Blanc au Marrons
(Chestnut Puree with Whipped Cream)

The French love chestnuts and use them at every opportunity. This celestial combination shows their subtle flavor and character to great advantage.

1 1/2 pounds chestnuts
3 cups milk
1 piece vanilla bean, 1 inch long, split
1/2 cup water
1/3 cup honey
2 tablespoons butter
1/2 teaspoon cinnamon
1 cup heavy cream, whipped
ground nutmeg

Boil chestnuts in enough water to cover for 8 minutes. Drain. While still hot, shell and peel. (There should be about 3 cups shelled chestnuts.) Place peeled chestnuts in a heavy-bottom saucepan with enough milk to cover. Add vanilla bean and cook until chestnuts are mealy and tender, 20 to 30 minutes. Discard vanilla bean. Force chestnuts through a food mill, using some of the hot cooking liquid to moisten, if necessary.

Combine water and honey in a small saucepan. Cook, uncovered, for 8 minutes. Then blend with pureed chestnuts, beating vigorously with a wooden spoon to make a thick paste. Cool. Stir in butter. Force mixture through a ricer, letting strands fall freely onto a large chilled serving plate to form a mound. Dust lightly with cinnamon. Spoon whipped cream over top third of mound to resemble a snowcapped mountain. Sprinkle with a little nutmeg and chill until serving time.

6 servings

Sauces and Glazes

English Custard Sauce (Hot or Cold)

4 egg yolks
1/3 cup light honey
2 teaspoons vanilla extract
1½ cups light cream
½ cup heavy cream, whipped (optional)

In a medium-size bowl beat egg yolks, honey, and vanilla until mixture is light and thick.

Place light cream in a medium-size saucepan and bring to a boil slowly. Pour hot cream slowly into egg yolk mixture, beating constantly. Transfer mixture to saucepan and stir over low heat until it coats the back of a spoon.

For fluffy sauce add whipped cream. For hot serving, fold whipped cream into hot sauce and serve over bread puddings, steamed puddings, or cobblers. For cold serving, chill sauce, fold in whipped cream, and serve over chilled fresh fruit.

Yields 2 cups

Cherry Sauce

Sour cherries are not always available, but they make the best sauce. If you have plenty of freezer space, make the sauce in quantity when cherries are in season and freeze in small containers, ready for use.

2 cups fresh sour cherries, pitted
3 tablespoons honey
2 teaspoons cornstarch
¼ cup water

Place cherries in a blender and process at medium speed until chopped but not pureed.

Place chopped cherries in a small saucepan. Add honey and stir over low heat until just below boiling.

Mix cornstarch and water, and add to cherries. Cook slowly until thick and smooth.

Serve hot over steamed puddings or dessert crepes, or chill and serve cold over ice cream, puddings, custards, pancakes, or waffles.

Yields about 2 cups

NOTE: Any kind of cherries may be used for sauce — sweet, Oxheart, or Bing — but if you substitute sweet cherries, be sure to use less sweetening, or none at all, according to your taste.

Lemon Sauce

¼ cup honey
1 tablespoon cornstarch or arrowroot*
1 cup boiling water
2 tablespoons butter
3 tablespoons lemon juice
1 teaspoon lemon rind

Combine honey and cornstarch or arrowroot in a small saucepan and blend well.

Very slowly add boiling water, stirring constantly. Simmer for 5 minutes. Remove from heat and stir in butter, lemon juice, and lemon rind.

Serve hot over molasses cake, steamed puddings, baked apples, or apple dumplings, or chill and serve cold over fruit tarts.

Yields about 1½ cups

*NOTE: If arrowroot is used, sauce cannot be reheated.

Raspberry Sauce

> 2 cups fresh raspberries, or 2 packages (10
>   ounces each) frozen raspberries
> 3 tablespoons honey
> 2 teaspoons cornstarch
> ¼ cup water

In a small saucepan combine raspberries and honey. Stir over low heat until just below boiling.

Mix cornstarch and water and add to berry-honey mixture. Cook slowly until thick and smooth, 5 to 7 minutes. Strain sauce through a coarse sieve.

Serve hot over crepes or custards, or chill and serve cold over pancakes, ice cream, or fresh fruit.

Yields about 2 cups

Rhubarb Dessert Sauce

This is a good sauce to know about, for it will perk up the flavor of a bland custard or cake and turn vanilla ice cream into something special.

> 2 cups ½-inch chunks rhubarb, cut across
>   stem fibers
> ½ cup orange juice
> 1 teaspoon orange rind
> ½ teaspoon ground cinnamon
> ⅓ cup honey
> 1 tablespoon prepared jam from a red fruit

Combine rhubarb, orange juice, orange rind, and cinnamon in a heavy stainless steel or enameled saucepan. Cover and cook over medium heat until rhubarb begins to get tender, about 10 minutes. Stir in honey and jam and cook over medium-high heat, stirring gently, until thickened. Try to keep rhubarb in distinct pieces. Serve either warm or chilled.

Yields 1½ cups

Almond Glaze

> 3 tablespoons butter, softened
> ¾ cup honey
> 1 tablespoon heavy cream
> ½ teaspoon almond extract

Beat together butter and honey in a small bowl. Beat in cream and almond extract. Pour over cake or coffee cake and refrigerate.

Yields about 1 cup

Apricot Glaze

> 2 cups chopped apricots
> 1 thin slice lemon with peel, chopped
> ⅓ cup honey

In a medium-size saucepan combine apricots, lemon, and honey. Heat slowly over low heat until honey is dissolved and fruit becomes juicy. Pour mixture into a blender and process at medium speed until completely pureed. Return to saucepan and cook slowly for 5 to 8 minutes, stirring so glaze will not scorch.

Brush over dessert crepes or cakes while warm, or chill and use as an icing for carrot cake or a filling for cookies.

Yields 1¾ cups

Red Currant Glaze

2 cups red currants
1 to 2 tablespoons water
$1/_3$ cup honey

Place currants in a small saucepan. With a fork crush currants against side of pan. Add just enough water to keep fruit from scorching. Cover and cook over low heat for about 5 minutes. Strain through a dampened cheesecloth jelly bag. Do not squeeze or press bag.

When all juice is extracted, pour juice into a heavy-bottom saucepan. Add honey and boil over medium heat for about 8 minutes.

Chill and serve cold as a topping for fruit tarts or cheese pies, or add to custards or ice cream for flavor.

Yields about 1 cup

Raspberry Glaze

½ cup honey
½ cup water
2 cups crushed fresh raspberries

Boil honey and water together slowly for about 12 minutes. Add berries and cook for another minute. Cool.

Chill and serve cold as a topping for fruit tarts or as a filling for cookies or layer cakes.

Yields about 2 cups

Pineapple Glaze

1 cup finely chopped fresh pineapple
1 tablespoon honey

In a small saucepan cook pineapple with honey over low heat for 12 to 15 minutes, or until slightly thickened and syrupy.

Chill and serve cold as a topping for cheese pies, torten, tarts, and pancakes, or as a filling for cookies.

Yields about 1 cup

Cakes, Cookies, and Confections

Cakes, cookies, and confections are among the most adaptable desserts. They can be created as stunning centerpieces for special occasions, or they can be the plain and simple goodies that serve so well as everyday desserts and snacks. Elaborate or modest, these items all reach new heights when made with natural ingredients.

Cakes

Making cakes is usually a simple process, even for an inexperienced cook, but it is important to pay close attention to the recipe directions. Begin by reading a recipe through, to make sure you have all the ingredients and understand how much time and effort will be involved. The measurements are given as precisely as possible, so follow them for best results. Measure all ingredients carefully. Although fancy equipment is not necessary, measuring cups and spoons, and small and large bowls are essential.

Use only the best-quality and freshest ingredients when you make a cake. Generally speaking, ingredients should be brought to room temperature before mixing for best results. Eggs will have greater volume, and butter will cream faster and become fluffier. However, if eggs must be separated, it is easier to do so before they reach room temperature.

Always make sure you have the proper type and size pan required for the recipe. The wrong-size pan can affect the cooking time and the texture of the cake. When the pan is too big, for example, the batter spreads out more than it should, so it bakes faster and doesn't rise well; when the pan is too small, the batter bakes more slowly because it is too tightly confined, and the rising cake will spill over the pan for the same reason. If the recipe calls for a preheated oven, be sure to follow the directions, and check the accuracy of the oven temperature.

Pay close attention to the mixing procedure called for in each cake recipe, such as *beating, blending,* and *creaming* (see Cake Mixing Terms, page 667). These steps are usually given in the order necessary for the most desirable results. Unless a recipe specifies otherwise, the batter is usually beaten just long enough to blend the ingredients evenly. Overbeating will give a dense-textured cake, and underbeating can cause the cake to be too coarse or have large holes in it. In general, it should take no longer than eight to ten minutes to add all the ingredients and blend them. With a little experience you will be able to tell when the beaten batter is just right, by its texture and appearance.

Types of Cakes

By tradition there are three categories of cakes, and these are determined by the type of leavening used for each.

Butter or *creamed cakes* are made with butter or vegetable oil and are leavened with baking powder or baking soda. If baking soda (which is alkaline) is used, molasses, sour milk, yogurt, or another acid ingredient must also be included in the recipe to neutralize the taste of the baking soda and to start the leavening process. (See Leavenings for Quick Breads, page 356.)

Angel food or *sponge cakes* made from light, foamy batters rely on the leavening power of egg whites. They contain no oil or butter and are ideal for those on fat-restricted diets. Sponge cakes contain only the fat from egg yolks, added separately from the beaten whites.

Torten are not as mysterious as their reputation makes them out to be, but they are unusual. They differ from other cakes in the use of cake or bread crumbs or ground nuts instead of flour as a base. They are enriched by the addition of egg yolks, but lightened by egg whites, and they contain no other added fat such as butter.

Cake Mixing Terms

Beating is mixing ingredients vigorously in a circular motion, using a long wooden spoon, a wire whisk, or an electric mixer.

Blending is mixing two or more ingredients together until an even and consistent mixture is attained.

Creaming is commonly done to butter alone or butter with a second ingredient. It is done by working the ingredients vigorously with a long wooden spoon or an electric mixer until a pale, fluffy, creamy mixture is attained.

Folding always refers to a slow and careful manual mixing of ingredients, often beaten egg whites with batter, so that the individual texture of each is maintained in the mixture.

Procedure for Making Cakes

For most cake recipes the combined dry ingredients are added alternately with the liquid ingredients to the mixture of creamed butter or oil, honey, and egg. This is an efficient way to blend ingredients without overmixing, so the result is an even-textured cake.

First, using butter that is at room temperature (about 70°F), cream it by repeatedly working it against the side of a large bowl with the back of a wooden spoon or by beating it at low speed with an electric mixer until it is a creamy, light color. Next, add the honey (warmed to make it flow and blend more easily), and beat with a wire whisk or at medium speed. The mixture should be smooth and a little thinner than the consistency of whipped cream.

The eggs — whole or the beaten yolks — are added next, slowly or one at a time. Beat them in until the mixture is thick, fluffy, and quite pale in color. At this point there is no need to worry about overbeating the batter, so beat it at high speed for several minutes to get the desired color and texture (usually specified in the recipe).

The flour and other dry ingredients, which have been combined and lightened by sifting or by stirring with a wire whisk, are added to the batter next, alternately with the liquid ingredients. (The dry ingredients may be combined in another bowl beforehand, so that they are ready to be added.) Begin this step by slowly adding a third of the flour mixture and beating it in at low speed. Add half the liquid, then another third of the flour mixture. Mix after each addition until mixture is just smooth. Complete the process with the second half of the liquid and the rest of the dry ingredients. Stop beating before you add each new ingredient and use a rubber spatula to scrape the sides of the bowl.

After the flour has been added, it is important to guard against hard or long beating of the batter, for overbeating develops the flour's gluten, resulting in a very dense-textured cake. Blend just until the batter is smooth.

If carob is used in a recipe, it can be added either in powdered form, as is cocoa, or as a syrup, which blends easily into the batter (see Basic Carob Syrup, page 737).

The last step is to gently fold the beaten egg whites into the batter by hand, using a wooden spoon or a rubber spatula, never with an electric mixer. Use a folding, vertical, circular motion and do not overfold.

Cake Tips

- At high altitudes be especially careful not to overbeat egg whites and incorporate too much air into the batter. Raise the cake's baking temperature by 25°F.
- Most cake batters can be baked as cupcakes. The baking time differs according to the size of the cupcakes. Follow the same procedure as for cakes for buttering and flouring muffin tins, or line tins with paper cups. Fill cups one-half to two-thirds full.
- Lightly dust nuts, dried fruit, and lumpy ingredients with flour to keep them from sinking to the bottom of the batter. Fold them into the batter just before baking.
- Warmed honey is easier to measure accurately and is more readily creamed with butter and eggs. To warm honey before adding it to other ingredients, set the honey jar in a small pan of hot water for 15 to 20 minutes.
- If making cakes with unbleached white flour, enrich the flour according to the Cornell Formula (see page 347) for a more nutritious product.

Pans

Angel food and sponge cakes and torten are usually baked in ungreased tube pans with removable rims. The center tube provides support for these very light and airy batters as they rise. If the pan has any traces of grease, clean it well and dry it, or the batter will not rise properly.

Layer cakes are best baked in pans with straight sides. For butter and creamed cakes the bottom of the pan is usually buttered or oiled, then lightly dusted with flour. Medium-weight, shiny baking pans distribute heat evenly and give a light, nicely browned cake crust. Dark or discolored pans may cause cakes to brown too much or to burn. If using glass baking dishes, remember to lower the baking temperature by 25°F, but bake for the same time.

Pour or spoon the batter into the pans, spreading it toward the sides and into the corners. Leave the center slightly lower to guarantee a level, flat-topped cake. Fill the pans about two-thirds full with batter.

Baking

The oven should be preheated to the desired temperature before the cake is put in. Unless the recipe directs otherwise, turn the oven on just before mixing the cake. This avoids interruption during mixing and ensures enough time for the oven to be heated sufficiently when the batter is ready.

Cakes should be browned nicely and evenly and begin to pull away from the pan's sides when done. To test whether a cake is done, insert a wooden pick into the center of the cake. The pick should come out clean with no batter adhering to it. If unsure, gently press the top of the cake; it should be spongy and show no fingerprints.

Removing Cakes from Pans

Most cakes should be removed from the pans soon after baking, or they will become soggy and difficult to remove. Butter cakes should be allowed to cool in the pan for about 5 minutes after being removed from the oven. Cakes that are exceptionally rich should stay in the pan for 10 to 15 minutes. Use a knife to loosen the cake from the sides of the pan and remove it carefully. Allow the cake to cool top-side up on a wire rack.

Angel food and sponge cakes should be cooled thoroughly upside down in the pan before being removed. Loosen the edges of the cake with a knife, and turn it out bottom-side up onto a cake plate.

Unless the recipe directs otherwise, allow cakes to cool completely before frosting or filling them.

How to Recognize and Remedy What Went Wrong with Your Cake

Problem	Possible Cause
Cracked top	Too much flour; oven temperature too high
Too-dark color	Too much sweetener; oven temperature too high; overbaked
Low volume	Too much shortening or liquid; oven temperature too low; pan too big
Sunken top	Too much shortening, sweetener, or leavening; too little liquid; underbaked
Coarse grain	Too little liquid; undermixed; too much shortening; oven temperature too low
Dense texture	Overmixed; too much liquid
Gaping holes	Too much egg; too little sweetener; uneven mixing
Dry	Too much leavening; over-baked; too little sweetener
Soggy	Too much shortening or liquid; undermixed; overbaked
Tough	Too little shortening; too much egg; overmixed; overbaked
Crumbly	Too much shortening; undermixed

Storing Cakes

Store cakes in covered containers away from other foods which might absorb moisture. Most cakes can be frozen, but it is best not to frost or fill cakes that are to be frozen. Wait until just before serving them, after they have defrosted.

Cheesecakes

Cheesecakes, rich and delicate, are prepared from a sweetened mixture of fresh cheese, eggs, and flavorings. The cheese may be made from whole, low-fat, or skim milk. Cream cheese, ricotta, and cottage cheese are the most commonly used cheeses, their richness depending on their butterfat content. Cream, sour cream, or yogurt may be added to the cheese mixture for smoothness and to lighten the cake.

Eggs thicken and bind the other ingredients, giving cheesecake its characteristic texture. They may be separated, the beaten egg whites folded in at the end to lighten the cake.

Flour, cornstarch, or gelatin may also be used to thicken and stabilize the cake's moisture. Gelatin, used only in unbaked cheesecakes, must first be softened in cold liquid, then dissolved over hot water. Too much gelatin will give a rubbery texture to the cake.

Honey, molasses, and maple syrup may all be used to sweeten. The amount of liquid used in the recipe is very easily adjusted to accommodate the liquid state of the sweetener.

Springform pans are usually used for cheesecakes with crusts. This makes the cake easy to remove from the pan without breaking the cake.

Baking time and temperature depend on the creaminess of the cake. The creamier the cake, the shorter the time it is baked. When the cake looks set and begins to pull away from the pan's edges, it is done.

Cheesecakes are very delicate and apt to crack, so they must be cooled slowly. A common practice is to allow the cake to remain in the turned-off oven for 1½ to 2 hours while it slowly reaches room temperature. It should then be covered and refrigerated. It can also be frozen.

Cake Frostings and Fillings

Some cakes are fine just as they are, without frostings or fillings. But frostings and fillings can add extra appeal to an ordinary cake, making it suitable for a special occasion. Frostings and fillings are simple to make and usually can be whipped up in the time it takes for the cake to bake.

Frostings are usually made with a high proportion of sweetener blended with rich ingredients such as butter, cream, sour cream, or yogurt. They may also be enriched with egg yolk or flavored with carob, nuts, peanut butter, lemon or orange rinds, or innumerable other natural flavorings.

Icing Requirements

Top and sides	1 9-inch-round cake	¾ cup
Top and sides	2 9-inch-round cake layers	1½ cups
Top and sides	3 9-inch-round cake layers	2¼ cups
Top and sides	9 × 5-inch loaf	1-1½ cups
Top	1 8-inch-square cake	½-¾ cup
Top	9 × 13-inch cake	1½ cups
Top	16 large or 24 small cupcakes	1-1½ cups
For filling	10 × 15-inch jellyroll	2 cups

Boiled icings are a traditional type of frosting based on a procedure for making what is known as Italian meringue—beating a hot syrup into beaten or unbeaten egg whites. These icings are very easily made with honey instead of sugar, usually with *unbeaten* egg whites. They will be soft, fluffy, and light but not quite as stiff as sugar frostings. All the ingredients, including the egg whites, may be put into the top of a double boiler and beaten with a wire whisk or a rotary beater while the mixture cooks. When it is ready, the frosting should be stiff enough to stand in peaks.

Use icings promptly to get the best out of them. If you must store a prepared icing, do so for as short a time as possible in a well-sealed container in the refrigerator.

Before applying an icing, make sure the cake is thoroughly cooled. Then lightly brush off any crumbs so the icing will not be lumpy. Place the first cake layer top-side down on a plate. Arrange wedges of wax paper just under the edge of the bottom layer, all around the cake, allowing them to extend over the plate's edge so they catch any drippings and keep the plate clean. (Remove the wax paper when the icing has set.)

Cover the first layer with frosting or filling almost to the edge. Place the second layer top-side up on top of this. First frost the sides with a rubber spatula or frosting knife, working the frosting from the bottom to the top. The frosting should touch the wax paper. Then pour all the remaining frosting on top of the cake. With sweeping strokes, spread it out to meet the sides. Use the frosting knife or the back of a teaspoon to stroke decorative swirls or scrolls into the icing.

Cookies

You can make good-tasting sweets in the form of cookies and bars using all sorts of natural food ingredients. Rolled oats, nonfat dry milk, wheat germ, yogurt, raisins, seeds, and nuts are just some of the nutritious extras that can be added to cookies.

They are perfect as desserts or snacks and ideal in lunches for work or school or for picnics.

There are four basic types of cookies:

Drop cookies are made from a fairly soft dough. You usually use one level teaspoon of dough for each cookie. If the dough doesn't drop easily from the spoon, push it off with your finger or another spoon. Allow plenty of space between cookies on the baking sheet because they spread as they bake.

Refrigerator cookies are popular because they are so easy to prepare. Also called sliced cookies, they are made from a dough that is chilled until firm enough to be cut into thin slices and baked. The dough is shaped into rolls 1½ to 2 inches in diameter, then wrapped in wax paper or plastic wrap or packed tightly into a rectangular pan. When the dough is firm, unwrap it or remove it from the pan, and slice it into rounds, squares, or oblongs from ⅛ to ½ inch thick, and bake as directed.

Bar cookies are baked in the pan. Pour the batter 1½ inches deep into buttered pans. Designated pan sizes should be observed because the wrong size will change the texture of the bar. These cookies can be cut into small bars or squares while still warm, then stored in the baking pan, covered, or transferred to airtight cookie tins when cooled.

Rolled cookies are the type in which the dough is rolled flat and often cut into shapes with cookie cutters.

Making cookies can be quick and easy. The ingredients may simply be stirred together, or creamed as for cakes, or mixed as for pastries. Using honey in place of sugar, as we do in this book, yields softer batters and doughs that are still suitable for most types of cookies.

It is up to the cook to decide on the texture of the cookies—thick and chewy or thin and crispy. Whole wheat pastry flour yields a cookie dough that spreads out during baking to produce thin, delicate cookies. Regular whole wheat flour yields a firmer cookie that holds its shape while baking. The amount of flour used will also affect the texture of the cookie. You may find it necessary to add more flour to some recipes because the freshness and absorbency of flours vary.

Using butter as the shortening yields the most flavorful cookie, but oil is an economical and suitable substitute, especially in recipes where strong flavorings such as cinnamon, cloves, or aniseeds are to be used.

Chilling cookie doughs is not absolutely necessary, but it makes them more manageable. Cookie dough can be made several days in advance and chilled until ready for use. You also may freeze cookie dough.

Baking Sheets

Cookies bake best on flat sheets made of heavy material. Cookies may also be baked on top of an overturned roasting pan if you do not have baking sheets. Unless a recipe specifies otherwise, butter or oil the sheet or use liquid lecithin. If you use lecithin, you may mix it with equal parts of vegetable oil for easier spreading. Usually one coating will last for a whole batch of cookies.

Place cookies of even sizes at least one inch apart on the sheet. Be sure there are at least two inches between the baking sheet edges and the oven walls so the heat can circulate freely. It is best to put just one baking sheet in the oven at a time, but if you choose to put in two, stagger them to opposite sides.

Cookies may be baked on parchment paper. Fit the baking sheet with a piece of it, and arrange the cookies on the paper. When they are baked, slide the whole sheet of paper onto a wire rack to cool. Cool the baking sheet slightly before placing another piece of parchment and more cookies on it. Parchment paper can be wiped clean with a paper towel and reused.

Baking Time

Although cookie dough is softer with a liquid sweetener than with sugar, it will bake similarly. The baking times will vary for different types of cookies, but all should be baked until the edges are just beginning to brown. Drop cookies take 12 to 15 minutes to bake. When done they should be delicately browned, with firm edges. Bar cookies take a little longer—18 to 20 minutes—and are done when the dough springs back when you press it lightly.

Some cookies may not actually look done when in the oven, even though they are, so be careful not to overbake them. If the cookies do not seem to be browning around the edges, lightly lift one with a spatula to check for browning underneath.

With cookies it is best to underbake because they dry out quickly. When the cookies are completely cooled, if they are too soft or sticky, you can allow them to dry at room temperature for several hours, or you can pop them back into the oven for three to five minutes.

After cookies have been baked, use a large spatula to move them carefully to a wire rack to cool. Bar cookies may be cut while still warm, but they should be left in the baking pan until cooled. Cookies are still fragile when warm, so handle them gently and never stack them on top of each other until completely cooled, or they will stick together.

Storing Baked Cookies

Allow cookies to cool completely before storing them between layers of plastic wrap or wax paper in a tightly covered can or jar. If you plan to keep the cookies for longer than a week, store them in the refrigerator. Cookies tend to improve in flavor after a few days' storage in an airtight container. Do not store more than one kind of cookie in the same tin because flavors tend to mingle. Baked cookies can also be frozen.

Cookie Tips

- If a cookie recipe calls for nuts, use any kind you enjoy. For a change of flavor and for added nutrition, try sunflower seeds, sesame seeds, wheat germ, or bran in addition to or in place of nuts.
- Freshen stale cookies by heating them in the oven for about five minutes at 325°F.
- When making different types of cookies, choose those that complement each other with various textures and flavors but that also make the most efficient use of the ingredients at hand.
- Bar cookies and most drop cookies are firm and moist and suitable for travel. Very delicate, crisp, wafer cookies are flimsy and crumble easily, so do not select these for that purpose.

Confections

Homemade candy will never have the professional uniform appearance of the store-bought product, but it will taste great and be a lot of fun to make.

Crystalline candies such as fudges and fondants are very difficult to make with all natural ingredients. The honey used in place of the sugar never loses its stickiness, to permit the proper texture that sugar gives. Using maple syrup instead of honey solves part of this problem, but maple syrup still lacks the ability to crystallize properly.

Noncrystalline candies such as taffies, brittles, and chewy candies are less difficult to make with natural ingredients. These usually contain butter, cream, and other ingredients that do not require crystal formation of sugar for a manageable consistency. Using honey, molasses, or maple syrup, they can be made in a wide variety of delicious flavors.

Cool, dry weather is ideal for candy making, as candy tends to become grainy in warm, sticky weather. If you must cook candy on a rainy day, cook it at 2°F higher temperature than that called for in the recipe.

Select a deep, heavy pot that is large enough to hold four or five times the amount of combined recipe ingredients. This will ensure against the candy's boiling over, which it has a tendency to do.

Since timing is such an important factor in candy making, a candy thermometer is often used. Although color and consistency can also indicate when the candy is done, it is advisable for inexperienced candy makers to use the most reliable method of testing. The thermometer and the cold-water test are the most trustworthy.

Procedure for Testing Candy

Never put a cold thermometer directly into boiling syrup. Either heat it first in water brought slowly to the boiling point, or stand the thermometer in the candy mixture before you start cooking and leave it there. The bulb must be completely covered with syrup yet must not touch the bottom of the pan. When the candy reaches the required temperature, remove the thermometer and put it where it can cool gradually before you wash it.

To apply the cold-water test, when the candy is nearly ready, remove the pan from the heat so the cooking will stop. Fill a cup or small bowl with cold water. Drop about one-half teaspoon of the syrup into the cold water and, if necessary, shape it with your fingers into a ball. Test for the degree of hardness according to the following stages:

Soft ball (234 to 238°F): The ball of candy flattens out somewhat.

Medium-soft ball (238 to 240°F): The ball of candy just barely holds its shape.

Firm ball (244 to 250°F): The ball of candy is firm but not hard.

Hard ball (265°F): The ball of candy is very firm and hard.

Hard crack (270 to 310°F): The syrup separates into threads when poured into the cup. The ball of candy is brittle when you tap it against the side of the cup. (Candies made with honey will not reach this stage.)

Cakes

Basic Sponge Cake,
Sponge Roll, or Ladyfingers

> 6 eggs, separated
> 1 tablespoon grated orange rind
> ½ cup orange juice
> ½ cup plus 2 tablespoons honey, warmed
> 1⅓ cups whole wheat pastry flour
> 1 teaspoon cream of tartar

Preheat oven to 325°F.

In a large bowl beat egg yolks at high speed of electric mixer for about 5 minutes. Add orange rind and orange juice, and beat for another 5 minutes. Gradually beat in ½ cup honey, 1 tablespoon at a time. Continue to beat until mixture is very thick and smooth, 12 to 15 minutes. Do not underbeat—the lightness of this sponge cake depends on this beating process.

Sift flour and fold into egg yolk mixture. Set aside.

In a large bowl beat egg whites until foamy, then add cream of tartar and beat until mixture forms soft peaks. Gradually add remaining honey and beat until mixture is stiff but not dry. Gently fold egg white mixture into egg yolk mixture, using a rubber spatula.

For a 3-layer sponge cake: Pour batter into 3 unbuttered 8-inch-round baking pans, and bake for 20 to 22 minutes, or until tops of layers are lightly browned. Cool cake completely before removing from pans. Ice as desired.

For a sponge roll: Place a sheet of parchment or wax paper in a 12 × 15-inch jellyroll pan. Pour in dough and bake for about 20 minutes. Remove from oven, loosen edges of cake, and invert on a clean dish towel. Roll up the cake (with parchment or wax paper still in place) and cool on a wire rack. To fill, unroll, remove paper, and spread with filling. Then reroll carefully and place on serving dish, seam-side down.

For ladyfingers: Place a piece of parchment paper on a baking sheet and drop batter by tablespoons onto paper, forming fingers about ¾ inch by 3 inches, spaced 2 inches apart. Bake for about 10 minutes. Cool for 5 minutes, then remove from paper, and place on a wire rack to cool completely. This yields 30 ladyfingers.

About 15 servings

Almond Cake with Orange-Spice Syrup

Syrup
½ cup honey
2 cups orange juice
1 stick of cinnamon
4 whole cloves

Cake
½ cup butter
¼ cup honey
3 eggs
½ teaspoon almond extract
1 cup whole wheat flour
½ teaspoon baking soda
½ cup chopped blanched almonds

To make the syrup: Combine honey, orange juice, cinnamon, and cloves in a heavy-bottom pot, and bring to a simmer over medium heat. Simmer gently for 15 minutes. Remove spices and cool.

To make the cake: Preheat oven to 350°F. Butter and flour an 8-inch-square baking pan.

Cream butter in a large bowl until light and fluffy. Gradually add honey and continue beating at medium speed of electric mixer for 2 minutes. Beat in eggs one at a time just until blended. Blend in almond extract.

Combine flour, baking soda, and nuts, and then slowly stir into creamed mixture. Pour batter into prepared pan and bake for 35 minutes, or until a wooden pick inserted into center comes out clean.

Remove from oven and set pan on a wire rack. Cut cake into squares, and pour cooled syrup over entire cake. Serve when cool.

9 servings

Angel Food Cake

10 egg whites, at room temperature
1½ teaspoons cream of tartar
1¼ teaspoons almond extract
½ cup clover honey, warmed
1 cup whole wheat pastry flour, sifted

Rinse a large bowl in warm water and dry thoroughly. Put egg whites in bowl and beat with a wire whisk until foamy. Then add cream of tartar, and continue to beat until whites are stiff but not dry. Add almond extract. Gradually fold in honey. (Do not beat.) Sprinkle flour by tablespoons over whites, using a spatula to fold flour into mixture. Do not overmix.

Spoon batter gently into an unbuttered 9- or 10-inch tube pan. (Angel food cake pan should not be used for other baking in which oil or butter is used.) Cut through the batter gently to remove any bubbles.

Set oven temperature at 325°F. Place cake on middle rack and bake for 1 hour. Turn off heat and leave cake in oven for 15 minutes.

Remove from oven and invert pan on a wire rack to cool. When cake is cool, run a thin knife between it and pan to loosen. Shake gently. Cake should drop to rack.

8 to 10 servings

Apple-Maple Coffee Cake

2½ cups sifted whole wheat pastry flour
1 teaspoon baking soda
½ cup butter
1 egg
½ cup maple syrup
¾ cup buttermilk
1½ to 2 apples, peeled, cored, and sliced
2 tablespoons dried currants
½ cup coarsely chopped walnuts or pecans
½ cup maple sugar
½ teaspoon ground cinnamon
¼ teaspoon ground cloves
¼ teaspoon ground nutmeg
½ cup butter, melted

Preheat oven to 375°F. Butter a 7 × 11-inch or 9-inch-square baking pan.

Combine flour and baking soda in a large bowl. Cut in butter with your fingers or a pastry blender until mixture resembles coarse crumbs.

In a small bowl combine egg, maple syrup, and buttermilk. Pour into flour mixture and beat just until smooth. Pour batter into prepared pan. Arrange apple slices on top. Sprinkle currants and nuts evenly over apples.

Combine maple sugar and spices, and sprinkle evenly on top of fruit and nuts. Drizzle melted butter over coffee cake and bake for 25 minutes.

Remove from oven and let cool slightly before cutting and serving.

9 to 12 servings

Apricot Upside-Down Skillet Cake

    3 tablespoons butter
    1 cup honey
    2 cups peeled halved apricots
    ¼ cup chopped walnuts
    ½ cup butter or vegetable oil
    2 eggs
    1 teaspoon vanilla extract
    ¼ cup buttermilk or yogurt
    ½ teaspoon baking soda
    1¾ cups whole wheat pastry flour

Melt butter over low heat in a heavy-bottom skillet with a tight-fitting lid, or in an electric skillet set at 250°F. Then stir in ⅓ cup honey, and simmer until well mixed and beginning to thicken. Arrange apricots cut-side down over mixture. Cover with nuts.

Preheat oven to 250°F (if using skillet).

In a large bowl cream butter or oil and ⅔ cup honey together. Then beat in eggs one at a time just until blended. Add vanilla.

Combine buttermilk or yogurt with baking soda and add to creamed mixture. Add flour and mix well.

Pour batter over apricots, spreading evenly. If using skillet, cover and bake for 40 to 50 minutes. If using electric skillet, cover (with vent open) and cook for 40 to 50 minutes.

Remove immediately by inverting a large cake plate over skillet and turning whole assembly upside down. Serve warm or cold, topped with sour cream, if desired.

    6 to 8 servings

Blueberry Cake

    2 eggs, separated
    ⅛ teaspoon cream of tartar
    ½ cup plus 1 tablespoon honey
    ½ cup butter
    1 teaspoon vanilla extract
    1½ cups sifted whole wheat flour
    ½ cup sifted whole wheat pastry flour
    1 teaspoon baking soda
    1 cup buttermilk
    1½ cups fresh blueberries, dusted with
        2 tablespoons whole wheat pastry flour

Preheat oven to 350°F. Butter and flour a 9-inch-square baking pan.

In a large bowl beat egg whites until foamy, and then add cream of tartar. Add 1 tablespoon honey gradually, and continue beating at high speed of electric mixer until egg whites are stiff but not dry. Set aside.

Cream butter in a large bowl until light and fluffy. Gradually pour in ½ cup honey, and continue beating at medium speed for 2 minutes. Beat in egg yolks one at a time. Beat in vanilla.

In a small bowl combine flours and baking soda and add slowly to creamed mixture, alternating with buttermilk. Add ¼ of the egg whites to batter and blend well. Fold in remaining whites and then blueberries. Pour batter into prepared pan and bake for 50 minutes, or until a wooden pick inserted into center comes out clean.

Remove from oven and let cool in pan for 10 minutes on a wire rack. Remove from pan and serve warm, or cool completely on rack. Serve with Lemon Sauce (page 663).

    9 servings

Buttermilk-Carob Cake

    2 cups whole wheat flour
    1 teaspoon baking soda
    ½ cup butter
    ⅔ cup honey
    1 teaspoon vanilla extract
    3 eggs, separated
    ¼ cup Basic Carob Syrup (page 737)
    1 cup buttermilk

Preheat oven to 350°F. Butter and flour two 9-inch-round baking pans.

Sift together flour and baking soda.

Cream butter in a large bowl. Then add honey and beat until light and fluffy. Add vanilla. Lightly beat egg yolks, add to mixture, and beat thoroughly. Stir in carob syrup. Alternately mix dry ingredients and buttermilk into wet ingredients in small amounts, beating well.

Beat egg whites until stiff but not dry, and fold into batter. Pour batter into prepared pans and bake for 30 to 35 minutes, or until a wooden pick inserted into center comes out clean.

Remove from oven and cool in pans for 5 minutes. Then cool completely on wire racks.

    10 to 12 servings

Butter-Pecan Chiffon Cake

2 tablespoons butter
½ cup coarsely chopped pecans
8 egg whites
½ teaspoon cream of tartar
2¼ cups sifted whole wheat pastry flour
1 teaspoon baking soda
½ cup vegetable oil
5 egg yolks
⅔ cup buttermilk
¾ cup honey
2 teaspoons vanilla extract

Preheat oven to 325°F. Line bottom of a 10-inch tube pan with wax paper.

Melt butter in a small skillet. Add nuts and brown them very lightly for about 5 minutes over medium heat. Drain on paper towels.

Beat egg whites until foamy, then add cream of tartar, and continue beating until stiff but not dry. Set aside.

In a large bowl combine flour, baking soda, oil, egg yolks, buttermilk, honey, and vanilla. Beat until smooth and then stir in nuts. Blend ¼ of the egg whites into batter. Then fold in remaining whites. Pour batter into pan and bake for 1 hour, or until a wooden pick inserted into center comes out clean.

Remove from oven and invert pan on a wire rack to cool completely. Remove cake from pan and serve plain, or frost with Seven-Minute Frosting (page 697) and dust with ground pecans.

10 to 12 servings

Carob-Potato Cake

The hot mashed potatoes may seem odd as an ingredient in a dessert cake, but you will be pleased by the moisture they impart to the finished product.

2 medium-size potatoes
½ cup butter
½ cup honey
3 eggs
1 teaspoon vanilla extract
2 cups sifted whole wheat pastry flour
⅓ cup sifted powdered carob
1 teaspoon baking soda
1 teaspoon ground cinnamon
1 teaspoon ground nutmeg
⅓ cup buttermilk

Cook potatoes in enough water to cover. Drain and mash.

Preheat oven to 350°F. Butter and flour two 8-inch-round baking pans, a 9-inch-square pan, or a 7 × 11-inch pan.

Cream butter in a large bowl until light and fluffy. Gradually add honey and continue beating at medium speed of electric mixer for 2 minutes. Beat in eggs one at a time just until blended. Add vanilla and ⅔ cup of the hot mashed potatoes and blend well.

In a separate bowl combine flour, carob, baking soda, and spices. Gradually blend into creamed mixture alternately with buttermilk. Pour batter into prepared pans and bake for 35 to 40 minutes, or until a wooden pick inserted into center comes out clean.

Remove from oven and set pans on wire racks for 10 minutes. Remove cake from pans and let cool completely on racks. Ice with Seven-Minute Frosting (page 697) or Carob Buttercream Frosting (page 695).

10 to 12 servings

Variation:
■ Omit spices, substitute orange juice for buttermilk, and add 1 tablespoon grated orange rind.

Carob Pound Cake

4 eggs, separated
¾ cup honey
1 cup butter
3 tablespoons buttermilk
1 teaspoon vanilla extract
1½ cups sifted whole wheat pastry flour
¼ cup sifted powdered carob
1 teaspoon baking soda

Preheat oven to 300°F. Butter and flour a 5 × 9-inch loaf pan or an 8- or 9-inch tube pan.

Beat egg whites until foamy, then gradually add ¼ cup honey, and continue beating at high speed of electric mixer until soft peaks form. Set aside.

In a large bowl cream butter until light and fluffy. Gradually add ½ cup honey and continue beating at medium speed for 5 minutes. Beat in egg yolks one at a time just until blended. Beat in buttermilk and vanilla.

In a separate bowl combine flour, carob, and baking soda. Add ¼ of the flour mixture at a time to batter, beating each time just until blended. Add ½ of the egg whites at a time, beating just until blended. Pour batter into prepared pan and bake for 1½ hours, or until a wooden pick inserted into center comes out clean.

Cool in pan on wire racks for 10 minutes, then remove from pan and let cool completely on racks. Serve plain or dusted with Coconut Sugar (page 698) or finely ground nuts.

8 to 10 servings

Carrot Cake

2 eggs
½ cup honey or maple syrup, warmed
¾ cup vegetable oil
¼ cup buttermilk
1½ cups grated carrots (about ½ pound)
½ cup chopped pecans, almonds, or walnuts
1¼ cups whole wheat pastry flour
1 teaspoon baking soda
1 tablespoon ground cinnamon

Preheat oven to 300°F. Butter an 8-inch-square baking pan.

In a large bowl beat eggs. Add honey or maple syrup, oil, and buttermilk, and beat until well blended. Stir in carrots and nuts.

In a separate bowl sift together flour, baking soda, and cinnamon. Fold into carrot mixture and mix well but do not beat. Pour batter into prepared pan and bake for 1 hour.

Remove from oven and allow to cool for 10 minutes. Cover with Apricot Glaze (page 664) and allow to cool completely.

6 to 8 servings

Cream-Walnut Cake

½ cup butter
½ cup honey
3 eggs
1 teaspoon vanilla extract
2 cups sifted whole wheat pastry flour
1 teaspoon baking soda
1 cup sour cream
½ cup coarsely chopped black walnuts, dusted with 2 tablespoons whole wheat pastry flour

Preheat oven to 350°F. Butter and flour two 8-inch-round baking pans, a 9-inch-square pan, or a 7 × 11-inch pan.

Cream butter in a large bowl until light and fluffy. Gradually add honey and continue beating at medium speed of electric mixer for 2 minutes. Beat in eggs one at a time just until blended. Add vanilla.

In a separate bowl combine flour and baking soda and slowly blend into creamed mixture, alternating with sour cream. Stir in nuts.

Pour batter into prepared pans and bake for 30 minutes, or until a wooden pick inserted into center comes out clean.

Remove cake from oven and cool in pans for 10 minutes on wire racks. Remove from pans and let cool completely on racks. Frost with White Frosting (page 698) or Seven-Minute Frosting (page 697), and sprinkle top with finely ground black walnuts.

10 to 12 servings

Variation:
■ Substitute almonds for walnuts, and almond extract for vanilla.

Crumb Coffee Cake

This old-fashioned breakfast cake is sometimes called Krum Kuchen *and is often baked in a piecrust, similar to shoo-fly pie and funny cake. Try it both ways—you may have a preference.*

2 cups whole wheat pastry flour, sifted
½ cup butter
½ cup plus 2 tablespoons honey
2 eggs, beaten
1 teaspoon baking soda
½ cup buttermilk

Preheat oven to 375°F. Butter an 8-inch-square baking pan.

In a large bowl combine flour and butter, and crumb well with a fork. Then add 2 tablespoons honey and blend. Take out 1 cup of crumbs and reserve. Add eggs and remaining honey.

In a small bowl dissolve baking soda in buttermilk and stir into flour mixture. Pour batter into prepared pan, top with reserved crumbs, and bake for about 30 minutes, or until a wooden pick inserted into center comes out clean.

8 servings

Eggless Spice Cake

½ cup butter, melted
⅓ cup molasses
⅓ cup honey
1 cup buttermilk
3½ cups sifted whole wheat pastry flour
1 teaspoon baking soda
2 teaspoons ground allspice
1 teaspoon ground cinnamon
½ cup dried currants, dusted with 1 tablespoon
    whole wheat pastry flour

Preheat oven to 350°F. Butter and flour two 8-inch-round baking pans, a 9-inch-square pan, or a 7 × 11-inch pan.

Combine butter, molasses, honey, and buttermilk in a large bowl and beat well.

Combine flour, baking soda, and spices, and gradually add to batter, beating just enough to combine. Stir in currants. Pour batter into prepared pans and bake for 30 minutes, or until a wooden pick inserted into center comes out clean.

Remove from oven and let cool in pans for several minutes. Then remove from pans and allow to cool completely on wire racks. Frost with Lemon Icing (page 696).

10 to 12 servings

Génoise

What could be simpler than the five ingredients called for in this recipe? The challenge is in achieving the classic lightness by following the instructions for assembly carefully.

½ cup butter
6 eggs
½ cup honey
1 teaspoon vanilla extract
1 cup sifted whole wheat pastry flour

Preheat oven to 350°F. Butter and flour two 8-inch-round baking pans.

In a small skillet clarify butter (see page 140 for directions). Set aside to cool.

Place eggs, honey, and vanilla in a large bowl, and whisk to combine ingredients. Place over simmering water for several minutes, until mixture is barely lukewarm, stirring occasionally. With an electric mixer beat at high speed for 10 minutes, or until mixture has tripled in volume.

Place flour back into sifter and hold over batter. Gradually sift in flour while folding it in with a wide rubber spatula. Slowly pour in butter and fold in. Pour batter into prepared pans. Place pans on a baking sheet and bake for 20 to 25 minutes, or until cake is golden brown, is springy to the touch, and has pulled away slightly from the sides of pans.

Remove from oven and cool in pans for 5 to 10 minutes on wire racks. Then remove from pans and cool completely on racks. Use as 2 layers, or split and use as 4 layers. Frost with Buttercream Frosting (page 695) or Soft Meringue Topping (page 440) and fill with Cherry Sauce (page 663), Raspberry Sauce (page 664), or cold English Custard Sauce (page 663).

8 to 12 servings

Golden Almond Shortcake

Here is an opportunity to try some new flours in an old standard. This cake is best if served soon after it is baked and still a bit warm.

½ cup amaranth flour, barley flour, or finely
    ground millet
1 cup whole wheat pastry flour
1½ teaspoons baking powder
1 egg
3 tablespoons honey
3 tablespoons milk
1 teaspoon vanilla extract
½ cup butter
½ cup almonds, toasted

Preheat oven to 425°F. Butter and flour a 9-inch-square baking pan.

In a medium-size bowl mix together flours and baking powder.

In a separate bowl mix egg and honey together with a wire whisk. Gradually whisk in milk and vanilla.

Using a pastry blender, 2 knives, or a food processor, cut butter into flour mixture until mixture resembles coarse crumbs. Coarsely chop almonds and add to flour mixture. Stir in liquid ingredients. Work quickly. Do not mix more than is necessary. Scrape dough into prepared pan and bake for about 15 minutes, or until lightly browned.

Cool slightly. Cut into serving-size pieces. Split each piece as it is removed from pan. Spoon a layer of sliced fruit onto bottom half of each piece and replace top half. Top with more fruit and whipped cream and serve immediately.

6 to 8 servings

Golden Layer Cake

    3 eggs, separated
    ¼ teaspoon cream of tartar
    4 tablespoons honey
    1 teaspoon vanilla extract
    ⅔ cup sifted whole wheat pastry flour

Preheat oven to 350°F. Butter an 8½ × 4½-inch loaf pan.

In a large bowl beat egg whites until foamy, and then add cream of tartar. Beat at medium speed of electric mixer until soft peaks form. Then gradually blend in 1 tablespoon honey. Beat at high speed until whites are stiff but not dry. Set aside.

Lightly beat egg yolks in a large bowl. Then gradually blend in remaining 3 tablespoons honey, and beat for 5 minutes at medium speed, or until thick and lemon colored. Add vanilla. Beat in flour. Beat in ¼ of the egg whites, and then fold in remaining whites. Pour batter into prepared pan and bake for 30 minutes, or until a wooden pick inserted into center comes out clean.

Remove cake from oven and let cool in pan on a wire rack for 10 minutes. Remove from pan and let

cool completely on rack. Slice cake into 3 layers. Fill and frost with Buttercream Frosting (page 695).

6 to 8 servings

Jam-Spice Cake

The blackberry jam is beaten right into the batter of this rich and nutty party cake.

    ½ cup butter
    ½ cup honey
    3 eggs
    1 cup blackberry jam
    2½ cups sifted whole wheat pastry flour
    1 teaspoon baking soda
    1 teaspoon ground allspice
    1 teaspoon ground cinnamon
    1 teaspoon ground nutmeg
    1 teaspoon ground cloves
    ⅓ cup buttermilk
    ½ cup coarsely chopped walnuts or pecans, dusted with 1 tablespoon whole wheat pastry flour
    ½ cup raisins or chopped dates, dusted with 1 tablespoon whole wheat pastry flour

Preheat oven to 350°F. Butter and flour two 8-inch-round baking pans, a 9-inch-square pan, or a 7 × 11-inch pan.

Cream butter in a large bowl until light and fluffy. Gradually add honey and continue beating at medium speed of electric mixer for 2 minutes. Beat in eggs one at a time just until blended. Beat in jam.

In a separate bowl combine flour, baking soda, and spices, and add slowly to creamed mixture, beating just until blended. Quickly beat in buttermilk. Fold in nuts and fruit. Pour batter into prepared pans and bake for 30 to 35 minutes, or until a wooden pick inserted into center comes out clean.

Remove from oven and let cool in pans for 10 minutes. Then remove from pans and allow to cool completely on wire racks. Serve plain or frost with Seven-Minute Frosting (page 697), if desired.

10 to 12 servings

Meringue-Nut Cake

6 egg whites
½ teaspoon cream of tartar
½ cup honey, warmed
1 teaspoon vanilla extract
½ teaspoon almond extract
1½ cups blanched almonds or hazelnuts, lightly toasted
2 tablespoons cornstarch

Preheat oven to 300°F. Butter and flour 2 baking sheets. Using an 8-inch-round baking pan as guide, draw around rim with tip of a rubber spatula. Make 3 of these circles on baking sheets. Other shapes may be made as desired.

Place egg whites in a large bowl, and beat at low speed of electric mixer until foamy. Add cream of tartar. Increase speed to medium and beat until soft peaks form. Gradually add honey and increase speed to high. Continue beating until whites are stiff but not dry. Add vanilla and almond extracts.

Finely grind nuts and combine with cornstarch. Sprinkle 4 or 5 tablespoons at a time over egg whites and fold in.

Using a pastry bag with a plain tip or a spoon, distribute batter within shapes outlined on baking sheets. Spread tops evenly with a long spatula so that cakes are the same thickness all over. Bake for 30 to 35 minutes, or until nicely browned.

Remove from oven and set baking sheets on wire racks until cake is cool enough to slide off sheets. Fill layers with Buttercream Frosting (page 694). Decorate top and sides with more frosting or with whipped cream, Coconut Sugar (page 698), or grated carob.

8 to 10 servings

Mocha Molasses Cake

½ cup butter
½ cup honey
½ cup molasses
2 eggs
2¼ cups sifted whole wheat pastry flour
1 teaspoon baking soda
½ teaspoon ground cloves
½ teaspoon ground cinnamon
½ teaspoon ground nutmeg
½ teaspoon ground ginger
½ cup Postum
⅔ cup raisins, dusted with 2 tablespoons whole wheat pastry flour
⅔ cup coarsely chopped walnuts or pecans, dusted with 2 tablespoons whole wheat pastry flour

Preheat oven to 350°F. Butter and flour two 8-inch-round baking pans, a 9-inch-square pan, or a 7 × 11-inch pan.

Cream butter in a large bowl until light and fluffy. Gradually add honey and molasses, and continue beating at medium speed of electric mixer for 2 minutes. Beat in eggs one at a time just until blended.

In a separate bowl combine flour, baking soda, and spices well, and slowly blend into creamed mixture alternately with Postum. Fold in raisins and nuts. Pour batter into prepared pans and bake for 35 to 40 minutes, or until a wooden pick inserted into center comes out clean.

Remove from oven and let cool in pans for 10 minutes. Then remove from pans and allow to cool completely on wire racks. Serve plain or frost with Buttercream Frosting (page 695).

10 to 12 servings

Nut Torte

In less than an hour you can take this cake from cracking the eggs to serving the slices—and most of that time is oven time, freeing you for other activities.

5 eggs, separated
⅓ cup honey
1 teaspoon vanilla extract
1¼ cups ground nuts (Brazil, walnut, hazelnut, or any firm nut)

Preheat oven to 350°F.

In a medium-size bowl beat egg whites until stiff but not dry.

Beat egg yolks in a large bowl, then beat in honey, vanilla, and nuts. Fold in egg whites, then turn batter into a buttered 9-inch-square or 9-inch-round baking pan, and bake for 10 minutes. Reduce heat to 325°F, and continue to bake for about 25 minutes, or until a wooden pick inserted into center comes out clean.

Cool for 10 minutes before removing from pan. Serve warm or cold with Cherry Sauce (page 663), Raspberry Sauce (page 664), or whipped cream.

4 to 6 servings

Orange-Walnut Cake

1 cup butter
1 cup honey
4 eggs
3 cups sifted whole wheat pastry flour
1 teaspoon baking soda
2 tablespoons grated orange rind
½ cup orange juice
1 cup coarsely chopped walnuts, dusted with
    2 tablespoons whole wheat pastry flour

Preheat oven to 350°F. Butter and flour an 8-inch springform or 10-inch tube pan.

Cream butter in a large bowl until light and fluffy. Gradually add honey and continue beating at medium speed of electric mixer for 2 minutes. Beat in eggs one at a time just until blended.

In a separate bowl combine flour, baking soda, and orange rind and slowly blend into creamed mixture alternately with orange juice. Fold in walnuts. Pour batter into prepared pan and bake for 40 to 50 minutes, or until a wooden pick inserted into center comes out clean.

Remove from oven and let cool in pan for 10 minutes. Then remove from pan and allow to cool completely on a wire rack. Frost with Seven-Minute Frosting (page 697) or dust with Coconut Sugar (page 698).

10 to 12 servings

Peach Upside-Down Cake

¼ cup butter
⅔ cup honey
1 teaspoon ground cinnamon
    dash of nutmeg
2 cups sliced peaches
1 cup plus 1 tablespoon whole wheat flour
1 teaspoon baking soda
¼ cup vegetable oil
½ cup buttermilk
1 tablespoon grated lemon rind
1 teaspoon vanilla extract
1 egg

Preheat oven to 350°F.

Melt butter in an 8-inch-square pan. Add ⅓ cup honey, cinnamon, and nutmeg and mix. Make sure mixture coats bottom of pan. Arrange peaches over butter mixture.

Combine flour and baking soda in a medium-size bowl. Set aside.

In a separate bowl mix remaining honey, oil, buttermilk, lemon rind, and vanilla. Add to flour mixture, mix well, and then add egg. When completely blended, pour over peaches in pan. Bake for 30 minutes.

Remove from pan immediately by inverting onto a serving plate.

6 to 8 servings

Peanut Butter Cake

Youngsters love the idea of this cake that incorporates one of their favorite foods, but the delicious overtone of peanut flavor makes it a treat for everyone.

½ cup butter
⅔ cup honey
3 eggs
1 teaspoon vanilla extract
½ cup peanut butter
2¼ cups sifted whole wheat pastry flour
1 teaspoon baking soda
1 cup buttermilk

Preheat oven to 350°F. Butter and flour 2 8-inch-round baking pans, a 9-inch-square pan, or a 7 × 11-inch pan.

Cream butter in a large bowl until light and fluffy. Gradually add honey and continue beating at medium speed of electric mixer for 2 minutes. Beat in eggs one at a time just until blended. Beat in vanilla and peanut butter.

In a separate bowl combine flour and baking soda and slowly beat into creamed mixture alternately with buttermilk, mixing only enough to blend. Pour batter into prepared pans and bake for 30 minutes, or until a wooden pick inserted into center comes out clean.

Remove from oven and let cool in pans on wire racks for 10 minutes. Then remove from pans and allow to cool completely on racks. Frost with Basic Carob Icing (page 694).

10 to 12 servings

Pound Cake

1 cup butter
1 cup honey, warmed
4 eggs
2 to 2¼ cups whole wheat pastry flour
½ teaspoon baking soda
⅔ cup sour cream
1 teaspoon vanilla extract

Preheat oven to 300°F. Butter and flour a large tube pan or a 9 × 5-inch loaf pan.

Cream butter in a large bowl. Add honey and blend well. Add eggs one at a time, beating well.

In a separate bowl mix flour and baking soda. Add to butter mixture alternately with sour cream and blend well. Fold in vanilla. Pour batter into prepared pan and bake for about 1½ hours, or until lightly browned.

Cool in pan on a wire rack for 10 minutes, then remove from pan and let cool completely on rack.

8 servings

Poppy Seed Cake

This is a generous cake with a lovely flavor that seems to appeal to just about everyone.

4 eggs, separated
¼ teaspoon cream of tartar
½ cup butter
⅔ cup honey
⅔ cup poppy seeds
2¼ cups sifted whole wheat pastry flour
1 teaspoon baking soda
½ teaspoon ground cinnamon
¼ teaspoon ground nutmeg
¼ teaspoon ground cloves
⅔ cup buttermilk
¼ cup lemon juice (1 lemon)
½ cup dried currants, dusted with 1 tablespoon
   whole wheat pastry flour

Preheat oven to 350°F. Butter and flour two 8-inch-round baking pans.

Beat egg whites at high speed of electric mixer until foamy. Add cream of tartar and continue beating

at high speed until stiff but not dry. Set aside.

In a large bowl cream butter until light and fluffy. Gradually add honey and continue beating at medium speed for 2 minutes. Beat in egg yolks one at a time just until blended. Beat in poppy seeds.

Combine flour, baking soda, and spices and gradually blend into creamed mixture alternately with buttermilk and lemon juice. Beat just until smooth. Beat in ¼ of the egg whites. Then fold in remaining egg whites. Fold in currants. Pour batter into prepared pans and bake for about 30 minutes, or until a wooden pick inserted into center comes out clean.

Remove from oven and let cool in pans on wire racks for about 15 minutes. Then remove from pans and cool completely on racks. Spread Vanilla Pastry Cream (page 699) or fruit jam between layers. Frost with whipped cream or Carob Ripple Frosting (page 695).

8 to 10 servings

Rice Flour Sponge Cake

A good all-purpose cake that can be served to those who must avoid wheat products.

5 eggs, separated
¼ cup molasses
1 teaspoon vanilla extract
½ cup brown rice flour
¼ teaspoon baking soda
¼ cup honey, warmed

Preheat oven to 325°F. Butter a 9-inch-square or 9-inch-round baking pan.

In a large bowl beat egg yolks until thick and lemon colored. Add molasses and vanilla.

In a separate bowl combine flour and baking soda, mixing to distribute soda evenly. Set aside.

In another bowl beat egg whites until soft peaks form. Add honey gradually, while continuing to beat, until stiff but not dry.

Stir flour mixture into egg yolk mixture. Then fold in ¼ of the egg whites until well blended. Fold remaining egg whites into batter. Pour into prepared pan. Bake for 25 minutes.

Cool in pan on a wire rack for 5 minutes. Remove cake carefully by running a spatula around the edge and underneath. When cool, spread with Almond Icing (page 694).

6 servings

Swedish Tea Ring

Serve this cake to top off an elegant brunch or as the centerpiece of a full-dress tea.

Cake
½ cup milk, scalded
2 tablespoons butter
2 tablespoons honey
½ cup water
1 tablespoon dry yeast
1 egg
3 cups whole wheat flour

Filling
10 pitted dried prunes
¼ cup prune juice
¼ teaspoon ground cinnamon
1 tablespoon lemon juice
2 tablespoons honey

Glaze
1 tablespoon honey
¼ teaspoon vanilla extract
2 tablespoons nonfat dry milk

To make the cake: In a large bowl combine milk, butter, and honey. Cool to lukewarm by adding water. Add yeast and mix well. Blend in egg, then cover and let stand in a warm place for about 10 minutes. Add flour and mix until dough is well blended and soft. Roll out into a 14 × 12-inch rectangle.

To make the filling: Soak prunes in hot water for 15 minutes. Drain, reserving soaking water. Put prunes in a blender with about ¼ cup reserved liquid and puree. Simmer prune puree, prune juice, cinnamon, lemon juice, and honey until thick. Cool.

Spread filling evenly on rolled dough. Roll up dough lengthwise, pinching seams closed with your fingers, and place on oiled baking sheet. Twist dough to form ring and join ends. With scissors, cut deep slashes about 1 inch apart. Turn each piece on its side,

cut-edge up. Cover with a cloth and let rise in a warm place until light, about 45 minutes.

Preheat oven to 350°F.

Bake for 30 minutes.

To make the glaze: Combine honey, vanilla, and dry milk. Drizzle over still-warm tea ring.

Makes 1

Tropical-Fruit Cake

Add extra dimension to the standard banana cake with coconut, almonds, and orange juice.

½ cup butter
½ cup honey
3 eggs
½ cup mashed banana (1 small banana)
½ cup unsweetened shredded coconut
1 teaspoon almond extract
2¼ cups sifted whole wheat pastry flour
1 teaspoon baking soda
½ cup finely chopped blanched almonds
½ cup orange juice

Preheat oven to 350°F. Butter and flour two 8-inch-round baking pans, a 9-inch-square pan, or a 7 × 11-inch pan.

Cream butter in a large bowl until light and fluffy. Gradually add honey and continue beating at medium speed of electric mixer for 2 minutes. Beat in eggs one at a time just until blended. Beat in banana, coconut, and almond extract.

In a separate bowl combine flour, baking soda, and almonds, and gradually blend into creamed mixture alternately with orange juice. Beat just until smooth. Pour batter into prepared pans and bake for 30 minutes, or until a wooden pick inserted into center comes out clean.

Remove from oven and let cool in pans on wire racks for about 15 minutes. Then remove from pans and cool completely on wire racks. Spread Vanilla Pastry Cream (page 699) or whipped cream and banana slices between layers, and dust top with Coconut Sugar (page 698), or ice with White Frosting (page 698).

8 to 10 servings

Walnut Torte

2 cups walnuts
4 eggs, separated
¼ cup plus 2 tablespoons honey
1 teaspoon vanilla extract

Preheat oven to 350°F. Butter a 9-inch-square or 9-inch-round baking pan.

Grind walnuts, ½ cup at a time, in a blender.

In a small bowl beat egg whites until stiff but not dry, then set aside.

Beat egg yolks in a large bowl. Then beat in honey and vanilla. Mix in ground nuts. Fold in egg whites. Turn batter into prepared pan and bake for 10 minutes. Then reduce heat to 325°F, and continue to bake for about 25 minutes longer, or until a wooden pick inserted into center comes out clean.

Cool in pan for 10 minutes and then remove from pan. Serve warm or cold with Cherry Sauce (page 663) or Raspberry Sauce (page 664).

6 servings

Yeast Cake

1/3 cup warm water
2 tablespoons plus 1 teaspoon honey
1 tablespoon dry yeast
½ cup butter
4 eggs
1/3 cup warm milk
2 cups sifted whole wheat pastry flour
¼ cup blanched almonds, toasted

In a small bowl combine water and 1 teaspoon honey, then stir in yeast. Let stand in a warm place for 5 to 10 minutes, or until foamy.

In a large bowl cream butter until light and fluffy. Slowly add remaining honey and continue beating at medium speed of electric mixer for 2 minutes. Beat in eggs one at a time just until blended. Add yeast mixture, milk, and flour, and beat until well blended. Cover bowl with a dampened cloth or plastic wrap, and let rise in a warm place until doubled in bulk, about 1½ hours.

Generously butter a 10-cup tube pan, ring mold, or Bundt or Kugelhopf pan.

Finely grind nuts, then sprinkle over all surfaces of pan.

When batter has doubled, stir briskly to expel air. Pour into prepared pan. Cover and let rise again until doubled in bulk, about 1 hour.

Preheat oven to 400°F.

Bake cake for 30 minutes, or until it becomes golden and begins to pull away from sides of pan.

Remove from oven and let cool in pan on a wire rack for 10 minutes. Then remove from pan and let cool completely on rack. Slice cake into 3 or 4 thin layers. Fill layers with chilled Vanilla Pastry Cream (page 699) and top with Apricot Glaze (page 664).

10 to 12 servings

Yogurt Coffee Cake

Here is a moist and flavorful breakfast cake with the topping baked right into it!

Topping
2 tablespoons honey, warmed
2 teaspoons ground cinnamon
2 tablespoons whole wheat flour
¾ cup chopped nuts

Cake
½ cup butter
½ cup honey, warmed
2 eggs
1 1/3 cups whole wheat flour
1 teaspoon baking soda
1 cup yogurt
1 teaspoon vanilla extract

Preheat oven to 350°F. Butter and flour a 9-inch-square baking pan.

To make the topping: In a small bowl combine honey, cinnamon, flour, and nuts.

To make the cake: Cream butter in a large bowl. Add honey and eggs and mix well.

Sift together flour and baking soda, and then fold into batter along with yogurt and vanilla. Pour ½ of the cake batter into prepared pan. Cover with ½ of the topping, then add remaining batter, and top with remaining topping. Bake for about 45 minutes, or until a wooden pick inserted into center comes out clean.

Cool slightly and cut into squares. Serve warm or cold.

8 servings

Cupcakes

Almond-Fig Treats

    8 ounces dried figs, chopped
    1 cup boiling water
1½ cups whole wheat pastry flour
    1 teaspoon baking powder
    1 teaspoon baking soda
    ¼ cup sour cream
    ¼ cup butter, softened
    ½ cup honey, warmed
    2 eggs
    1 cup chopped almonds

Preheat oven to 375°F. Line muffin tins with paper cups.

In a small bowl soak figs in boiling water for 15 minutes. Drain and discard water.

Sift together flour, baking powder, and baking soda.

In a large bowl beat together sour cream, butter, honey, and eggs for 5 minutes. On low speed of electric mixer, gradually beat ½ of the flour mixture into sour cream mixture. Gradually beat in ½ of the figs. Beat in remaining flour, then remaining figs. Fold in almonds. Spoon into prepared tins and bake for 20 minutes, or until a wooden pick inserted into center comes out clean.

Cool in tins for 5 minutes. Then remove from tins and cool completely on wire racks.

Makes 1 to 1½ dozen

Apricot Cupcakes

1½ cups whole wheat pastry flour
    1 cup soy flour
    2 teaspoons baking powder
    ½ cup butter, softened
    ½ cup honey
    4 eggs
    ¼ cup milk
   ⅓ cup orange juice
    1 cup chopped dried apricots

Preheat oven to 325°F. Butter muffin tins or line with paper cups.

Sift together flours and baking powder.

In a large bowl beat butter and honey, adding eggs one at a time and beating until light. Add ¼ of the flour mixture and beat. Add ½ of the milk and beat.

Repeat. Add additional ¼ of the flour mixture and beat. Add orange juice and beat.

Toss apricots in remaining flour and fold into batter. Spoon batter into prepared tins, and bake for 20 to 25 minutes, or until a wooden pick inserted into center comes out clean.

Cool in tins for 5 minutes. Then remove from tins and cool completely on wire racks. Frost with White Frosting (page 698).

Makes 1 to 1½ dozen

Banana Crunch Cupcakes

This may well be the only crunchy banana cupcake you will ever experience. It is a nice surprise for those used to characteristic banana cake texture.

    ½ cup rolled oats
   ⅓ cup date sugar
    2 tablespoons butter, melted
    ½ teaspoon ground cinnamon
    ½ cup butter, softened
    ½ cup honey
    ¼ cup yogurt
    3 eggs
    1 cup mashed bananas
    1 teaspoon vanilla extract
1¼ cups oat or whole wheat flour
    ¾ cup soy flour
    2 teaspoons baking soda
    ½ cup chopped walnuts

Preheat oven to 325°F. Butter muffin tins or line with paper cups.

In a small bowl mix together oats, date sugar, melted butter, and cinnamon.

In a large bowl beat together softened butter and honey. Beat in yogurt, eggs, bananas, and vanilla.

In a separate bowl sift together flours and baking soda. Gradually add dry ingredients to liquid ingredients, mixing well. Fold in nuts. Spoon batter into muffin tins, and sprinkle each cupcake with date sugar mixture. Bake for 20 to 25 minutes, or until a wooden pick inserted into center comes out clean.

Cool in tins for 5 minutes. Then remove from tins and cool completely on wire racks. Frost with Buttercream Frosting (page 695).

Makes 1 to 1½ dozen

Carob Cupcakes

 1 egg
 ½ cup sifted powdered carob
 ½ cup butter, softened
 1½ cups whole wheat pastry flour
 ½ cup sour cream, yogurt, or buttermilk
 1 teaspoon baking soda
 ½ cup honey, warmed
 ½ cup hot water

Preheat oven to 375°F. Butter a 12-cup muffin tin or line with paper cups.

Place ingredients in a large bowl in order given. Do not mix until last item has been added and then beat well. Fill muffin tin ⅔ full and bake for 20 to 25 minutes, or until a wooden pick inserted into center comes out clean.

Cool in tins for 5 minutes. Then remove from tins and cool completely on wire racks. Frost with White Frosting (page 698).

Makes 1 dozen

Chewy Prune Cupcakes

 2 cups pitted dried prunes
 1 cup whole wheat pastry flour
 ⅔ cup soy flour
 1 tablespoon baking powder
 ¼ cup butter, softened
 ½ cup honey
 6 eggs, separated
 2 teaspoons vanilla extract

Preheat oven to 350°F. Butter muffin tins or line with paper cups.

Cut prunes into small pieces with kitchen shears. Shake prunes in enough flour just to coat.

Sift together flours and baking powder.

In a large bowl beat together butter and honey. Beat in egg yolks one at a time. Mix in vanilla.

Beat egg whites until stiff but not dry. Blend egg whites into butter mixture alternately with flour mixture. Fold in prunes. Spoon batter into muffin tins and bake for 20 minutes, or until a wooden pick inserted into center comes out clean.

Cool on wire racks, then remove from tins.

Makes 1 to 1½ dozen

Chunky Apple Cupcakes

The apple chunks are softened some by the baking, but they are still firm enough to retain their identity and provide welcome texture surprises.

 1½ cups whole wheat flour
 ¾ cup soy flour
 1 teaspoon ground cinnamon
 2 teaspoons baking powder
 1 teaspoon baking soda
 ½ cup butter, softened
 ¼ cup vegetable oil
 ½ cup honey
 ½ cup sour cream
 2 eggs
 1½ cups cubed peeled apples
 ½ cup chopped walnuts

Preheat oven to 325°F. Butter muffin tins or line with paper cups.

In a large bowl sift together flours, cinnamon, baking powder, and baking soda.

In another bowl beat together butter, oil, and honey. Beat in sour cream and eggs. Gradually blend with dry ingredients. Fold in apples and nuts. Spoon batter into muffin tins and bake for 20 to 25 minutes, or until a wooden pick inserted into center comes out clean.

Cool for 5 minutes in tins. Then remove from tins and cool completely on wire racks.

Makes 1 to 1½ dozen

Coconut Cakes

 1¾ cups whole wheat pastry flour
 2 teaspoons baking powder
 1 teaspoon baking soda
 ½ cup honey
 ¼ cup sour cream
 ⅓ cup butter, softened
 ¾ cup milk
 3 egg whites
 1 teaspoon almond extract
 3 cups grated fresh coconut

Preheat oven to 350°F. Butter a 12-cup muffin tin or line with paper cups.

In a large bowl sift together flour, baking powder, and baking soda.

In another bowl beat together honey, sour cream, and butter. Add to flour mixture, along with milk, beating at low speed of electric mixer for 2 minutes. Add egg whites and almond extract, beating for another 2 minutes. Fold in coconut. Spoon batter into tin and bake for 20 to 25 minutes, or until a wooden pick inserted into center comes out clean.

Cool for 5 minutes in tin. Then remove from tin and cool completely on wire racks. Frost with Vanilla-Cream Cheese Frosting (page 697).

Makes 1 dozen

Honey-Almond Cakes

2½ cups whole wheat pastry flour
1 teaspoon baking soda
1 teaspoon baking powder
½ cup butter, softened
½ cup vegetable oil
⅔ cup honey
¼ cup yogurt
2 eggs
½ teaspoon almond extract
1 cup sliced almonds
¼ cup honey, warmed

Preheat oven to 325°F. Butter muffin tins.
Sift together flour, baking soda, and baking powder.
In a large bowl beat together butter, oil, and honey. Add yogurt and beat in. Add eggs and almond extract, and continue to beat for 2 minutes. Stir in flour mixture. Fold in almonds. Spoon batter into tins and bake for 20 minutes, or until a wooden pick inserted into center comes out clean.

Brush cupcakes with warmed honey, and broil 6 inches from heat for 1 to 2 minutes. Cool slightly before removing from tins.

Makes 1 to 1½ dozen

Lemon Cupcakes

2 cups whole wheat pastry flour
½ cup soy flour
1 tablespoon baking powder
2 teaspoons baking soda
¼ cup butter, softened
¼ cup vegetable oil

⅔ cup honey
2 tablespoons sour cream
2 eggs, beaten
¼ cup milk
¼ cup plus 2 tablespoons lemon juice
½ teaspoon grated lemon rind
½ cup chopped walnuts

Preheat oven to 325°F. Butter muffin tins or line with paper cups.
Sift together flours, baking powder, and baking soda.
In a large bowl beat together butter, oil, honey, sour cream, and eggs. Add milk and flour mixture, beating until batter is smooth. Beat in lemon juice. Fold in lemon rind and nuts. Spoon batter into tins and bake for 20 to 25 minutes, or until a wooden pick inserted into center comes out clean.

Cool in tins for 5 minutes. Then remove from tins and cool completely on wire racks.

Makes 1 to 1½ dozen

Luscious Lemon-Filled Cupcakes

1¾ cups whole wheat pastry flour
1 tablespoon baking powder
¼ teaspoon ground nutmeg
¼ cup plus 2 tablespoons butter, softened
½ cup honey, warmed
8 egg yolks, lightly beaten
1 tablespoon lemon juice
½ cup milk
Lemon Filling (page 699)

Preheat oven to 325°F. Butter muffin tins or line with paper cups.
Sift flour with baking powder and nutmeg.
In a large bowl beat together butter and honey for 3 minutes. Add egg yolks and continue to beat until fluffy. Mix in lemon juice. Add flour mixture and milk alternately, beating well after each addition. Using ½ of the batter, fill tins ⅓ full. Add 1 teaspoon lemon filling to each cupcake, top with remaining batter, and bake for 20 to 25 minutes.

Cool in tins for 5 minutes. Then remove from tins and cool completely on wire racks.

Makes 1 to 1½ dozen

Marble Cupcakes

1¾ cups whole wheat flour
1 tablespoon baking powder
1 teaspoon baking soda
½ cup butter, softened
¼ cup vegetable oil
¾ cup honey
5 eggs, separated
½ cup carob chips
2 tablespoons water

Preheat oven to 350°F. Butter muffin tins or line with paper cups.

Sift together flour, baking powder, and baking soda.

In a large bowl beat together butter, oil, and ½ cup honey for 3 minutes. Beat in egg yolks, one at a time.

Beat egg whites until stiff but not dry.

Mix ½ of the flour mixture into butter mixture. Fold in ½ of the egg whites. Mix in remaining flour mixture and fold in remaining egg whites.

In top of a double boiler, melt carob and remaining ¼ cup honey with 2 tablespoons water. Fold melted carob into batter so that it streaks batter. Spoon into tins and bake for 20 minutes, or until a wooden pick inserted into center comes out clean.

Cool for 5 minutes in tins. Then remove from tins and cool completely on wire racks.

Makes 1 to 1½ dozen

Orange Blossom Cupcakes

1½ cups whole wheat flour
¾ cup soy flour
2 teaspoons baking powder
½ cup honey
¼ cup butter, softened
¼ cup vegetable oil
2 eggs
¼ cup light cream
¼ cup orange juice
½ teaspoon orange extract
1 navel orange, chopped

½ cup orange juice (optional)
½ cup honey (optional)

Preheat oven to 350°F. Butter a 12-cup muffin tin or line with paper cups.

Sift together flours and baking powder.

In a large bowl beat together ½ cup honey, butter, and oil. Beat in eggs, and then cream, ¼ cup orange juice, and orange extract. Gradually mix dry ingredients into liquid ingredients. Fold in oranges. Spoon batter into tin and bake for 25 minutes, or until a wooden pick inserted into center comes out clean.

Cool for 5 minutes in tin. Then remove from tin and cool completely on wire racks.

If desired, mix together ½ cup orange juice and ½ cup honey in a small saucepan. Bring to a boil, reduce heat, and simmer until slightly thickened, about 5 minutes. Dip tops of cupcakes in this glaze.

Makes 1 dozen

Pineapple-Carrot Cupcakes

3 to 4 carrots, shredded
2¼ cups whole wheat flour
2 teaspoons baking soda
2 teaspoons baking powder
1½ teaspoons ground cinnamon
½ cup vegetable oil
3 eggs, beaten
¼ cup sour cream
¾ cup honey
1 teaspoon vanilla extract
1 cup unsweetened flaked coconut
1 cup unsweetened crushed pineapple

Steam carrots for about 5 minutes, or until soft.

Preheat oven to 350°F. Butter and flour muffin tins or line with paper cups.

In a large bowl sift together flour, baking soda, baking powder, and cinnamon. Add oil, eggs, sour cream, honey, and vanilla, mixing after each addition. Beat by hand for 1 minute. Fold in carrots, coconut, and pineapple. Spoon batter into tins and bake for 25 minutes, or until a wooden pick inserted into center comes out clean.

Cool in tins for 5 minutes. Then remove from tins and cool completely on wire racks.

Makes 1 to 1½ dozen

Strawberry Swirl Cupcakes

1½ cups whole wheat pastry flour
1 teaspoon baking powder
1 teaspoon baking soda
½ teaspoon ground cinnamon
¼ cup plus 2 tablespoons butter, softened
¼ cup sour cream
½ cup honey
3 eggs
½ cup strawberry jam

Preheat oven to 350°F. Line a 12-cup muffin tin with paper cups.

Sift together flour, baking powder, baking soda, and cinnamon.

In a large bowl beat together butter, sour cream, and honey. Beat in eggs one at a time. Mix dry ingredients into liquid ingredients with a spoon. Spoon batter into prepared tin. Place ½ teaspoon strawberry jam in center of each cupcake, and bake for 20 minutes, or until a wooden pick inserted into center comes out clean.

Cool in tin for 5 minutes. Then remove from tin and cool completely on wire racks.

Makes 1 dozen

Sweet Tahini Cupcakes

¾ cup soy flour
1 cup whole wheat flour
1 teaspoon baking soda
1 teaspoon baking powder
½ cup vegetable oil
¾ cup tahini (sesame butter)
½ cup sour cream
2 eggs
¾ cup honey
1 teaspoon vanilla extract

Preheat oven to 325°F. Butter muffin tins or line with paper cups.

Sift together flours, baking soda, and baking powder.

In a large bowl beat together oil, tahini, sour cream, eggs, and honey. Mix in vanilla. Slowly mix dry ingredients into liquid ingredients. Spoon batter into tins and bake for 20 to 25 minutes, or until a wooden pick inserted into center comes out clean.

Cool in tins for 5 minutes. Then remove from tins and cool completely on wire racks.

Makes 1 to 1½ dozen

Fruitcakes

Holiday Fruitcake

4 large eggs, beaten
¾ cup honey
½ cup vegetable oil
3 tablespoons grated orange rind
2 cups whole wheat flour
½ cup sesame seeds
1½ cups raisins
½ cup sunflower seeds
1½ cups chopped walnuts
1 cup slivered almonds
1 cup chopped dried figs
1 cup quartered dates
½ cup chopped dried apples
½ cup coarsely chopped hazelnuts
½ cup quartered dried apricots

Preheat oven to 300°F. Generously oil a small ring mold or 9 × 5-inch loaf pan.

Mix eggs, honey, oil, orange rind, and flour together in a large bowl until smooth. Add remaining ingredients and mix well. Turn mixture into prepared pan and bake for about 1 hour and 20 minutes, or until cake springs back when lightly pressed with a finger.

Cool in pan on a wire rack for 30 minutes. Remove from pan and cool completely on rack.

Makes 1

No-Bake Holiday Fruitcake

A rich—very rich—cake that never sees the inside of an oven. It should be parceled out sparingly since each slice is so full of good things.

   1 cup orange juice
   ¼ to ½ cup honey
   ¼ to ½ cup maple syrup
   ½ cup thinly sliced dried apricots
   ½ cup thinly sliced dried peaches
   ½ cup thinly sliced dried pears
   1 cup chopped dried apples
   ½ cup halved dried cherries
   ½ cup sliced dried figs
   1 cup sliced dates
   1 cup golden raisins
   ¼ cup Candied Citrus Rind, Orange (page 691)
   ¼ cup Candied Citrus Rind, Lemon (page 691)
   2 tablespoons reserved syrup from Candied Citrus Rind
   ¾ cup butter, melted
   1 teaspoon vanilla extract
   ¼ teaspoon almond extract
   1 cup pecan halves
   ½ cup ground pecans
   2 cups finely ground almonds
   ¾ cup fine whole grain bread crumbs
   ½ teaspoon ground cinnamon
   ¼ teaspoon ground nutmeg
   ¼ teaspoon ground cloves
   pecan halves
   blanched almonds

Bring orange juice, honey, and maple syrup to a boil in a medium-size saucepan. Add apricots, peaches, pears, apples, and cherries. Stir well, remove from heat, cover, and let stand for 30 minutes.

Transfer mixture to a large bowl. Add figs, dates, raisins, citrus rind and reserved syrup, butter, vanilla and almond extract, and 1 cup pecan halves. Mix together, making sure fruits and nuts are well coated with flavored liquids.

Combine ground nuts, bread crumbs, and spices. Work these dry ingredients into moist ones. Dough will be sticky. When mixture is well combined, pat it into a wax paper-lined 9 × 5-inch loaf pan, pushing it down into all four corners. Press nuts or other desired items into top to decorate. Cover and refrigerate.

Fruitcake will be firm enough to cut the next day but is best when flavors are allowed to mellow for a week or more.

Makes 1

NOTE: You can keep fruitcake in loaf pan or remove it and rewrap it. If wrapping in foil, first wrap in wax paper because the acid from the citrus could react with the foil.

Always slice and serve this fruitcake cold. It becomes soft and sticky at room temperature.

Old-fashioned Dark Christmas Fruitcake

   1 cup raisins
   1 cup chopped dates
   ½ cup chopped dried figs
   3 cups chopped assorted dried fruits (apples, peaches, apricots, pears, and cherries)
   ¼ cup Candied Citrus Rind, Orange (page 691)
   2 tablespoons Candied Citrus Rind, Lemon (page 691)
   1 cup broken walnuts
   1 cup slivered almonds
   1 cup apple cider
   1¼ cups honey
   ½ cup buttermilk
   4 cups whole wheat flour
   2 teaspoons baking soda
   2 teaspoons ground cinnamon
   ½ teaspoon ground nutmeg
   ½ teaspoon ground allspice
   ½ teaspoon ground mace
   1 cup butter, softened
   ¼ cup unsulfured molasses
   4 eggs, separated
   1 cup grape jam

A day ahead combine the fruits, citrus rind, and nuts in a large bowl. Mix in cider and 1 cup honey until all fruit is coated. Cover and let soak at room temperature overnight.

Drain excess liquid from fruit mixture and add it to buttermilk.

Preheat oven to 300°F. Butter a 10-inch tube pan (one with a removable tube works best), line it with wax paper or parchment, and then butter paper.

Combine flour, baking soda, and spices.

Cream butter, molasses, and remaining honey in

a large bowl. Beat in egg yolks one at a time and then beat in jam.

Beat egg whites until stiff but not dry.

Add flour mixture to creamed mixture alternately with buttermilk, beating well after each addition. Stir in drained fruits and nuts, and then fold in egg whites. Spoon batter into prepared pan.

Place a pan of hot water on bottom of oven. Bake cake for 2 hours, or until it springs back when pressed lightly with a finger. (Cover top of cake with foil if it is browning too much.)

Remove from oven and cool completely before removing from pan. Then invert cake on a plate and peel off wax paper. Cool, then store cake in refrigerator in an airtight container, or wrap it in wax paper and then foil. Allow it to mellow for at least 3 weeks. If desired, glaze cake with Fruitcake Glaze (see opposite) before serving.

Makes 1

Candied Citrus Rind
(Lemon or Orange)

> 1 medium-size orange or 1 large lemon
> ½ cup honey

Squeeze juice from orange or lemon and reserve. Scrape remaining pulp out of rind, leaving a clean shell. Slice rind into very thin strips, about 1/16 inch thick and ½ to 1 inch long.

Add water to orange juice to equal ½ cup, if necessary, or to lemon juice to equal 1/3 cup. Combine juice, honey, and rind in a 1-quart saucepan. Bring to a boil, lower heat, and allow to remain at a steady, easy boil, uncovered, for about 30 minutes. As mixture cooks, the boil will become foamy. Lower heat as liquid cooks down, and stir frequently. The rind should turn shiny and translucent when finished.

Remove from heat and immediately press excess syrup from rind through a sieve. Reserve syrup for use in recipes. Cut a piece of wax paper 18 inches long. Lay pieces of candied rind on wax paper, one by one, with about ½-inch space between them. Leave a 1½- to 2-inch border along side edges.

Allow to dry for about 2 hours. If not using citrus immediately, roll up wax paper, twist ends, and store in an airtight container until ready to use.

Makes ½ cup orange rind or 1/3 cup lemon rind

Fruitcake Glaze

> 2 cups apple juice or cider
> 1 cup maple syrup
> ¼ cup dried apricots

Combine ingredients, bring to a boil in a 2-quart pot, and continue to boil for 30 minutes. Turn the heat down gradually as liquid evaporates, but always keep syrup boiling. Remove apricots and use as desired. Boil syrup for another 20 minutes, or until it drips in sheets from a metal spoon. During this last time period syrup will be foamy. Stir it occasionally.

To glaze fruitcake, have cake at room temperature or slightly cooler, and the glaze hot so that it flows on the cake. Use a pastry brush to apply glaze. It will be sticky. After cake is well coated, set nuts or other decorations, if desired, on cake. Allow glaze to dry well at room temperature before wrapping or serving.

Yields about 1½ cups

NOTE: For holiday decorating, cut out a paper stencil of some holiday symbol, place this on the cake after glaze has been applied, and dust over it with ground almonds. Press nuts in lightly with your fingers and carefully remove stencil.

Cheesecakes

Basic Cheesecake Crust

> 1¼ cups graham cracker, zwieback, vanilla
> wafer, or cake crumbs
> ¼ cup butter, melted
> 2 tablespoons honey (optional)

Butter a 9-inch springform pan.

Place crumbs in a medium-size bowl. Combine butter and honey (if used) and pour over crumbs. Mix well. Press onto bottom and 1 inch up sides of prepared pan. Chill.

Makes 1

Variations:
Spiced Cheesecake Crust: Add ½ teaspoon ground spice, such as cinnamon, nutmeg, or ginger.

Rich Nut Crust: Substitute ¼ cup ground walnuts or pecans for ¼ cup crumbs.

Rich Cheesecake Crust

1 cup sifted whole wheat pastry flour
2 tablespoons honey
1 teaspoon grated lemon rind
1 egg yolk
½ cup butter, softened

Preheat oven to 400°F. Butter a 9-inch spring-form pan.

Combine ingredients in a medium-size bowl and blend well with your fingers. Press onto bottom and 1 inch up sides of prepared pan. Prick with a fork. Bake for 10 minutes, or until golden. Cool in pan on a wire rack.

Makes 1

Almond Cheesecake

1 Rich Cheesecake Crust (see above)
1 pound cream, Neufchatel, ricotta, or cottage
    cheese
⅔ cup honey
4 eggs
2 teaspoons vanilla extract
1 teaspoon almond extract
2 cups sour cream

Chill crust. Have all other ingredients at room temperature.

Preheat oven to 350°F.

Place cheese in a large bowl and cream well. If using cottage cheese, puree in a food mill or blender. Gradually beat in ⅓ cup honey. Add eggs, one at a time, mixing well after each addition. Stir in 1 teaspoon vanilla and ½ teaspoon almond extract. Pour batter into prepared crust and bake for 25 to 30 minutes, or until set. While cheesecake is baking, mix sour cream and remaining ⅓ cup honey, 1 teaspoon vanilla, and ½ teaspoon almond extract.

Remove cheesecake from oven and increase heat to 500°F. Very slowly spread sour cream mixture over baked batter. Return to oven and bake for 5 minutes more. Cool on a wire rack, then chill.

Remove rim from pan. Serve plain or with whipped cream, and decorate with ground almonds or grated carob.

Makes 1

Italian Nesselrode Cheesecake

Crust
¼ cup butter
1 cup finely ground millet
    grated rind of 1 lemon
1 egg yolk
1 tablespoon honey

Filling
1 cup raisins
1 cup honey
1 pound well-drained ricotta cheese
4 eggs, separated
2 tablespoons cornstarch
½ teaspoon grated whole nutmeg
1½ teaspoon vanilla extract
3 tablespoons brown rice, cooked

To make the crust: In a medium-size bowl cut butter into millet with 2 knives or a pastry blender until mixture resembles coarse crumbs. Add remaining ingredients and blend well. Form into a ball, flatten slightly, wrap in plastic wrap, and chill in refrigerator until dough is firm enough to manage, about 30 minutes. Then roll out dough on a flat surface, between lightly floured sheets of wax paper or plastic wrap, to a 10-inch circle. Fit carefully into a 9-inch springform pan, using fingers to press dough over bottom and against sides of pan. Refrigerate until ready to use. Then bake for 15 minutes at 350°F.

To make the filling: Simmer raisins and honey in a small saucepan over medium heat until raisins are plumped, about 15 minutes. Remove raisins with a slotted spoon and allow honey and raisins to cool.

In a large bowl beat together ricotta, honey, and egg yolks until smooth and creamy. (A food processor or blender is helpful.) Stir in cornstarch, nutmeg, and vanilla. Blend in rice and raisins.

Preheat oven to 350°F.

Beat egg whites until stiff but not dry. Carefully fold into cheese mixture and pour into prepared crust.

Bake for 45 to 60 minutes, or until golden brown and set. Cool thoroughly on a wire rack, then chill. For best flavor refrigerate for several hours or overnight before serving.

Remove rim from pan. Decorate with whipped cream and dusting of nutmeg.

Makes 1

Lemon Cheesecake

½ cup whole grain bread crumbs
½ teaspoon ground cinnamon
4 eggs, separated
1½ teaspoons grated lemon rind
½ teaspoon grated orange rind
    juice of ½ lemon
½ cup plus 2 tablespoons honey
1½ cups low-fat cottage cheese
¼ cup buttermilk
1½ tablespoons vanilla extract
3 tablespoons triticale or whole wheat flour
2 cups fresh strawberries

Butter bottom and sides of a 9-inch springform pan. Combine bread crumbs and cinnamon. Sprinkle mixture into pan and coat sides lightly, allowing excess to coat bottom in an even layer. Press bottom gently.

In a small bowl beat egg yolks until thick and lemon colored. In a large bowl beat egg whites until stiff but not dry.

Preheat oven to 350°F.

In a food processor or blender process all remaining ingredients, except ¼ cup honey and strawberries, until smooth and creamy. Carefully fold in egg yolks, then fold in egg whites. Pour batter into prepared pan.

Bake for 40 minutes, or until puffed and set. Turn off oven and open door for 1 minute to reduce heat. Close door and allow cheesecake to remain in oven for another hour. Then refrigerate for several hours or overnight.

Remove rim from pan. Just before serving, dip strawberries in remaining honey to glaze each one, and arrange attractively on top of cheesecake.

Makes 1

Rich Cheesecake

1 Basic Cheesecake Crust (page 691)
4 eggs, separated
½ teaspoon cream of tartar
½ cup plus 2 tablespoons honey
1 pound cream, Neufchatel, ricotta, or cottage
    cheese
2 tablespoons whole wheat pastry flour
1 cup sour cream or yogurt

1 teaspoon vanilla or almond extract
3 tablespoons lemon or orange juice
1 teaspoon grated lemon or orange rind

Chill crust. Have all other ingredients at room temperature.

Preheat oven to 350°F.

In a large bowl beat egg whites until foamy, add cream of tartar, and beat at high speed of electric mixer, gradually adding 2 tablespoons honey. Beat until stiff but not dry.

In another large bowl beat cheese until soft. Gradually beat in ½ cup honey and flour. Add egg yolks, one at a time, beating well after each addition. Add sour cream or yogurt, vanilla or almond extract, lemon or orange juice, and lemon or orange rind and blend. Fold in egg whites until just combined. Pour batter into prepared crust.

Bake for 1¼ hours. Turn off oven and let cake stand in oven for 30 minutes more. Cool on a wire rack, then chill.

Remove rim from pan, and serve plain or decorate with whipped cream, ground nuts, or Cheesecake Fruit Topping (see below).

Makes 1

Variation:

Carob Cheesecake: Add 2 tablespoons Basic Carob Syrup (page 737) to batter with ½ cup honey and flour.

Cheesecake Fruit Topping

2 cups fresh strawberries, blueberries, or
    cherries, or sliced apricots or peaches
4 tablespoons water
2 tablespoons honey
1 tablespoon unflavored gelatin or agar flakes

Combine 1 cup fruit with 2 tablespoons water and bring to a boil. Puree in a blender or food processor.

Combine puree with honey and bring to a boil.

Sprinkle gelatin or agar flakes over remaining 2 tablespoons water and let stand for 5 minutes. Then add to heated fruit puree. Stir and cook until dissolved. Cool mixture and then chill until slightly thickened.

Place remaining 1 cup fruit on top of cheesecake. Pour glaze over fruit. Chill thoroughly.

Frostings and Fillings

Almond Icing

    2 cups blanched almonds
    2 tablespoons butter, softened
    1/3 cup honey
    1/4 to 1/3 cup milk or light cream
    1 teaspoon vanilla extract

Grind almonds in a blender to a fine flour. Place in a medium-size bowl. Add butter, honey, 1/4 cup milk or cream, and vanilla. Mix well. If icing is too thick, add more milk or cream.

    Yields 2 cups

Apricot-Walnut Frosting

    3 tablespoons honey
    1 teaspoon vanilla extract
    3 egg yolks
    1/2 cup butter
    1/4 cup finely chopped dried apricots
    1/4 cup finely chopped walnuts

In a large bowl blend honey and vanilla, mixing in egg yolks one at a time. Blend in butter. Fold in apricots and walnuts. Refrigerate until thickened but not set.

    Yields about 1 1/2 cups

NOTE: Keep this icing refrigerated. Raw egg yolks are susceptible to spoilage if left long at room temperature.

Banana Cream Frosting

    1 cup heavy cream
    1/2 teaspoon lemon juice
    1/2 teaspoon vanilla extract
    1 large ripe banana

In a large bowl whip cream until dry, gradually mixing in lemon juice and vanilla. Put banana through a potato ricer right into whipped cream. Fold in. Use immediately.

    Yields about 2 cups

Golden Egg Icing

    4 egg yolks
    1/2 teaspoon cream of tartar
    2 tablespoons very cold water

    2 1/2 tablespoons lemon juice
    2/3 cup honey
    1/4 teaspoon grated lemon rind (optional)

Heat all ingredients except rind in top of a double boiler. Beat until fluffy and thick, 5 to 6 minutes. Fold in rind, if used. Refrigerate until icing reaches spreading consistency.

    Yields about 1 1/2 cups

NOTE: Keep this icing refrigerated. Raw egg yolks are susceptible to spoilage if left long at room temperature.

Basic Carob Icing

    1/3 cup sifted powdered carob
    3 tablespoons water
    3 tablespoons honey
    3 ounces cream cheese
    1/2 cup chopped walnuts or pecans (optional)

Combine carob, water, and honey in a small saucepan. Mix well and place over low heat. Simmer for 5 minutes, stirring constantly with a wire whisk.

Remove from heat and beat in cream cheese. Add nuts (if used). Cool slightly before spreading over cake.

    Yields 1 1/4 cups

NOTE: For a thinner creamier icing add 1 tablespoon light cream along with cream cheese.

Basic Honey Icing

    1/2 cup honey
    8 ounces cream cheese, or 1 cup cottage cheese
    1/2 teaspoon vanilla extract

With an electric mixer beat all ingredients in a large bowl until thick and creamy, about 5 minutes. Spread immediately over cooled cake. If desired, top with chopped nuts, coconut, or chopped dried apricots.

    Yields 1 1/2 cups

Broiled Coconut Icing

    2 tablespoons butter, softened
    3 tablespoons honey
    1/2 cup unsweetened shredded coconut

Mix all ingredients. Spread over warm freshly baked cake. Place cake under broiler for about 5 minutes, or until icing is bubbly and slightly browned. (Watch carefully so coconut does not burn.)

    Yields 1/2 to 3/4 cup

Buttercream Frosting

This is a basic icing that accepts a variety of flavorings and can be used for innumerable purposes.

¼ cup plus 2 tablespoons butter
¼ cup honey
2 egg yolks
1 tablespoon vanilla extract

In a large bowl cream butter until smooth. Gradually beat in honey, then egg yolks and vanilla. Beat at medium speed for 5 minutes, or until smooth. Chill frosting until it is cool but can still be spread.

Buttercream frosting can be stored in refrigerator or freezer. Bring to spreading consistency before using.

Yields 1½ cups

NOTE: Keep this icing refrigerated. Raw egg yolks are susceptible to spoilage if left long at room temperature.

Variations:

Almond Buttercream Frosting: Use only 2 teaspoons vanilla plus ½ teaspoon almond extract.

Carob Buttercream Frosting: Replace vanilla with 2 tablespoons Basic Carob Syrup (page 737).

Lemon Buttercream Frosting: Replace vanilla with 1 tablespoon lemon juice and 1 tablespoon grated lemon rind.

Mocha Buttercream Frosting: Replace vanilla with 1 tablespoon Basic Carob Syrup (page 737) and 1 tablespoon Postum.

Orange Buttercream Frosting: Replace vanilla with 1 tablespoon orange juice and 1 tablespoon grated orange rind.

Caramel Frosting

½ cup honey
¼ cup butter
¼ cup light cream
1/3 cup chopped pecans, almonds, or walnuts (optional)

In a medium-size saucepan boil honey over very low heat for 4 minutes, or until thick and dark golden in color. (Watch carefully so it does not scorch.) Add butter and beat until butter melts completely. Remove from heat, add cream, and continue to beat until mixture is slightly cooled but still warm. Spread immediately over top of cake, and allow excess icing to run down sides of cake. Sprinkle with nuts, if used.

Yields 1 cup

Carob Ripple Frosting

8 ounces cream cheese, softened
¾ cup plus 2 tablespoons honey
1½ teaspoons vanilla extract
¾ cup carob chips
2 tablespoons butter

In a medium-size bowl beat together cream cheese, ¾ cup honey, and vanilla.

In top of a double boiler, melt carob, butter, and 2 tablespoons honey, stirring constantly. Add 1/3 of the carob mixture to cream cheese mixture, beating until smooth. Frost cake.

Heat remaining carob in top of double boiler, gradually adding enough water so carob is just pourable. Dribble over top of frosted cake in lines about an inch apart. Draw through lines with a sharp knife, about an inch apart, across dribbled lines of carob, alternating direction to make ripples.

Yields about ¾ cup

Crème Chantilly

1 cup heavy cream
1 tablespoon light honey
1 teaspoon vanilla extract

Place cream in a large metal bowl over ice. Beat with a wire whisk until almost stiff. Add honey and vanilla. Beat cream until it holds its shape.

Yields 2 cups

Date-Nut Icing

½ cup date sugar
½ cup hot water
3 egg whites, at room temperature
¾ cup nonfat dry milk
¼ cup ground pecans

In a small saucepan heat sugar and water for 5 minutes, stirring constantly. Set aside to cool.

In a large bowl beat egg whites until stiff but not dry. Slowly mix in date sugar syrup and nonfat dry milk, beating briefly. Mix in pecans. Refrigerate until icing reaches spreading consistency.

Yields about 2 cups

NOTE: Keep this icing refrigerated. Raw egg whites are susceptible to spoilage if left long at room temperature.

Lemon Icing

¼ cup honey, warmed
2 tablespoons lemon juice
⅛ teaspoon cream of tartar
1 egg white
1 teaspoon grated lemon rind

In top of a double boiler, mix honey, lemon juice, cream of tartar, and egg white. Beat for several minutes, then place over boiling water and beat until mixture forms soft peaks, 5 to 8 minutes. Remove from heat and beat until thick enough to spread. Fold in lemon rind.

Yields 1½ cups

NOTE: This is a soft icing and cake should be used the day it is iced or icing might soak into cake.

Monkey Frosting

The banana is the source for the odd name of this delicious and versatile icing.

½ teaspoon vanilla extract
8 ounces cream cheese, softened
1 large ripe banana
½ cup unsweetened flaked coconut

In a medium-size bowl mix vanilla into cream cheese. Put banana through potato ricer right into mixture. Mash in. Fold in coconut.

Yields about 1½ cups

Orange-Cream Cheese Frosting

8 ounces cream cheese, softened
⅓ cup orange juice
1 tablespoon honey
½ teaspoon orange extract
¼ teaspoon grated orange rind
¼ teaspoon ground cinnamon

Blend together all ingredients in a blender. Refrigerate until frosting reaches spreading consistency.

Yields about 1½ cups

Peach Topping

This is an interesting and light choice for a plain pound cake or sponge cake.

1 cup peach preserves
2 teaspoons lemon juice
½ teaspoon vanilla extract
½ cup nonfat dry milk

In a small saucepan heat peach preserves, lemon juice, and vanilla. Strain them. Add dry milk to mixture, and cool before using. Topping will be thin.

Yields about 1 cup

Peanut Butter Frosting

¼ cup milk or light cream
½ cup peanut butter
½ cup honey
2 tablespoons vegetable oil

Heat milk or cream in a medium-size saucepan. Do not allow to boil. Add peanut butter, honey, and oil. Blend well with a wire whisk over very low heat for about 5 minutes. Cool slightly before spreading over cake.

Yields 1¼ cups

Peanut-Coconut Frosting

½ cup peanut butter
8 ounces cream cheese, softened
⅓ cup honey
3 tablespoons milk
¾ cup unsweetened flaked coconut

In a medium-size bowl cream together peanut butter, cream cheese, honey, and milk. Fold in coconut.

Yields about 2½ cups

NOTE: For a thinner, creamier frosting, add more milk along with the cream cheese.

Pineapple Frosting

3 ounces cream cheese, softened
1 can (8 ounces) unsweetened crushed
    pineapple, drained, with juice reserved
½ teaspoon vanilla extract
1 teaspoon honey

In a medium-size bowl beat together cream cheese, 2 tablespoons reserved pineapple juice, vanilla, and honey. Fold in pineapple and refrigerate until thick enough to spread.

Yields about 1 cup

Pistachio-Whipped Cream Frosting

½ teaspoon unflavored gelatin
1 tablespoon cold water
1 cup heavy cream
2 tablespoons honey
½ teaspoon almond extract
½ cup ground pistachios

Soften gelatin in cold water for 5 minutes, and then heat in a small saucepan until dissolved. Set aside to cool.

In a large bowl beat cream until it stands in peaks, gradually mixing in honey, almond extract, and gelatin. Fold in pistachios and frost cake immediately.

Yields about 1½ cups

Raspberry Frosting

8 ounces cream cheese, softened
½ cup raspberry preserves
1 teaspoon vanilla extract
2 tablespoons nonfat dry milk

In a medium-size bowl beat all ingredients together. Refrigerate until frosting reaches spreadable consistency.

Yields 1½ cups

Ricotta-Almond Icing

1 cup ricotta or cottage cheese
2 tablespoons butter, softened
¼ to ⅓ cup honey
½ cup slivered almonds, toasted

In a large bowl beat together cheese and butter. Add honey and beat until smooth. Spread on cake and cover with almonds.

Yields 1½ cups

Seven-Minute Frosting

3 egg whites
⅔ cup honey
1 teaspoon vanilla extract

Place egg whites and honey in top of a double boiler over hot, but not boiling, water. Beat with a rotary beater, or an electric beater at low speed, while water comes to a boil. Continue to beat for 7 minutes, or until mixture forms soft peaks. Remove from heat, add vanilla slowly, and continue beating until frosting is stiff enough to hold its shape.

Yields about 3 cups

Strawberry Icing

¼ cup honey (if using fresh strawberries)
4 egg yolks
½ cup butter, softened
½ cup strawberry preserves, or 1 cup fresh
        strawberries
¼ cup nonfat dry milk
3 strawberries, sliced

In a blender or food processor blend honey (if used) with egg yolks, one at a time. Blend in butter, strawberry preserves or strawberries, and dry milk. Refrigerate until thickened. Decorate frosted cake or cupcakes with sliced strawberries.

Yields 1½ cups

NOTE: Keep this icing refrigerated. Raw egg yolks are susceptible to spoilage if left long at room temperature.

Vanilla-Cream Cheese Frosting

1 cup butter, softened
8 ounces cream cheese, softened
½ cup honey
2 egg yolks
1½ teaspoons vanilla extract

In a large bowl beat together butter and cream cheese. Beat in honey, adding egg yolks one at a time. Stir in vanilla.

Yields about 2 cups

NOTE: Keep this icing refrigerated. Raw egg yolks are susceptible to spoilage if left long at room temperature.

Whipped Carob Frosting

1 teaspoon unflavored gelatin, softened in 1
    tablespoon cold water
1 tablespoon sifted powdered carob
1½ tablespoons honey
1 cup heavy cream

In a small saucepan heat softened gelatin, carob,
and honey until dissolved, adding water if needed. Set
aside and let cool to lukewarm.

In a medium-size bowl whip cream until stiff
peaks form, gradually mixing in gelatin mixture.

Yields about 2 cups

White Frosting

1 cup Coconut Sugar (see below)
2 tablespoons butter, softened
¼ cup warm milk or light cream
½ teaspoon vanilla extract
2 tablespoons maple syrup or honey

Blend ingredients thoroughly in a large bowl.
Immediately spread on cooled cake.

Yields 1½ cups

Yogurt Boiled Frosting

2 eggs
1 egg yolk
¾ cup yogurt
¼ cup butter (optional)
¾ cup honey
½ teaspoon vanilla extract

Combine eggs, egg yolk, yogurt, butter (if used),
and honey in top of a double boiler. Place over boiling
water and cook, stirring constantly, until thickened,
about 5 minutes. Remove from heat, add vanilla, and
allow to cool before spreading on cooled cake.

Yields about 1¾ cups

Coconut Sugar

1 cup unsweetened dried coconut

Place coconut in a blender or coffee mill and
process at medium speed until coconut is very fine.
Store in a sealed jar and use in place of powdered
sugar to dust cakes and cookies.

Yields 1 cup

Apple Filling

*Try this between layers of a spice cake or a
plain pound cake. It also makes a tasty topping for
vanilla ice cream.*

4 tart apples
1¾ cups water
⅓ cup honey
2 tablespoons cornstarch, dissolved in ¾ cup
    water
1½ tablespoons butter
½ teaspoon ground cinnamon

Peel, core, and dice apples. In top of a double
boiler, but over direct heat, cook apples in 1 cup water
until tender but not mushy. Add honey. Stir cornstarch
into apples and cook until thick, stirring constantly.
Add butter and cinnamon. Then place top of double
boiler over simmering water, and cook for another 10
minutes, stirring constantly. Cool before using.

Yields about 3 cups

Creamy Fruit Filling

1 cup heavy cream
2 tablespoons honey
¾ cup diced peaches, crushed fresh raspberries,
    crushed fresh strawberries, whole fresh
    blueberries, or crushed unsweetened
    pineapple

In a large bowl whip cream until stiff, gradually
mixing in honey. Fold in fruit.

Yields about 2½ cups

Creamy Vanilla Filling

½ cup honey
3 tablespoons cornstarch
1 cup milk
1 cup light cream
4 egg yolks, lightly beaten
1 teaspoon vanilla extract

Place honey in a medium-size saucepan.

Combine cornstarch and milk in a jar with a
tight-fitting lid, and shake until smooth. Stir into
honey. Add cream and bring mixture to a boil over
medium heat, stirring constantly, until thickened.

Mix a little hot mixture into egg yolks. Add egg yolks to saucepan. Cook for another 2 minutes, stirring constantly. Stir in vanilla and allow to cool before using.

Yields about 2½ cups

Date Filling

½ cup date sugar
¾ cup water
½ cup honey
2 tablespoons lemon juice
1 tablespoon butter

Place date sugar, water, and honey in a medium-size saucepan. Bring to a boil and boil for 4 minutes, stirring constantly. Add lemon juice and butter and blend. Cool in refrigerator before using.

Yields about 1½ cups

Lemon Filling

2 tablespoons cornstarch, dissolved in 1 cup cold water
½ cup honey
2 egg yolks, lightly beaten
¼ cup lemon juice
1 teaspoon butter

Place dissolved cornstarch and honey in a medium-size saucepan. Cook, stirring constantly, until thickened.

Add a little hot mixture to egg yolks. Add egg yolks to saucepan and cook for 2 minutes, stirring constantly. Add lemon juice and butter. Stir until butter melts. Cool before using.

Yields about 1½ cups

Lemon-Curd Filling or Spread

Lemon curd is a popular English lemon butter that can be used in many ways: as a spread for toast at teatime, a filling for meringues, cakes, and sponge rolls, or as a dessert pudding (decorated with whipped cream).

½ cup butter
½ cup honey, warmed
grated rind of 2 lemons (4 tablespoons)
juice of 3 lemons (½ cup)
6 eggs, beaten

In top of a double boiler, combine all ingredients and mix well. Set over boiling water and cook, stirring constantly with a wooden spoon, for 15 to 20 minutes, or until mixture is thick and smooth. Cool and store in a jar in refrigerator.

Yields about 2½ cups

Orange Filling

⅓ cup honey
2½ tablespoons cornstarch
¾ cup orange juice
½ cup water
1 tablespoon lemon juice
¼ teaspoon ground cinnamon
2 tablespoons butter

Place honey in a small saucepan.

Combine cornstarch and ¼ cup orange juice in a jar with a tight-fitting lid, and shake until smooth. Add to honey and stir in remaining orange juice, water, and lemon juice. Bring mixture to a boil over medium heat and boil, stirring constantly, until thickened. Stir in cinnamon and butter, and cook until butter melts. Cool before using.

Yields about 1½ cups

Vanilla Pastry Cream

3 eggs
3 tablespoons whole wheat pastry flour
2 tablespoons light honey
1 envelope unflavored gelatin
1 teaspoon vanilla extract
¾ cup milk
1 cup heavy cream, whipped

Separate 2 eggs. Combine egg, 1 egg yolk, flour, and honey in a large bowl and beat thoroughly. Add gelatin and beat again.

Place vanilla and milk in a 1½-quart saucepan, and slowly bring them to a boil. Remove from heat at once, and pour into egg mixture, stirring constantly.

Transfer egg and milk mixture to saucepan, and stir over low heat until it just comes to a boil. Remove saucepan from heat and place over a bowl of ice. Continue to stir mixture with a wire whisk until it cools and thickens.

Beat egg whites until they form soft peaks, and fold into egg and milk mixture. Then add whipped cream, one spoonful at a time, beating vigorously with whisk after each addition. The mixture should be medium thick, smooth, and creamy.

Yields about 2 cups

Cookies

Applesauce Yummies

    2 cups sifted whole wheat flour
    1 teaspoon baking powder
    ½ teaspoon baking soda
    1 teaspoon ground cinnamon
1½ cups rolled oats
    1 cup unsweetened applesauce
    ½ cup honey
    ½ cup butter, softened
    1 egg, beaten
    1 teaspoon vanilla extract
    1 cup carob chips (optional)

Preheat oven to 375°F. Oil a baking sheet.

In a large bowl sift together flour, baking powder, baking soda, and cinnamon.

In a medium-size bowl mix oats and applesauce.

In a medium-size bowl beat together honey and butter, mixing in egg. Mix butter mixture with oats and applesauce. Stir in vanilla and then add to flour mixture. Fold in carob (if used). Drop by teaspoons onto prepared baking sheet and bake for 10 to 12 minutes, or until edges begin to brown. Remove from baking sheet and cool on wire racks.

Makes about 4 dozen

Banana Drops

    1 cup whole wheat flour
    1 teaspoon baking soda
    1 teaspoon ground nutmeg
1½ cups cornmeal
    ½ cup honey
    ¾ cup butter, softened
    1 egg
    ¼ cup sour cream
    3 large very ripe bananas, mashed
    ¹/₃ cup chopped peanuts

In a large bowl sift together flour, baking soda, and nutmeg. Stir in cornmeal.

In a medium-size bowl beat together honey and butter. Beat in egg and then sour cream. Mix into flour mixture. Chill for 2 hours or overnight.

Preheat oven to 350°F. Oil a baking sheet.

Add bananas and peanuts, blending well. Drop by teaspoons onto prepared baking sheet and bake for 10 to 15 minutes, or until lightly browned. Remove from baking sheet and cool on wire racks.

Makes about 3 dozen

Biscotti
(Italian Nut Cookies)

In the households of Italy, biscotti are always at hand—to be served at the morning meal, with wine or coffee when friends visit, or as a wholesome snack for children and adults at any time. This recipe gives one of the many possible variations on this classic cookie.

    1 cup hazelnuts
    ½ cup butter, at room temperature
    ¼ cup plus 2 tablespoons honey
    2 eggs
1½ cups whole wheat flour
    2 teaspoons baking powder

Preheat oven to 350°F.

Roast hazelnuts (see page 401). Grate ½ of the nuts in a nut grater; leave remaining nuts whole.

Beat butter and honey in a large bowl with an electric mixer at medium speed until light. Add eggs, one at a time, beating well after each addition. Mix together flour, grated nuts, and baking powder, and then add gradually to butter mixture. Beat on low speed until blended. Stir in whole nuts. Dough will be soft.

Divide dough in half. Spoon onto an oiled baking sheet, forming each half into a 12-inch-long strip, 2 to 2½ inches wide. Shape with lightly floured spoon and fingertips.

Bake for 15 minutes, or until light golden brown. Remove from oven, cut on a diagonal into about ½-inch-thick slices, turn each slice on its side, and bake for another 10 to 15 minutes, or until slightly toasted and golden.

Remove slices to a wire rack and let cool completely. These keep well in a tightly covered container. Flavor improves after a few days.

Makes about 3 dozen

Carob Meringues with Buttercream Filling

½ cup honey
¼ cup water
2 tablespoons sifted powdered carob
6 egg whites, at room temperature
½ teaspoon cream of tartar
½ teaspoon vanilla extract

Filling
3 egg yolks
$1/_3$ cup butter, softened
2½ tablespoons honey
¼ cup heavy cream
½ teaspoon vanilla extract

Preheat oven to 350°F. Line a baking sheet with parchment paper.

In a large saucepan bring honey, water, and carob to hard ball stage (see page 673). Remove from heat.

In a large bowl beat egg whites and cream of tartar until soft peaks form. Slowly add carob syrup, beating constantly for 5 minutes. Mix in vanilla. Drop by tablespoons onto prepared baking sheet, making an indentation in center of each with a spoon, and bake on middle shelf of oven until firm and browned, about 10 minutes. Remove from baking sheet and cool on wire racks.

To make the filling: In a medium-size bowl beat together egg yolks and butter. Add honey and continue to beat until well blended. Beat in cream and vanilla to a creamy consistency.

Place a little filling in indentation of each cooled meringue just before serving.

Makes about 2 dozen

NOTE: Keep Buttercream Filling refrigerated. Raw egg yolks are susceptible to spoilage if left long at room temperature.

Carrot Cookies with Orange Frosting

1 pound carrots
¾ cup butter, softened
½ cup honey, warmed
1 egg, beaten
1 teaspoon vanilla extract
2 cups oat flour
2 teaspoons baking powder
¾ cup unsweetened shredded coconut
Orange Frosting (see below)

Cook carrots in enough water to cover. Drain and mash.

Preheat oven to 350°F. Oil a baking sheet.

In a large bowl mix butter, honey, 1 cup of the mashed carrots, egg, and vanilla.

Sift together flour and baking powder. Combine with butter mixture and fold in coconut. Drop by the spoonful onto prepared baking sheet, pressing to flatten, and bake for 15 minutes, or until lightly browned. Remove from baking sheet and cool on wire racks before frosting.

Makes about 2 dozen

Orange Frosting

½ cup honey, warmed
1 cup nonfat dry milk
¼ cup orange juice
½ teaspoon orange extract, or 1 teaspoon grated orange rind

Beat all ingredients together until blended. Allow to stand for 15 minutes before frosting cookies.

Yields 1½ cups

Chinese Almond Cookies

    2 cups whole wheat pastry flour
    1 teaspoon baking powder
    ⅔ cup butter
    1 egg
    ⅓ cup honey, warmed
    2 teaspoons almond extract
    1 cup apricot jam (optional)
    1 egg yolk, beaten
    24 whole almonds

Preheat oven to 350°F.

In a medium-size bowl sift together flour and baking powder and cut in butter with 2 knives or a pastry blender, or combine flour, baking powder, and butter in a food processor and process for 5 to 10 seconds, or until mixture is consistency of cornmeal.

In a small bowl beat egg, adding honey and almond extract. Add to flour mixture and mix thoroughly, or add to food processor and process for 15 to 20 seconds, or until dough forms a ball. Wrap dough with plastic wrap and refrigerate for 1 hour.

Roll dough into 1-inch balls, and flatten on unoiled baking sheet, pressing with back of a spatula. Place a teaspoon of jam (if used) in center of each cookie. Brush around jam to edges with beaten egg yolk. Place almond in center of each cookie, pressing point of almond down so it sticks into cookie dough, and bake until lightly browned, about 15 minutes. Remove from baking sheet and cool on wire racks.

Makes about 2 dozen

Cranberry-Raisin Cookies

    3 cups raisins
    ½ cup white grape juice
    ¼ cup butter, softened
    ½ cup honey
    2 eggs, beaten
    2 tablespoons sour cream
    1½ cups whole wheat pastry flour
    1½ teaspoons baking soda
    2 teaspoons ground cinnamon
    1 teaspoon ground nutmeg
    ½ teaspoon ground cloves
    1 cup fresh or frozen chopped cranberries

Preheat oven to 325°F. Oil a baking sheet.

In a small bowl plump raisins in grape juice.

In a large bowl beat together butter and honey, adding eggs and sour cream.

Sift together flour, baking soda, cinnamon, nutmeg, and cloves. Stir gradually into butter mixture. Add raisins and grape juice. Fold in cranberries. Drop by teaspoons onto prepared baking sheet, and bake until lightly browned, 12 to 15 minutes. Remove from baking sheet and cool on wire racks.

Makes about 3 dozen

Fennel Cookies

The mild licorice flavor in these cookies is more subtle than anise, yet clearly present.

    1 cup butter, softened
    1 cup honey
    2 eggs, beaten
    1 teaspoon vanilla extract
    1 tablespoon crushed fennel seeds
    1 cup finely chopped walnuts
    4 cups whole wheat pastry flour
    2 tablespoons baking powder

In a large bowl beat together butter, honey, eggs, and vanilla. Add fennel and nuts. Sift flour and baking powder gradually into mixture while beating. Blend well and roll dough into 1½-inch-thick roll. Wrap with plastic wrap and refrigerate for 4 hours.

Preheat oven to 350°F. Oil a baking sheet.

Cut dough into ⅛-inch rounds and bake until lightly browned, 8 to 10 minutes. Remove from baking sheet and cool on wire racks.

Makes about 4 dozen

Fruit-Filled Cookies

    1 egg
    ⅓ cup vegetable oil
    ⅓ cup honey
    2 tablespoons nonfat dry milk
    ½ teaspoon baking soda
    2 tablespoons buttermilk
    ½ teaspoon vanilla extract

1 cup whole wheat pastry flour
¼ cup Apricot Glaze (page 664) or Raspberry
    Glaze (page 665)

In a large bowl beat egg with oil, honey, dry milk, and baking soda dissolved in buttermilk. Stir in vanilla. Add flour and mix thoroughly. Chill for several hours.

Preheat oven to 325°F. Oil a baking sheet.

Drop batter by teaspoons onto prepared baking sheet. With a small spoon make a well in center of each cookie, and fill with about ¼ teaspoon fruit glaze. Bake for 12 to 15 minutes. Remove from baking sheet and cool on wire racks.

Makes about 2½ dozen

Hanukkahgelt Cookies

Jewish children are treated to goodies during the celebration of the Festival of Lights, and this cookie is a sweet reward.

1 cup butter
1½ cups honey
¼ cup sour cream
4 cups whole wheat flour
2 teaspoons baking soda
1 teaspoon ground cinnamon
½ teaspoon ground cloves
½ teaspoon ground allspice
¼ cup apple juice
¼ cup nonfat dry milk

Preheat oven to 350°F. Oil a baking sheet.

Beat together butter and 1 cup honey in a large bowl. Fold in sour cream.

Sift together flour, baking soda, cinnamon, cloves, and allspice. Combine with butter mixture. Roll dough into a ball and refrigerate for 1 hour.

Roll out dough on a floured surface to ¼-inch thickness. Cut into shapes with a cookie cutter, and place on prepared baking sheet. Bake for 8 to 10 minutes. Remove from baking sheet and cool on wire racks.

Cook ½ cup honey, apple juice, and dry milk to soft ball stage (see page 673). Cool and frost cooled cookies.

Makes about 3 dozen

Ginger Cookies

⅓ cup butter, softened
⅔ cup molasses
1 egg, beaten
2½ cups whole wheat flour
1 teaspoon baking soda
2 teaspoons ground cinnamon
1 teaspoon ground ginger

Preheat oven to 375°F. Oil a baking sheet.

Combine butter and molasses in a large bowl and beat until fluffy. Add egg, beating it into mixture thoroughly.

Combine flour, baking soda, and spices, and then add to liquid ingredients, beating just enough to mix dough thoroughly. Chill dough in refrigerator for several hours.

Roll out dough on a floured surface to thickness of ⅛ inch. Cut dough into shapes, using cookie cutters, and place on prepared baking sheet. Bake for 5 minutes, or until cookies are brown on bottom and firm to the touch. Remove from baking sheet and cool on wire racks.

Makes about 4 dozen

Kirsebaerkugler
(Danish Cookies)

½ cup butter, softened
½ cup honey
1 egg, beaten
1 teaspoon vanilla extract
2 cups sifted whole wheat pastry flour
24 pitted dates
½ cup Coconut Sugar (page 698)

Preheat oven to 350°F.

Beat together butter and honey in a large bowl. Beat in egg and vanilla. Sift flour into mixture and blend well to make dough. Roll some dough around each date to form a ball. Roll balls in coconut, and bake on unoiled baking sheet for 8 to 10 minutes, or until lightly browned. Remove from baking sheet and cool on wire racks.

Makes 2 dozen

Lemon Cookies

2 eggs, separated
2 tablespoons honey or maple syrup
    grated rind of 1 lemon
¼ cup sifted whole wheat pastry flour
2 tablespoons potato starch*
1 teaspoon ground almonds

Preheat oven to 325°F. Line a baking sheet with parchment paper.

In a large bowl cream together egg yolks and honey or maple syrup until very smooth and thick. Add lemon rind.

Combine flour, potato starch, and almonds, and add to egg yolk mixture. Beat well.

Beat egg whites until stiff but not dry. Fold into batter. Drop by rounded teaspoons onto prepared baking sheet, about 2 inches apart, and bake for about 18 minutes, or until edges begin to brown. Remove from baking sheet and cool on wire racks.

Makes about 3 dozen

*Potato starch is available in natural foods stores.

Linzer Cookies

½ cup butter, softened
¼ cup molasses
¼ cup honey
1 egg yolk
1 teaspoon vanilla extract
1½ cups whole wheat pastry flour
¾ cup amaranth flour, barley flour, or finely
    ground millet
1 teaspoon baking powder
¾ cup finely chopped pecans
36 pecan halves, or ¼ cup fruit preserves

Cream butter in a large bowl. Slowly beat in molasses and honey. Beat in egg yolk and vanilla. Continue beating until mixture is light and fluffy.

Mix flours and baking powder together. Add to butter mixture, ½ cup at a time, stirring no more than is necessary to blend mixtures. Working quickly, knead in pecans. Divide dough in half. Pat each half into a circle 1 inch thick. Wrap in wax paper and refrigerate until chilled, about 2 hours. It is important to keep dough chilled. While working, keep unused portions of dough and dough scraps refrigerated.

Preheat oven to 350°F. Lightly oil a baking sheet.

Gently roll out first dough circle on a lightly floured surface to ¼ inch thick. Cut into shapes with cookie cutters. If making preserve-filled cookies, use round cookie cutters, and cut a small round hole in center of ½ of the cookies.

Transfer cookies to baking sheet. If not filling cookies, press a pecan half into each cookie. Bake for 6 to 10 minutes, or until cookies brown lightly around edges. Remove from baking sheet and cool on wire racks. Repeat with remaining dough circle.

Knead dough scraps into a ball, flatten, and roll out. Cut into diamonds or rectangles and bake. The rerolled cookies have a less delicate texture.

If making filled cookies, spread preserves in a thin layer on whole cookies, and press cookies with holes on top.

Makes about 3 dozen pecan cookies or 1½ dozen filled cookies

Maple-Almond Kisses

2 egg whites
⅓ cup maple syrup
½ teaspoon vanilla extract
¼ cup finely chopped almonds

Preheat oven to 275°F. Line a baking sheet with foil or unglazed brown paper.

In a large bowl beat egg whites until soft peaks form. Gradually beat in maple syrup, continuing to beat until whites are stiff but not dry. Fold in vanilla and almonds. Drop by teaspoons onto prepared baking sheet and bake for 45 minutes. Reduce heat to 250°F and bake for 10 minutes more. Allow kisses to cool on baking sheet, then remove gently. Foil or paper can be peeled off.

Makes about 2½ dozen

Molasses Icebox Cookies

3 cups whole wheat flour
½ teaspoon baking soda
⅓ cup honey
½ cup butter, melted
1 egg, beaten
2½ teaspoons molasses
½ teaspoon vanilla extract

Preheat oven to 350°F. Oil a baking sheet.

Sift together flour and baking soda into a large bowl.

Combine honey, butter, egg, molasses, and vanilla. Mix into flour mixture. Roll dough into a 2-inch-wide log. Wrap with plastic wrap and refrigerate for about 4 hours.

Cut into ¼-inch rounds and bake on prepared baking sheet for 8 to 10 minutes, or until lightly browned. Remove from baking sheet and cool on wire racks.

Makes about 3 dozen

No-Grain Coconut Cookies

2 eggs, beaten
½ cup honey
2 cups unsweetened shredded coconut

Preheat oven to 350°F. Oil a baking sheet.

Combine eggs and honey in a medium-size bowl. Add coconut and mix well. Drop by teaspoons onto prepared baking sheet. Bake for 10 minutes, or until lightly browned. Remove from baking sheet and cool on wire racks.

Makes about 3 dozen

Oatmeal-Honey Wafers

2 eggs, beaten
½ cup vegetable oil
¾ cup honey
1 teaspoon almond extract
1 cup nonfat dry milk
3 cups rolled oats

Preheat oven to 325°F. Oil a baking sheet.

Combine eggs, oil, and honey in a medium-size bowl. Add almond extract and dry milk and stir to blend. Add oats and mix well. Drop by teaspoons onto prepared baking sheet, about 2 inches apart. Bake for 10 to 12 minutes, or until wafers are brown around edges. Remove wafers carefully with a spatula and cool on wire racks.

Makes about 3 dozen

Oatmeal Lace Cookies

These cookies are very thin, very rich, but a little hard to handle. However, they are so good you'll agree they are worth the effort.

1 cup rolled oats
1 egg
¾ cup honey, warmed, or ¼ cup maple syrup
    plus ½ cup honey
1 teaspoon vanilla extract
½ cup butter, melted

Preheat oven to 350°F. Line a baking sheet with parchment paper.

Place oats in a blender and process for a few minutes, until they become a coarse flour. Set aside.

In a medium-size bowl combine egg, honey, maple syrup (if used), and vanilla. Beat until well combined. Add butter and continue to beat until smooth. Stir in oats. Drop by ½ teaspoons onto prepared baking sheet, about 3 inches apart. (They will spread while baking.) Bake for 12 minutes. Remove from baking sheet and cool on wire racks.

Makes 3½ to 4 dozen

Orange Cookies

½ cup butter
½ cup honey, warmed
1 egg
1 tablespoon grated orange rind
⅓ cup orange juice
¾ teaspoon baking soda
2 to 2¼ cups whole wheat pastry flour

In a large bowl combine butter, honey, egg, and orange rind. Mix well. Add orange juice, baking soda, and flour, combining thoroughly. Let dough stand for 15 minutes.

Preheat oven to 350°F.

Drop dough by teaspoons onto unoiled baking sheet, 2 inches apart. (Dough spreads during baking.) Bake for 8 to 10 minutes, or until edges begin to brown. Remove from baking sheet and cool on wire racks.

Makes 3½ to 4 dozen

Peanut Butter Cookies

½ cup butter, softened
½ cup peanut butter
⅔ cup honey, warmed
½ teaspoon vanilla extract
1 egg
1½ cups whole wheat flour
¾ teaspoon baking soda
1 cup chopped peanuts

In a large bowl combine butter, peanut butter, honey, vanilla, and egg. Beat thoroughly.

Stir together flour and baking soda. Add to peanut butter mixture and blend. Add peanuts and mix. Chill dough several hours or overnight.

Preheat oven to 325°F. Oil a baking sheet.

Drop dough by level tablespoons onto prepared baking sheet and bake for 10 to 15 minutes, or until lightly browned. Let stand for a few minutes on baking sheet before removing to wire racks to cool.

Makes 5 dozen

Pecan-Amaranth Tassies

Amaranth flour adds a special touch to the pastry of this popular, sweet snack.

Pastry
⅔ cup whole wheat flour
⅓ cup amaranth flour
¼ cup butter
4 ounces cream cheese
1 egg yolk

Filling
2 eggs, beaten
2 tablespoons butter, melted
⅓ cup honey
2 tablespoons molasses
1 teaspoon vanilla extract
½ cup finely chopped pecans
2 tablespoons amaranth, popped*
¼ cup finely chopped dried pineapple (optional)

36 pecan halves

To make the pastry: Combine flours in a medium-size bowl. Cut in butter until mixture resembles coarse crumbs. Working quickly, knead in cream cheese and egg yolk. Handle dough as little as possible.

Divide dough into 2 equal balls. Place each ball in middle of a large sheet of wax paper. With palm of your hand, press dough out to a square approximately ½ inch thick. Wrap dough in wax paper and chill thoroughly for 3 to 4 hours in refrigerator or for 30 to 40 minutes in freezer.

Turn dough out onto a floured surface and flour top of dough. Roll dough out until ⅛ inch thick, and cut into 3-inch circles with a biscuit cutter.

Lightly butter miniature muffin tins. Ease each circle of dough into a cup of the tin, forming small pastry shells. Sides should be lightly scalloped. Refrigerate while you prepare filling.

To make the filling: Combine eggs, butter, honey, molasses, vanilla, chopped pecans, amaranth, and pineapple (if used) in a large bowl. Fill pastry shells almost to their tops. Decorate each with pecan half. Bake for 15 minutes. Reduce temperature to 250°F and bake for 10 minutes more. Remove tassies from tins immediately, and cool on wire racks.

Makes 3 dozen

*To pop amaranth: Heat a wok or heavy skillet (without oil) until very hot. Add 1 tablespoon amaranth and stir with a pastry brush to keep from burning. When all the seeds have popped, empty into a bowl and repeat with remaining seeds.

Pecan Cookies

½ cup butter
⅓ cup vegetable oil
¼ cup honey, warmed
¼ cup maple syrup
2 to 2½ cups whole wheat pastry flour
2 teaspoons vanilla extract
1 cup chopped pecans
48 pecan halves

Preheat oven to 325°F.

In a large bowl cream butter, oil, honey, and maple syrup until smooth. Stir in flour. Add vanilla and chopped pecans and mix well.

Form dough into 1-inch balls, place on an unoiled baking sheet, and press pecan half lightly into center of each, flattening cookie slightly in process. Bake for 15 to 20 minutes, or until light brown. Remove from baking sheet and cool on wire racks.

Makes 4 dozen

NOTE: Storing these cookies for a few days in an airtight container or freezing them improves their flavor.

Pignoli-Almond Treats

½ cup honey, warmed
1 tablespoon almond paste
4 eggs
¼ cup sour cream
2½ teaspoons almond extract
2¼ cups whole wheat pastry flour
½ teaspoon baking powder
½ teaspoon baking soda
3 ounces cream cheese, softened
2 tablespoons honey
¼ cup pine nuts

Preheat oven to 350°F. Oil and flour a baking sheet.

In a large bowl beat together honey, almond paste, and eggs for 5 minutes. Beat in sour cream and 1½ teaspoons almond extract.

Sift together flour, baking powder, and baking soda and stir into batter. Drop by spoonfuls onto prepared baking sheet, flattening slightly with back of a spoon, and bake for 10 to 12 minutes, or until edges begin to brown. Remove from baking sheet and cool on wire racks.

Beat together cream cheese, 2 tablespoons honey, and 1 teaspoon almond extract. Frost cooled cookies and decorate with pine nuts. Store, covered, in refrigerator.

Makes about 4 dozen

Pineapple Surprises

4 cups sifted whole wheat pastry flour
2 teaspoons baking powder
1 teaspoon baking soda
1 cup butter, softened
½ cup honey
2 eggs, beaten
½ teaspoon vanilla extract
1 cup sour cream
2 tablespoons cornstarch
2 cups unsweetened crushed pineapple

Sift together flour, baking powder, and baking soda.

Cream together butter and honey in a large bowl. Mix eggs and vanilla into butter mixture. Stir in sour cream. Add dry ingredients gradually, blending well. Refrigerate for 1 hour to harden.

In a small saucepan combine cornstarch and pineapple. Cook, stirring constantly, until mixture thickens. Set aside to cool.

Preheat oven to 375°F. Oil a baking sheet.

On a floured surface roll dough to thickness of about ⅛ inch. Cut dough with 3-inch-round cookie cutter. Place ½ of the rounds on prepared baking sheet. Place about 1 teaspoon pineapple on each round, and cover with remaining rounds, pinching edges together tightly. Lightly score tops of cookies and bake for 8 to 10 minutes, or until lightly browned. Remove from baking sheet and cool on wire racks.

Makes about 3 dozen

Spicy Raisin Drop Cookies

3 cups whole wheat flour
1 teaspoon baking powder
1 teaspoon ground ginger
1½ teaspoons ground cinnamon
1 cup butter
¾ cup honey
1 egg
1 teaspoon vanilla extract
2 cups raisins
½ cup chopped nuts

Preheat oven to 375°F. Oil a baking sheet.

Sift together flour, baking powder, ginger, and cinnamon.

In a large bowl beat together butter, honey, eggs, and vanilla. Mix dry ingredients into butter mixture. Fold in raisins and nuts. Drop by teaspoons onto prepared baking sheet and bake for 10 to 12 minutes, or until lightly browned. Remove from baking sheet and cool on wire racks.

Makes about 2 dozen

Sunshine Snacks

¼ cup butter, softened
½ cup honey
½ cup tahini (sesame butter)
¾ cup sesame seeds, toasted
1½ teaspoons vanilla extract
1¾ cups whole wheat flour
1 teaspoon baking powder

In a large bowl beat together butter, honey, and tahini. Mix in sesame seeds and vanilla.

Sift together flour and baking powder, and mix into sesame batter. Form dough into a roll about 12 inches long. Wrap tightly with plastic wrap, and refrigerate for about 8 hours.

Preheat oven to 350°F. Oil a baking sheet.

Cut dough into ¼-inch slices, place on prepared baking sheet, and bake for 8 to 10 minutes, or until lightly browned. Remove from baking sheet and cool on wire racks.

Makes about 3 dozen

Thanksgiving Pumpkin Cookies

½ cup honey
½ cup butter, softened
1 egg, beaten
1 cup mashed cooked pumpkin
1 teaspoon vanilla extract
2 teaspoons baking powder
½ teaspoon baking soda
2 cups sifted whole wheat pastry flour
1 teaspoon ground allspice
1 teaspoon ground cinnamon
1 cup raisins
1 cup chopped nuts

Preheat oven to 375°F.

Cream together honey and butter in a large bowl. Add egg and pumpkin, mixing well. Add vanilla.

Sift together baking powder, baking soda, flour, allspice, and cinnamon. Gradually mix into butter mixture. Fold in raisins and nuts. Drop by teaspoons onto unoiled baking sheet, flatten with back of a spoon, and bake until lightly browned, 8 to 10 minutes. Remove from baking sheet and cool on wire racks.

Makes about 2 dozen

Turkish Treats

1 cup butter, softened
⅓ cup honey
2 egg yolks, lightly beaten
1 teaspoon almond extract
2 cups whole wheat flour
½ cup currant jelly

Preheat oven to 350°F. Lightly oil a baking sheet.

Beat together butter and honey in a large bowl. Add egg yolks and beat. Mix in almond extract. Sift flour into mixture, blending well.

Roll dough into balls about the size of walnuts, and place on prepared baking sheet, flattening with a spoon and making indentations in tops. Place about ½ teaspoon jelly in each indentation and bake for 12 to 15 minutes, or until lightly browned. Remove from baking sheet and cool on wire racks.

Makes about 3 dozen

Zucchini-Raisin Cookies

For those who thought there was nothing more to do with zucchini, this cookie is a pleasant revelation—a moist, chewy sweet.

1 cup butter, softened
¾ cup honey, warmed
2 eggs
¼ cup sour cream
1 teaspoon ground cinnamon
1 teaspoon ground cloves
2 cups whole wheat pastry flour
1 teaspoon baking soda
2 cups rolled oats
2 cups raisins
1½ cups chopped seeded zucchini

Preheat oven to 350°F. Oil a baking sheet.

In a large bowl beat together butter, honey, eggs, sour cream, cinnamon, and cloves.

Sift together flour and baking soda, and mix with liquid ingredients. Fold in oats, raisins, and zucchini. Drop by teaspoons onto prepared baking sheet and bake until golden, 10 to 12 minutes. Remove from baking sheet and cool on wire racks.

Makes about 4 dozen

Carob Brownies

This is a favorite at Rodale's Fitness House dining room.

    1 cup sifted powdered carob
    ²/₃ cup vegetable oil
    ½ cup honey
    4 eggs
    1 cup finely ground peanuts
    5 tablespoons rye flour
    1 cup chopped walnuts
    2 teaspoons vanilla

Preheat oven to 325°F. Oil a 9-inch-square baking pan.

In a small bowl combine carob, oil, and honey.

In a large bowl beat eggs until light. Beat in carob mixture. Stir in ground peanuts and flour and mix well. Mix in nuts and vanilla. Spread batter evenly in prepared pan and bake for 30 minutes, or just until surface is firm to the touch. Remove from oven and cool for about 10 minutes. Cut into squares.

Makes about 16

NOTE: If using ground roasted peanuts, decrease oil to ¹/₃ cup.

Butterscotch Brownies

    2 eggs
    2 tablespoons vegetable oil
    1 tablespoon molasses
    ²/₃ cup honey
    2 teaspoons vanilla extract
    ¹/₃ cup finely ground raw peanuts
    ½ cup nonfat dry milk
    ²/₃ cup whole wheat flour
    ½ cup chopped walnuts

Preheat oven to 350°F. Oil a 9-inch-square baking pan.

Beat eggs in a medium-size bowl until light. Add oil, molasses, honey, and vanilla and mix.

In a large bowl combine ground peanuts, dry milk, flour, and walnuts. Stir liquid ingredients into dry ingredients. Spread batter evenly in prepared pan and bake for 30 minutes, or just until surface is firm to the touch. Remove from oven and cool before serving.

Makes about 16

Fig Bars

Most modern youngsters have never seen this all-time favorite in any guise but a supermarket package. It can be made at home, of course, and the product is superior.

    Filling
    12 ounces dried figs
    ¹/₃ cup honey
    1 tablespoon lemon juice
    2 tablespoons water
    2 tablespoons orange juice

    Dough
    ½ cup butter, softened
    ½ cup honey
    1 egg
    ½ teaspoon grated lemon rind
    1 tablespoon lemon juice
    3 cups whole wheat flour
    1 teaspoon baking powder
    ½ teaspoon baking soda

To make the filling: Grind figs in a meat grinder or food processor.

In a small saucepan combine figs, honey, lemon juice, water, and orange juice. Cook over low heat for 10 minutes, stirring occasionally. Remove from heat and set aside to cool.

To make the dough: In a large bowl cream butter and honey together until light and fluffy. Add egg and mix well. Stir in lemon rind and juice. Add flour, baking powder, and baking soda to butter mixture, mixing well. Divide dough in half.

Press ½ of the dough into bottom of an oiled 9 × 13-inch baking pan. Spread fig filling evenly over dough. Roll out remaining dough between wax paper into 9 × 13-inch rectangle. Lay this dough over top of filling, pressing down to seal.

Preheat oven to 400°F.

Bake for 12 to 15 minutes, or until dough springs back when pressed lightly with a finger. Cool and cut into 1½ × 2-inch bars.

Makes about 4½ dozen

High-Protein Brownies

²/₃ cup butter
4 eggs, beaten with ½ cup honey
1 cup sifted powdered carob
¼ cup soy grits plus ¼ cup water, or ²/₃ cup okara
  (soy pulp)
½ cup finely ground peanuts
½ cup whole wheat flour
1 cup chopped walnuts
2 teaspoons vanilla extract

Preheat oven to 325°F.

Place butter in a 10-inch-square baking pan, and set pan in preheating oven until butter melts.

Sift carob into a medium-size bowl. Stir melted butter into carob, mixing thoroughly.

If using soy grits, combine them with water. Add soy grits or okara to carob mixture along with eggs and honey and mix well. Stir in ground peanuts, flour, walnuts, and vanilla. Pour into pan and bake for 25 to 30 minutes, or just until surface of brownies is firm to the touch. Do not overbake. Remove pan from oven and cool on a wire rack. Cut into squares while warm.

Makes about 2 dozen

Peanut Butter Bars

½ cup butter, softened
½ cup plus 3 tablespoons honey, warmed
1 egg
1 cup peanut butter
½ teaspoon baking soda
½ teaspoon vanilla extract
1 cup whole wheat pastry flour
1 cup rolled oats
¼ cup plus 2 tablespoons Basic Carob Syrup
  (page 737)

Preheat oven to 350°F. Butter a baking sheet or an 11 × 14-inch baking pan.

In a large bowl mix together butter, ½ cup honey, egg, ½ cup peanut butter, baking soda, vanilla, flour, and oats. Spread batter on prepared baking sheet or in prepared pan, and bake for 20 to 25 minutes, or until lightly browned.

Meanwhile, mix carob syrup, 3 tablespoons honey, and remaining ½ cup peanut butter in a small bowl. Beat or stir until smooth.

When batter has finished baking, remove from oven and spread immediately with carob mixture. Cool and cut into bars.

Makes about 6½ dozen

Walnut Bars

1 egg
½ cup honey, warmed
½ teaspoon vanilla extract
¾ cup whole wheat flour
½ teaspoon baking soda
¾ cup chopped walnuts

Preheat oven to 325°F. Butter a 7 × 11-inch baking pan.

In a medium-size bowl beat egg with honey and vanilla.

Combine flour and baking soda, and add to liquid ingredients. Mix well. Spread batter in prepared pan, sprinkle nuts over top, and bake for about 25 minutes, or until batter springs back when pressed lightly with a finger. Cut into squares or bars while still warm.

Makes about 3 dozen

Confections

Almond Caramels

1½ cups honey
2 tablespoons butter, softened
2 cups heavy cream
1 teaspoon almond extract
1½ cups chopped almonds

Butter an 8-inch-square baking pan.

Cream together honey and butter in a deep heavy-bottom pot. Mix in 1 cup cream. Boil until mixture reaches soft ball stage (see page 673).

Gradually mix in remaining cream, and boil until mixture reaches hard ball stage.

Remove from heat. Add almond extract and nuts. Pour into prepared pan. Allow to stand at room temperature for about 8 hours.

With a sharp buttered knife cut caramel into 1-inch squares. Wrap individually.

Makes about 4 dozen

Assorted Bonbons

A welcome holiday gift for adults, as well as an easy way to wean children from excessive intake of poor-quality store-bought candies.

½ cup honey
1 teaspoon vinegar
2 tablespoons water
1 teaspoon sifted powdered carob (optional)
1½ teaspoons vanilla extract
8 ounces cream cheese, softened

Combine honey, vinegar, water and carob (if used) in a deep heavy-bottom pot, and cook to hard ball stage (see page 673).

Mix in vanilla and cream cheese. Set aside to cool. Then refrigerate until very stiff.

Shape mixture into balls about ½ inch in diameter. Place on wax paper and push down slightly to flatten bottoms. Cover with another piece of wax paper and refrigerate for 8 hours. Wrap individually.

Makes about 3 dozen

Variations:

▪ Roll in ground nuts after forming balls.
▪ Use almond extract instead of vanilla.
▪ Use orange extract instead of vanilla and omit carob.
▪ Use orange rind, omit carob, and roll in unsweetened shredded coconut.

Caramel-Cashew Chews

1 cup honey
2 tablespoons lemon juice
1 tablespoon butter
1½ cups cashews

In a deep heavy-bottom pot boil honey, lemon juice, and butter to hard ball stage (see page 673). Set aside to thicken.

When mixture is quite stiff, stir in cashews and let stand until very firm.

Drop with a buttered teaspoon onto a heavily buttered baking sheet. Wrap chews separately and store in an airtight container in refrigerator.

Makes about 2 dozen

Carob-Coconut Figs

12 large dried figs, stems cut off
2 tablespoons ground almonds
3 tablespoons unsweetened flaked coconut
1 tablespoon grated carob
1 tablespoon honey, warmed

Preheat oven to 350°F.

Push in stem ends of figs to form pockets.

Combine almonds, coconut, carob, and honey. Stuff figs with mixture. Pinch openings together over stuffing and bake for 10 minutes. Cool before serving.

Makes 1 dozen

Coco-Date-Nut Confections

2 cups finely chopped dates
¼ cup honey
½ cup water
½ teaspoon vanilla extract
1 cup finely chopped walnuts or pecans
1½ cups unsweetened grated coconut

In a deep heavy-bottom pot cook dates, honey, and water over low heat, stirring constantly, until thick, about 5 minutes. Remove from heat. Add vanilla, nuts, and coconut.

When mixture has cooled to workable temperature, form into 1-inch balls, and place on wax paper. Store in refrigerator or freezer. Serve at room temperature.

Makes about 3 dozen

Coconut Kisses

½ cup honey
½ cup peanut butter
¼ cup nonfat dry milk
1 teaspoon vanilla extract
2 cups unsweetened shredded coconut

Preheat oven to 300°F. Oil a baking sheet. (Do not use butter.)

In a large bowl combine honey, peanut butter, dry milk, and vanilla. Fold in coconut. Drop by teaspoons onto prepared baking sheet and bake for 10 minutes. Cool on a wire rack.

Makes about 2½ dozen

Date Balls

2 cups chopped dates
½ cup butter
½ cup honey
1 egg, beaten
1 teaspoon vanilla extract
2 cups chopped sunflower seeds
¼ cup unsweetened shredded coconut

Mix dates, butter, honey, egg, and vanilla in a deep heavy-bottom pot. Bring to a rolling boil and boil for 1 minute. Cool.

Mix in seeds. Form mixture into 1-inch balls and roll in coconut. Store in refrigerator.

Makes about 3 dozen

Divinity

As long as there are church socials and bake sales—and people with a sweet tooth—this old-time confection will continue to be popular. It makes a dandy confection to have around at holiday time.

¾ cup honey
¼ cup water
1 teaspoon vinegar
1 egg white
½ cup chopped pecans
½ teaspoon vanilla extract
30 pecan halves

In a deep heavy-bottom pot cook honey, water, and vinegar to firm ball stage (see page 673).

While mixture is cooking, beat egg white until stiff but not dry. When syrup is at firm ball stage, pour it very slowly into egg white, beating continually until creamy, light, and firm. Mix in chopped nuts and vanilla.

Drop by teaspoons onto buttered wax paper, or spread in a buttered 8-inch-square pan. When partly cooled, cut into squares. Press a pecan half into center of each piece.

Makes 2½ dozen

High-Energy Bar

A convenient carry-along version of granola-style cereal. Nice to take on car trips or hikes and good for the lunch box, too.

2 cups Almond Crunch cereal (page 305)
2 eggs, beaten

Preheat oven to 300°F. Lightly oil a baking sheet.

In a medium-size bowl combine cereal and eggs. Mix thoroughly. Spread carefully on prepared baking sheet, pressing into oblong shape, about 6 inches by 8 inches and ¼ inch thick. Press firmly to be sure bars will hold together. With a sharp knife cut mixture into bars 1½ inches wide and 2 inches long. Bake for 20 minutes.

Remove from oven and allow to cool for 5 minutes, then break apart (or recut). Cool completely, wrap individually, and store in a covered container.

Makes 15

Peanut Butter Balls

½ cup honey, warmed
1 cup peanut butter

½ cup nonfat dry milk
½ cup Basic Carob Syrup (page 737)
 1 teaspoon honey
 2 tablespoons butter

In a medium-size bowl mix honey, peanut butter, and ¼ cup dry milk. Work into a smooth paste and roll into small balls. Chill.

In a small saucepan mix carob syrup, ¼ cup dry milk, honey, and butter. Place over low heat and stir until well blended. Remove from heat.

Dip peanut butter balls into hot carob mixture, drop onto buttered wax paper, and chill. Store in refrigerator.

Makes about 1½ dozen

Peanut Butter-Stuffed Prunes

¼ cup peanut butter
¼ cup chopped dates
¼ cup chopped cashews
¼ cup sunflower seeds
 2 tablespoons honey
1½ teaspoons orange juice
20 large dried prunes

In a large bowl combine all ingredients except prunes.

Using tip of a knife, slit prunes, remove pits, and open prunes wide enough to stuff each with a rounded teaspoon of peanut butter mixture. Fill prunes until mixture is used up. Chill until firm. Store in a covered container in refrigerator.

Makes about 1½ dozen

Pralines

This is a version of the confection closely associated with New Orleans, in which the honey brings a different texture to the product.

½ cup honey
½ cup buttermilk
½ teaspoon baking soda
 1 tablespoon butter
¾ cup broken pecans

In a deep heavy-bottom pot mix honey, buttermilk, and baking soda. Cook over high heat for 5 minutes. Add butter and continue to cook, stirring frequently, to soft ball stage (see page 673). Remove from heat and cool for 5 minutes.

Beat with an electric mixer until creamy. Add nuts. Immediately drop by tablespoons onto buttered wax paper. For storing, wrap each praline in plastic wrap.

Makes 1 dozen

Sesame Squares

⅓ cup honey
⅓ cup peanut butter
¾ cup nonfat dry milk
¾ cup sesame seeds
¼ cup raisins
¼ cup unsweetened shredded coconut

Mix together all ingredients in a large bowl. Spread in an 8-inch-square baking pan and refrigerate for 4 hours. Cut into 1-inch squares.

Makes about 5 dozen

Pies and Pastries

Although all desserts are intended to give pleasure, none seems to do it so completely as a fancy pie or pastry, created to tempt the eye as well as the taste buds. A well-made pastry is also prized for its versatility. It can enfold, encase, or be layered with so many delightful fillings. A golden brown piecrust alone can be beautifully enhanced by tangy fruits, fluffy creams, rich custards, and light chiffons. Some very light pastries can be rolled, coiled, or piped, and partnered with a variety of nut, fruit, or jamlike fillings.

Although there are numerous types of pastry, they are all based on a mixture of flour, shortening, and water. In traditional baking, several types of pastry are especially familiar, such as short crust, puff, chou, phyllo, and strudel. Though all of these have similar qualities, they differ from each other in the proportions of ingredients used and the different ways the ingredients are treated during mixing.

For example, puff pastry differs from a basic short-crust pastry in that a type of flour that has a lower gluten content must be used in order to keep the puff pastry especially tender. This factor is imperative as insurance against toughness. A chou pastry behaves differently still, because some of the very same ingredients that are used in short-crust and puff pastries are heated at certain stages of its mixing process. Strudel and phyllo pastries are the most elastic of pastries — able to be stretched thin enough, they say, so a newspaper can be read through them.

The success of these types of pastries relies heavily on flours that are refined or low in gluten-forming protein. The bran content of whole wheat flour, which is not refined and is high in gluten, gives a texture too heavy for these doughs. It is possible to produce a tender, tasty pastry with whole wheat pastry flour, but it will be coarser and somewhat heavier than any made with refined white flour. Rolled oats, brown rice flour, and other whole grain flours may be used along with whole wheat pastry flour for added flavor, nutrition, and varying textures.

Piecrusts

The golden rule in making a good pastry crust is to handle the dough as little and as quickly as possible. Overworking the dough promotes too much gluten formation, which is undesirable in pastry making, unlike bread making. For this reason the shortening used is cut into the flour, usually with two knives (crisscross fashion), a fork, or a pastry blender, until the texture of coarse cornmeal is achieved. When you must finally handle the dough, do so lightly, incorporating as much air as possible. Flaky, tender crust is the objective of this attentive care.

Butter is the best choice of shortening for a soft, tender piecrust, but an all-butter dough may be difficult to manage. A combination of butter and oil is recommended for easier handling. Sometimes cheese — ricotta, cottage, or cheddar — or sour cream is added for an especially rich dough.

714

Ice water is added to the shortening-flour mixture to keep the shortening firm, resulting in less gluten development and a flakier crust. Always add water gradually in small quantities, and only add as much as is necessary to hold the dough together. The dough should form a ball and no longer stick to the sides of the bowl when it contains enough water.

Sweetener may be added to some pastry doughs for crispness and better browning, and tart and strudel pastries usually require some sweetness in the dough to complement the filling, but basic short-crust pie pastry is not sweetened, as a rule.

Eggs enrich and add color to pastry dough. The whole egg may be used or, for extra richness, just the yolk. Egg pastry doughs are quite batterlike and elastic due to the egg protein. Like sweetener, eggs are generally not added to pie pastry.

Pie plates come in various sizes: The most common size is a 9-inch plate.

Filled piecrusts should never be baked in shiny plates, which reflect heat, or a soggy undercrust will result. For tender, browned undercrusts the best materials are heat-resistant glass plates, darkened tin, or enamelware. For pies with very juicy fillings, such as fruit pies, a pan with a trough is often used to catch the juices that will inevitably boil up during baking.

Easy Method for Making a Lattice Top

Roll out the dough for the top piecrust into an oblong. Cut it into strips one-half inch wide with a knife or, for a fancy edge, with a pastry cutter. Lay strips across the filling, parallel to each other approximately an inch apart. Turn the pie slightly and, instead of laying the top strips perpendicular (at right angles) to the bottom layer of strips, lay them diagonally (on a slant). This gives the impression that the strips are woven without actually weaving them. Lay a strip of pastry all around the rim of the plate, covering the ends of the other strips. Crimp this strip to make an attractive edge all around the pie.

When making a baked piecrust for a pie that takes a cooked filling, prick the pastry with a fork in several places before baking, to prevent buckling due to steam while it is in the oven. Placing a handful of dried beans on the bottom will also check any warping. Remove the beans two to three minutes before the crust is done.

Sometimes piecrusts that are to be baked with their fillings are baked "blind" or *à blanc* for several minutes. This means they are partially baked to set the dough and reduce its absorbency.

Rolling a Piecrust

When all the ingredients cohere into a ball that is not too sticky or too stiff, the dough is ready for rolling. If you are making a double-crust pie, divide the dough into two balls. Chilling the dough was traditionally done to make it more manageable for rolling, but cooks today consider this an unnecessary step. If you do chill the dough, for any reason, allow it to return to room temperature before rolling.

A pastry cloth and roller stocking are sometimes used to avoid using extra flour. The cloth permits you to pick the dough up, then transfer it to the plate. However, if you use a smooth surface such as marble or Formica, these are unnecessary.

Roll the dough from the center out, keeping it circular and stroking as little as possible. Roll the dough to about one-eighth-inch thickness and wide enough to extend about two inches over the sides of the pie plate. Patch any tears carefully by pinching the dough together and rolling over the patch so it is unnoticeable.

When the dough has been rolled to the right size, you can ease it into the pie plate by flopping half of it over the rolling pin and gently lifting the other half with an outspread hand. Arrange it gently and trim off the excess dough by running a knife around the edge of the plate. If making a single-crust pie, form a decorative fluted edge by pinching the rim of the crust all around the circumference with your thumb and forefinger.

Double-Crust Pies

For a double-crust pie it is not necessary to prick the bottom crust; the weight of the filling prevents air bubbles from forming. When the bottom crust is in place and the filling has been added, neatly trim the overhanging dough. Then roll out the top crust to extend two inches over the circumference of the pan.

It is necessary to form vents in the top crust so that steam can escape, otherwise the underside of the crust will become soggy. You can do this in several ways. One way is to fold the rolled-out top crust in quarters and cut slits in the two straight folded edges with a knife or scissors. Another way is to pierce the top crust in several places with a knife or fork after it has been positioned over the filling. If you do not wish to cut slits in the crust, you can form a steam vent by inserting the wide end of a pastry tip in the middle of the top crust. Do so after the crust has been positioned and sealed. Be sure to remove the circle of dough that will be cut out by the pastry tip.

To position the top crust on the pie, you can fold the rolled-out dough in quarters, carefully place it on top of the filled bottom crust, and unfold. Trim the overhanging dough with a knife and gently press the top and bottom crusts together to seal them tightly. Crimp the edges with a fork or your fingers to reinforce the seal. This will keep the juices from seeping out during baking.

Pressed Piecrust

If you find you have great difficulty rolling a crust, you may prefer the never-fail pressed piecrusts. Instead of rolling the dough, press it into the pie plate with your fingers, working it onto the bottom and sides as evenly as possible. When the pressed crust is in place, use the bottom of a flat cup or glass to smooth the dough and set it firmly into the pie plate. A pressed crust will not be as thin or flaky as a rolled one.

Crumb pastries used for pressed piecrusts are very easy to make. They are not really pastries, but they are often used as shells for cream or cheesecake fillings. Crumb crusts can be made from finely crumbled cake or cookies. The crumbs are usually bound with melted butter or oil and are pressed into a pie plate. Dry cereal, shredded coconut, wheat germ, or ground nuts or seeds may also be added to the crumb mixture.

Glazing

Top piecrusts may be glazed to enhance their appearance. The glaze gives an attractive color and luster to the crust. Piecrust glaze is usually made from egg yolk or egg white, mixed with milk or water. It should be applied lightly with a pastry brush just before the pie is baked.

Sometimes a bottom crust is glazed to help waterproof it against any seepage of filling.

Tart Shells

Individual tart shells may be made the same way as piecrusts. They can be used with the same fillings or with fresh, uncooked fruit topped with cream. Divide the dough from any single piecrust recipe into four parts. Roll each section to a six-inch circle. Position the circles of dough over the cups of overturned muffin tins, and prick holes in the dough with a fork. Bake for eight to ten minutes at 450°F. Remove the tart shells and allow them to cool before filling them.

Pie Fillings

Some fillings are baked along with the piecrust; some are cooked separately, then added to the baked piecrust. Fruit fillings are usually baked with the piecrust. For apple pies try to select apples that have tender skins unsprayed with insecticides. This way you need not peel away the valuable nutrients in the skin. A light sprinkling of lemon juice over apples before baking adds a nice tang.

The top crusts of fruit pies have a tendency to fall in the center because of excess moisture. For this reason the fruit mixture is usually thickened with flour or cornstarch. Generally two tablespoons of either whole wheat flour or cornstarch per two cups of fresh, uncooked fruit is sufficient thickener. You may also sprinkle some dry cookie or cake crumbs on the bottom of the piecrust before adding the filling.

Custard fillings are generally baked with the piecrust. They may contain fruits, nuts, or coconut in the mixture. To prevent this type of pie from becoming soggy, cool it as soon as it comes out of the oven. Place it on a wire rack or an inverted colander so the air can circulate freely. Custard pies should not be stored for longer than one day.

If eaten promptly, cream pies do not become soggy because the filling is always placed in a prebaked piecrust. However, if left overnight, the crust may absorb the filling's moisture.

Meringue

When preparing meringue sweetened with honey, it is necessary to follow the recipe directions very carefully. When a meringue has been prepared as a pie topping, be sure to spread it over the filling while the filling is still warm. A cold filling can cause meringue to "weep." Spread the meringue to the very edges of the pie for a good seal. It should be about an inch thick and spread in peaks, never flat, to permit the oven heat to touch more surface.

In spreading the meringue on the pie, use a knife or spatula which has been dipped in cold water, to permit the meringue to slip off it easily.

Do not bake the meringue too long. At 425°F bake for 8 minutes; at 375°F bake for 10 to 15 minutes or until light brown. Serve the pie as soon as possible after the meringue has been baked. (See Meringues, page 426.)

Baking Pies

Baking time and temperature are as important as the correct plate size for piecrusts, so make sure they are as accurate as possible, using an oven thermometer if necessary. Off center, toward the back of the oven is usually the best place to position a pie for an even browning. If baking two pies at once, stagger them on two different racks and do not allow them to touch the oven walls.

If the piecrust seems to be browning too quickly, cover the crimped edges with aluminum foil. A done piecrust should be golden brown. A single piecrust will have browned, crisp edges and the filling, if custard, should be well set.

Most pies should be cooled for several minutes on a wire rack before being cut. Others must be chilled, and some merely need to reach room temperature before being served.

Pies

Barley-Oat Piecrust

  1 cup barley flour
  1 cup oat flour
  1/3 cup vegetable oil
  1/4 cup plus 2 tablespoons ice water

Preheat oven to 400°F. Prepare a 9-inch pie plate by brushing bottom and sides lightly with oil.

Sift flours into a medium-size bowl. Mix oil and ice water and stir into dry ingredients with a fork. Stir until a ball is formed.

Press onto bottom and sides of prepared pie plate, or roll out on a flat surface between 2 pieces of wax paper and line pie plate, making high edge around outside. Prick with fork and bake for 10 to 12 minutes. Cool on a wire rack.

Makes 1

Basic Pressed Piecrust

  3/4 cup rolled oats
  3/4 cup whole wheat pastry flour
  1/4 cup unsweetened shredded coconut
  1/3 cup vegetable oil
  2 tablespoons ice water

Place oats in a blender and blend into coarse flour. Transfer to a large bowl. Add flour and coconut and mix well. Blend in oil and then ice water.

Preheat oven to 425°F.

Press dough onto bottom and sides of a buttered 9-inch pie plate to about 1/8-inch thickness. Prick with a fork and bake for 12 to 15 minutes. Cool on a wire rack.

Makes 1

Basic Rolled Piecrust

1¼ cups whole wheat pastry flour
3 tablespoons butter
2 to 3 tablespoons vegetable oil
2 to 3 tablespoons ice water

Measure flour into a medium-size bowl. Cut butter into flour with a fork or pastry blender. Add oil slowly and continue to cut or mix until dough looks crumbly. Slowly add ice water, while mixing, until you can gather dough into a ball.

Place dough on a piece of floured wax paper on a flat surface. Flatten dough with your hand, sprinkle a little flour over it, cover with another piece of wax paper, and roll out to form a circle about 12 inches in diameter, ⅛ to ¼ inch thick.

Remove top piece of wax paper; invert a buttered 9-inch pie plate over dough; turn plate, dough, and remaining piece of wax paper right-side up; remove wax paper; and line plate with dough. Flute edges or simply trim away excess dough with a knife.

If recipe calls for a baked crust, prick dough with a fork and bake for 12 to 15 minutes at 425°F. Cool on a wire rack.

Makes 1

Mixed Grains Piecrust

This is not a sweet pastry crust. Use for a quiche or a main dish pie.

½ cup millet meal (whole millet coarsely ground in a blender)
¼ cup corn flour
½ cup whole wheat pastry flour
¼ cup butter, melted, or safflower oil
2 to 3 tablespoons ice water

Mix millet meal and corn flour together and toast in a small dry skillet over medium heat, stirring constantly, until mixture begins to give off nutty aroma. Remove from heat, turn into a medium-size bowl, and stir in whole wheat flour. Slowly pour butter or oil over mixture while mixing with a fork or pastry blender. Add water and mix thoroughly. This crust does not gather neatly into a ball; it must be pressed into pie plate.

Preheat oven to 350°F. Butter a 9-inch pie plate.

Press small pieces of dough next to each other in pie plate until bottom and sides are evenly covered. Prick with a fork and flute edges. Prebake for quiche for 5 to 10 minutes before adding filling. Crust firms up when it bakes.

Makes 1

Crumb Piecrust

2 cups fine cookie crumbs
1 tablespoon honey
3 tablespoons butter, melted
3 tablespoons vegetable oil

Combine crumbs, honey, butter, and oil and mix thoroughly. Reserve ½ cup crumb mixture for topping. Press remaining crumbs onto bottom and sides of a buttered 9-inch pie plate.

Chill for 20 minutes or bake immediately at 325°F for about 10 minutes. Cool on a wire rack.

Add filling, top with reserved crumbs, if desired, and chill again before serving.

Makes 1

Oat and Rice Flaky Pastry

¾ cup oat flour
¾ cup brown rice flour
¼ cup plus 2 tablespoons butter
1 tablespoon vegetable oil
1 to 2 tablespoons ice water

Preheat oven to 400°F. Sprinkle a 9-inch pie plate lightly with flour.

Combine flours in a medium-size bowl. Cut in butter with 2 knives or a pastry blender. Add oil gradually, working it in with your fingers. Then add ice water. Knead dough briefly until water is distributed evenly.

Press onto bottom and sides of prepared pie plate, or roll out on a flat surface between well-floured sheets of wax paper and line pie plate, making a high fluted edge around outside. If baking without filling, prick with a fork and bake for 10 to 12 minutes. Cool on a wire rack.

Makes 1

Rich Piecrust

½ cup ricotta cheese
⅓ cup butter
1¼ cups whole wheat pastry flour

Combine cheese, butter, and flour in a medium-size bowl and toss together gently to form dough. Chill.

When ready to fill pie, press onto bottom and sides of a 9-inch pie plate.

Makes 1

Sour Cream Piecrust

1¼ cups whole wheat pastry flour
¼ cup butter
¼ to ⅓ cup cold sour cream

Place flour in a medium-size bowl. Cut in butter, leaving mixture in coarse lumps. Add sour cream a little at a time so that no more is added than is necessary to hold dough together. Chill for 30 minutes or more.

When ready to fill pie, roll out dough on a flat surface to ¼-inch thickness and line a buttered 9-inch pie plate.

Makes 1

Apple Pie

pastry for 2 Basic Rolled Piecrusts (page 718)
7 cups sliced apples
1 tablespoon tapioca
¼ cup molasses
1 egg
½ teaspoon ground cinnamon
½ teaspoon vanilla extract

Preheat oven to 400°F.
Roll out ½ of pastry on a flat surface and line a 9-inch pie plate. Fill dough with apples. Mix together remaining ingredients and pour over apples. Roll out remaining dough and place over filling. Trim, seal, and crimp edges. Make several steam vents in top crust with a knife or fork.

Bake for 15 minutes, then reduce heat to 350°F and bake for 30 minutes more. Cool on a wire rack.

Makes 1

Variations:

Peach, Pear, or Plum Pie: Substitute 6 cups fruit for 7 cups apples.

Apple-Cheese Pie in Coconut Crust

Crust
1 cup unsweetened shredded coconut
½ cup wheat germ
2 tablespoons butter, melted

Filling
4 cups thinly sliced apples
½ teaspoon ground cinnamon
2 tablespoons butter, softened
3 eggs
¼ cup honey
4 ounces cream cheese
1 teaspoon vanilla extract

Topping
⅔ cup whole wheat pastry flour
¼ teaspoon ground cinnamon
1 tablespoon butter
1 tablespoon vegetable oil
2 teaspoons honey
1 tablespoon finely chopped walnuts

To make the crust: Spread thin layer of coconut on a baking sheet and bake at 350°F for 7 minutes, or until toasted. Then combine coconut with wheat germ and butter in a medium-size bowl. Toss with 2 forks until coconut is thoroughly coated with butter. Press mixture firmly onto bottom and sides of a 9-inch pie plate. Cover and refrigerate until firm.

To make the filling: Toss apples with cinnamon, then arrange apples on bottom of crust. Cream butter, eggs, and honey together. Add cream cheese and vanilla and blend just until smooth. Pour over apples.

Preheat oven to 350°F.

To make the topping: Mix flour, cinnamon, butter, oil, honey, and walnuts. Sprinkle on top of pie. Bake for 45 minutes, or until apples are tender. Cool on a wire rack, and then refrigerate.

Makes 1

Apple-Peach Pie

pastry for 2 Basic Rolled Piecrusts (page 718)
1 teaspoon lemon juice
1 tablespoon water
3 cups thinly sliced peeled apples
3 cups thinly sliced peeled peaches
1/3 cup honey
1 egg, beaten
3 tablespoons whole wheat flour
1 teaspoon ground cinnamon
1/2 teaspoon ground nutmeg
1 tablespoon butter

Preheat oven to 425°F.

Roll out 1/2 of pastry on a flat surface and line a 9-inch pie plate.

Mix lemon juice and water and toss with apples and peaches in a large bowl. Mix together honey, egg, flour, cinnamon, and nutmeg. Toss with fruit and fill dough. Dot filling with butter. Roll out remaining dough and place over filling. Trim, seal, and crimp edges. Make several steam vents in top crust with a knife or fork.

Bake for 40 minutes. Serve warm, or cool on a wire rack, then refrigerate.

Makes 1

Apricot Chiffon Pie

2 cups dried apricots
2 cups water
2 teaspoons unflavored gelatin
2 tablespoons cold water
3 egg yolks
1/3 cup honey
1 tablespoon lemon juice
3 egg whites, at room temperature
1/8 teaspoon vanilla extract
1 baked Basic Rolled Piecrust (page 718)

Cook apricots in 2 cups water for 20 minutes, making sure water does not all boil away. Then puree apricots and water in a blender or food processor.

Soften gelatin in cold water for 3 minutes.

In top of a double boiler, beat egg yolks, gradually mixing in honey, lemon juice, and pureed apricots. Cook until barely thickened, about 5 minutes. Pour in gelatin and continue to cook until it dissolves. Set aside to cool until thick but not set.

Beat egg whites until stiff but not dry, adding vanilla. Fold into apricot mixture. Turn into piecrust and refrigerate until set.

Makes 1

Banana Cream Pie

2 cups milk
1/4 cup plus 1 tablespoon cornstarch
1/4 cup honey, warmed
2 egg yolks, lightly beaten
1 tablespoon butter
1/2 teaspoon vanilla extract
3 large or 4 small ripe bananas
1 baked Basic Rolled Piecrust (page 718)
1 cup heavy cream, whipped

Pour 1 1/2 cups milk into top of a double boiler. Combine remaining milk with cornstarch and add to milk in double boiler. Add honey and cook, stirring constantly, until well thickened. Blend small amount of hot milk mixture into egg yolks, then add egg yolks to double boiler and stir well. Cook for 1 minute longer. Remove from heat and add butter and vanilla. Cool.

Slice bananas into piecrust. (Bottom should be well covered with about 3 layers of banana.) Cover immediately with cooled custard. Top with whipped cream.

Makes 1

Berry Pie

pastry for 2 Basic Rolled Piecrusts (page 718)
4 cups fresh berries (blackberries, blueberries, cherries, cranberries, currants, elderberries, gooseberries, huckleberries, juneberries, loganberries, raspberries, or strawberries)
1/4 cup tapioca
1/4 cup plus 1 tablespoon honey*
2 tablespoons butter, melted
1/2 teaspoon ground cinnamon or nutmeg (optional)

Preheat oven to 450°F.

Roll out 1/2 of pastry on a flat surface and line a 9-inch pie plate.

In a medium-size bowl mix berries, tapioca, honey, butter, and cinnamon or nutmeg (if used). Pour mixture into dough. Roll out remaining dough and place over filling. Trim, seal, and crimp edges. Make several steam vents in top crust with a knife or fork.

Bake for 15 minutes, then reduce heat to 350°F and bake for 45 to 60 minutes more. Cool to room temperature on a wire rack before serving.

Makes 1

*For cherries, cranberries, gooseberries, or any very tart berries add 3 tablespoons more honey and, if desired, ½ cup raisins.

Black and White Pie

    ⅓ cup plus 1 tablespoon honey
    2 tablespoons cornstarch
    ¼ cup water
    2 egg yolks, lightly beaten
    1¾ cups milk
    2 teaspoons unflavored gelatin
    3 tablespoons cold water
    1 teaspoon almond extract
    ¼ cup carob chips
    2 tablespoons butter
    1 baked Basic Rolled Piecrust (page 718)
    2 egg whites, at room temperature
    ¼ teaspoon cream of tartar

Place ⅓ cup honey in a large saucepan. Dissolve cornstarch in ¼ cup water and add to honey. Beat egg yolks with milk and mix into honey. Bring to a boil over medium heat, stirring constantly. Remove ½ of mixture and set aside.

Soften gelatin in cold water for 3 minutes. Add to hot mixture in saucepan, mixing well. Add almond extract. Cool in refrigerator until thickened but not set.

In top of a double boiler, melt carob and butter. Stir into reserved ½ of pie filling. Cool slightly and turn into piecrust.

Beat egg whites, cream of tartar, and 1 tablespoon honey until stiff but not dry. Fold into refrigerated gelatin mixture and place on top of carob in piecrust. Chill until firm. If desired, top pie with whipped cream just before serving.

Makes 1

Blackberry-Pineapple-Tapioca Pie

    pastry for 2 Basic Rolled Piecrusts (page 718)
    3 cups fresh or frozen and thawed blackberries
    1 cup unsweetened shredded pineapple
    ¼ cup honey
    3 tablespoons quick-cooking tapioca
    ½ teaspoon grated lemon rind
    2 tablespoons butter

Preheat oven to 450°F.

Roll out ½ of pastry on a flat surface and line a 9-inch pie plate.

Mix together blackberries, pineapple, honey, tapioca, and lemon rind. Allow to stand for 30 minutes, stirring occasionally.

Pour blackberry mixture into dough and dot with butter. Roll out remaining dough and place over filling. Trim, seal, and crimp edges. Make several steam vents in top crust with a knife or fork.

Bake for 15 minutes, then reduce heat to 350°F and bake for another 25 to 30 minutes. Serve warm, or cool on a wire rack, then refrigerate. Top with vanilla ice cream, if desired.

Makes 1

Blueberry Custard Pie

    Custard
    2 tablespoons honey
    2 tablespoons cornstarch
    1 cup milk
    2 eggs, beaten
    1 tablespoon butter
    1 teaspoon vanilla extract

    1 baked Basic Rolled Piecrust (page 718)

    Topping
    ¼ cup honey
    1 tablespoon cornstarch
    ¼ cup water
    1 teaspoon lemon juice
    1½ cups blueberries (other berries may be substituted)

To make the custard: Using a wire whisk, combine honey, cornstarch, and milk in top of a double boiler, but not over heat. Add eggs and cook, stirring constantly, over boiling water until thick, about 5 minutes. Remove from heat and add butter and vanilla. Cool and spread over piecrust.

To make the topping: Combine honey and cornstarch in a large saucepan. Add ¼ cup water and mix with wire whisk until smooth. Cook mixture over medium heat until slightly thick. Then add lemon juice and berries, and stir and cook for 5 minutes more. Cool and spread over custard. Chill before serving.

Makes 1

Buttermilk-Fruit Pie

    pastry for 1 Basic Rolled Piecrust (page 718)
    ½ cup butter, softened
    1 cup honey
    3 eggs, separated
    3 tablespoons cornstarch
    1½ cups buttermilk
    1 teaspoon grated lemon rind
    1 tablespoon lemon juice
    1½ cups cooked sliced peeled peaches or plums
        ground nutmeg

Preheat oven to 350°F.

Roll out pastry on a flat surface and line a 9-inch pie plate.

In a large bowl beat butter, honey, and egg yolks together until combined. Dissolve cornstarch in buttermilk and add to butter mixture, along with lemon rind and juice. Mix in fruit.

Beat egg whites until stiff but not dry and fold in carefully. Turn filling into piecrust and decorate with nutmeg.

Bake for 20 minutes, then reduce heat to 300°F and continue to bake for 15 to 20 minutes, or until filling is set. Cool on a wire rack before serving.

    Makes 1

Carob Pie

    pastry for 1 Basic Rolled Piecrust (page 718)
    4 ounces carob
    3 tablespoons butter
    ½ cup honey
    1½ cups light cream or milk
    ½ cup whole wheat pastry flour
    1 teaspoon vanilla extract
    3 eggs, beaten
    1 cup unsweetened flaked coconut
    ½ cup chopped walnuts

Preheat oven to 350°F.

Roll out pastry on a flat surface and line a 9-inch pie plate.

In top of a double boiler, melt carob, butter, and honey. Remove from heat.

In a jar with a tight-fitting lid, shake cream or milk and flour until smooth. Place in a large bowl and beat in carob mixture, adding vanilla and eggs. Stir in coconut and nuts. Turn into dough.

Bake until knife inserted into center comes out clean, about 35 minutes. Cool on a wire rack before serving.

    Makes 1

Carrot-Coconut Pie

    pastry for 1½ Basic Rolled Piecrusts
        (page 718)
    2 cups pureed cooked carrots
    ½ cup honey
    1 tablespoon butter, melted
    1 teaspoon ground cinnamon
    ½ teaspoon ground allspice
    1 cup light cream or milk
    3 eggs, beaten
    1 teaspoon vanilla extract
    1 cup unsweetened shredded coconut

Roll out pastry on a flat surface and line a 9-inch deep dish pie plate. Prick dough with a fork, weight bottom with dried beans, and bake at 425°F for 5 minutes. Set aside to cool.

Preheat oven to 450°F.

In a large mixing bowl combine carrots and honey. Stir in butter, cinnamon, and allspice. Add cream or milk a little at a time, mixing well. Stir in eggs, vanilla, and coconut. Turn into piecrust.

Place in preheated oven, reduce heat to 350°F, and bake until pie is almost set in center, 50 to 60 minutes. Serve warm, or cool on a wire rack, then refrigerate.

    Makes 1

Cherry-Berry Pie

    pastry for 2 Basic Rolled Piecrusts (page 718)
    3 cups fresh sour cherries, pitted
    1 cup fresh blackberries
    ¼ cup honey, warmed

1 tablespoon butter
¾ cup water
3 tablespoons cornstarch
¼ cup cold water
3 egg yolks, lightly beaten

Preheat oven to 450°F.

Roll out ½ of pastry on a flat surface and line a 9-inch pie plate.

Combine cherries, blackberries, honey, butter, and water in a large saucepan. Simmer, stirring constantly, until fruit softens.

Shake together cornstarch and cold water in a jar with a tight-fitting lid until smooth. Add to saucepan and cook, stirring until mixture thickens. Mix 2 tablespoons fruit into egg yolks, then mix egg yolks into saucepan and continue cooking, stirring constantly, for 2 more minutes. Turn into dough. Roll out remaining dough and place over filling. Trim, seal, and crimp edges. Make several steam vents in top crust with a knife or fork.

Bake for 10 minutes, then reduce heat to 325°F and bake for 20 to 25 minutes more. Cool on a wire rack before serving.

Makes 1

Coconut Cream Pie

2 cups milk
1 cup unsweetened shredded coconut
3 egg yolks
¼ cup honey, warmed
2 tablespoons butter, softened
2 teaspoons vanilla extract
¼ cup whole wheat flour
1 baked Basic Rolled Piecrust (page 718)
¼ cup unsweetened shredded coconut, toasted

Mix ½ cup milk with 1 cup coconut. Heat remaining milk in a large heavy saucepan.

Mix egg yolks, honey, butter, and vanilla in a medium-size bowl. Stir in flour and mix thoroughly.

Pour about ½ cup hot milk into mixture. Stir well, then pour into saucepan. Cook over medium heat until thick and smooth, stirring constantly.

Remove from heat and add coconut-milk mixture. Stir until well blended. Pour into piecrust and cool. Decorate with toasted coconut and chill until ready to serve.

Makes 1

NOTE: Fresh coconut can be used for filling in this pie. It is not necessary then to soak coconut in milk; simply omit that step and use only 1¾ cups milk for custard. For decoration use dried coconut—it is easier to toast.

Coconut-Lime Pie

Crust
2 cups unsweetened flaked coconut
¼ cup butter, softened

Filling
½ cup honey
1 envelope unflavored gelatin
4 egg yolks, lightly beaten
½ cup lime juice
½ cup water
4 egg whites, at room temperature
½ teaspoon cream of tartar

Preheat oven to 325°F.

To make the crust: Mix together coconut and butter. Press onto bottom and sides of a 9-inch pie plate. Bake for 20 to 25 minutes, then set on a wire rack to cool.

To make the filling: In a medium-size saucepan combine honey, gelatin, and egg yolks. Stir in lime juice and water, and bring to a boil over medium heat, stirring constantly. Remove from heat and pour into a medium-size bowl. Refrigerate until thickened but not set.

Beat egg whites until they form soft peaks, adding cream of tartar. Fold into lime mixture and turn into piecrust. Refrigerate until set.

Makes 1

Cranberry-Pear Pie

pastry for 2 Basic Rolled Piecrusts (page 718)
3 cups fresh cranberries
¾ cup honey
⅓ cup cornstarch
½ cup water
2½ cups coarsely sliced peeled pears (3 medium-size pears)
½ cup chopped walnuts

Roll out ½ of pastry on a flat surface and line a 9-inch pie plate.

Place cranberries in a medium-size saucepan. Bring to a boil in enough water to cover, and cook for 4 minutes. Add honey.

In a small bowl combine cornstarch with water and stir until dissolved. Add to cranberries. Simmer, stirring constantly, until mixture thickens. Remove from heat and stir in pears and walnuts. Pour into dough.

Preheat oven to 400°F.

Roll out remaining pastry and cut into strips. Make a lattice on top of pie filling (see page 715). Bake for 40 to 45 minutes. Cool on a wire rack.

Makes 1

Fig-Walnut Pie with Orange Sauce

Crust
5 egg whites
1 cup ground dried figs
1 cup ground walnuts
¼ teaspoon ground cinnamon

Sauce
8 ounces cream cheese
½ cup orange juice
1 teaspoon grated orange rind
¼ cup honey

Preheat oven to 375°F. Butter a 9-inch pie plate.

To make the crust: Beat egg whites in a large bowl until stiff but not dry. Gently fold in figs, walnuts, and cinnamon. Pour into prepared pie plate and bake for 25 minutes, or until lightly browned. Chill.

To make the sauce: Place cream cheese, juice, rind, and honey in a blender and process until smooth. Pour over baked meringue shell.

Makes 1

Fresh Fruit-Cheese Pie

Crust
1 cup chopped walnuts
½ cup butter, softened
¾ cup whole wheat flour
½ cup date sugar
½ teaspoon vanilla extract

Filling
4 cups fresh fruit (peaches, apples, nectarines, or other fruit)
1 cup yogurt
1 cup small-curd cottage cheese
½ cup unsweetened crushed pineapple
¼ cup unsweetened shredded coconut

Preheat oven to 350°F. Butter a 9-inch pie plate.

To make the crust: In a medium-size bowl blend nuts, butter, flour, date sugar, and vanilla together with a fork. Press onto bottom and sides of prepared pie plate. Bake for 10 to 15 minutes, or until lightly browned. Cool on a wire rack.

To make the filling: Cut fruit into bite-size pieces and place in piecrust. Process yogurt, cottage cheese, and pineapple in a blender until smooth. Pour mixture over fruit. Sprinkle with coconut. Chill for several hours before serving.

Makes 1

Fresh Pear Pie

Crust
1 cup chopped walnuts
½ cup butter, softened
¾ cup whole wheat flour
½ cup date sugar
½ teaspoon vanilla extract

Filling
4 ripe pears, cored
1 cup nonfat dry milk

1 cup warm water
2 tablespoons arrowroot
¼ cup honey

pear slices

Preheat oven to 350°F. Butter a 9-inch pie plate.

To make the crust: In a medium-size bowl blend nuts, butter, flour, date sugar, and vanilla together with a fork. Press onto bottom and sides of prepared pie plate. Bake for 10 to 15 minutes, or until lightly browned. Cool on a wire rack.

To make the filling: Place pears in a blender and puree until smooth. Place pureed pears in a large saucepan. Add nonfat dry milk, warm water, arrowroot, and honey and cook over low heat, while stirring, until smooth and thickened. Pour mixture into piecrust. Chill for several hours. Decorate with pear slices.

Makes 1

Ginger Peachy Pie with Streusel Topping

pastry for 1 Basic Rolled Piecrust (page 718)
⅔ cup plus 2 teaspoons whole wheat flour
⅓ cup date sugar
⅓ cup butter
½ cup unsweetened shredded coconut
¼ cup honey
2 teaspoons lemon juice
4 cups thinly sliced peeled peaches
¼ teaspoon ground ginger

Roll out pastry on a flat surface and line a 9-inch pie plate.

Mix ⅔ cup flour with date sugar in a medium-size bowl. Cut in butter with a pastry blender or 2 knives until mixture is texture of cornmeal. Mix in coconut and refrigerate.

Preheat oven to 450°F.

Mix together honey and lemon juice. Toss with peaches. Place ½ of peaches in dough. Mix 2 teaspoons flour with ginger. Sprinkle ½ on peaches in piecrust. Place remaining peaches on top. Sprinkle with remainder of flour and ginger. Top with date sugar mixture.

Bake for 10 minutes, then reduce heat to 350°F and bake for another 20 to 25 minutes. Cool on a wire rack.

Makes 1

Green Grape Dream Pie

2 cups milk
¼ cup plus 1 tablespoon cornstarch
¼ cup honey
3 egg yolks, lightly beaten
1 tablespoon butter
1 teaspoon vanilla extract
1 baked Basic Rolled Piecrust (page 718)
30 seedless green grapes, halved
¾ cup peach preserves

In a jar with a tight-fitting lid, shake 1 cup milk with cornstarch until smooth. Place in top of a double boiler. Add remaining milk and honey and cook, stirring constantly, until mixture thickens. Stir some of the thickened milk into egg yolks. Add egg yolks to top of double boiler and stir constantly until very thick, about 1 minute. Add butter and vanilla, stirring for another minute. Cool, then pour into piecrust.

Completely cover top of custard with grapes, placing them cut-side down. In a blender process preserves until smooth. Brush grapes with preserves. Refrigerate until ready to serve.

Makes 1

Italian Cheese Pie

pastry for 1 Basic Rolled Piecrust (page 718)
1½ pounds ricotta cheese
¼ cup chopped roasted almonds
4 eggs
¼ cup honey
1 teaspoon vanilla extract
ground cinnamon

Roll out pastry on a flat surface and line a 9-inch pie plate.

Preheat oven to 375°F.

Put ricotta through a sieve into a large bowl. Add almonds. Set aside.

Beat eggs and honey until foamy. Add vanilla. Blend with ricotta mixture until smooth. Pour mixture into pastry.

Bake for about 45 minutes, or until filling is firm. Cool on a wire rack. Decorate with cinnamon just before serving.

Makes 1

Lemon Chiffon Pie

1 envelope unflavored gelatin
¼ cup cold water
4 eggs, separated
½ cup honey, warmed
½ cup lemon juice
1 teaspoon grated lemon rind
1 baked Crumb Piecrust (page 718)
½ cup heavy cream, whipped
¼ cup chopped nuts

Soak gelatin in cold water.

In top of a double boiler, but not over heat, beat egg yolks. Add honey, lemon juice, lemon rind, and gelatin mixture. Place over hot water and cook until thickened, stirring constantly. Cool.

Beat egg whites until stiff but not dry. Fold into batter and spoon into piecrust. Serve topped with whipped cream and chopped nuts.

Makes 1

Lemony Nut Pastry with Orange Custard Filling

Crust
1 cup chopped walnuts
½ cup butter, softened
¾ cup whole wheat flour
½ cup date sugar
½ teaspoon vanilla extract

Filling
2 navel oranges
½ cup lemon juice
½ cup orange juice
1 teaspoon grated lemon rind
1 teaspoon grated orange rind
4 eggs
¼ cup butter
½ cup nonfat dry milk
¼ cup warm water
¼ cup honey

½ cup wheat germ
½ teaspoon ground nutmeg

Preheat oven to 350°F. Butter a 9-inch pie plate.

To make the crust: In a medium-size bowl blend nuts, butter, flour, date sugar, and vanilla together with a fork. Press onto bottom and sides of prepared pie plate. Bake for 10 to 15 minutes, or until lightly browned. Cool on a wire rack.

To make the filling: Peel oranges and separate into segments. Place citrus juices and rinds in a large saucepan. Add eggs and beat together until light and foamy. Add butter, nonfat dry milk, warm water, and honey and cook over low heat until thickened, stirring constantly to prevent burning. Remove from heat. Gently fold in oranges.

Preheat oven to 350°F.

Pour filling into piecrust. Sprinkle with wheat germ and then top with nutmeg. Bake for about 25 minutes. Cool on a wire rack before serving.

Makes 1

Mincemeat Pie

pastry for 2 Basic Rolled Piecrusts (page 718)
4 cups Mincemeat (see below)

Preheat oven to 450°F.

Roll out ½ of pastry on a flat surface and line a 9-inch pie plate. Add mincemeat to dough. Roll out remaining dough and place over mincemeat. Trim, seal, and crimp edges. Make several steam vents in top crust with a knife or fork.

Bake for 10 minutes, then reduce heat to 350°F and bake for 20 to 25 minutes more. Cool on a wire rack before serving.

Makes 1

Mincemeat

1 pound stewing beef, trimmed of fat
2 cups water
4 pounds cooking apples, cored and quartered
½ cup butter or suet
1 unpeeled orange, quartered
1 unpeeled lemon, quartered
1¼ cups honey
1 cup orange juice or water
2½ cups raisins
1¾ cups dried currants

½ teaspoon ground cinnamon
¼ teaspoon ground cloves
¼ teaspoon ground mace

In a large saucepan combine beef with water. Cover and simmer for 2 hours, or until meat is tender. Drain and cool.

Using coarse blade of a meat grinder, grind beef, apples, butter or suet, orange, and lemon. In an 8-quart pot mix ground meat mixture with remaining ingredients. Cover and simmer on low heat for 2 hours. If mincemeat is too moist, remove lid after 2 hours of cooking and cook until desired consistency is obtained.

Yields 12 cups

Minty Apricot Pie

pastry for 2 Basic Rolled Piecrusts (page 718)
4 cups sliced peeled apricots
1 tablespoon water
1 teaspoon lemon juice
2 tablespoons cornstarch
¼ cup honey, warmed
2 teaspoons minced fresh mint
1 egg yolk, lightly beaten

Preheat oven to 350°F.
Roll out ½ of pastry on a flat surface and line a 9-inch pie plate.
Toss together apricots, water, and lemon juice in a large bowl. Mix cornstarch into honey until dissolved. Toss mint with apricots. Add honey and toss again. Pile fruit into dough. Roll out remaining dough and place over filling. Trim, seal, and crimp edges. Make several steam vents in top crust with a knife or fork. Brush with egg yolk.
Bake until fruit is soft, about 45 minutes. Serve warm, or cool on a wire rack, then refrigerate.

Makes 1

Nectarine Meringue

6 nectarines
½ cup orange juice
½ cup dried currants
¼ cup wheat germ
¼ teaspoon ground cinnamon

4 egg whites
1 tablespoon honey
⅓ cup sliced almonds

Slice nectarines thin, leaving skin intact. Remove pits. Place nectarines in a 2-quart saucepan with orange juice and currants. Cover and cook over low heat for 5 minutes. Remove from heat.
Preheat oven to 400°F. Butter a 9-inch pie plate.
Sprinkle wheat germ over sides and bottom of pie plate. Place nectarine mixture over wheat germ. Sprinkle with cinnamon.
Beat egg whites and honey until stiff but not dry. Cover nectarine mixture completely with meringue and carefully stick in almonds. Bake for 5 minutes, or until brown. Cool on a wire rack before serving.

Makes 1

No-Bake Cheese Pie

Crust
½ cup pitted dates
½ cup unsweetened shredded coconut
½ cup walnuts
¼ teaspoon ground cinnamon

Filling
1 pound cream cheese
1½ cups yogurt
1 can (8 ounces) unsweetened crushed pineapple, drained
¼ cup chopped walnuts

Butter a 9-inch pie plate.
To make the crust: Place dates, coconut, walnuts, and cinnamon in a food processor or blender. Process until slightly chopped. Press onto sides and bottom of prepared pie plate. Chill.
To make the filling: Blend cream cheese in a large bowl until smooth. Fold in yogurt. Add pineapple carefully, stirring just until blended. Pour into chilled piecrust.
Chill for several hours, or until firm. Sprinkle with walnuts.

Makes 1

Orange Puff Pie

> pastry for 1½ Basic Rolled Piecrusts (page 718)

2 tablespoons cornstarch
¼ cup water
1½ cups chopped navel oranges
¼ cup honey, or more to taste
1 tablespoon butter, softened
3 tablespoons whole wheat pastry flour
¾ cup cottage cheese
3 eggs, beaten
½ cup milk
½ teaspoon vanilla extract

Preheat oven to 425°F.

Roll out pastry on a flat surface and line a 9-inch deep dish pie plate.

Blend cornstarch and water in a medium-size saucepan. Stir in oranges and boil, stirring constantly, until thick. Chill.

In a medium-size bowl beat together honey and butter. Beat in flour and cottage cheese. Gradually beat in eggs and then milk. Add vanilla and blend.

Spread orange mixture on bottom of pastry. Pour cheese mixture over it.

Bake for 15 minutes, then reduce heat to 325°F and bake for another 45 minutes, or until center is puffy. Cool on a wire rack before serving.

Makes 1

Peachy Cheese Tart

> *Crust*
½ cup date sugar
½ cup butter, softened
½ teaspoon vanilla extract
¾ cup whole wheat pastry flour
1 cup chopped pecans

> *Filling*
2 cups sliced peaches
1 tablespoon lemon juice
1 pound cream cheese
2 eggs
¼ cup honey
1 teaspoon vanilla extract
½ teaspoon ground cinnamon
¼ cup butter

Preheat oven to 350°F. Butter a 9-inch pie plate.

To make the crust: Beat date sugar, butter, and vanilla together until well blended. Add flour and chopped pecans. Mix well. Press onto bottom and sides of prepared pie plate.

To make the filling: Mix peaches with lemon juice to prevent discoloration.

Beat cream cheese in a large bowl until smooth. Add eggs and then honey, beating until light and fluffy. Add vanilla and cinnamon.

Pour cheese mixture into piecrust. Place peaches carefully over cheese mixture and dot with butter.

Bake for 45 to 50 minutes. Cool on a wire rack, then refrigerate until serving time.

Makes 1

Pecan Pie

> pastry for 1 Basic Rolled Piecrust (page 718)

1 to 1½ cups pecan halves
3 eggs
¼ cup butter, melted
½ cup molasses
½ cup honey
1 teaspoon vanilla extract
few drops vinegar

Preheat oven to 350°F.

Roll out pastry on a flat surface and line a 9-inch pie plate. Place pecans on dough, arranging them so that those on top are right-side up (curved side facing up).

Beat eggs, then add remaining ingredients, mixing well to combine. Pour filling over pecans.

Bake for 30 minutes, or until a knife inserted into center comes out clean. Cool on a wire rack before serving.

Makes 1

Perfect Plum Pie

> pastry for 2 Basic Rolled Piecrusts (page 718)

1 tablespoon lemon juice
1 tablespoon water
3½ pounds purple plums, pitted
½ cup honey, warmed
3 tablespoons tapioca
1 teaspoon ground allspice
2 tablespoons butter
1 cup heavy cream

Roll out ½ of pastry on a flat surface and line a 9-inch pie plate.

Mix together lemon juice and water and sprinkle over plums in a large bowl. Mix honey, tapioca, and allspice. Toss with plums and allow to stand for 15 minutes, stirring occasionally.

Preheat oven to 425°F.

Turn filling into dough and dot with butter. Roll out remaining dough and place over filling. Trim, seal, and crimp edges. Make several steam vents in top crust with a knife or fork.

Bake for 15 minutes, then reduce heat to 350°F and bake for another 20 to 25 minutes.

Whip cream. Serve pie warm with dollop of cream on each portion.

Makes 1

Persimmon Pie

    pastry for 1 Basic Rolled Piecrust (page 718)
    4 eggs
    ½ cup plus 2 tablespoons honey
    2 cups light cream or milk
    2 cups persimmon pulp, pureed (6 persimmons)
    1 teaspoon vanilla extract
    1 cup sour cream
    1 tablespoon white grape juice

Preheat oven to 425°F.

Roll out pastry on a flat surface and line a 9-inch pie plate.

Beat eggs well. Beat in ½ cup honey. Add cream or milk, persimmon, and vanilla, beating until blended. Pour into dough.

Bake for 10 minutes, then reduce heat to 350°F and bake until set, about 25 minutes. Cool well on a wire rack.

Mix sour cream, grape juice, and remaining honey and spread on top of pie. Serve immediately.

Makes 1

Pineapple-Pear Tart

    pastry for 1½ Basic Rolled Piecrusts
       (page 718)
    8 ounces cream cheese, softened

    ¼ cup plus 1 tablespoon pineapple juice
    2 tablespoons honey
    1 teaspoon vanilla extract
    24 slices unsweetened pineapple
    3 pears, peeled, halved, and cored
    1 strawberry
    ½ cup peach preserves

Preheat oven to 400°F.

Roll out pastry on a flat surface and line a 12-inch-round pizza pan. Prick dough with a fork, weight with dried beans, and bake until lightly browned, about 12 minutes.

In a medium-size bowl beat cream cheese, ¼ cup pineapple juice, honey, and vanilla until smooth. Spread on piecrust. Return to oven for 5 minutes, then cool on a wire rack.

Place a row of pineapple around outer edge of crust. Arrange pears in circle in middle. Place strawberry in center of pie.

In a small saucepan heat preserves and 1 tablespoon pineapple juice. Brush fruit with preserves and refrigerate tart until ready to serve.

Makes 1

Pumpkin Pie

    pastry for 1 Basic Rolled Piecrust (page 718)
    ½ teaspoon ground ginger
    1 teaspoon ground cinnamon
    1½ cups pureed pumpkin
    3 cups milk or light cream
    3 eggs, beaten
    ¼ cup honey
    1 tablespoon molasses
    1 teaspoon vanilla extract

Preheat oven to 450°F.

Roll out pastry on a flat surface and line a 9-inch pie plate.

Add seasonings to pumpkin. Place milk or cream and eggs in a large bowl. Stir in pumpkin mixture, honey, molasses, and vanilla. Pour filling into dough.

Bake for 10 minutes, then reduce heat to 350°F and bake for 30 minutes longer. Cool on a wire rack before serving.

Makes 1

Raspberry Chiffon Pie

1½ cups finely chopped peanuts plus 3
tablespoons butter, softened, or 1 baked
Basic Rolled Piecrust (page 718)
1 envelope unflavored gelatin
2 tablespoons honey
½ cup water
1½ cups fresh or frozen and thawed raspberries
1½ cups sour cream

Thoroughly mix peanuts and butter, press onto
bottom and sides of a 9-inch pie plate, and chill until
firm; or set Basic Rolled Piecrust aside to cool.

Mix gelatin, honey, and water in a small saucepan.
Allow to stand for 3 minutes. Then place over medium
heat, stirring constantly, until gelatin dissolves and
mixture just comes to a boil.

In a food processor or blender process gelatin
until foamy. Add raspberries, and puree. Fold in sour
cream and refrigerate until thickened but not set. Then
turn into piecrust and chill until set.

Makes 1

Ricotta-Pineapple Pie

Crust
1½ cups pine nuts
1 tablespoon honey
1 tablespoon butter, melted

Filling
1 cup pine nuts
1 tablespoon arrowroot
4 eggs
2 cups ricotta cheese
1 cup unsweetened crushed pineapple
½ teaspoon vanilla extract
½ teaspoon ground cinnamon

To make the crust: Place pine nuts and honey in a
blender and process until nuts are coarse. Add butter
and mix. Press onto bottom and sides of 9-inch
pie plate.

Preheat oven to 375°F.

To make the filling: Mix pine nuts with arrowroot.
In a large bowl beat eggs until fluffy. Mix in cheese,
pineapple, and vanilla. Fold in nuts. Pour into piecrust
and sprinkle with cinnamon.

Bake for 40 to 45 minutes. Cool on a wire rack.

Makes 1

Spicy Fig Pie

pastry for 1 Basic Rolled Piecrust (page 718)
3 tablespoons butter, softened
½ cup honey
2 tablespoons lemon juice
8 eggs, beaten
1 teaspoon ground cinnamon
½ teaspoon ground nutmeg
1½ cups chopped dried figs
¼ cup raisins
2 tablespoons whole wheat flour
½ cup chopped nuts

Preheat oven to 425°F.

Roll out pastry on a flat surface and line a 9-inch
pie plate. Prick dough with a fork, weight it with dried
beans, and bake for 5 minutes. Cool on a wire rack.

Reduce heat to 375°F.

Beat together butter and honey, adding lemon
juice, eggs, cinnamon, and nutmeg while beating.
Shake figs and raisins in just enough flour to barely
coat. Stir into batter. Stir in nuts. Turn into piecrust
and bake until center is set, about 40 minutes. Cool on
a wire rack before serving.

Makes 1

Strawberry-Banana Pie

2 cups fresh or frozen and thawed strawberries,
quartered
¾ cup water
¼ cup plus 1 teaspoon honey
2 tablespoons cornstarch
½ teaspoon ground cinnamon
½ teaspoon vanilla extract
1 large banana
1 baked Basic Rolled Piecrust (page 718)

In a medium-size saucepan simmer strawberries,
½ cup water, and ¼ cup honey for 5 minutes. Shake
cornstarch and ¼ cup water in a jar with a tight-fitting
lid until smooth. Slowly add to strawberries, cooking
until mixture thickens. Stir in cinnamon and vanilla.

When strawberry mixture has cooled slightly, thinly slice banana into piecrust. Pour strawberries over bananas. Refrigerate until set.

When ready to serve, top with whipped cream, if desired.

Makes 1

Strawberry-Cheese Refrigerator Pie

Crust
¼ cup butter
2 cups unsweetened shredded coconut

Filling
2 cups fresh strawberries
1 cup yogurt
8 ounces cream cheese
2 tablespoons honey

½ cup pecan halves, toasted

Preheat oven to 300°F.

To make the crust: Place butter and coconut in a medium-size bowl. Lightly toss with a fork until well mixed. Press evenly onto bottom and sides of a 9-inch pie plate. (Do not go up to rim.) Bake for 25 minutes, or until lightly browned. Cool on a wire rack.

To make the filling: Place strawberries, yogurt, cream cheese, and honey in a blender. Blend until smooth, then pour into piecrust.

Decorate top with pecan halves. Chill until served.

Makes 1

Sweet Potato-Nut Pie

4 medium-size sweet potatoes
pastry for 1 Basic Rolled Piecrust (page 718)
⅔ cup plus 3 tablespoons honey
½ teaspoon ground ginger
½ teaspoon ground cinnamon
½ teaspoon ground nutmeg
3 eggs
1½ cups light cream or milk
3 tablespoons butter
½ cup chopped walnuts

Cook sweet potatoes in enough water to cover. Drain and mash.

Preheat oven to 425°F.

Roll out pastry on a flat surface and line a 9-inch pie plate.

In a food processor mix sweet potatoes, ⅔ cup honey, ginger, cinnamon, nutmeg, eggs, and cream or milk. Pour into dough.

Place in preheated oven, reduce heat to 350°F, and bake until center is barely firm, about 50 minutes. Remove from oven and cool on a wire rack.

In a small saucepan melt butter. Add 3 tablespoons honey and bring to a boil. Remove from heat. Stir in walnuts and pour on top of pie. Just before serving, top with whipped cream, if desired.

Makes 1

Tofu Cheese Pie

pastry for 1 Crumb Piecrust (page 718)
2 tablespoons cornstarch
¼ cup cold water
2 eggs
½ cup honey
2 teaspoons vanilla extract
1 cup tofu, drained
1 cup creamed cottage cheese
¼ teaspoon grated lemon rind
2 teaspoons lemon juice
⅓ cup butter, melted

Topping
1 cup sour cream
1 tablespoon honey, or more to taste
1 teaspoon vanilla extract (optional)

Press pastry onto bottom and sides of a 9-inch pie plate.

Preheat oven to 350°F.

Place cornstarch and cold water in a blender and process until smooth. Add remaining ingredients, except topping ingredients, and blend until very smooth. Pour into pastry.

Bake for 30 to 40 minutes. Center may still be a bit soft, but it is important to avoid overcooking pie. A knife inserted into center should *not* come out entirely clean. Remove pie and cool on a wire rack for about 5 minutes before adding topping.

To make the topping: Stir together all ingredients and pour over top of pie. Return to a 350°F oven for no more than 5 minutes. Cool on a wire rack, then refrigerate before serving.

Makes 1

Yogurt-Raisin Pie

> pastry for 1 Basic Rolled Piecrust (page 718)
> 3 eggs
> 1/3 cup honey
> 1½ cups yogurt
> 1½ cups raisins, chopped
> ¼ teaspoon ground nutmeg
> 1½ tablespoons lemon juice

Preheat oven to 450°F.

Roll out pastry on a flat surface and line a 9-inch pie plate.

Beat eggs. Add honey and continue to beat until light. Fold in yogurt. Then add raisins, nutmeg, and lemon juice, and mix lightly but thoroughly. Pour mixture into dough.

Bake for 10 minutes, then reduce heat to 350°F and bake for 35 minutes longer. Cool on a wire rack before serving.

Makes 1

Zucchini Custard Pie

> 4 medium-size zucchini
> 4 egg yolks
> ¼ cup honey
> ½ teaspoon vanilla extract
> 1 cup nonfat dry milk
> ½ cup warm water
> ½ teaspoon ground cinnamon
> 1 baked Basic Rolled Piecrust (page 718)

Preheat oven to 350°F.

Grate and then squeeze all liquid out of zucchini.

In a 2-quart saucepan place egg yolks, honey, vanilla, nonfat dry milk, and warm water. Cook over low heat, stirring constantly, until thickened. Remove from heat. Add cinnamon and zucchini and blend. Pour into piecrust.

Bake for 20 minutes, or until custard is set. Cool on a wire rack, then chill.

Makes 1

Pastries
Cream Puffs

> 1 cup water
> ½ cup butter
> 1 cup whole wheat or rye flour
> 4 eggs

Preheat oven to 400°F. Lightly butter a baking sheet.

Bring water and butter to a boil in a medium-size saucepan. Remove pan from heat. Add flour all at once, stirring hard with a wooden spoon. Reduce heat and continue to cook dough, stirring constantly, for 1 to 2 minutes to make sure flour is cooked. Cool slightly.

Transfer dough to a large bowl. Add eggs, one at a time, beating well after each addition. Drop dough by the teaspoon onto prepared baking sheet, leaving 1 inch between puffs.

Bake for 25 to 30 minutes, or until cream puffs are quite firm. Loosen carefully with a spatula and cool on wire racks away from drafts. Store in a cool dry place until time to split and fill. Filling should be done just before serving, to prevent cream puffs from getting soggy.

Makes about 72 small or 10 large

NOTE: Cream puffs can be filled with any of the sweet fillings in Frostings and Fillings (page 694). Or for a savory filling see Dips and Spreads (page 78).

Date-Nut Pastries

Dough
1 tablespoon dry yeast
1 cup warm water
3 tablespoons butter, melted
1 tablespoon honey
1 egg
3 cups whole wheat flour

Topping
½ cup finely chopped walnuts
½ cup finely chopped dates
1 tablespoon grated lemon rind
1 teaspoon ground cinnamon
2 tablespoons honey

To make the dough: Dissolve yeast in warm water in a large bowl, and set aside to proof. Then add butter and honey. Blend in egg, then add flour and mix until dough is well blended and soft. Place in an oiled bowl, cover with a cloth, and allow to rise for 1 hour in a warm place.

Butter a baking sheet.

Roll out dough on a well-floured board to a ¼-inch-thick rectangle and fit onto prepared baking sheet.

To make the topping: Mix nuts, dates, lemon rind, cinnamon, and honey. Spread mixture evenly over dough.

Cut into 1½-inch squares. Cover with a damp cloth and let rise again in a warm place until doubled in bulk, about 25 minutes.

Preheat oven to 400°F.

Bake for 15 minutes. Cool on a wire rack before serving.

Makes 3½ dozen

Fruit Danish

Dough
½ cup milk, scalded
¼ cup butter or vegetable oil
1 tablespoon honey
½ cup cold water
1 tablespoon dry yeast
1 egg
3 cups whole wheat flour

Topping
½ cup whole grain bread crumbs
2 tablespoons honey
¼ teaspoon ground cinnamon
1 egg white, lightly beaten
1/3 cup chopped cooked fruit (apricots, prunes, raisins, or other fruit)

To make the dough: In a large bowl mix milk, butter or oil, and honey. Cool to lukewarm by adding ½ cup cold water. Stir in yeast, then beat in egg, cover, and let stand in a warm place for 10 to 15 minutes.

Add flour and knead until dough is well blended and soft. Shape into 12 buns.

Butter a baking sheet.

To make the topping: Combine bread crumbs, honey, and cinnamon. Dip each bun first in egg white, then in crumb mixture.

Place buns on prepared baking sheet, cover with a cloth, and let rise in a warm place until light, about 45 minutes.

Preheat oven to 375°F.

Press deep indentation into center of each bun. Place about 1 teaspoon fruit into each indentation. Bake for 25 minutes. Cool on wire racks.

Makes 1 dozen

Beverages

An invitation to stop for a drink is an invitation to relax for a few minutes, a time to share a pleasant conversation with a friend. Whatever you choose to serve will be welcome—on a cold afternoon a cup of hot herb tea, after the movies a milk shake so thick the straw stands straight up, on a lazy summer day an invigorating vegetable concoction.

Aside from their social value, beverages play an important role in maintaining good health. To be at your best you should drink eight to ten glasses of fluids a day. Your need increases when you are exposed to hot weather, when you are very active, and when you are sick. It makes sense to keep your pantry and refrigerator well stocked with ingredients for tasty beverages; that way it is easy to respond to your body's demand for fluids in varied and interesting ways.

Fruit Beverages

Sweet or tangy, pulpy or clear, fruit-based drinks are a welcome treat at any time. At breakfast plain fruit juices provide the perfect start to your day. Whipped with milk, fruit juices make a healthy pick-me-up or satisfying snack at any time. And once you have sampled the cozy goodness of hot, mulled apple cider or a zippy punch with pineapple juice, you will want to try a greater variety of fruit beverages, hot as well as cold.

Most fruit drinks are rich in vitamins and minerals, so you can also think of them as a simple and delicious way to supplement your nutrition. For example, orange juice and grapefruit juice are rich in vitamin C, and apricot nectar is loaded with vitamin A. These and many other juices are also excellent sources of potassium.

Whenever possible, serve freshly processed fruit juices. They are sweeter and more delicately flavored than frozen or canned ones. This is particularly true of the citrus juices. Refrigerated in a covered pitcher or jar, fresh fruit juices will keep for several days.

Juicing citrus fruits is easy. Start with very ripe, almost overripe, fruit—then simply squeeze. Other fruits can be processed in a juicer (follow the manufacturer's directions).

When a juicer is not available, use one of two alternate methods: Simmer the fruit, tightly covered, in a very small amount of water (or in its own juice) in a heavy stainless steel, glass, or enameled pot. (Avoid aluminum pots since they react with the acid in the fruit to produce off-flavors and colors.) When the fruit is tender, press it through two layers of cheesecloth or through a sieve or food mill. Straining through cheesecloth will give you the clearest juice. Save the pulp for making preserves (see Jams and Jellies, page 779, sauces, or leathers (see Fruit Leather, page 787). Or for a quick, pulpier juice somewhat diluted in flavor, you can simply process peeled and chopped fresh fruit with a small amount of water in a blender. One cup of cubed fruit blended with one-quarter cup of water will yield about three-quarters cup of juice.

Juices from apples, apricots, melons, grapes, peaches, sweet cherries, pears, pineapples, and

734

some berries are sweet enough as they are. Sometimes, a bit of grated rind and a squeeze of juice from an orange, lemon, or lime will give too-sweet juices a welcome touch of tartness and help to preserve a fresh color as well. Juices from sour cherries, cranberries, currants, plums, and rhubarb look for a touch of honey to relieve the puckery effect.

Blends of two or more juices, herb teas, and other liquids often have intriguing flavors. Be careful in planning combinations because some mixtures, such as orange juice added to a red juice, can result in a murky brown or gray color; pineapple juice added to a red juice can turn the blend blue.

If you add ice and/or carbonated mineral water to any of these drinks, be wary of diluting the juice too much. Carbonated mineral water loses its fizz quickly, so pour it in at the last possible moment before serving.

For a fine finishing touch to a colorful fruit drink, add one of these garnishes: iced fruits in various shapes (whole, halves, wedges, chunks, balls, slices, twists), fruit kabobs, fruit stick stirrers, cinnamon stick stirrers (especially for hot drinks), or citrus wheels stuck with whole cloves (especially for hot drinks).

Punch for a Crowd

- Allow two to three half-cup servings of punch for each guest.
- Chill all ingredients and equipment before mixing the punch.
- Use large blocks of ice; they will melt more slowly than small cubes.
- To avoid diluted punch, use frozen blocks of juice instead of water.
- Eliminate garnishes that interfere with ladling the punch.
- Fill cups or glasses only two-thirds full to avoid embarrassing spills.

Vegetable Juices

Tomato juice is still the favorite vegetable juice, but carrot, spinach, cabbage, celery, and cucumber juices are rapidly gaining in popularity. Spike any of these with green pepper, parsley, watercress, sprouts, or garlic to add even more flavor and food value. Or combine two or more vegetable juices, such as carrot and celery, to create tasty blends.

You can juice vegetables with the same ease that you juice fruits, but be sure to have an abundant supply of very ripe, fresh vegetables on hand before you start. It takes about one pound of carrots to get a cup of juice; one pound of spinach yields only half of a small glass of juice. For a drink with body, use a juicer (follow the manufacturer's directions) to pulverize the fibers; then serve the drink unstrained, thick, and rich with pulp. (If you use a blender, you must add liquid as you process the vegetable.) For thinner juices, cook the vegetables and press them through a sieve. Serve hot or cold, and garnish with lemon slices, celery sticks, or carrot swizzles.

Vegetable juices will keep fresh for several days if refrigerated in a covered container. For longer storage, can or freeze them.

Milk Drinks

Milk-based beverages, from frothy, cold, fruit-flavored shakes to hot, vanilla-honey-laced potables, are American favorites. Few can resist their rich, sweet taste. On top of that, milk is wonderfully good for you since it is rich in calcium and in protein. Add eggs, wheat germ, and fruit, and you transform milk into a meal in a glass with an even better balance of nutrients.

Fat gives milk its smooth texture but adds calories as well. Mixing skim milk with an equal portion of whole milk reduces the number of troublesome calories with just a hint of change in body. Using only skim milk cuts calories even more.

Nothing could be simpler than whipping up cold milk and fruit shakes. A blender works best, making a foamy, thoroughly mixed drink in a matter of seconds. When combining milk and an acid fruit puree or juice, gradually pour the fruit into the milk rather than vice versa. Slowly adding the acid source lessens the chance that the milk might curdle. To make a frosted milk shake, beat ice cream together with the milk and fruit. If you crave a float, drop in a scoop of ice cream after the fruit and milk are blended together.

Create a Milk and Fruit Shake

Experiment with the following suggested combinations to make your own milk shake recipe. To prepare: Place the chilled milk, one of the fruits or juices, and the suggested flavoring in a blender or food processor. Process for one to two seconds, until smooth, then serve immediately. Each combination of milk, fruit, and flavoring makes one serving.

Milk	Fruit or Juice	Flavoring
1 cup	¼ cup chopped apples	1 or 2 drops mint extract
1 cup	¼ cup chopped apricots	dash of ground cinnamon
1 cup	¼ cup chopped avocados	½ teaspoon honey and 1 thin slice lemon
1 cup	⅓ cup mashed bananas	1 thin slice orange
1 cup	½ cup blueberries, raspberries, or strawberries	1 thin slice lemon
1 cup	½ cup chopped melon	1 thin slice lime
½ cup	½ cup orange juice	1 or 2 drops almond extract
1 cup	½ cup chopped papayas	1 thin slice orange
1 cup	¼ cup chopped peaches	dash of ground nutmeg
1 cup	½ cup chopped pears	1 or 2 drops mint extract
1 cup	¼ cup pineapple juice	1 teaspoon maple syrup
½ cup	½ cup prune juice	1 thin slice lemon

For hot drinks, warm milk cautiously over low heat or in the top of a double boiler. (Milk scorches very easily.) To prevent a skin from forming on hot milk, stir frequently with a wire whisk. Heat milk only until you see steam rising from the pan. Never boil milk; it spoils the taste.

Right before serving, add a special touch to milk drinks by dusting them with ground cinnamon, nutmeg, or nuts; with grated orange or lemon rind; or with carob shavings. Use fruit kabobs or cinnamon sticks as stirrers in place of spoons.

Carob-Flavored Drinks

Carob, or St. John's bread, has a rich brown color and a delicate sweetness that suggests mild milk chocolate so that many people use it in place of cocoa and chocolate. Yet carob imparts its own unique and delicious flavor to beverages.

Carob has several advantages over cocoa and chocolate. Since carob is naturally sweet, there is no need to use sugar to mask bitterness as with cocoa and chocolate. When added to milk, carob subtly boosts the calcium level of the drink with its own calcium content. Cocoa and chocolate, on the other hand, have no calcium. Another nice thing about carob—unlike cocoa and chocolate it has no caffeine.

You can buy unsweetened carob in chips that look similar to chocolate chips and in powder that is either raw or roasted. Roasting brings out its full, rich flavor. Carob is sold in most natural foods stores and in many supermarkets. Store it in a tightly covered container in a cool, dry place.

Use carob as a syrup when adding it to beverages. This will prevent graininess and speed thorough mixing. It is easy to prepare and can be used in a multitude of other dishes as well, in place of bitter or unsweetened chocolate. (If you wish to convert one of your own recipes that calls for melted semisweet chocolate, use the recipe on page 737, adding ¼ cup honey and, if you wish, 2 tablespoons butter.)

Basic Carob Syrup

    1 cup sifted powdered carob
    1 cup water

In a small saucepan mix carob and water. Bring to a boil over very low heat, stirring constantly to avoid scorching and lumping. Cook for 5 to 8 minutes, or until syrup is completely smooth. Cool.

Store syrup in a covered jar in refrigerator. It will keep for weeks.

Yields about 1½ cups

Cocoa- and Chocolate-Flavored Drinks

Cocoa and chocolate come from roasted cacao beans. There is only a small difference between the two: Chocolate has added cocoa butter (fat) and often contains added sugar as well. Abundant carbohydrates and fats make cocoa and chocolate easy to digest and high in calories. Both foods contain the stimulants theobromine and caffeine, plus oxalic acid which reduces the amount of calcium absorbed by the body.

The cooking principles for cocoa and chocolate are the same. Neither blends easily with liquids; for a lump-free mixture it helps to whirl the ingredients in a blender. Also, it is best to heat them over hot water instead of over direct heat, since both readily scorch.

Herb Teas

Herb teas (called tisanes by the French) make light, calorie-free substitutes for the standard cup of tea. Served clear and sparkling over ice, they lend a refreshing lift on a hot summer's day. In the winter a piping hot cup of herb tea perks up the spirit in a low period and soothes the senses when you come in from the cold. Most herb teas (maté is an exception) have no caffeine.

Natural foods stores and some of the larger supermarkets carry dried herbs for making tea. Of course, your own garden—indoor or outdoor—is the best source for fresh herbs. Make tea from fresh herbs immediately after harvesting, or dry the herbs for later use (see Drying Fresh Herbs, page 48). Store dried herbs in airtight jars in a cool, dry place.

Characteristics of Selected Herb Teas

Herb	Taste and Scent of Brewed Tea
Alfalfa	bland, grassy
Aniseed	licoricelike, strong, spicy, aromatic
Basil	clovelike, aromatic
Bay	fragrant, slightly bitter
Bergamot	citruslike, fragrant
Birch	similar to wintergreen
Borage	similar to cucumber
Burnet	cool, similar to cucumber
Camomile	strong, aromatic, applelike
Caraway	warm, sweet, biting
Catnip	bitter, aromatic, minty
Cinnamon	warm, sweet-pungent, fragrant
Clove	strong, pungent, spicy
Clover	strong
Dandelion	slightly bitter
Elder	honeylike, slightly bitter
Fennel	aniselike
Fenugreek	celerylike, hint of burnt sugar
Ginger	hot, spicy-sweet
Ginseng	pleasant, rootlike
Goldenrod	warm, mild, aniselike
Hawthorn	sweet, astringent
Hops	bitter
Horehound	bittersweet, musky
Hyssop	bitter, minty
Lavender	aromatic, mild
Lemon balm	pungent, lemony, refreshing, fragrant
Lemon verbena	lemony
Licorice	bittersweet
Linden	sweet, fragrant
Mallow	mild, sweet
Marigold	bitter, similar to saffron
Marjoram	warm, sweet, slightly oily, tangy
Meadowsweet	sweet, delicate
Mugwort	strong
Mullein	sweet
Nutmeg	warm, spicy, slightly sharp
Peppermint	pungent, refreshing, minty
Raspberry	aromatic
Rose	sweet, astringent, aromatic

[continued]

Characteristics of Selected Herb Teas—
Continued

Herb	*Taste and Scent of Brewed Tea*
Rosemary	fresh, clean, tangy, hint of ginger and camphor
Sage	slightly bitter, peppery, pungent, distinctive
Sarsaparilla	bitter, licoricelike
Savory	peppery, hint of camphor
Spearmint	fragrant, sharp
Strawberry	cool
Thyme	warm, aromatic
Wintergreen	pleasant, warm

You can prepare herb teas by decoction or by infusion. To decoct an herb: Boil one ounce of the herb's roots, bark, or seeds in three cups of fresh water for 30 minutes, uncovered; then strain. This will give you about two cups of concentrated herb tea. It can be diluted to the preferred strength by adding fresh, boiling water or ice cubes.

To infuse an herb: Bring fresh water to a rapid boil. For every five to six ounces of water (standard teacup size), add one-quarter to one-half teaspoon of the dried leaves or flowers and steep for three to ten minutes. (If the herb is fresh or very mild, use one-half to one tablespoon of leaves or flowers.) Keep the pot or teapot covered to retain heat. Strain out the herb as soon as the tea has reached the desired strength. A well-prepared cup of herb tea is crystal clear.

Herb coolers and frappés are simple to make. For the coolers, infuse herbs in one of three ways. Steep the leaves or flowers for three to ten minutes in hot water, cool to room temperature, and refrigerate. Or steep overnight in a container of cold water in the refrigerator. Or steep in a covered pitcher of cold water placed in warm sunlight for two to four hours, then refrigerate. Mint leaves, orange slices, and pineapple sticks make colorful, refreshing garnishes. To make a frappé: Process one cup of iced herb tea, one tablespoon of honey, and some cracked ice in a blender. Pour into a frosted glass, garnish, and serve while foamy.

Flavor Herb Teas with Fruit

Fruit-flavored herb teas, served hot or cold, are a healthful alternative to coffee and black tea. Try the combinations below to find your favorite.

To prepare: Combine the fruit or juice with the flavoring, and add it to the hot herb tea. Serve immediately or cool and add ice. Each combination makes one serving.

Brewed Herb Tea (1 cup)	*Fruit or Juice*	*Flavoring*
Aniseed	¼ cup mashed bananas	1 drop mint extract
Camomile flower	¼ cup papaya juice	2 drops mint extract
Cardamom seed	¼ cup mashed avocados	¼ teaspoon honey
Fennel seed	1 teaspoon apricot syrup	1 drop almond extract
Linden blossom	2 tablespoons grape juice	1 thin slice lemon
Peppermint leaf	¼ cup pineapple juice	dash of ground nutmeg
Sage leaf	1 tablespoon lime juice	1 teaspoon honey
Spearmint leaf	¼ cup apple juice	dash of ground cinnamon

Tea

The Chinese were the first to brew leaves, making the piping hot cups of clear, slightly astringent beverage we call tea. Gradually its use spread to the Middle East, to Europe, and then to America, courtesy of the English colonists.

The three basic types of tea—black, green, and oolong—come from the same tea plant. For black tea the leaves are allowed to ferment before they are dried. Leaves for green tea are dried immediately after they are picked, before they have a chance to ferment. And leaves for oolong tea are partially fermented, then dried. Black tea leaves make a hearty brew with a rich, full, amber color. Green tea leaves give a pale, greenish yellow beverage of distinctive flavor. Oolong tea leaves produce a drink with a subtle flavor and bouquet and a light, brownish green color.

When buying tea, you will notice that some teas are labeled *pekoe* and *orange pekoe* as well as black, green, or oolong. The terms *pekoe* and *orange pekoe* refer to the size of the tea leaves, not to the variety or the flavor.

Tea can be bought in packages of loose leaves or in packages that contain premeasured tea bags for making individual cups of tea. After opening the package, transfer the loose tea or tea bags to a container with a tight-fitting lid. Stored this way, tea will retain its fresh taste for up to six months.

Tea, like coffee, has no calories and no nutrients if served without milk, lemon, or honey. Like coffee, too, it contains caffeine (sometimes referred to as theine). The amount of caffeine in a cup of tea is usually less than that contained in a similar-size cup of coffee (see Caffeine Content table, below).

Caffeine Content of Selected Beverages

Beverage	Caffeine Content in 1 Cup (milligrams)
Cocoa	6-42
Coffee	
Brewed	90-120
Brewed decaffeinated	2-5
Instant	40-108
Instant decaffeinated	2-8
Substitute (cereal or legume)	0
Herb tea (excluding maté)	0
Tea (black, green, or oolong)	
Bag	68-100
Instant	24-31
Loose-leaf	30-48

Brewing Tea

China, glass, or pottery teapots are the best for making tea since they retain heat while the tea is steeping. A tea cozy over the pot will keep it warm for serving.

To brew hot tea: Use one teaspoon of tea leaves or one tea bag for every five to six ounces (about three-quarters cup) of fresh, rapidly boiling water (soft water is best). It is imperative that the water be fresh since reheated water, or water that has been standing, will make flat tea. Boiling water is necessary to extract the full tea flavor. Avoid hard water—it reacts with the chemicals in tea to form an unattractive, grayish precipitate. Steep the tea for three to five minutes (steeping it longer will only make the tea bitter); then remove the leaves and serve the tea. For optimum flavor never steep the leaves more than once. Serve hot tea accompanied with lemon wedges or garnished with fresh mint leaves.

Iced tea is a favorite beverage among Americans, especially during the summer months. To make sparkling iced tea: Double the quantity of tea and steep as for hot tea; then pour over ice cubes. Or double the quantity of tea and steep in cold water for eight hours. Or use the regular quantity of tea and steep in cold water in the sun for three to four hours. Garnish iced tea with slices of lemon or fresh sprigs of mint.

Coffee and Coffee Substitutes

Throughout the world customary ways of serving coffee differ almost as much as peoples and their cultures differ. The French favor café au lait— half hot coffee and half hot milk, while the Syrians are partial to boiled coffee with cracked cardamom and orange blossom water. Although the Viennese and the Italians both enjoy strong coffee, the Viennese like to top theirs with whipped cream. The Greeks and the Turks take pleasure in sipping a boiled, very strong and sweet, almost syruplike coffee. Here in the United States most people prefer a mild, light brew served plain or with a touch of cream and sugar.

Coffee is a slightly bitter, full-bodied, highly aromatic beverage. When served without sugar, milk, or cream, it has no calories and no nutrients. Coffee is a brew that makes people feel peppy and alert. The stimulation comes from caffeine—a mild, addictive drug that sometimes causes insomnia, nervousness, high blood pressure, and other health problems.

Coffee is also available chemically decaffeinated. A good blend of decaffeinated coffee tastes much like regular coffee.

NOTE: The use of any chemical in processing a food is of concern to health-conscious people because its long-term effects on the body are unpredictable. Regarding coffee, official evaluations of safety vary periodically, so each individual must weigh the advantages of a decaffeinated drink against the possible safety concerns of the decaffeinating process.

Chicory, as a ground roasted tap root, is a popular addition to coffee in the southern United States. Coffee with chicory added has less caffeine, looks darker, tastes less bitter, and costs less than coffee made entirely from coffee beans. To form your own blend, replace up to one-half of the required amount of ground coffee with chicory. You can also brew chicory by itself; the drink has a rich, caramel, semisweet taste.

Coffeelike beverages (imitation coffees) made from ground roasted cereals or legumes are excellent-tasting substitutes for coffee, and they are free of caffeine. These coffees can be brewed and served in the same manner as real coffee. (Recipes for imitation coffees are given at the end of this chapter.)

Brewing Coffee and Coffee Substitutes

There is no secret to brewing good coffee, whether real or imitation. Start with the proper grind—regular (coarse), drip (medium), or fine—of your favorite blend. The grind you select should be the one best suited to the method of brewing. Use regular in a percolator, drip in a drip pot, and fine in a vacuum pot. Be certain you use the freshest coffee or coffee substitute possible. The staler the product is, the less its aroma and flavor.

Always use a scrupulously clean pot for brewing coffee. The oils of true coffee tend to become rancid and will surely taint the flavor of the freshly brewed beverage. To remove the tenacious oils from previous brewings, use baking soda dissolved in warm water or a cleaner especially formulated for cleaning coffee makers. You may find it necessary to use a small brush to scrub small openings and seams.

Porcelain, stoneware, glass, enameled, or stainless steel coffee makers are best for brewing since they do not affect the taste of the beverage. Aluminum, on the other hand, imparts a distinctive metallic flavor. Also, the brew will taste better if you make a full pot rather than half a pot.

Since hard or chemically softened water affects the taste of coffee and coffee substitutes, too, try to locate a source of pure soft water for brewing that ideal cup. For each three-quarters cup of fresh water, use two level tablespoons of ground roasted coffee beans or coffee substitute.

Once the water and grounds start brewing, time the process carefully and do not let the liquid boil. Prolonged brewing and high heat bring out tannic acid, which makes a bitter-tasting and murky-looking coffee.

When the brew is done, remove the grounds and throw them away. Serve the drink immediately or hold it at serving temperature for no longer than one hour. Both real and imitation coffee taste better if kept warm instead of being reheated.

Methods of Brewing

There are many ways of brewing coffee and coffee substitutes.

Drip: Beverages made in this way have the best flavor and are the least bitter since the grounds are in the hot water for only a short period of time. Place a clean filter in the drip pot and add the necessary amount of fresh grounds. Pour a measured amount of boiling water over the grounds. When dripping stops, the beverage is ready to serve.

Perked: Because the very hot water circulates through the grounds several times, perked beverages are likely to be somewhat bitter. Pour a measured amount of cold water in the percolator bottom (be sure the water level is below the basket) and put the grounds in the percolator basket. Place the percolator over high heat. The moment the water starts to perk, reduce the heat and allow the beverage to perk slowly for six to eight minutes. When it is done, remove the basket and serve.

Vacuum-method: The product of this method is slightly bitter since the grounds are in contact with the hot water for several minutes. Fill the lower bowl with the correct amount of water and put the unit over medium heat. Place a wet filter in the upper bowl and add the grounds. Insert the upper bowl into the lower one. When the water has risen into the upper bowl, stir the water and the grounds thoroughly. Remove the pot from the heat after one to three minutes.

Steeped: This is sometimes called boiled coffee. It is best reserved for camping trips or for other times when equipment is limited since steeping makes the most bitter beverage of all the methods. Put the necessary quantity of water in a saucepan, bring it to a boil, and stir in the grounds. Cover the pan and keep it over the lowest possible heat for five to ten minutes. Settle the grounds before serving by adding eggshells or beaten egg whites, or pour the beverage through a sieve.

Espresso: Use the espresso grind and a special espresso pot. To make the coffee, follow the directions that come with the pot.

Iced: Make double-strength brew (use twice as many grounds or half as much water) and pour the hot brew over a glassful of ice. Or make regular-strength brew and pour it over ice cubes which are also made of regular-strength brew.

Storing Coffee

- Keep a sealed can of ground coffee in a cool place for up to one year.
- Tightly cover an opened container of ground coffee and store it in the refrigerator. For optimum freshness the coffee should be used within one week.
- Keep whole coffee beans in the refrigerator for a maximum of three weeks, or store them in the freezer for longer periods. For the best flavor and aroma, grind small batches as you are ready to use them.
- Store brewed coffee in a covered container in the refrigerator for no more than one day. Of course, when reheated, it will lack the taste and aroma of freshly brewed coffee.

Fruit Beverages

Carob-Orange Cooler

1 cup orange juice
1 tablespoon sifted powdered carob
dash of vanilla extract

Combine ingredients in a blender and process until smooth. Pour over crushed ice in a tall glass and serve immediately.

1 serving

Hot Cranberry Grog

1 cup fresh cranberries
½ cup water
1 tablespoon honey
¾ cup pineapple juice
¼ teaspoon ground allspice
¼ teaspoon whole cloves
dash of ground nutmeg
1 stick of cinnamon, ½ inch long

In a medium-size saucepan combine all ingredients. Place over medium heat and bring to a boil. Reduce heat, cover, and simmer for 15 minutes. Pour mixture through a strainer and serve immediately.

2 servings

Cranberry-Syrup Shake

1 cup milk
¼ cup plus 2 tablespoons Cranberry Syrup (see below)

Combine milk and syrup in a blender and process until smooth.

1 serving

Cranberry Syrup

2 cups fresh cranberries
2 cups water
2 tablespoons honey

In a medium-size saucepan combine berries and water and boil together over low heat for 5 minutes, or until berries have popped open.

Pour through a strainer and press with the back of a spoon to extract all juice; discard pulp. (This will yield about 2 cups juice.) Return juice to saucepan, add honey, and simmer for 10 minutes. Do not overcook or syrup will jell. Store in refrigerator.

Yields 1½ cups

Fruit-Nut Whiz

3 cups orange or apple juice
12 to 16 fresh strawberries
½ cup chopped cashews, almonds, or pecans
2 cups cubed melon

Place all ingredients in a blender and process until smooth. Serve immediately.

6 servings

Ginger-Peach Froth

4 large peaches
4 cups milk
½ teaspoon ground ginger
2 tablespoons honey

Peel and pit peaches (reserve skin for garnish). Place peaches in a blender. Add milk, ginger, and

honey and blend to a froth. Serve at once in stemmed goblets. Garnish with a thin curl of reserved peach skin.

6 servings

Hot Mulled Pineapple Juice

6 cups pineapple juice
1 stick of cinnamon, 2 inches long
dash of ground cloves

Combine pineapple juice, cinnamon, and cloves in a medium-size saucepan and bring to a boil over medium heat. Reduce heat, cover, and simmer for 20 minutes to blend flavors. Remove from heat and discard cinnamon stick. Serve warm in individual mugs.

6 to 8 servings

Limeade

2 teaspoons honey
2½ cups water
½ cup lime juice

In a medium-size saucepan boil honey and ½ cup water for 5 minutes. Add lime juice and remaining 2 cups water and stir. Chill before serving.

2 to 4 servings

Mint Jewel

1 cup mint sprigs
½ cup lemon juice
grated rind of 1 lemon
2 cups water
¾ cup honey
½ cup orange juice
½ cup pineapple juice

In a medium-size bowl crush mint (reserve a few leaves for garnish). Add lemon juice and rind and marinate for 30 minutes.

In a medium-size saucepan simmer water and honey together for about 7 minutes to make a syrup.

Pour syrup over mint mixture. Then add orange juice and pineapple juice. Strain, cool, and then chill.

When ready to serve, pour into tall stemmed glasses and garnish with reserved mint leaves.

6 servings

Natural Fruit Soda

2 tablespoons frozen orange, grapefruit, or grape juice concentrate, or to taste
1 cup carbonated mineral water, chilled

In a small bowl or pitcher add juice concentrate to mineral water and stir until dissolved. Pour over crushed ice in a tall glass and serve immediately.

1 serving

Orangeade

¼ cup honey
4 cups water
5 oranges
1 lemon

In a medium-size bowl dissolve honey in water. Squeeze juice from 4 oranges and lemon, then add to honey and water. Slice remaining orange into rounds. Pour juice mixture over cracked ice or ice cubes. Garnish with orange slices.

6 servings

Orange-Cashew Cooler

½ cup crushed cashews
4 cups water
¼ cup honey
4 cups orange juice

Place all ingredients in a blender and process until combined. Strain and chill before serving.

8 servings

Party Lemonade

8 cups water
¾ cup honey
1 cup lemon juice
1 orange, sliced
1 cup cubed fresh pineapple

Heat water in a medium-size saucepan and stir in honey. Add remaining ingredients, stir, and chill. Pour over cracked ice or ice cubes and serve.

8 servings

Raspberry Shrub

1 cup fresh or frozen raspberries*
½ cup ice water
1 slice lemon, with rind, ¼ inch thick
1 teaspoon honey
mint sprig

In a blender combine raspberries, water, lemon, and honey and process until smooth. Then chill.

When ready to serve, pour into a sherbet or parfait glass and garnish with mint sprig.

1 serving

*If frozen berries are used, it is not necessary to thaw them since a shrub should be served very cold.

Watermelon Whiz

4 cups diced watermelon
1 cup apricot juice
¼ cup lime juice
2 to 3 tablespoons honey (optional)
lime slices

In a blender liquefy watermelon. Add juices and honey (if used). Whiz briefly and pour into tall glasses. Garnish with lime slices.

6 servings

Punches

Cinnamon-Spice Bouquet for Punches and Teas

This bouquet can be used to flavor 2½ to 3 quarts of punch or tea.

> 1 stick of cinnamon, 1 inch long
> 8 to 10 whole cloves
> ½ whole nutmeg, cracked

Combine spices in a stainless steel tea ball, or place them in a piece of cheesecloth or nylon net, tied closed.

Add to punch before chilling or to hot water when steeping tea. Remove spices when desired flavor has been obtained.

Ginger-Spice Bouquet for Punches and Teas

You can enhance the flavor of 2½ to 3 quarts of punch or tea by adding this bouquet.

> 1 slice peeled ginger root, ½ inch long
> 1 cluster of star anise
> 1 teaspoon dried lemon or orange rind

Crush ginger root with the back of a spoon. Then place ginger root, anise, and citrus rind in a stainless steel tea ball, or combine them in a piece of nylon net or cheesecloth and use string to tie it closed.

Add to punch before chilling or to hot water when steeping tea. When desired flavor has been extracted, remove spices and discard.

Festive Tropical Punch

The iced fruit mold, made a day ahead, highlights this special punch.

> 1 cup chopped fresh pineapple
> 1 cup pineapple juice
> 1 cup fresh raspberries, blueberries, or grapes
> 5 cups water
> 1 cup lemon juice
> ½ cup honey
> ½ teaspoon almond extract
> 2 cups watermelon juice or puree
> 2 cups papaya juice

> 1 bottle (28 ounces) chilled carbonated mineral water
> ½ cup unsweetened shredded coconut
> ¼ cup ground blanched almonds
>   mint sprigs or fresh flowers

The day before the punch is to be served, select an attractively shaped 1-quart mold or bowl. Combine pineapple, pineapple juice, berries or grapes, and 1 cup water. Pour into mold and place in freezer.

Next day, combine lemon juice, honey, and remaining 4 cups water in a large saucepan. Bring to a boil and stir until honey is dissolved. Transfer to a large bowl and cool.

Stir in almond extract, watermelon juice or puree, and papaya juice. Mix well and chill.

When ready to serve, pour punch and mineral water into a punch bowl. Stir to mix. Remove iced fruit mold from freezer and unmold into center of punch bowl. Sprinkle coconut and almonds over floating mold. Garnish with mint sprigs or flowers.

Yields about 4 quarts

Grape and Citrus Punch

> 4 cups grape juice
> 4 cups Party Lemonade (page 743) or Limeade (page 742)
> 4 cups orange juice

Mix all ingredients thoroughly. Serve over ice in a punch bowl.

Yields 3 quarts

Variations:
■ Add 2 cups carbonated mineral water just before serving.
■ Place a small scoop of vanilla ice cream in each glass of punch.

Raspberry-Lemon Punch

> 4 cups fresh raspberries
> 2 cups warm water
> ½ cup honey
> ½ cup lemon juice
> 8 cups carbonated mineral water
>   lemon slices

Place raspberries in a medium-size saucepan with 1 cup warm water, bring to a boil, and simmer for 10 minutes. Then puree mixture in a blender and press through a sieve to remove seeds.

Pour remaining warm water into a large bowl and stir in honey until dissolved. Add lemon juice, mineral water, strained berry mixture, and ice to chill. Serve in individual glasses with ice and a generous slice of lemon.

Yields about 3 quarts

Regal Purple Punch

    4 cups grapefruit juice
    4 cups grape juice
    1 bottle (28 ounces) carbonated mineral water
       lemon slices

In a large pitcher combine grapefruit juice and grape juice. Chill.

Just before serving, pour juice mixture over ice in a punch bowl, add mineral water, and stir well. Garnish with lemon slices.

Yields about 3 quarts

Rhubarb Juice Punch

    Rhubarb Juice (see below)
    1/3 cup honey
    ½ cup orange juice
    1/3 cup lemon juice
    1 bottle (28 ounces) carbonated mineral water

Combine rhubarb juice and honey in a large saucepan. Bring to a boil and continue to gently boil for 5 minutes. Cool. Then add orange juice and lemon juice and chill thoroughly.

Just before serving, pour punch over ice in a punch bowl and stir in mineral water.

Yields about 3 quarts

Rhubarb Juice

    5 cups chopped rhubarb
    5 cups water
    2/3 cup honey

In a large saucepan combine rhubarb, water, and honey. Cook over medium heat for about 12 minutes, or until fruit is soft. Strain mixture through cheesecloth. Discard pulp and store juice in a tightly covered jar in refrigerator.

Yields 2 quarts

Rosemary Bridal Punch

    2 cups honey
    16 cups water
    2 cups lemon juice
    3 tablespoons fresh rosemary
    8 cups fresh strawberries
    2 cups lime juice
    1 bottle (28 ounces) carbonated mineral water

In a medium-size saucepan combine honey with 4 cups water, ¼ cup lemon juice, and rosemary. Bring to a boil, then remove from heat and steep for 5 minutes. Strain out rosemary and transfer liquid to a large bowl. Cool.

Meanwhile, slice strawberries, force them through a fine sieve, and add to cooled liquid. Then stir in remaining water, lime juice, and remaining lemon juice. Pour over ice in a punch bowl, add mineral water, and serve.

Yields 9 quarts

Sparkling Grape Punch

    1 orange
       juice of 1 lemon
    1 lemon, thinly sliced
    2 bottles (25 ounces each) sparkling red grape
       juice
    ¼ cup honey
    1 bottle (28 ounces) carbonated mineral water

Cut rind of orange in a spiral with a vegetable peeler. Squeeze juice out of orange.

In a large bowl or pitcher combine orange and lemon juices, orange rind spiral, and lemon slices. Add grape juice and honey. Stir until honey is completely dissolved and then chill for 4 to 6 hours.

Just before serving, add mineral water and pour over ice in a large punch bowl.

Yields about 2½ quarts

Spicy Holiday Punch

¼ cup honey
1 cup water
3 sticks of cinnamon, each 2 inches long
1 teaspoon whole cloves
2 cups Cranberry Syrup (page 742)
1½ cups pineapple juice
½ cup lemon juice
1 bottle (28 ounces) carbonated mineral water
   pineapple slices and lemon slices pierced with whole cloves (optional)

In a medium-size saucepan combine honey with water, cinnamon, and cloves. Bring to a boil and continue to boil gently for 5 minutes. Remove cinnamon and cloves. Transfer liquid to a large bowl and chill. Then add cranberry syrup, pineapple juice, and lemon juice.

Just before serving, pour punch over ice in a punch bowl and add mineral water. If desired, garnish with pineapple and lemon slices.

Yields about 2 quarts

Tart Fruit Juice Punch

4 cups apricot juice
4 cups cranberry juice
4 cups grapefruit juice
4 cups pineapple juice
   mint sprigs and orange slices

Mix juices together and chill. Pour mixture over ice in a punch bowl, and garnish with mint sprigs and orange slices.

Yields 4 quarts

Vegetable Beverages

Cucumber Frappé

3 large cucumbers
3 cups yogurt
¼ cup chopped fresh parsley
¼ cup chopped fresh mint
9 ice cubes

Cut 6 slices from 1 cucumber and reserve for garnish. Peel, seed, and chop remaining cucumbers.

Place yogurt, parsley, and mint in a blender and process until smooth. Add cucumbers, a small amount at a time, and process until well blended. Add ice cubes and blend until crushed. Serve garnished with reserved cucumber slices.

6 servings

Dill-Cucumber Drink

1 cup sliced peeled cucumbers
1 stalk celery, coarsely chopped
½ teaspoon chopped fresh dill
½ teaspoon soy sauce
1 cup buttermilk

Combine all ingredients in a blender and process until smooth. Chill.

1 serving

Variation:
   Dill-Cabbage Drink: Substitute 1 cup chopped cabbage for the cucumbers.

Emerald Isle

$1/3$ cup chopped fresh parsley
  6 cups pineapple juice
10 leaves lettuce, chopped
$1/3$ cup chopped celery leaves
$1/3$ cup watercress

Process all ingredients in a blender until liquefied. Chill before serving.

6 servings

Onion-Apple Bracer

½ cup chopped peeled apples
¼ cup chopped sweet onions
1 stalk celery, coarsely chopped
1 thin slice lime
1 cup water

Combine ingredients in a blender and process until smooth.

2 servings

Tomato-Herb Cocktail

   3 cups tomato juice
   2 slices lemon
   4 leaves cabbage, chopped
   1 sprig parsley
     pinch of dried basil
     pinch of dried marjoram

Place all ingredients in a blender and process until smooth.

6 servings

Tomato Kick

   3 cups tomato juice
   1 tablespoon green pepper juice
   1 sprig parsley
   1 scallion
   1 stalk celery, with leaves
   1 tablespoon lemon juice
   ½ teaspoon grated horseradish, or to taste

Process all ingredients except horseradish in a blender until liquefied. Before serving, season to taste with horseradish.

4 servings

Tomato-Lime Cooler

   ¼ cup Poultry Stock (page 110)
   ¾ cup tomato juice
   ⅛ teaspoon honey
   2 teaspoons lime juice
   ⅛ teaspoon soy sauce
     dash each of celery powder, dried basil, and
      cayenne pepper
     celery stalk, with leaves

In a small pitcher combine stock, tomato juice, honey, lime juice, soy sauce, and seasonings. Mix well and then chill.

When ready to serve, strain and pour over ice cubes in a tall glass. Garnish with celery stalk.

1 serving

Tomato Tempter

   1 cup diced tomatoes
   2 cups cold milk
   1 tablespoon lemon juice
   1 teaspoon chopped onions or dash of onion
     juice
     dash of hot pepper sauce

Process ingredients in a blender until smooth. Pour into glasses and serve immediately.

4 servings

Zucchini-Vegetable Refresher

   2 tablespoons olive oil
   1 cup thinly sliced onions or leeks (white and
     pale green parts only)
   3 cups diced zucchini
1 to 2 medium-size potatoes, diced
   1½ cups thinly sliced carrots
   1½ teaspoons chopped fresh tarragon
   2 tablespoons chopped fresh dill
   2 cups Poultry Stock (page 110)
     cold milk, for thinning

Heat oil in a large saucepan. Add onions or leeks and stir. Add remaining vegetables, one at a time, stirring occasionally. Add tarragon, 1 tablespoon dill, and stock and bring to a boil. Reduce heat, cover, and simmer until vegetables are tender, stirring occasionally. Remove from heat and cool. Place vegetables and liquid in a blender and process until smooth. Chill thoroughly.

Before serving, add just enough milk to thin beverage, pour into mugs, and garnish with remaining dill.

6 servings

Milk Drinks

Banana Eggnog

1 egg
1 tablespoon maple syrup
1 banana, diced
1 cup milk

Combine egg, maple syrup, and banana in a blender and process until smooth. Add milk and process for another few seconds or until well mixed. Chill.

2 servings

Banana Tang

1 large banana
1 cup cold milk
¼ cup yogurt
   dash of ground nutmeg, ground cinnamon, or finely chopped walnuts

In a blender process banana, milk, and yogurt until smooth and foamy. Pour into chilled glasses, sprinkle with nutmeg, cinnamon, or walnuts, and serve immediately.

1 to 2 servings

Variations:
Peach Tang: Substitute 2 large peaches, peeled and chopped, for banana.
Strawberry Tang: Substitute ⅔ cup chopped fresh strawberries for banana.

Carob-Banana Milk

3 cups milk
1 teaspoon honey
1 tablespoon Basic Carob Syrup (page 737)
½ medium-size banana

Process ingredients in a blender until smooth and serve.

2 to 4 servings

Carob Demitasse

2 tablespoons water
2 tablespoons sifted powdered carob
2 tablespoons honey
1 cup skim milk
   whipped cream
   ground cinnamon

In a small saucepan heat water, carob, and honey together until carob is dissolved, stirring to make a smooth mixture. Add milk and bring to a boil. Serve immediately in demitasse cups, garnished with whipped cream and cinnamon.

2 to 4 servings

Carob-Mint Drink

1 cup milk
2 teaspoons sifted powdered carob
¼ teaspoon mint extract

Combine all ingredients in a blender and process until smooth.

1 serving

Carob Eggnog

2 tablespoons honey
2 eggs, separated
5 tablespoons sifted powdered carob
4 cups milk, scalded

Topping
1 teaspoon honey
½ cup heavy cream, whipped
   sifted powdered carob

In top of a double boiler, combine honey and egg yolks and beat. Add carob, then slowly stir in milk. Cook over hot but not boiling water, stirring constantly, until mixture coats a spoon. Cool.

In a small bowl beat egg whites until soft peaks form. Fold into carob mixture until thoroughly blended. Chill for 4 hours.

To make the topping: Fold honey into whipped cream. Top each serving of chilled eggnog with a dollop of whipped cream and sprinkle with carob.

6 servings

Carob-Raisin Shake

1 cup skim milk
3 tablespoons golden raisins*
2 teaspoons sifted powdered carob

Combine 1/3 cup of milk, raisins, and carob in a blender. Process until raisins are completely pureed. Add remaining milk and process until mixture is smooth. Serve immediately.

1 serving

*Dark raisins may be used, but the color of the drink will be less attractive.

Coconut-Wheat Germ Daybreaker

¾ cup soymilk
¼ cup unsweetened grated coconut
1 egg
½ cup orange or pineapple juice
2 teaspoons wheat germ

Combine all ingredients in a blender and process until smooth. Serve immediately.

1 serving

Date Shake

1 cup yogurt
1 cup milk
4 ice cubes
12 pitted dates, or to taste
4 almonds, ground

Process ingredients thoroughly in a blender. Chill and serve.

2 servings

Honey Eggnog

3 cups milk
4 eggs
3 tablespoons honey
freshly ground nutmeg

Process milk, eggs, and honey in a blender until smooth. Garnish with nutmeg.

4 to 6 servings

Hot Carob-Granola Drink

2/3 cup very hot water
¼ cup nonfat dry milk
½ cup Granola (page 307)
2 teaspoons sifted powdered carob
⅛ teaspoon vanilla extract
whipped cream (optional)

Combine all ingredients, except whipped cream, in a blender and process until smooth. If desired, top with a dollop of whipped cream and garnish with a little extra granola. Serve immediately.

1 serving

Kefir, Citrus, and Banana Froth

The slightly acidic edge kefir has makes it an excellent companion for the citrus in this recipe, and the banana smoothes it all.

2 cups kefir (page 448)
juice of 1 lime (about 1 tablespoon)
juice of 2 oranges (about 1 cup)
grated rind of 1 orange
1 banana
6 ice cubes
2 tablespoons wheat germ
2 teaspoons vanilla extract
3 to 4 tablespoons honey

Combine all ingredients in a blender and process until ice cubes have broken up and drink is thick and frothy.

2 to 4 servings

Low-Cal Milk Shake

1 cup water
¼ cup nonfat dry milk
2 teaspoons maple syrup
¼ cup pineapple, strawberries, peaches,
bananas, or apricots

Combine all ingredients in a blender and process until frothy and smooth.

1 serving

Milk and Honey

3 tablespoons honey
4 cups warm milk
sifted powdered carob

In a medium-size bowl mix honey and milk together until honey is dissolved. Pour into mugs and garnish with carob.

4 servings

Peach-Soymilk Shake

2 medium-size peaches, peeled and pitted
1 teaspoon vanilla extract
2 tablespoons honey
1½ cups soymilk

Place all ingredients in a blender and process until well mixed. Serve chilled.

1 to 2 servings

Peanut Butter-Carob Shake

⅔ cup water
2 tablespoons nonfat dry milk
1 tablespoon sifted powdered carob
1 tablespoon peanut butter
½ teaspoon maple syrup or honey (optional)

Combine all ingredients in a blender and process until peanut butter is thoroughly blended.

1 serving

Piima Fruit Shake

The piima makes this a thick and tangy treat, highlighting the fruit.

1 egg
1 cup chopped orange segments, chopped fresh
pineapple, or chopped bananas
1 teaspoon honey (optional)
½ cup piima (page 448)

In a blender combine egg, fruit, and honey (if used). Process until smooth. Then fold in piima, pour into a tall glass, and serve immediately.

1 serving

Sunflower Breakfast Shake

1 slice ripe fresh pineapple, 2 inches thick
1 cup soymilk
¼ cup sunflower seeds
1 tablespoon golden raisins

Combine ingredients in a blender and process until smooth. Chill before serving.

1 serving

Herb Teas

Camomile-Peppermint Tea

1 teaspoon dried camomile blossoms
1 teaspoon dried peppermint
2 cups boiling water
ground cinnamon
orange slices

Combine camomile and peppermint, add boiling water, and steep for 5 minutes. Top each serving with a dash of cinnamon and an orange slice.

2 to 3 servings

Ginger Tea Drink

1 tablespoon molasses
⅛ teaspoon ground ginger
2 teaspoons lemon juice
2 cups water

In a small saucepan combine molasses, ginger, lemon juice, and water. Bring to a boil, then remove from heat, cover, and steep for 5 minutes. Serve immediately, or chill and serve over ice.

2 to 3 servings

Spearmint-Ginseng Tea

1 teaspoon crushed dried spearmint
¼ teaspoon powdered ginseng root
1 cup boiling water
1 cup orange juice
    lemon slices pierced with whole cloves

Combine spearmint and ginseng, add boiling water, and steep for 5 minutes. Add orange juice and mix well. Top each serving with a lemon slice.

2 to 3 servings

Spiced Mint Tea

¼ cup water
2 tablespoons honey
2 tablespoons chopped fresh mint
⅛ teaspoon ground allspice
¼ cup lemon juice
½ cup orange juice
2 cups boiling water

In a small saucepan boil water and honey together for 5 minutes. Add mint and allspice and steep for 10 minutes. Strain. Then add lemon juice, orange juice, and boiling water. Serve hot or chilled.

3 to 4 servings

Coffee Substitutes

Roasted Bulgur Beverage

¼ cup bulgur
2 cups water

In a coffee mill coarsely grind bulgur.
Place ground bulgur on a baking sheet and roast in a 250°F oven for about 25 minutes, or until deep golden brown. Stir occasionally to brown evenly.
Brew with water, using the coffee-making method of your choice. Serve immediately.

2 servings

Roasted Split Pea Beverage

¼ cup dried split peas
2 cups water

In a coffee mill coarsely grind split peas.
Place ground split peas on a baking sheet and roast in a 250°F oven for about 15 minutes, or until deep brown. Stir occasionally to brown evenly.
Brew with water, using the coffee-making method of your choice. Serve immediately.

2 servings

Toasted Sesame Seed Beverage

¼ cup sesame seeds
2 cups water

In a small dry skillet toast sesame seeds over medium heat for about 20 minutes, or until dark golden brown.
Grind seeds very briefly in a coffee mill and then brew with water, using the coffee-making method of your choice. Serve immediately.

2 servings

Preservation

Preserving your own food is a marvelous way to capture the bounty of summer for savoring throughout the cold and barren winter months. Whether you freeze, can, dry, pickle, or make jams and jellies, foods put up at home save money, taste great, and retain much of the nutrition found in fresh foods. The time it takes to preserve foods at home is time well spent.

Freezing

Freezing is a simple, quick way of preserving most of the goodness—nutrients, taste, texture, color—of fresh foods by slowing the growth of damaging bacteria, molds, and yeasts. And the investment in equipment, other than buying and running the freezer, is minimal.

For top-quality frozen foods, consider the following guidelines for maintaining your freezer and its food supply:

- Use a thermometer to check periodic temperature fluctuations. The freezer should maintain 0°F or less since changes cause deterioration of food quality.
- Freeze foods rapidly because quick freezing helps preserve the texture of foods by keeping ice crystals small. To aid rapid freezing, set the temperature to -10°F or less the night before freezing large quantities of food. Prepare only what can be frozen in 24 hours. As a rule, the maximum amount is two to three pounds for each cubic foot of freezer space. Place containers near the cold walls of the freezer and leave space between them to allow cold air to circulate.
- Leave an appropriate amount of headspace in the containers to allow for expansion, otherwise containers or seals break during freezing. Too much space, on the other hand, allows air, which dries the food, to enter the containers.
- Plan to use food before its quality is diminished by being too long in the freezer. The timetables in this and other sections provide guidelines to optimum storage times. Maintaining a current list of foods in the freezer and labeling each package with the freezing date, the type of food, and the quantity will aid in keeping up a steady turnover.

Freezer Malfunctions and Power Failures

If your freezer stops working, slow the thawing of frozen foods with one or more of these measures:

- Do not open the freezer. Even in hot weather, food will stay frozen for about two days in a freezer that is full.
- Use dry ice to keep food frozen for longer than two days. If the freezer is half full, the ice will keep the food frozen for an additional two days; if nearly full, it will keep the food frozen for an extra three to four days. Allow approximately 2½ pounds for each cubic foot of freezer space. Put the ice on cardboard over the food; keep the room well ventilated; and never touch dry ice with your bare hands.
- Transfer food to a commercial locker if dry ice is unavailable.

752

Freezer Materials

Many materials, both rigid and flexible, are suitable for freezer containers. Select a size that holds the amount you would use for one meal.

Made from metal, plastic, glass, or heavily waxed cardboard, rigid containers work best for liquid and semiliquid foods. Choose containers with straight sides instead of those with necks, since foods can slide easily through wide openings while still partially frozen. Also, square containers stack better and use space more efficiently than round ones. Though reusable rigid containers initially cost more than flexible disposable ones, the rigid types are often cheaper in the long run. For dry foods use flexible containers of heavy foil, cellophane, heavy plastic, or laminated paper, or use a wrap made of one of these materials.

Either freezer tape or masking tape works well to seal casserole dishes and packages wrapped in foil, cellophane, heavy plastic, or laminated paper. Wire twisters covered with paper are useful for closing heavy plastic bags. Carefully press out air before sealing flexible packages, and be certain the seal is secure. Exposure to air during freezing will cause freezer burn (dry, tasteless, tough spots).

Gummed labels and colored tapes make good labels. Mark them with crayons, ball-point, or felt-tipped pens.

Defrosting the Freezer

To keep your freezer working most efficiently, defrost it when the ice buildup on the sides reaches one-half-inch thickness. Ice thicker than that makes the freezer work too hard to maintain 0°F or less.

To defrost: Turn off the freezer and quickly wrap the food in several layers of paper to prevent thawing. Once the ice has melted, clean the freezer with a solution of one tablespoon baking soda to one quart lukewarm water. Allow the freezer to dry before starting it; then run it for 30 minutes before returning the food. As you put the packages of food in the freezer, wipe them with a dry cloth.

Drugstore Wrap

- Cut wrap (foil, cellophane, heavy plastic, laminated paper) large enough to go around the food 1½ times. Place food in the center of the wrap.
- Bring together the long edges of the paper over the food and fold over one inch. Crease the fold, and fold again. Continue folding until the wrap is close to the food. Press the wrap to force out the air.
- Fold the ends to form points. Then fold the ends under and toward each other. Pull tight and seal all edges with tape.

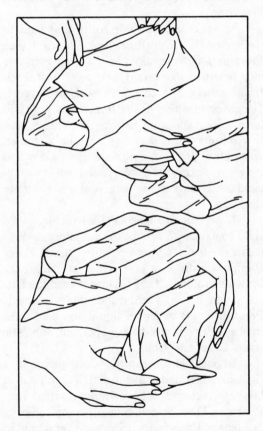

Freezing Fruits

Most fruits—bananas are an exception—freeze fairly successfully. (Once frozen, bananas are useful only for pureeing in drinks or for baked goods.) Select only choice, blemish-free, ripe fruits for freezing; then wash, dry, peel, and cut as you would for serving fresh.

You can freeze most fruits in any of three different packs: dry, unsweetened, or with syrup. Choose the type of pack that best suits the way you intend to use the fruit. Dry packs and unsweetened packs work well for fruits that are destined for the oven or stove top. Both these packs have a shorter storage time than the syrup pack. A light syrup benefits fruits to be served uncooked by allowing them to retain good shape and texture. Fruits in syrup also store nicely for a long time.

To pack dry: Sprinkle fruits that tend to darken with an antibrowning solution (see Preventing Discoloration, below), but skip this step for fruits that retain their color well. Pack fruits loosely in a container, seal, and freeze. Generally speaking, fruits frozen this way will form a solid block on freezing. To ensure that frozen fruits will shake freely from the container, spread fruit pieces in a single layer on a tray and freeze. When they are frozen, pack them in a semi-rigid container or freezer bag, seal, and return to the freezer.

To pack unsweetened: Place fruit pieces in a rigid container and shake the container to pack down the fruits without crushing them. Cover the fruits with juice or water containing anti-browning solution if needed (see Preventing Discoloration, below), leaving adequate headspace. Press the fruits under the liquid and hold them in place with crumpled wax paper, foil, or plastic wrap. Cover and seal.

To pack with syrup: Put fruit pieces in a rigid container and shake to settle; then pour in honey syrup and antibrowning solution (see Preventing Discoloration, below), leaving sufficient headspace. Press fruits under syrup and hold in place with crumpled wax paper, foil, or plastic wrap. Cover and seal.

Preventing Discoloration

Several kinds of fruit—apples, apricots, cherries, peaches, plums—become dark and brown with exposure to air and during storage and thawing. Slow browning by dipping pieces cut for dry

pack in a solution of one-quarter cup lemon juice or one to two tablespoons rose hip concentrate in one gallon water. (Alternatively, one-half teaspoon ascorbic acid powder, crystals, or crushed tablets to make 1,500 milligrams to four cups liquid can be used.) For syrup pack add a small amount of acid to the syrup.

Honey Syrup for Freezing Fresh Fruits

For a thin syrup: Dissolve one cup honey in three cups boiling water. For a medium syrup: Dissolve two cups honey in two cups boiling water. Chill before adding to fruits.

Freezing Vegetables

Most vegetables (except cabbage, celery, cucumbers, eggplant, potatoes, radishes, salad greens, scallions, and whole tomatoes, which lose characteristic texture during storage) freeze well, retaining good color, fresh flavor, and sufficient body. Freeze only fresh, tender vegetables of peak quality.

Wash, peel, and cut vegetables the same as you do when serving them fresh. Sort according to size; then blanch most vegetables (see below); cool quickly; drain; and pack. (See Freezing Vegetables table, page 759, for instructions on preparation and packing of vegetables for freezing.) Chill first batches in the refrigerator while processing others; freeze when several batches are ready. (This is best done within one hour of blanching.)

Blanching

Blanching destroys the enzymes that mature, or age, vegetables even during freezing; thus it helps to keep the vegetables in prime condition. Blanching can be done either in boiling water or with steam.

To blanch in boiling water: Fill an eight- to ten-quart pot with at least one gallon of water to blanch a pound of vegetables. Bring the water to a rapid boil; then lower into the water a wire basket, strainer, or piece of cheesecloth containing one pound or less of vegetables. (The water should return to boiling within a minute. If it takes longer, use a smaller amount of vegetables in the next batch.) Cover the pot and start timing immediately (see Freezing Vegetables table, page 759); do not overcook. For even heat penetration, shake the basket occasionally. As soon as the time is up, stop the cooking promptly. Remove the vegetables and put them in water chilled with one pound of ice, or hold under cold running water. Chill the vegetables until the pieces are cool to the center. Drain the vegetables and pat dry.

To steam blanch: Fill a large pot with one to two inches of water; put a rack over the water; then bring the water to a full boil. Place vegetables in a basket in a single layer and lower the basket onto the rack. Cover the pot with a tight-fitting lid to hold in the steam, and immediately start timing. Steam blanching takes one-half to one minute longer than blanching in water (see Freezing Vegetables table, page 759) and fewer vegetables can be blanched at a time. Occasionally shake the basket to distribute the heat evenly. When blanching is done, quickly stop the cooking. Hold the vegetables under cold running water or submerge them in water cooled by one or more trays of ice cubes. When the pieces are chilled to the center, drain and pat dry.

NOTE: Several kinds of vegetables—beets, green peppers, mushrooms, onions, pumpkins, winter squashes—are not blanched before freezing; instead, they require special handling. For these vegetables, follow the preparation directions in Freezing Vegetables table, page 759.

Freezing Herbs

Freezing is an excellent way to preserve the delightful flavor and aroma of garden-fresh herbs. Since frozen herbs have the same potency as fresh herbs, use about twice as much as when a recipe calls for dried herbs.

To retain the best color and flavor, blanch the herbs before freezing. Tie each two to three stalks into a bunch, then dip the bunches into boiling water for one minute. Next, quickly chill them in ice water. Pat dry with clean toweling.

After blanching, remove the leaves from the stalks, and wrap five large leaves or one tablespoon small leaves in a small piece of plastic wrap. Repeat until all the leaves are packaged. Overwrap each package with foil and spread in a single layer on a tray. Freeze, then bundle frozen packages in a plastic bag. To use the herbs, mince the leaves while frozen.

Herbs are also handy when frozen in ice cube trays. After blanching, remove the leaves from the stems and mince the leaves. Put one tablespoon leaves in each ice cube compartment, fill with water, and freeze. Once frozen, bundle the cubes in a plastic bag. To use the herbs, simply add a cube to a soup, sauce, stew, or casserole. If a recipe such as a salad calls for herbs without liquid, thaw the cube in a small strainer over a small bowl. Reserve the liquid for a soup, stew, or sauce. It will add a hint of herb flavor and aroma.

Freezing Meats

By removing excess bone and fat from cuts of meat, you can use freezer space wisely. Save the bones to prepare a concentrated stock which can be frozen in ice cube trays (see Stocks, page 100). Wrap chops and patties in individual portions or in small groups with a piece of wax paper between each layer for easy separation. For retaining the best quality during freezing, follow recommended storage times (see Home Storage of Meat table, page 466).

Freezing Poultry

Poultry halves, quarters, and disjointed parts take up less freezer space than whole birds. Use plastic freezer bags or other flexible freezer materials to wrap poultry carefully. Pad the bone tips with foil or freezer wrap to prevent them from breaking through the package, and separate pieces with foil or other freezer material so that they may be broken apart for quicker thawing and cooking. When freezing whole birds, *never* stuff first. For optimum quality use poultry within the recommended storage times (see the table Freezer Storage Time, page 756) and thaw carefully.

Freezer Storage Time for Fish and Poultry

Food	Maximum Storage Time (months)
Fish	
Codfish, flounder, haddock, halibut, pollack	6
Mullet, ocean perch, sea trout, striped bass	3
Ocean perch (Pacific)	2
Salmon steak	2
Sea trout, dressed	3
Striped bass, dressed	3
Whiting, drawn	4
Crab meat	
Dungeness	3
King	10
Shrimp	12
Poultry	
Chicken	
Cut-up	9
Livers	3
Whole	12
Duck, whole	6
Goose, whole	6
Turkey	
Cut-up	6
Whole	12

Freezing Fish

Although fish is tastiest when fresh, it can be frozen for a short time. Immediately after catching or buying fish, freeze it in freezer wrap, in a block of ice, or with an ice glaze.

To freeze in freezer wrap: Use the standard drugstore wrap (see page 753) to cover dressed whole fish, fish fillets, or fish steaks. After wrapping, seal with tape.

To freeze in a block of ice: Fill a loaf pan, wax carton, or coffee tin with cold water. Insert the fish and freeze. If using a pan, you can remove the pan once the water has frozen and wrap the block in freezer packaging material. Seal.

To freeze with an ice glaze: Freeze dressed whole fish unwrapped. Then dip the frozen fish in very cold water and return the fish to the freezer. Repeat until the glaze is one-eighth to one-quarter inch thick. Wrap in freezer wrap and seal.

Thaw fish in the refrigerator to prevent excessive loss of juice. Fish that is dry tends to be tough.

Freezing Prepared Foods

Since many casseroles, braised dishes, soups, and stews freeze very nicely, they are excellent dishes to make in quantity and then put in the freezer in meal-size portions for future use. Frozen cooked dishes will have the most flavor and best texture if you consider the following factors during the initial preparation and cooking.

• Freezing and reheating tends to soften foods, so undercook vegetables, pastas, whole grains, legumes, and meats during the initial cooking. Cool quickly to stop the cooking.

• Seasonings change—some intensify, others diminish—during freezing, so season lightly at first and adjust when reheating.

• Fats blend very poorly when reheated, so use fats sparingly.

• Sauces thickened with flour tend to separate after thawing. Stir while reheating.

• The textures of hard-cooked egg whites, mayonnaise, and potatoes change drastically during storage. Add those foods after thawing the dishes they are to be part of.

• Cold foods freeze more quickly than hot ones. The results are fewer and smaller ice crystals and better texture. To cool hot, cooked casseroles quickly, chill in a pan of ice water.

When packing prepared dishes for freezing, pack food tightly to remove air spaces, and allow sufficient headspace for expansion. Seal casserole lids with tape and overwrap, or line the casserole dish with foil. If lining with foil, cut the liner to extend over the sides of the dish. (There should be enough foil to fold over the contents after the food has frozen.) When the contents have frozen, lift them and foil from the dish and close the foil using the drugstore wrap (see page 753). The dish is now free for another use. Reheating is simple: Peel off the foil and place the frozen block back in the casserole.

Freezing Dairy Foods and Eggs

Milk, foods made from milk, and eggs can be frozen, though their texture suffers somewhat. Freeze milk products in their original containers and thaw them slowly in the refrigerator. Remove eggs from their shells before freezing. (See Freezing Eggs and Dairy products table, page 764.)

Refreezing

As a general rule, if a food is safe to eat, it is safe to refreeze. Foods can be refrozen safely if they have been kept cold (40°F or less) and still contain a few ice crystals. Do not refreeze any food that has warmed to room temperature or that has been left for two or more hours at room temperature. Of course, raw foods that have been frozen, thawed, and then cooked can be refrozen easily and safely.

Since refreezing results in lowered quality, keep storage time short to prevent further deterioration of flavor and texture. Baked goods such as plain breads, cakes, and cookies are an exception. They can be thawed and refrozen without loss of quality.

Thawing Foods

For the best taste and texture, thaw only the amount of food needed for a single meal and use the food promptly. Also, follow the thawing recommendations discussed in the appropriate chapters and sections of this book to retain nutrients, preserve quality, and ensure safety.

When reheating cooked foods (either frozen or thawed), use the original cooking temperature or the one suggested in the Freezing Precooked Foods table (page 761). A meat thermometer

inserted in the center of the food should register 180°F when the food is ready for serving.

Not Every Food Freezes Well

A few foods are unsuitable for freezing because their texture and flavor change radically during freezing and thawing. The following table lists these foods and the changes that occur when they are frozen.

Foods That Do Not Freeze Well

Food	Change That Occurs During Freezing
Breaded and fried foods	Both become soggy.
Buttermilk, yogurt, custard, cottage cheese	These dairy products separate into solids and liquids.
Cake, with custard and pudding fillings	Cake becomes soggy as filling separates into solids and liquid.
Cream cheese	Texture becomes dry and crumbly.
Eggs Hard-cooked	White becomes tough and rubbery.
In shell	Shells crack; yolks are unstable.
Frostings, boiled	Surface becomes weepy.
Gelatin	Surface becomes weepy.
Mayonnaise	Oil separates from solids.
Meats, cured	Salt and fat cause poor freezing and result in quick rancidity.
Potatoes, white, boiled	Texture becomes mealy.
Poultry, stuffed at home	Dressing may not freeze quickly enough to prevent bacteria from multiplying rapidly.
Salad greens, cucumbers, radishes	Crisp vegetables become limp.

Freezing Fruits

Fruits	Preparation	Type of Pack*
Apples		
Sauce	Prepare sauce (see page 620). Pack.	Pack with or without honey and lemon juice to taste.
Slices	Peel, core, and slice. Pack or tray freeze.†	Pack dry or sweeten with 2-4 tablespoons honey. To prevent darkening, mix 2 tablespoons lemon juice or 1 teaspoon rose hip concentrate with honey.
Berries		
Blackberries Blueberries Raspberries	Wash and dry thoroughly. (Or pack unwashed and wash immediately before using.) Pack or tray freeze.†	Pack dry.
Strawberries	Wash and hull. Slice or leave whole. Pack whole berries and slices. Tray freeze† whole berries, if desired.	Pack dry if whole. Sweeten with thin honey syrup (see page 754) if sliced.
Cantaloupes	Cut flesh in slices, cubes, or balls. Pack or tray freeze.† (For best texture eat while partially frozen.)	Pack dry or mix with lemon juice and honey.
Cherries		
Sour	Wash, stem, and pit. Pack or tray freeze.†	Pack dry or mix with a small amount of honey.
Sweet	Wash, stem, and pit. Pack or tray freeze.†	Pack moistened with lemon juice or rose hip concentrate.
Cranberries	Wash, sort, and drain. Pack or tray freeze.†	Pack dry.
Peaches	Wash, peel, and pit. Leave in halves or slice. Pack.	Pack with thin honey syrup (see page 754) and a small amount of lemon juice or rose hip concentrate.
Pineapples	Pare and remove eyes. Slice, dice, or cut in wedges. Pack.	Pack in own juice or thin honey syrup (see page 754).
Plums	Wash and pit. Pack.	Pack with 2 tablespoons lemon juice or 1 teaspoon rose hip concentrate per pint. Sweeten with honey.
Rhubarb	Discard leaves. Wash stalks and cut away woody ends. Slice in 1-inch pieces. Pack or tray freeze.†	Pack dry, or cook and pack in thin honey syrup (see page 754).

NOTE: The recommended maximum storage time for all home-frozen fruits is 1 year. For best quality use within a shorter time.

*Allow for the appropriate headspace. For fruit and liquid, purees, and juices using a container with a wide opening: pint, ½ inch; quart, 1 inch. Using a container with a narrow opening: pint, ¾ inch; quart, 1½ inches. For fruit without liquid: all containers ½ inch.

†To tray freeze: Spread fruit in a single layer on a tray and freeze. When fruit is frozen, put it in a semirigid container or freezer bag. Seal and return to freezer.

Freezing Vegetables

Vegetable	Preparation	Blanching Time—Boiling* (minutes)
Asparagus	Wash thoroughly; cut off tough part of stalk. Leave in spear lengths to fit container or cut in 1-inch pieces. Blanch.†	thin stalks—2 medium stalks—3 thick stalks—4
Beans Green and Wax	Wash; snap ends. Leave whole, cut in 1-inch lengths, or cut in French style (julienne). Blanch.†	3
Lima	Shell and sort according to size. Blanch.†	small beans—2 medium beans—3 large beans—4
Beets	Wash and sort according to size. Trim tops, leaving ½ inch of stems. Cook in boiling water until tender, 25-50 minutes. Cool in cold water. Remove skins and cut into cubes or slice. Pack with ½-inch headspace, seal, and freeze.	No blanching; beets are completely cooked before freezing.
Broccoli	Soak to remove insects and worms. Pare stems if tough and discard woody parts. Slice lengthwise so that heads are no more than 1½ inches across. Blanch.† Pack with heads in alternate directions.	3
Brussels sprouts	Discard outer leaves. Wash; inspect for insects. Sort according to size. Blanch.†	small heads—3 medium heads—4 large heads—5
Carrots	Remove tops. Wash and peel. Leave small carrots whole. Cut large ones into lengthwise strips, thin "penny" slices, or ¼-inch cubes. Blanch.†	whole—5 cubes or slices—2 strips—2
Cauliflower	Discard outer leaves. Trim and separate into florets about 1½ inches across. Soak to remove insects and worms. Blanch.†	3
Corn Kernels	Husk, remove silk, and rinse. Blanch. Cool quickly and drain. Cut kernels from cob with a sharp knife. Pack, leaving ½-inch headspace, seal, and freeze.	4

NOTE: The recommended maximum storage time for all home-frozen vegetables is 8 months. For best quality use within a shorter time.

*Add 1-2 minutes if blanching in steam.

†After blanching, cool quickly and drain. Pack, leaving ½-inch headspace. Seal and freeze. Or spread on a tray to freeze; then put in container, seal, and freeze.

[*continued*]

Freezing Vegetables—*Continued*

Vegetable	Preparation	Blanching Time—Boiling* (minutes)
Corn (*continued*) On the cob	Husk, remove silk, and rinse. Blanch; cool quickly. Drain and dry. Spread on tray and freeze. Wrap in moisture-resistant material. Seal and freeze.	½–1¾-inch diameter—7 1¾–2-inch diameter—9 over 2-inch diameter—11
Greens	Wash and remove large, tough stems. Blanch† in small batches to prevent matting.	beet, mustard, turnip greens, kale, chard—2 spinach—1½
Mushrooms	Wash and trim. Divide into stems and caps, leave whole, or slice. Sauté lightly in butter, 3-5 minutes. Cool and package in meal-size amounts.	No blanching; mushrooms are sautéed instead.
Onions	Dice, pack, and seal.	No blanching necessary.
Peas	Shell and sort. Blanch.†	1½
Peppers, green	Wash; remove seeds and membranes. Halve, slice, or dice. Freeze. (Peppers frozen without blanching may be used in uncooked foods. Blanched† peppers are easier to pack.)	halves—3 slices—2 diced—1
Pumpkins	Wash, cut in large sections, and remove seeds. Steam, pressure-cook, or bake until tender (see Selecting, Storing, and Using Vegetables table, page 192). Remove rind and discard. Mash or sieve pulp. Cool and pack with ½-inch headspace. Seal and freeze.	No blanching; pumpkin is cooked before freezing.
Squashes Summer Winter	Wash and slice in ½-inch pieces. Blanch.† Same as for pumpkin.	3
Tomatoes Juice	Wash and cut out stems. Slice or quarter. Simmer for 5 minutes. Sieve and cool. Pour into containers, allowing 1½-inch headspace. Seal and freeze.	No blanching; juice is cooked before freezing.
Stewed	Wash and remove stems. Peel and cut into quarters. Cover and cook until tender, 5-10 minutes. Cool. Pack, leaving 1-inch headspace. Seal and freeze.	No blanching; tomatoes are cooked before freezing.
Vegetables, mixed	Prepare and blanch each according to recommendations. Mix, pack, and seal.	See individual recommendations.

*Add 1-2 minutes if blanching in steam.

†After blanching, cool quickly and drain. Pack, leaving ½-inch headspace. Seal and freeze. Or spread on a tray to freeze; then put in container, seal, and freeze.

Freezing and Using Precooked Foods

Food	Preparation	Approximate Storage Time	Thawing and Using
Breads			
Quick			
Biscuits and muffins	Cool completely; wrap individually in foil or place in plastic bags.	3-6 months	Thaw at room temperature for 1 hour, or heat frozen, in foil, at 300°F for 20 minutes.
Fruit and nut	Cool completely; wrap in plastic wrap, foil, or place in plastic bags.	3-6 months	Thaw in package at room temperature for 45 minutes. Or warm in foil, when thawed, at 400°F for 10 minutes.
Waffles	Bake to light brown, cool, and wrap individually in foil or place in plastic bags.	1-2 months	Remove from package and heat in toaster.
Yeast			
Baked	Cool completely; wrap in foil or place in plastic bags.	6-8 months	Thaw at room temperature for 45 to 60 minutes. Reheat in foil at 400°F for 10 minutes.
Unbaked	Wrap in plastic wrap.	3-4 weeks	Thaw at room temperature before rising and baking.
Cakes			
Angel, chiffon, sponge (unfrosted)	Cool completely; place in plastic bags. Store with rigid protective covering to prevent crushing.	2 months	Thaw at room temperature; unwrap and heat at 350°F for 10 minutes.
Fruit, pound (unfrosted)	Cool completely; wrap in plastic wrap or place in plastic bags.	12 months	Thaw in package at room temperature for about 1 hour.
Layer (frosted and filled)	It is best to freeze frosting and cake separately. However, if desired, freeze the frosted cake on a flat pan, unwrapped to harden frosting first. Then wrap and freeze in plastic wrap and place in rigid container for protection.	4-6 months	Thaw in refrigerator. Remove wrapping before thawing to prevent it from sticking to frosting.
Cookies			
All (except meringue), baked	Package when completely cool in rigid containers with layers of freezer paper. Crush some paper to fill spaces, so cookies do not break.	6-12 months	Thaw in package at room temperature for about 1 hour.
Refrigerator, unbaked	Shape prepared dough for slicing. Wrap in freezer paper and seal. (Label with baking directions.)	3-6 months	Slice frozen dough using sharp knife— or thaw slightly if too hard to slice. Bake in frozen state.

[continued]

Freezing and Using Precooked Foods—*Continued*

Food	Preparation	Approximate Storage Time	Thawing and Using
Danish pastries, doughnuts, unfilled éclairs, cream puffs	Cool completely and pack individually in foil; overwrap in plastic bag.	3 months	Remove as needed from plastic bag. Keep in foil and heat frozen in 400°F oven for 10-15 minutes.
Desserts			
Fruit pies and cheesecakes, baked	Cool completely; wrap tightly in foil or place in plastic bags. Store with rigid protective covering to prevent crushing.	3 months	Remove wrapping and thaw at room temperature or in refrigerator.
Fruit pies, unbaked	Prepare pie as for baking. Do not cut vents in top crust. Freeze before packaging. Wrap in foil. Store in carton, or top with second plate turned upside down. Tape edges and wrap in foil.	4 months	Remove wrapping. Cut vents in upper crust. Bake frozen for 15-20 minutes at 450°F, then 375°F for about 30 minutes.
Mousses and cold soufflés	Prepare recipe in freezerproof serving dishes. Cover tightly with foil. Use inverted foil pan, or make foil collar, to protect delicate surface.	1 month	Thaw in refrigerator for 8 hours.
Pastry shells, unbaked	Flat sheets: Place on baking sheet or foil-wrapped cardboard. Separate each layer with double-wax-paper layer; wrap flat in foil (handle carefully—they are very brittle). Piecrusts: Shape the pastry in plates; prick with fork; separate with wax paper. Place empty pie plate inside top shell to eliminate air. Wrap in foil or place in plastic bags.	4-6 months	Remove each sheet as needed. Place on pie plate and thaw for 15 minutes at room temperature before shaping. Shape, prick with fork, and bake unfilled at 425° for 15 minutes. Remove wrapping. Bake frozen at 475°F for 8 to 10 minutes.
Meals			
Casseroles, unbaked	Prepare, except for final baking. Place foil or wrap inside casserole. Fill, seal, and freeze. When frozen, remove contents from casserole or pan, store in freezer, and reuse casserole.	4-6 months	Remove wrapping, return to pan. Add any topping at this point, such as cheese or bread crumbs. Cover and bake frozen at 350°F for 1½-2 hours, depending on size.
Whole	Choose foods that will retain quality for about the same length of time. Prepare as either: individual servings—wrap separately in foil and assemble packages in a plastic bag; or sectioned foil trays—covered with foil.	4 months	Do not thaw before heating. Reheat foil-wrapped foods in 400°F oven for 20-30 minutes. Do not remove foil cover. Heat in 400°F oven for 20-30 minutes. For crisp foods, uncover the portion of tray to be crisped for last 10 minutes.

Freezing and Using Precooked Foods—*Continued*

Food	Preparation	Approximate Storage Time	Thawing and Using
Cooked meat and poultry			
Large pieces	Trim excess fat; wrap snugly.	4-6 months	To serve cold, thaw in package in refrigerator. To reheat, unwrap and bake frozen in 350°F oven for 1 hour.
Slices	Cool, cover with gravy, then package.	4-6 months	Reheat in 350°F oven for 30 minutes or until gravy bubbles.
Meat loaf	If baked, cool and package in foil after removing from pan. If unbaked, leave in pan lined with foil. Freeze. Remove pan and store meat loaf in freezer.	3 months	To serve cold, thaw baked loaf in refrigerator. To serve hot, unwrap unbaked frozen loaf and return it to pan. Bake at 350°F for 1½ hours.
Cooked Shellfish (crab, lobster, shrimp)	Remove meat from shells and pack to top of rigid container. (Slightly tough when cooked and frozen.)	3-6 months	To serve cold, thaw in container in refrigerator. Or use in cooked dish from frozen state or slightly thawed. Thaw in refrigerator for cold shrimp and cooked dishes. Do not overcook.
Pizza	Prepare as usual, but do not bake. Cool, wrap in plastic wrap or foil on cardboard base.	1 week	Remove wrapping. Bake frozen at 450°F for 20 minutes.
Sandwiches, closed or open-faced	Use fillings that freeze well—meat, poultry, spreads, nut pastes. Do not use raw vegetables or hard-cooked egg whites. Wrap sandwiches individually in foil, plastic wrap, or plastic bags. Open-faced sandwiches can be frozen on foil-wrapped cardboard, then overwrapped in plastic.	1-2 months	Thaw at room temperature for 3-3½ hours. Sandwiches packed in a lunchbox in the morning will be ready to eat by lunch. (Pack cold sandwiches near a fresh fruit to keep chilled.) Partially frozen sandwiches can be toasted in the oven.
Sauces, glazes, syrups	Pack serving-size portions in plastic containers or jars. Leave ½-1-inch headspace.	6 months when using fresh fruit; 1 month when using fruit juices, flavorings, and pudding mixtures	Heat in top of double boiler, or thaw in container in refrigerator.
Soups	Whenever possible, freeze soup stocks to conserve space and add to other ingredients. Package meal-size portions in rigid containers, allowing ½-inch headspace, or freeze stocks in ice cube trays and package in plastic bags for individual soups and sauces.	1-2 months	Heat in frozen state. If concentrated, add liquid.

Freezing Eggs and Dairy Products

Food	Preparation	Approximate Storage Time	Thawing and Using
Eggs			
Whole (1 egg = 3 tablespoons; 5 eggs = 1 cup)	Lightly beat yolks and whites with a fork. Do not incorporate too much air. Add 1 teaspoon honey for each cup of eggs to stabilize. Freeze in ice cube trays. When frozen, remove cubes and package in plastic bags.	6-9 months	Thaw in refrigerator or at room temperature. Use promptly in any recipe that calls for whole eggs and honey.
Whites (1 egg white = 2 tablespoons)	For uniform texture, pass egg whites through a strainer. Freeze in ice cube trays. When frozen, remove cubes and package in plastic bags.	6-12 months	Thaw in refrigerator or at room temperature. Thawed egg whites will remain fresh in refrigerator for 2-3 days. Egg whites thawed at room temperature produce greater volume when beaten.
Yolks (1 egg yolk = 1½ tablespoons; 14 yolks = 1 cup)	Strain fork-beaten yolks. Add 1 teaspoon honey for each cup of yolks to stabilize. Freeze in ice cube trays. When frozen, remove cubes and package in plastic bags.	6-9 months	Thaw in refrigerator or at room temperature. Use promptly. To make up 1 egg from separately frozen whites and yolks, mix 1 tablespoon yolk and 2 tablespoons egg white.
Milk	Either whole or skim milk can be frozen, but whole milk tends to separate when thawed. Freeze in the unopened paper carton that the milk comes in if there is room at the top for expansion. If repackaging, allow 2-inch headspace.	1 month (Can be kept 3-4 months, but there will be a quality change.)	Thaw in refrigerator.
Cream			
Heavy	Pasteurized cream containing at least 36 percent butterfat can be frozen but whipping quality will be impaired and cream will tend to separate. Freeze small amounts in rigid containers. Leave ½-inch headspace. Freeze only enough for immediate use after thawing.	3-6 months	Thaw in refrigerator.

Freezing Eggs and Dairy Products—*Continued*

Food	Preparation	Approximate Storage Time	Thawing and Using
Heavy, whipped	Whip cream in chilled bowl until stiff enough to hold shape. Drop by spoonfuls (or squeeze through pastry tube to form rosettes) onto baking sheet lined with wax paper. Place in freezer until solid. Pack in rigid container, separating layers with foil.	3-6 months	Frozen whipped cream mounds do not need defrosting when used on hot drinks or warm desserts. Allow a few minutes to soften at room temperature when using on cold desserts.
Light	Light cream can be frozen but tends to separate when thawed. Freeze small amounts in rigid containers. Leave ½-inch headspace. Freeze only enough for immediate use after thawing.	3 months	Thaw in refrigerator.
Sour	Sour cream can be frozen but will separate when thawed. It also curdles very easily in cooking. Freeze small amounts in rigid containers. Leave ½-inch headspace. Freeze only enough for immediate use after thawing.	3 months	Thaw in refrigerator.
Yogurt	Yogurt can be whipped and frozen with fruit and honey, much like ice cream. Unwhipped yogurt that has been frozen and thawed is best used for cooking.	3 months	Allow whipped yogurt to soften slightly at room temperature so that it can be served easily. Thaw unwhipped yogurt in refrigerator.
Ice Cream	If original container is used to freeze ice cream, overwrap with foil. As ice cream is used, press foil or plastic wrap against the cut surface. For homemade ice cream, pack in rigid well-washed container. Allow ½-inch headspace. Ice cream becomes grainy during long storage, and surface, when covered improperly, becomes gummy.	1-2 months	Allow to soften slightly at room temperature so it can be scooped out more easily.

[*continued*]

Freezing Eggs and Dairy Products—*Continued*

Food	Preparation	Approximate Storage Time	Thawing and Using
Butter	Salted, unsalted, or home-churned butter must be over-wrapped in plastic wrap or foil.	6 months	Thaw in refrigerator.
Cheeses			
Cottage cheese	Homemade, pasteurized, skim milk cottage cheese should be washed. Add cream at time of serving. Freeze commercial cottage cheese in original container and overwrap in foil. Both types may separate when thawed.	4-6 months	Thaw in refrigerator.
Cream cheese	Overwrap in foil. Becomes crumbly when thawed. Best used in dips or cheesecakes.	4 months	Thaw in refrigerator.
Hard or semihard cheeses (such as blue, cheddar, Swiss)	Cut in ¼- or ½-pound pieces; overwrap in foil. On thawing, hard and semihard cheeses become crumbly and lose flavor. Use in cooking or crumbled in salad dressing.	6 months	Thaw in refrigerator. Bring to room temperature before serving.
Soft cheeses (such as Brie, Camembert)	Overwrap in foil. May crumble slightly when thawed.	4 months	Thaw in refrigerator. Bring to room temperature before serving.

Canning

Long before effective freezers were available to homeowners, canning was a popular method of preserving food at home. In many areas of the country, canning is still the primary way of storing produce from a bountiful garden.

Canning preserves food by using heat to destroy the enzymes and organisms—molds, yeasts, bacteria—that cause spoilage. The containers are then sealed to prevent new organisms from entering. If you follow the procedures recommended by home economists at the United States Department of Agriculture and described in this section, your canned foods will be free of *Clostridium botulism* bacteria and be very safe to eat.

NOTE: *Clostridium botulism* bacteria grow in low-acid foods in airtight containers and produce a deadly toxin. Use a pressure canner to raise the temperature of the food to 240°F and destroy the spores of the bacteria. High-acid foods (tomatoes and most fruits) can safely be canned in only boiling water.

Canning Equipment

The following equipment helps simplify safe canning:

jar tongs—This tool is extremely useful for lifting jars from the water when processing is done.

ladle—A large soup ladle facilitates spooning hot jams and liquids into jars.

long-handled spoon—This type of spoon permits stirring of large quantities of food.

slotted spoon—One of these is ideal for draining the excess liquid from hot vegetables when spooning them into canning jars.

widemouthed funnel—This funnel speeds filling the jars and reduces spills on the rim and outside edges of the jars.

water bath canner—A canner of this type is suitable for processing fruits and vegetables high in acid (such as tomatoes). Select one with a rack and a tight-fitting lid. Be certain the canner is large enough that the jars will not touch and deep enough that the jars will be submerged two inches below the surface of the water. Also, the canner should have a flat bottom with no more than two inches overhang around the circumference of the burner and be no more than four inches wider than the burner where it will be used. Too much overhang will result in poor processing of the jars around the outer edge of the canner.

pressure (steam) canner—This canner is a must for processing all foods that are low in acid: most vegetables, meats, poultry, fish, soups, and stews. Select a pressure canner that has a rack, a lid with a rubber seal, a safety valve, and a petcock (vent). The canner should be designed to maintain ten pounds of pressure. Check the pressure gauge before starting to can (a maximum thermometer is available from County Extension home economists for this purpose) and have it repaired if it is more than four pounds off. If less, adjust during processing. (A pressure saucepan can be used if you are canning small amounts. Because the saucepans heat and cool more quickly, add 20 minutes to all processing times.)

jars—Containers made of tempered glass and manufactured especially for home canning are best. Never use jars left over from commercially made peanut butter, mayonnaise, or pickles—they may crack during processing and their seals may not be tight. Each year examine your canning jars for cracks or chips before using them, and discard any that are damaged.

caps—Select either the porcelain-lined zinc caps with rubber rings or the two-piece screw band with flat, metal self-sealing lids. Generally speaking, the self-sealing lids are preferred because they result in the fewest seal failures. Never reuse rubber rings or metal self-sealing lids since the sealing compound is good for one use only. If you plan to use new rubber rings left over from a previous year's canning, check them for resilience. Fold each ring in half or pleat it. Examine the folds and reject any rings showing cracks or softness. Also reject any that do not spring back when released.

Preparation of Foods for Canning

Select foods at peak quality, then wash all fruits and vegetables thoroughly to remove dirt and surface pesticides. Peel and cut each food according to the recommendations in the tables that begin on page 770. Handle foods quickly and gently to avoid bruising or other damage, and prepare only as much food as you can process at one time.

Preparing Jars and Lids

After checking the jars to be sure there are no chips, cracks, or sharp edges that will prevent an airtight seal or cause breakage, wash the jars and lids in hot, soapy water. Rinse well and leave them in hot, clear water until you are ready to use them. Keeping the jars hot will help prevent cracking from sudden temperature changes when piping hot food is poured into them. Sterilizing, however, is not necessary since processing will sterilize both the jars and the food. If you are using rubber rings, keep them wet until they are placed on the jars.

Packing the Jars

There are two safe ways of packing food into jars: hot pack and raw pack (sometimes called cold pack). Hot pack is the preferred method since it removes air from food tissues and results in a slower loss of quality during storage.

Hot pack: Heat foods to the boiling point in water, juice, or syrup; then pack the hot foods loosely in the jars and pour in the boiling liquid to surround the pieces and cover them completely. Most foods with liquid should be packed to one-half inch from the top of the jar, but corn, lima beans, and peas should be packed only to one inch from the top since they will expand somewhat during processing.

Raw (cold) pack: Put raw, unheated foods directly into the jars. Pack tightly since the pieces of food will shrink during processing; then pour in enough boiling water, juice, or syrup to surround the pieces and cover them. (Meat and poultry are packed raw without liquid.) Use the same headspace that is allowed for the hot pack.

After packing the jars with food and liquid, run a narrow spatula between the food and the sides of the jar to remove air bubbles. Next, wipe the rim and threads of the jar clean. The jars are now ready for capping and processing.

Honey Syrup for Canning Fresh Fruits

Fruits canned in juice or plain water are delightfully tasty, and they are safe to eat, too, since a sweetener is added primarily for flavor. But for slightly better shape and color, as well as sweeter flavor, pack fruit pieces in a light honey syrup. To make syrup for 6 to 12 pints of fruit, blend two cups light honey with four cups very hot water; stir well.

Closing the Jars

If using the two-piece screw bands with metal lids, place each lid with the sealing compound next to the glass. Screw the metal band down firmly, but do not use extreme force. After processing, no further tightening is needed. The screw bands can be removed when the jars have cooled for 12 to 24 hours.

If using the porcelain-lined zinc caps with rubber rings, fit each wet ring on the jar shoulder but do not stretch the ring. Screw the porcelain cap down firmly; then turn it back one-quarter inch. As soon as the processing is done, screw the cap firmly to complete the seal.

Using a Water Bath Canner

A boiling water canner is useful for processing foods high in acid: fruits, tomatoes, pickles, jams, and jellies. For all other foods use a pressure (steam) canner.

Place the rack on the bottom of the canner; then fill the canner half full with hot water. Over high heat bring the water to a boil for hot-packed foods and almost to a boil for raw-packed foods. Next, lower all the jars to the rack, leaving enough room between the jars for the water to circulate. Add boiling water until the jars are covered by one to two inches of liquid, but do not pour the water directly onto the jars. Cover the canner and return the water to a gentle boil. Start timing the processing when the water begins to boil, and add more boiling water as needed to keep the water one to two inches above the jars. (See the table on page 770 for processing times.) As soon as the processing is complete, remove the jars.

Safe Canning

Putting up your own food is safe as well as enjoyable if you take a few simple precautions. Avoid spoilage and contamination with botulism toxin by always using recommended procedures and equipment. Never use the open-kettle method of canning foods. (In this method food is cooked in an open pot, then packed into jars with no further processing.) Never process in the oven, slow cooker, or microwave. Do not skimp on processing time, and do not overpack, since it can result in underprocessing. Avoid canning combinations of food. If you must can mixtures, use the processing time for the food that requires the longest time and highest temperature. Do not can overripe foods; their acid content is often very low.

CAUTION: If foods are not correctly processed, deadly botulism spores can grow in airtight jars of low-acid foods. Always process foods at the recommended temperature and for the recommended length of time.

Using a Pressure Canner

A pressure canner is essential for processing all low-acid foods and combinations of foods: vegetables, meats, poultry, fish, soups, and stews. Follow the manufacturer's directions for using the canner, as well as consulting the general directions given in this section.

Put the rack on the bottom of the canner and fill the canner with two to three inches of hot water. Place the jars of food on the rack, leaving space for water and steam to circulate between each jar and between the jars and the sides of the canner. Fasten the cover securely; then heat the water to the boiling point and exhaust the canner for ten minutes. Close the vent or put on the weighted gauge. Begin timing the processing when the gauge reaches ten pounds of pressure or the weighted gauge jiggles or rocks. (See the table on page 773 for processing times.) Regulate the heat so that the weight moves two to three times a minute, and process at ten pounds of pressure for the entire time. When the processing time is up, remove the canner from the heat and let the pressure return to zero. This will take 30 to 60 minutes, depending on the size of the canner. Open the vent slowly (do not open before the pressure drops!), cautiously remove the lid from the canner, and take out the jars.

Cooling the Jars

As soon as processing is done, remove the hot jars from the canner. Set them upright on a wire rack or folded cloth. (Do not open the jars to add more liquid if it has boiled down.) Leave room between the jars (two to three inches) for air to circulate, yet keep them away from drafts since sudden coolness can crack the jars. After 24 hours, remove the screw bands and store the jars of food.

Testing the Seal

The common two-piece screw band and metal lid is self-sealing, but the other types of caps are not. If you have used a cap that does not self-seal, complete the seals, following the manufacturer's directions, as soon as you remove the jars from the canner.

After the jars have cooled for at least 12 hours, check the seal. Test the two-piece screw bands and metal lids by pressing the center of each lid. If the center has a slight dip and will not move, the jar is sealed. An alternate test is to tap the center of the lid with a spoon. The resulting ring should be clear if the seal is good. Yet, a dull sound may or may not mean the seal is bad, since food touching the lid can cause dullness. Test the jars with zinc caps and rubber rings by looking at the caps; they are sealed if the caps are low in the center.

If any of the jars has a poor seal, the food can be refrigerated and used within two days or reprocessed. To reprocess, empty the jar and, using a clean jar and new metal lid, repeat all the steps in processing. Reprocessing will lower the quality of the canned food, however.

Storing Home-Canned Foods

As a rule, canned foods stored in a cool (below 70°F), dry, dark place will keep very nicely for up to a year. But foods kept in damp, hot, very cold, or bright areas can deteriorate in six months or less. Dampness can corrode the metal lids and cause leakage or allow entry of bacteria; freezing temperatures can change good texture to mushiness and damage seals; sunlight and heat can cause fading and loss of flavor and texture.

Using Home-Canned Foods

Serve fruits which are high in acid straight from the jar or use them to create tasty cooked dishes. But boil low- and non-acid foods — meats, poultry, and most vegetables — for 10 minutes (boil corn and spinach for 20 minutes) before tasting them. If foods foam, produce off-odors, or do not look right during or after boiling, discard them *without* tasting.

Home-canned foods make delightful soups, stews, and casseroles. Take care, however, not to cook them more than necessary since canned foods are extensively cooked during processing.

Detecting Spoilage

Even with careful preparation, home-canned foods spoil occasionally. Before opening jars, check them for cracks and for loose, bulging, or leaky lids; after opening, check contents for off-colors or odors, mold, sediment, slime, or soft texture. Discard any foods that look suspicious — do not taste them! Reject also any that spurt or fizz when opened.

Processing High-Acid Foods (Fruits and Tomatoes) in Boiling Water Bath

Food	Type of Pack	Preparation*	Processing Time† (minutes)	
			Pints	Quarts
Apples Slices	hot	Peel, core, and slice. To slow darkening, place in 1 gallon water with 2 tablespoons vinegar. Drain and rinse. Boil for 5 minutes in water, juice, or light syrup (see page 768). Stir occasionally to prevent burning. Pack in jars, leaving ½-inch headspace. Cover with hot syrup or water to ½ inch of top.	15	20
Applesauce	hot	Prepare apple slices as above and simmer until tender, about 20 minutes. Stir frequently to prevent burning. For chunky style pack in jars; for smooth style press through strainer or food mill and then pack. (Or follow recipe on page 620 and pack while hot.) Leave ½-inch headspace.	15	15
Apricots		See peaches. Peeling can be omitted for apricots.		
Berries (except strawberries‡) Blackberries Dewberries Loganberries Raspberries Blueberries Currants Elderberries Gooseberries Huckleberries	raw	Cap and stem. Pack in jars to ½ inch of top, shaking berries down gently. Cover with boiling juice, light syrup (see page 768), or water, leaving ½-inch headspace.	15	15
	hot	Drain well after washing. Add ¼ cup honey to each quart currants, elderberries, or huckleberries. Cover and bring to a boil. Blanch blueberries or gooseberries for 15–30 seconds. Cool and drain. For all berries, pack in jars, leaving ½-inch headspace.	15	15
Cherries (Sour or sweet)	raw	Stem, remove pits. Sweet cherries can be left un-pitted, but sour cherries are best when pitted. For unpitted cherries, prick skin with a sharp knife to prevent splitting during processing. Pack cherries in jars, shaking cherries down gently. Cover with boiling juice or light syrup (see page 768) to ½ inch of top.	20	25
	hot	Prepare cherries as above. For each quart sweet cherries, add ⅛ cup honey plus ¼ cup water; for each quart sour cherries, add ¼ cup honey plus ½ cup water. Bring to a boil. Pack in jars, leaving ½ inch headspace.	15	15

*Wash all fruit carefully as the first step in preparation.
†At altitudes of 2,000 feet, add 2 minutes processing time to all times specified for 20 minutes or less. For specified times of more than 20 minutes, add 4 minutes to processing times. At higher altitudes still more time is needed.
‡Strawberries are best when frozen or preserved as jams.

Processing High-Acid Foods (Fruits and Tomatoes) in Boiling Water Bath—*Continued*

Food	Type of Pack	Preparation*	Processing Time† (minutes) Pints	Quarts
Fruit juices	hot	Prepare juice (see page 734). Reheat to simmering, and pack in jars, allowing ¼-inch headspace.	15	15
Fruit purees	hot	Prepare puree. Press simmered fruit (see page 609) through strainer or food mill. Reheat to simmering and pack in jars, leaving ¼-inch headspace.	15	15
Nectarines		See peaches.		
Peaches	raw	To remove skins, dip in boiling water until skins are loosened, for ½–1 minute; then dip in cold water. Slip off skins; remove pits; and cut in halves or slices. To prevent darkening, place in 1 gallon water with 2 tablespoons vinegar. Drain and rinse. Pack in jars (halves with cut-side down) and shake fruit down. Cover with boiling light syrup (see page 768), leaving ½-inch headspace.	25	30
	hot	Prepare as above. Bring to a boil in light syrup (see page 768). Pack in jars and cover with syrup, leaving ½-inch headspace.	20	25
Pears	hot	Peel pears, cut in half lengthwise, and core. To prevent darkening, place in 1 gallon water with 2 tablespoons vinegar. Drain and rinse. Boil pears for 5 minutes in light syrup (see page 768). Pack in jars. Place cut-side down and fill in layers. Cover with boiling syrup to ½ inch of top.	20	25
Plums	raw	Stem. To can whole, prick skins with table fork to prevent splitting. Or halve and pit freestone varieties. Pack firmly in jars and cover with boiling light syrup (see page 768) to ½ inch of top.	20	25
	hot	Prepare as above. Heat plums in boiling light syrup (see page 768). Pack in jars and cover with boiling syrup to ½ inch of top.	20	25
Rhubarb	hot	Cut stalks into ½-inch pieces. Add ¼ cup honey to each quart rhubarb and let stand to draw out juice. Bring to a boil. Pack in jars to ½ inch of top.	15	15

*Wash all fruit carefully as the first step in preparation.
†At altitudes of 2,000 feet, add 2 minutes processing time to all times specified for 20 minutes or less. For specified times of more than 20 minutes, add 4 minutes to processing times. At higher altitudes still more time is needed.

[continued]

Processing High-Acid Foods (Fruits and Tomatoes) in Boiling Water Bath—*Continued*

Food	Type of Pack	Preparation*	Processing Time† (minutes)	
			Pints	Quarts

Tomatoes§
  Whole or
  pieces
	raw	Dip in boiling water for 15–30 seconds to split skins, then dip in cold water. Slip off skins and remove cores. Leave whole, or cut in halves or quarters. Pack in jars, pressing gently to fill spaces, or add hot tomato juice. Do *not* add water. Leave ½-inch headspace. Add 4 teaspoons lemon juice or ½ teaspoon powdered citric acid per quart to low-acid tomatoes.	35	45

	hot	Prepare as above. Quarter and bring to a boil, stirring to prevent sticking. Pack boiling hot in jars, leaving ½-inch headspace. Add 4 teaspoons lemon juice or ½ teaspoon powdered citric acid per quart to low-acid tomatoes.	35	45
Juice	hot	Remove stems and trim off bruised or discolored spots. Quickly cut about 1 pound tomatoes into quarters and place directly into a large pot. Bring immediately to a boil. Crush pieces and add additional freshly cut pieces slowly to boiling mixture. Crush new pieces once boiling resumes. Keep mixture boiling constantly and vigorously while adding remaining tomato pieces. Simmer for 5 minutes after all tomato pieces have been added. Press hot cooked tomatoes through a sieve or food mill to remove skins and seeds. Reheat to a boil. Pour immediately into jars, leaving ¼-inch headspace.	35	35
Juice blend with vegetables	hot	To 18 pounds freshly crushed and simmering tomatoes, add no more than 3 cups of any combination of finely chopped celery, onions, carrots, or sweet peppers. Simmer for 20 minutes, then press through a sieve or food mill to remove skins and seeds. Bring to a boil. Pour immediately into jars leaving ½-inch headspace.	35	35
Sauce, plain	hot	Prepare and press tomato juice as above. Simmer until sauce reaches desired consistency. Reduce volume by ⅓ for a thin sauce and by ½ for a thick one. Pour into jars, leaving ¼-inch headspace.	35 (thin) 20 (thick)	35 (thin) 20 (thick)
Sauce with vegetables	hot	Prepare the same as juice blend with vegetables (see above). After pressing the juice, simmer it until its volume is reduced by ½.	35	35
Sauce with meat		See Processing Low-Acid Foods in Pressure Canner table, page 775.		

*Wash all fruit carefully as the first step in preparation.
†At altitudes of 2,000 feet, add 2 minutes processing time to all times specified for 20 minutes or less. For specified times of more than 20 minutes, add 4 minutes to processing times. At higher altitudes still more time is needed.
§Can only high-quality tomatoes. Never can soft, decayed, cracked, moldy, or spotted ones, or those picked from dead vines or vines damaged by frost.

Processing Low-Acid Foods (Vegetables, Fish, Meat, and Poultry) in Pressure Canner

Food	Type of Pack	Preparation*	Processing Time with 10 Pounds Pressure† (minutes)	
			Pints	Quarts
Asparagus	raw	Trim off tough scales and stems, wash a second time, and leave whole or cut into 1-inch pieces. Pack tightly in jars, taking care not to crush. Cover with boiling water to 1 inch of top.	25	30
	hot	Prepare as above. Cover with boiling water and simmer for 2-3 minutes. Pack loosely in jars (do not press or shake down) leaving 1-inch headspace. Cover with fresh boiling water to 1 inch of top.	25	30
Beans Snap (green, string, wax)	raw	Trim ends. Cut or snap into 1-inch pieces. Pack tightly in jars, leaving 1-inch headspace. Cover with boiling water to 1 inch of top.	20	25
	hot	Prepare as above. Cover with boiling water and boil for 5 minutes. Pack in jars, leaving 1-inch headspace. Cover with fresh boiling water to 1 inch of top.	20	25
Lima (butter)	raw	Shell young tender beans. Pack loosely in jars (do not press or shake down). For small beans fill pints to 1 inch of top and quarts to 1½ inches; for large beans fill pints to 1 inch of top and quarts to 1¼ inches. Cover with boiling water to 1 inch of top.	40	50
	hot	Prepare as above. Cover with boiling water and bring to a boil. Pack loosely in jars, leaving 1-inch headspace. Cover with fresh boiling water to 1 inch of top.	40	50
Beets	hot	Cut off tops, but retain 1 inch of stem. Do not cut off root. Cover with boiling water, and simmer until skins slip off easily, 15-25 minutes. Trim stems and roots and slip off skins. Leave small beets whole, cut medium or large beets into ½-inch cubes or slices, and cut very large beets into ½-inch cubes. Pack in jars, leaving 1-inch headspace. Cover with fresh boiling water to 1 inch of top.	30	35
Carrots	raw	Peel carrots and slice or dice. Pack tightly in jars, leaving 1-inch headspace. Cover with boiling water to 1 inch of top.	25	30
	hot	Prepare as above. Cover with boiling water, then bring to a boil. Pack in jars, leaving 1-inch headspace. Cover with cooking liquid to 1 inch of top.	25	30

*Wash all vegetables carefully as the first step in preparation, except where otherwise noted.
†Process at 11 pounds pressure for the same amount of time at altitudes of 2,000 feet if using a pressure canner with a dial gauge. At higher altitudes, process at still higher pressure. If using a canner with a weighted gauge, no adjustment is necessary.

[continued]

Processing Low-Acid Foods (Vegetables, Fish, Meat, and Poultry) in Pressure Canner— Continued

Food	Type of Pack	Preparation*	Processing Time with 10 Pounds Pressure† (minutes)	
			Pints	Quarts
Corn				
Cream style	raw	Husk corn and remove silk. Wash. Cut corn from cob at center of the kernel, and scrape cob. Pack in pint jars, leaving 1-inch headspace. Cover with boiling water to 1 inch of top.	95	Not recommended.
	hot	Prepare as above. To each quart of corn, add 1 pint boiling water, and heat to boiling. Pack in pint jars, leaving 1-inch headspace.	85	Not recommended.
Whole kernel	raw	Husk corn and remove silk. Wash. Cut corn from cob at $2/3$ the depth of the kernel. Pack loosely in jars (do not press or shake down), leaving 1-inch headspace. Cover with boiling water to 1 inch of top.	55	85
	hot	Prepare as above. Blanch for 3 minutes in boiling water. Cool corn and cut kernels from cob. To each quart of kernels, add ½ pint hot water. Bring to a boil. Pack hot corn mixture in jars, leaving 1-inch headspace.	55	85
Mixed vegetables	hot	Prepare vegetables in manner described under each vegetable. Mix, cover with boiling water, and boil for 3 minutes. Drain; pack in jars, allowing 1 inch headspace. Cover with fresh boiling water to 1 inch of top.	Time according to vegetable requiring longest processing.	Time according to vegetable requiring longest processing.
Mushrooms	hot	Trim stems and discolored parts. Wash thoroughly to remove all dirt. Rinse in clean water. Leave small mushrooms whole; slice medium and large ones. Steam for 4 minutes or heat gently for 10 minutes with added liquid in covered pan. Pack in jars, leaving 1-inch headspace. For good color retention add ⅛ teaspoon crystalline ascorbic acid per pint. Cover with fresh boiling water to 1 inch of top.	45	Not recommended.
Peas				
Sweet green	raw	Shell and wash peas. Pack loosely in jars (do not press or shake down), leaving 1-inch headspace. Cover with boiling water to 1 inch of top.	40	40
	hot	Prepare as above. Cover with boiling water; return to a boil. Pack loosely in jars, leaving 1-inch headspace. Cover with fresh boiling water to 1 inch of top.	40	40

*Wash all vegetables carefully as the first step in preparation, except where otherwise noted.
†Process at 11 pounds pressure for the same amount of time at altitudes of 2,000 feet if using a pressure canner with a dial gauge. At higher altitudes, process at still higher pressure. If using a canner with a weighted gauge, no adjustment is necessary.

Processing Low-Acid Foods (Vegetables, Fish, Meat, and Poultry) in Pressure Canner— *Continued*

Food	Type of Pack	Preparation*	Processing Time with 10 Pounds Pressure† (minutes)	
			Pints	Quarts
Sugar snap (edible pods)	raw	Trim ends. Leave whole or cut in 1-inch pieces. Pack in jars, leaving 1-inch headspace. Cover with boiling water to 1 inch of top.	20	35
	hot	Prepare as above. Cover with boiling water and cook for 5 minutes. Pack in jars. Cover with fresh boiling water, leaving 1-inch headspace.	20	25
Potatoes Cubed	hot	Peel and cut into 1-inch cubes. Cook immediately in boiling water and drain. Pack in jars, leaving 1-inch headspace. Cover with fresh boiling water to 1 inch of top.	35	40
Whole (1-2 inch diameter)	hot	Prepare as above. Cook in boiling water for 10 minutes. Drain and pack in jars, leaving 1-inch headspace. Cover with fresh boiling water to 1 inch of top.	30	40
Pumpkins	hot	Slice off stem end, remove seeds, and peel. Cut into 1-inch cubes and boil for 2 minutes in water. Pack in jars, allowing 1-inch headspace. Cover with cooking liquid (and boiling water if necessary to completely fill) to 1 inch of top.	55	90
Spinach and other greens	hot	Can only top-notch, tender fresh greens. Rinse until greens are free of grit; drain. Remove tough ribs and stems. Steam until well wilted, 3-5 minutes. Pack loosely in jars, leaving 1-inch headspace. Cover with boiling water to 1 inch of top.	70	90
Squashes, winter		See pumpkins.		
Tomato sauce with meat	hot	Prepare sauce according to favorite recipe. Pack in jars, leaving 1-inch headspace.	60	75
Fish	raw	Use only firm, fresh fish. Bleed well. Wash thoroughly. Pack in jars, leaving 1-inch headspace. Cover with boiling water to 1 inch of top.	100	100

*Wash all vegetables carefully as the first step in preparation, except where otherwise noted.
†Process at 11 pounds pressure for the same amount of time at altitudes of 2,000 feet if using a pressure canner with a dial gauge. At higher altitudes, process at still higher pressure. If using a canner with a weighted gauge, no adjustment is necessary.

[*continued*]

Processing Low-Acid Foods (Vegetables, Fish, Meat, and Poultry) in Pressure Canner—
Continued

Food	Type of Pack	Preparation*	Processing Time with 10 Pounds Pressure† (minutes)	
			Pints	Quarts
Meat Ground, chopped	hot	Choose fresh, high-quality chilled meat. With venison, add 1 part high-quality pork fat to 3 or 4 parts venison before grinding. Shape chopped meat into patties or balls; cut cased sausage in 3-4-inch links. Cook until lightly browned. Ground meat may be sautéed without shaping. Remove excess fat. Pack hot in jars, leaving 1-inch headspace. Cover with boiling meat stock, tomato juice, or water to 1 inch of top.	75	90
Strips, cubes	raw	Choose high-quality chilled meat. Remove excess fat and large bones. Place meat in jars, leaving 1-inch headspace. Do not add liquid.	75	90
	hot	Prepare meat as above. Precook meat until rare by roasting, stewing, or browning in a small amount of fat. Pack in jars, leaving 1-inch headspace. Cover with boiling stock, meat drippings, water, or tomatoes to 1 inch of top.	75	90
Poultry	raw	Choose freshly killed and dressed animals. (Older chickens are more flavorful than fryers.) Dressed poultry should be chilled for 6-12 hours before canning. Remove excess fat. Cut chicken into pieces suitable for cooking or canning. Pack loosely in jars (do not press or shake down), leaving 1¼-inch headspace. Do not add liquid.	65 (with bones) 75 (without bones)	75 (with bones) 90 (without bones)
	hot	Prepare as above. Boil, steam, or bake until about ⅔ done. Pack hot pieces in jars, leaving 1¼-inch headspace. Cover with boiling stock to 1 inch of top.	65 (with bones) 75 (without bones)	75 (with bones) 90 (without bones)
Soups with fish, meat, or poultry	hot	Prepare each ingredient: brown or boil meat, fish, or poultry; cook vegetables. Combine with stock, tomatoes, or water to cover; then boil for 5 minutes. Do not add flour, cornstarch, or other thickeners. Season lightly, if desired, since some seasonings change during processing. Fill jars about ½ full with solid mixture. Add remaining liquid, leaving 1-inch headspace. Prior to serving, add thickeners and seasonings, as desired.	60	75

*Wash all vegetables carefully as the first step in preparation, except where otherwise noted.
†Process at 11 pounds pressure for the same amount of time at altitudes of 2,000 feet if using a pressure canner with a dial gauge. At higher altitudes, process at still higher pressure. If using a canner with a weighted gauge, no adjustment is necessary.

Pickling

Often, even after you have put up endless rows of colorful pints and quarts of fruits and vegetables, your garden continues to offer more of the same wonderful foods. When this happens next year, try pickling some foods and treat your family and guests to a delightful change of taste.

Almost any food can be pickled, but cucumbers, sweet peppers, green tomatoes, and corn are among the best and most popular. Though pickled foods are preserved in a salt brine or spiced vinegar solution, remember that they must also always be canned.

Kinds of Pickles

There are four classic types of pickled foods.

Fresh-pack or quick-process pickles: Very easy to prepare at home, these pickles made from whole or sliced vegetables can be processed either with or without salt. In the salt method, the foods (cucumbers are most common, but beets, cauliflower, green beans, and okra are also pickled in this manner) are soaked in a low-salt brine for several hours or overnight, then drained and processed with boiling vinegar, spices, and herbs. In a no-salt method that some cooks use, the foods are initially cooked with a spiced vinegar, then packed and processed immediately. Alternatively, the foods are first packed in the jars, next the spiced vinegar is poured in, and then the processing is done. Pickles made without salt tend to have a soft texture and sharp vinegar flavor.

NOTE: Studies have shown that excessive salt intake can cause hypertension and other related health problems in susceptible people, hence the interest in a salt-free pickling process.

Fruit pickles: To make these pickles, whole fruits such as peaches, pears, and watermelon rind are simmered in a spicy, sweet-sour syrup, then packed and processed.

Relishes: Mixed fruits and vegetables which have been chopped into small pieces, seasoned, and then cooked, packed, and processed make up this broad category of pickled foods. Hot and spicy, or sweet and spicy, relishes include condiments of all types: catsup, chili sauce, chowchow, chutneys, corn relish, and piccalilli.

Brined pickles: Cabbage (for sauerkraut) and cucumbers are the vegetables usually preserved by curing in a brine. The curing process takes about three weeks in either a low-salt or high-salt brine. After curing, the pickles are packed and processed.

Pickling Ingredients

Fruits and vegetables: Although cauliflower, corn, cucumbers, green beans, green tomatoes, onions, peaches, pears, sweet peppers, and watermelon rind are among the fruits and vegetables most commonly pickled, almost any tender one of top quality is a good choice. For the crispest, most flavorful pickled foods, allow no more than 24 hours (preferably less) to elapse between picking and processing; and refrigerate the produce immediately after picking if it will not be processed within an hour.

When possible, select slightly underripe produce; it will result in crisper pickles than if ripe or overripe produce is used. Avoid moldy or badly bruised produce since off-flavor and mushy texture cannot be overcome by seasoning, curing, or processing. And do not use waxed cucumbers or green peppers; the waxed skin will not absorb the brine. To reduce chances of rot, do use cucumbers with a short piece of the stem left on the fruit.

Wash fruits and vegetables gently but thoroughly under running water. Drain on clean, dry towels and tenderly blot dry. Remove any blossoms since they are frequently the source of softening.

Vinegar: Cider vinegar or any other vinegar with a mild flavor makes tasty pickles. But cider vinegar and red wine vinegar discolor light vegetables and fruits such as cauliflower, onions, and pears. Choose white distilled vinegar (it has a somewhat sharp, pungent taste) for those vegetables, to preserve the integrity of the color.

Whichever vinegar you choose, be absolutely certain its acidity is 4 to 6 percent. Any less acid can almost guarantee spoilage and dangerous eating. If you find the pickles too sour with the recommended acidity, add sweetener, but never dilute the vinegar.

Honey: Light honeys such as clover and alfalfa are mild in flavor and excellent for pickling. Unfortunately, honey changes color and flavor when boiled as many recipes suggest. To prevent these changes, alter the recipe. Instead of boiling the honey, vinegar, and spices together, boil only the vinegar and spices. Then add the honey to the vinegar-spice mixture and bring the syrup to a *very* brief boil. Add the syrup quickly to the pickles.

Herbs and spices: Fresh herbs and spices lend the most flavor to pickled foods. Tie whole leaves and seeds in a cheesecloth bag or stainless steel spice ball for easy removal before pickles are packed. Spices left in the jar through processing can cause off-flavors and dark pickles. Ground spices, too, tend to darken pickles, so avoid using them.

Water: Soft water (either natural or artificially softened) is best for attractive-looking pickles. Iron or sulfur in hard water will darken pickles; calcium and other salts can interfere with the fermentation process and often cause a white scum or precipitate.

Equipment

Most of the equipment required for pickling is inexpensive and already stocked in the average kitchen. The few essential specialty items that run into more money, such as a canner and jars, can be used repeatedly.

For heating and mixing the vinegar-spice liquid, use a stainless steel, unchipped enameled, or glass saucepan. Avoid aluminum and never use copper, brass, iron, or galvanized pans or utensils. These metals can react with the strong acid of the vinegar and cause unwanted color and taste changes as well as form poisonous compounds.

In the preparation of the fruits and vegetables, use standard household utensils. Some items you will find helpful are: a cutting board, paring knife, food grinder, ladle, wooden spoon, tray, tongs, and measuring equipment.

For the actual canning process you will need jars and a canner, along with other equipment (see Canning Equipment, page 766). When selecting a canner for pickling, choose the boiling water bath type. It is currently considered acceptable for canning pickled foods since these foods have an increased acid content from the added vinegar.

Packing and Processing Pickled Foods

The packing and processing steps for pickled foods are identical to those for plain, high-acid fruits and vegetables, although the liquid used in pickling is a spiced vinegar instead of water, juice, or syrup. Be sure the spiced vinegar surrounds each piece of food.

Process pickled foods for 10 to 15 minutes using the boiling water bath method (see Using a Water Bath Canner, page 768). Follow the canning instructions for testing the seal and noting signs of spoilage (see page 769).

Food Safety and Pickling

Fresh-pack pickles made from corn, cucumbers, green peppers, green tomatoes, or zucchini are canned by the water bath process in order to retain crispness, even though these low-acid foods would normally be canned in the pressure canner as a safety measure (see Canning, page 766). The vinegar added during pickling therefore has a dual role: It must acidify the foods to make them safe for water bath processing and add flavor as well. Unfortunately, scientists are no longer certain that traditional home pickling recipes, especially those made without salt, acidify adequately. Without a vote of confidence on safety from those who are charged with making such judgments, we believe such techniques should be avoided entirely.

Storing Pickled Foods

Pickled foods are tastiest when the flavor is allowed to develop for at least three weeks before the jars are opened. Store pickled foods, like other canned items, in a cool, dry, dark place.

What Happened to the Pickles?

Problem	Possible Cause
Soft or slippery	Vinegar solution too weak; foods not kept submerged in the pickling liquid
Dark	Water contains iron or sulfur; ground spices were used
Hollow and float	Cucumbers pickled too long after picking
Shriveled	Vinegar solution has too much acid or sweetener
Faded	Pickles kept too long or exposed to bright light during storage

Jams and Jellies

Jams, jellies, conserves, marmalades, preserves, fruit butters—all lend a sweet, delicate touch to any luncheon or dinner. Easy to make, they provide a wonderful way to use up and preserve an overabundance of luscious fruits. Best of all, jams and jellies, with their rich, jewellike hues, make lovely special gifts for friends and family.

Equipment

Several pieces of equipment simplify the preparation of jams and jellies:

large pot—This item is essential. Select an eight- to ten-quart pot that will hold four times the volume you will be cooking, since jellies foam when boiled rapidly. The pot should have a heavy, flat bottom.

jelly bag and stand (or cheesecloth and colander, or fruit press)—For crystal-clear jellies a jelly bag is needed for straining the fruit juices.

jelly (candy or deep-fat) thermometer—A thermometer takes the guesswork out of making jams and jellies. It is especially important when no commercial pectin is used.

jellmeter—A graduated glass tube with an opening at each end, a jellmeter is handy for measuring pectin levels in juices.

jelly glasses (or canning jars)—Glasses or straight-sided containers work well for jellies and can be sealed with paraffin. Canning jars with lids are best used for jams, preserves, conserves, and marmalades since paraffin seals tend to loosen on these products.

other useful kitchen equipment—quart measure, measuring cups and spoons, paring knives, food grinder, food mill, bowls, wire basket or colander, long-handled spoon, ladle, and household scale.

Jam and Jelly Ingredients

To jell, all jellies and jams require fruit, acid, pectin, and a sweetener in proper proportions. Other ingredients such as nuts are simply tasty extras.

Fruit: The main ingredient, fruit provides the characteristic flavor, color, and aroma for each jam and jelly. It also gives some of the pectin and acid needed to make a gel. Fruits that are firm yet just barely ripe are the richest in pectin and acid. But those low in pectin will still make good jams and jellies if combined with fruits high in pectin or combined with extracted pectin. Fruits high in pectin are: tart blackberries, boysenberries, Concord grapes, crab apples, cranberries, green gooseberries, loganberries, plums, fresh prunes, quinces, red currants, sour guavas, and tart apples. Those low in pectin are: apricots, blueberries, cherries, figs, peaches, pears, pineapples, raspberries, and strawberries.

Acid: Both flavor and gel formation benefit from the acid in fruit. If the acid level of the fruit is low, lemon juice is commonly added.

Pectin: A natural component of fruit, pectin is necessary for gel formation. For fruits low in pectin and fully ripe, commercial liquid or powdered pectin can be added to aid jelling. (Directions for use are on the package.) But most commercial pectins contain some sucrose (sugar) and require substantial quantities of sugar to set. Alternatives to commercial pectin include low-methoxyl pectin (see below) and homemade pectin (see opposite).

Using Low-Methoxyl Pectin

Low-methoxyl pectin differs from both commercial and natural pectins because it requires calcium salts instead of sugar to form a gel. The beauty of using this pectin is, therefore, that you are free to add as little or as much sweetening as you want. Best of all, jelly making with low-methoxyl pectin is simple. For information on where to obtain low-methoxyl pectin, see Appendix 4.

Prepare crushed fruit for jam or juice for jelly as usual, and place it in a large saucepan over medium heat. Bring it just to a boil.

Measure one-eighth cup honey (or to taste) and one-half teaspoon low-methoxyl pectin for each cup fruit or juice, and mix them well in a small bowl. Pour the mixture into the boiling fruit; stir until the honey and pectin are completely dissolved. Combine one-eighth teaspoon calcium salts with one-quarter cup water, then add one teaspoon of this solution for each cup fruit or juice. Stir quickly until well mixed. Remove one tablespoon of the jam or jelly to a cold plate, and chill briefly in the freezer to test whether it has jelled. Add juice or calcium salts, if necessary, to adjust consistency. Ladle into jars, adjust seals, and process in a boiling water bath for 15 minutes (see Canning, page 766).

Sweetener: Honey makes a pleasant-tasting change from the sugar traditionally used in making homemade jellies and jams. But there are some differences between the two. Sugar acts as a preservative and helps to firm the fruit, to produce a clear, bright color, and to heighten sweetness without changing the fruity flavor. Honey, too, is a preservative, but it gives a loose texture, slightly dark color, and mild honey flavor to the gel. In addition, honey tastes sweeter than sugar, so the amount of sweetener called for in a recipe must be reduced. Whenever possible, use a recipe specially developed for honey, since direct replacement usually does not give satisfactory results. Also, recipes for jams, preserves, and conserves made with honey give the most pleasing products; jellies made with honey are often disappointingly loose. When using honey, add it near the end of the cooking period to achieve maximum fruity flavor.

Make Your Own Pectin

Using homemade pectin, often called apple jelly stock, or extract, is one way to boost pectin levels without adding commercial pectin. To make pectin, choose mature apples that are rich in pectin and acid as well as abundant and inexpensive.

Wash four pounds of apples carefully, and cut them into thin slices (include the peel and core since both contain pectin). Put the apples and four pints of water in a large pot. Cover the pot and bring the water to a boil. Simmer rapidly for 20 minutes. Without squeezing, strain off the free-running juice through one thickness of cheesecloth or a jelly bag. Reserve the liquid and return it to the pot. Heat the juice until it is reduced by half. Test the pectin by using the pectin test (see page 781).

Use this pectin immediately for blending with other fruit juices to make jelly or jam, or preserve it by canning or freezing for future use. To can, seal and process for 15 minutes in a boiling water bath (see Canning, page 766). Six to eight tablespoons of homemade pectin replaces approximately one tablespoon of commercial liquid or powdered pectin in most recipes.

Making Jams and Jellies

The preliminary preparation of fruits destined for jams and jellies is the same as for table use. Simply wash the fruit thoroughly but gently, and pat dry. Use a cutting board and sharp knife, a grinder, or a blender to chop the fruit into small pieces.

NOTE: Fruits chopped in a grinder or blender tend to turn dark faster than those chopped by hand.

Extracting Juice

To extract juice, prepare the fruit as directed in the recipe. As a rule, berries are crushed without heating, while other fruits are chopped, then heated. Take care not to overcook the fruit; too much heat destroys pectin. Put the prepared fruit in a damp jelly bag or fruit press. The clearest jelly comes from juice that has dripped through a jelly bag without pressing. Though you get more juice with pressing, pressed juice tends to be cloudy. Re-strain pressed juice through a damp jelly bag or a double thickness of cheesecloth without squeezing.

Pectin Test

When making jellies without added pectin, use one-quarter underripe fruit, which has a high pectin content, and three-quarters fully ripe fruit. The underripe fruit helps assure jelling; the fully ripe fruit provides the best flavor.

These jellies require less sweetener per cup of fruit juice than do those with added pectin. If you know the amount of pectin in the fruit juice, you can determine how much sweetener you actually need. Use one of the following pectin tests to estimate the amount of pectin.

Jellmeter test: Pour fruit juice through the graduated glass tube (jellmeter). The rate of flow through the tube gives an estimate of the amount of pectin in the juice.

Alcohol test: Mix one tablespoon denatured (grain or ethyl) alcohol with one tablespoon extracted juice. Stir slightly to mix. Juices rich in pectin will form one transparent, firm, jellylike mass. Those low in pectin will form two or more small jellylike masses or particles. *(Never taste the alcohol mixture. It is poisonous!)*

Use a low ratio of sweetener to juice if the pectin level is high, and a slightly higher ratio if the pectin level is low.

Cooking the Fruit Mixture

For best results, carefully follow the directions given in your favorite jelly or jam recipe. And consider these pointers for fine-tuning your skills:

- Do not double or triple the recipe. Best results come from preparing a single batch at a time.
- Cook jams and jellies in a heavy pot over low heat to prevent scorching.
- Start timing the cooking as soon as the mixture comes to a rapid boil that cannot be stirred down.
- Skim off the foam that forms on the surface, as it will detract from the appearance of the finished product.
- Remove whole spices immediately after cooking to prevent darkening of conserves.
- Seal jams, preserves, marmalades in canning jars with screw bands and metal lids, and process for 15 minutes (see Using a Water Bath Canner, page 768). Jellies can often be safely sealed with paraffin, but in humid climates even these are more satisfactorily canned (see Sealing Jelly Jars with Paraffin, page 782).
- Gently shake jars of jams, preserves, and marmalades several times during cooling to distribute the fruit evenly. Also, use mostly fully ripe fruit since it is less likely to float to the top.

Testing for Jelling Point

A well-made jelly holds its shape when released from a mold, yet it is tender enough to cut with a spoon. Also, good jelly has a fresh fruit flavor, never a caramelized sugar taste. To determine when a jelly has reached the jelling point, use one of these three tests:

Temperature test: This is probably the most accurate test, but to get a reliable reading, it is essential that you know the boiling point for water in your area. Check the temperature of boiling water shortly before making the jelly; then cook the jelly mixture to a temperature 8°F higher than the boiling point of the water. At this point, the mixture should jell nicely when cool.

Sheet Test: This test requires a watchful eye. It is very popular but not entirely dependable. With a cool metal spoon scoop up a small amount of the boiling jelly mixture and raise it about a foot above the pot away from the steam. Quickly tip the spoon and let the jelly run off the side. If the syrup forms two drops that flow together and fall from the spoon as a sheet, the jelly is probably done. If it slides from the spoon as separate drops, cook the mixture a little longer, then test again.

Freezer Test: During this test the hot jelly mixture should be removed from the heat. Put a few drops of the jelly on a cold plate; then chill in the freezer for a few minutes. If the mixture jells, it is done.

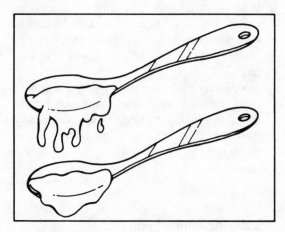

Sealing Jelly Jars with Paraffin

Hot paraffin is tricky to handle but will form a good, though not airtight, seal on jellies that have a smooth surface. Use an old saucepan or a small, clean metal can when working with paraffin. And always melt it in a double-boiler arrangement over an inch or two of water since paraffin can easily burst into flames. Heat the paraffin just until it melts. If too hot, paraffin will shrink from the sides of the jelly glasses as the jelly and the paraffin cool.

When the paraffin has melted, cautiously spoon one tablespoon of it onto the hot jelly mixture. Tilt the glass so that the paraffin flows over the entire surface and touches the glass at all points of seal. Prick any bubbles that appear. Use only one thin layer (one-eighth inch thick) of paraffin. Thick layers become brittle and pull from the sides of the glasses. When the jelly is cool and the paraffin hard, cover the glasses to protect them from dust.

Storing Jams and Jellies

The brilliant colors of homemade jams and jellies are very sensitive to bright light. To prevent fading in your jams and jellies, store them in a dark place. If you choose a spot that is also cool and dry, the overall quality of the unopened jars will stay high for up to a year. Once opened, jams and jellies should be stored in the refrigerator.

Uncooked jams will keep nicely in the freezer for a year. After thawing and opening an uncooked jam, store it in the refrigerator and use it within three weeks.

Jams and Jellies

Peach Jam

4 pounds peaches, peeled and pitted
¼ cup lemon juice
½ cup mild honey, or more to taste
¼ cup tapioca flour or starch*

Chop or coarsely grind peaches, blending with lemon juice. You should have 4 cups. Place fruit and lemon juice in a 6- to 8-quart saucepan, bring to a boil over medium heat, stirring constantly, and cook until peaches are very soft.

Stir, then slowly add honey, blending well. Add more honey if desired. Continue stirring and return to a full rolling boil. Add tapioca flour or starch and cook over medium heat, while stirring, until thickened, about 10 to 15 minutes.

Ladle into pint or ½-pint jars and process for 15 minutes in a boiling water bath (see Canning, page 766). When cool, check seals.

Yields 3 pints

*Tapioca flour or starch is available in oriental grocery stores.

Strawberry Jam

4 cups crushed fresh strawberries
½ cup orange blossom honey
¼ cup maple syrup
2 tablespoons tapioca flour or starch*
2 tablespoons water

In a large saucepan bring berries, honey, and syrup to a boil. Reduce heat to medium and cook until mixture is reduced by ⅓. You should have 3 cups.

Dissolve tapioca flour or starch in water. Stir into berries and cook until mixture thickens. Do not overcook. Ladle into ½-pint jars, seal, and process for 15 minutes in a boiling water bath (see Canning, page 766). When cool, check seals.

Yields 1½ pints

*Tapioca flour or starch is available in oriental grocery stores.

Apple Jelly

4½ pounds apples
¾ cup honey for each cup juice

Remove stems and dark spots from apples. Quarter but do not pare or core. Place apples in a 6- to 8-quart pot, add just enough water to half cover, and cook over low heat until soft, about 1 hour. Drain, using a jelly bag. (You will get more juice if you squeeze the bag, but it will make a cloudy jelly.)

Measure juice and pour into a large saucepan. Add honey. Boil until a good jelly test is obtained. Ladle into hot sterilized glasses and cover with paraffin.

Variation:

Mint Jelly: Just before removing apple jelly from heat, add a few mint leaves (about ¼ cup mint leaves to 1 quart juice) and a bit of natural green coloring. Stir, remove leaves, and ladle jelly into hot sterilized glasses. Cover with paraffin. This makes an attractive and delicious jelly to serve with lamb.

Yields 1½ cups

Butters

Apricot Butter

4 pounds apricots, chopped
½ cup honey
¼ teaspoon ground cinnamon
¼ teaspoon ground nutmeg

Puree apricots in batches in a blender. Then place in a Dutch oven or slow cooker. Add honey, cinnamon, and nutmeg. Cover and cook over low heat for 4 hours. (If butter is not as thick as desired, cook longer with lid off, stirring often.) Ladle into ½-pint jars, seal, and process for 15 minutes in a boiling water bath (see Canning, page 766). When cool, check seals.

Yields 4½ pints

Baked Apple Butter

18 pounds apples
8 cups water
1½ cups honey
juice and grated rind of 3 lemons
2 teaspoons ground cinnamon
1 teaspoon ground cloves
1 teaspoon ground allspice

Core and quarter apples. Place in 2 10- to 12-quart pots or 1 canning kettle and add water. Simmer for 1½ hours.

Preheat oven to 300°F.

Put apple pulp through a strainer, blender, or food mill and pour back into original pot (if it is ovenproof) or into a roasting pan. Add honey, lemon juice, rind, and spices.

Place apple pulp mixture in oven and cook slowly, stirring occasionally. It will take several hours — perhaps overnight — for butter to thicken sufficiently.

When thick enough for your taste, remove from oven and ladle into pint jars, seal, and process for 15 minutes in a boiling water bath (see Canning, page 766). When cool, check seals.

Yields about 4 pints

Yellow Peach Butter

>   6 cups sliced yellow peaches
>   ¾ cup water
>   ¼ cup lemon juice
>   10 whole cloves
>   1 stick of cinnamon, 2 inches long
>   1¼ cups honey

Combine peaches, water, and lemon juice in a large heavy-bottom saucepan. Cover and simmer until peaches are soft, about 10 to 15 minutes. Place in a blender and process to a puree. Return to saucepan. Add cloves and cinnamon and continue to cook, uncovered, over low heat to desired consistency, stirring occasionally. Remove cloves and cinnamon. Stir in honey. Immediately ladle into ½-pint jars, seal, and process in a boiling water bath for 15 minutes (see Canning, page 766). When cool, check seals.

Yields 1½ pints

Conserves and Preserves

Sweet Cherry Conserve

>   4 unpeeled medium-size oranges
>   2 cups water
>   8 cups pitted fresh sweet cherries
>   1½ to 2 cups honey, or to taste
>   ¾ cup lemon juice
>   1½ teaspoons ground cinnamon
>   12 whole cloves
>   2 cups pecan halves or walnut quarters

Slice oranges thinly and remove seeds.

Place orange slices in a large saucepan and add water. Cover and simmer until tender, about 10 minutes. Add cherries, honey, lemon juice, cinnamon, and cloves. Simmer, covered, for 30 minutes. Add nuts. Immediately ladle into pint jars, seal, and process in a boiling water bath for 15 minutes (see Canning, page 766). When cool, check seals.

Yields 4 pints

Ginger and Pear Conserve

>   3 pounds Seckel pears (21 to 24)
>   ½ unpeeled orange

>   1 tablespoon chopped peeled ginger root or 1
>   piece ginger root, about 1½ inches square,
>   peeled
>   ½ cup honey
>   1 tablespoon lemon juice

Peel, core, and slice pears. Remove seeds from orange and chop finely. If desired, chop half the amount of peeled and cored pears in a blender along with orange. Make a spice bag of cheesecloth, and put ginger into it.

In a large saucepan combine pears and orange, spice bag, honey, and lemon juice. Cover, bring slowly to a simmer, and cook until pears are tender. Remove cover and continue to cook, stirring occasionally, until desired consistency is reached. Immediately ladle into ½-pint jars, seal, and process for 15 minutes in a boiling water bath (see Canning, page 766). When cool, check seals.

Yields about 1½ pints

Fresh Strawberry Preserves

>   2 cups water
>   1 envelope unflavored gelatin
>   2 cups sliced fresh strawberries (about 1 quart
>   whole strawberries)
>   1 teaspoon lemon juice
>   ⅓ cup honey

Pour 1 cup water into a large saucepan and sprinkle gelatin over it. Let stand for 5 minutes.

In a blender puree ½ the berries with 1 cup water, lemon juice, and honey. Add remaining berries and pureed mixture to saucepan. Heat just to a boil, stirring constantly. Ladle into ½-pint jars and refrigerate. For longer keeping, freeze.

Yields about 2 pints

Drying

Drying, one of the oldest ways of preserving food, is being rediscovered by people who want a low-cost, energy-efficient method of putting up fresh fruits, vegetables, and herbs. Meanwhile, backpackers, cyclists, and the like are also discovering the benefits of dried foods, which are light in weight, wholesome, and easy to prepare.

Drying preserves food by removing 80 to 90 percent of the water that enzymes and spoilage organisms—molds, yeasts, bacteria—thrive on. Because so much water has been removed, dried foods take up one-sixth to one-third the storage space of whole foods, yet all their goodness remains. Actually, dried foods without rehydration, when compared by weight to whole foods, have more calories, flavor, and nutrients.

Equipment

To dry foods at home, you will need a solar dryer, an electric dehydrator, or an oven. Several Rodale Press books—*Stocking Up* (1977), *Solar Food Dryer* (1981), and *Home Foods Systems Catalog* (1980), among others—have excellent directions for constructing a dryer yourself. These books also give pointers on selecting commercially made dehydrators.

Drying indoors with controlled heat has several advantages. Drying goes on day and night, unaffected by the weather. Controlled-heat dryers shorten the drying time and extend the drying season to include late-maturing fruits and vegetables. Best of all, foods dried this way have better color and flavor and rehydrate more effectively.

Preparation for Drying

For full-flavored dried fruits and vegetables, select those that are ripe and of peak quality. Wash the produce thoroughly and peel the varieties with thick skins. To hasten drying, cut the produce into small pieces or slice it very thinly. Keep the size of the pieces uniform so that drying is even. Blanch the produce, then loosely place it on drying trays in single layers. (For specific instructions see Drying table, page 788.)

Blanching

Blanching aids the retention of quality in dried foods in three ways. It hastens drying by softening the exterior of the food, making it easier for moisture to escape; it stops the action of enzymes which can cause quality to deteriorate during storage; and it facilitates rehydration.

To blanch produce for drying, follow the general steam-blanching directions for freezing (see Blanching, page 754), but shorten the length of the blanching time slightly since pieces of food cut for drying are exceptionally small and thin. Likewise, the chilling step mentioned for freezing can be skipped because foods are heated somewhat during drying. Without chilling to stop the blanching process, however, it is easy to over-blanch. Again, compensate by reducing the blanching time.

Preventing Discoloration

Some fruits—apples, apricots, bananas, nectarines, peaches, pears—tend to discolor when sliced. You can preserve the color by soaking the slices in a solution of one tablespoon lemon juice to one quart water. Soak the fruits for five minutes, then drain them and spread on trays to dry.

Drying Methods

Whether drying in the sun or with controlled heat, try to keep the heat at 140°F for at least two-thirds of the drying time. Build the heat up slowly from 120°F so that the outside of the food will not harden and inhibit the release of moisture from the center. Stir the food often (every 30 to 60 minutes) to keep drying even.

To dry in the oven: Place food directly on oven racks, one piece deep, or, if the slats are too far apart, cover the racks with nylon mesh or cheesecloth and then put the food on top of the cloth. Trays made of wooden slats and mesh, such as those used for drying in the sun, are best if additional trays are needed. Separate the trays by placing three-inch blocks of wood at each corner when stacking them in the oven. Leave the door ajar and use a small fan to aid air circulation.

To dry in the sun: Use a well-designed solar collector dryer with good ventilation and covers to protect the food from insects. Start early in the day and dry in full sun on days when the humidity is low. Bring the food in at night to avoid dampness from night dew. Drying should be as quick as possible (about two days), to avoid decomposition, but not so rapid that the food scorches.

Testing Dryness

Too much moisture left in dried foods will permit mold to grow during storage, so check foods carefully every day during the drying process. Select a few pieces from the trays, allowing them to cool before testing since hot foods often seem to contain more moisture than they really have. In general, appropriately dried fruits will have no moisture when cut and squeezed. They will feel leathery and be resilient. Well-dried vegetables are brittle and tough and rattle when stirred on the trays. (See Drying table, page 788.)

Pasteurizing and Conditioning Dried Foods

Once the food is dried, pasteurize it to ensure that no insect eggs will hatch or harmful spoilage organisms will develop. Pasteurizing is necessary since the low heat used in drying is not high enough to kill contaminants. To pasteurize, spread the dried food one inch thick on baking sheets or trays and heat for 10 to 15 minutes in a preheated 175°F oven. Cool the food thoroughly.

After pasteurizing the food, condition it by putting it in an open container in a warm, dry area. Cover the container loosely to keep curious insects and animals out. During the next four days, stir the contents several times to bring drier pieces in contact with the more moist ones. In that way, moisture content will be evenly distributed. When conditioning has been done, the food is ready for storage.

NOTE: If the food seems too moist after conditioning, return it to the dryer until the proper consistency is reached.

Storing Dried Foods

If stored under the right conditions, dried fruits will retain good quality for up to a year and vegetables for up to four months. Keep dried foods in tightly closed jars or insect-resistant plastic bags in a cool, dry place. If appropriate shelf space is not available, put dried foods in the freezer. Resist the temptation to store the colorful jars or bags in an area exposed to bright light, because light fades dried foods readily. Instead, protect the foods by placing the containers in brown bags or by wrapping containers in foil.

Using Dried Foods

Dried foods are scrumptious when eaten out of hand or used in hearty vegetable stews, refreshing cold fruit soups, and satisfying casseroles. Fairly crisp dried fruits and vegetables can be ground into flour and used as flavorful, nutritious additions to crackers, cookies, quick breads, yeast breads, and pancakes. (For every cup of flour called for in a recipe, you can replace up to one-quarter cup with finely ground fruit or vegetable flour.)

For some dishes, dried foods give the nicest texture and flavor when rehydrated before use, but for others dried foods work well while still dry. Soups and stews, for example, have so much liquid that rehydration can be skipped. However, casseroles are usually light in liquid so that rehydration before combining ingredients is best. Except for uncooked dishes such as salads, which need fresh ingredients, any dish takes herbs in the dry state beautifully. Baked goods, on the other hand, are enhanced by plumped berries, raisins, and currants.

To rehydrate fruits and vegetables: Put food into a saucepan; then pour in enough boiling water to just cover the food (too much water will dilute the flavor). Next, cover the pan and place it over low heat—keep the water hot but not boiling. Rehydration will be uneven, so stop the process when most of the food is ready. (For several suggested rehydration times, see Rehydration table, page 790.)

Fruit Leather

A variation of dried fruit slices, fruit leather is fruit pulp (from juicing apples, apricots, peaches, prunes, or other fruit) which is dried to form a naturally sweet, confectionlike food that will keep in good condition for one year or more. Fruit leather can be made from almost any fruit or any combination of fruits.

Apricot, Peach, or Nectarine Leather

8 pounds apricots, peaches, or nectarines, pitted
1½ cups pineapple juice
¼ cup honey, or more to taste
3 teaspoons almond extract (optional)

Place fruit and pineapple juice in a large heavy pot. Cover, and cook over low heat until soft. Pour fruit into a strainer and catch juice in a small bowl. Drain juice well, lifting fruit from sides of strainer to allow all the juice to run out freely. (The more juice strained out, the quicker the process of leather making.) Can or freeze juice for later use, or drink it fresh.

Put fruit through a blender, food mill, or sieve, removing skins for a smooth product, or use skins as part of pulp for the leather. Sweeten pulp with honey and add almond extract (if used). Pulp should be as thick as apple butter or more so. Spread it on lightly oiled baking sheets, or on baking sheets covered with freezer paper or plastic wrap, so that it is ¼ inch thick. If it is much thicker than this, it will take very long to dry. Place baking sheets in a low oven or food dryer. If using an oven, turn control to warm (120°F) and leave oven door slightly open to allow moisture to escape. (Pulp should dry in about 12 hours in oven.)

When leather is dry enough to be lifted or gently pulled from baking sheets, place leather on wire racks so that it can dry on both sides. Dust lightly with cornstarch or arrowroot when all stickiness has disappeared. Then stack in layers with freezer paper, wax paper, or foil between each sheet. Cover with freezer paper, wax paper, or foil and store in a cool dry place.

Makes 4 pieces, about 10 × 5 inches each

Apple Leather

8 pounds apples, peeled and cored
1½ cups apple cider
½ to 1 cup honey
ground cinnamon, cloves, and/or nutmeg, to taste (optional)

Cut apples into pieces and put through a grinder. In a large bowl catch juice which runs from grinder and return it to ground apples. (A blender may also be used. It mashes a limited number of apple pieces at a time, but there is no escaping juice.)

Place ground apples and juice in a large heavy pot and add 1 cup apple cider. (Apples are drier than other fruits and will scorch as they are heated if no liquid is added to pot.) Place pot over low heat and bring apples to a boil. Add more cider if needed to prevent apples from sticking to bottom of pot. Add honey when mixture looks somewhat clear and is boiling well. Then add spices (if used).

When mixture reaches consistency of a very thick sauce, remove from heat and put through a grinder, blender, or food processor. Return to heat and cook to consistency of thick applesauce. Spread pulp on oiled baking sheets, or on baking sheets lined with freezer paper or plastic wrap, so that it is about ¼ inch thick. Dry apple pulp as directed in recipe for Apricot, Peach, or Nectarine Leather (see opposite). When it can be lifted from baking sheets, place on wire racks so that it can dry on both sides. Dust leather lightly with cornstarch or arrowroot when all stickiness has disappeared. Wrap and store as for Apricot, Peach, or Nectarine Leather.

Makes 4 pieces, about 10 × 5 inches each

Drying Fruits and Vegetables

Food	Preparation	Characteristics after Drying
Apples	Use firm fruit; peel, core, and slice; blanch for 4 minutes.	soft, pliable, slightly tough
Apricots	Use ripe fruit; pit and slice; dip in ascorbic acid solution; blanch for 4 minutes.	soft, pliable
Artichokes	Use only tender hearts; trim leaves, cut in halves; blanch for 5 minutes.	brittle
Asparagus	Trim scales and ends; no slicing; blanch for 5 minutes.	very tough to brittle
Avocados	Drying not recommended.	
Bananas	Slice; dip in ascorbic acid solution; no blanching.	pliable to crisp
Beans		
Green	Use tender beans; French cut; blanch for 6 minutes.	brittle, crisp
Lima	Shell and wash; blanch for 5 minutes.	hard, brittle
Beets	Remove tops and roots; slice; blanch until tender.	tough to brittle
Blackberries	Drying not recommended.	
Blueberries	Remove stems; blanch to break skins.	leathery, pliable, similar to raisins
Broccoli	Trim tough stalks; split large stalks; blanch for 4 minutes.	crisp, brittle
Brussels sprouts	Drying not recommended.	
Cabbage	Core and shred; blanch for 2 to 3 minutes.	brittle
Carrots	Peel; slice; blanch for 4 minutes.	tough to brittle
Cauliflower	Use only florets; remove from core; split stems; blanch for 3 minutes.	crisp, slightly browned
Celery	Trim base; cut into ½-inch slices; blanch for 1 minute.	very brittle
Cherries	Remove stems; cut in half and pit; blanch for 1 minute.	leathery, pliable, similar to raisins
Coconuts	Drain milk; remove meat from shell; grate or slice; no blanching.	leathery to crisp
Corn	Husk ears and remove silk; cut from cob; blanch for 5 minutes.	dry, brittle
Cucumbers	Peel; slice; blanch for 1 minute.	crisp
Dates	No pretreatment necessary.	leathery, deep russet color

Drying Fruits and Vegetables—*Continued*

Food	Preparation	Characteristics after Drying
Eggplants	Peel; cut into ½-inch slices; blanch for 4 minutes.	leathery to brittle
Figs	Cut in half to shorten drying; no blanching.	leathery
Garlic	Peel; cut into thin pieces; no blanching.	crisp
Grapefruit rind	Scrape out bitter white part; no blanching.	crisp
Grapes, seedless	Blanch long enough to split skins.	raisins
Horseradish	Trim tops; grate or slice; no blanching.	brittle
Lemon rind	Scrape out bitter white part; no blanching.	crisp
Lettuce	Drying not recommended.	
Mushrooms	Trim woody portion from stem; cut into ½-inch slices; blanch for 3 minutes. Warning: Do not dry poisonous mushrooms.	leathery to crisp
Nectarines	Use mature fruit; pit and slice; blanch for 2 minutes.	leathery, pliable
Okra	Cut off tips; slice; blanch for 5 minutes.	tough to brittle
Onions	Remove skin and trim bulb ends; dice; no blanching.	brittle
Orange rind	Scrape out bitter white part; no blanching.	crisp
Papayas	Remove seeds; peel and slice; no blanching.	leathery to crisp
Parsnips	Trim tops; peel and slice; blanch for 5 minutes.	tough to brittle
Peaches	Use ripe fruit; blanch to remove skins; pit and slice; dip in ascorbic acid solution.	soft, pliable, leathery
Pears	Use ripe fruit; peel; blanch for 2 minutes.	soft, pliable, leathery
Peas	Use fresh peas; shell; blanch for 3 minutes.	wrinkled, brittle

Peppers
    Chili
    Green
	
	Wear rubber gloves; dice; blanching optional.
	Dice; blanching optional.
		
		leathery to brittle
		leathery to brittle

Pineapples	Use ripe fruit; peel and core; blanch for 1 minute.	leathery, not sticky
Plums	Cut in ⅛-inch slices; no blanching.	leathery, pliable

Potatoes
    Sweet
    White
	
	Grate, slice, or dice; blanch for 3 minutes.
	Peel; grate, slice, or dice; blanch for 6 minutes.
		
		tough to brittle
		crisp, brittle

[*continued*]

Drying Fruits and Vegetables—*Continued*

Food	Preparation	Characteristics after Drying
Pumpkins	Remove stems, seeds, and fibrous tissue; peel outer layer; blanch for 3 minutes.	very tough to brittle
Radishes	Drying not recommended.	
Raspberries	Drying not recommended.	
Rhubarb	Trim and slice diagonally; blanch until tender but not soft.	tough to crisp
Spinach	Trim leaves; blanch until slightly wilted.	crisp, crumbles easily
Squashes		
Summer	Cut into thin slices; no peeling; blanch for 3 minutes except when making chips.	leathery to brittle
Winter	Drying not recommended.	
Strawberries	Remove stems; cut into halves or thirds; blanch for 1 minute.	leathery, pliable
Tangerine rind	Scrape out bitter white part; no blanching.	crisp
Tomatoes	Slice; blanch for 3 minutes.	leathery
Turnips	Remove tops and roots; slice; blanch for 5 minutes.	very tough to brittle

Approximate Water and Rehydration Time Needed for Some Popular Dried Vegetables

Dried Vegetable	Quantity (cups)	Water (cups)	Rehydration Time (minutes)	Yield (cups)
Beans, green	¾	2	45	2½
Cabbage	1	1	40	1½
Corn	1	2	50	2¾
Greens	3	1½	15	1½
Squashes, summer	1	1	40	1
Tomatoes	1	1	30	1
Vegetables, mixed (for soup)	⅛	1	10	1

Appendix 1
Summary of Major Nutrients

A diet high in a variety of nutrients is essential for good health. Most unprocessed foods— vegetables, meats, fruits, grains, fish, poultry, dairy products, nuts—are excellent sources of nutrition, and a potpourri of those foods should be included in your diet every day. Excessively processed foods lack important nutrients. For the best in food values and flavor, choose unprocessed foods at every opportunity.

The following table highlights the major nutrients necessary for optimum health, along with some of the best food sources for each nutrient. Check the table, too, for food preparation techniques that minimize nutrient loss.

Nutrient	Good Food Sources	Kitchen Preparation	Health Functions
Carbohydrates	fruits, vegetables, whole grain products	Store in cool area. Avoid prolonged cooking at high temperatures.	Energy supply. Metabolic role in utilization of fats and proteins. Muscle contraction. Conduction of nerve impulses.
Fats	dairy products, fish, meats, nuts, poultry, seeds, vegetable oils, whole grain products	Store in cool area. Avoid cooking at high temperatures. Avoid reheating and reusing. Avoid lengthy storage.	Concentrated energy source. Carrier of fat-soluble vitamins. Fuel reserve for body. Protein-sparing action. Regulation of uptake and excretion of nutrients by cells. Insulator against temperature changes. Slows emptying time of stomach and delays onset of sensation of hunger.

NOTE: Other important elements in the diet include biotin, chloride, choline, chromium, copper, fiber, fluoride, iodine, manganese, pantothenic acid, phosphorus, selenium, sodium, vitamin K, and water.

Nutrient	Good Food Sources	Kitchen Preparation	Health Functions
Protein	dairy products; eggs; fish; meats; poultry; legumes,* nuts, seeds, and whole grain products when combined with dairy products or with each other	Avoid extreme heat.	Growth, repair, and maintenance of tissues. Regulation of body processes. Formation of enzymes and hormones. Regulation of water balance. Maintenance of chemical neutrality (neither acid nor alkaline). Formation of antibodies.
Vitamins Vitamin A	apricots; broccoli; dark green leafy vegetables; fish-liver oils; liver; yellow, orange, and red vegetables such as carrots, pumpkins, and winter squash	Cook or process in covered utensils. Avoid frying at high temperatures. Avoid over-exposure to air.	Smooth, healthy-looking skin. Resistance to infection and other diseases. Normal vision. Healthy mucous membranes.
Vitamin B_1 (thiamine)	brewer's yeast, dark green leafy vegetables, lean meats, legumes,* nuts, sunflower seeds, variety meats,† wheat germ, whole grain products	Cook in a minimum of water, or steam. Avoid prolonged cooking at high temperatures. Avoid using baking soda with B_1 foods except as a leavening agent in baked products.	Emotional stability. Energy. Memory.
Vitamin B_2 (riboflavin)	almonds, asparagus, broccoli, dairy products, eggs, variety meats,† wheat germ, whole grain products, wild rice	Cook in a minimum of water, or steam. Cut vegetables into large pieces rather than small. Avoid overexposure to light. Cook in covered pots.	Enzyme functions in the metabolism of proteins, sugars, and fats. Essential for growth.
Vitamin B_6 (pyridoxine)	bananas, brewer's yeast, buckwheat flour (dark), hazelnuts, peanuts, poultry, rice, salmon, sunflower seeds, tomatoes, variety meats,† wheat germ, whole grain products	Avoid excessive processing and refining when possible. (Freezing, canning, and milling result in substantial reduction of B_6.) Cook in a minimum of water.	Production of antibodies. Elimination of excess fluids in premenstrual women. Emotional stability. Healthy skin. Central nervous system regulation.
Vitamin B_{12} (cyano-cobalamin)	eggs, fish, meats, milk, variety meats†	Avoid cooking at high temperatures.	Normal growth. Healthy nervous system. Normal red blood cell formation.

*Legumes include peas, beans, peanuts, and lentils.
†Variety meats include liver, heart, and kidney.

Nutrient	Good Food Sources	Kitchen Preparation	Health Functions
Folacin (folate)	asparagus, brewer's yeast, broccoli, dark green leafy vegetables, legumes,* liver, nuts, onions, tempeh, wheat germ, whole grain products	Avoid cooking at high temperatures. Process and cook in a minimum of water, or steam. Avoid overexposure to light. Avoid storing at room temperature.	New red blood cell production. Found in the most rapidly growing tissues, such as bone marrow, alimentary tract lining, or tumors.
Niacin	brewer's yeast, fish, legumes,* poultry, variety meats,† whole grain products	Niacin is very stable in heat, light, acid, alkali, and oxygen. Little is lost in normal food processing and preparation.	Reduced blood cholesterol levels. Mental and emotional health. Aids metabolism of carbohydrates, fats, and amino acids.
Vitamin C (ascorbic acid)	broccoli, brussels sprouts, cabbage, cantaloupes, cauliflower, citrus fruits and their juices, currants, dark green leafy vegetables, green peppers, persimmons, pimientos, strawberries, tomatoes	Avoid excessive processing— eat foods raw or minimally cooked when possible. Cook in a minimum of water, or steam. Avoid prolonged cooking. Avoid soaking vegetables in water. Cut foods into large pieces rather than small. Avoid overexposure to air and light. Avoid storing at room temperature.	Formation of teeth and bones. Bone-fracture healing. Wound and burn healing. Resistance to infection and other diseases. Collagen formation.
Vitamin D	fish-liver oils, herring, mackerel, salmon, sardines, tuna	Avoid overexposure to air.	Bone structure. Remineralization of mature bone. Facilitates the absorption and utilization of calcium and phosphorus.
Vitamin E	almonds, corn oil, hazelnuts, olive oil, peanuts, safflower oil, sesame oil, soybean oil, sunflower seeds, wheat germ, wheat germ oil	Avoid overexposure to air. Avoid deep frying. Avoid freezing.	Healthy red blood cells, heart, and skeletal muscles. Possible retardation of the aging process through protection of body fats from oxidation. Helps fight effects of air pollutants such as lead, mercury, ozone.

*Legumes include peas, beans, peanuts, and lentils.
†Variety meats include liver, heart, and kidney.

Nutrient	Good Food Sources	Kitchen Preparation	Health Functions
Minerals Calcium	almonds; brewer's yeast; broccoli; dark green leafy vegetables; hazelnuts; milk, cheese, and most dairy products; salmon; soybeans; tempeh; tofu; watercress	Cook in a minimum of water, or steam. Avoid excessive processing and refining when possible. Avoid discarding outer leaves of vegetables when possible.	Blood clotting. Normal functioning of nerve tissues. Normal pulse and cardiac contraction. Formation and growth of bones and teeth.
Iron	apricots, blackstrap molasses, brewer's yeast, dark green leafy vegetables, eggs, legumes,* nuts, sunflower seeds, variety meats,† wheat germ, whole grain products	Simmer (rather than boil) in a minimum of water, or steam. Avoid prolonged cooking. Use vegetable stocks for soups or gravies when possible.	Blood formation. Transporting of oxygen within the body.
Magnesium	brown rice, dark green leafy vegetables, molasses, nuts, peas, soybeans, tofu, whole grain products	Cook in a minimum of water, or steam. Avoid excessive processing and refining when possible.	Biological reactions within the cell. Conduction of nerve impulses. Normal muscle contraction. Healthy heart, muscles, nerves, brain, kidneys, liver, and other organs. Maintenance of normal basic metabolism.
Potassium	apples, apricots, avocados, bananas, beef, blackstrap molasses, brewer's yeast, broccoli, chicken, halibut, oranges, peanuts, potatoes, raisins, sesame seeds, sunflower seeds, tomatoes, tuna, wheat germ	Cook in a minimum of water. Avoid excessive processing and refining when possible. Retain meat drippings, remove fat, and use remaining liquid for gravies.	Biological reactions within the cell. Healthy kidneys, heart, and skeletal muscles.
Zinc	beef, cheese, eggs, fish, green beans, lamb, lima beans, meats, nuts, wheat germ, whole grain products	Cook in a minimum of water. Retain meat drippings, remove fat, and use remaining liquid for gravies.	Production and growth of new healing cells. Healthy skin. Numerous enzyme actions throughout the body. Carbon dioxide exchange. Normal maintenance of vitamin A blood levels.

*Legumes include peas, beans, peanuts, and lentils.
†Variety meats include liver, heart, and kidney.

Appendix 2
Caloric Content of Some Common Foods

Food	Amount	Calories
BEVERAGES		
Alcoholic		
Beer	12 ounces	151
Whiskey, gin, rum, vodka, etc.		
80 proof	1½ ounces	97
86 proof	1½ ounces	105
Wine		
Dessert	3½ ounces	141
Table	3½ ounces	87
Fruit drinks and juices		
Apple juice	6 ounces	87
Apricot nectar	6 ounces	107
Cocoa, in 1 cup water	1 ounce	102
Cranberry juice cocktail	6 ounces	124
Grape juice	6 ounces	125
Lemonade	6 ounces	81
Orange juice	6 ounces	84
Prune juice	6 ounces	148
Soda		
Club	12 ounces	0
Cola	12 ounces	144
Cream	12 ounces	160
Fruit-flavored	12 ounces	171
Ginger ale	12 ounces	113
Tonic	12 ounces	113
Vegetable juices		
Tomato juice cocktail	6 ounces	38
Vegetable juice cocktail	6 ounces	31

Food	Amount	Calories
BREADS		
Biscuits	2	206
Boston brown bread	1 slice	95
Crackers		
Butter	5	87
Cheese	10	150
Cheese-peanut butter sandwiches	4	139
Graham	1	55
Rye wafers	5	112
Saltines	4	48
Italian	1 slice	56
Muffins, blueberry	1	112
Pancakes, from mix, with milk and eggs	1 (6-inch diameter)	164
Pizza, with cheese topping	1 slice	153
Pretzels, thin	5	117
Rolls, hard	1	156
Rye	1 slice	61
Stuffing, bread	½ cup	208
Waffles, from mix, with milk and eggs	1 (7-inch diameter)	206
White	1 slice	76
Whole wheat	1 slice	67

Food	Amount	Calories
CONDIMENTS		
Jams and preserves	1 tablespoon	54
Marmalade	1 tablespoon	51
Mayonnaise	1 tablespoon	101
Olives, mission	5 large	44
Salad dressing, commercial	1 tablespoon	66
Sauerkraut	½ cup	21
DAIRY FOODS		
Cheeses		
Blue or Roquefort	1 ounce	104
Camembert	1 ounce	85
Cheddar	1 ounce	113
Cottage, creamed	6 ounces	180
Swiss	1 ounce	104
Cream		
Sweet	1 tablespoon	32
Whipped	1 tablespoon	27
Sour, cultured	1 tablespoon	25
Ice cream, vanilla	½ cup	127
Milk, whole	6 ounces	119
Yogurt, low-fat, plain	1 cup	113
DESSERTS		
Cakes		
Chocolate, with icing	1 small piece	277
Fruitcake	1 slice (1 ounce)	114
Gingerbread	1 piece (3 × 3 × 2 inches)	371
Pound cake	1 slice (1 ounce)	142
Sponge cake	1 slice (2 ounces)	196
Cookies		
Assorted	6	250
Brownies, with nuts	1 (3 × 3 × 1 inch)	97
Chocolate chip	1	51
Fig bars	1	50
Gingersnaps	1	29
Macaroons	1	90
Marshmallow	1	74
Oatmeal, with raisins	1	59
Oreo-type	1	50
Raisin, biscuit-type	1	67
Sugar wafers	1 large	44
Vanilla wafers	1 large	19
Cream puffs, filled	1	303

Food	Amount	Calories
Custard, baked	1 cup	305
Doughnuts	1	164
Gelatin dessert, made with water	1 cup	142
Pies		
Apple	1 piece (⅛ pie)	302
Banana custard	1 piece (⅛ pie)	252
Blueberry	1 piece (⅛ pie)	286
Boston cream	1 piece (⅛ pie)	208
Coconut custard	1 piece (⅛ pie)	268
Lemon meringue	1 piece (⅛ pie)	268
Mince	1 piece (⅛ pie)	320
Pecan	1 piece (⅛ pie)	431
Pumpkin	1 piece (⅛ pie)	241
Puddings		
Bread, with raisins	½ cup	248
Chocolate	½ cup	193
Rice, with raisins	½ cup	194
Tapioca cream	½ cup	111
EGGS		
Hard-cooked	1 large	82
FATS AND OILS		
Butter	1 pat	36
Margarine	1 pat	36
Oils, vegetable	1 tablespoon	120
FISH (*see also* Shellfish)		
Bluefish, broiled or baked with butter	6 ounces	270
Fish sticks, breaded	6 ounces	300
Flounder, baked with butter	6 ounces	342
Halibut, broiled with butter	6 ounces	288
Salmon		
Baked, with butter	6 ounces	312
Sockeye, canned	3 ounces	145
Sardines, canned (drained)	1 can	187
Tuna, canned		
Oil-packed		
Drained	6½ ounces	309
With oil	6½ ounces	530
Water-packed	6½ ounces	234

Food	Amount	Calories
FRUITS		
Apples	1 medium-size	80
Applesauce	½ cup	116
Apricots		
Fresh	3	55
Dried	¼ cup	85
Avocados	½	188
Bananas	1	101
Blueberries		
Fresh	½ cup	45
Frozen, sweetened	½ cup	121
Cherries, fresh	10	47
Citrus		
Grapefruit	½	40
Oranges	1	65
Tangerines	1	46
Dates	5	110
Grapes, seedless	10	34
Mangoes	1	152
Muskmelons		
Cantaloupe	½	82
Casaba	1 wedge ($^1/_{10}$ melon)	38
Honeydew	1 wedge ($^1/_{10}$ melon)	49
Nectarines	1	88
Peaches		
Fresh	1	58
Dried	5 large halves	190
Pears, Bartlett	1	100
Pineapple		
Fresh	2 slices	88
Canned, with syrup	2 slices	156
Plums	1	32
Prunes	5	137
Raisins	$^1/_3$ cup	124
Watermelon	1 wedge (4 inches thick)	111
GRAINS AND GRAIN PRODUCTS		
Amaranth, cooked	1 ounce	109
Brown rice, cooked	½ cup	116
Cornmeal, degermed, cooked	3½ ounces	50
Oatmeal, cooked	1 cup	132
Wheat bran	1 ounce	60
Wheat germ, toasted	6 tablespoons	138
LEGUMES		
Dried beans		
Mung, sprouted	1 cup	37

Food	Amount	Calories
Navy		
Baked, Boston-style, with pork	1 cup	311
Cooked	1 cup	224
Soybeans		
Cooked	1 cup	234
Tofu	1 piece (2½ × 2¾ × 1 inch)	86
Lentils, cooked	1 cup	212
Peanuts		
Roasted in shell	10	105
Peanut butter	1 tablespoon	94
Peas		
Black-eyed, cooked	1 cup	174
Split, cooked	1 cup	232
MEATS*		
Beef		
Corned	3 ounces	316
Ground		
Regular	3 ounces	245
Lean	3 ounces	185
Pot roast		
Lean and fat	6 ounces	490
Lean only	5 ounces	280
Rib roast		
Lean and fat	6 ounces	750
Lean only	5.4 ounces	375
Steak		
Round, broiled		
Lean and fat	6 ounces	440
Lean only	4.8 ounces	260
Sirloin, broiled		
Lean and fat	6 ounces	660
Lean only	4 ounces	230
Lamb chops, lean	2 (5.2 ounces)	280
Pork		
Bacon	2 slices	86
Chops, lean and fat	2 thick (3.5 ounces each)	520
Ham		
Boiled	2 ounces	135
Cured, lean and fat	6 ounces	490
Roast, lean and fat	6 ounces	620
Sausage	1 patty (2 ounces before cooking)	129
Veal		
Cutlet, medium fat	6 ounces	370
Roast, medium fat	6 ounces	460

*All meat values are for cooked meat.

Food	Amount	Calories
Luncheon meats		
Bologna	2 ounces	170
Liverwurst	3 ounces	265
Salami	3 ounces	145
Variety meats		
Gizzard, chicken,		
simmered	6 ounces	253
Heart		
Beef, braised	6 ounces	323
Calf, braised	6 ounces	354
Liver		
Beef, fried	6 ounces	390
Calf, fried	6 ounces	448
Poultry, simmered	6 ounces	283
Sweetbreads, calf, braised	6 ounces	288
Tongue, beef, braised	6 ounces	415
Tripe	6 ounces	220

NUTS AND SEEDS

Food	Amount	Calories
Almonds	about 11	85
Brazil nuts	6 large	185
Cashews, roasted in oil	about 14 large	159
Pecans	10 halves	124
Pumpkin seeds	1 ounce	157
Sesame seeds	1 ounce	161
Sunflower seeds	1 ounce	160
Walnuts, English	14 halves	185

PASTA

Food	Amount	Calories
Macaroni, with cheese	1 cup	430
Noodles	½ cup	100
Spaghetti, with meatballs, tomato sauce, and Parmesan cheese	1 cup	332

POULTRY AND GAME

Food	Amount	Calories
Chicken		
Chicken à la king	1 cup	468
Chicken and noodles	1 cup	367
Chicken fricassee	1 cup	386
Fried (including bone)	½ breast, 2 drumsticks (7.5 ounces)	335
Roasted, flesh, skin, and giblets	½ pound	549
Roasted, white meat only	½ pound	413
Duck, roasted, flesh and skin	6 ounces	558
Goose, roasted, flesh and skin	6 ounces	756
Rabbit, stewed, flesh	6 ounces	371
Turkey, roasted, white and dark meat	6 ounces	324

Food	Amount	Calories
SHELLFISH (*see also* Fish)		
Crab, deviled	1 cup	451
Lobster, cooked	1 cup	138
Oysters, raw	3 ounces	57
Scallops, breaded and fried	6⅔ ounces	367
Shrimp, french-fried	3 ounces	192

SWEETENERS

Food	Amount	Calories
Honey	1 tablespoon	64
Molasses, blackstrap	1 tablespoon	43
Sugar, granulated	1 tablespoon	48
Syrups, table blend	1 tablespoon	60

VEGETABLES

Food	Amount	Calories
Amaranth, raw greens	1 cup	20
Asparagus, cooked	4 spears	12
Beans, cooked		
Green	1 cup	31
Lima	1 cup	189
Beets, cooked	1 cup	218
Broccoli, cooked	1 cup	40
Brussels sprouts, cooked	½ cup	28
Cabbage, cooked	1 cup	31
Carrots		
Raw	1	30
Cooked, sliced	½ cup	24
Cauliflower, cooked	½ cup	14
Celery	1 large stalk	7
Corn		
Cooked on the cob	1 ear	70
Canned	½ cup	70
Cucumbers	1 small	25
Eggplant, cooked and diced	1 cup	38
Kale, cooked	½ cup	22
Lettuce	1 head	72
Mushrooms, sliced	½ cup	10
Onions, sliced	¼ cup	11
Peas, cooked	⅓ cup	41
Peppers, green	1 large	36
Potatoes		
Baked	1 large	145
French fried	10 (4 inches long)	214
Mashed, with milk and butter	½ cup	99
Radishes	5 medium-size	4
Spinach, cooked	1 cup	41
Squash, summer, cooked	1 cup	25
Tomatoes	1	40
Turnips, cooked, cubed	½ cup	18
Vegetables, mixed	½ cup	58
Watercress	1 cup	7

Appendix 3
Sodium Content of Some Common Foods

Food	Amount	Sodium (milligrams)
BEVERAGES		
Coffee		
Brewed	1 cup	2
Instant		
Regular	1 cup	1
Decaffeinated	1 cup	1
With chicory	1 cup	7
Substitute	1 cup	3
Fruit drinks		
Sweetened		
Lemonade	1 cup	50
Orangeade	1 cup	35
Other fruit	1 cup	0
Unsweetened, all flavors	1 cup	0
Fruit juices		
Apple cider or juice	1 cup	5
Apricot nectar	1 cup	9
Citrus		
Grapefruit juice		
Canned	1 cup	4
Frozen, diluted	1 cup	5
Lemon or lime juice		
Canned	1 cup	2
Frozen, diluted	1 cup	4
Orange juice		
Canned	1 cup	5
Frozen, diluted	1 cup	5
Tangerine juice	1 cup	2

Food	Amount	Sodium (milligrams)
Grape juice, bottled	1 cup	8
Peach nectar	1 cup	10
Pear nectar	1 cup	8
Pineapple juice	1 cup	5
Prune juice	1 cup	5
Mineral water, imported	1 cup	42
Tea		
Brewed	1 cup	1
Instant	1 cup	2
Vegetable juices		
Tomato juice		
Regular	1 cup	878
Low-sodium	1 cup	9
Vegetable juice cocktail	1 cup	887
BREADS		
Biscuits, baking powder	1	175
Corn	1 ounce	176
Cracked wheat	1 slice	148
Crackers, whole wheat	1	30
French	1 slice	116
Mixed-grain	1 slice	138
Muffins, English	1 medium-size	293
Pita	1	132
Pumpernickel	1 slice	182
Rye	1 slice	139
Whole wheat	1 slice	132

Food	Amount	Sodium (milligrams)	Food	Amount	Sodium (milligrams)
CONDIMENTS			Cottage		
			Creamed	1 ounce	114
Baking powder	1 teaspoon	339	Dry-curd, unsalted	1 ounce	4
Baking soda	1 teaspoon	821	Low-fat, 1 percent	1 ounce	115
Catsup			Low-fat, 2 percent	1 ounce	115
Regular	1 tablespoon	156	Cream	1 ounce	84
Low-sodium	1 tablespoon	3	Edam	1 ounce	274
Chili powder	1 teaspoon	26	Feta	1 ounce	316
Garlic			Gouda	1 ounce	232
Powder	1 teaspoon	1	Gruyère	1 ounce	95
Salt	1 teaspoon	1,850	Limburger	1 ounce	227
Horseradish, prepared	1 tablespoon	198	Monterey Jack	1 ounce	152
Meat tenderizer			Mozzarella	1 ounce	106
Regular	1 teaspoon	1,750	Part-skim	1 ounce	132
Low-sodium	1 teaspoon	1	Muenster	1 ounce	178
Mustard, prepared	1 teaspoon	65	Parmesan, grated	1 tablespoon	528
Onion			Provolone	1 ounce	248
Powder	1 teaspoon	1	Romano	1 ounce	340
Salt	1 teaspoon	1,620	Roquefort	1 ounce	513
Parsley, dried	1 tablespoon	6	Swiss		
Pepper, black	1 teaspoon	1	Cheese food,		
Relish, sweet	1 tablespoon	124	pasteurized process	1 ounce	440
Salad dressings			Pasteurized process	1 ounce	388
Blue cheese	1 tablespoon	153	Unprocessed	1 ounce	74
French	1 tablespoon	92	Cream		
Mayonnaise	1 tablespoon	78	Sweet		
Russian	1 tablespoon	133	Fluid, all types	1 tablespoon	6
Salt	1 teaspoon	1,938	Whipped	1 tablespoon	4
Sauces			Sour, cultured	1 tablespoon	6
Soy	1 tablespoon	1,029	Milk		
Worcestershire	1 tablespoon	206	Fluid		
Tomato paste	1 cup	77	Whole and skim	1 cup	122
Tomato sauce	1 cup	1,498	Whole, low-sodium	1 cup	6
Vinegar	½ cup	1	Buttermilk, cultured		
Yeast, dry	1 tablespoon	1	Salted	1 cup	257
			Unsalted	1 cup	122
			Canned		
			Evaporated		
			Whole	1 cup	266
DAIRY FOODS			Skim	1 cup	294
Cheeses			Sweetened, condensed	1 cup	389
American			Dry		
Cheese food, cold pack	1 ounce	274	Nonfat		
Cheese spread,			Regular	½ cup	322
pasteurized process	1 ounce	381	Instant	1 cup	373
Pasteurized process	1 ounce	406	Buttermilk	½ cup	310
Blue	1 ounce	396	Milk desserts		
Brick	1 ounce	159	Custard, baked	1 cup	209
Brie	1 ounce	178	Ice cream		
Camembert	1 ounce	239	Custard, French	1 cup	84
Cheddar	1 ounce	176	Strawberry	1 cup	77
Colby	1 ounce	171	Vanilla	1 cup	112

Food	Amount	Sodium (milligrams)
Milk desserts *(continued)*		
Puddings		
Tapioca, cooked	½ cup	130
Vanilla	½ cup	83
Yogurt		
Plain		
Regular	1 cup	105
Low-fat	1 cup	159
Skim-milk	1 cup	174
With fruit	1 cup	133
DESSERTS		
Cookies		
Macaroon	2	14
Oatmeal	1	77
Raisin	2	55
EGGS		
Whole	1	59
White	1	50
Yolk	1	9
FATS AND OILS		
Butter		
Regular	1 tablespoon	116
Unsalted	1 tablespoon	2
Whipped	1 tablespoon	74
Oils, vegetable (including corn, olive, and soybean)	1 tablespoon	0
FISH (*see also* Shellfish)		
Bluefish		
Baked with butter	3 ounces	87
Breaded, fried	3 ounces	123
Bonito, canned	3 ounces	437
Codfish, broiled with butter	3 ounces	93
Eel, raw	3 ounces	67
Flounder (and other flat fish, including sole), baked with butter	3 ounces	201
Haddock, breaded, fried	3 ounces	150
Halibut, broiled with butter	3 ounces	114
Herring, smoked	3 ounces	5,234
Mullet, breaded, fried	3 ounces	83
Ocean perch, fried	3 ounces	128
Rockfish, baked	3 ounces	57

Food	Amount	Sodium (milligrams)
Salmon		
Broiled with butter	3 ounces	99
Canned		
Salt added		
Pink	3 ounces	443
Red	3 ounces	329
Silver	3 ounces	298
Without salt added	3 ounces	41
Sardines, canned (drained)	3 ounces	552
Shad, baked with butter	3 ounces	66
Tuna, canned		
Light meat, chunk		
Oil-packed	3 ounces	303
Water-packed	3 ounces	288
White meat (albacore)		
Chunk, low-sodium	3 ounces	34
Solid		
Oil-packed	3 ounces	384
Water-packed	3 ounces	309
FRUITS		
Apples		
Raw or baked	1	2
Frozen, slices	1 cup	28
Frozen, scalloped	1 cup	45
Dried, sulfured	1 cup	210
Applesauce, canned		
Sweetened	1 cup	6
Unsweetened	1 cup	5
Apricots		
Fresh	3	1
Canned		
Peeled	1 cup	27
Unpeeled	1 cup	10
Dried	1 cup	12
Avocados	1	22
Bananas	1	2
Berries		
Blackberries (boysenberries)		
Fresh	1 cup	1
Canned	1 cup	3
Blueberries		
Fresh	1 cup	1
Canned	1 cup	2
Raspberries		
Fresh	1 cup	1
Frozen	1 cup	3
Strawberries		
Fresh	1 cup	2
Frozen	1 cup	6

Food	Amount	Sodium (milligrams)	Food	Amount	Sodium (milligrams)
Cherries			**Prunes**		
Fresh	1 cup	1	Cooked	1 cup	8
Frozen	1 cup	3	Dried	5 large	2
Canned	1 cup	10	Raisins, seedless	1 cup	17
Citrus			**Rhubarb**		
Grapefruit			Cooked, sugared	1 cup	5
Fresh	½	1	Frozen	1 cup	5
Frozen, unsweetened	1 cup	6	Watermelon	1/16	8
Canned, sweetened	1 cup	4			
Kumquats	1	1	**GRAINS AND GRAIN PRODUCTS**		
Lemons	1	1	Barley, pearled, cooked	1 cup	6
Oranges	1	1	Brown rice, cooked	1 cup	10
Tangelos	1	1	Corn, grits, cooked	1 cup	1
Tangerines	1	1	**Popcorn**		
			Plain	1 cup	1
Cranberries	1 cup	1	With oil and salt	1 cup	175
Cranberry sauce	1 cup	75	Oatmeal, regular or quick	¾ cup	1
Currants			Wheat bran	¼ cup	3
Fresh	1 cup	3	Wheat germ, toasted	¼ cup	1
Dried	1 cup	10			
Dates, dried	10	1	**LEGUMES**		
Figs					
Fresh	1	2	Dried beans, canned		
Canned	1 cup	3	Baked, Boston-style	1 cup	606
Dried	1	2	With or without pork	1 cup	928
Fruit cocktail, canned	1 cup	15	Kidney	1 cup	844
Grapes, Thompson seedless	10	1	Dried beans, cooked		
Mangoes	1	1	Chick-peas	1 cup	13
Muskmelons			Great Northern	1 cup	5
Cantaloupe	½	24	Kidney	1 cup	4
Casaba	1 wedge (1/5 melon)	34	Lima	1 cup	4
			Navy	1 cup	3
Honeydew	1 wedge (1/5 melon)	28	Pinto	1 cup	4
			Soybeans	1 cup	4
Nectarines	1	1	Miso		
Papayas	1	8	Red	¼ cup	3,708
Peaches			White	¼ cup	2,126
Fresh	1	1	Tofu	¼ pound	9
Frozen	1 cup	10	Lentils, cooked	1 cup	4
Canned	1 cup	15	**Peanuts**		
Dried, uncooked	1 cup	10	Dry roasted, salted	1 cup	986
Pears			Roasted, salted	1 cup	601
Fresh	1	1	Spanish, salted	1 cup	823
Canned	1 cup	15	Unsalted	1 cup	8
Dried	1 cup	10	Peanut butter, commercially ground		
Pineapple			Smooth or crunchy	1 tablespoon	81
Fresh	1 cup	1	Low-sodium	1 tablespoon	1
Canned	1 cup	7	**Peas**		
Plums			Black-eyed, cooked	1 cup	12
Fresh	1	1	Split, cooked	1 cup	5
Canned	1 cup	10			

Food	Amount	Sodium (milligrams)	Food	Amount	Sodium (milligrams)
MEATS			**PASTA**		
Beef			Macaroni or spaghetti, cooked	1 cup	2
Cooked, lean	3 ounces	55	Noodles, cooked	1 cup	2
Corned					
Cooked	3 ounces	802	**POULTRY AND GAME**		
Canned	3 ounces	893	**Chicken, roasted**		
Dried, chipped	1 ounce	1,219	Breast with skin	½ breast	69
Lamb, cooked, lean	3 ounces	58	Drumstick with skin	1 drumstick	47
Pork			Duck, roasted, flesh and skin	½ duck	227
Fresh, cooked, lean	3 ounces	59	Goose, roasted, flesh and skin	½ goose	543
Cured			Rabbit, cooked, flesh	¼ pound	70
Bacon			Turkey, small, roasted		
Cooked	2 slices	274	Breast with skin	½ breast	182
Canadian	1 slice	394	Leg with skin	1 leg	195
Ham	3 ounces	1,114			
Salt pork, raw	1 ounce	399	**SALADS**		
Sausage			**Bean**		
Pork	1 link	168	Marinated	½ cup	104
Pork and beef	1 patty	217	Canned	½ cup	537
Veal, cooked, lean	3 ounces	69	Carrot-raisin	½ cup	97
Variety meats			Coleslaw	½ cup	68
Gizzard, poultry, simmered	1 ounce	17	Macaroni	½ cup	507
Heart			Potato	½ cup	625
Beef, braised	1 ounce	29			
Calf, braised	1 ounce	32	**SHELLFISH** (*see also* Fish)		
Poultry, simmered	1 ounce	14			
Kidney, beef, braised	1 ounce	71	**Clams, raw**		
Liver			Hard	3 ounces	174
Calf, fried	1 ounce	33	Soft	3 ounces	30
Pork, simmered	1 ounce	14	Crab		
Poultry, simmered	1 ounce	16	Canned, drained	3 ounces	425
Sweetbreads, calf, cooked	1 ounce	32	Steamed	3 ounces	314
Tongue, beef, braised	1 ounce	17	Lobster, boiled	3 ounces	212
Tripe	1 ounce	13	Oysters		
			Raw	3 ounces	113
NUTS AND SEEDS			Fried	3 ounces	174
			Frozen	3 ounces	323
Almonds			Scallops		
Salted, roasted	1 cup	311	Raw	3 ounces	217
Unsalted, slivered	1 cup	4	Steamed	3 ounces	225
Brazil nuts	1 cup	1	Shrimp		
Cashews			Raw	3 ounces	137
Dry roasted, salted	1 cup	1,200	Fried	3 ounces	159
Roasted in oil	1 cup	21	Canned	3 ounces	1,955
Chestnuts	1 cup	10			
Hazelnuts	1 cup	2	**SWEETENERS**		
Peanuts (*see* Legumes)					
Pecans	1 cup	1	Corn syrup, light and dark	1 tablespoon	16
Pistachios	1 cup	6	Honey	1 tablespoon	Trace
Sunflower seeds	1 cup	44	Maple syrup	1 tablespoon	5
Walnuts, English	1 cup	3			

Food	Amount	Sodium (milligrams)	Food	Amount	Sodium (milligrams)
Molasses			Cabbage		
Blackstrap	1 tablespoon	19	Green		
Light	1 tablespoon	3	Raw	1 cup	8
Sugars			Cooked	1 cup	16
Brown	1 tablespoon	4	Red, raw	1 cup	18
Granulated	1 tablespoon	Trace			
Powdered	1 tablespoon	Trace	Carrots		
			Raw	1	34
VEGETABLES			Frozen	3.3 ounces	43
			Canned		
Artichokes			Regular	1 cup	386
Whole, cooked	1 medium	36	Low-sodium	1 cup	58
Hearts, frozen	3 ounces	40			
Asparagus			Cauliflower		
Raw	1 spear	1	Raw	1 cup	17
Frozen	4 spears	4	Cooked	1 cup	13
Canned			Frozen	1 cup	18
Regular	4 spears	298			
Low-sodium	1 cup	7	Celery, raw	1 stalk	25
Beans			Chard, cooked	1 cup	143
Italian			Chicory	1 cup	6
Frozen	3 ounces	4	Collards		
Canned	1 cup	913	Cooked	1 cup	24
Lima			Frozen	3 ounces	41
Cooked	1 cup	2	Corn		
Frozen	1 cup	128	Cooked	1 ear	1
Canned	1 cup	456	Frozen	1 cup	7
Low-sodium	1 cup	7	Canned		
Snap			Cream-style		
Cooked	1 cup	5	Regular	1 cup	671
Frozen	3 ounces	3	Low-sodium	1 cup	5
Canned			Vacuum-packed	1 cup	577
Regular	1 cup	326	Whole kernel		
Low-sodium	1 cup	3	Regular	1 cup	384
Bean sprouts, mung			Low-sodium	1 cup	2
Raw	1 cup	5	Cucumbers	7 slices	2
Canned	1 cup	71	Dandelion greens, cooked	1 cup	46
Beets			Eggplant, cooked	1 cup	2
Cooked	1 cup	73	Endive, raw	1 cup	7
Canned			Kale		
Sliced	1 cup	479	Cooked	1 cup	47
Low-sodium	1 cup	110	Frozen	3 ounces	13
Harvard	1 cup	275	Kohlrabi, cooked	1 cup	9
Pickled	1 cup	330	Leek	1 bulb	1
Beet greens, cooked	1 cup	110	Lettuce	1 cup	4
Broccoli			Mushrooms		
Raw	1 stalk	23	Raw	1 cup	7
Frozen	1 cup	35	Canned	2 ounces	242
Brussels sprouts			Mustard greens		
Raw	1 medium-size	1	Raw	1 cup	11
			Cooked	1 cup	25
Frozen	1 cup	15	Frozen	3 ounces	25
In butter sauce	3.3 ounces	421	Okra, cooked	10 pods	2

Food	Amount	Sodium (milligrams)	Food	Amount	Sodium (milligrams)
Onions			Spinach		
Mature, dry	1 medium-size	10	Raw	1 cup	49
			Cooked	1 cup	94
Scallions	2 medium-size	2	Frozen	3.3 ounces	65
			Canned		
Parsley, raw	1 tablespoon	2	Regular	1 cup	910
			Low-sodium	1 cup	148
Parsnips, cooked	1 cup	19	Squash		
			Summer		
Peas, green			Cooked	1 cup	5
Cooked	1 cup	2	Canned	1 cup	785
Frozen	3 ounces	80	Winter		
Canned			Baked, mashed	1 cup	2
Regular	1 cup	493	Frozen	1 cup	4
Low-sodium	1 cup	8	Sweet potatoes		
			Baked or boiled in skin	1	20
Peppers			Canned		
Hot, raw	1 pod	7	Regular	1	48
Sweet, raw or cooked	1 pod	9	Low-sodium	1 serving	27
			Candied	1	42
Potatoes			Tomatoes		
Baked or boiled	1 medium-size	5	Raw	1	14
			Cooked	1 cup	10
Canned	1 cup	753	Canned		
Mashed, with milk and salt	1 cup	632	Whole	1 cup	390
Au gratin	1 cup	1,095	Stewed	1 cup	584
			Low-sodium	1 cup	16
Pumpkin, canned	1 cup	12	Turnip greens, cooked	1 cup	17
Radishes	4 small	2	Vegetables, mixed		
Rutabaga, cooked	1 cup	8	Frozen	3.3 ounces	45
Sauerkraut, canned	1 cup	1,554	Canned	1 cup	380
Shallot	1	3			

Appendix 4
Mail-Order Sources

Dairy Supplies

American Supply House
Box 1114
Columbia, MO 65205

Offers a good line of cultures.

The Coburn Co.
Box 147
Whitewater, WI 53190

Offers a large selection of dairy equipment.

Countryside General Store
103 N. Monroe St.
Waterloo, WI 53594

Offers a variety of home dairy, cheese-making, and ice cream supplies, as well as pasteurizers and separators.

Cumberland General Store
Route 3
Crossville, TN 38555

Offers a large selection of home dairy supplies and ice cream-making equipment.

Hamilton R & R Sales
319 S. Broadway
New Ulm, NM 56073

Offers a good line of cultures.

Homecraft
111 Stratford Center
Winston-Salem, NC 27104

Offers a variety of cheese-making supplies.

The International Yogurt Co.
628 North Doheny Dr.
Los Angeles, CA 90069

Carries buttermilk, acidophilus, and kefir cultures.

New England Cheesemaking Supply Co.
Box 85
Ashfield, MA 01330

Offers a large selection of cheese-making supplies, presses, cultures, and books.

Flours and Grains

Arrowhead Mills, Inc.
Box 866
Hereford, TX 79045

Offers a large selection of whole grains, dried beans, nuts, seeds, and cereals. Catalog available.

Birkett Mills
P.O. Box 440A
Penn Yan, NY 14527

Offers a large selection of whole grain flours and buckwheat groats, including several grades of roasted buckwheat or kasha.

Butte Creek Mill
402 Royal Ave. N
Eagle Point, OR 97524

Offers a large selection of whole grain flours, cereals, and dried beans.

Calloway Gardens Country Store
Highway 27
Pine Mountain, GA 31822

Offers a complete line of whole grains. Free catalog available.

East West Journal
17 Station St.
Brookline, MA 02146

Offers a large selection of whole grains. Catalog available.

Edwards Mill
School of the Ozarks
Point Lookout, MO 65726

Offers stone-ground whole grain flours, including cornmeal.

Erewhon Trading Co.
236 Washington St.
Brookline, MA 02146

Offers a complete line of whole grains, whole grain flours, dried beans, nuts and seeds, soyfood products, and sea vegetables. Catalog available.

Fangorn Organic Farm
Route 3, Box 141B
Rocky Mount, VA 24151

Offers whole grains, whole grain flours, and soyfood products.

Flory Brothers
841 Flory Mill Rd.
Lancaster, PA 17601

Offers a complete selection of whole grains and whole grain flours, including potato flour.

Great Valley Mills
Quakertown, PA 18951

Offers a complete line of whole grains and whole grain flours.

Grover Co.
2111 S. Industrial Park Ave.
Tempe, AZ 85282

Offers a complete selection of whole grains, including triticale, rye, buckwheat, and millet. Also supplies sprouting seeds.

Hodgson Mill Enterprises, Inc.
P.O. Box 126
Gainsville, MO 65655

Offers a large selection of whole grain flours.

Homestead Flour
911 W. Camden Rd.
Montgomery, MI 49255

Offers whole grain flours, yellow cornmeal, and soybeans.

Kenyon's Grist Mill
Usquepaugh, RI 02836

One of the largest suppliers of stone-ground white cornmeal.

Letoba Farm Foods
Box 180, Route 3
Lyons, KS 67554

Offers whole grains, whole grain flours, dried beans, oils, herbs and spices, and sea vegetables.

New Hope Mills
R.R. 2
Moravia, NY 13118

Offers whole grain flours (including soy flour),
rolled oats, and buckwheat grits.

Old Mill of Guilford
Box 623, Route 1
Oak Ridge, NC 27310

Offers a large selection of whole grain flours
(including barley and millet flours) and yellow
and white grits.

Shiloh Farms
Box 97, Highway 59
Sulphur Springs, AR 72768

Offers a complete selection of whole grains, whole
grain flours (including triticale flour), nuts and
seeds, dried beans, and natural sweeteners. Free
catalog available.

Vermont Country Store
Weston, VT 05161

Offers a large selection of whole grains, whole
grain flours, nut and seed butters, and natural
sweeteners.

Walnut Acres
Penns Creek, PA 17862

Offers a complete selection of whole grains, whole
grain flours (including amaranth and sorghum
flours), dried beans, cereals, nuts and seeds,
soyfood products, herbs and spices, oils and
vinegars, and low-methoxyl natural sweeteners.

Wilson Milling Co.
P.O. Box 481
LaCross, KS 67548

Offers whole grain flours and wheat berries. Price
list available upon request.

Herbs and Spices

Attar Herbs & Spices
Playground Rd.
New Ipswich, NH 03071

Offers a large selection of dried herbs and spices.

Calico Herbs, Inc.
P.O. Box 68
Old England Rd.
Ipswich, MA 01938

Offers a selection of dried herbs and a few herb
blends.

Caprilands Herb Farm
534 Silver St.
Coventry, CT 06238

Offers a variety of dried herbs, spices, and teas,
as well as herb plants and seeds.

The Country Herbery
P.O. Box 1573
Auburn, CA 95603

Offers a selection of dried herbs, spices, and some
spice blends.

Country Herbs
3 Maple St.
Stockbridge, MA 01262

Offers dried herbs, spices, and herb blends, as
well as a large selection of annual and perennial
plants and some seeds.

Cricket Hill Herb Farm, Ltd.
Glen St.
Rowley, MA 01969

Offers a selection of dried herbs, spices, teas,
and herb blends, as well as an extensive selection
of herb plants. Catalog available for a fee.

The Dutch Mill Herb Farm
Route 2, Box 190
Forest Grove, OR 97116

Offers dried herbs.

Flintridge Herbs & Spindles & Things
Route 1, Box 187
Sister Bay, WI 54234

Offers an extensive selection of dried herbs and spices, as well as annual and perennial herb plants and seeds. Catalog available for a fee.

Fragrant Fields
Route 2, Box 199
Dongola, IL 62926

Offers dried herbs, spices, and teas, as well a large selection of perennial and annual herb plants.

Harvest Health, Inc.
1944 Eastern Ave. SE
Grand Rapids, MI 49507

Offers a large selection of dried herbs and spices.

Herbal Effect
Box 6
Carmel Valley, CA 93924

Offers a large selection of dried herbs and spices.

Herbally Yours, Inc.
P.O. Box 26
Changewater, NJ 07831

Offers a selection of dried herbs, herb and spice blends, and tea blends.

The Herbary and Potpourri Shop
P.O. Box 543
Childs Homestead Rd.
Orleans, MA 02653

Offers a large variety of dried herbs, spices, herb blends, and a few herb teas, as well as herb plants. Catalog available for a fee.

The Herb Cottage
Washington Cathedral
Mount Saint Alban
Washington, DC 20016

Offers a variety of dried herbs and spices, as well as herb seeds.

Hickory Hollow Herbs
Route 1, Box 52
Peterstown, WV 24963

Offers dried herbs and spices and herb teas, as well as many annual and perennial seeds.

Hilltop Herb Farm, Inc.
P.O. Box 1734
Cleveland, TX 77327

Offers an extensive selection of dried herbs, spices, and herb blends, as well as perennial herb plants and annual and perennial herb seeds. Catalog available for a fee.

Indiana Botanic Gardens
P.O. Box 5
Hammond, IN 46325

Offers a selection of dried herbs, spices, and teas. Catalog available for a fee.

Misty Morning Farm
2220 W. Sisson Rd.
Hastings, MI 49058

Offers dried herbs, as well as an extensive variety of annual and perennial herb plants and seeds.

Nichols Garden Nursery
1190 North Pacific Highway
Albany, OR 97321

Offers a large selection of dried herbs, spices, herb blends, and tea blends, as well as herb seeds and perennial herb plants.

The Rosemary House
120 S. Market St.
Mechanicsburg, PA 17055

Offers a selection of dried herbs, spices, and herb teas, as well as annual and perennial herb seeds and perennial herb plants. Catalog available for a fee.

Sanctuary Seeds
2388 W. 4th
Vancouver, BC Y6K 1P1

Offers a large variety of dried herbs, as well as annual and perennial seeds.

Smile Herb Shop
4908 Berwyn Rd.
College Park, MD 20740

Offers a selection of dried herbs, spices, herb teas, herb seeds, and herb plants.

The White Pine Co.
Box 3512
Madison, WI 53704

Offers dried herbs, herb blends, and teas. Catalog available for a fee.

Wide World of Herbs
11 St. Catherine St. E
Montreal, PQ H2X 1K3

Offers a large variety of dried herbs and spices.

Yankee Peddler Herb Farm
Route 1, Box 251A
Burton, TX 77835

Offers a large selection of dried herbs, spices, and tea blends, as well as herb seeds. Catalog available for a fee.

Kitchen Equipment

Bazaar de la Cuisine
1003 Second Ave.
New York, NY 10022

Offers a complete selection of international cookware and bread-baking accessories. Catalog available.

Bridge Co.
212 E. 52nd St.
New York, NY 10022

Offers a fine selection of unusual cooking and baking utensils.

Casa Moneo Spanish Imports
210 W. 14th St.
New York, NY 10011

Carries tortilla-making equipment. Catalog available for a fee.

Dean & Deluca
121 Prince St.
New York, NY 10012

Carries a variety of specialty equipment.

Hoffritz
515 W. 24th St.
New York, NY 10011

Offers a complete selection of cutlery. Catalog available for a fee.

Katagiri
224 E. 59th St.
New York, NY 10022

Carries Japanese specialty equipment.

H. Roth & Son
1577 1st Ave.
New York, NY 10028

Offers a large selection of kitchen equipment.
Catalog available.

Williams-Sonoma
P.O. Box 3792
San Francisco, CA 94119

Offers a large selection of cooking equipment
and specialty food equipment, including ice cream
molds. Catalog available.

Natural Sweeteners

Brookman Farms
Box 157, R.R. 2
South Dayton, NY 14138

Produces maple syrup in pints, quarts, half
gallons, and gallons. Price list available.

Brookside Farm
Tunbridge, VT 05077

Produces Grade A and Grade B maple syrup
in pints, quarts, and gallons. Free price list
available.

Clark Hill Sugary
Canaan, NH 03741

Produces maple syrup in pints, quarts, and half
gallons. Free brochure available.

Shiloh Farms
Box 97, Highway 59
Sulphur Springs, AK 72768

Carries a variety of natural sweeteners. Free
catalog available.

Vermont Country Store
Weston, VT 05161

Offers natural sweeteners.

Walnut Acres
Penns Creek, PA 17862

Carries low-methoxyl natural sweeteners.

Sea Vegetables

Chico San, Inc.
P.O. Box 810
Chico, CA 95926

Carries sea vegetables, as well as soyfood
products, nuts and seeds, dried beans, and herbs
and spices. Free catalog available.

Erewhon Trading Co.
236 Washington St.
Brookline, MA 02146

Carries sea vegetables, as well as whole grains,
whole grain flours, dried beans, nuts and seeds,
and soyfood products. Catalog available.

Katagiri
224 E. 59th St.
New York, NY 10022

Offers a variety of sea vegetables, as well as
Japanese specialty equipment.

Letoba Farm Foods
Box 180, Route 3
Lyons, KS 67554

Carries sea vegetables, as well as dried beans,
herbs and spices, oils, whole grains, and whole
grain flours.

Index

Boldface *page numbers indicate entries in tables.*